Gynecologic Oncology

NOTICE

Medicine is an ever-changing science. As new research and clinical experience broaden our knowledge, changes in treatment and drug therapy are required. The authors and the publisher of this work have checked with sources believed to be reliable in their efforts to provide information that is complete and generally in accord with the standards accepted at the time of publication. However, in view of the possibility of human error or changes in medical sciences, neither the authors nor the publisher nor any other party who has been involved in the preparation or publication of this work warrants that the information contained herein is in every respect accurate or complete, and they disclaim all responsibility for any errors or omissions or for the results obtained from use of the information contained in this work. Readers are encouraged to confirm the information contained herein with other sources. For example and in particular, readers are advised to check the product information sheet included in the package of each drug they plan to administer to be certain that the information contained in this work is accurate and that changes have not been made in the recommended dose or in the contraindications for administration. This recommendation is of particular importance in connection with new or infrequently used drugs.

Gynecologic Oncology

Clinical Practice & Surgical Atlas

Beth Y. Karlan, MD

Director, Women's Cancer Program
Samuel Oschin Comprehensive Cancer Institute and Division
    of Gynecologic Oncology
Board of Governors Chair in Gynecologic Oncology
Department of Obstetrics and Gynecology
Cedars-Sinai Medical Center
Professor, Obstetrics and Gynecology
David Geffen School of Medicine at UCLA
Los Angeles, California

Robert E. Bristow, MD, MBA

The Philip J. DiSaia Prestigious Chair in Gynecologic Oncology
Professor and Vice-Chair for Clinical Affairs
Department of Obstetrics and Gynecology
Director, Division of Gynecologic Oncology
University of California, Irvine
Orange, California

Andrew J. Li, MD

Co-Director, Women's Reproductive Cancers Center of Excellence
Samuel Oschin Comprehensive Cancer Institute
Department of Obstetrics and Gynecology
Cedars-Sinai Medical Center
Health Sciences Associate Clinical Professor, Obstetrics and Gynecology
David Geffen School of Medicine at UCLA
Los Angeles, California

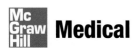 **Medical**

New York Chicago San Francisco Lisbon London Madrid Mexico City
Milan New Delhi San Juan Seoul Singapore Sydney Toronto

Gynecologic Oncology: Clinical Practice and Surgical Atlas

Copyright © 2012 by The McGraw-Hill Companies, Inc. All rights reserved. Printed in China. Except as permitted under the United States Copyright Act of 1976, no part of this publication may be reproduced or distributed in any form or by any means, or stored in a data base or retrieval system, without the prior written permission of the publisher.

1 2 3 4 5 6 7 8 9 0   CTP/CTP   17 16 15 14 13 12

ISBN 978-0-07-174926-8
MHID 0-07-174926-8

This book was set in Adobe Garamond by Cenveo Publisher Services.
The editors were Alyssa Fried and Peter J. Boyle.
The production supervisor was John Williams.
Project management was provided by Sandhya Gola, Cenveo Publisher Services.
The illustration manager was Armen Ovsepyan; the illustrator was Erin Frederikson.
The designer was Diana Andrews; the cover design is by Pehrsson Design. The lower image of cervical cancer cells is by Steve Gschmeissner/Photo Researchers, Inc.
China Translation & Printing Services, Ltd., was printer and binder.

Library of Congress Cataloging-in-Publication Data

Gynecologic oncology : clinical practice and surgical atlas / [edited by] Beth
   Y. Karlan, Robert E. Bristow, Andrew J. Li. — 1st ed.
         p. ; cm.
     Includes bibliographical references and index.
     ISBN 978-0-07-174926-8 (hardback : alk. paper)
     I. Karlan, Beth Y. (Beth Young)   II. Bristow, Robert E.   III. Li, Andrew J.
     [DNLM: 1. Genital Neoplasms, Female—diagnosis—Atlases.   2. Genital Neoplasms,
   Female—therapy—Atlases.   3. Gynecologic Surgical Procedures—methods—Atlases. WP 17]
   616.99′465—dc23

                                                                    2012007123

McGraw-Hill books are available at special quantity discounts to use as premiums and sales promotions, or for use in corporate training programs. To contact a representative please e-mail us at bulksales@mcgraw-hill.com.

Dedication

This textbook and all of our professional accomplishments would not be possible without the enduring support of our families. We dedicate this effort to our understanding spouses, Scott, Michelle, and Cathy; our high-spirited children, Matthew and Jocelyn Karlan, Jackson, Chloe, and Haley Bristow, Jason, Lucas, and Evan Li; and to our loving parents, Beverly and Stanley Young, Lynn and Lonnie Bristow, and Chien and Marian Li, who raised us with passions for caring and eternal learning. Our many teachers and mentors provided us with the knowledge and skills to care for women with gynecologic cancers and motivated us to continue pushing the therapeutic envelope until cures are within our grasp. Our colleagues—physicians, scientists, nurses, and other professionals—work shoulder to shoulder with us, and support, challenge, motivate, and make us laugh when it is most needed. And most importantly, this book is dedicated to the legions of women with gynecologic cancer, both living and in our memories, who have taught us tenacity, selflessness, and courage. We hope that this text will educate future generations of clinicians and scientists whom we can enlist on our journey to end cancer as a threat to women.

Contents

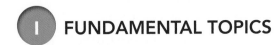

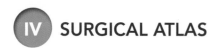

IV SURGICAL ATLAS

Contributors

Nadeem R. Abu-Rustum, MD
Attending Gynecology Service
Department of Surgery
Memorial Sloan-Kettering Cancer Center
New York, New York
Chapter 28

Addie Alkhas, MD
Fellow
Department of Gynecologic Oncology
National Capital Consortium in Gynecologic Oncology
Washington, DC
Chapter 23

Ronald D. Alvarez, MD
Professor and Director
Division of Gynecologic Oncology
Department of Obstetrics and Gynecology
University of Alabama at Birmingham
Birmingham, Alabama
Chapter 12

Malaika Amneus, MD
Assistant Professor
Department of Obstetrics and Gynecology
David Geffen School of Medicine at UCLA
Los Angeles, California
Chapter 16

M. William Audeh, MD, MS
Associate Clinical Professor of Medicine
David Geffen School of Medicine at UCLA
Los Angeles, California
Chapter 15

David M. Boruta II, MD
Assistant Professor
Department of Obstetrics and Gynecology
Harvard Medical School
Boston, Massachusetts
Chapter 25

Wendy R. Brewster, MD, PhD
Associate Professor and Director
Center for Women's Health Research
Department of Obstetrics and Gynecology
University of North Carolina
Lineberger Comprehensive Cancer Center
Chapel Hill, North Carolina
Chapter 1

Jubilee Brown, MD
Associate Professor
Department of Gynecologic Oncology and
    Reproductive Medicine
University of Texas M.D. Anderson Cancer Center
Houston, Texas
Chapter 14

Jay W. Carlson, DO
Clinical Associate Professor
Department of Obstetrics and Gynecology
Des Moines University
Des Moines, Iowa
Chapter 32C

Jori S. Carter, MD
Instructor and Clinical Fellow
Division of Gynecologic Oncology
University of Minnesota Medical School
Minneapolis, Minnesota
Chapter 4

Lee-may Chen, MD
Professor
Edward C. Hill, MD, Endowed Chair
Division of Gynecologic Oncology
Department of Obstetrics, Gynecology, and
    Reproductive Sciences
UCSF Helen Diller Family Comprehensive Cancer Center
San Francisco, California
Chapter 18

Dennis S. Chi, MD
Professor
Gynecology Service
Department of Surgery
Memorial Sloan-Kettering Cancer Center
New York, New York
Chapter 30

Junzo Chino, MD
Assistant Professor
Department of Radiation Oncology
Duke University
Durham, North Carolina
Chapter 10

ix

David E. Cohn, MD
Professor
Department of Obstetrics and Gynecology
Ohio State University Medical Center
Columbus, Ohio
Chapter 12

Robert L. Coleman, MD
Professor and Vice Chair, Clinical Research
Department of Gynecologic Oncology
University of Texas M.D. Anderson Cancer Center
Houston, Texas
Chapter 21

Allan Covens, MD, FRCSC
Professor
Department of Obstetrics and Gynecology
Division of Gynecologic Oncology
University of Toronto
Toronto, Ontario
Chapter 26

Catherine M. Dang, MD
Associate Director
Wasserman Breast Cancer Risk Reduction Program
Department of Surgery
Cedars-Sinai Medical Center
Los Angeles, California
Chapter 15

Summer B. Dewdney, MD
Assistant Professor
Division of Gynecologic Oncology
Rush University Medical Center
Chicago, Illinois
Chapter 29

Bojana Djordjevic, MD
Assistant Professor
Department of Pathology and Laboratory Medicine
University of Ottawa, Ottawa Hospital
Ottawa, Ontario
Chapter 6

Lisa A. dos Santos, MD
Gynecologic Oncology Fellow
Department of Surgery
Memorial Sloan-Kettering Cancer Center
New York, New York
Chapter 28

Levi S. Downs Jr, MD, MS
Associate Professor and Director
Division of Gynecologic Oncology
Obstetrics, Gynecology and Women's Health
University of Minnesota
Minneapolis, Minnesota
Chapter 4

Eric L. Eisenhauer, MD
Assistant Professor
Department of Obstetrics and Gynecology
Division of Gynecologic Oncology
Ohio State University
Columbus, Ohio
Chapter 24

John C. Elkas, MD, JD
Associate Clinical Professor
Department of Obstetrics and Gynecology, Inova Campus
Virginia Commonwealth University
Falls Church, Virginia
Chapter 23

Pedro F. Escobar, MD
Director of Minimally Invasive Surgery and Robotics
Section of Gynecologic Oncology
Department of Obstetrics and Gynecology
Cleveland Clinic
Cleveland, Ohio
Chapter 31

Jeffrey M. Fowler, MD
John G. Boutselis Professor in Gynecologic Oncology
Department of Obstetrics and Gynecology
Ohio State University
Columbus, Ohio
Chapter 24

Michael Frumovitz, MD, MPH
Associate Professor
Department of Gynecologic Oncology
University of Texas M.D. Anderson Cancer Center
Houston, Texas
Chapter 31

Barbara A. Goff, MD
Professor and Director
Division of Gynecologic Oncology
Department of Obstetrics and Gynecology
University of Washington
Seattle, Washington
Chapter 32A

Laura J. Havrilesky, MD, MHSc
Associate Professor
Department of Obstetrics and Gynecology
Duke University Medical Center
Durham, North Carolina
Chapter 10

Christine H. Holschneider, MD
Associate Professor
Department of Obstetrics and Gynecology
David Geffen School of Medicine at UCLA
Los Angeles, California
Chapter 16

Marilyn Huang, MD, MS
Fellow
Department of Gynecologic Oncology and
    Reproductive Medicine
University of Texas M.D. Anderson Cancer Center
Houston, Texas
Chapter 6

Warner K. Huh, MD
Associate Professor
Department of Obstetrics and Gynecology
University of Alabama at Birmingham
Birmingham, Alabama
Chapter 5

David A. Iglesias, MD
Fellow
Department of Gynecologic Oncology and
    Reproductive Medicine
University of Texas M.D. Anderson Cancer Center
Houston, Texas
Chapter 6

Fady Khoury-Collado, MD
Fellow
Gynecology Service, Department of Surgery
Memorial Sloan-Kettering Cancer Center
New York, New York
Chapter 30

Kenneth H. Kim, MD
Fellow and Clinical Instructor
Department of Obstetrics and Gynecology
University of Alabama
Birmingham, Alabama
Chapter 5

Sarah H. Kim, MD, MSCE
Assistant Professor
Surgical Oncology
Fox Chase Cancer Center
Philadelphia, Pennsylvania
Chapter 27

Wui-Jin Koh, MD
Professor of Radiation Oncology
Seattle Cancer Care Alliance
University of Washington Medical Center and
    School of Medicine
Seattle, Washington
Chapter 19

Thomas C. Krivak, MD
Assistant Professor
Director, Gynecologic Oncology Fellowship
Division of Gynecologic Oncology
Magee-Women's Hospital of the University of
    Pittsburgh Medical Center
Pittsburgh, Pennsylvania
Chapter 32B

Nita K. Lee, MD
Assistant Professor of Obstetrics and Gynecology
University of Chicago Medical Center
Chicago, Illinois
Chapter 17

Gary S. Leiserowitz, MD, MS
Professor, Associate Vice Chair, and Chief
Division of Gynecologic Oncology
Department of Obstetrics and Gynecology
UC Davis Medical Center
Sacramento, California
Chapter 7

Charles F. Levenback, MD
Professor
Department of Gynecologic Oncology
Medical Director
Gynecologic Oncology Center
University of Texas M.D. Anderson Cancer Center
Houston, Texas
Chapter 9

Douglas A. Levine, MD
Associate Attending Surgeon
Gynecology Service
Department of Surgery
Memorial Sloan-Kettering Cancer Center
New York, New York
Chapter 2

William J. Lowery, MD
Gynecologic Oncology Fellow
Division of Gynecologic Oncology
Duke University Medical Center
Durham, North Carolina
Chapter 10

Karen H. Lu, MD
Professor
Department of Gynecologic Oncology and
    Reproductive Medicine
University of Texas M.D. Anderson Cancer Center
Houston, Texas
Chapter 6

Ursula A. Matulonis, MD
Medical Director, Associate Professor of Medicine
Harvard Medical School
Medical Director of Gynecologic Oncology
Dana-Farber Cancer Institute
Boston, Massachusetts
Chapter 20

Mark Milam, MD, MPH
Assistant Professor
Obstetrics, Gynecology, and Women's Health
University of Louisville
Louisville, Kentucky
Chapter 9

Susan C. Modesitt, MD
Associate Professor and Director
Gynecologic Oncology Division
Obstetrics and Gynecology Department
University of Virginia Health System
Charlottesville, Virginia
Chapter 14

Mark A. Morgan, MD
Chief, Section of Gynecologic Oncology
Department of Surgery
Fox Chase Cancer Center
Philadelphia, Pennsylvania
Chapter 27

Howard G. Muntz, MD
Clinical Associate Professor
Department of Obstetrics and Gynecology
University of Washington School of Medicine
Seattle, Washington
Chapter 32A

Christa I. Nagel, MD
Gynecologic Oncology Fellow
Department of Obstetrics and Gynecology
Division of Gynecologic Oncology
University of Texas Southwestern Medical Center
Dallas, Texas
Chapter 11

Sameer A. Patel, MD
Assistant Clinical Professor
Department of Surgical Oncology
Division of Plastic and Reconstructive Surgery
Fox Chase Cancer Center
Philadelphia, Pennsylvania
Chapter 27

Matthew A. Powell, MD
Assistant Professor
Department of Obstetrics and Gynecology
Washington University School of Medicine
St. Louis, Missouri
Chapter 29

Pedro T. Ramirez, MD
Associate Professor
Department of Gynecologic Oncology
University of Texas M.D. Anderson Cancer Center
Houston, Texas
Chapter 31

Peter G. Rose, MD
Professor and Director
Section of Gynecologic Oncology
Women's Health Institute
Cleveland Clinic
Cleveland, Ohio
Chapter 3

Paul J. Sabbatini, MD
Associate Attending Physician
Gynecologic Medical Oncology Service
Department of Medicine
Memorial Sloan-Kettering Cancer Center
New York, New York
Chapter 21

Ritu Salani, MD, MBA
Assistant Professor
Department of Obstetrics and Gynecology
Ohio State University
Columbus, Ohio
Chapter 11

Lindsay R. Sales, MD
Resident in Radiation Oncology
University of Washington Medical Center
Seattle, Washington
Chapter 19

John O. Schorge, MD
Associate Professor
Department of Obstetrics, Gynecology and Reproductive
    Biology
Harvard Medical School
Chief, Gynecologic Oncology
Vincent Obstetrics and Gynecology Service
Massachusetts General Hospital
Boston, Massachusetts
Chapter 25

Leigh G. Seamon, DO, MPH
Assistant Professor
Obstetrics and Gynecology
Division of Gynecologic Oncology
University of Kentucky, Markey Cancer Center
Lexington, Kentucky
Chapter 32C

Angeles Alvarez Secord, MD
Associate Professor
Department of Obstetrics and Gynecology
Division of Gynecologic Oncology
Duke University Medical Center
Durham, North Carolina
Chapter 13

Gregory P. Sfakianos, MD
Fellow
Department of Obstetrics and Gynecology
Division of Gynecologic Oncology
Duke University Medical Center
Durham, North Carolina
Chapter 13

Ie-Ming Shih, MD, PhD
Professor
Departments of Pathology and Oncology
Johns Hopkins Medical Institutions
Baltimore, Maryland
Chapter 13

Diljeet K. Singh, MD, DrPH
Assistant Professor
Department of Obstetrics and Gynecology
Northwestern University Feinberg School of Medicine
Chicago, Illinois
Chapters 8 and 22

Pamela T. Soliman, MD, MPH
Assistant Professor
Department of Gynecologic Oncology
University of Texas M.D. Anderson Cancer Center
Houston, Texas
Chapter 6

David Starks, MD
Gynecologic Oncology Fellowship
Division of Gynecologic Oncology
Cleveland Clinic Foundation
Cleveland, Ohio
Chapter 3

Paniti Sukumvanich, MD
Assistant Professor
Division of Gynecologic Oncology
Magee-Women's Hospital of the University of Pittsburgh
    Medical Center
Pittsburgh, Pennsylvania
Chapter 32B

Edward J. Tanner III, MD
Gynecologic Oncology Fellow
Department of Surgery
Memorial Sloan-Kettering Cancer Center
New York, New York
Chapter 30

Krishnansu S. Tewari, MD
Associate Professor
Department of Gynecologic Oncology
University of California, Irvine
Orange, California
Chapter 1

Renata Urban, MD
Assistant Professor
Department of Obstetrics and Gynecology
Division of Gynecologic Oncology
University of Washington Medical Center
University of Washington School of Medicine
Seattle, Washington
Chapter 18

Danielle Vicus, MD, FRCSC
Assistant Professor
Division of Gynecologic Oncology
Division of Surgical Oncology
Toronto Sunnybrook Health Sciences Centre
University of Toronto
Toronto, Ontario
Chapter 26

Vivian E. Von Gruenigen, MD
Chair
Department of Obstetrics and Gynecology
Summa Akron City Hospital
Medical Director
Women's Health Services
Summa Health System
Akron, Ohio
Chapter 22

Joan L. Walker, MD
George Lynn Cross Research Professor and Chief
Section of Gynecologic Oncology
Department of Obstetrics and Gynecology
University of Oklahoma, HSC
Oklahoma City, Oklahoma
Chapter 33

S. Diane Yamada, MD
Associate Professor and Chief
Section of Gynecologic Oncology
Department of Obstetrics and Gynecology
University of Chicago Medical Center
Chicago, Illinois
Chapter 17

Bin Yang, MD, PhD
Associate Professor
Pathology and Laboratory Medicine Institute
Cleveland Clinic Lerner College of Medicine
Cleveland, Ohio
Chapter 3

Angela J. Ziebarth, MD
Fellow
Department of Gynecologic Oncology
University of Alabama at Birmingham
Birmingham, Alabama
Chapter 5

Preface

Gynecologic oncology has experienced remarkable advances over the last decade. Scientific discovery has unraveled many of the underpinnings and molecular origins of reproductive tract cancers. Clinical trials and meticulous data analyses have elucidated the natural history and led to evidence-based therapeutic advances. Targeted therapies, vaccines, and immunotherapies have been added to our armamentarium, and important roles for complementary medicine and supportive care have been recognized. Surgical innovation has revolutionized the approach to gynecologic cancers resulting in both smaller and larger surgeries that can now be performed with improved outcomes under safer operative conditions.

With this backdrop, the time is right to take a fresh look at the practice of gynecologic oncology. This new reference presents fundamental and emerging information in a comprehensive and accessible format. Recognized experts address individual gynecologic cancers and other relevant topics. Clinical practice guidelines are highlighted and the diagnosis, management, and treatment of specific reproductive tract malignancies are emphasized. Acknowledging access to electronic databases, only the most relevant and recent references are highlighted, as well as a few classic articles. A key component of this reference is the surgical atlas, which illustrates essential procedures in gynecologic oncology in a step-by-step fashion.

The reference is organized into four sections. Fundamental and overarching topics such as genetics, clinical trial design, and diagnostic modalities are covered in the first section. Specific reproductive tract disease sites and conditions are individually addressed next. These chapters are presented in a uniform format including epidemiology, pathology, diagnosis, staging, treatment, and outcomes. The focus is on evidence-based practice guidelines and the critical supporting data. The clinical management topics in the third section include perioperative and critical care, as well as principles of chemotherapy, radiation therapy, and targeted and immunotherapies. All the chapters include many figures, tables, color photos, and other illustrations that highlight important concepts and conditions while improving comprehension and learning. The last quarter of the text is devoted to the step-by-step surgical atlas. Ovarian, uterine, cervical, vulvar, and vaginal procedures are meticulously illustrated. In addition, minimally invasive surgical procedures, staging, and advanced cytoreductive procedures are described and illustrated in detail. This comprehensive treatment of gynecologic oncology positions this reference as the definitive resource in the field.

Gynecologic Oncology: Clinical Practice and Surgical Atlas will be useful to all physicians involved in the diagnosis and management of gynecologic cancers. Reproductive tract malignancies remain a significant aspect in the daily clinical practice of obstetrician-gynecologists and other providers of women's health care. Our goal is to become the authoritative resource for gynecologic oncology and to impact women's health care.

Part I | Fundamental Topics

1 Epidemiology of Gynecologic Cancers, Clinical Trials, and Statistical Considerations

Wendy R. Brewster and Krishnansu S. Tewari

EPIDEMIOLOGY OF GYNECOLOGIC CANCERS

The burden of cancer on our population is expected to rise sharply over the next 20 years. This is the result of the aging and growth of the world's population, alongside an increasing adoption of cancer-causing behaviors, particularly smoking and increasing obesity. Overall, cancer incidence is expected to increase by 45% between 2010 and 2030, with the greatest increase borne by older adults and minorities. By 2030, approximately 70% of all cancers will be diagnosed in older adults, and 28% of all cancers will be diagnosed in minorities.[1] Resources will be required to effect and optimize cancer prevention, screening, and early detection. Meaningful improvements in cancer therapy and/or prevention strategies will be required to prevent a dramatic increase in the number of cancer deaths over the next 20 years.

Uterine Corpus Cancer

Endometrial cancer is the most common gynecologic cancer and the fourth most common cancer of women in the United States; 43,470 new cases diagnosed are predicted for 2010, with 7950 deaths.[2] A 50-year old woman in the United States has a 1.3% probability of being diagnosed with endometrial cancer before age 70 years.

Eighty-seven percent of all endometrial cancers are of endometrioid histology. The most common nonendometrioid histology is papillary serous (10%),

followed by clear cell (2%-4%), mucinous (0.6%-5%), and squamous cell (0.1%-0.5%). Some non-endometrioid endometrial carcinomas behave more aggressively than the endometrioid cancers such that even women with clinical stage I disease often have extrauterine metastasis at the time of surgical evaluation.[3] Features of type 1 (endometrioid) carcinoma include increased exposure to estrogen (nulliparity, early menarche, chronic anovulation, and unopposed exogenous estrogen), obesity, and responsiveness to progesterone therapy. Patients more often are white, younger in age, present with a low-grade cancer, and have a better prognosis. The precursor to this malignancy is endometrial hyperplasia. Type 1 endometrial cancers often have a phosphatase and tensin homolog (*PTEN*) mutation and a higher incidence of microsatellite instability. In contrast, type 2 endometrial cancers are unrelated to estrogen exposure and occur in older, thinner women. The most common forms of type 2 endometrial cancer include uterine papillary serous carcinoma and clear cell carcinoma. Uterine papillary serous cancers are aggressive, with an increased incidence of p53 and HER-2/*neu* overexpression.

Risk factors for endometrial cancer include diabetes, obesity, hypertension, nulliparity, polycystic ovarian syndrome, unopposed estrogen therapy, tamoxifen usage, infertility or failure to ovulate, and late menopause.[4] A number of studies have reported a positive association between diabetes and incidence of mortality from endometrial cancer.[5] Diabetes mellitus (both types 1 and 2) has been associated with up to a 2-fold increased risk of endometrial cancer.

Adult overweight/obesity is one of the strongest risk factors for endometrial cancer. In affluent societies, adult obesity accounts for approximately 40% of the endometrial cancer incidence.[6] In postmenopausal women, adiposity is thought to enhance endometrial cancer risk through the mitogenic effects of excess endogenous estrogens that are produced in the adipose tissue through aromatization of androgens. In addition, obesity is accompanied by increased bioavailable estrogen as a result of decreased sex hormone–binding globulin concentration.[6] Although obesity increases endometrial cancer risk independent of other factors, it is not associated with stage or grade of disease.[7]

Tamoxifen citrate is an antiestrogen agent that binds to estrogen receptors but acts as a weak estrogen agonist in postmenopausal endometrial tissue. A spectrum of endometrial abnormalities is associated with its use (including polyps and hyperplasia). Endometrial carcinoma is also associated with long-term tamoxifen treatment.[8]

Endometrial Hyperplasia

In a nested case-control retrospective review of predominantly white participants from Kaiser Permanente Northwest, in the northwest of the United States, the average age at the time of diagnosis of endometrial hyperplasia was 52 years. The endometrial carcinoma risk among women with non-atypical endometrial hyperplasia—who represent the majority of all endometrial hyperplasia diagnoses—is 3 times higher than that of the average population. The risk of endometrial cancer among women with atypical hyperplasia (27.5%) is 21 times higher than the average population risk. The absolute and cumulative risk of progression are represented in Figures 1-1 and 1-2. Cumulative 20-year progression risk among women who remain at risk for at least 1 year is less than 5% for non-atypical endometrial hyperplasia but is 28% for atypical hyperplasia.[9] A Gynecologic Oncology Group (GOG) prospective cohort study designed to estimate the prevalence of concurrent carcinoma in patients who have a biopsy diagnosis of atypical endometrial hyperplasia found that the prevalence of carcinoma in hysterectomy specimens was 42.6%.[10]

Hormonal Therapy

Menopausal estrogen therapy (ET) increases the risk of endometrial cancer in postmenopausal women; however, the risk of endometrial cancer varies with the duration, dose, and type of estrogen used. It is generally believed that daily use of low-dose progestin opposes the effect of exogenous and endogenous estrogen on the endometrium, resulting in a lower risk of endometrial cancer. The California Teachers Study

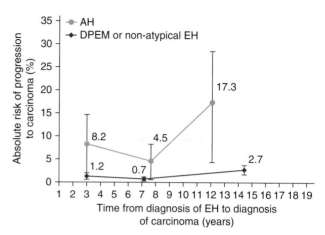

FIGURE 1-1. Absolute risk of subsequent endometrial carcinoma by endometrial hyperplasia (EH) type at index biopsy over intervals of 1 to 4, 5 to 9, and 10 to 19 years. Vertical bars indicate 95% CIs. Data points are plotted at the mean time to diagnosis within each time interval. Size of data points is proportional to the number of case patients diagnosed with endometrial carcinoma during that time interval. AH, atypical hyperplasia; DPEM, disordered proliferative. (Reproduced, with permission, from Lacey JV Jr, Sherman ME, Rush BB, et al. Absolute risk of endometrial carcinoma during 20-year follow-up among women with endometrial hyperplasia. *J Clin Oncol.* 2010;28(5):788-792.)

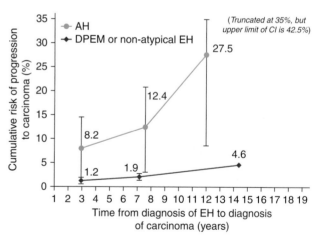

FIGURE 1-2. Cumulative risk of subsequent endometrial carcinoma by endometrial hyperplasia (EH) type at index biopsy. Vertical bars indicate 95% CIs. Data points are plotted at the mean time to diagnosis within each time interval. Size of data points is proportional to the number of case patients diagnosed with endometrial carcinoma during that time interval. AH, atypical hyperplasia; DPEM, disordered proliferative endometrium. (Reproduced, with permission, from Lacey JV Jr, Sherman ME, Rush BB, et al. Absolute risk of endometrial carcinoma during 20-year follow-up among women with endometrial hyperplasia. *J Clin Oncol.* 2010;28(5): 788-792.)

cohort analyzed the association between long-term hormonal therapy use and endometrial cancer risk and the modifying effect of body mass index (BMI) in a case-control study. Long-term (≥ 10 years) use of ET, sequential estrogen–progesterone therapy (with < 10 days per month of progestin), and continuous combined estrogen and progesterone therapy (≥ 25 days/month of progestin) were all associated with an elevated risk of endometrial cancer (odds ratio [OR], 4.5; 95% confidence interval [CI], 2.5-8.1; OR, 4.4; 95% CI, 1.7-11.2; and OR, 2.1; 95% CI, 1.3-3.3, respectively). The risk associated with short-term use was elevated only for ET preparations. The association for continuous combined estrogen–progesterone therapy was confined to thinner women (BMI < 25 kg/m^2). Among heavier women (BMI ≥ 25 kg/m^2), use of continuous combined estrogen–progesterone therapy was associated with a nonsignificant reduction in risk. These findings confirm that long-term use of ET, sequential estrogen–progesterone therapy, or continuous combined estrogen–progesterone therapy among normal-weight women is associated with increased risk of endometrial cancer.[11]

Genetics of Endometrial Cancer

A somatic mutation or deletion of the *PTEN* tumor suppressor gene has been reported in approximately 40% and 40% to 76%, respectively, of endometrial adenocarcinomas.[12] It is well established that estrogen increases endometrial cancer risk, whereas progesterone opposes the estrogen effects. *PTEN* regulates proliferation, growth, and apoptosis in a phosphatidylinositol-3-OH kinase (PI3K)–dependent pathway. Genetic variation in the progesterone receptor gene region is associated with endometrial cancer risk.[13]

Lynch Syndrome (Hereditary Nonpolyposis Colorectal Cancer)

Individuals with Lynch syndrome, also called hereditary nonpolyposis colorectal cancer (HNPCC), are at an increased risk for colorectal cancer, endometrial cancer, and other associated cancers such as gastric cancer, ovarian cancer, urothelial cancer, hepatobiliary tract cancer, brain cancer, cancer of the small intestine, pancreatic cancer, and particular skin cancers. HNPCC-associated cancers are caused by defects in DNA mismatch repair genes. Lynch syndrome is primarily due to germline mutations in one of the DNA mismatch repair genes, mainly hMLH1 or hMSH2 and less frequently hMSH6 and rarely hPMS2.[14] These genetic defects in the DNA mismatch repair system result in microsatellite instability and the absence of protein expression in the tumor. Currently,

Table 1-1 Amsterdam Criteria II and Revised Bethesda Guidelines

Amsterdam Criteria II
There should be at least 3 relatives with colorectal cancer (CRC) or with a Lynch syndrome–associated cancer: cancer of the endometrium, small bowel, ureter, or renal pelvis.
• One relative should be a first-degree relative of the other 2
• At least 2 successive generations should be affected
• At least 1 tumor should be diagnosed before the age of 50 years
• FAP should be excluded in the CRC case if any
• Tumors should be verified by histopathologic examination

Revised Bethesda Guidelines
1. CRC diagnosed in a patient aged < 50 years
2. Presence of synchronous, metachronous colorectal or other Lynch syndrome–related tumors,[a] regardless of age
3. CRC with MSI-H phenotype diagnosed in a patient aged <60 years
4. Patient with CRC and a first-degree relative with a Lynch syndrome–related tumor,[a] with 1 of the cancers diagnosed at age <50 years
5. Patient with CRC with ≥ 2 first-degree or second-degree relatives with a Lynch syndrome–related tumor,[a] regardless of age

FAP, familial adenomatous polyposis; MSI-H, high probability of microsatellite instability.
[a]Lynch syndrome–related tumors include colorectal, endometrial, stomach, ovarian, pancreas, ureter, renal pelvis, biliary tract and brain tumors, sebaceous gland adenomas and keratoacanthomas, and carcinoma of the small bowel.
Reproduced, with permission, from Vasen HF, Möslein G, Alonso A, et al. Guidelines for the clinical management of Lynch syndrome (hereditary non-polyposis cancer). *J Med Genet.* 2007;44(6):353-362.

the diagnosis of Lynch syndrome is based on either clinical (revised Amsterdam criteria) or molecular criteria. The Bethesda Guidelines were revised in 2004 to include extra-colonic tumors to improve the sensitivity of detecting families with Lynch syndrome and to determine which individuals should have microsatellite instability or immunohistochemical testing of their tumors (Table 1-1). Low BMI, age less than 50 years, and positive family history have all been identified as risk factors in endometrial cancer patients who might benefit from HNPCC screening.[15]

Uterine Sarcomas

Uterine sarcomas are rare tumors of the uterus that comprise 4% to 9% of all invasive uterine cancers and 1%

of female genital tract malignancies.[16] Carcinosarcoma, previously referred to as malignant mixed mullerian tumor, is a biphasic neoplasm composed of distinctive and separate, but admixed, malignant-appearing epithelial and mesenchymal elements. The sarcomatous components are heterogeneous, and almost all are high grade. The homologous components of carcinosarcoma are usually spindle cell sarcoma without obvious differentiation; many resemble fibrosarcomas or pleomorphic sarcomas. The most common heterologous elements are malignant skeletal muscle or cartilage resembling either pleomorphic rhabdomyosarcoma or embryonal rhabdomyosarcoma. Carcinosarcomas comprise almost half of all uterine sarcomas. One-third of all cases are diagnosed at an advanced stage. Up to 37% of patients with carcinosarcomas have a history of pelvic irradiation. These tumors tend to occur in younger women, often contain heterologous elements, and are found at advanced stage. Carcinosarcomas are highly aggressive tumors and are fatal in the vast majority of cases.

After excluding carcinosarcoma, leiomyosarcoma is the second most common subtype of uterine sarcoma; however, it accounts for only 1% to 2% of uterine malignancies. Most occur in women over 40 years of age who usually present with abnormal vaginal bleeding (56%), palpable pelvic mass (54%), and pelvic pain (22%).[16] The vast majority of uterine leiomyosarcomas are sporadic. These are very aggressive tumors, even when diagnosed at an early stage. Patients with germline mutations in fumarate hydratase are believed to be at increased risk for developing uterine leiomyosarcomas as well as uterine leiomyomas.[17]

The next common subset of uterine sarcomas, termed endometrial stromal tumors, are divided into 3 groups: endometrial stromal nodule, low-grade endometrial stromal sarcoma, and undifferentiated endometrial sarcomas. Endometrial stromal nodules can occur in women at any age. Patients with endometrial stromal nodules have an excellent prognosis and can be cured by hysterectomy.[16] Endometrial stromal sarcomas are indolent tumors with a favorable prognosis. They occur in women between 40 and 55 years of age. Some cases have been reported in patients with ovarian polycystic disease, after estrogen use, or tamoxifen therapy. In contrast, undifferentiated endometrial sarcomas have very poor prognosis. Endometrial stromal tumors often contain estrogen and progesterone receptors. However, the prognostic implication of these findings is uncertain.[18]

Cervical Cancer

Cervical cancer is the second most frequent cancer in women worldwide and the principal cancer in most developing countries, where 80% of the cases occur.[19] During the years 1973 and 1997, cervical

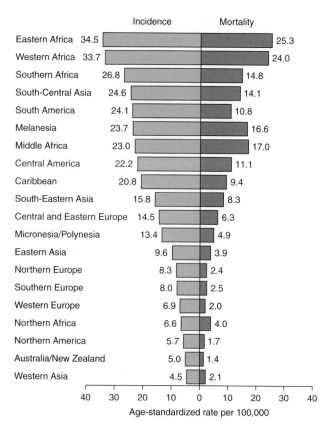

FIGURE 1-3. Age-standardized cervical cancer incidence and mortality rates by world area. (Reproduced, with permission, from Jemal A, Bray F, Center MM, Ferlay J, Ward E, Forman D. Global cancer statistics. *CA Cancer J Clin.* 2011;61(2):69-90.)

cancer rates decreased in most parts of the world. Incidence rates are almost 2-fold higher in less-developed compared with more-developed countries (19.1 and 10.3 per 100,000 person-years, respectively). The incidence is highest in Africa and Central/South America (approximately 29 per 100,000 person-years) and lowest in Oceania and North America (approximately 7.5 per 100,000 person-years).[19] India, the second most populous country in the world, accounts for 27% (77,100) of the total cervical cancer deaths[1] (Figure 1-3). In the United States, cervical cancer is the third most common gynecologic cancer of women. For 2010, 12,200 new cases and 4210 deaths were predicted.[2]

The search for an infectious etiology of cervical cancer dates back to observations made centuries ago, when the Greeks and Romans observed that genital warts were associated with sexual promiscuity and regarded them as infectious. In 1842, Rigoni-Stern, an Italian physician in Verona, observed the higher frequency of cervical cancer among married women, prostitutes, and widows than among virgins or nuns. Subsequently, the medical literature displayed reports of rare malignant conversion of condylomata acuminate into squamous cell carcinoma. In 1976, 2 morphologically distinct human papilloma virus (HPV) lesions were described in the uterine cervix, known currently as a flat and an inverted condyloma. Koilocytes were identified. These new HPV lesions were shown to be frequently associated with concomitant cervical intraepithelial neoplasia (CIN) and carcinoma in situ (CIS) lesions and occasionally with invasive cervical carcinomas as well. Harald zur Hausen identified HPV16 DNA in cervical cancers in 1983 and then identified HPV18 in 1984 by Southern blot hybridization. He was awarded the Nobel Prize in Medicine in 2008 for his research on the role of the papilloma virus in cervical cancer. Cervix cancer is the result of the progression of a clone of persistently infected cells from intraepithelial neoplasia to invasive disease.

More than 200 genotypes of HPV have been identified, and approximately 30 types of HPV specifically cause anogenital infections.[20] HPV is classified into high-risk and low-risk virus types, depending on its ability to cause malignancy in the infected epithelium. The high-risk types (16, 18, 31, 33, 45, 51, 52, 58) are associated with more than 90% of cervical cancers. HPV16 accounts for approximately half of all cervical cancers, whereas HPV18 is involved in another 10% to 20%.

Age-specific HPV prevalence in women over the age of 30 years generally declines from a peak at younger ages; however, the prevalence remains consistently above 20% in many low-resource regions. In middle-aged women (age 35-50 years), maximum HPV prevalence differs across geographical regions: Africa (approximately 20%), Asia/Australia (approximately 15%), Central and South America (approximately 20%), North America (approximately 20%), Southern Europe/Middle East (approximately 15%), and Northern Europe (approximately 15%). Women aged 30 years and older who test negative for carcinogenic HPV with cytologically normal Pap tests are at an extremely low risk for incipient precancer of the cervix over the next 10 years.[21]

In the United States, the prevalence of HPV in women 14 to 59 years is estimated to be 27%, with the highest prevalence (44.8%) among women aged 20 to 24 years. The overall prevalence of HPV among females aged 14 to 24 years is 33.8%. This prevalence corresponds to 7.5 million females with HPV infection[22] (Figure 1-4). The acquisition of HPV occurs soon after sexual initiation and typically resolves very quickly. HPV acquisition is associated with nonpenetrative sexual activity, but much less frequently than with sexual intercourse. Risk factors for HPV infection are primarily related to sexual behavior, including the

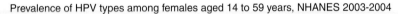

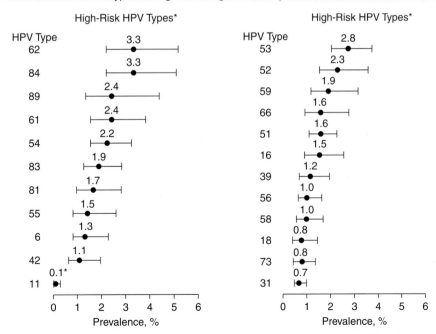

FIGURE 1-4. Prevalence of human papilloma virus (HPV) types among females aged 14 to 59 years. (Reproduced, with permission, from Dunne EF, Unger ER, Sternberg M, et al. Prevalence of HPV infection among females in the United States. *JAMA.* 2007;297(8):813-819.)

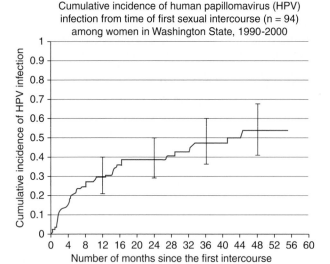

Cumulative incidence of human papillomavirus (HPV) infection from time of first sexual intercourse (n = 94) among women in Washington State, 1990-2000

FIGURE 1-5. Cumulative incidence of human papilloma virus from time of first sexual intercourse. (Reproduced, with permission, from Winer RL, Lee SK, Hughes JP, Adam DE, Kiviat NB, Koutsky LA. Genital human papillomavirus infection: incidence and risk factors in a cohort of female university students. *Am J Epidemiol.* 2003;157(3):218-226.)

number of sex partners, introduction of new partners, lifetime history of sex partners, and partner's sexual history[23] (Figure 1-5).

The risk factors for cervical neoplasia and HPV infection are very similar. The risk factors are a high number of lifetime sexual partners, young age at first sexual activity, sexual contact with high-risk individuals, and early age at first pregnancy. However, the lifetime number of sexual partners is the major determinant of acquisition of oncogenic HPV.[24] HPV types 16, 18, and 33 seropositivity is strongly correlated with the lifetime number of sexual partners but reaches a plateau at 6 to 10 lifetime partners, with an overall seroprevalence for HPV types 16, 18, and 33 of 53%. The probability of infection per any sexual act and the difference in infection per HPV type are unknown.

Studies on the association between the age at sexual debut on HPV positivity are few. However, there is a weak, nonsignificant excess of HPV positivity in women who started having intercourse before age 15 after adjustment for the number of sexual partners.[24] Interpretation of the effect of lifetime number of sexual partners and age at first intercourse on cervical cancer risk is made difficult by the fact that these variables do not fully describe a woman's risk profile for HPV infection. In many of the study populations reviewed, most women reported only 1 sexual partner. For these women, the risk of exposure to HPV—and consequently of developing cervical cancer—chiefly depends on the lifetime number of sexual partners of their husband/partner.[25]

HPV infection is most prevalent in young women and adolescents, and the lower prevalence of HPV infection in older women as compared with younger women has been found to be independent of sexual behavior. Infection with high-risk HPV is more common than with low-risk types. It is possible that infections acquired at later ages have a greater potential for progression in women who have accumulated more years of exposure to known progression cofactors. It is also possible that, biologically, adolescent young women may be more susceptible to infection. The prevalence of HPV infection ranges from 28% to 36% in women younger than 25 years and 2% to 4% in women older than 45 years.[26]

Genital HPV is primarily associated with sexual intercourse; however, nonpenetrative sexual contact, such as genital–genital contact, can also result in HPV transmission.[26] HPV can be cleared even after 1 to 3 years of persistence, and the risk of developing cancer and its precursor, CIN 3, requires at least several years of viral persistence.[27] Screening programs to identify CIN have significantly reduced the morbidity and mortality of this disease (Figure 1-6).

Oral Contraceptives

HPV16 infection alone is probably insufficient to cause cervical cancer, and several possible cofactors have been identified, including the steroid hormones. Steroid hormones are proposed to act with human papillomaviruses as cofactors in the etiology of cervical cancer. A few mechanisms have been proposed whereby use of hormonal contraceptives might affect the development of HPV infection and risk of cervical neoplasia. Steroid hormone–activated nuclear receptors (NRs) are thought to bind to specific DNA sequences within transcriptional regulatory regions on the HPV DNA to either increase or suppress transcription of dependent genes.[28] Hormones may inhibit the immune response to HPV infection. Hormone-related mechanisms may influence the progression from premalignant to malignant cervical lesions by promoting integration of HPV DNA into the host genome, which results in deregulation of E6 and E7 expression. Hormones influence cervical epithelial differentiation and maturation. HPV gene expression and cellular proliferation is increased by estrogen and progestin in vitro.

Several but not all epidemiologic studies have identified oral contraceptive (OC) use as a cofactor in cervical carcinogenesis among HPV high-risk type DNA-positive women.[29] In the studies that demonstrate an association between women with oncogenic HPV and hormonal contraceptive use, there was no increase in the risk of cervical neoplasia for the duration of OC use for up to 4 years. However, use of OCs for longer than 5 years was significantly associated with cervical neoplasia

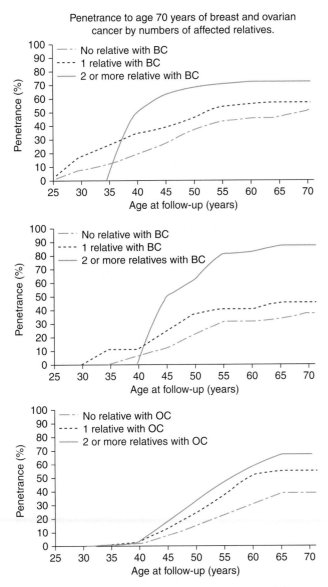

Penetrance to age 70 years of breast and ovarian cancer by numbers of affected relatives.

FIGURE 1-6. Penetrance to age 70 years of breast cancer (BC) and ovarian cancer (OC) by numbers of affected relatives. (Reproduced, with permission, from Metcalfe K, Lubinski J, Lynch HT, et al. Hereditary Breast Cancer Clinical Study Group. Family history of cancer and cancer risks in women with *BRCA1* or *BRCA2* mutations. *J Natl Cancer Inst.* 2010;102(24):1874-1878.)

(OR, 3.4; 95% CI, 2.1-5.5). OC use for longer than 5 years increased risk for invasive cervical cancer 4-fold (OR, 4.0; 95% CI, 2.0-8.0) and risk for carcinoma in situ 3-fold (OR, 3.4; 95% CI, 2.1-5.5).[29]

Cervical Cancer and Parity

Parity has been consistently associated with cervical carcinogenesis. Traumatic, nutritional, and immunologic mechanisms for this association have been postulated.

High parity maintains the transformation zone on the ectocervix for many years, and hormonal changes induced by pregnancy may also affect the immune response to HPV and influence risk of persistence or progression.[29]

Cervical Adenocarcinoma

Most cancers of the uterine cervix are of squamous cell histology. Although the incidence of squamous cell carcinomas of the cervix is in decline, cervical adenocarcinoma has risen in recent years.[30] Whereas smoking and high parity have been associated with increased risk of squamous cell carcinoma, there is none or an inverse association with adenocarcinoma. More than 3 lifetime sexual partners is a risk factor for adenocarcinoma (OR, 2.1; 95% CI, 1.1-4.0), and obesity seems to be a risk factor for adenocarcinoma, but not for squamous cell carcinoma.[31] Hormonal factors, both endogenous (ie, parity) and exogenous (ie, use of hormonal contraceptives), are cofactors in the pathogenesis of cervical adenocarcinoma.

Although HPV16 remains the most common viral type in both histologic types, a greater percentage of glandular malignancies contain HPV18 DNA as the sole infective agent. An analysis of 8 case-control studies of cervical cancer conducted in 8 countries with a range in the incidence of cervical cancer showed that the prevalence of HPV18 in adenocarcinomas (39%) is statistically significantly greater than that in squamous cell carcinoma (18%).[30]

Ovarian Cancer

Germ Cell Tumors

Teratomas are neoplasms containing tissue from all 3 germ cell layers. Mature cystic teratomas, commonly called dermoid cysts, are the most common benign germ cell tumors of the ovary in women of reproductive age. They arise from primordial germ cells and comprise dysgerminomatous and nondysgerminomatous tumors, including yolk sac tumors (endodermal sinus tumors), immature teratomas, mixed germ cell tumors, pure embryonal carcinomas, and nongestational choriocarcinomas.[32] In 85% of women the presenting signs and symptoms include abdominal pain and a palpable pelvic-abdominal mass. Approximately 10% of patients present with acute abdominal pain mimicking appendicitis, usually caused by rupture, hemorrhage, or torsion of the ovarian tumor. Less common signs and symptoms include abdominal distension (35%), fever (10%), and vaginal bleeding (10%). A small proportion of patients exhibit isosexual precocity related to human chorionic gonadotropin (hCG) production by the tumor.[33] Dysgerminoma is

Table 1-2 Classification of Germ Cell Cancers

I. Primitive germ cell tumors
- A. Dysgerminoma
- B. Yolk sac tumor
  1. Polyvesicular vitelline tumor
  2. Glandular variant
  3. Hepatoid variant
- C. Embryonal carcinoma
- D. Polyembryoma
- E. Nongestational choriocarcinoma
- F. Mixed germ cell tumor, specify components

II. Biphasic or triphasic teratoma
- A. Immature teratoma
- B. Mature teratoma
  1. Solid
  2. Cystic, dermoid cyst
  3. Fetiform teratoma, homunculus

III. Monodermal teratoma and somatic-type tumors associated with biphasic or triphasic teratoma
- A. Thyroid tumor group
- B. Carcinoid group
- C. Neuroectodermal tumor group
- D. Carcinoma group
- E. Melanocytic group
- F. Sarcoma group
- G. Sebaceous tumor group
- H. Pituitary-type tumor group
- I. Retinal anlage tumor group
- J. Others

Modified from the World Health Organization histologic classification of tumors of the ovary. (Tavassoli FA, Deville P. *Pathology and Genetics of Tumours of the Breast and Female Genital Organs.* Lyon, France: International Agency for Research on Cancer; 2003.)

one of the most common ovarian neoplasms noted in pregnancy. In patients examined because of primary amenorrhea, it is not infrequently associated with gonadal dysgenesis and a gonadoblastoma (Table 1-2).

Malignant ovarian germ cell tumors have specific tumor markers that can aid in diagnosis and management and are very chemosensitive. Yolk sac tumor and choriocarcinoma are the prototypes of α-fetoprotein (AFP) and hCG production, respectively. Both embryonal carcinoma and polyembryoma may produce hCG and AFP, the former more commonly. A small percentage of dysgerminomas produce low levels of hCG related to the presence of multinucleated syncytiotrophoblastic giant cells, and approximately one-third of immature teratomas produce AFP. Mixed germ cell tumors may produce either, both, or none, depending on the type and quantity of elements present. Occasionally, other serum tumor markers, such as lactic dehydrogenase, may be elevated in patients with malignant ovarian germ cell tumors, particularly dysgerminoma.[33]

Approximately 60% to 70% of cases are International Federation of Gynecologic Oncology (FIGO) stage I or II, 20% to 30% are stage III, and stage IV is relatively uncommon. Bilateral ovarian involvement is uncommon, even when metastatic disease is present. Bilateral involvement occurs in approximately 10% to 15% of dysgerminoma patients.[33] With optimal therapy, the prognosis is excellent, and most patients may retain reproductive function. For those with early-stage disease, cure rates approach 100%, and for those with advanced-stage disease, cure rates are reportedly at least 75%.

Ovarian Stromal Tumors

Sex cord–stromal tumors account for approximately 7% of all malignant ovarian neoplasms, and their extreme rarity represents a limitation in our understanding of their natural history, management, and prognosis.[33] The incidence in developed countries varies from 0.4 to 1.7 patient cases per 100,000 women. Most of these occur in perimenopausal women, but they may occur at any age. The juvenile granulosa cell tumors represent approximately 5% of granulosa cell neoplasms. The reported 5-year survival rate for patients with stage I granulosa cell tumors ranges from 75% to 95%, with the majority of studies demonstrating a greater than 90% survival rate.[34]

One hypothesis for the development of granulosa cell tumors is that the degeneration of follicular granulosa cells after oocyte loss and the consequent compensatory rise in pituitary gonadotrophins may induce irregular proliferation and eventually granulosa cell neoplasia. This hypothesis is consistent with the observation that most granulosa cell tumors occur soon after menopause, when a similar situation of oocyte depletion and high levels of gonadotrophins are observed. However, this explanation cannot be applied to those tumors developing during the reproductive years or even before menarche[34] (Table 1-3).

Pelvic Serous Carcinoma

There is ongoing debate about the cell of origin of pelvic serous carcinomas (defined as tumors of serous histology arising in the ovary, fallopian tube, or peritoneum). There are 2 possible origins under consideration: (1) carcinogenesis of the ovarian surface epithelium, mullerian inclusions, or endometriosis in the ovary, or (2) carcinogenesis of the distal fallopian tube epithelium.

Ovarian Cancer/Fallopian Tube Cancer

Ovarian/fallopian cancer is the eighth most common cancer among both white and African American

Table 1-3 Classification of Sex Cord–Stromal Ovarian Tumors

Classification
Granulosa stromal cell tumors
Granulosa
Adult type
Juvenile type
Tumors in the thecoma-fibroma group
Thecoma
Fibroma-fibrosarcoma
Sclerosing stromal tumor
Sertoli-Leydig cell tumors, androblastomas
Sertoli
Leydig
Sertoli-Leydig
Well differentiated
Intermediate differentiation
Poorly differentiated
With heterologous elements
Retiform
Mixed
Gynandroblastoma
Sex cord tumor with anular tubules
Unclassified

Reproduced, with permission, from Colombo N, Parma G, Zanagnolo V, Insinga A. Management of ovarian stromal cell tumors. *J Clin Oncol.* 2007;25(20):2944-2951.

women and the fifth most common cause of cancer death in the United States.[2] Ovarian cancer represents the sixth most commonly diagnosed cancer in women across the world. It is the second most common gynecologic malignancy in the United States, with a death toll of 13,850 annually.[2] Parity, OC use, and hysterectomy substantially reduce epithelial ovarian cancer risk.[35] Epithelial ovarian cancer risk is reduced with earlier age at menopause, per year of being pregnant, for shorter time intervals between menarche and menopause, and per-year reduction in total menstrual life span.[36]

Obesity and Physical Activity

Obesity is a risk factor for many hormonally related malignancies, including endometrial and postmenopausal breast cancer. Approximately 30% of patients with ovarian cancer are overweight, and 12% are obese. A meta-analysis of 28 eligible studies found consistent epidemiologic evidence that the risk of ovarian cancer increases with increasing BMI. The pooled effect estimate for adult obesity was 1.3 (95% CI, 1.1-1.5), with a smaller increased risk for overweight women (OR, 1.2; 95% CI, 1.0-1.3).[37]

Physical activity may also influence ovarian cancer risk through a reduction in chronic inflammation or anovulation and thereby potentially reduce ovarian cancer risk.[38] A meta-analysis of 12 studies of recreational physical activity and risk of epithelial ovarian cancer provided summary estimates of 0.79 (95% CI, 0.70-0.85) for case-control studies and 0.81 (95% CI, 0.57-1.17) for cohort studies for the risk of ovarian cancer associated with highest versus lowest levels of recreational physical activity.[37]

Hereditary Ovarian Cancer

Hereditary breast and ovarian cancer (HBOC) due to mutations in breast cancer 1 gene *BRCA1* and breast cancer 2 gene *BRCA2* occurs in all ethnic and racial populations and is the most common cause of hereditary forms of both breast and ovarian cancer. The *BRCA1* gene is located on 17q21 and has a total length of approximately 100 kilobyte (kB). *BRCA1* is believed to contribute to the maintenance of chromosomal stability. The *BRCA2* gene is located on 13q12.3. It has a total length of 70 kB. *BRCA2* binds to the DNA-repair protein Rad51 at the BRC repeat regions and contributes to the maintenance of chromosomal stability and to homologous recombination.

Three distinct clinical patterns of cancer have been noted in the families of women with ovarian cancer:

1. Ovarian cancer in association with breast cancer
2. Ovarian cancer alone
3. Ovarian cancer in association with cancers of the colon, rectum, endometrium, stomach, urothelium, and pancreas, and the hereditary nonpolyposis colon cancer syndrome (Lynch syndrome)

Ashkenazi Jewish women have a substantially elevated risk of HBOC because of a high frequency of *BRCA1/2* mutations, which are mainly attributable to 3 well-described founder mutations: 2 of which are in the *BRCA1* gene (187delAG and 5385insC, also known as 185delAG and 5382insC, respectively) and 1 of which is in the *BRCA2* gene (6174delT).[39] The lifetime risks for ovarian cancer are estimated to be in the range of 28% to 66% for a *BRCA1* mutation and 16% to 27% for a *BRCA2* mutation.[40]

A prospective multinational cohort study modeled the influence of a family history of cancer on the risks of breast and ovarian cancer for 3011 women with a deleterious mutation in *BRCA1* or *BRCA2*. Compared with *BRCA1* mutation carriers with no first- or second-degree relative with ovarian cancer, those with ≥2 first- or second-degree relatives with ovarian cancer were statistically significantly more likely to develop ovarian cancer in the follow-up period. For women with a *BRCA1* mutation, the risk of ovarian cancer increased by 61% for each first- or second-degree relative with fallopian or ovarian cancer (multivariable hazard ratio [HR] = 1.61; 95% CI, 1.21-2.14; P = .001)[40] (Figure 1-6).

It is recommended that women with inherited *BRCA1* or *BRCA2* (*BRCA1/2*) mutations undergo risk-reducing salpingo-oophorectomy (RRSO) to reduce their cancer risk, generally by age 40 years or after the completion of childbearing.[41] RRSO is highly effective in reducing ovarian and fallopian tube cancers in both *BRCA1* and *BRCA2* mutation carriers and in those with and without prior breast cancer. In *BRCA1* mutation carriers, RRSO is associated with a 70% reduction in the risk of ovarian cancer in those without prior breast cancer and an 85% reduction in those with prior breast cancer.[42] There is some evidence that short-term use of hormone replacement therapy after RRSO does not negate the reduction in breast cancer risk conferred by RRSO.[43] Women with *BRCA1/2* mutations who have markedly increased risks of breast and ovarian cancer have a different risk and benefit profile; therefore, issues of timing and the safety of hormone therapy are important.

Primary Peritoneal Cancer

Primary peritoneal cancer (PPC) arises in the tissue that lines the abdominal cavity and pelvic cavity. It is an uncommon disease that shares many histopathologic and clinical characteristics with epithelial ovarian cancer (EOC), but PPC is distinguished by the absence of a malignant/invasive ovarian mass. It is uncertain whether PPC is a distinct disease from EOC or if they share common origin(s). Features shared by both PPC and EOC include the preponderance of serous histology, the advanced stage at diagnosis for the majority of women, and similar responsiveness to platinum/taxane chemotherapy. The similarities of these cancers as well as cancers of the fallopian tubes have led to the suggestion that each of these cancer types develops from a common cell lineage, the embryonic Mullerian system.[44] Recent findings implicate the fallopian tube fimbria as a possible site of origin of cancers previously characterized as "ovarian" carcinomas (Figure 1-7). Expression profiling studies have shown that high-grade epithelial cancers cluster separately from

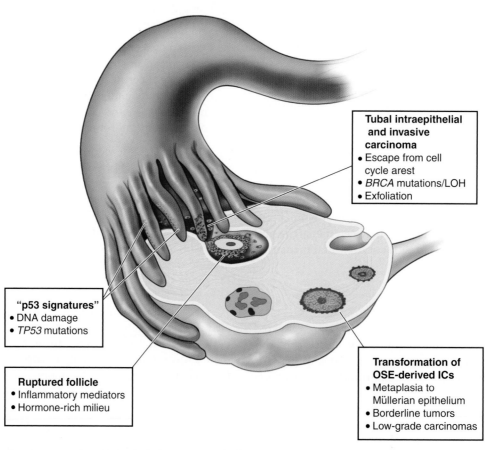

Tubal intraepithelial and invasive carcinoma
- Escape from cell cycle arest
- *BRCA* mutations/LOH
- Exfoliation

"p53 signatures"
- DNA damage
- *TP53* mutations

Ruptured follicle
- Inflammatory mediators
- Hormone-rich milieu

Transformation of OSE-derived ICs
- Metaplasia to Müllerian epithelium
- Borderline tumors
- Low-grade carcinomas

FIGURE 1-7. Carcinogenesis of epithelial ovarian carcinoma. LOH, loss of heterozygosity; OSE, ovarian surface epithelium; ICs, invasive carcinomas.

low-grade carcinomas and borderline tumors.[45] This leads to the classification of ovarian cancers into type 1 tumors, which are low grade and slowly developing (including endometrioid, mucinous, and low-grade serous), and type 2 tumors, which are rapidly progressing, high-grade serous carcinomas. High-grade tumors are associated strongly with *TP53* mutations, whereas low-grade tumors are associated with mutations in *KRAS*, *BRAF*, *PTEN*, and *CTNNB1/β-catenin*.[46]

Vulva/Vaginal Cancer

Vulvar cancers are a rare malignancy of the female genital tract. The incidence of invasive and in situ vulvar carcinoma has been increasing at a rate of 2.4% per year, and the National Cancer Institute has identified vulvar cancer as 1 of 12 cancers with rising incidence. Epidemiologic factors that have been associated with the development of vulvar cancer include granulomatous infection, herpes simplex virus, and human papillomavirus.

Vaginal Cancers

Although the majority of squamous cell cancers of the vulva are associated with HPV infection, a small proportion of vaginal cancers are clear cell adenocarcinomas that have been linked to intrauterine exposure to maternal diethylstilbestrol (DES) use. Chronic vaginitis, prior hysterectomy for benign disease, endometriosis, and cervical irradiation have also been cited as predisposing factors for vaginal cancers.[47]

DES is a synthetic estrogen that was prescribed to pregnant women from the 1940s to 1970s in order to prevent pregnancy-associated complications, including miscarriage. This drug was administered to almost 3 million women in the United States. Among women exposed prenatally to the drug, several adverse health effects have been observed before age 30 years, such as clear cell adenocarcinoma of the vagina and cervix. In a European study of cancer risk in a large cohort of 12,091 DES daughters, with long-term follow-up, the risk of clear cell adenocarcinoma of the vagina and cervix was statistically significantly increased (standardized incidence ratio = 24.23; 95% CI, 8.89-52.74); the elevated risk persisted above 40 years of age.[48]

HPV has been associated with vulvar and vaginal cancer and vulvar intraepithelial neoplasia (VIN) and vaginal intraepithelial neoplasia (VAIN). HPV DNA in VIN and vulvar cancerous lesions has been reported to vary from 0% to 89%. The largest series of HPV DNA types analyzed from surgical samples in a cohort of 241 German women with lower genital tract intraepithelial neoplasia demonstrated that 92% of the VIN2/3, VAIN2/3 samples were HPV positive.[49] Overall, however, HPV16/18 contributes to 84.0% of VIN3 and 65.1% of VAIN3.

Extramammary Paget Disease

Most cases of vulvar extramammary Paget disease are primary; that is, they arise within the epidermis, and very few are associated with cutaneous sweat glands. Vulvar extramammary Paget disease has been described in association with endometrial, endocervical, and vaginal as well as vulvar cancers.

Gestational Trophoblastic Neoplasia

Gestational trophoblastic diseases consist of a group of neoplastic disorders arising from placental trophoblastic tissue after normal or abnormal fertilization. Inclusive are hydatidiform moles (partial and complete), choriocarcinoma, placental site trophoblastic tumors, and epithelioid trophoblastic tumors. Estimates from studies conducted in North America, Australia, New Zealand, and Europe have shown the incidence of hydatidiform mole to range from 0.57 to 1.1 per 1000 pregnancies, whereas studies in Southeast Asia and Japan have suggested an incidence as high as 2.0 per 1000 pregnancies. The 2 established risk factors that have emerged are extremes of maternal age and prior molar pregnancy. Advanced or very young maternal age has consistently correlated with higher rates of complete hydatidiform mole. Compared with women aged 21 to 35 years, the risk of complete mole is 1.9 times higher for women both >35 years and <21 years as well as 7.5 times higher for women >40 years. The risk of repeat molar pregnancy after 1 mole is approximately 1%, or approximately 10 to 20 times the risk for the general population. Familial biparental hydatidiform mole (FBHM) is a maternal-effect autosomal recessive disorder in which recurrent pregnancy failure with molar degeneration occurs. Several women affected with FBHM have previously been shown to have biallelic mutations in the *NLRP7* gene (*NALP7*).[50] Subsequent pregnancies in women diagnosed with this condition are likely to be complete hydatidiform moles.

CLINICAL TRIAL DESIGN AND STATISTICAL CONSIDERATIONS

The design, execution, and analysis of results from clinical trials in oncology have resulted in a robust body of evidence-based medicine in gynecologic oncology. Evidence-based practice requires statistically valid trial design to produce clinically relevant and meaningful conclusions. An overview of the concepts in clinical trial design and the methods of statistical analysis are described next. Many volumes have been written on this topic, and the interested reader is referred to these references.[51,52]

Methodology and End Points

Randomization

The use of nonrandomized controls in clinical trials results in differential bias in the selection of patients as a consequence of physician choice, self-selection by patients, and varied referral patterns. The use of random treatment assignment to form the control group minimizes selection biases that otherwise make their way into phase 3 clinical trials. In addition, randomization balances the arms of a trial with respect to prognostic variables (both known and unknown). Although randomization helps to ensure an unbiased evaluation of the relative efficacies and tolerabilities of the treatment regimens under investigation, it should be emphasized that this process does not ensure that a given study will include a representative sample of all patients with the disease in question. Finally, randomization forms the basis for statistical analyses—specifically, the basis for an assumption-free statistical test of the equality of treatments. When properly executed, the randomized controlled clinical trial provides the strongest evidence of the clinical efficacy of preventative procedures and therapeutic regimens in the oncologic arena.

The most common methods of randomization include simple, block, stratified, and unequal randomization.

Simple Randomization. This is equivalent to tossing a coin for each subject that enters a trial (eg, heads = chemotherapy drug A; tails = chemotherapy drug A plus investigational target agent B). This method is simple and easy to implement, and the treatment assignment is completely unpredictable. Unfortunately, simple randomization may lead to imbalanced treatment assignment. Even if treatment is balanced at the end of a trial, it may not be balanced at some time during the trial. This is particularly important if a trial is monitored during the process of conduct of the entire trial. Imbalanced randomization reduces statistical power.

Block Randomization. If patient characteristics change over time (eg, patients accrued earlier experience a decrease in performance status), early imbalances cannot be corrected. Block randomization may be used to address this issue. This method divides potential patients into 2 blocks, and then each block is randomized such that a certain number of patients are allocated to A and a certain number are allocated to B. Blocks are then chosen randomly. This method ensures equal treatment allocation within each block if the complete block is used.

Stratified Randomization. As discussed previously, an imbalanced randomization in numbers of subjects reduces statistical power. Importantly, however, an imbalance in prognostic factors will also render a clinical trial inefficient in estimating treatment effect. A trial may not be valid if it is not well balanced across prognostic factors. For example, in a trial of advanced endometrial cancer, with 6 patients with FIGO stage IIIC1 disease, there is 22% chance of 5-1 or 6-0 split by block randomization only. Stratified randomization is the solution to achieve balance within subgroups: use block randomization separately for FIGO stage IIIC1 and other advanced FIGO stages.

Unequal Randomization. Most randomized trials allocate equal numbers of patients to experimental and control groups. This is the most statistically efficient randomization ratio because it maximizes statistical power for a given total sample size. However, when a clinical trial is designed to allocate fewer patients to the placebo or to a no-treatment arm, a randomization ratio of 2:1 may be used with only a modest loss in statistical power. Generally, a randomization ratio of 3:1 will lose considerable statistical power, and more extreme randomization ratios are not useful in oncology.

Placebo

A placebo is an inactive drug used in a control group in place of the actual treatment. If a drug is being evaluated, the inactive vehicle or carrier is used alone so it is as similar as possible in appearance and in administration to the active drug. Placebos are used to blind investigators and the patients to which group the patient is allocated. Placebos are usually not used in front-line oncology clinical trials but may be used in studies of consolidation therapy for patients in clinical remission for whom an investigational agent is being studied to determine whether recurrence can be prevented or further delayed. Placebo-controlled trials are never appropriate when a highly effective or potentially curative therapy is available for a patient unless the trial allows the patient to receive the new treatment/placebo in addition to the potentially curative therapy.

The use of placebos in cancer clinical trials becomes particularly important when studying biologic agents. Although most antineoplastic drugs cause obvious tumor shrinkage, many targeted therapies slow tumor growth but may not cause decrease in tumor size. Testing such drugs requires that the trial has a control group so that investigators can determine whether stabilization of tumor growth is an effect of the novel agent or just reflects tumor biology.

Blinding

Because human behavior is influenced by what we know and believe, in research there is a particular risk of expectation influencing findings. This occurs most often when there is some level of subjectivity in assessment, and this can lead to biased results. Such bias is not due to deliberate deception but is rather the result of human nature and even prior held beliefs about the area of study.

Blinding is a method to reduce bias by preventing investigators and/or patients involved in a clinical trial from knowing the hypothesis being investigated, the case-control classification, the assignment of individuals or groups, or the different treatments being provided. In oncology clinical trials, blinding is often used for treatment allocation. Blinding reduces bias by preserving symmetry in the investigator's measurements and assessments.

Blinding patients to treatment in a randomized control trial is particularly important when the response criteria are subjective (eg, alleviation of pain). Conversely, blinding of the cancer center staff caring for patients in a randomized trial to treatment allocation minimizes possible bias in patient management in assessing disease status. As an example, the decision to withdraw a patient from a study or to adjust drug dosage could easily be influenced by knowledge of the treatment arm a patient has been assigned to. In a double-blind trial, neither the patient nor the oncologist and her/his team have knowledge of the treatment assignment.

Stratification

A more detailed discussion on the importance of stratification is warranted. As discussed previously, it is important to stratify the randomization to ensure equal distribution of important prognostic factors when they are known. Through block randomization, a separate randomization list is created for each stratum of patients. Balancing each list is important so that each block of patients within a given stratum will result in treatment groups containing equal numbers of patients. The sequence of treatment assignments is random within each block. Investigators designing clinical trials in oncology must make every effort to limit stratification to those factors that have been definitely shown to have independent prognostic effects. Ideally, these factors will have been identified and/or validated in previous prospective clinical trials. If 2 factors are closely correlated with outcome in the same direction, only 1 factor needs to be included in the stratification. Stratification helps to maintain balance for interim analyses, especially in trials in which sample sizes may be limited. Furthermore, stratification allows for the performance of subsequent subset analyses at the conclusion of a clinical trial.

Sample Size and Power Analysis

Sample size planning is predicated on the assumption that at the conclusion of the protocol-specified follow-up

period, statistical analyses between the control arm and the investigational arm(s) may be able to detect a statistically significant difference for a primary end point. Clinical trials in oncology should be large enough to detect reliably the smallest possible differences in the primary end point with therapy that has clinical benefit.

The *power* of a study is its ability to detect a true difference in outcome between the reference (ie, control) arm and the investigational arm(s). Typically, a power set at 80% accepts the likelihood of 20% of missing such a real difference (ie, a false-negative result). The threshold P value is defined by the chosen *level of significance*, which sets the likelihood of detecting a treatment effect when no effect exists (ie, a false-positive result). A result with a P value above the specified threshold indicates that an observed difference may be due to chance alone, whereas those with a P value below the threshold suggest that the intervention has a real effect. In most trials, the level of significance is set at 5% (ie, $P = .05$), and therefore the investigator is prepared to accept a 5% chance of erroneously reporting a significant effect. A 1-sided significance level represents the probability, by chance alone, of obtaining a difference as large as and in the same direction as that actually observed. A 2-sided significance level is usually twice the 1-sided significance level and represents the probability of obtaining by chance a difference in either direction as large in absolute magnitude as that actually observed. A 2-sided significance level of .05 is widely accepted as a standard level of evidence.

The *underlying event rate* in the population under study must be established from previous studies, including observational cohorts. The *treatment effect* is the difference between the rate of the event in the control arm and the rate in the investigational arm and can be expressed as an absolute difference or as a relative reduction. It is critical that a clinical trial be designed to identify a realistically modest treatment effect; otherwise, small real reductions are rendered statistically nonsignificant. Finally, sample size must be adjusted for other factors, including *patient compliance* with their allocated treatments. It is often not possible to predict lack of compliance, and this is a source of a major limitation in sample size calculations.

Factorial Designs

One method to answer 2 different questions in a clinical trial is to design the study using a 2 × 2 factorial design. In such a trial, there are 4 treatment allocations. The sample size of a 2 × 2 factorial trial is computed, assuming there is no interaction between the 2 factors under investigation. The Bayesian model suggests that in designing a 2 × 2 factorial trial in which interactions are unlikely but cannot be excluded, the sample size should be increased by at least 30% as compared with a simple 2-arm clinical trial for detecting the same size of treatment effects. This makes the trial more feasible than doing a true 4-arm randomized trial in which the sample size would need to be doubled.

Therapeutic Equivalence

Therapeutic equivalency or therapeutic equivalency trials are problematic. In these clinical trials, the objective is to determine whether a new treatment is therapeutically equivalent to an established effective treatment. Additionally, these trials may be used to determine whether a new treatment is effective relative to no treatment. Unfortunately, it is not possible to demonstrate therapeutic equivalence, and at best one can establish that results are only consistent with differences in efficacy within specified limits. In point of fact, the failure to reject the null hypothesis may be the result of inadequate sample size rather than a demonstration of equivalence.

Large sample sizes are needed to establish that differences in efficacy are within narrow limits, and this in turn is predicated on the degree of effectiveness of the active control. Stated differently, the limits within which a difference in efficacy is bounded depends on the precision with which the effectiveness of the active control is estimated. For these reasons, therapeutic equivalence trials are neither feasible nor interpretable unless there is strong quantifiable evidence (ie reproducible, consistent) for the effectiveness of the active control.

Non-Inferiority Trials

Non-inferiority trials are designed to demonstrate that the effect of a new treatment is not worse than that of an active control by more than a specified margin. Lack of protection from bias by blinding and the difficulty in specifying the non-inferiority margin are 2 inherent weaknesses of such trials. Non-inferiority trials may be required in those oncologic scenarios in which it would not be ethical to include a placebo group.

As discussed previously, it is fundamentally impossible to prove that 2 treatments have exactly equivalent effects. Therapeutic equivalence trials are designed to show that the effects differ by no more than a tolerable amount or equivalence margin. In therapeutic equivalence trials, if the effects of the 2 treatments differ by more than the equivalence margin in either direction, then equivalence does not hold. Conversely, non-inferiority trials aim to show that the investigational arm is not worse than the active control by more than the equivalence margin.

Intention-to-Treat Analysis

Intention to treat (ITT) is an analysis based on the initial treatment allocation in a clinical trial, rather than on the treatment that is ultimately administered. ITT is a tool that eliminates misleading artifacts that may arise during the conduct of a clinical trial. As an example, if patients with more refractory, chemoresistant disease tend to drop out at a higher rate, a completely ineffective treatment may appear to be providing benefits if the investigator only evaluates the "healthier" group that completed treatment and ignores those that discontinued the study. Therefore, in ITT, each subject who begins treatment is considered part of the trial, whether they complete protocol-specified therapy or not. ITT analyses are also performed to avoid the effects of crossover, which may also break the randomization.

Because ITT adheres to the randomization allocation, it is widely recognized as the most valid analytic approach for superiority trials that involve long-term endpoint follow-up. Although ITT may be viewed as overly conservative, most investigators acknowledge that a positive ITT analysis of a superiority trial is convincing evidence of efficacy.

Per-Protocol Analysis

Unlike ITT (discussed in the preceding section), per-protocol analysis (PP) analyzes only patients who complete the entire clinical trial on the protocol-specified arm they were assigned to on enrollment. In other words, PP restricts the comparison of treatment arms to ideal patients (ie, those who adhere perfectly to the clinical trial instructions as stipulated in the protocol). Therefore, PP attempts to determine the biological effect of a new drug/therapy, but by restricting analysis to a selected patient population, PP is unable to demonstrate the practical value of a new drug/therapy. Because PP excludes data from patients with major protocol violations, these exclusionary data sets can substantially bias results in either direction.

Interim Analysis

An interim analysis allows for early stopping of a clinical trial if large differences between treatment arms are recognized. This strategy not only conserves time and resources, but can reduce patient exposure to inferior treatment and/or life-threatening toxicities. Implicit in the performance of an interim analysis is whether an ongoing clinical trial can realistically answer its primary objective(s). Among the factors that are considered when performing an interim analysis are the following:

1. Accrual rate
2. Rate of life-threatening/severe adverse events

3. Is the projected outcome of the therapeutic arm(s) comparable with that of previous experience in the population under study?
4. Is/are there significant difference(s) between the treatment arms that exceed the differences defined by the statistical guidelines of the protocol?

Any 1 of the above 4 factors can lead to early termination of an ongoing clinical trial.

Data Safety and Monitoring Board

The Data and Safety Monitoring Board (DSMB) is an independent group of experts who evaluate patient safety and efficacy data during an ongoing clinical trial. The DSMB typically comprises at least 1 biostatistician and clinicians knowledgeable about the disease under study. In some cases, an ethicist and/or a representative from a patient advocacy group may be included. A DSMB is particularly important for clinical trials that are double-blinded in order to allow for someone to oversee the conduct of the study and the results as they become available. In addition, a meeting of a DSMB may also be called when the results of a mid-trial safety analysis indicate that a predetermined threshold for specific adverse events has been crossed. Early termination of a study may therefore be based on safety concerns, futility, or overwhelming benefit.

Safety. Although the DSMB may recommend termination of a study based on interim safety data suggesting the more common occurrence of serious/life-threatening adverse events in the investigational arm, this is only done after a careful evaluation of the risk-to-benefit ratio. If the resulting improvement in survival outweighs serious adverse events (provided the adverse events do not lead to death), the DSMB may not close the study. However, the primary mandate of the DSMB is to protect patient safety.

Futility. During an interim analysis, if it is determined that none of the experimental arms are likely to outperform the control arm, the DSMB may recommend early closure of the trial. Crossing the futility boundary may be one of the most common reasons to close a trial.

Overwhelming Benefit. In the very rare situation in which the investigational arm demonstrates undeniable superiority to the control arm, early termination may be recommended. The statistical evidence for overwhelming benefit must be very high.

Hypothesis Testing and Confidence Limits

Hypothesis testing allows investigators to evaluate data on the basis of the probability or improbability of observing the results obtained. Four possible outcomes are allowed by hypothesis testing:

1. The null hypothesis is rejected when it is false.
2. The null hypothesis is rejected when it is true (type I or α error).
3. The null hypothesis is accepted when it is true.
4. The null hypothesis is accepted when it is false (type II or β error).

It should be recognized that items 2 and 4 in the preceding list are errors that can lead to the erroneous adoption of certain hypotheses.

A *confidence interval* (CI) is a range around a measurement that conveys how precise the measurement is. The CI denotes the range of values within which the true prevalence or percentage lies with a specified degree of assurance. The most frequently used confidence interval for clinical trial data is the 95% confidence interval for the mean treatment difference.

If the study design used to compute the 95% confidence interval is used over and over again with the same patient population, drug dosages, and schedule, 95% of the time the interval will contain the true parameter value. A 95% confidence interval will either contain the true parameter value of interest or it will not (thus the probability of containing the true value is either 1 or 0).

Hazard Ratios

The hazard ratio (HR) is derived from the Cox proportional hazards model. The HR provides a statistical test of treatment efficacy and an estimate of the relative risk of events of interest to oncologists. If the event of interest is a complication, the HR describes the relative risk of the complication on the basis of comparison of event rates. Hazard ratios have also been used to describe the outcome of therapeutic trials where the question is to what extent investigational therapy can improve progression-free survival (PFS) and/or overall survival (OS). The HR, however, does not always accurately portray the degree of improvement in that patients may have a longer PFS and/or OS, but the HR does not convey information about the absolute length of improvement.

End Points

Examples of commonly used end points include response rate (RR), duration of response, disease-free survival (DFS), PFS, and OS.

DFS is used to analyze the results of treatment for localized disease that renders a patient apparently disease-free. Examples of such treatment include surgery alone or surgery plus adjuvant therapy. With DFS, the event is relapse rather than death, in that the people who experience relapse are still alive but are no longer disease-free. Because in the majority of cases patients survive for at least some time after relapse, the curve for OS looks better than that for DFS for the same population under study. PFS, on the other hand, is a tool used to analyze the results of treatment of advanced disease. The event for PFS is that the disease progresses or worsens. Similarly, duration of response is used to analyze the results of treatment for advanced disease with the event being tumor progression. Duration of response measures the length of the response only in those patients who responded.

Survival Curves

Two methods may be used to create a survival curve. With the *actuarial method*, the x-axis is separated into regular intervals (eg, months or years), and survival is calculated for each interval. The resulting graph will only step at the regular specified intervals. Actuarial analysis should be performed when the actual date of a survival event is unknown and is also useful for population-based death rates and DFS. With the *Kaplan-Meier (K-M) method*, survival is recalculated every time a patient dies. The K-M method is actually preferable for most oncologic trials as well as for analyzing postoperative survival. It is used when the actual date of the end point(s) is/are known. End points not reached are treated as censored at the date of last follow-up for the analysis. K-M analysis is undertaken at each survival event, death, or censoring, and the graphs will step at each failure time and may or may not be drawn to show the location of censored observations. The term *life-table analysis* may be applied to both the actuarial and K-M methods.

Forest Plots

Forest plots are designed to illustrate the relative strength of treatment effects in multiple scientific studies addressing the same question. These charts were originally developed as a means of graphically representing a meta-analysis of the results of randomized controlled trials. Forest plots are commonly presented with 2 columns. In the left-hand column, the names of the studies appear, and in the right-hand column, there is a plot to measure effect (eg, an odds ratio) for each of these studies (often represented by a square) incorporating confidence intervals represented by horizontal lines. The area of each square is proportional to the study's weight in the meta-analysis. A vertical line representing no effect is also plotted. If the confidence intervals for individual studies overlap with this line, it demonstrates that at the given level of confidence, their effect sizes do not differ from no effect for the individual study. This also applies to the meta-analyzed measure of effect: If the points of the

diamond overlap the line of no effect, then the overall meta-analyzed result cannot be said to differ from no effect at the given level of confidence.

Multivariate Analysis

Multivariate analysis is based on the statistical principle of analysis of more than 1 statistical variable at a time. Two examples of multivariate analysis from recently published phase 3 randomized trials appear later.

Meta-Analysis

In statistics, a *meta-analysis* combines the results of several studies that address a set of related research hypotheses. The general aim of a meta-analysis is to more powerfully estimate the true effect size as opposed to a smaller effect size derived in a single study under a given single set of assumptions and conditions. Meta-analyses are often, but not always, important components of a *systematic review* procedure. Here it is convenient to follow the terminology used by the Cochrane Collaboration and use *meta-analysis* to refer to statistical methods of combining evidence, leaving other aspects of *research synthesis* or *evidence synthesis*, such as combining information from qualitative studies, for the more general context of systematic reviews.

Evaluation of New Agents for Clinical Use

Phase 1 Clinical Trials

Phase 1 clinical trials are designed to determine toxicity profiles and the appropriate dose for use in phase 2 trials. Patients enrolled on phase 1 trials must have normal organ function, but their cancers are considered untreatable with standard therapy. Multiple dose levels are used in these studies, with 3 to 6 patients treated at each dose level. If no dose-limiting toxicity (DLT) is observed at a given dose level, the dose is escalated for the next cohort. If the incidence of DLT is greater than 33% at a given dose, then the dose escalation stops. The phase 2 dose is the highest dose for which the incidence of DLT is less than 33%. Phase 1B trials have been advanced in the clinical arena to study the association of targeted therapy dose estimation with both toxicity and immunologic effect.

A limitation of a phase 1 trial is that patients may be exposed to subtherapeutic doses of new drugs. In addition, these trials may not provide critical information about interpatient variability and cumulative toxicity. This is due to the fact that unlike phase 2 and phase 3 trials, phase 1 studies have smaller numbers, and a given trial may contain patients with multiple different tumor types.

Phase 2 Clinical Trials

It is imperative that phase 2 trials be conducted in cohorts of patients who are likely to benefit from the investigational agent but for whom no effective therapy is available. Patients enrolled on these studies should have excellent performance status and have had minimal prior exposure to chemotherapy. For patients with chemo-sensitive malignancies, such as ovarian cancer, new drugs should be evaluated in populations with no more than 1 prior treatment for metastatic disease. Adherence to the principle of studying novel agents first in favorable populations limits exposure of patients with more advanced disease to inactive therapy for whom the incidence of toxic effects are higher.

For phase 2 trials evaluating single agents, response rate is an appropriate end point. It should be recognized that because phase II trials do not have an internal control, any conclusions drawn regarding survival are purely speculative. A 2-stage design is a common method used in phase 2 trials. During the first stage of the trial, if fewer than a specified number of responses are obtained among the first predetermined number of patients treated, then the study is terminated and the drug is rejected. If the drug meets its response rate goal with the first stage, then the study is continued into the second stage to accrue the full number of patients assigned.

Phase 2 studies are sometimes divided into phase 2A and phase 2B trials. Phase 2A clinical trials are specifically designed to assess dosing requirements, whereas phase 2B studies are designed to study efficacy.

Randomized phase 2 studies are designed as randomized clinical trials in which subjects receive a drug and others receive standard treatment or a placebo. Randomized phase 2 trials require fewer patients than randomized phase 3 trials.

Phase 3 Clinical Trials

Survival and quality of life are appropriate end points for phase 3 clinical trials. It is important for the results of phase 3 trials to be applicable to patients seen in the community outside of clinical research centers. For this reason, phase 3 trials are often multi-institutional and include community physician participation. This allows for generalization and therefore applicability of the conclusions reached at the end of the trial. Importantly, tumor shrinkage is usually not an appropriate end point for phase 3 trials because it may have little or no relation to patient benefit.

Phase 4 Clinical Trials

Phase 4 clinical trials involve safety surveillance of a drug after it has received approval by the US Food and Drug Administration (FDA) to be marketed. This is known as *pharmacovigilance*. The implementation of a phase 4 study may be a requirement of regulatory authorities or may be undertaken by the industry sponsor for competitive marketing or for other reasons (eg, effect of the drug on the conduct of pregnancy). The safety surveillance is designed to detect any rare or long-term adverse effects over a much larger patient population and longer time period than was possible during the phase 1 to 3 clinical trials. Harmful effects discovered by phase 4 trials may result in a drug being no longer sold or restricted to certain uses.

Clinical Trial Mechanics

There are 3 types of clinical trials. Hypothesis-driven, investigator-initiated studies may be conducted at ≥ 1 institution but originate usually from a single investigator and are often paid through a successful intramural or extramural funding program, the latter of which may include a corporate sponsor or even the National Institutes of Health. Industry-sponsored protocols are developed within a pharmaceutical company by a medical science officer and scientific committee and are then rolled out to different institutions for consideration of participation. Cooperative group trials are developed through coordinated communication among many committees both internally and externally. Cooperative group trials of the Gynecologic Oncology Group are supported through National Cancer Institute funding and may also receive support through an independent sponsor through provision of novel agent(s) being tested in the trial.

The clinical trial protocol includes the *Study Objectives*, which are followed by the *Background and Rationale* sections. These passages describe the state of the science leading up to the development of the protocol as a strategy to answer the questions proposed. Detailed eligibility criteria as well as specific conditions/scenarios that make a patient ineligible (eg, prior treatment of recurrent disease with chemotherapy) are listed. The randomization procedure is carefully detailed.

The treatment plan for each arm of the trial is provided, with details on the storage and administration of each agent. Treatment modifications for hematologic and nonhematologic toxicity are then listed for each agent separately. Study parameters are provided and tabulated to indicate the timing of various interventions and evaluations (eg, quality of life survey, hematologic profile, translational research specimens). Study duration, monitoring, and finally statistical considerations are described fully. The statistical section contains hypothesis modeling and sample size calculations based on the end points being studied. Additionally, a plan for monitoring of unacceptable toxicity in the experimental arms provides the number of events for each investigational arm that needs to occur before a meeting of the DSMB is called. Finally, the schedule for an interim analysis is also included. Reporting of results of a prospective randomized phase 3 trial to the FDA may be preceded by a public announcement by the sponsor (ie, pharmaceutical company), which often coincides with unblinding of subjects if the trial was blinded. At this point the sponsor has the option to prepare an application to the FDA for registration of the agent under investigation. The application is first reviewed by the Oncology Drugs Advisory Board, which will submit their recommendation to the FDA regarding the label.

BIOSTATISTICAL TERMS

Absolute Risk: The probability or chance that a person will have a medical event. Absolute risk is expressed as a percentage. It is the ratio of the number of people who have a medical event divided by all of the people who could have the event because of their medical condition.

Association: A relationship. In research studies, association means that 2 characteristics (sometimes also called variables or factors) are related so that if one changes, the other changes in a predictable way. An association does not necessarily mean that one variable causes the other.

Bias: Any factor, recognized or not, that distorts the findings of a study. In research studies, bias can influence the observations, results, and conclusions of the study and make them less accurate or believable.

Blinding: A way of making sure that the people involved in a research study—participants, clinicians, or researchers—do not know which participants are assigned to each study group. Blinding is used to make sure that knowing the type of treatment does not affect a participant's response to the treatment, a health care provider's behavior, or assessment of the treatment effects.

Cohort Study: A clinical research study in which people who presently have a certain condition or receive a particular treatment are followed over time and compared with another group of people who are not affected by the condition.

Confidence Interval: A statistical estimate of how much the study findings would vary if other different people participated in the study. A confidence interval is defined by 2 numbers, one lower than the result found in the study and the other higher than the study's result. The size of the confidence interval is the difference between these 2 numbers.

Confounding: Confounding is a mixing or blurring of effects that occurs when a researcher attempts to relate an exposure to an outcome but actually measures the effect of a third factor (the confounding variable).

Control Group: The group of people who do not receive the treatment being tested. The control group might receive a placebo, a different treatment for the disease, or no treatment at all.

Effect Modification: This occurs when the association between the exposure and disease varies by levels of a third factor.

Heterogeneity: Differences among research studies. Heterogeneity can apply to either the way the studies were conducted, the methodologies used in the studies, or differences in the way people respond to the treatment. Research reports may describe different types of heterogeneity.

Hypothesis: The scientific idea that led to the research study.

Incidence: The number of new cases developing in a population of individuals at risk during a specified time period. The cumulative incidence is the number of new cases during a given time period/total population at risk. The incidence rate is the number of new cases during given time period/total person-time of observation (ie, person-years).

Likelihood Ratio: A way of comparing the probability that the test result would occur in people with the disease as opposed to occurring in people without the disease.

Measurements of Scale: Variables differ in terms of how well they can be measured.

- Nominal variables. Examples: sex, ethnicity, smoking status, family history of disease
- Ordinal variables. This requires a ranking of the variables. Examples: stage at presentation, socioeconomic status
- Interval variables. This allows for rank order and calculation of size differences. Example: age at diagnosis, survival time

Meta-Analysis: A meta-analysis is a statistical process that combines the findings from individual studies.

Negative Predictive Value: The likelihood that people with a negative test result would not have a condition. The higher the value of the negative predictive value, the more useful the test is for predicting that people do not have the condition.

Odds Ratio: The chance of an event occurring in one group as compared with the chance of it occurring in another group. The OR is a measure of effect size and is commonly used to compare results in clinical trials.

P **Value**: A mathematical technique to measure whether the results of a study are likely to be true. *Statistical significance* is calculated as the probability that an effect observed in a research study is occurring because of chance. Statistical significance is usually expressed as a *P* value. The smaller the *P* value, the less likely it is that the results are due to chance (and more likely that the results are true). Researchers generally believe that results are probably true if the statistical significance is a *P* value less than .05 ($P < .05$).

Positive Predictive Value: The likelihood that a person with a positive test result would actually have the condition for which the test is used. The higher the value of the positive predictive value, the more useful the test is for predicting that the person has the condition.

Pretest Probability: The probability that a person has a particular disease before any test results are obtained. The pretest probability for large groups of people (eg, the population of a city) is the same as the prevalence of the disease in that group.

Prevalence: The frequency with which a disease or condition occurs in a group of people. Prevalence is calculated by dividing the number of people who have the disease or condition by the total number of people in the group.

Risk: The chance that something will happen.

Relative Risk: Ratio of risk of disease in exposed individuals to the risk of disease in nonexposed individuals.

RR = 1, no association between exposure and disease

RR > 1, positive association between exposure and disease

RR < 1, negative association between exposure and disease

Sensitivity: The ability of a test to identify correctly people with a condition. A test with high sensitivity will nearly always be positive for people who have the condition (the test has a low rate of false-negative results). Sensitivity is also known as the true-positive rate.

Specificity: The ability of a test to identify correctly people without a condition. A test with high specificity will rarely be wrong about who does NOT have the condition (the test has a low rate of false-positive results). Specificity is also known as the true-negative rate.

Validity: Whether a test or technique actually measures what it is intended to measure. Validity can refer to an individual measurement or to the design and approach taken in a clinical research study. When referring to a single measurement, validity means the accuracy of the measurement.

REFERENCES

1. Jemal A, Bray F, Center MM, Ferlay J, Ward E, Forman D. Global cancer statistics. *CA Cancer J Clin.* 2011;61(2):69-90.

2. Jemal A, Siegel R, Xu J, Ward E. Cancer statistics, 2010. *CA Cancer J Clin.* 2010;60(5):277-300.

3. Mendivil A, Schuler KM, Gehrig PA. Non-endometrioid adenocarcinoma of the uterine corpus: a review of selected histological subtypes. *Cancer Control.* 2009;16(1):46-52.

4. Karageorgi S, Hankinson SE, Kraft P, De Vivo I. Reproductive factors and postmenopausal hormone use in relation to endometrial cancer risk in the Nurses' Health Study cohort 1976-2004. *Int J Cancer.* 2010;126(1):208-216.

5. Friberg E, Mantzoros CS, Wolk A. Diabetes and risk of endometrial cancer: a population-based prospective cohort study. *Cancer Epidemiol Biomarkers Prev.* 2007;16(2):276-280.

6. Chang SC, Lacey JV Jr, Brinton LA, et al. Lifetime weight history and endometrial cancer risk by type of menopausal hormone use in the NIH-AARP diet and health study. *Cancer Epidemiol Biomarkers Prev.* 2007;16(4):723-730.

7. Reeves KW, Carter GC, Rodabough RJ, et al. Obesity in relation to endometrial cancer risk and disease characteristics in the Women's Health Initiative. *Gynecol Oncol.* 2011;121(2):376-382.

8. Vogel VG, Costantino JP, Wickerham DL, et al. Update of the national surgical adjuvant breast and bowel project study of tamoxifen and raloxifene (STAR) P-2 trial: preventing breast cancer. *Cancer Prev Res (Phila).* 2010;3(6):696-706.

9. Lacey JV Jr, Sherman ME, Rush BB, et al. Absolute risk of endometrial carcinoma during 20-year follow-up among women with endometrial hyperplasia. *J Clin Oncol.* 2010;28(5):788-792.

10. Trimble CL, Kauderer J, Zaino R, et al. Concurrent endometrial carcinoma in women with a biopsy diagnosis of atypical endometrial hyperplasia: a Gynecologic Oncology Group study. *Cancer.* 2006;106(4):812-819.

11. Razavi P, Pike MC, Horn-Ross PL, Templeman C, Bernstein L, Ursin G. Long-term postmenopausal hormone therapy and endometrial cancer. *Cancer Epidemiol Biomarkers Prev.* 2010;19(2):475-483.

12. Mutter GL, Lin MC, Fitzgerald JT, et al. Altered PTEN expression as a diagnostic marker for the earliest endometrial precancers. *J Natl Cancer Inst.* 2000;92(11):924-930.

13. Lee E, Hsu C, Haiman CA, et al. Genetic variation in the progesterone receptor gene and risk of endometrial cancer: a haplotype-based approach. *Carcinogenesis.* 2010;31(8):1392-1399.

14. Umar A, Boland CR, Terdiman JP, et al. Revised Bethesda Guidelines for hereditary nonpolyposis colorectal cancer (Lynch syndrome) and microsatellite instability. *J Natl Cancer Inst.* 2004;96(4):261-268.

15. Lu KH, Schorge JO, Rodabaugh KJ, et al. Prospective determination of prevalence of Lynch syndrome in young women with endometrial cancer. *J Clin Oncol.* 2007;25(33):5158-5164.

16. D'Angelo E, Prat J. Uterine sarcomas: a review. *Gynecol Oncol.* 2010;116(1):131-139.

17. Ylisaukko-oja SK, Kiuru M, Lehtonen HJ, et al. Analysis of fumarate hydratase mutations in a population-based series of early onset uterine leiomyosarcoma patients. *Int J Cancer.* 2006;119(2):283-287.

18. Li AJ, Giuntoli RL 2nd, Drake R, et al. Ovarian preservation in stage I low-grade endometrial stromal sarcomas. *Obstet Gynecol.* 2005;106(6):1304-1308.

19. Kamangar F, Dores GM, Anderson WF. Patterns of cancer incidence, mortality, and prevalence across five continents: defining priorities to reduce cancer disparities in different geographic regions of the world. *J Clin Oncol.* 2006;24(14):2137-2150.

20. Munoz N, Bosch FX, de Sanjose S, et al. Epidemiologic classification of human papillomavirus types associated with cervical cancer. *N Engl J Med.* 2003;348(6):518-527.

21. Kjaer S, Hogdall E, Frederiksen K, et al. The absolute risk of cervical abnormalities in high-risk human papillomavirus-positive, cytologically normal women over a 10-year period. *Cancer Res.* 2006;66(21):10630-10636.

22. Dunne EF, Unger ER, Sternberg M, et al. Prevalence of HPV infection among females in the united states. *JAMA.* 2007;297(8):813-819.

23. Winer RL, Lee SK, Hughes JP, Adam DE, Kiviat NB, Koutsky LA. Genital human papillomavirus infection: incidence and risk factors in a cohort of female university students. *Am J Epidemiol.* 2003;157(3):218-226.

24. Vaccarella S, Franceschi S, Herrero R, et al. Sexual behavior, condom use, and human papillomavirus: pooled analysis of the IARC human papillomavirus prevalence surveys. *Cancer Epidemiol Biomarkers Prev.* 2006;15(2):326-333.

25. International Collaboration of Epidemiological Studies of Cervical Cancer. Cervical carcinoma and sexual behavior: collaborative reanalysis of individual data on 15,461 women with cervical carcinoma and 29,164 women without cervical carcinoma from 21 epidemiological studies. *Cancer Epidemiol Biomarkers Prev.* 2009;18(4):1060-1069.

26. Tarkowski TA, Koumans EH, Sawyer M, et al. Epidemiology of human papillomavirus infection and abnormal cytologic test results in an urban adolescent population. *J Infect Dis.* 2004;189(1):46-50.

27. Moscicki AB, Ma Y, Wibbelsman C, et al. Risks for cervical intraepithelial neoplasia 3 among adolescents and young women with abnormal cytology. *Obstet Gynecol.* 2008;112(6):1335-1342.

28. Wu MH, Chan JY, Liu PY, Liu ST, Huang SM. Human papillomavirus E2 protein associates with nuclear receptors to stimulate nuclear receptor- and E2-dependent transcriptional activations in human cervical carcinoma cells. *Int J Biochem Cell Biol.* 2007;39(2):413-425.

29. Moreno V, Bosch FX, Munoz N, et al. Effect of oral contraceptives on risk of cervical cancer in women with human papillomavirus infection: the IARC multicentric case-control study. *Lancet.* 2002;359(9312):1085-1092.

30. Castellsague X, Diaz M, de Sanjose S, et al. Worldwide human papillomavirus etiology of cervical adenocarcinoma and its cofactors: implications for screening and prevention. *J Natl Cancer Inst.* 2006;98(5):303-315.

31. Altekruse SF, Lacey JV Jr, Brinton LA, et al. Comparison of human papillomavirus genotypes, sexual, and reproductive risk factors of cervical adenocarcinoma and squamous cell carcinoma: Northeastern United States. *Am J Obstet Gynecol.* 2003;188(3):657-663.

32. Weinberg LE, Lurain JR, Singh DK, Schink JC. Survival and reproductive outcomes in women treated for malignant ovarian germ cell tumors. *Gynecol Oncol.* 2011;121(2):285-289.

33. Gershenson DM. Management of ovarian germ cell tumors. *J Clin Oncol.* 2007;25(20):2938-2943.

34. Colombo N, Parma G, Zanagnolo V, Insinga A. Management of ovarian stromal cell tumors. *J Clin Oncol.* 2007;25(20):2944-2951.

35. Moorman PG, Palmieri RT, Akushevich L, Berchuck A, Schildkraut JM. Ovarian cancer risk factors in African-American and white women. *Am J Epidemiol.* 2009;170(5):598-606.

36. Collaborative Group on Epidemiological Studies of Ovarian Cancer, Beral V, Doll R, Hermon C, Peto R, Reeves G. Ovarian cancer and oral contraceptives: collaborative reanalysis of data from 45 epidemiological studies including 23,257 women with ovarian cancer and 87,303 controls. *Lancet.* 2008;371(9609):303-314.

37. Olsen CM, Green AC, Whiteman DC, Sadeghi S, Kolahdooz F, Webb PM. Obesity and the risk of epithelial ovarian cancer: a systematic review and meta-analysis. *Eur J Cancer.* 2007;43(4):690-709.

38. Campbell KL. Exercise and biomarkers for cancer prevention studies. *J Nutr.* 2007;137(1 suppl):161S-169S.

39. Petrucelli N, Daly MB, Feldman GL. Hereditary breast and ovarian cancer due to mutations in BRCA1 and BRCA2. *Genet Med.* 2010;12(5):245-259.

40. Metcalfe K, Lubinski J, Lynch HT, et al. Family history of cancer and cancer risks in women with BRCA1 or BRCA2 mutations. *J Natl Cancer Inst.* 2010;102(24):1874-1878.

41. Domchek SM, Friebel TM, Garber JE, et al. Occult ovarian cancers identified at risk-reducing salpingo-oophorectomy in a prospective cohort of BRCA1/2 mutation carriers. *Breast Cancer Res Treat.* 2010;124(1):195-203.

42. Heemskerk-Gerritsen BA, Kriege M, Seynaeve C. Association of risk-reducing surgery with cancer risks and mortality in BRCA mutation carriers. *JAMA.* 2010;304(24):2695; author reply 2695-2696.

43. Eisen A, Lubinski J, Gronwald J, et al. Hormone therapy and the risk of breast cancer in BRCA1 mutation carriers. *J Natl Cancer Inst.* 2008;100(19):1361-1367.

44. Dubeau L. The cell of origin of ovarian epithelial tumours. *Lancet Oncol.* 2008;9(12):1191-1197.

45. Bonome T, Lee JY, Park DC, et al. Expression profiling of serous low malignant potential, low-grade, and high-grade tumors of the ovary. *Cancer Res.* 2005;65(22):10602-10612.

46. Levanon K, Crum C, Drapkin R. New insights into the pathogenesis of serous ovarian cancer and its clinical impact. *J Clin Oncol.* 2008;26(32):5284-5293.

47. Insinga RP, Liaw KL, Johnson LG, Madeleine MM. A systematic review of the prevalence and attribution of human papillomavirus types among cervical, vaginal, and vulvar precancers and cancers in the united states. *Cancer Epidemiol Biomarkers Prev.* 2008;17(7):1611-1622.

48. Verloop J, van Leeuwen FE, Helmerhorst TJ, van Boven HH, Rookus MA. Cancer risk in DES daughters. *Cancer Causes Control.* 2010;21(7):999-1007.

49. Hampl M, Sarajuuri H, Wentzensen N, Bender HG, Kueppers V. Effect of human papillomavirus vaccines on vulvar, vaginal, and anal intraepithelial lesions and vulvar cancer. *Obstet Gynecol.* 2006;108(6):1361-1368.

50. Hayward BE, De Vos M, Talati N, et al. Genetic and epigenetic analysis of recurrent hydatidiform mole. *Hum Mutat.* 2009;30(5):E629-E639.

51. Green S, Crowley J, Benedetti J, Smith A. *Clinical Trials in Oncology.* 2nd ed. Boca Raton, FL: Chapman and Hall/CRC; 2002.

52. Piantadosi S. *Clinical Trials: A Methodologic Perspective.* New York, NY: John Wiley & Sons; 1997.

2 Genetics and Biology of Gynecologic Cancers

Douglas A. Levine

All cancer is genetic, meaning that all cancers have a genetic basis and result from an accumulation of mutations or other genetic defects. Cancer can be caused by many different factors, but all cancers function through genetic mutation or other alterations. Most cancers occur when the normal functioning of a single cell in a tissue of origin goes awry. The old tenet of cancer being an imbalance of growth and death still holds true, but over the years, we have learned much about the causes and details of how this growth/death dichotomy becomes muddled. For some, cancer will have an inherited origin passed down through generations; for others it will be a newly developed, or de novo, mutation obtained by the tissue of origin to turn normal tissue into cancer. Many of the cancer-causing genes can be grouped into categories of tumor suppressors and oncogenes. There are a number of cancer syndromes that predispose to the development of gynecologic malignancies. In some cases, environmental factors may increase the risk of certain cancer types.

PRINCIPLES OF CANCER MOLECULAR GENETICS

Oncogenes

Oncogenes are cancer drivers that have the ability to initiate tumor formation when turned on, most commonly by mutations. Before a gene becomes an oncogene or develops the ability to transform normal cells to malignant cells, it is referred to as a proto-oncogene,

or a gene with oncogenic potential. In addition to mutation, proto-oncogenes can transform into oncogenes through structural rearrangements such as translocations, duplications, or splice variants, as well as overexpression of the gene product. Genes can function as oncogenes through increasing protein activity or by losing the ability to suppress negative regulators of growth. The first oncogene, src, was discovered in chickens. *RAS* and *MYC* were other early oncogenes found to regulate transcription and affect cell proliferation. Since then, many other oncogenes, which are often activated by somatic mutations, have been discovered. An example of a more recently discovered oncogene is *PIK3CA*, which is activated by cell surface receptor tyrosine kinases and regulates AKT activation, cell growth, and survival (Figure 2-1). Through sequence analysis of various human tumors, *PIK3CA* mutations in multiple human tumors were identified.[1] Remarkably, most of these mutations were clustered at a limited number of nucleotide positions, termed *hotspots*, making them useful for cancer diagnostics and therapeutics. Mutations in related genes such as *PIK3R1* and *PIK3R2*, which encode the regulatory and structural subunits of the PI3K protein, have also been identified. Currently, there are many drugs designed to target various subunits of PI3K that have the potential for effectiveness in tumors with activating PI3K mutations and others. Other regulatory genes, such as microRNAs, can function as oncogenes by promoting cancer development and growth. MicroRNAs usually negatively regulate gene expression, but if they release their normal negative inhibition, unsuppressed growth

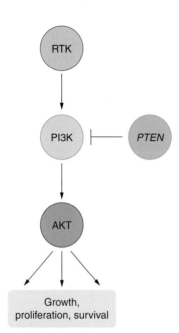

FIGURE 2-1. Schematic diagram of PI3K signaling. *PTEN* is a tumor suppressor gene inhibiting the pathway. Classically, both copies of *PTEN* need to be lost to release this inhibition and allow for uncontrolled AKT activity, as is seen in many solid tumors. *PTEN* can be lost through a combination of mutation, methylation, and deletion. *PIK3CA* encodes a catalytic subunit of PI3K. A single activating mutation in 1 copy of *PIK3CA* is necessary to activate AKT and result in uncontrolled growth, as it is an oncogene. (Reprinted [modified] by permission from Macmillan Publishers Ltd: Oncogene [Yuan TL, Cantley LC. PI3K pathway alterations in cancer: variations on a theme. *Oncogene.* 2008;27:5497-5510], copyright 2008.)

can result in oncogenic activity. Thus a gene can have direct or indirect oncogenic potential (Figure 2-2).

Tumor Suppressor Genes

Tumor suppressor genes (TSGs) are genes that have normal inhibitory function that, when lost, permit cell transformation or tumor growth. Unlike oncogenes, which promote growth when activated, TSGs require complete inactivation in order to fully release inhibitory activity. Classically, this has been referred to as the "two-hit hypothesis," in which both copies of a TSG need to be lost in order to release inhibitory function sufficiently to promote cancer development and growth. The loss of both copies, or alleles, of a TSG can occur by 2 mutations developing over time, such that the first mutation increases the likelihood of developing a second mutation.

Alternatively, first copy of a TSG can be inactivated by mutation, and the second copy can be inactivated by a separate mechanism such as methylation,

structural rearrangement, or loss of heterozygosity. *BRCA1* is a good example of a TSG in that both alleles are lost in ovarian tumors. Interestingly, this has not been uniformly shown to be the case for breast cancer.[2] Commonly mutated TSGs include *PTEN*, which suppresses activation of the PI3K/AKT pathway; *RB1*, the retinoblastoma gene; *APC* in colon cancer; and the most commonly mutated TSG, *TP53*, which is mutated in nearly all serous ovarian cancers and approximately half of most other epithelial malignancies. When 1 copy of a TSG is lost, such as when a *BRCA1* mutation is inherited from a parent, this is termed *haploinsufficiency*. The functional impact of haploinsufficiency is unclear and likely varies between tissue types and biologic circumstances, but in some cases it may predispose to loss of the second allele.

Mismatch Repair Proteins

Mismatch repair (MMR) proteins help to correct normal errors in DNA replication. Every time a cell divides, its DNA undergoes replication, which is not a perfect process. In fact, when DNA is replicating, errors occur 1 in every 10^6 to 10^8 nucleotides. Considering the size of the human genome, many errors occur. Thus mechanisms to repair DNA replication errors must be robust. Most errors in replication are repaired during the replication process itself through a mechanism called *proofreading*. However, some errors persist after replication and are fixed through MMR. MMR is one of several DNA repair mechanisms. In general, DNA repair mechanisms can be grouped into 2 classes: those that repair single-strand DNA breaks and those that repair double-strand DNA breaks.

Mechanisms that repair single-strand DNA damage include base excision repair, nucleotide excision repair, and MMR. MMR is the only mechanism of single-strand repair that repairs undamaged, misaligned DNA primarily due to errors of replication. The MMR proteins that are most commonly mutated in gynecologic cancer syndromes are MLH1 and MSH2. MMR mutation leads to greater errors of DNA replication in repetitive regions of the genome within tumors. This phenomenon is referred to as *microsatellite instability* (MI), in which short repeat regions undergo expansion or contraction in the number of repetitive elements. It is particularly common in endometrial and colorectal cancers. MI can be detected by sequencing DNA from normal tissues (such as blood) and comparing it with malignant tissues. When the malignant tissue has greater or fewer repetitive elements than the normal tissue, this is referred to as MI. In addition to MI developing as a consequence of MMR mutations, which can often be inherited, MI can also develop from somatic changes, such as methylation of the MLH1 promoter.

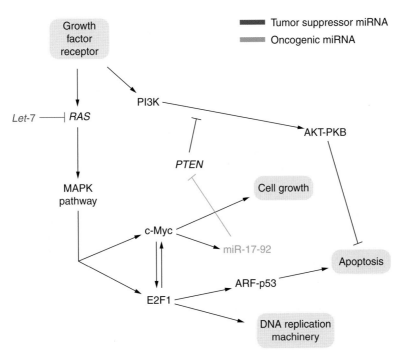

FIGURE 2-2. MicroRNAs can function as oncogenes or tumor suppressor genes. Let-7 inhibits the *RAS* oncogene and therefore is functioning as a TSG. When lost, it would release its inhibition, and the *RAS* oncogene would be active, as happens in many malignancies. The miR17-92 cluster of microRNAs functions as an oncogene in that it inhibits the TSGs *PTEN*. *PTEN* normally inhibits AKT activity, but when inhibited itself, the PI3K/AKT pathway is activated/no longer inhibited, and cancer can develop or progress. (Reprinted from Hammond SM. MicroRNAs as oncogenes. *Curr Opin Genet Dev.* 2006;16:4-9, with permission from Elsevier.)

Inheritance Patterns

Inheritance refers to traits or genes obtained from parents and can be referred to as hereditary or inherited. Traditional inheritance patterns are autosomal dominant, autosomal recessive, and sex- (or X-) linked. Dominant inheritance occurs when the trait or gene is functional or active by inheriting a single copy from either parent. Dominantly inherited traits have a 50% chance of being passed down to each offspring. *BRCA1/2* mutations are a good example of a dominantly inherited trait in that each offspring has a 50% chance of inheriting the mutation from a single parent who carries the mutation. Recessive patterns of inheritance are less common and require inheritance of a trait or gene from each parent, as 2 affected alleles are required for disease manifestation. X-linked traits can be inherited from either parent, but recessive traits are manifest in males, who only carry one X chromosome, whereas dominant traits would be manifest equally in males and females. Recessive X-linked traits require inheritance from each parent for manifestation. All inherited traits or mutations do not manifest themselves. The genetic composition of mutations or other variations are referred to as *genotypes*, and the manifestation of

these mutations or traits are referred to as *phenotypes*. All mutations (or mutated genotypes) do not result in a disease phenotype; this phenomenon is referred to as *incomplete penetrance*, in which the diseased gene is only manifest in a subset of people. For most biologic situations, we do not understand the factors (or modifiers) that affect penetrance. Consider a *BRCA1* mutation that confers a lifetime risk of 40% for ovarian cancer, meaning that not everyone with a *BRCA1* inherited mutation develops ovarian cancer. The penetrance of a *BRCA1* mutation for ovarian cancer is approximately 40%. The patterns of inheritance refer to the germline, or every cell in your body. When you inherit a mutation from a parent, it is present in every cell of your body. A disease-causing mutation may not cause disease in every cell of your body, but it is present in every cell of your body. This is in contrast to *somatic mutations*, which are not inherited but develop within the host and are commonly found in cancer. Many germline mutations will predispose to somatic mutations, which can function as the "second hit" to inactivate a TSG and initiate tumor formation. This distinction between germline events or mutations and somatic mutations is key to understanding what tumor-causing mechanisms are inherited and which develop de novo.

BIOLOGY OF GYNECOLOGIC CANCER

Endometrial Cancer

Endometrial cancers are broadly classified into 2 groups. Type 1 tumors are of endometrioid histology and are directly related to estrogen excess. Most commonly, the excess estrogen is derived from adipocytes and thus is more frequent in obese women. Many years ago, the most common source of exogenous estrogen was unopposed ingested estrogen, before combination hormone replacement therapy was prescribed. The initial report from the *New England Journal of Medicine* in 1975 identified a 4.5-fold increased risk of endometrial cancer in users of unopposed estrogens.[3] Once the link between unopposed estrogen and endometrial cancer was established, hormone replacement therapy began including progestins for women who had their uterus in place. Other causes of unopposed estrogen include polycystic ovarian syndrome, in which anovulation leads to metabolic and hormonal derangements, which increase the risk of endometrial cancer in premenopausal women.[4]

Type 2 tumors are of more aggressive histologic subtypes, with the prototypic tumor being of serous histology. The etiology of type 2 tumors is less understood, but they have a higher propensity for recurrence and likely benefit from adjuvant treatment after surgical resection. These tumors are not associated with obesity and have no specific epidemiologic predilection, although they appear more common in nonobese women. Other aggressive type 2 histology subtypes include carcinosarcoma and clear cell (Table 2-1).

Pathology of Type 1 and Type 2 Endometrial Carcinoma

Type 1 endometrioid tumors follow a natural progression from normal endometrium to endometrial hyperplasia (with or without atypia) followed by invasive cancer. A premalignant lesion within regions of endometrial hyperplasia has been recently identified and termed *endometrial intraepithelial neoplasia* (EIN). EIN is associated with a far greater increase in endometrial cancer risk than simple endometrial hyperplasia. The risk of progression from a precursor lesion to endometrial carcinoma increases with greater complexity and nuclear atypia. From the most recent comprehensive review, the risk of progression to invasive endometrial cancer was < 1% for simple hyperplasia without atypia, 7% to 9% for either simple hyperplasia with atypia or complex hyperplasia without atypia, and 20% for complex hyperplasia with atypia. These risks are all approximately doubled in the presence of EIN.[5]

Type 2 serous tumors do not have a logical and stepwise progression from a well-defined precursor

Table 2-1 Comparison Between Type 1 and Type 2 Endometrial Cancers

	Type 1	Type 2
Clinical Features		
Risk factors	Unopposed estrogen	Age
Differentiation	Well differentiated	Poorly differentiated
Histology	Endometrioid	Serous, clear cell
Stage	I/II	III/IV
Prognosis	Favorable	Not favorable
Endometrial lining	Atrophic	Hyperplastic
Characteristic Molecular Features		
Ploidy	Diploid	Aneuploid
P53 overexpression	No	Yes
PTEN mutations	Yes	No
Microsatellite instability	Yes	No

lesion to invasive carcinoma. Often, uterine serous carcinoma can be confined to a small endometrial polyp, yet present with metastatic disease, at the time of comprehensive surgical staging. A precursor lesion has been identified and termed *endometrial intraepithelial carcinoma* (EIC). EIC has been specifically associated with uterine serous tumors and uterine carcinosarcomas that contain a serous epithelial component and can be found adjacent to most established uterine serous carcinomas.[6] Epidemiologic studies suggest that nearly 50% of apparently uterine-confined disease have spread beyond the uterus at the time of diagnosis.[7] Unlike type 1 tumors, which typically develop in a background of hyperplasia, type 2 tumors, particularly serous tumors, develop in a background of relative endometrial atrophy, with uterine polyps or other focal changes occurring at the site of tumorigenesis. These tumors also lack the presence of hormone receptors commonly seen in type 1 tumors.

Endometrial carcinosarcoma is an aggressive type 2 tumor that was initially thought to be 2 tumor types that collided at a well-defined interface. Subsequent molecular studies clearly proved that these tumors arise through clonal evolution where a given malignant epithelial cell undergoes differentiation into 2 histologically distinct lineages. Thus these tumors have traditionally been considered as a subset of uterine sarcomas, but in fact, they represent poorly differentiated and divergent epithelial tumors with sarcomatous differentiation.[8] If any part of the sarcomatous component contains cell types that are not native to the uterine corpus, this is referred to as a heterologous differentiation. If all cell types are commonly seen within the uterus, this is referred to as a homologous differentiation. In several well-designed studies, it has been reported that patients with endometrial carcinosarcomas having heterologous differentiation have a worse outcome as compared with patients having homologous differentiation for both early- and late-stage disease.[9]

Genetics of Type 1 and Type 2 Endometrial Carcinoma

In addition to the well-defined histologic progression of type 1 endometrioid tumors, the genetics of type 1 tumors are also fairly well understood. It is thought that *PTEN*, a tumor suppressor gene that negatively regulates the PI3K/AKT pathway, is lost early in the neoplastic process. In fact, *PTEN* mutations have been found in the preneoplastic EIN lesions. *PTEN* loss can occur through a number of mechanisms, including somatic mutation, promoter methylation, or deletion. In the uncommon Cowden syndrome, which includes development of hamartomas and increased risks of endometrial, breast, renal, thyroid, and possibly colorectal malignancies, *PTEN* mutation is present in the germline (and thus is inherited). Subsequent to *PTEN* loss, additional mutations are accumulated that also frequently occur in the PI3K/AKT pathway. *PIK3CA* encodes the catalytic subunit of the PI3K enzyme and contains activating mutations in approximately 25% of endometrioid and serous tumors. Interestingly, mutations in this gene are often identified at the same genetic position, or at the same nucleotide, and are therefore termed *hotspot mutations*. These types of hotspot mutations in *PIK3CA* and other genes can be easily detected through modern laboratory assays such as mass spectrometry and are therefore good targets for both diagnostics and therapeutics. In fact, there are many *PIK3CA* inhibitors being developed and in early-phase clinical trials. The regulatory and structural units of the PI3K enzyme are encoded by the genes *PIK3R1* and *PIK3R2*, both of which are also frequently mutated in type 1 cancers.

Mutations in *FGFR2* were first reported in 2007 and are present in 10% to 15% of type 1 tumors.[10] This finding has clinical relevance, as there are small-molecule inhibitors of *FGFR2* in addition to other targets. High-grade type 1 endometrial tumors, like other high-grade solid tumors, have fairly frequent mutations in *TP53*, in the order of 50%. Other commonly mutated genes include *CTNNB1*, *KRAS*, and occasionally *AKT1*. Type 1 tumors also have a 20% to 25% frequency of MI, which can be easily detected through a consensus panel of 5 microsatellite markers and has been adopted

as a reference set by the National Cancer Institute.[11] The clinical significance of MI in endometrial cancer is unclear, with studies demonstrating both improved and worse outcomes in the setting of MI. For colorectal cancer, it is well established that MI tumors have an improved clinical course.[12]

The lack of well-defined progression from normal histology to cancer for type 2 tumors is also reflected in the genetics of these lesions. EIC is thought to be the precursor lesion, which overexpresses and contains mutations in *TP53*. *TP53* mutation is also found in 80% to 90% of uterine serous carcinomas, in contrast to the low frequency in low-grade endometrioid type 1 tumors and modestly higher frequency in high-grade type 1 tumors. Type 2 tumors are also characterized by the lack of MI and a very low frequency of *KRAS*, *PTEN*, and *CTNNB1* mutations. There is a similar frequency of mutations in *PIK3CA*, offering the possibility that PI3K-targeted therapy may be equally successful in type I and type 2 tumors. *TP53* mutations are also commonly seen in uterine carcinosarcomas but occur at low frequency in clear cell tumors.[13]

Lynch Syndrome

First described by Henry T. Lynch, this syndrome commonly includes malignancies of the uterus, colon, stomach, and ovary.[14] Less frequent malignancies that are part of this syndrome include small bowel, upper urinary tract, brain, and biliary tract. Lynch syndrome is primarily caused by an inherited germline mutation in one of several MMR genes: *MLH1*, *MSH2*, and less often *MSH6*, *PMS1*, and *PMS2*. The syndrome was initially divided into 2 subtypes—Lynch I and Lynch II—based on whether or not extracolonic tumors were included in a given pedigree. It was quickly realized that the genetic basis of these 2 subtypes was similar, and the syndrome was commonly referred to as hereditary nonpolyposis colorectal cancer syndrome (HNPCC). This was due mostly to the fact that the predominant malignancy was colon cancer. However, this name soon became a misnomer when the high frequency of endometrial cancer was identified in women. Furthermore, the colons within which the colorectal tumors developed as part of HNPCC did in fact contain multiple colonic polyps in many cases; however, the extent of the polyposis was far less than that seen in the related familial adenomatous polyposis (FAP) syndrome, in which a great many polyps are found throughout the colon due to a germline mutation in *APC*. One main difference in the risk of colorectal cancer between these 2 syndromes is that the risk of colorectal cancer with FAP is nearly 100%, but the risk of colorectal cancer in HNPCC is approximately 80% and occurs at a later onset than with FAP. For these reasons, HNPCC is no longer an accurate description of the clinical and genetic syndrome, and Lynch syndrome (without any further distinction between type I and type II) is now the preferred terminology.

Pathogenesis and Pathology

Lynch syndrome is due to inherited mutations in 1 of 5 MMR genes. *MLH1* and *MSH2* are the most commonly mutated genes in this syndrome. These defects lead to faulty DNA repair and increased risk of malignancy. In women, endometrial cancer and colon cancer have an equal likelihood of being the sentinel malignancy in this syndrome. In women with Lynch syndrome, the lifetime risk of colon cancer and endometrial cancer are both approximately 50%, in contrast to the risk of colon cancer in men, which is 50% greater.[15,16] The mean age of endometrial cancer diagnosis in Lynch syndrome patients is approximately 45 years, as compared with a mean age of 62 years for endometrial cancer in general. In women under 50 years of age with endometrial cancer, the likelihood of having Lynch syndrome as determined by a germline mutation in one of the MMR genes is 9%.[17] Young patients with Lynch syndrome tend to have a lower body mass index than young patients with sporadic endometrial cancer. Immunohistochemical markers are now robustly available for testing for the absence (abnormal) of expression in *MLH1*, *MSH2*, *MSH6*, and *PMS2*.

The absence of MMR protein expression is indicative of MI, but a fair portion of these cases may be due to promoter methylation of *MLH1* and not an inherited germline mutation, which is the only circumstance diagnostic of Lynch syndrome. If immunohistochemistry (IHC) only is applied to endometrial cancer patients younger than 50 years of age, 25% to 35% of tumors have been found to lack normal IHC staining, which increases when considering only nonobese women. Nonetheless, approximately one-third to one-half of these cases may be due to MI without a true germline mutation secondary to epigenetic/methylation silencing.[18,19] The lifetime risk of Lynch syndrome–associated ovarian cancer ranges from 8% to 12%. Ovarian cancers appear to be moderate to high grade, mostly epithelial in nature, and, unlike sporadic ovarian cancer, predominately stage I or II. Endometrial cancer is diagnosed synchronously in approximately 20% of Lynch syndrome patients with ovarian cancer. The mean age of ovarian cancer diagnosis in Lynch syndrome patients is approximately 43 years, as compared with a mean age of 63 years for ovarian cancer in general.[20] Women with synchronous ovarian and endometrial cancer have a 7% risk of having Lynch syndrome[21] (Figure 2-3).

Endometrial tumors associated with Lynch syndrome are more commonly found in the lower uterine

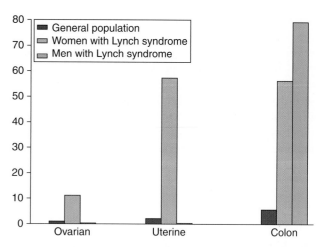

FIGURE 2-3. Lifetime risk for colon, endometrial, and ovarian cancer in individuals with Lynch syndrome compared with the general population. (Reproduced, with permission, from Schmeler KM, Lu KH. Gynecologic cancers associated with Lynch syndrome/HNPCC. *Clin Transl Oncol.* 2008;10:313-317.)

segment and are more often poorly differentiated and deeply invasive, with a higher mitotic rate and more tumor-infiltrating lymphocytes (TILs).[22] However, a comprehensive review comparing Lynch-associated endometrial cancer with sporadic endometrial cancer and *MLH1* promoter methylated tumors found a similar frequency of non-endometrioid histologies between groups, but the *MLH1* methylated tumors were more likely to be undifferentiated.[23] This review also found similar frequencies of myometrial invasion, high stage, and TILs. Many centers have adopted pathologic screening approaches to identify patients who may have Lynch syndrome and should be referred for genetic counseling. These varied algorithms typically start with standard IHC directed toward the 4 common MMR proteins: MLH1, MSH2, MSH6, and PMS2 in women under the age of 50 years with endometrial cancer, those with a family history suggestive of Lynch syndrome, or in patients with characteristic tumor morphology such as lower uterine segment involvement and prominent TILs. If MLH1 immunostaining is absent/lost, a follow-up assay is performed for MLH1 methylation, as this is a common cause of both MLH1 loss and MI, but is not inherited or associated with Lynch syndrome. If there is IHC loss in any of the tested proteins and no evidence of MLH1 promoter methylation, patients should then be referred for genetic counseling and consideration of germline testing for inherited mutations in these 4 genes. At any time, if there is high clinical suspicion, patients should be referred for genetic counseling, regardless of screening test results.

Screening and Prevention

Ovarian and endometrial screening is recommended for women with Lynch syndrome in addition to all screening recommended for both sexes. Physical examination, CA-125 measurements, and transvaginal sonography should be performed twice yearly and begin at age 30 to 35 years. This screening approach is the standard for women at high risk for ovarian cancer and will also identify gross abnormalities within the uterine cavity based on sonography. However, this screening approach has never been proven to reduce the risk of death from these diseases; nonetheless, it appears reasonable and awaits full validation and, in the absence of better screening approaches, is currently the best management scheme. Because this approach will not fully evaluate the uterine cavity for early lesions, annual endometrial sampling/biopsy is also recommended. For women who have completed childbearing, risk-reducing total hysterectomy with bilateral salpingo-oophorectomy is recommended. This approach reduces the risk of ovarian and endometrial cancer to approximately zero. In one study, the incidence of endometrial cancer in a control group was 33% compared with none in the risk-reducing hysterectomy group. The incidence of ovarian cancer in a control group was 5% compared with none in the risk-reducing salpingo-oophorectomy group.[24] Colonoscopy should be performed every 1 to 2 years for at-risk patients.

Endometrial Cancer in Young Women

Endometrial cancer diagnosed in young women presents a difficult clinical dilemma. Because the mean age of endometrial cancer diagnosis is 63 years, "young women" can be characterized as those under the age of 50 or even 40 years. For early noninvasive endometrial cancer, conservative therapy may be appropriate for women who have not yet completed childbearing. The specific algorithms and outcomes are beyond the scope of this section; however, a portion of these patients will present with synchronous ovarian cancer or develop metachronous ovarian cancer. Clearly, young women with endometrial cancer are candidates for genetic counseling and Lynch syndrome testing. Recent data suggest that fewer than 10% of women with synchronous endometrial and ovarian cancer have Lynch syndrome, suggesting other pathobiology for women with these synchronous tumors, of which only half are under the age of 50 years at diagnosis.[21] Young, normalweight women with endometrial cancer appear to have a relatively high incidence of infertility and/or irregular menstrual cycles, likely due to anovulation, which may also contribute to the increased risk of endometrial cancer.[25]

Approximately one-quarter of the normal weight, young women with endometrial cancer also had a synchronous ovarian cancer. Most of the synchronous ovarian tumors are of endometrioid histology, suggesting a possible field effect or link through endometriosis, as most sporadic ovarian cancer is of serous histology. Approximately 15% of the obese young women with endometrial cancer also had a synchronous ovarian cancer, suggesting greater frequency and possible different pathoetiology of synchronous ovarian cancer in young women with endometrial cancer based on body mass index and associated hormonal dysfunction. Additional studies have confirmed the approximate 25% incidence of synchronous ovarian cancer in young women with endometrial cancer.[26]

Synchronous endometrioid histologies have been associated with more favorable outcomes. These findings suggest that synchronous ovarian cancers develop in young women with endometrial cancer at a high rate for reasons that are not entirely clear, but this should be discussed with patients considering conservative management of early endometrial cancer. Risk-reducing salpingo-oophorectomy and hysterectomy should be considered for these patients once childbearing is complete.

Ovarian Cancer

The majority of ovarian cancers are epithelial in nature; a small percentage of them are sarcomas, and even fewer are germ cell or sex–cord stromal tumors. These uncommon tumors will be discussed elsewhere in the text. The most common histologic subtypes of epithelial ovarian cancer are serous, endometrioid, clear cell, and mucinous. Transitional cell tumors were described as an epithelial subtype, but more recently, they have been considered a simple epithelial variant and not a separate histologic subtype as originally thought.

Epithelial tumors of serous histology were thought to arise from the ovarian surface epithelium. Two common hypotheses of their origin are based on incessant or repeated ovulation and excessive hormonal stimulation. The first hypothesis implicates the ovarian surface epithelium and repeated cycles of ovulatory damage and repair. This hypothesis is supported by data that late menarche, early menopause, multiparity, and oral contraceptive use all decrease the risk of ovarian cancer. However, the reduction in the number of ovulatory cycles does not account for the associated magnitude of risk reduction. The evidence to support a hormonal basis of ovarian cancer arises from several areas. Lower gonadotropin levels, present during pregnancy and oral contraceptive use, reduce the risk of ovarian cancer. Women with polycystic ovarian disease, who have increased circulating androgens, are at an increased risk of developing ovarian cancer. Inclusions cysts, which have also been proposed to be the precursor cell to ovarian cancer, are found within the cortex of the ovary in close proximity to the vasculature,

CHAPTER 2

circulating hormones, and follicular cysts, which have high levels of androgen.[27] Therefore, although ovulation and hormones have been directly linked to ovarian tumorigenesis, there are insufficiencies that fail to fully explain epidemiologic findings, suggesting a different set of biochemical, anatomic, and hormonal interactions, which will be discussed later.

Ovarian cancers have been broadly classified into 2 groups. Type 1 tumors are of endometrioid, mucinous, clear cell, and low-grade serous histology and thought to arise from ovarian cysts and secondary mullerian sites, such as endometriosis. These tumors appear to progress in a stepwise fashion from benign to borderline or atypical to malignant and invasive tumors. In this regard, various precursor lesions can be potentially identified and used for screening or prevention as appropriate. Type 2 tumors are more aggressive and contain high-grade serous tumors. These tumors most likely have a precursor lesion within the fallopian tube (discussed later) and metastasize early, present at an advanced stage, and account for most deaths from this disease. High-grade endometrioid tumors were thought to be a small subset of the more aggressive, advanced-stage ovarian epithelial tumors, but recent work has suggested that when IHC is incorporated into the diagnostic algorithm, many high-grade endometrioid tumors are morphologic variants of high-grade serous carcinoma, and only a few high-grade endometrioid tumors truly represent progression from a low-grade endometrioid tumor.[28,29] Carcinosarcoma is another aggressive type 2 histology subtype, but is relatively uncommon (Table 2-2).

Pathology of Type 1 and Type 2 Ovarian Carcinoma

Type 1 ovarian tumors include endometrioid, mucinous, clear cell, and low-grade serous tumors. Most of these tumors develop in a stepwise fashion from a precursor borderline or low malignant potential (LMP) tumor. They are often confined to the ovary at the time of diagnosis and infrequently spread beyond the ovary, as compared with the more aggressive type 2 ovarian tumors. Type 1 serous tumors are uniformly low grade. Many will present in association with a borderline tumor. Borderline/LMP tumors contain branched glandular serous cells, and a subset of these tumors have a greater papillary architecture, referred to as *micropapillary*. Micropapillary tumors are thought to have a greater propensity for metastasis and association with frank invasion.

There is some controversy regarding whether to consider early invasive borderline tumors to be low-grade serous carcinoma or persistent borderline tumors, simply with a focus of microinvasion. Either naming scheme applied to these tumors describes the

Table 2-2 Comparison Between Type 1 and Type 2 Ovarian Cancers

	Type 1	Type 2
Clinical Features		
Precursor lesion	Ovarian cyst, endometriosis	Distal fallopian tube, ovarian surface epithelium
Differentiation	Well differentiated	Poorly differentiated
Histology	Endometrioid, clear cell	Serous
Stage	I/II	III/IV
Prognosis	Favorable	Not favorable
Characteristic Molecular Features		
P53 overexpression	No	Yes
BRCA1/2 mutations	No	Yes
PTEN, BRAF, KRAS, PIK3CA mutations	Yes	No
Genomic instability	No	Yes

same histologic morphology and portends a higher likelihood of metastasis, recurrence, and progression to fully invasive low-grade serous carcinoma.[30,31] Microinvasion and micropapillary architecture are the 2 most reproducible findings associated with decreased long-term outcomes in borderline/LMP tumors.

Mucinous tumors of the ovary are extremely rare. In the past, many gastrointestinal tumors metastatic to the ovary had been misclassified as primary ovarian mucinous neoplasms.[32] Although IHC can assist with the differential diagnosis of an ovarian versus a gastrointestinal primary, anatomic features may be most helpful. When IHC is performed, primary ovarian mucinous tumors preferentially express CK7 over CK20 and are negative for nuclear CTNNB1 (β-catenin). Features favoring metastatic disease include bilateral involvement, surface involvement, signet ring cells, and small size. Mucinous tumors that are bilateral and of any size or unilateral and smaller than 13 cm are mostly metastatic tumors to the ovary. Tumors that are unilateral and larger than or equal to 13 cm in size are mostly primary ovarian malignancies. This algorithm correctly classified 98% of the primary ovarian tumors and 82% of the metastases.[33] These findings are further confirmed by a recent cooperative group study.[34]

Of all potential advanced-stage mucinous ovarian neoplasms, approximately one-third are found to be primarily from the ovary, and the remainder are tumors metastatic to the ovary. Advanced mucinous tumors of both types have a worse overall survival than ovarian serous tumors, likely due to relative chemoresistance to standard agents. Classic pseudomyxoma peritonei, traditionally thought to be associated with metastatic mucinous ovarian neoplasms, is in fact uniformly associated with appendiceal neoplasms, with the rare exception of an appendiceal neoplasm that arises in the setting of a mature cystic teratoma of the ovary. Primary ovarian mucinous tumors are uniformly low grade at presentation and can grow to be quite large before metastasizing.

Borderline *endometrioid tumors* are often found in association with invasive endometrioid ovarian carcinoma, which is typically low grade at diagnosis and confined to the ovary. As with mucinous ovarian tumors, endometrioid ovarian carcinomas can be large at presentation, yet without evidence of metastasis to other organs. These tumors are also frequently seen in association with endometriosis, suggesting a pathogenic link between the 2 processes. Morphologically, these tumors resemble similar low-grade tumors of the endometrium. Pure borderline endometrioid tumors without invasive components follow an entirely benign course. *Clear cell ovarian tumors* represent a unique subset of type 1 tumors. They are similar to other type 1 ovarian tumors in that they can be large and unilateral at presentation, are often associated with a borderline clear cell tumor, and are commonly confined to the ovary at diagnosis. They are different from the other type 1 tumors in that they are high-grade lesions. These tumors are typically composed of hobnail cells with clear cytoplasm.

Type 2 high-grade serous tumors do not have a logical and stepwise progression from a well-defined precursor lesion to invasive carcinoma. High-grade serous tumors represent the vast majority of all serous ovarian invasive carcinomas. These tumors are generally at an advanced stage at presentation, with 94% of these tumors presenting at stage III or IV. These tumors are morphologically heterogeneous with marked nuclear atypia, frequent papillae, and intermittent presence of psammoma bodies. They are often gland forming, but can also present in a solid, sheet-like arrangement.

Genetics of Type 1 and Type 2 Ovarian Carcinoma

Type 1 ovarian tumors have well-defined molecular abnormalities. *Low-grade serous carcinomas* have frequent and mutually exclusive *KRAS* and *BRAF* mutations and rare mutation in either *ERBB2* or *TP53* (< 10%). Both *KRAS* and *BRAF* mutations occur in

approximately 30% of low-grade serous carcinomas and their precursor borderline serous tumor. Low-grade tumors have much less chromosomal instability than high-grade tumors.[35] *Primary ovarian mucinous tumors* are rare, and anatomic findings, discussed previously, best differentiate ovarian from gastrointestinal mucinous tumors. *KRAS* mutations are common in mucinous ovarian tumors, present in up to 50% of cases.[36] *Endometrioid ovarian carcinomas* harbor various mutations in well-known oncogenes and tumor suppressors. Mutations in *KRAS* and *BRAF* are present in approximately 10% of endometrioid tumors, and *PTEN* mutations are present in approximately 20%. Mutations in *CTNNB1* (β-catenin) have been reported in up to 60% of low-grade endometrioid tumors. Mutations in these genes have also been found in precursor lesions of LMP tumors. The striking overlap between the mutational spectrum of low-grade endometrioid ovarian tumors and endometrioid tumors of the endometrium suggests a shared etiology, which is likely mediated through the process of endometriosis. Recently, next-generation sequencing of RNA (RNA-seq) from ovarian tumors identified common mutations in 2 novel genes: *ARID1A* and *PPP2R1A*. *ARID1A* mutations were identified in 30% of endometrioid ovarian tumors and are thought to function as a tumor suppressor. *PPP2R1A* mutations have been identified in approximately 10% of ovarian endometrioid tumors and are thought to function as oncogenes.[37,38] Endometrioid tumors fail to express *WT-1* and often have MI, in contrast to the more common high-grade serous tumors. *Clear cell ovarian carcinomas* also have mutations in *ARID1A* and *PPP2R1A*. These mutations were first identified in clear cell tumors.[39,40] *ARID1A* mutations are present in approximately 50% of ovarian clear cell tumors, and *PPP2R1A* mutations are present in 5% to 10%.[37,38] Clear cell carcinomas also have mutations in *PTEN*, *KRAS*, and *TP53*, but at low frequency. Interestingly, for a high-grade tumor, clear cell carcinomas have a relatively low frequency of chromosomal instability. Clear cell carcinomas frequently overexpress *HNF-1B* and, similar to endometrioid tumors, have no overexpression of *WT-1* or *TP53*.

The discussion of type 2 tumors will be limited to *high-grade serous carcinomas*. Carcinosarcomas of the ovary are rare. They are part of the type 2 spectrum, have frequent *TP53* mutations, and, like carcinosarcomas of the endometrium, are thought to be morphologic variants of serous tumors. It has been known for some time that high-grade serous carcinomas have frequent mutations in *TP53*. In fact, high-grade serous carcinomas may be the solid tumor with the highest frequency of *TP53* mutations, besides certain inherited cancer syndromes. It is now well established that *TP53* mutations can be identified in greater than

95% of high-grade serous carcinomas of the ovary.[41] Although the majority of type 2 serous tumors develop as de novo high-grade lesions with early loss of *TP53*, there are rare cases in which high-grade serous tumors can be molecularly characterized as arising from previously established low-grade serous tumors.[42]

Some of the earlier molecular genetic studies of high-grade serous carcinoma have been hampered by the inclusion of other subtypes of epithelial ovarian carcinoma. As evident from the previous sections, epithelial ovarian cancer is a heterogeneous group of diseases, a fact only fully recognized of late. Germline and somatic mutations in *BRCA1* and *BRCA2* are also relatively common in high-grade serous carcinomas. Germline mutations in each gene are present in 6% to 8% of high-grade serous carcinomas, and somatic mutations in each gene are present in approximately 3% of cases. Beyond these molecular findings, there are few recurrently mutated genes in high-grade serous carcinomas, a finding determined by The Cancer Genome Atlas (TCGA) pilot project in ovarian carcinoma, which was recently completed. TCGA comprehensively sequenced the whole exome of more than 300 high-grade serous carcinomas of the ovary and found few genes mutated in more than 5% of the samples other than *TP53*, *BRCA1*, and *BRCA2* (tcga.cancer.gov). Copy number alterations are found in most high-grade serous carcinomas throughout the genome, making high-grade serous carcinoma one of the most genomically complex solid tumors. Recurrent amplifications are found in *CCNE1*, *PIK3CA*, *KRAS*, and *MYC*. Focal deletions have been identified in *PTEN*, *RB1*, *NF1*, and *CDKN2A*. High-grade serous carcinomas commonly overexpress both *TP53* and *WT-1*.

Origins of Ovarian Carcinoma

It is well established and logical that type 1 tumors originate in a stepwise fashion from precursor lesions such as borderline tumors and endometriotic lesions. However, the origins of type 2 tumors remain elusive. Few precursor lesions have been identified on the ovarian surface epithelium, which has been the putative site of origin for high-grade serous carcinoma. In many other solid tumors, such as colorectal cancer, the normal tissue of origin histologically resembles the malignant counterpart and undergoes a stepwise progression from normal to cancer. In the ovary, which is lined by a single-cell layer of modified mesothelium, there is little resemblance to high-grade serous carcinoma, which frequently displays a great degree of papillary architecture prior to becoming diffusely solid or anaplastic. Furthermore, the ovarian surface is, embryologically, a modified mesothelial layer of peritoneum, and the ovary itself is a mesonephric

structure, both unlike established high-grade serous carcinoma, which has a Mullerian phenotype. The uterus and fallopian tubes are true Mullerian structures developing, embryologically, from the Mullerian ducts in the absence of Mullerian inhibitory factor. When risk-reducing bilateral salpingo-oophorectomy became common for women with germline mutations in *BRCA1* or *BRCA2* (discussed later), occult "ovarian" cancers were identified in a small portion of cases. Interestingly, these occult tumors occurred predominantly in the distal fallopian tube and not on the surface of the ovary. To date, unifocal tubal carcinoma has not been reported in the proximal fallopian tube. These findings led investigators to examine the distal fallopian tube as a site of origin for epithelial ovarian cancer. To assist with these efforts, new processing methods for the fallopian tube were established to comprehensively section and evaluate the entire fimbria and perform better interrogation of the remainder of the fallopian tube. This technique is referred to as SEE-FIM[43] (Figure 2-4).

As the distal fallopian tube was further interrogated, a putative precursor lesion, called serous tubal intraepithelial carcinoma (STIC), was identified. STIC lesions are characterized by nuclear atypia, epithelial layering, overexpression of *TP53*, increased proliferation as measured by Ki-67, and lack of stromal invasion. When these lesions are clearly invading underlying stroma, they can be classified as truly invasive

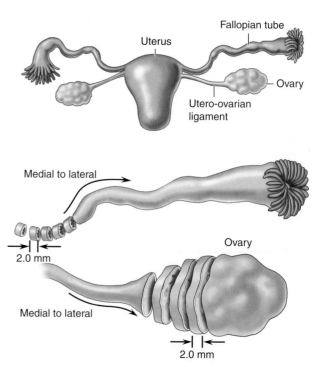

FIGURE 2-4. Suggested procedure for processing risk-reducing salpingo-oophorectomy specimens.

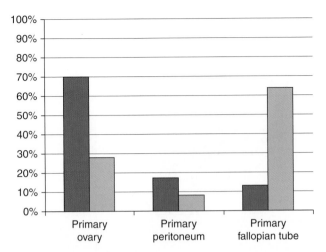

FIGURE 2-5. Comparison of frequency distribution of high-grade serous carcinomas in pelvic (nonuterine) sites based on criteria for primary site origin. Dark blue: Conventional criteria, regardless of the presence of tubal intraepithelial carcinoma (TIC). Light blue: Conventional criteria ± TIC (cases with TIC were classified as being of primary fallopian tube origin and cases without TIC were classified as either an ovarian, peritoneal, or tubal primary tumor based on conventional criteria). (Reproduced, with permission, from Przybycin CG, Kurman RJ, Ronnett BM, et al. Are all pelvic [nonuterine] serous carcinomas of tubal origin? *Am J Surg Pathol.* 2010;34:1407-1416.)

malignancies. STIC lesions or invasive carcinoma has been found in 3% to 8% of all risk-reducing salpingo-oophorectomy specimens. Molecular evidence supports the relationship between STIC and invasive serous carcinoma. In 2 surveys of advanced serous carcinoma, STIC lesions were identified in the fallopian tubes of approximately 50% of cases[44,45] (Figure 2-5). In addition, identical *TP53* lesions have been identified in both the STIC lesions and established invasive carcinomas in the same patients.

It has been suggested that ovarian inclusion cysts may be sites of serous ovarian carcinogenesis. The data to support this theory are the identification of both intraepithelial carcinoma within ovarian inclusion cysts as well as regions of aneuploidy within pathologically normal tissue.[27] The inclusion cyst hypothesis is consistent with the fallopian tube hypothesis in that fallopian tube epithelium can be shed onto the ovarian surface and later incorporated into the inclusion cyst during ovulation and surface repair. Additionally, immunomarkers, such as PAX8, found within fallopian tube epithelium, have also been found in the ovarian inclusion cysts, but not on the ovarian surface epithelium.[46] Taken together, these data suggest that the distal fallopian tube is a likely site of origin for approximately 50% of all serous carcinomas, suggesting that pelvic serous carcinoma (PSC) may be a

better term for previously presumed "ovarian" carcinoma (Figure 2-6). Where do the other half of PSCs originate? It is possible that there is an additional site of origin, or that all PSCs originate in the distal fallopian tube, yet we are only able to identify a precursor lesion in half of cases. The preneoplastic or early neoplastic cell could be shed onto the ovary or peritoneum early in the carcinogenic process, preventing the ability to identify a true precursor lesion within the fallopian tube. Further experimental evidence will be required to answer these important questions.

Hereditary Breast and Ovarian Cancer Syndrome

Mutations in *BRCA1* and *BRCA2* are known to increase the lifetime risks of breast and ovarian carcinoma. In the early 1990s, *BRCA1* and *BRCA2* were identified, cloned, and sequenced. Mutations in these genes were initially found in families with early-onset breast cancer. *BRCA1* is the breast cancer 1 gene, and its naming has also been ascribed to the location where it was first identified: Berkeley, California. Since its identification, we have learned that *BRCA1* increases the risk of both breast and ovarian cancer, whereas *BRCA2* increases the risks of these 2 cancers among others. Both genes function as classic tumor suppressors, and in the case of hereditary breast and ovarian cancer syndrome, the first allele is mutated in the germline, and the second allele is typically inactivated through loss of heterozygosity, epigenetic silencing through methylation of the *BRCA1* promoter, or rarely, a second somatic mutation. Both genes play important roles in maintaining genomic stability, and loss of either impairs the ability of DNA to repair damage. These genes play a critical role in homologous recombination, which is the most efficient mechanism to repair double-strand DNA damage that is often introduced through cytotoxic chemotherapy (Figure 2-7).

When homologous recombination is deficient, the cell must use other less efficient mechanisms of repair, such as nonhomologous end joining (NHEJ) or microhomology-mediated end joining (MMEJ). Both NHEJ and MMEJ are more error-prone mechanisms of double-strand DNA repair than homologous recombination. Therefore, under the stress of chemotherapy, homologous recombination–deficient cells, such as those found in *BRCA*-associated tumors, are less likely to survive. Other genes that are thought to participate in homologous recombination include *PTEN*, *ATM*, *ATR*, *PALB2*, *RAD51*, and the Fanconi Anemia genes. Mutations and deletions in these genes are individually less common in high-grade serous carcinomas than *BRCA1/2* mutations, but when all potential homologous recombination defects are considered together, nearly 50% of high-grade serous carcinomas

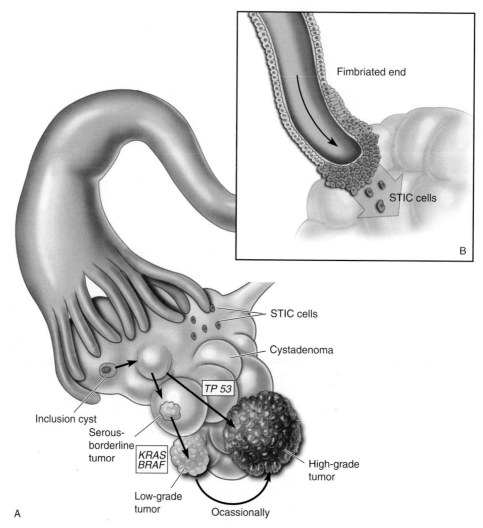

FIGURE 2-6. Proposed development of low-grade (LG) and high-grade (HG) serous carcinoma. A. One mechanism involves normal tubal epithelium that is shed from the fimbria, which implants on the ovary to form an inclusion cyst. Depending on whether there is a mutation of *KRAS/BRAF/ERRB2* or *TP53*, an LG or HG serous carcinoma develops, respectively. LG serous carcinoma often develops from a serous borderline tumor, which, in turn, arises from a serous cystadenoma. Another mechanism involves exfoliation of malignant cells from an STIC that implants on the ovarian surface, resulting in the development of an HG serous carcinoma. **B.** A schematic representation of direct dissemination or shedding of STIC cells onto the ovarian surface on which the carcinoma cells ultimately establish a tumor mass that is presumably arising from the ovary. Of note, there may be stages of tumor progression that precede the formation of an STIC.

have defective homologous recombination, a concept supported by experimental evidence.[47]

Penetrance

BRCA1 and *BRCA2* germline mutations are uncommon in the general population, with an estimated frequency of approximately 0.1%. In certain ethic groups and geographic regions, however, germline mutations are more common. The most well-studied population are the Ashkenazi Jews, who carry 2 common founder mutations in *BRCA1* (185delAG, 5382insC) and 1 in *BRCA2* (6174delT). Founder mutations are mutations that originally arose in a single individual and then spread through a closely knit population. The Ashkenazi Jewish population is rife with these mutations due to repetitive occurrences of population contraction and expansion such as the Spanish Inquisition, the Holocaust, and the crusades and pogroms. The prevalence of *BRCA1/2* founder mutations in the Ashkenazi Jewish population is approximately 2.5%. Other populations, such as French Canadians, Icelanders, Turks, Pakistanis, and certain ethnic groups in Africa, also have *BRCA1/2* founder mutations. Icelanders, for example, are geographically isolated, allowing for the enrichment of founder mutations over time.

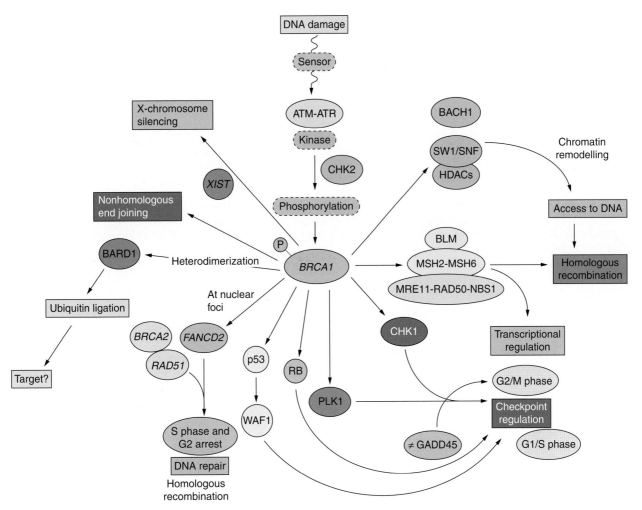

FIGURE 2-7. The *BRCA1* network. *BRCA1* is an important component of pathways that regulate DNA repair, cell-cycle progression, ubiquitylation, and transcriptional regulation. (Reprinted by permission from Macmillan Publishers Ltd: Nat Rev Cancer [Narod SA, Foulkes WD. *BRCA1* and *BRCA2*: 1994 and beyond. *Nat Rev Cancer*. 2004;4:665-676], copyright 2004.)

BRCA1 germline mutations confer a lifetime risk of approximately 40% for ovarian cancer and 60% to 80% for breast cancer. The general population risk for ovarian cancer is approximately 1.5%. *BRCA1* mutations also greatly increase the risk of fallopian tube and peritoneal cancer, but because these cancers are uncommon, the lifetime risks remain low. Due to the fallopian tube hypothesis discussed previously, it is likely that these lifetime risks will change due to changes in diagnostic criteria for ovarian and tubal carcinoma. *BRCA2* germline mutations confer a lifetime risk of approximately 20% for ovarian cancer and 60% to 80% for breast cancer (Figure 2-8). These mutations also increase the risks of fallopian tube and peritoneal cancer as well as cancers of the prostate, pancreas, melanoma, stomach, and biliary tract.

Whether or not *BRCA1/2* mutations increase the risk of endometrial cancer, endometrial serous cancer in particular, is debatable, with published studies finding evidence both for and against such an association. *BRCA1/2* somatic mutations are each found in approximately 3% of high-grade serous carcinomas. In Ashkenazi Jewish women with high-grade serous carcinoma, the likelihood of identifying a germline *BRCA1/2* mutation is 30% to 40%. In all women with high-grade serous carcinoma, the prevalence of germline *BRCA1/2* mutations is approximately 15%, leading some academic centers to recommend genetic testing for all women with high-grade serous carcinoma. Members of families at high risk for breast or ovarian cancer should undergo genetic testing. These families generally include multiple members with breast and/or ovarian cancer, often at an early age of onset. Specific testing guidelines can be found from various professional organizations, the National Cancer Institute, and the National Comprehensive Cancer Network (nccn.org).

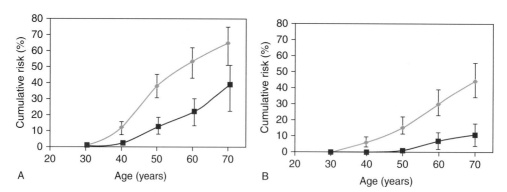

FIGURE 2-8. Lifetime risks of breast (♦) and ovarian cancer (■) of *BRCA1* (A) and *BRCA2* carriers (B). (Reprinted from Antoniou A, Pharoah PD, Narod S, et al. Average risks of breast and ovarian cancer associated with *BRCA1* or *BRCA2* mutations detected in case Series unselected for family history: a combined analysis of 22 studies. *Am J Hum Genet.* 2003;72:1117-1130, with permission from Elsevier.)

Pathology and Clinical Course

Ovarian tumors that develop in *BRCA1/2* mutation carriers are uniformly high-grade serous carcinomas. There have been reports of transitional cell and endometrioid tumors in this population, but with the inclusion of IHC, these tumors are not considered morphologic variants of high-grade serous carcinoma. Greater than 90% of *BRCA*-associated ovarian tumors have been reported to be high-grade serous carcinomas, with 1% to 2% reported as endometrioid, transitional, or mucinous. The non-serous tumors are likely to be serous variants, as mentioned, or incidental metastases from non-ovarian primary sites such as gastrointestinal tumors. Most cases present at an advanced stage, as is seen with most high-grade serous carcinomas. The mean age at diagnosis for *BRCA1*- and *BRCA2*-associated cases is 54 and 62 years, respectively, compared with the mean age of 63 years for sporadic cases. Thus *BRCA1*-associated cases are diagnosed approximately 10 years earlier than sporadic cases, but *BRCA2*-associated cases are diagnosed at the same age as sporadic cases.

Although women with *BRCA1/2* cases are more likely to develop ovarian cancer, as discussed previously, multiple studies have confirmed that, when diagnosed with high-grade serous carcinoma, these patients have a more favorable clinical course. It seems that the superior outcomes seen in *BRCA*-associated cases are due to an improved response to platinum-based chemotherapy. Because these tumors have defective homologous recombination repair, they are more likely to respond to the DNA damaging agents, such as platinum drugs and now possibly poly (ADP ribose) polymerase (PARP) inhibitors. Multiple studies have demonstrated a 50% to 100% longer overall survival in *BRCA* heterozygotes with high-grade serous carcinoma compared with sporadic high-grade serous carcinoma and an approximately 50% improvement in progression-free survival.

It is not clear whether tumors that obtain somatic *BRCA1* or *BRCA2* mutations will have a similarly improved survival as those with germline mutations, but this is a logical, yet unproven, conclusion. It is also not entirely clear if the improved outcomes seen in *BRCA*-associated tumors are completely independent of age at diagnosis, which is also a consistently identified factor associated with improved outcome. Some studies have found mutation status and age to be independent predictors of outcome, others have not, and others still have not assessed this relationship. The distinction between outcomes specifically related to *BRCA1*-associated versus *BRCA2*-associated tumors also remains murky because most studies have combined both mutation types to increase statistical power. However, considering the differences in clinical features, such as age at onset, and different biologic functions, the possibility remains that the clinical course could be different. As more consortia are created to study these issues, reliable answers should be forthcoming.

The role of *BRCA* promoter methylation, present in 10% of high-grade serous carcinomas, in clinical outcome and response to therapy remains unclear. The most recent and largest analysis performed by TCGA has confirmed that *BRCA* promoter methylation is not associated with an improved overall survival compared with sporadic cases, both of which are not as favorable as *BRCA*-associated cases. Unlike *BRCA*-associated ovarian cancer, *BRCA*-associated breast cancers are more likely to be triple negative, node positive, and aggressive, resulting in a general worse outcome for *BRCA*-associated breast cancer.

Prevention

Because germline testing can readily identify carriers of *BRCA1* and *BRCA2* mutations, ovarian cancer prevention can be considered in these women, and it is highly effective. Risk-reducing bilateral salpingo-oophorectomy is strongly recommended for ovarian cancer risk reduction in known carriers of germline *BRCA1* or *BRCA2* mutations. Multiple studies have demonstrated an 80% to 90% reduction in ovarian cancer risk in mutation carriers who had risk-reducing bilateral salpingo-oophorectomy as compared with those who had not. This procedure also reduces the risk of estrogen receptor–positive breast cancer. The earlier the procedure is performed, the greater the magnitude of risk reduction for both breast and ovarian cancer. This procedure also reduces the risk of fallopian tube cancer, as the fallopian tubes are (and should be) removed along with the ovaries.

All risk-reducing salpingo-oophorectomy procedures should be performed through minimally invasive approaches, unless there are extenuating circumstances. This procedure, when performed properly, will result in a small residual portion of the interstitial fallopian tube remaining in the uterine cornu. Although previously thought to potentially increase the risk of subsequent fallopian tube cancer, multiple studies have now confirmed that fallopian tube cancer develops in the distal fallopian tube or fimbria, and no cases of fallopian tube cancer developing in the interstitial portion of the tube have been reported. The association between *BRCA* germline mutations and the risk of uterine serous carcinoma is more controversial, with studies both supporting and refuting this association. No definitive data have yet been published to strongly support the role of hysterectomy at the time of risk-reducing salpingo-oophorectomy for the sole purpose of reducing the risk of potential *BRCA*-associated uterine serous carcinoma. There are often other medical, oncologic, and gynecologic reasons to consider hysterectomy at the time of risk-reducing salpingo-oophorectomy, and the risks and benefits of an associated hysterectomy must be evaluated individually. A small ongoing lifetime risk of primary peritoneal cancer persists after risk-reducing bilateral salpingo-oophorectomy (approximately 2%-3%).

Cervical Cancer

Cervical cancer is one of the greatest gynecologic cancer problems worldwide. Improvements have been made through screening and prevention with vaccination. Cervical cancer is a unique gynecologic malignancy in that more than 90% of cases can be etiologically linked to infection with the human papillomavirus (HPV). There are more than 100 types of papillomaviruses, which are double-stranded DNA viruses. Multiple types can infect the lower gynecologic tract, but only certain ones have been found to cause cervical cancer. The genome of HPV contains various open reading frames (ORFs). ORF E6 and E7 are oncoproteins that have the ability to integrate into host cells and are necessary for malignant transformation.[48] HPV infection alone is not sufficient for malignant transformation, as many HPV infections are cleared spontaneously or progress into dysplasia but not cancer. The immune system mediates the host's ability to clear HPV infections and regress dysplastic lesions. HPV also contains 2 capsid proteins that allow for type-specific vaccine production.

REFERENCES

1. Samuels Y, Wang Z, Bardelli A, et al. High frequency of mutations of the PIK3CA gene in human cancers. *Science*. 2004;304(5670):554.
2. King TA, Li W, Brogi E, et al. Heterogenic loss of the wild-type *BRCA* allele in human breast tumorigenesis. *Ann Surg Oncol*. 2007;14(9):2510-2518.
3. Smith DC, Prentice R, Thompson DJ, et al. Association of exogenous estrogen and endometrial carcinoma. *N Engl J Med*. 1975;293(23):1164-1167.
4. Pillay OC, Te Fong LF, Crow JC, et al. The association between polycystic ovaries and endometrial cancer. *Hum Reprod*. 2006; 21(4):924-929.
5. Baak JP, Mutter GL, Robboy S, et al. The molecular genetics and morphometry-based endometrial intraepithelial neoplasia classification system predicts disease progression in endometrial hyperplasia more accurately than the 1994 World Health Organization classification system. *Cancer*. 2005;103(11):2304-2312.
6. Sherman ME, Bitterman P, Rosenshein NB, et al. Uterine serous carcinoma. A morphologically diverse neoplasm with unifying clinicopathologic features. *Am J Surg Pathol*. 1992;16(6): 600-610.
7. Boruta DM 2nd, Gehrig PA, Fader AN, et al. Management of women with uterine papillary serous cancer: a Society of Gynecologic Oncology (SGO) review. *Gynecol Oncol*. 2009;115 (1):142-153.
8. McCluggage WG. Uterine carcinosarcomas (malignant mixed Mullerian tumors) are metaplastic carcinomas. *Int J Gynecol Cancer*. 2002;12(6):687-690.
9. Ferguson SE, Tornos C, Hummer A, et al. Prognostic features of surgical stage I uterine carcinosarcoma. *Am J Surg Pathol*. 2007;31(11):1653-1661.
10. Pollock PM, Gartside MG, Dejeza LC, et al. Frequent activating FGFR2 mutations in endometrial carcinomas parallel germline mutations associated with craniosynostosis and skeletal dysplasia syndromes. *Oncogene*. 2007;26(50):7158-7162.
11. Boland CR, Thibodeau SN, Hamilton SR, et al. A National Cancer Institute Workshop on Microsatellite Instability for cancer detection and familial predisposition: development of international criteria for the determination of microsatellite instability in colorectal cancer. *Cancer Res*. 1998;58(22):5 248-5257.
12. Vilar E, Gruber SB. Microsatellite instability in colorectal cancer—the stable evidence. *Nat Rev Clin Oncol*. 2010;7(3): 153-162.
13. An HJ, Logani S, Isacson C, et al. Molecular characterization of uterine clear cell carcinoma. *Mod Pathol*. 2004;17(5):530-537.
14. Lynch HT, Shaw MW, Magnuson CW, et al. Hereditary factors in cancer. Study of two large midwestern kindreds. *Arch Intern Med*. 1966;117(2):206-212.
15. Aarnio M, Sankila R, Pukkala E, et al. Cancer risk in mutation carriers of DNA-mismatch-repair genes. *Int J Cancer*. 1999;81(2):214-218.

16. Meyer LA, Broaddus RR, Lu KH. Endometrial cancer and Lynch syndrome: clinical and pathologic considerations. *Cancer Control.* 2009;16(1):14-22.

17. Lu KH, Schorge JO, Rodabaugh KJ, et al. Prospective determination of prevalence of lynch syndrome in young women with endometrial cancer. *J Clin Oncol.* 2007;25(33): 5158-5164.

18. Matthews KS, Estes JM, Conner MG, et al. Lynch syndrome in women less than 50 years of age with endometrial cancer. *Obstet Gynecol.* 2008;111(5):1161-1166.

19. Walsh MD, Cummings MC, Buchanan DD, et al. Molecular, pathologic, and clinical features of early-onset endometrial cancer: identifying presumptive Lynch syndrome patients. *Clin Cancer Res.* 2008;14(6):1692-1700.

20. Watson P, Bützow R, Lynch HT, et al. The clinical features of ovarian cancer in hereditary nonpolyposis colorectal cancer. *Gynecol Oncol.* 2001;82(2):223-228.

21. Soliman PT, Broaddus RR, Schmeler KM, et al. Women with synchronous primary cancers of the endometrium and ovary: do they have Lynch syndrome? *J Clin Oncol.* 2005;23: 9344-9350.

22. Garg K, Soslow RA. Lynch syndrome (hereditary non-polyposis colorectal cancer) and endometrial carcinoma. *J Clin Pathol.* 2009;62(8):679-684.

23. Broaddus RR, Lynch HT, Chen LM, et al. Pathologic features of endometrial carcinoma associated with HNPCC: a comparison with sporadic endometrial carcinoma. *Cancer.* 2006;106(1): 87-94.

24. Schmeler KM, Lynch HT, Chen LM, et al. Prophylactic surgery to reduce the risk of gynecologic cancers in the Lynch syndrome. *N Engl J Med.* 2006;354(3):261-269.

25. Schmeler KM, Soliman PT, Sun CC, et al. Endometrial cancer in young, normal-weight women. *Gynecol Oncol.* 2005;99(2): 388-392.

26. Walsh C, Holschneider C, Hoang Y, et al. Coexisting ovarian malignancy in young women with endometrial cancer. *Obstet Gynecol.* 2005;106(4):693-699.

27. Pothuri B, Leitao MM, Levine DA, et al. Genetic analysis of the early natural history of epithelial ovarian carcinoma. *PLoS One.* 2010;5:e10358.

28. Gilks CB, Ionescu DN, Kalloger SE, et al. Tumor cell type can be reproducibly diagnosed and is of independent prognostic significance in patients with maximally debulked ovarian carcinoma. *Hum Pathol.* 2008;39(8):1239-1251.

29. Madore J, Ren F, Filali-Mouhim A, et al. Characterization of the molecular differences between ovarian endometrioid carcinoma and ovarian serous carcinoma. *J Pathol.* 2010;220(3): 392-400.

30. Kurman RJ, Shih IeM. Pathogenesis of ovarian cancer: lessons from morphology and molecular biology and their clinical implications. *Int J Gynecol Pathol.* 2008;27(2):151-160.

31. McKenney JK, Balzer BL, Longacre TA. Patterns of stromal invasion in ovarian serous tumors of low malignant potential (borderline tumors): a reevaluation of the concept of stromal microinvasion. *Am J Surg Pathol.* 2006;30(10):1209-1221.

32. Soslow RA. Histologic subtypes of ovarian carcinoma: an overview. *Int J Gynecol Pathol.* 2008;27(2):161-174.

33. Yemelyanova AV, Vang R, Judson K, et al. Distinction of primary and metastatic mucinous tumors involving the ovary: analysis of size and laterality data by primary site with reevaluation of an algorithm for tumor classification. *Am J Surg Pathol.* 2008;32(1):128-138.

34. Zaino RJ, Brady MF, Lele SM, et al. Advanced stage mucinous adenocarcinoma of the ovary is both rare and highly lethal: a Gynecologic Oncology Group study. *Cancer.* 2011;117(3):554-562.

35. Kuo KT, Guan B, Feng Y, et al. Analysis of DNA copy number alterations in ovarian serous tumors identifies new molecular genetic changes in low-grade and high-grade carcinomas. *Cancer Res.* 2009;69(9):4036-4042.

36. Gemignani ML, Schlaerth AC, Bogomolniy F, et al. Role of KRAS and BRAF gene mutations in mucinous ovarian carcinoma. *Gynecol Oncol.* 2003;90(2):378-381.

37. McConechy MK, Anglesio MS, Kalloger SE, et al. Subtype-specific mutation of PPP2R1A in endometrial and ovarian carcinomas. *J Pathol.* 2011;223(5):567-573.

38. Shih IeM, Panuganti PK, Kuo KT, et al. Somatic mutations of PPP2R1A in ovarian and uterine carcinomas. *Am J Pathol.* 2011;178(4):1442-1447.

39. Wiegand KC, Shah SP, Al-Agha OM, et al. ARID1A mutations in endometriosis-associated ovarian carcinomas. *N Engl J Med.* 2010;363(16):1532-1543.

40. Jones S, Wang TL, Shih IeM, et al. Frequent mutations of chromatin remodeling gene ARID1A in ovarian clear cell carcinoma. *Science.* 2010;330(6001):228-231.

41. Ahmed AA, Etemadmoghadam D, Temple J, et al. Driver mutations in TP53 are ubiquitous in high grade serous carcinoma of the ovary. *J Pathol.* 2010;221(1):49-56.

42. Dehari R, Kurman RJ, Logani S, et al. The development of high-grade serous carcinoma from atypical proliferative (borderline) serous tumors and low-grade micropapillary serous carcinoma: a morphologic and molecular genetic analysis. *Am J Surg Pathol.* 2007;31(7):1007-1012.

43. Medeiros F, Muto MG, Lee Y, et al. The tubal fimbria is a preferred site for early adenocarcinoma in women with familial ovarian cancer syndrome. *Am J Surg Pathol.* 2006;30(2): 230-236.

44. Kindelberger DW, Lee Y, Miron A, et al. Intraepithelial carcinoma of the fimbria and pelvic serous carcinoma: evidence for a causal relationship. *Am J Surg Pathol.* 2007;31(2): 161-169.

45. Przybycin CG, Kurman RJ, Ronnett BM, et al. Are all pelvic (nonuterine) serous carcinomas of tubal origin? *Am J Surg Pathol.* 2010;34(10):1407-1416.

46. Auersperg N. The origin of ovarian carcinomas: a unifying hypothesis. *Int J Gynecol Pathol.* 2011;30(1):12-21.

47. Mukhopadhyay A, Elattar A, Cerbinskaite A, et al. Development of a functional assay for homologous recombination status in primary cultures of epithelial ovarian tumor and correlation with sensitivity to poly(ADP-ribose) polymerase inhibitors. *Clin Cancer Res.* 2010;16(8):2344-2351.

48. zur Hausen H. Papillomaviruses causing cancer: evasion from host-cell control in early events in carcinogenesis. *J Natl Cancer Inst.* 2000;92(9):690-698.

3 Diagnostic Modalities

David Starks, Bin Yang, and Peter G. Rose

In the field of gynecologic oncology, the various diagnostic modalities available serve as invaluable tools in the diagnosis, management, staging, treatment, and monitoring of gynecologic malignancies. Technological advances in existing modalities such as ultrasound, computed tomography (CT), and magnetic resonance imaging (MRI) have furthered their utility as diagnostic and management instruments, while the indications for newer imaging modalities such as 2-(18F)-fluoro-2-deoxy-D glucose (FDG) positron emission tomography (PET)/CT continue to expand. The use of tumor markers in identifying disease and molecular pathology in confirming which specific disease exists is presented. Because of the important role played by these diagnostic tools, the gynecologic oncologist must possess at least a passing familiarity with the basic science underlying these diagnostic instruments, as well as understand their advantages and limitations in imaging the spectrum of gynecologic cancers. Not all diagnostic modalities are useful or appropriate in evaluating the different and varied gynecologic cancers. Furthermore, the impact of diagnostic studies in the field of gynecologic oncology is ever expanding as newer technological developments become available to the clinician who must understand how to translate these advancements into improved patient care. Finally, as cost-effectiveness becomes an ever more important driver of health care decision making, it behooves the gynecologic oncologist to understand the various diagnostic tools in his armamentarium in order to use them to maximal effect.

IMAGING MODALITIES

Diagnostic imaging is an expanding field that has replaced radiology and now encompasses numerous new and varied technologies.

Ultrasound

Ultrasound is the most widely used imaging modality in the field of gynecology and is often the initial radiologic study used in the evaluation of pelvic abnormalities. Ultrasound technology uses a hand-held transducer containing *piezoelectric crystals* capable of emitting high-frequency sound waves that are projected into the patient's body. Emitted frequencies range from 7.0 to 8.0 MHz, used in transabdominal scanning, and up to 9.0 MHz is generally used in transvaginal ultrasound (TVUS). Higher-frequency sound waves result in improved image resolution, but reduced tissue penetration. The piezoelectric crystals serve as both the emitter and receiver of the sound waves. As the wave encounters tissue surfaces, it is both reflected and transmitted. The reflected wave returns to the transducer, where it is converted into an electrical signal, which is termed an *echo*, and the signal is amplified and converted into different shades of gray based on the degree of amplification. Stronger echoes are perceived as whiter shades, whereas weaker echoes are assigned darker shades.

Doppler ultrasonography can be added to basic ultrasound studies in order to evaluate vascular structures and blood flow. Doppler ultrasonography uses the principles of the *Doppler Effect*, which states that a moving object will emit a wavelength with differing frequencies and lengths based on whether the object is moving toward or away from the source emitting the sound wave. The sound waves emitted by the ultrasound transducer are reflected by vascular structures being studied, and objects moving toward the transducer emit a high-frequency, short-wavelength echo, whereas objects moving away from the transducer emit a low-frequency, long-wavelength echo. Based on these frequencies and wavelengths, the ultrasound transducer is able to determine the velocity of flow in the vascular structure and generate a Doppler waveform. Color-flow Doppler, by convention, assigns flow toward the transducer as red and flow away from the transducer as blue, but this assignment is arbitrary and can be reversed by the ultrasonographer.

The strengths of ultrasound technology includes its relative ubiquity and low cost, as well as a high safety profile due to the absence of ionizing radiation. The weaknesses of ultrasound include its reliance on the skill and experience of the operator, the need for a high degree of training in order to obtain a necessary degree of competence, the inability of the sound waves to penetrate gas or bone, and difficulty in visualizing midline organs due to the obscuring effect of overlying bowel gas or patient obesity and body habitus.

Indications for performing ultrasound studies in the field of gynecologic oncology include the initial evaluation of the endometrial lining in the setting of postmenopausal bleeding; evaluating and describing the nature of pelvic and adnexal masses, identifying and diagnosing gestational trophoblastic disease, and playing an important role in the performance of ultrasound-guided biopsies and percutaneous drainage procedures conducted by interventional radiologists.

Computed Tomography

High-resolution CT scans are an invaluable tool for the gynecologic oncologist, and use of CT scans in the field is extensive. Indeed, CT scans are probably the most frequently used imaging technique ordered by gynecologic oncologists and the second most common imaging study after ultrasound in the field of gynecology. CT scans offer the oncologist a noninvasive means of evaluating the extent and spread of metastatic disease and provide guidance in surgical planning, detecting disease recurrence and progression, and detecting lymph node involvement. CT scans also play a role in interventional radiology, permitting accurate biopsies and drainage procedures to occur.

CT scanners use x-ray beams that are rotated about a patient in a 180-degree arc. Laying directly opposite of the beam emitters are sets of crystal detectors,

2 to 10 mm in size, that capture the emitted photons and measure tissue absorption. This information is then processed by a computer that generates a 2-dimensional cross-sectional representation of the anatomic structure under radiologic evaluation. In order to generate clearer and more diagnostic images, contrast medium is often used to enhance the discrepancy in tissue absorption and densities. Contrast medium may be given to patients either orally, intravenously, or rectally, and care must be used when administering contrast to patients with a known iodine allergy or renal dysfunction.

The advantages of CT scans include a short period of time required for scanning; minimization of the dependency on operator skill, thus leading to a high degree of reproducibility, and a high degree of spatial and anatomic resolution. More recent modifications in CT technology have led to further improvement in image resolution and visualization. For example, helical CT combines continuous patient transport through a scanner with a single row detector array that generates a spiraling projection of x-rays. This is a dynamic modification of the traditional CT, in which the patient remains stationary while being scanned. Helical CT decreases the scanning time required for a patient, decreases the volume of contrast dye that needs to be administered for improved resolution, and provides more images from several different angles, thus generating higher image quality. Helical CT also has improved detection of smaller lesions that are difficult to detect with conventional CT. Movement artifacts such as peristalsis in the intestines or interference from patient breathing are minimized, allowing for improved image resolution. Another modification of conventional CT is the multidetector CT scanner (MDCT), which uses the same basic principles of helical scanning, but uses a multiple-row detector array instead of a single-row detector array. Current scanners use 16-, 32-, or 64-slice systems that create a cross-sectional slice thickness of 1 to 2 mm, yielding images with even higher spatial resolution and improved image quality.

The disadvantages of CT scans include the use of ionizing radiation, which has led to a growing concern of an increased risk of radiation-associated cancers. A recent study concluded that for a 40-year-old female patient being evaluated by a routine CT of the abdomen and pelvis with contrast, the chance of developing cancer is 1 in 870, as compared with 1 in 470 for a woman 20 years of age and 1 in 1400 for a woman 60 years of age.[1] Caution must be used in interpreting these findings and those from similar studies. The risk of cancer to the individual patient from having a CT scan performed is small, even with the use of high-dose radiation. This risk is often outweighed by the benefits accrued from CT scans that are truly indicated, but the growing awareness in the medical community of this risk of cancer secondary to radiation has led to an effort to minimize nonindicated or multiple scans. Other disadvantages of CT include the fact that patient body habitus, as well as implanted metallic devices and prostheses, can obscure and degrade image quality, leading to the generation of a nondiagnostic scan.

Magnetic Resonance Imaging

MRI scanners produce a magnetic field that aligns hydrogen nuclei within the patient. An intermittent radiofrequency pulse is emitted from the scanner, which alters the alignment of these hydrogen nuclei. When the radiofrequency pulse is discontinued, the hydrogen nuclei return to their original alignment, releasing a quantity of energy in the process. The amount and rate of energy released is wholly dependent on the property of the tissues containing the hydrogen nuclei. The longitudinal relaxation time is termed *T1*, and in T1-weighted images, fluid appears dark and fat appears white. In the transverse relaxation time, termed *T2*, fluid has a white appearance. In contrast to CT, MRI does not use ionizing radiation, but instead relies on magnetic fields and radiofrequencies. The paramagnetic element gadolinium is used as a contrast agent in MRI, and in comparison with the iodine-containing contrast agents used in CT, gadolinium has a much lower rate of adverse reactions and allergies. Recent studies of gadolinium have established an association with nephrogenic systemic fibrosis (NSF) in patients with a history of acute renal failure and end-stage renal disease. The American College of Radiology (ACR) has published guidelines for the use of gadolinium in patients at risk for the development of NSF.[2] The ACR recommends that before the administration of gadolinium, a recent glomerular filtration rate (GFR) (in the last 6 weeks) be obtained for any patient with a history of renal disease, age greater than 60 years, history of hypertension or diabetes, or history of severe hepatic disease or liver transplantation. Although patients with stage I or stage II chronic renal disease do not require any special consideration, patients with stage III or V disease (GFR <30 mL/min/1.73 m^2) need to be referred to a nephrologist for evaluation before gadolinium administration and potential dialysis after the performance of an MRI.

The advantages of MRI include the use of nonionizing radiation and non–iodine-containing contrast agents. MRI can penetrate calcified material such as bone without significant attenuation in the signal or loss of image resolution. MRI also has remarkable soft tissue resolution. Recent advances have shortened the imaging time required to obtain scans, as well as created techniques for imaging the heart and blood vessels without the need for contrast agents.

The disadvantages of MRI include the expense of scans, issues with motion artifacts, and the inability of patients with metallic implants and prosthesis, such as pacemakers and artificial joints, to be placed inside an MRI scanner. Many patients experience episodes of anxiety or claustrophobia inside MRI scanners and may require anxiolytics to be fully compliant during scanning.

The role of MRI in gynecologic oncology is still being elaborated, but it can serve as a useful adjunct in determining the extent of local and distant tumor spread in gynecologic malignancies and also has great sensitivity and specificity in the evaluation of vaginal and vulvar cancers.

Positron Emission Tomography

PET scans have developed an important role in the diagnosis and management of a number of different malignancies, including gynecologic cancers. PET scans use a radiochemical tracer, most commonly FDG, which is preferentially taken up by malignant cells due to their increased rate of glycolysis. This means that PET scans are capable of detecting the early biochemical abnormalities associated with malignancy, before the development of the structural and tissue changes caused by malignancies that are necessary for cancer detection by other imaging techniques.[3] Combining FDG-PET with CT in a single scanning device has allowed the images obtained by both modalities to be fused, generating images in which areas of increased FDG uptake are superimposed on CT images, providing anatomical localization.

The advantages of PET scans are largely due to their ability to detect the early abnormalities associated with tumor growth and recurrence. Their disadvantages include the current high cost of both the PET scanner, as well as the cost of the scan. These costs are often not covered by a patient's insurance, except in a few indicated conditions such as staging cervical cancer. PET scans have a high false-negative rate in evaluating lesions that are less than 1.0 cm in size or in detecting malignancies with low metabolic activity. Furthermore, areas of inflammation can result in false-positive results.

The role of FDG-PET CT in the management of gynecologic cancers is still being elaborated. It currently has a role in the staging of cervical cancer, as well as monitoring for recurrence of cervical cancer. PET may also be useful in the detection of recurrent ovarian and endometrial cancer, but more study is needed before greater clinical application is undertaken.

Image-Guided Percutaneous Biopsies

The use of percutaneous biopsy, performed by interventional radiology using either CT or ultrasound guidance, to assist in the diagnosis of a pelvic mass continues to develop and is not without controversy. Biopsies may be obtained with the use of 16- or 18-gauge needles or through the use of 1.0- to 1.8-mm Surecut needles (UK Biopsy Ltd., Halifax, Great Britain) in order to obtain a core biopsy. Clinicians have raised concerns that biopsies of cystic ovarian lesions may have a high false-negative rate and a low diagnostic accuracy, while increasing a patient's risk for procedure-related tumor seeding and contamination of the peritoneum due to rupture or leakage of the cystic mass. It may be that the concern for peritoneal seeding of malignancy is theoretical at best, but the current clinical consensus in the management of a cystic ovarian lesion is for surgical management of the lesion, either by laparoscopy or laparotomy, rather than through percutaneous biopsies. The use of percutaneous biopsies to aid in the diagnosis of solid pelvic masses is less controversial and may be of benefit, especially in cases of widespread metastatic disease. The concern for intraperitoneal seeding does not appear to have the same risk for tumor leakage that seems inherent in performing a biopsy in a cystic lesion. Ascites is often a common finding in the setting of advanced malignancy, but the sensitivity of performing cytology on ascites appears to be 60%. With solid tumors, it is possible to obtain larger tissue samples by core biopsy, permitting immunohistochemical studies and molecular profiling to be performed. A recent study by Hewitt et al[4] examined 149 women with suspected ovarian cancer undergoing a biopsy of an adnexal mass by either CT or ultrasound guidance using an 18-gauge needle. The diagnostic rate was 90% for CT and 91% by ultrasound, with only 1 hemorrhagic complication documented in the series. The authors argued that percutaneous biopsy was safe and could be considered as a replacement for surgical intervention in the initial management and diagnosis of malignancy. Such conclusions are currently preliminary at best, and surgical management and diagnosis of pelvic masses is still considered to be the standard of care.

IMMUNOHISTOPATHOLOGY

Immunohistochemistry is a method for localizing specific antigens in tissue or cells based on antigen-antibody recognition. In the past 3 decades, a laundry list of antibodies has been developed with tissue specificity. Immunohistochemistry has enormous impact on the accuracy of pathologic diagnosis. We briefly summarize the current application of immunohistochemistry in facilitating the accurate diagnosis of gynecologic neoplasms, with focus on malignant epithelial neoplasms.

Cervix: p16 Is a Surrogate Biomarker for High-Grade Cervical Dysplasia

High-risk human papilloma virus (HPV), most commonly 16 or 18, is responsible for the majority of cervical cancers. Development of invasive cervical cancer is preceded by HPV-related cervical dysplasia, known as cervical intraepithelial neoplasia (CIN). CIN can be low grade (CIN1) or high grade (CIN2-3). Detection of high-grade cervical dysplasia by Pap smear and subsequent tissue biopsy is critical in the identification and treatment of precursor lesions for the prevention of cervical cancer. Unfortunately, the reproducibility of diagnosis of CIN2 in pathologic samples is not good. Therefore, the identification of surrogate markers for HPV infection and, more importantly, evidence of molecular changes leading to cervical cancer would be of vital importance in the discrimination between low-grade and high-grade dysplasia.

These HPV types encode 2 proteins, E6 and E7, that are oncogenic by their inhibition of tumor suppressor genes. This results in uninterrupted cellular replication and malignant transformation of some infected cervical cells.[5] Integration of HPV DNA into the cells is the prerequisite step for the expression of the oncoproteins E6 and E7, which subsequently degrades tumor suppressor proteins such as *p53* and pRb. HPV E7 protein expression results in degradation of pRb protein, which normally inhibits the transcription of *p16* (CDKN2A).

Diffuse *p16* expression has reliably been shown to be a surrogate biomarker for CIN2-3. However, there are approximately less than 30% of CIN1 lesions also expressing *p16* with a expressing *p16* with a focal and patchy pattern. Recent studies indicated that approximately 20% of *p16*-positive CIN1 progress to high-grade lesions as compared with none of the *p16*-negative CIN1 lesions within a 12-month follow-up period. Diffuse and full thickness of the *p16* immunostaining pattern is a hallmark of high-grade CIN and is a very useful ancillary tool in those challenging cases in differentiating CIN2 from CIN1 and from immature squamous metaplasia.

Diffuse expression of *p16* is also seen in adenocarcinoma in situ (AIS) of the cervix. Again, this expression correlates with the involvement of high-risk HPV in the development of these lesions. Detection of *p16* is helpful in the diagnosis of cervical AIS to distinguish AIS from endometriosis and tubo-endometrial metaplasia. The latter has a focal and discontinuous staining pattern that is distinct from the disuse and continuous staining pattern in AIS lesions. Additionally, *p16* aids in the differential diagnosis of endometrioid adenocarcinoma of the endometrium with endocervical adenocarcinoma. A diffuse *p16* staining pattern is typically seen in endocervical adenocarcinoma, but is rarely seen in endometrioid adenocarcinoma. However, it should be emphasized that *p16* immunostaining alone has no role in the differential diagnosis between endocervical adenocarcinoma and serous adenocarcinoma of the endometrium because diffuse *p16* staining pattern can be seen in both types of cancer.

Vulva: p16 and p53 Expression in Vulvar Intraepithelial Neoplasia

There are 2 types of vulvar intraepithelial neoplasia (VIN), classic (usual) and simplex (differentiated) types, based on histopathologic features and distinct molecular pathogenetic pathways. The most common precursor for vulvar squamous cell cancers is the classic or usual type of VIN, which is associated with HPV infection. These tumors are seen in younger patients who often have a history of cervical HPV infection. It has shown that tumor suppressor protein *p16* has been overexpressed in the majority of high-grade VINs. The staining pattern is diffuse and full thickness of the dysplastic epithelium. The molecular mechanism for overexpression of *p16* in the classic type of VIN is analogous to that seen in HPV-associated cervical CIN.[6] Furthermore, unlike simplex VIN, classical VIN is rarely associated with *p53* overexpression.

Simplex (differentiated) type of VIN is less frequently seen clinically and tends to be seen in older patients with no association of HPV infection. These lesions often arise in a background of lichen sclerosis. Histopathologically, recognition of simplex VIN and differentiating it from benign squamous hyperplasia can be challenging. Furthermore, these lesions are not as commonly detected before the development of invasive disease. This is thought to reflect both the difficulty in clinical and pathologic diagnosis of this lesion and the fact that it is thought to have a short time to progression to invasive disease.

Simplex VIN and keratinizing squamous cell vulvar cancers have consistently been strongly associated with *p53* mutations. It has been shown that approximately two-thirds of simplex VIN lesions display overexpression of *p53* immunohistochemically. *p53* immunostaining is a useful ancillary tool in making the distinction between simplex VIN and benign vulvar lesions. However, caution must be taken when dealing with a lesion with morphology and a *p53* immunostaining discrepancy. Because *p53* deletion is seen in some of the simplex VINs, a negative *p53* immunostaining should not prevent the diagnosis if morphologically convincing.

Immunoprofile of Extramammary Paget Disease

Extramammary Paget disease (EMPD) is an unusual diagnosis characterized by the presence of Paget cells proliferating within the intraepidermis. Vulvar Paget disease can be primary or secondary. Primary disease is that which originates from the epidermis or skin appendages, and secondary disease is that which represents extension of a visceral carcinoma to the vulva, most commonly rectal or urologic carcinomas. The clinical and histologic appearance of primary and secondary EMPD is similar, and thus differentiation can be a challenge. The prognostic implications between the 2 diagnoses are significant. Primary EMPD is usually a locally confined lesion, and the clinical outcomes are substantially better. Secondary EMPD, on the other hand, represents the spread of visceral tumor onto the vulvar skin and has a substantially worse prognosis. Therefore, accurate clinical diagnosis is very important in this disorder. Molecular markers have recently been found to be of utility in the distinction between primary and secondary EMPD and may have utility in aiding with diagnosing these lesions.

Cytokeratins (CKs) have utility in the detection of certain cancers. CK20 is associated with colorectal adenocarcinomas. It has also been correlated with the presence of a primary colorectal adenocarcinoma associated with secondary EMPD. Furthermore, CK20 staining was not seen in primary EMPD. CK7, on the other hand, has been consistently seen in primary EMPD and sometimes in secondary EMPD, although not as frequently. Therefore, a vulvar Paget disease possessing the immunoprofile of CK7–/CK20+ should prompt an aggressive search for an underlying malignancy, such as colorectal cancer.

Gross cystic disease fluid protein (GCDFP)-15 is a glycoprotein expressed in apocrine epithelial cells. GCDFP-15 has been found in primary EMPD, and its absence is correlated with the presence of secondary EMPD.[7] The immunohistochemical detection of carcinoembryonic antigen (CEA) has also been found to be of value in EMPD. The value of CEA staining seems to be in differentiating EMPD from superficial spreading melanoma and not in the separation of primary and secondary EMPD, although negative CEA staining is seen more commonly in secondary EMPD.

Endometrium

Based on the degree of malignancy and prognosis, endometrial carcinoma is divided into type 1 and type 2 cancers. Type 1 cancer includes endometrioid and mucinous adenocarcinoma, whereas type 2 encompasses serous and clear cell adenocarcinoma.

Loss of *PTEN* in Type 1 Endometrial Carcinoma

In type 1 cancers, loss of expression of pTEN protein due to point mutations and promoter methylation is the most frequent genetic alterations observed. *PTEN* is a tumor suppressor gene located on chromosome 10q23. The *PTEN* gene encodes a dual-specificity phosphatase with a role in cell cycle arrest and promotion of apoptosis via phosphatidylinositol-(3,4,5)-triphosphate (PIP3). Immunohistochemically, the majority of endometrioid and mucinous adenocarcinomas have negative immunoreactivity to pTEN antibody compared with adjacent benign endometrium. Because loss of pTEN is an early molecular event during endometrial carcinogenesis, lack of pTEN immunoreactivity has in recent years become the important biomarker in identifying the precursor lesion of endometrial intraepithelial neoplasia and a small subset of higher-grade endometrioid adenocarcinomas acquiring *p53* mutations at a late stage.[8] Therefore, *p53* immunostaining alone does not distinguish between serous adenocarcinoma and grade 3 endometrioid adenocarcinoma harboring a *p53* alteration.

p53, p16, and IMP3 Expression in Type 2 Endometrial Carcinoma

Type 2 cancers are often characterized by *p53* mutations. *p53* is a tumor suppressor gene and is the most commonly mutated gene in human cancers. *p53* protein product binds to DNA and upregulates transcription of genes, which act to halt the cell cycle and assist with DNA repair or initiate apoptosis if repair is not possible. Anti-*p53* antibody reacts with both wild-type and mutant *p53* proteins. However, because the half-life of wild-type *p53* protein in cells is only less than 20 minutes, it rarely detects *p53* immunoreactivity in most normal cells. In contrast, because the majority of mutant *p53* proteins have greater than 16 hours of half-life, its accumulation can be easily seen immunohistochemically in malignant cells. Approximately 90% of serous adenocarcinomas demonstrate *p53* mutation and accumulation of *p53* immunohistochemically. Different from type 1 cancers, *p53* mutation is an early genetic event in serous adenocarcinoma. It has been shown that up to 80% of endometrial intraepithelial carcinomas (EIC) contain mutations in *p53*. Therefore, immunohistochemical detection of *p53* overexpression is a very useful biomarker in identifying and confirming early precursors of EIC in endometrial biopsy or curettage specimens. Approximately 30% to 40% of clear cell adenocarcinomas harbor *p53* mutations.

Overexpression of *p16* protein is also seen in serous adenocarcinoma of the endometrium or the ovary. Overexpression of *p16* in serous adenocarcinoma is not linked to HPV infection. The underlying molecular mechanism is still largely unresolved. Because both cervical adenocarcinoma and serous adenocarcinoma can share high nuclear grade histopathologically, and overexpression of *p16* is found in both cervical adenocarcinoma and serous adenocarcinoma, another layer of challenge in the differential diagnosis of the 2 is added. When the issue arises, application of both *p16* and *p53* immunostains helps in resolving the issue. Serous adenocarcinoma will be strongly positive both for *p53* and *p16*, whereas cervical adenocarcinoma will be positive for *p16* but negative for *p53*.

IMP3 is an oncoprotein that is mainly expressed in fetal and malignant tissues and rarely in adult benign tissues. *IMP3* has been found to be involved in cell growth, adhesion, and migration. Strong *IMP3* staining has been demonstrated in 86% to 94% of serous adenocarcinoma, as opposed to only 3% to 28% of endometrioid adenocarcinoma. Furthermore, 50% of clear cell cancers also stain positive for *IMP3*. Expression of *IMP3* is also seen in 89% of EICs, indicating its involvement in early carcinogenesis.

Ovarian Epithelial Cancers

There are 5 types of ovarian epithelial cancer, each with distinct cell types and clinicopathologic features and treatment options: (1) papillary serous carcinoma (PSC), (2) clear cell carcinoma, (3) endometrioid carcinoma, (4) mucinous carcinoma, and (5) transitional cell carcinoma. Each type has its distinct pathogenesis and immunophenotypes.

p53 and *p16* Expression in Papillary Serous Carcinoma

p53 mutations are seen in approximately 70% of high-grade PSCs, but are rarely seen in low-grade PSCs.[9] *p16* is also expressed in high-grade PSC. The similar expression pattern of *p53* and *p16* in both endometrial and ovarian serous adenocarcinoma suggests an analogous pathway for carcinogenesis of these tumors.

Immunoprofile for Mucinous Adenocarcinoma

Mucinous adenocarcinoma, especially intestinal type, of the ovary can be morphologically indistinguishable from those derived from gastrointestinal tract. One of the most important issues clinically is to know whether a mucinous adenocarcinoma is primary ovarian cancer or secondary from other sites. Earlier studies indicate that the majority of colorectal cancer is CK7 negative and CK20 positive, whereas primary ovarian mucinous carcinoma is positive for both CK7 and CK20. Therefore, a CK7-negative mucinous adenocarcinoma is likely metastasized from the colorectum, and a CK-positive mucinous adenocarcinoma is likely an ovarian primary, if endocervical adenocarcinoma is excluded. The recent discovery of CDX2 expression in most of gastrointestinal cancers further facilitates the differential diagnoses. However, recent evidence of expression of CDX2 in some of the primary mucinous adenocarcinoma of the ovary and the expression of CK7 in some right-sided colon cancers further complicated the case. Therefore, although immunohistochemistry is in many situations helpful in the differential diagnosis, it is by no means a magic bullet. Clinicopathologic correlation is still crucial in rendering the correct diagnosis. Furthermore, CK7-negative and CK20-positive immunoprofile is also seen in mucinous adenocarcinomas of the lung, breast, pancreas, and stomach. Therefore, immunohistochemical findings must be put into a clinical context, and the expression of CK7 does not exclude that the ovarian tumor is secondary.

TUMOR MARKERS

Tumor markers are serologic substances that are produced by a malignancy or are abnormally elevated in response to the presence of a malignancy. They can be enzymes, growth factors, hormones, tumor antigens, receptors, and glycoconjugates. They play a role in screening, diagnosis, monitoring treatment response, and detecting disease recurrence. A large number of tumor markers have been investigated in recent years, but few have entered into clinical practice. This has largely been due to the fact that many of these tumor makers have poor specificity, which is defined as the proportion of patients without a cancer who have a negative test. Many of the current markers can be elevated in a number of conditions, both benign and malignant, contributing to their lack of specificity. With the development of new high-throughput approaches such as proteomics, which uses mass spectrometry (MS) techniques, a new interest has developed in investigating the patterns of tumor marker expression. Identification and describing these patterns offers the promise of the development of more sensitive and specific assays for various cancers and their histologic subtypes.

Cervical Cancer

No serum tumor markers exist or are being researched to screen for cervical cancer due to the success of Pap and HPV DNA-based screening programs. The few markers that were historically investigated were abandoned due to their low sensitivity and specificity. Several serologic markers have been assessed to play a potential role in determining prognosis, detecting recurrent disease, and monitoring treatment response. For example, squamous cell carcinoma antigen (SCCA) has moderate sensitivity when elevated in the setting of cervical cancer, but unfortunately has a low specificity, as SCCA levels may be elevated in a number of other squamous cell cancers, such as carcinoma of the head, neck, and lung. SCCA can also be elevated in benign conditions as well, such as psoriasis and eczema. However, there does appear to be a correlation of SCCA with prognosis and the clinical response of cervical cancer to treatment. Levels of SCCA above 1.1 ng/mL are associated with a poor prognosis. A recent study demonstrated that elevated levels of SCCA immediately after treatment with chemoradiation was predictive of distant recurrence.[10] Another study demonstrated that in patients being treated with chemoradiation, previously elevated SCCA levels normalized in 93% of patients at 1 month after treatment and in 96% of patients with a complete remission at 1 month. Although used in Europe and Japan, no US company has pursued licensing of this assay for use in the United States.

CA-125 is elevated in only approximately 21% of women with squamous cell carcinoma of the cervix and may correspond to prognosis, particularly if there is a decrease in preoperative CA-125 after treatment. The addition of other markers to CA-125, such as CEA and CA19-9, can increase the sensitivity of a tumor marker panel for detecting cervical cancer, but currently, obtaining these 3 tumor markers to manage a diagnosed cervical cancer is not considered to be standard of care.

CA-125 is elevated in 20% to 75% of patients with cervical adenocarcinoma and may reflect tumor stage, size, grade, presence of lymphovascular space involvement and lymph node involvement. A recent study of patients with adenocarcinoma of the cervix observed that in multivariate analysis, CA-125 was an independent prognostic factor for disease-free survival. The investigators also demonstrated that tumor necrosis factor receptor type I may potentially be the most useful marker in evaluating the prognosis of adenocarcinoma, particularly in early-stage disease.[11] Further research into the use of these particular tumor markers is warranted before their use can become widespread.

Endometrial Cancer

CA-125 is often elevated in patients with uterine serous carcinomas and advanced-stage endometrioid cancers, and obtaining CA-125 preoperatively has demonstrated a correlation with metastatic disease and extrauterine spread. However, CA-125 can be falsely positive, particularly after pelvic or abdominal radiation. Several other serologic markers, including CA15-3, CA19-9, CA72-4, cancer associated serum antigen, CEA, squamous-cell carcinoma antigen (SCCA), gamma-GT, urinary gonadotropin fragment (UGF), placental protein 4 and others, have been investigated as potential tumor markers but have been largely abandoned as viable candidates for either screening or clinically managing endometrial cancer. Other novel makers currently under investigation include the glycoprotein YKL-40, which, obtained preoperatively, may detect endometrial cancer and aid in determining prognosis. Higher levels of serum inhibins, particularly inhibin β-B (INH-β-B) was observed in grade 3 endometrial cancers compared with grade 2 cancers. In one study, inhibin α (INH-α) was an independent prognostic factor for progression-free survival, cause-specific survival, and overall-survival. Elevations in human kallikrein 6 may be overexpressed in patients with papillary serous endometrial cancer. Finally, pyruvate kinase M2, chaperonin 10, and α-1-antitrypsin performed well as a panel of biomarkers demonstrating a high sensitivity, specificity, and positive predictive value (PPV) in detecting endometrial cancer.[12] Testing of current biomarker candidates and the development of better tumor markers is ongoing.

Ovarian and Fallopian Tube Cancers

CA-125 is a 200-kilodalton (kDa) glycoprotein that is recognized by the OC-125 murine monoclonal antibody. It has 2 important antigenic domains: A is the domain-binding monoclonal antibody OC125; B is the domain binding monoclonal antibody M11. A number of assays exist for detecting serum CA-125; one of the most widespread is the second-generation heterologous CA-125 II assay, which uses both OC125 and M11 antibodies. The upper limit of normal of serum CA-125 of 35 U/mL was chosen because only 1% of healthy women had a value above this point. Levels can fluctuate, however, based on the phase of the menstrual cycle and is more often elevated if the woman is pre- versus postmenopausal. Eighty-five percent of women with epithelial ovarian cancer have a CA-125 level greater than 35 U/mL, with 25% to 50% of stage I patients having an elevated level and 90% of women with advanced-stage disease demonstrating an elevation in CA-125. The sensitivity of CA-125 is approximately 78%, with a specificity of 95% and a PPV of 82% based on both prospective and retrospective data. CA-125 is nonspecific and can be elevated in a number of other malignancies (cancers of the breast, colon, lung, and pancreas), benign conditions, endometriosis, pelvic inflammatory disease, and pregnancy. Finally, CA-125 is not a marker for nonepithelial ovarian malignancies, and low levels are common in borderline, endometrioid, clear cell, and mucinous epithelial tumors.

CA-125 is useful to measure treatment response, with the levels and pattern of CA-125 being monitored over time. In assessing treatment response, a decrease in CA-125 by 50% correlates with disease responsive to chemotherapy, whereas a doubling of CA-125 from baseline constitutes treatment failure and disease progression. A recent study found that CA-125 half-life and nadir concentration had independent prognostic value for disease-free and overall survival. The same investigative group recently demonstrated that a bi-exponential CA-125 decay was an indicator of poor prognosis after primary chemotherapy.[13] However, CA-125 is a poor marker of small-volume disease and can be falsely negative, as demonstrated in studies of second-look laparotomy after chemotherapy, which found active disease despite low or normal CA-125 levels.

CA-125 is a strong predictor of disease recurrence as well, and serial measurements are used to monitor patients for this indication. Serum elevations may be detectable 2 to 6 months before evidence of disease recurrence becomes visible on imaging studies.[14] A recent study demonstrated that in patients with a complete clinical remission, a progressive low-level increase in serum CA-125, from a baseline nadir, with an absolute increase of 5 to 10 U/mL, was strongly associated with disease recurrence. However, a recent randomized trial of early detection of recurrent disease with CA-125 failed to improve overall survival.[15] The only other marker with current US Food and Drug Administration approval for detection of recurrent ovarian cancer is HE4. A recent study demonstrated that HE4 correlated with a patient's clinical status in 76.2% of cases, which was not inferior to CA-125's correlation of 78.8%.[16] Use of both CA-125 and HE4 in a combined assay appears to increase sensitivity and maintain specificity in the detection of primary ovarian cancer in women with a newly diagnosed pelvic mass.

Although playing an important role in ovarian cancer surveillance strategies, the use of CA-125 as a screening tool remains investigational. Because of its lack of specificity, use of CA-125 alone as a screening tool is controversial. It has been reported that screening specificity can be increased with the addition of TVUS, improving specificity to 99.9% and PPV to 26.8% in postmenopausal women. However, the recent Prostate, Lung, Colorectal and Ovarian (PLCO) screening trial demonstrated the limitations of CA-125 and TVUS in screening for ovarian cancer. In this trial, 34,261 postmenopausal women were randomized to receive annual CA-125 and TVUS screening for 3 years, followed by 2 additional years of CA-125 monitoring. Women were referred to a gynecologic oncologist if either the CA-125 or TVUS were abnormal. The PPV for CA-125 was 3.7% and for TVS was 1%. If both were abnormal, the PPV was 23.5%, but more than 60% of ovarian malignancies would have been missed using this strategy. Finally, the sensitivity for detecting early-stage disease was notably low, with only 21% of detected ovarian cancers being either stage I or II.[17]

Improved screening PPV and specificity can be obtained by abandoning the use of a fixed cutoff of 35 U/mL and using the statistical Risk of Ovarian Cancer Algorithm (ROC), which uses a woman's age-specific incidence of ovarian cancer and CA-125 behavior over time to estimate a woman's risk of ovarian cancer. A prospective randomized trial of the ROC algorithm in 13,582 postmenopausal women demonstrated a high specificity of 99.8% and a PPV of 19% in detecting primary invasive epithelial ovarian cancer.[18] The ROC algorithm is currently being used in the UK Collaborative Trial of Ovarian Cancer Screening (UKCTOCS) study, which is ongoing at this time. In addition to CA-125, a large number of serum markers have been studied and evaluated, but very few have any relevance to the clinical realm due to poor sensitivity and specificity. CEA is elevated in endometrioid and Brenner tumors and occasionally in mucinous tumors. CA19-9 is expressed by mucinous ovarian cancers and cancers of the colon, but has low levels of expression in other epithelial ovarian cancers. A few of the tumor markers used in the diagnosis and management of nonepithelial ovarian cancers are detailed in Table 3-1.

Serum inhibin levels are elevated in sex–cord stromal tumors, especially granulosa cell tumors. Inhibin plays a role in the regulation of follicle-stimulating hormone secretion by the pituitary. It is composed of an α subunit and 1 of 2 β subunits (BA or BB). Although inhibin A and inhibin B levels can both be elevated in patients with granulosa cell tumors, an inhibin B level is elevated in a higher proportion of these tumors. A recent study evaluating the use of serum inhibin levels in 30 women with granulosa cell tumors demonstrated that the sensitivities and specificities for inhibin A were 67% and 100% and for inhibin B were 89% and 100%, respectively. The investigators also noted that inhibin A level was elevated before or at the time of first clinical recurrence in 58% of patients, whereas

Table 3-1 Tumor Markers Useful in Germ Cell Tumors of the Ovary

Germ Cell Tumor Type	AFP	hCG	LDH
Dysgerminoma			+
Endodermal sinus tumor	+		
Immature teratoma			
Embryonal carcinoma	+	+	
Choriocarcinoma		+	

AFP, α-fetoprotein; hCG, human chorionic gonadotropin; LDH, lactate dehydrogenase.

inhibin B level was elevated in 85%. The lead time from elevation of inhibin levels to clinical recurrence was estimated to be 11 months. Inhibin A and B levels were not elevated in any of the 17 patients who were postoperatively disease-free.[19]

Vulvar and Vaginal Cancers

The rarity of vulvar and vaginal cancers has made the investigation and development of useful tumor markers considerably difficult. There are a couple of novel markers under investigation, including carbonic anhydrase IX (CAIX), which may be elevated in vulvar cancer and may be correlated with recurrence-free survival compared with CAIX-negative tumors. CAIX overexpression may also correspond to tumor progression and inguinal lymph node metastasis. Overexpression of another marker, COX-2, may correspond with disease-specific survival in vulvar cancer. Other markers that have been investigated include tissue polypeptide-specific antigen, SCCA, and urinary gonadotropin fragment. No serologic marker to date has demonstrated sufficient sensitivity or specificity to play a role in screening or in detecting recurrent disease, or in directing clinical management. Due to the rarity of these 2 cancers, the creation of large trials sufficient to validate any tumor marker under current investigation seems doubtful.

IMAGING FOR SPECIFIC GYNECOLOGIC CANCERS

Cervical Cancer

Cancer of the uterine cervix is the third most common gynecologic malignancy in the United States, with 12,200 new cases and 4210 deaths expected in 2010. However, worldwide cervical cancer is the most common gynecologic cancer and among women is second only to breast cancer as the most common cancer. Staging of cervical cancer remains clinical, rather than surgical, due the high prevalence of disease in developing countries, where access to imaging technology and resources are limited. In the United States, radiologic studies are used for assistance in evaluating the extent of disease, monitoring treatment response, and detecting recurrent disease. Because most cases of cervical cancer are detected on physical examination or Pap smear, imaging studies play a limited role in the screening of cervical cancer.

Ultrasound

The role of ultrasound in the detection of primary cervical cancer is limited. Transrectal (TRUS) ultrasound permits better visualization of the cervix and detection of cervical malignancies than transabdominal or transvaginal ultrasound. Abnormal findings due to cervical canal obstruction by a mass, such as hematometra, can be detected on ultrasound, but overall its use in evaluating newly diagnosed cervical cancer is marginal.

TVUS or TRUS does not play a significant role in the evaluation of initial disease extent in cervical cancer. Ultrasound may be able to detect parametrial, pelvic sidewall, and bladder involvement by a cervical malignancy. However, the limited ability of ultrasound to appropriately visualize soft tissue planes, and its limited field of view compared with cross-sectional imaging modalities such as CT or MRI, has inhibited any meaningful use of ultrasound in the staging of cervical cancer.

The role of ultrasound in the detection of recurrent disease is obviously limited as well. Ultrasound's greatest utility in the setting of suspected recurrence is as a guidance modality for tissue biopsies in confirming disease recurrence. Transabdominal ultrasound can also detect hydronephrosis, indicating the need for ureteral stent placement in order to protect renal function. Ultrasound may also assist in the detection and management of complications related to disease status or treatment such as lymphocysts, abscesses, and fistulous tracts.

Computed Tomography

CT has no role in the primary detection of cervical cancer. CT has difficulty in direct tumor visualization and in distinguishing the interfaces between normal tissue and tumor. However, contrast-enhanced CT has had a long and well-established role in evaluating the extent of disease spread in cervical cancer. Although the staging of cervical cancer is still clinical, a staging system by CT has been proposed and correlated with the International Federation of Gynecology and Obstetrics (FIGO) staging system.[20] Of note, lymph node involvement is not considered to be part of the FIGO staging system, but detection of pelvic or para-aortic lymph node involvement, with lymph nodes larger than 1 cm in diameter in the short axis, correlates with stage IVB disease when using this system of evaluation with CT. This is important because the detection of lymphadenopathy has been shown both to affect prognosis and to alter potential clinical interventions. The reported accuracy of CT in detecting lymph node invasion is 83% to 85%, with a reported sensitivity ranging from 24% to 70%. CT can also be used to direct biopsies in the case of enlarged or suspicious nodes. Because cervical cancer is clinically staged, this text refers to evaluation of the extent of disease spread, rather than "staging," because according to FIGO criteria, no gynecologic cancer is staged through imaging modalities alone.

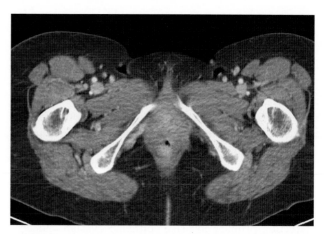

FIGURE 3-1. Cervical cancer on CT. Stage IB1 adenocarcinoma of the cervix. Enlarged cervical mass noted without invasion into the parametria or sidewall.

It is important to note that the sensitivity and specificity of CT in evaluating the spread of disease is constrained due to its inability to detect small tumors, invasion of the parametria (76%-80% accuracy), and early invasion of the rectum or bladder. Fifty percent of cervical tumors are isodense to the cervical stroma on CT, rendering the tumor practically invisible. When a cervical tumor is visible, it has a hypodense appearance due to necrosis and diminished vascularity (Figures 3-1 and 3-2). In a study of 172 patients, CT was compared with MRI and FIGO clinical staging in the pretreatment evaluation of invasive cervical cancer. In cases of advanced cervical cancer (stage ≥ IIB), the

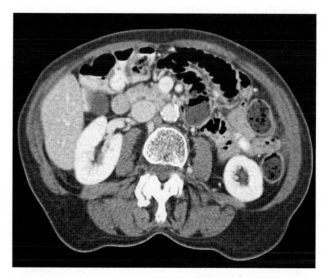

FIGURE 3-2. Cervical cancer on CT. Stage IB2 squamous cell carcinoma of the cervix. Enlarged aortocaval lymph node is noted, consistent with metastatic lymph node involvement.

sensitivity of CT was 42%, specificity was 82%, and negative predictive value (NPV) was 84%.[21] Although the accuracy of CT in evaluating disease spread is better than that of clinical examination, it appears to be greatly inferior to MRI. Multidetector CT (MDCT) may improve the diagnostic accuracy of conventional CT due to enhanced spatial and contrast resolution, but further investigation is warranted before MDCT could play a larger role in the staging process.

The most important and established role for CT is in the setting of post-treatment surveillance and the detection of recurrent disease. Currently CT is the imaging modality of choice for routine surveillance. Early detection of cervical cancer is essential in order to maximize the potential for salvage therapy such as radiotherapy or pelvic exenteration. The majority of recurrences are in the pelvis, including the vaginal cuff, parametrium, and the pelvic sidewall. Serial CT scans used in disease surveillance have a higher sensitivity and specificity in the detection of recurrent malignancy as compared with primary disease detection. CT also has improved detection and visualization of extrapelvic involvement by cervical cancer, including metastasis to the para-aortic nodes, liver, lungs, and abdomen. CT continues to have limitations in discriminating between postradiation changes, postsurgical fibrosis, and disease recurrence. In cases in which there is a high suspicion for disease recurrence, equivocal findings on CT may require either an MRI or obtaining a tissue specimen by fine-needle aspiration (FNA) or a core biopsy for a pathologic diagnosis of cervical cancer recurrence.

Magnetic Resonance Imaging

MRI is currently considered to be the most accurate imaging modality in the management of cervical cancer, playing key roles in pretreatment assessment, particularly in determining the tumor size and extent of local invasion, detecting lymph node involvement, evaluating response to therapy, and detecting disease recurrence. Although MRI is not routinely used in the primary screening of cervical cancer, it is considered to be the imaging modality of choice performed after the detection of cervical cancer by Pap smear and physical examination due to its superior soft tissue resolution capabilities (Figures 3-3, 3-4, and 3-5). T2-weighted images are particularly useful in the detection of cervical cancer, and it has been noted that the tumor has the appearance of a mass with an intermediate-signal intensity. Contrast-enhanced T1-weighted images can be helpful in detecting bladder or rectal wall invasion. However, non–contrast-enhanced T1-weighted images can pose difficulty in detecting the primary cervical lesion, which can be isointense to the surrounding normal cervix. The

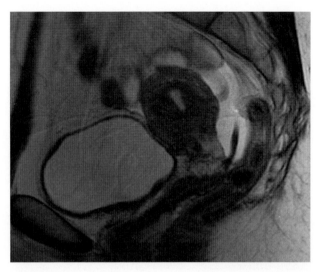

FIGURE 3-3. Cervical cancer on MRI. Stage IB1 squamous cell carcinoma of the cervix on T2-weighted MRI. Small areas of decreased enhancement are noted in the lower cervical stroma. This mass is confined to the cervical stroma, with no invasion of the parametria.

addition of gadolinium increases early enhancement of the primary tumor on T1-weighted images, rendering the malignancy more visible.

MRI appears to be superior to ultrasound, CT, and clinical examination in the evaluation of disease extent of cervical cancer. Like CT, MRI staging conventions correlate with the FIGO staging system. The overall staging accuracy of MRI is reported to be 77% to 93%, as compared with 69% in CT.

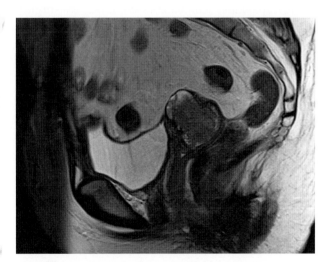

FIGURE 3-4. Cervical cancer on MRI. Stage IB1 squamous cell carcinoma of the cervical stump after a supracervical hysterectomy. T2-weighted MRI reveals a 3.7 cm heterogeneous enhancing mass. The mass is noted to disrupt the cervical stroma and invade the parametria on imaging.

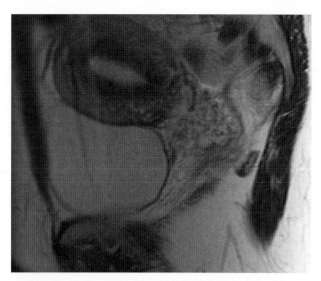

FIGURE 3-5. Cervical cancer on MRI. Stage IIB squamous cell carcinoma of the cervix on T2-weighted imaging. A 2.5 × 4.5 × 4.3 cm enhancing circumferential lobulated mass is noted to replace the cervix, with parametrial invasion noted on this T2-weighted MRI.

However, a recent prospective study conducted by the ACR Imaging Network and the Gynecologic Oncology Group demonstrated equivalence between MRI and CT in the preoperative staging of patients with early invasive cervical cancer. MRI was superior in the detection of parametrial invasion and visualization of the primary tumor. Furthermore, CT demonstrated greater interobserver variability compared with MRI.[21]

MRI is superior to clinical evaluation in determining the size of the primary tumor and has measurement capabilities comparable to those of surgical measurements. A retrospective study demonstrated size determination by MRI to be within 8 mm of histologic size in 95% of tumors larger than 10 mm. The accuracy of MRI in the detection of lymphadenopathy is reported to range from 76% to 100%, with a sensitivity ranging from 36% to 89.5%. This lower sensitivity is due to the inability of MRI to detect micrometastasis within normal-appearing lymph nodes. Nodes greater than 1.0 mm in the short-axis diameter are considered to be positive, as are findings of central necrosis, extracapsular extension, round shape, and soft tissue in the node with the same signal intensity as the tumor. A study using lymph node–specific contrast agent (ferumoxtran-10, an ultrasmall particles of iron oxide [USPIO]) increased the sensitivity of MRI in detecting lymph node involvement from 29% to 82% to 93% on a node-by-node basis and from 27% to 91% to 100% on a patient-by-patient basis without a loss in specificity. The accuracy of MRI in detecting parametrial involvement has been reported to range from 88% to 97%, with a sensitivity of 44% to 100% and a specificity of 80% to 97%. Finally, use of MRI as a staging modality has been found to be cost-effective because its use precludes the need for further imaging studies, diagnostic tests, or surgical procedures.[22]

Like CT, MRI plays an important role in the detection of disease recurrence. Recurrent tumor has an intermediate to high signal on T2-weighted images. MRI has several advantages over CT in the setting of post-treatment recurrence because of its ability to distinguish recurrence from post-treatment fibrosis due to surgery and radiation. One year after treatment, post-treatment fibrosis has a low-signal intensity on T1- and T2-weighted images, compared with the intermediate- to high-signal intensity of tumor on T2-weighed images. MRI has a reported sensitivity of 86% and specificity of 94% in detecting recurrent cervical cancer a year after treatment. Dynamic contrast-enhanced MRI is reported to have an accuracy of 85%, as compared with 64% to 68% in non–contrast-enhanced T2-weighted MRI. Functional imaging such as dynamic multiphase contrast-enhanced MRI and diffusion-weighted imaging have demonstrated an increased ability to distinguish recurrence from post-treatment changes even as early as in the first 6 months after treatment and may play an important role in detecting cervical cancer recurrence in the future.[23]

Positron Emission Tomography

There is no established role for FDG-PET in screening for primary cervical cancer. However, the role of FDG-PET in the staging and detection of recurrent disease has been well studied, and its use has become increasingly widespread, particularly after coverage for the initial staging of cervical cancer was approved by the Centers for Medicare and Medicaid Services. Lymph node involvement on imaging correlates with stage IVB disease, and one of the strengths of FDG-PET is its ability to detect lymphadenopathy. Prospective studies have demonstrated FDG-PET/CT to have a sensitivity of 75% to 100% and a specificity of 87% to 100% (Figures 3-6, 3-7, and 3-8). In early cervical cancer, FDG-PET/CT is reported to have a sensitivity of 72%, specificity of 99.7%, and a diagnostic accuracy of 99.3% (Figures 3-9 and 3-10). All undetected nodes were smaller than 0.5 cm in diameter; for nodes greater than 0.5 cm, the sensitivity of FDG-PET/CT was 100% and specificity was 99.6%. FDG-PET also improves initial staging because it is also able to detect distant extrapelvic disease, such as metastasis to the supraclavicular nodes. A meta-analysis of 15 studies on the use of FDG-PET in patients with cervical cancer reported a pooled sensitivity of 84% and specificity of 95% in the detection of aortic lymph node involvement and 79% to 99% in the detection of pelvic

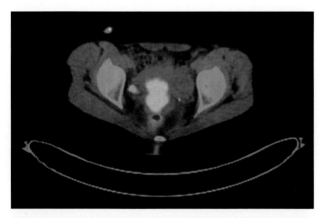

FIGURE 3-6. Cervical cancer on PET/CT. Stage IIIB squamous cell carcinoma of the cervix with marked hypermetabolic uptake of soft tissue lesion in the cervix.

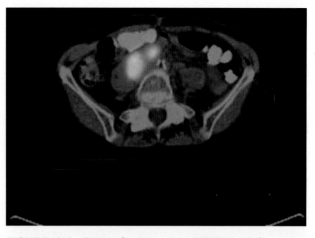

FIGURE 3-8. Cervical cancer on PET/CT. Right upper pelvic retroperitoneal mass noted with hypermetabolic uptake. Also noted is a hypermetabolic periaortic lymph node slightly caudal to the level of the renal veins, consistent with nodal metastasis.

lymph node involvement. This improvement in staging has been shown to significantly alter clinical and treatment decisions, including changing the therapeutic approach or initiating a treatment that was not previously planned.[24]

FDG-PET can also be used to monitor disease response to treatment and detect recurrent disease. A demonstration of a complete metabolic response post-treatment has been positively associated with survival in both prospective and retrospective studies. In a recent prospective study of patients treated with chemoradiation, the 3-year survival rate was 78% for patients who had a complete metabolic response on FDG-PET. The 3-year survival rate was 33% for a partial metabolic response and 0% for patient who had documented disease progression.[25] FDG-PET has a documented sensitivity of 80% for the detection of recurrent disease in asymptomatic women, as compared with a sensitivity of 100% in symptomatic women. A recent study evaluating the utility of FDG-PET in the detection of recurrence reported a sensitivity of 96%, specificity of 84%, and a diagnostic accuracy of 92%. Revised Response Evaluation Criteria In Solid

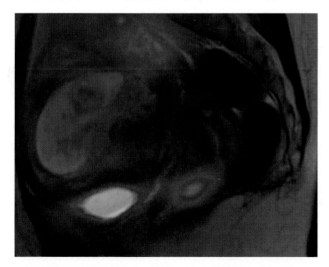

FIGURE 3-7. Cervical cancer on PET/CT. Exophytic, hypermetabolic mass arising from the anterior lip of the cervix and projecting into the upper vagina. The parametrium is normal without any obvious tumor involvement, and there are no pelvic side wall lymph nodes. The uterus is enlarged and contains a gestational sac with a single fetus. The patient was approximately 12 weeks pregnant at the time of this imaging.

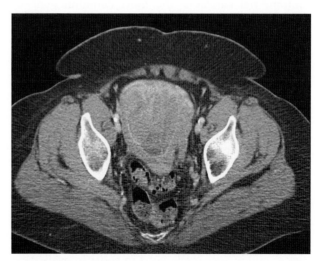

FIGURE 3-9. Uterine cancer on CT. Carcinosarcoma of the uterus demonstrating a heterogenous soft tissue mass filling the uterine cavity.

CHAPTER 3

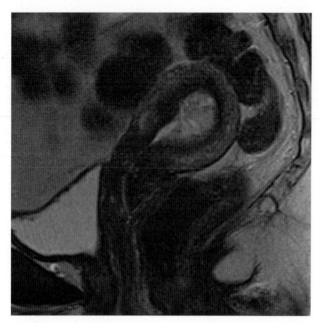

FIGURE 3-10. Uterine cancer on MRI. Stage IC endometrial adenocarcinoma of the uterus. Heterogenous thickened endometrium with partial enhancement on T2-weighted imaging.

Tumor (RECIST) that have been created, which include an interpretation of FDG-PET scans, demonstrating the widespread acceptance of FDG-PET in monitoring tumor response.[26] Further evaluation and larger prospective studies are still needed to fully elaborate the utility of FDG-PET in surveillance and recurrence detection.

Endometrial Cancer

Endometrial cancer is the most common gynecologic malignancy affecting women in the developed world. There are an estimated 43,470 new cases of cancer of the uterus and 7950 deaths expected in 2010. Most cancers of the uterus are detected at an early stage due to abnormal or postmenopausal bleeding, and when detected early, the overall survival rate is quite high. The symptoms of abnormal bleeding usually lead to a diagnosis by either endometrial biopsy or dilation and curettage (D&C). Often ultrasound is used in the initial assessment of patients with abnormal uterine bleeding as a means of evaluating the thickness of the endometrial lining, providing adjunctive information about the uterine anatomy. CT, MRI, and FDG-PET/CT have a very limited role in the screening of primary endometrial cancer and are generally used to assist in evaluating disease extent, monitoring treatment response, or in the detection of recurrent disease.

Ultrasound

Transvaginal ultrasound (TVUS) is the most common imaging modality ordered in the setting of peri- and postmenopausal bleeding. TVUS evaluation is invaluable in ruling out other possible causes of abnormal bleeding such as fibroids and polyps. TVUS also allows evaluation of the endometrial lining, which in a postmenopausal woman should be less than 5 mm in thickness. When a normal endometrial stripe is documented on TVUS, the risk of there being an underlying endometrial cancer ranges from 1% to 5.5%. A finding of an endometrial stripe with a thickness greater than 5 mm often leads to the performance of an endometrial biopsy (EMB) or D&C. However, in an asymptomatic patient, clinical judgment must be exercised, and thus clinical judgment must be exercised in evaluating such findings. Other studies have concluded that TVUS is much more sensitive in the detection of endometrial cancers and in triaging women into a subgroup of low-risk patients who do not require invasive follow-up studies such as EMB or D&C. However, the aggressive histologies of endometrial cancer (serous and clear cell) arise from atrophic endometrium and may have normal endometrial thickness necessitating histologic evaluation.

Saline infusion sonohysterography (SHG) appears to improve the diagnostic accuracy of TVUS in detecting endometrial cancer. The sensitivity of SHG is 89%, the specificity 46%, the PPV is 16%, and the NPV is 97%. However, there is a potential concern for seeding the peritoneal cavity with malignant cells, which in some cases has been reported in up to 7% of cases. The role of SHG in the evaluation of patients with abnormal uterine bleeding continues to evolve, but it is currently recommended as an adjunctive study when TVUS demonstrates a thickened endometrial lining but an EMB has a negative result for malignancy. Doppler ultrasound of uterine malignancies can demonstrate increased vascularity with vessels originating from multiple sources, in contrast to benign conditions such as polyps, which obtain their blood supply from a single artery. The vascular findings, which can also include an increase in the resistance index, are not considered to be particularly accurate in distinguishing benign from malignant endometrial conditions. Currently, Doppler ultrasound findings do not play any significant role in the primary screening for cancer of the uterus.

After the initial diagnosis of endometrial cancer has been made through a pathologic tissue diagnosis, the role of ultrasound in the further evaluation of endometrial cancer is limited. TVUS is significantly less accurate than MRI in detecting myometrial invasion, with an overall diagnostic accuracy of 60% to 76%. SHG may be slightly more accurate than TVUS in detecting myometrial invasion and cervical involvement by endometrial cancer. However, neither modality has found widespread acceptance or use in the staging or detection of recurrent endometrial cancer.

Computed Tomography

CT has no established role in the primary screening of endometrial cancer, although disease may be found incidentally on CT scans obtained for other indications. Detection of uterine cancer on noncontrast CT is difficult due to endometrial cancer's similar attenuation to the myometrium on imaging, rendering evaluation of the malignancy rather difficult. The administration of intravenous (IV) contrast improves the ability of CT to detect endometrial cancer because the tumor will demonstrate a low attenuation signal compared with the surrounding myometrium. Uterine cancer can appear as a hypodense mass with a smooth interface identified between the mass and the myometrium (Figure 3-9). Several studies have found that helical CT has improved sensitivity and specificity in the detection of myometrial and cervical invasion compared with conventional CT, although use of helical CT for this indication is not currently widespread.

Although the staging of endometrial cancer is surgical, CT can play an important role in the evaluation of the extent of disease. Criteria for the staging of endometrial cancer by CT have been proposed and are similar to FIGO classifications. CT is often used to detect myometrial invasion, pelvic sidewall or parametrial involvement, and lymphadenopathy. CT has a reported accuracy of 86% in the detection of extrauterine spread. Lymph nodes greater than 1 cm in the short axis or rounded nodes with a short-axis to long-axis ratio of >0.8 are considered to have tumor involvement. CT is also extremely accurate in the detection of malignant ascites, peritoneal implants, liver parenchyma involvement, and lung metastasis.

Endometrial cancer tends to recur most commonly at the vaginal cuff in women treated with surgery alone. Serial imaging is generally unnecessary in such patients, because they are subsequently treated with radiation therapy after the detection of disease recurrence. For patients previously treated with radiation, however, recurrence happens more commonly along the pelvic side wall or distantly. CT can play an important role in the early detection of distant recurrence, and because CT is commonly found in most medical centers, and is relatively inexpensive compared with MRI or FDG-PET/CT, it is the primary imaging modality used in the evaluation of recurrent endometrial cancer.

MRI

MRI does not have an accepted role in the initial evaluation of patients with abnormal uterine bleeding.

Because of its lower cost, ultrasound is the initial imaging modality of choice. However, MRI is considered to be the most accurate imaging modality in the staging of endometrial cancer due to its excellent resolution of the soft tissues of the pelvis (Figure 3-10). Although surgical staging is the gold standard in endometrial cancer, MRI can be used to evaluate the extent of disease in patients who are poor surgical candidates, in cases of type 2 endometrial cancer in which there is a high probability of nodal involvement, and in cases of suspected cervical involvement. Compared with TVUS or CT, it appears that MRI is currently the best imaging modality for the evaluation of cervical or parametrial extension of disease that warrants the performance of a radical hysterectomy. Several studies have demonstrated that contrast MRI has an overall staging accuracy higher than that of CT and TVUS. MRI has an 87% sensitivity and 91% specificity in evaluating myometrial invasion, an 80% sensitivity and 96% specificity in determining cervical involvement, and a 50% sensitivity and 95% specificity in determining lymph node involvement by endometrial cancer.

Like CT, MRI can also be used in the evaluation of recurrent endometrial cancer. After surgery alone, without adjuvant radiation therapy, vaginal recurrence is the most frequent site of disease recurrence. Vaginal recurrence appears as a high-signal-intensity mass on T2-weighted images. MRI can accurately determine vaginal tumor size and extravaginal disease extent, which correlates with a poor prognosis.[27]

FDG-PET/CT

The role of FDG-PET/CT in endometrial cancer screening, evaluation of disease extent or monitoring for recurrence, has not been established. Case reports of PET scans obtained in the evaluation of other cancers have incidentally detected uptake in uterus, which has led to the diagnosis of endometrial cancer. However, endometrial FDG uptake can be physiologic and is increased in the proliferative phase of the menstrual cycle. Despite the possibility of physiologic uptake, incidental abnormal uterine uptake warrants histologic evaluation. In evaluating disease extent, FDG-PET was compared with MRI in evaluating the depth of myometrial invasion in 22 patients with stage I disease, but neither was clearly superior. A recent study demonstrated that FDG-PET/CT had a similar sensitivity, specificity, and accuracy to MRI in the detection of primary disease, nodal involvement, and distant metastasis (Figure 3-11). Preoperative evaluation with FDG-PET/CT compared with MRI in patients who were subsequently surgically staged demonstrated a sensitivity of 90% for PET/CT compared with 92% for MRI; a specificity of 51% compared with 33%,

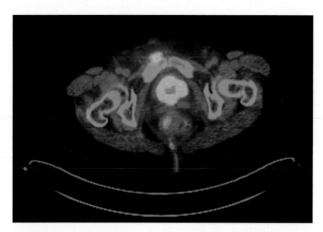

FIGURE 3-11. Uterine cancer on PET/CT. Stage IIIC endometrial adenocarcinoma with a soft tissue density noted in the distal portion of the right rectus muscle, consistent with metastatic disease.

respectively; and an accuracy of 85% for both imaging modalities. PET/CT had a nonsignificant trend in the increased detection of nodal metastasis over MRI and had 100% sensitivity and 93% specificity in detecting metastatic disease. The authors concluded that the primary benefit of PET/CT is in the detection of metastatic disease, although this imaging modality may play a future role in evaluating lymph node involvement in patients who are poor surgical candidates.[28]

There currently is no accepted role for FDG-PET in the preoperative evaluation of endometrial cancer. Its utility in the detection of recurrent disease is also an area of current investigation. A recent study by Chung[29] retrospectively evaluated 31 patients who had FDG-PET/CT performed for evaluation of recurrent endometrial cancer. They described the sensitivity of imaging to be 100%, with a specificity of 95% and an accuracy of 93%. These findings appeared to be similar in the detection of recurrent uterine sarcomas as well. A study demonstrated a sensitivity of 93%, specificity of 100%, and an accuracy of 95% for surveillance PET in evaluating symptomatic patients with a diagnosis of sarcoma, and a sensitivity of 88%, a specificity of 96%, and an accuracy of 93% in asymptomatic patients with a history of sarcoma. Evaluation with PET led to changes in clinical decision making in 33% of the patients in the study.[30]

Gestational Trophoblastic Disease

Ultrasound

Gestational trophoblastic disease (GTD) comprises a spectrum of rare placental abnormalities that includes hydatidiform mole, invasive mole, choriocarcinoma, placental site trophoblastic tumor, and epithelioid

trophoblastic tumor. The primary lesion, either a complete or incomplete mole, is usually detected by ultrasound, and ultrasound remains the imaging modality of choice for detection of primary lesions. Ultrasound also plays an important role in the subsequent monitoring of patients for persistent or recurrent disease. Molar pregnancies can be subdivided into complete and incomplete moles based on their genetic composition. Complete moles have a classical vesicular appearance on ultrasound described as a "snowstorm" appearance due to swelling of the chorionic villi. Fetal parts are largely absent. Detection of complete moles by ultrasound is best accomplished in the late first trimester or early second trimester, when the detection rate can be as high as 80%. However, improvements in TVUS have led to enhanced detection of molar pregnancies in the early first trimester as well.

Detection of partial moles by ultrasound is more difficult than detection of complete moles due to their less classic appearance on imaging. A recent retrospective study suggested that although the sensitivity and PPV of ultrasound in detecting complete moles was 95% and 40%, respectively, it was only 20% and 22%, respectively, for partial moles.[31] Occasionally a fetus with multiple congenital anomalies may be present, along with a placenta that may be enlarged and contain hydropic foci, but often the scan by itself is nondiagnostic.

The presence of bilateral theca-lutein cysts is another classic ultrasound finding in GTD that is detected on ultrasound. However, because of improved ultrasound technology and the earlier diagnosis of GTN, enlarged theca-lutein cysts are becoming rare. Ultrasound is used to follow patients who are suspected of having persistent GTD, as well as in the evaluation of choriocarcinoma or placental site trophoblastic tumor, and to look for retained trophoblastic tissue or local spread to the pelvis.

Computed Tomography

CT does not have a role in the primary evaluation of patients with suspected GTN (Figure 3-12). Its major use is in the detection of metastatic disease. Metastasis to the lungs is the most common site of spread in GTN due to embolization of trophoblastic tissue, and chest imaging is a standard component of a metastatic work-up. Chest imaging, either by chest x-ray or by CT, is required to rule out metastasis to the lungs. Although chest CT is more sensitive than chest x-ray in the detection of pulmonary metastasis, it is not predictive of outcomes. FIGO currently still recommends obtaining a chest x-ray, rather than a chest CT, in the evaluation of metastatic disease.[32] GTN can also metastasize to the liver, and metastases to the liver are often multiple, hypointense, and hemorrhagic. Metastasis to the brain may present as single or

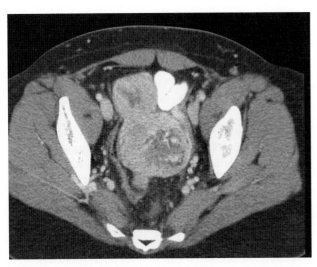

FIGURE 3-12. Gestational trophoblastic disease on CT. Enhancing heterogenous material noted in an enlarged uterus found to be a molar pregnancy on D&C. The imaging also demonstrates an exophytic lesion, consistent with a fibroid uterus.

multiple lesions, which are often hemorrhagic, and appear hyperintense on noncontrast CT scans. It is our practice to obtain CT scans of the head in patients with pulmonary metastasis.

Magnetic Resonance Imaging

MRI does not have a role in the evaluation and management of suspected GTN, and often MRI findings in primary disease can be nonspecific, making it difficult to distinguish GTN from an incomplete miscarriage. On MRI, GTN obliterates the normal uterine zonal anatomy, and tumors have a highly vascular appearance on T1- and T2-weighted images. Engorgement of the internal iliac vessels and increased tumor enhancement is noted with the use of gadolinium contrast. MRI can also detect extrapelvic extension, including spread of disease to the adnexa, parametria, and the vagina. It is the preferred imaging modality for the evaluation of metastatic disease to the vagina. Finally, patients treated with chemotherapy will have a noted decrease in uterine volume and tumor vascularity that is detectable with MRI. With treatment, normal uterine zonal anatomy will reappear on T2-weighted images, and intra-lesional hemorrhage may develop. By 6 to 9 months after treatment, the uterus should appear normal on both T1- and T2-weighted images, although persistent adnexal cysts may be evident.

Positron Emission Tomography

The data on the role of PET in the setting of GTN is limited to case reports and a few case series. FDG-PET may be useful in the diagnosis of metastatic disease, particularly when conventional imaging modalities fail to identify an occult malignancy. FDG-PET/CT was reported in one study to be more beneficial in 7 of 16 patients (43.8%) compared with CT alone in terms of detecting chemotherapy-resistant lesions, excluding false-positive lesions found on CT, and confirming complete responses to chemotherapy.[32] However, 2 scans were falsely negative, 1 scan was indeterminate, and 6 scans were of no benefit. Larger studies are required before FDG-PET can play a meaningful clinical role in the management of GTN.

Ovarian Cancer

Although ovarian cancer is the second most common gynecologic malignancy in the United States, it has the highest mortality rate of all gynecologic cancers. This is due to the fact that most ovarian cancers present at an advanced stage, usually stage III or stage IV. Early detection of ovarian cancer has continued to elude clinicians due to the current absence of any reliable screening modalities. The role of imaging in ovarian cancer is largely one of detection, staging, preoperative planning, and post-treatment surveillance.

Ultrasound

TVUS is the imaging modality of choice in the initial evaluation of a pelvic mass. Transabdominal ultrasound can play a limited role, especially in the evaluation of large masses that are displaced outside the pelvis, as well as in the documentation of ascites and hydronephrosis. Classic morphologic findings in pelvic masses that are concerning for malignancy include thick septations (>3 mm), internal papillations, loculations, solid masses, cystic lesions with solid components, and smaller cysts incorporated into the structure of larger cysts. These morphologic descriptors have a high sensitivity for malignancy, but a low specificity because some of these findings are also found in benign lesions and borderline tumors as well as invasive malignancy. Multiple studies have shown that when strict morphologic criteria are used in the evaluation of an adnexal mass, the PPV of ultrasound is 95% and the NPV is 99% in excluding malignancy.

The addition of color Doppler to the traditional ultrasound morphologic assessment may increase the diagnostic capability of ultrasound in evaluating an adnexal mass, but the benefit of the addition of duplex scanning remains controversial. The neovascularization associated with ovarian malignancy has led to the evaluation of the blood flow and vascular structures that support an adnexal mass. Several studies have demonstrated that malignancies often have an increase in vessel density and tortuosity, as well as low-resistance waveforms due to the absence of

CHAPTER 3

smooth muscle in the newly formed vascular support structures. It was initially thought that documentation of arteriovenous shunting and finding a resistance index cutoff of 0.4 and a pulsatility index of 1 were highly sensitive and specific for malignancy. However, such waveform findings have been frequently noted in benign conditions as well, especially in premenopausal women. However, a finding of low-resistance blood flow in a postmenopausal woman must always be viewed with suspicion. A combination of morphologic assessment with Doppler ultrasound may lead to an increase in the ability to discriminate between benign and malignant lesions. The addition of color Doppler to conventional ultrasound appeared to improve the specificity from 82% to 92% and the PPV from 63% to 97%. Doppler evaluation can provide adjunctive information to help classify a lesion as malignant rather than benign.

Because of the low prevalence of ovarian cancer in the general population, large-scale screening programs have proven to be unsuccessful and not cost-effective. The focus of most screening programs have been on women at high risk for developing ovarian cancer, especially those with a family history or genetic predisposition (*BRCA1* and *BRCA2*, *HNPCC*). Besides the low prevalence, another difficulty in creating an effective screening program is that ovarian cancer may have rapid growth and early spread outside of the ovary, making detection of early disease extremely difficult. A recent prospective study enrolled 25,327 women to receive an annual screening TVUS. The women enrolled were either asymptomatic women older than 50 years or women older than 25 years with a family history of ovarian cancer. The PPV for ultrasound was 27% and the sensitivity was 85%, and for those women detected by screening, the 5-year-overall survival was 77% compared with 49% for historical controls from the same institution.[33] Several issues exist with this study, including its lack of randomization, lack of a control group, and inclusion of many high-risk women, which argues that the PPV would presumably be lower in a group of average-risk women. Additionally, the percentage of expected *BRCA*-mutated patients is likely increased among high-risk women, and the improved survival of *BRCA*-mutated ovarian cancer patients is well known.

Screening protocols have been developed that attempt to combine a number of modalities, including ultrasound, serologic markers (CA-125), and physical examination. Two recent large trials have been conducted evaluating the impact of ovarian cancer screening on survival. The PLCO Cancer Screening Trial enrolled 34,261 healthy women with an age range of 55 to 74 years and randomly assigned them to have an annual CA-125 plus TVUS or "usual care." During the 4 years of screening, the PPV of a positive screening test was 1% to 1.3% for an abnormal TVUS, 3.7% for an abnormal CA-125, and 23.5% if both CA-125 and TVUS were abnormal.[34] The United Kingdom Collaborative Trial of Ovarian Cancer Screening enrolled 202,638 postmenopausal women with an age range of 50 to 74 years at an average risk for ovarian cancer.[35] These women were randomly assigned to a control group that received a pelvic examination only, an annual TVUS, or an annual CA-125 plus TVUS if an abnormal CA-125 was detected. The multimodality group had a significantly greater specificity (99.8%) and PPV (35.1%) compared with ultrasound alone (specificity of 98.2% and PPV of 2.8%). The sensitivity did not differ between the 2 groups. The effect of screening on mortality has not yet been reported.

In the United States, ultrasound is not typically used in the evaluation of disease extent of ovarian cancer. Transabdominal ultrasound is useful in the detection of ascites and in performing ultrasound-guided paracentesis. Ultrasound also has a limited role in the detection of recurrent ascites. Ultrasound may be used in suspected recurrent disease, assisting interventional radiologists in performing imaging-guided biopsies to obtain a tissue for cytologic diagnosis.

Computed Tomography

CT does not have a role in the primary screening of ovarian cancer, although incidental detection of adnexal malignancies is not an infrequent event. Ultrasound is considered to be the initial study of choice in the evaluation of adnexal masses, but CT can provide additional information when the initial ultrasound evaluation is indeterminate. One study demonstrated that in the case of an indeterminate ultrasound, CT had a sensitivity of 81% and a specificity of 87% in predicting a diagnosis of ovarian cancer. Advanced stage ovarian cancer on contrast-enhanced CT demonstrates cystic lesions that may have irregular borders, thickened walls, papillary projections, calcifications, and septations (Figure 3-13). Peritoneal implants, carcinomatosis, ascites, and pelvic organ and sidewall involvement can also be described on CT. The clinician must always have a high suspicion for metastatic tumor involvement from the gastrointestinal tract or the breast when evaluating CT scans demonstrating carcinomatosis, as these tumors may have a similar radiographic appearance.

Ovarian cancer is surgically staged, but CT can also assist in the process. CT can provide evidence of metastatic spread, involvement of abdominal and pelvic organs, and lymphadenopathy and permit some determination of the likelihood of performing optimal surgical cytoreduction. Numerous studies have suggested

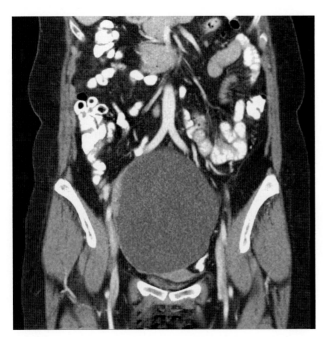

FIGURE 3-13. Ovarian cancer on CT. 13.9 × 9.3 × 10.9 cm fluid-filled mass found to be consistent with a high-grade ovarian cancer.

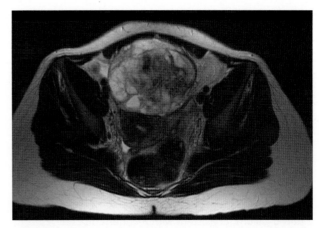

FIGURE 3-14. Ovarian cancer on MRI. Enlarged, complex, septated, adnexal mass on T2-weighted imaging.

that CT findings can predict suboptimal cytoreduction (Table 3-1). However the predictive value of CT varies by institution due to variations in surgical practice and aggressiveness.[36]

Lesions located in the mesentery, porta hepatis, liver, pelvic sidewall, and lymphadenopathy superior to the celiac axis may not be optimally resectable. Patients who have disease that may not be amenable to optimal debulking are often treated with neoadjuvant chemotherapy.

Although CT scans are routinely used in clinical trials in post-treatment surveillance, the optimal tumor marker and imaging algorithm is not established. According to the 2009 National Comprehensive Cancer Network guidelines, CT scans can be used as a surveillance tool whenever clinical indications such as patient symptoms or a rising CA-125 level warrant. CT has an estimated sensitivity of 59% to 83% and a specificity of 83% to 88% in detecting residual tumor and recurrence. Recurrence often presents as a pelvic mass, malignant ascites, peritoneal implants, carcinomatosis, and lymphadenopathy. It is important to note that CT has difficulty with visualization of lesions smaller than 1cm in size, and CT sensitivity decreases to 25% to 50% in such cases. Thus the clinician should consider the possibility of a false-negative CT scan in cases of symptomatic patients or in those patients with rising CA-125 levels. FDG-PET/CT may aid in evaluating such situations.[37]

Magnetic Resonance Imaging

MRI does not have a role in the primary screening of ovarian cancer. However, contrast-enhanced MRI does appear to have potential utility in the evaluation of adnexal masses that produced an indeterminate ultrasound study (Figure 3-14). In a meta-analysis examining patients with an indeterminate TVUS study, MRI with gadolinium contrast had the greatest accuracy of diagnosing ovarian cancer as compared with CT, Doppler ultrasound, or MRI without gadolinium contrast. The sensitivity of contrast-enhanced MRI was 81%, and the specificity was 98%. A prospective study of contrast-enhanced MRI used as a second imaging modality after an indeterminate ultrasound study of a pelvic mass demonstrated a sensitivity of 100% and specificity of 94%.

Surgical staging is considered the gold standard for management of early-stage ovarian cancer. Like CT, MRI can be used for pretreatment planning and assistance with determining whether optimal debulking is feasible. MRI can also be used in suboptimally debulked patients to evaluate multisite disease or areas of unresectable tumor. The accuracy of MRI in staging ovarian cancer, which is approximately 70% to 90%, is comparable to that of CT.

The use of MRI for post-treatment surveillance is not considered routine in most medical centers. MRI offers certain advantages over CT; it is safe to use in patients with iodine allergies, and MRI is better able to visualize disease recurrence in the vaginal vault, cul-de-sac, and the bladder base.

Positron Emission Tomography

FDG-PET currently does not have an accepted role in the primary evaluation of pelvic masses due to its expense. However, the ability of FDG-PET to detect

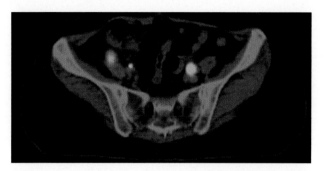

FIGURE 3-15. Ovarian cancer on PET/CT. Stage IIIC papillary serous ovarian cancer after multiple courses of chemotherapy. Patient noted to have hypermetabolic uptake in 2 pelvic lesions, consistent with recurrent disease.

early metabolic changes in tumors before the development of structural changes offers a promise for earlier detection of malignancy. A prospective study evaluated 101 patients with adnexal masses and a Risk of Malignancy Index >150 based on CA-125, ultrasound, and menopausal status who were referred for evaluation by FDG-PET/CT. The authors found that the sensitivity of FDG-PET/CT in the diagnosis of ovarian cancer was 100% and the specificity was 93%. They concluded that PET/CT should be considered an imaging modality of choice after a finding of a pelvic mass by ultrasound.[38]

Again, due to its cost, there is currently no established role for FDG-PET/CT in the initial evaluation of disease extent in ovarian cancer. However, a recent study demonstrated that the addition of FDG-PET to CT appears to increase the staging accuracy of CT from 89.7% to 94%, the sensitivity from 37.6% to 69.4%, and the specificity from 97.1% to 97.5% (Figures 3-15 and 3-16). Despite the more common use of CT scans in detecting recurrent disease, it appears that FDG-PET/CT may be the most accurate imaging technique. A study by Nam et al[39] found that

preoperative PET/CT was superior to pelvic ultrasound, CT, and pelvic MRI in the diagnosis of ovarian cancer and in the detection of metastatic disease. A meta-analysis comparing FDG-PET/CT with CT and MRI in the detection of recurrent disease found that FDG-PET/CT was more accurate than CT or MRI. The sensitivity of FDG-PET/CT was 91% and the specificity was 88%, whereas the sensitivity and specificity of CT was 79% and 84% and for MRI was 75% and 78%, respectively.[40] Although there appears to be evidence that FDG-PET/CT may be comparable, if not superior, to CT and MRI in the detection of recurrent ovarian cancer, its routine use is not currently standard of care.

Vulvar Cancer

Due to their rarity in Western populations, large prospective studies investigating the utility of various imaging modalities in vulvar and vaginal cancer are nonexistent. Vulvar cancer, with an incidence of 5% of gynecologic cancers, was by convention clinically staged until FIGO adopted a surgical staging system in 1988. Because of the emphasis placed by the FIGO system on the surgical-pathologic approach to staging vulvar cancer, imaging modalities have traditionally had a minimal role in the detection and evaluation of primary malignancies. Barium enemas, intravenous pyelograms, and, later, CT have been the traditional tools used to assist in management of especially large vulvar tumors that may have extended into adjacent organs, in cases of suspected metastatic disease, and in select cases of recurrent disease.

Ultrasound

The role of ultrasound in the detection and management of vulvar cancer has been extremely limited to date. A recent study demonstrated that ultrasound combined with fine-needle aspiration (FNA) was superior to CT in the detection of groin node metastasis. Ultrasound combined with FNA had a sensitivity of 80%, specificity of 100%, PPV of 93%, and NPV of 100%.

Magnetic Resonance Imaging

MRI has been shown to have some value in differentiating vulvar cancer recurrence from postradiation changes. In the setting of primary and recurrent vulvar cancer, MRI accurately determined the size of the vulvar lesion in 83% of patients.[41] Accuracy in staging of primary vulvar cancers was only 69.4%, and detection of groin lymph node metastasis was between 85% and 87%. The authors concluded that MRI might have a useful role as an adjunct in determining the size of a vulvar lesion and in detecting the presence of lymph node metastasis.

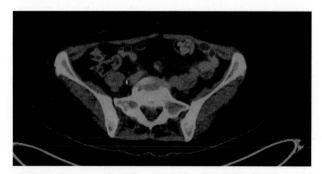

FIGURE 3-16. Ovarian cancer on PET/CT. Stage IIIC papillary serous ovarian cancer. Hypermetabolic nodule measuring 1.1×0.9 cm noted in the mesentery, consistent with metastatic disease.

Positron Emission Tomography

The role of FDG-PET in vulvar cancer has yet to be fully elucidated, but several small, early studies have indicated some promise. On a per-patient basis FDG-PET had a sensitivity of 80%, specificity of 90%, PPV of 80%, and a NPV of 90% for detecting groin node metastases. On a groin-to-groin basis, the sensitivity was 67%, specificity 95%, PPV 86%, and NPV 86%. FDG-PET was more accurate in the detection of extranodal disease than disease found only in the nodes. The authors concluded that PET was relatively insensitive in the detection of vulvar cancer metastatic to the inguinal lymph nodes and was not an adequate substitute for traditional lymph node dissection. However, FDG-PET may have an as yet undefined role in aiding radiation planning or as an adjunct to sentinel lymph node dissection. More research into the application and utility of FDT-PET in vulvar cancer is indicated based on the initial promise of this study.

Vaginal Cancer

Magnetic Resonance Imaging

Vaginal cancer has an incidence of 3% of gynecologic malignancies and is clinically staged. Both CT and MRI can be used for the detection of pelvic adenopathy and metastatic disease. Additionally, MRI provides information regarding tumor size and invasion of adjacent organs. This is important for radiation treatment planning and evaluating response to therapy. There appears to be no role for ultrasound in the setting of vaginal cancer.

Positron Emission Tomography

There are few studies examining the use of FDG-PET in the diagnosis and management of vaginal cancer. FDG-PET detected 100% of the primary vaginal lesions as compared with 43% detected by CT. FDG-PET detected metastasis to the groin and pelvic lymph nodes in 35% of patients as compared with 17% detected by CT. Although FDG-PET was superior to CT in the detection of vaginal lesions and metastasis, this was not correlated with a survival advantage. Further research into the utility of FDG-PET in the setting of vaginal cancer is warranted.

FUTURE DIRECTIONS

Gynecologic malignancies are clinically or surgically staged by established (periodically revised) systems. Although diagnostic imaging can play a role in the pretreatment determination of the extent of disease, "staging" by imaging is not considered to be standard of care. Ultrasound, as the least expensive imaging modality in gynecology, continues to play an important role in the detection and diagnosis of primary diseases, in particular endometrial and ovarian cancers, as well as in the management and surveillance of gestational trophoblastic diseases. CT continues to play the predominant role in the evaluation of most gynecologic malignancies, including determining the extent of metastatic disease and detection of recurrent disease. Newer imaging techniques, such as helical CT, have improved both the speed and imaging resolution of the traditional CT scanner. Concern has been raised in recent years about the level of radiation exposure to patients, particularly cancer patients who are subjected to repetitive CT scans as part of their post-treatment surveillance.

Due to the lack of ionizing radiation, its superior soft tissue resolution, and its multiplanar imaging capabilities, the use of MRI in the evaluation and management of pelvic malignancies continues to increase. Cost, slower scanning times, and patient anxiety during scans were some of the initial barriers to the more widespread use of MRI and are starting to be overcome. In particular, MRI appears to be superior in staging endometrial and cervical cancers as compared with CT and TVUS. Although CT and MRI both provide important information about nodal and distant metastasis, MRI provides more information about local disease extent, whereas CT provides more information about distant spread of disease. The addition of PET to CT provides information about biologic activity with the ability to provide anatomic localization, providing an additional component of information beyond simple anatomic dimensions. Further investigation with larger prospective trials in all pelvic malignancies is required to fully elaborate the role of FDG-PET, but the initial findings in a number of clinical settings—primary detection, staging, surveillance, and recurrence—have been extremely promising. Despite improvements in diagnostic imaging, serum tumor markers remain a safe and cost-effective way to monitor disease status and aid in determining when further diagnostic modalities may be indicated.

As we move into a more structured practice environment, issues of cost and cost-effectiveness will become ever more important considerations for the clinician. One of the ways in which cost-effectiveness will factor into the practice of gynecologic oncology will be in selecting the most accurate diagnostic modalities for evaluating and following patients. Although CT is the most commonly used imaging modality for diagnosing and following patients with gynecologic cancers, it has a number of limitations, including its reliance on ionizing radiation and reduced sensitivity and specificity in the detection of lymph node metastasis and early recurrent disease. MRI and PET-CT can compensate for some of the deficiencies inherent in CT technology, but their current expense and lack of coverage by most insurance companies limit their routine use except in select circumstances. Further prospective studies will be needed to determine how best to leverage these imaging modalities in the interest of improved patient care. In particular, MRI and PET-CT herald the advent of functional imaging and the promise of earlier detection of primary disease as well as recurrence. Such early detection may lead to a significant impact on disease incidence and mortality if earlier detection can be coupled with more effective treatment. Additional comparative studies will be necessary to determine the most accurate and cost-effective diagnostic algorithm if such potential benefits are to be realized.

REFERENCES

1. Smith-Bindman R, Lipson J, Marcus R, et al. Radiation dose associated with common computed tomography examinations and the associated lifetime attributable risk of cancer. *Arch intern Med.* 2009;169(22):2078-2086.

2. Kanal E, Barkovich AJ, Bell C, et al. ACR guidance document for safe MR practices: 2007. *AJR Am J Roentgenol.* 2007; 188(6):1447-1474.

3. Juweid ME, Cheson BD. Positron-emission tomography and assessment of cancer therapy. *N Engl J Med.* 2006;354(5):496-507.

4. Hewitt MJ, Anderson K, Hall GD, et al. Women with peritoneal carcinomatosis of unknown origin: efficacy of image-guided biopsy to determine site-specific diagnosis. *BJOG.* 2007;114:46-50.

5. Ledwaba T, Dlamini Z, Naicker S, et al. Molecular genetics of human cervical cancer: role of papillomavirus and the apoptotic cascade. *Biol Chem.* 2004;385(8):671-682.

6. van der Avoort IA, Shirango H, Hoevanaars BM, et al. Vulvar squamous cell carcinoma is a multifactorial disease following two separate and independent pathways. *Int J Gynecol Pathol.* 2006;25(1):22-29.

7. Liegl B, Leibel S, Gogg-Kamerer M, et al. Mammary and extra-mammary Paget's disease: an immunohistochemical study of 83 cases. *Histopathology.* 2007;50(4):439-447.

8. Mutter GL, Lin M-C, Fitzgerald JT, et al. Altered *PTEN* expression as a diagnostic marker for the earliest endometrial precancers. *J Natl Cancer Inst.* 2000;92(11):924-930.

9. Singer G, Stohr R, Cope L, et al. Patterns of *p53* mutations separate ovarian serous borderline tumors and low- and high-grade carcinomas and provide support for a new model of ovarian carcinogenesis: a mutational analysis with immunohistochemical correlation. *Am J Surg Pathol.* 2005;29(2):218-224.

10. Hirakawa M, Nagai Y, Inamine M, et al. Predictive factor of distant recurrence in locally advanced squamous cell carcinoma of the cervix treated with concurrent chemoradiotherapy. *Gynecol Oncol.* 2008;108(1):126-129.

11. Kotowicz B, Kaminska J, Fukseiwicz M, et al. Clinical significance of serum CA-125 and soluble tumor necrosis factor receptor type I in cervical adenocarcinoma patients. *Int J Gynecol Cancer.* 2010;20(4):588-592.

12. Dube V, Grigull J, DeSouza LV, et al. Verification of endometrial tissue biomarkers previously discovered using mass spectrometry-based proteomics by means of immunohistochemistry in a tissue microarray format. *J Proteome Res.* 2007;6(7):2648-2655.

13. Riedinger JM, Eche N, Basuyau JP, et al. Prognostic value of serum CA 125 bi-exponential decrease during first line paclitaxel/platinum chemotherapy: a French multicentre study. *Gynecol Oncol.* 2008;109(2):194-198.

14. Rustin GJ, van der Burg ME. A randomized trial in ovarian cancer (OC) of early treatment of relapse based on CA-125 levels alone versus delayed treatment based on conventional clinical indications: MRC OV05/EORTC 55955 trials. *Lancet* 2010;276(9747):1155-1163.

15. Rustin GJ, van der Burg ME, Griffin CL. Early versus delayed treatment of relapsed ovarian cancer (MRC OV05/EORTC 55955): a randomised trial. *Lancet.* 2010;376:1155-1163.

16. Allard WJ, Somers E, Theil R, Moore RG. Use of a novel biomarker HE4 for monitoring patients with epithelial ovarian cancer. *J Clin Oncol.* 2009;26(suppl). Abstract 5533.

17. Partridge E, Kreimer AR, Greenlee RT, et al. Results from four rounds of ovarian cancer screening in a randomized trial. *Obstet Gynecol.* 2009;113(4):775-782.

18. Menon U, Skates SJ, Lewis S, et al. Prospective study using the risk of ovarian cancer algorithm to screen for ovarian cancer. *J Clin Oncol.* 2005;23:7919-7926.

19. Mom CH, Engelen MJ, Willemse PH, et al. Granulosa cell tumors of the ovary: the clinical value of serum inhibin A and B levels in a large single center cohort. *Gynecol Oncol.* 2007;105(2):365-372.

20. Hancke K, Heilmann V, Straka P, et al. Pretreatment staging of cervical cancer: is imaging better than palpation? Role of CT and MRI in preoperative staging of cervical cancer: single institution results for 255 patients. *Ann Surg Oncol.* 2008;15(10):2856-2861.

21. Hricak H, Gatsonis C, Coakley FV, et al. Early invasive cervical cancer: CT and MR imaging in preoperative evaluation-ACRIN/GOG comparative study of diagnostic performance and interobserver variability. *Radiology.* 2007;245(2):491-498.

22. Rockall AG, Ghosh S, Alexander-Sefre F, et al. Can MRI rule out bladder and rectal invasion in cervical cancer to help select patients for limited EUA? *Gynecol Oncol.* 2006;101(2):244-249.

23. Padhani AR, Liu G, Koh DM, et al. Diffusion weighted magnetic resonance imaging as a cancer biomarker: consensus and recommendations. *Neoplasia.* 2009;11(2):102-125.

24. Chao A, Ho KC, Wang CC, et al. Positron emission tomography in evaluating the feasibility of curative intent in cervical cancer patients with limited distant lymph node metastases. *Gynecol Oncol.* 2008;110(2):172-178.

25. Schwarz JK, Siegel BA, Dehdashti F, Grigsby PW. Association of posttherapy positron emission tomography with tumor response and survival in cervical carcinoma. *JAMA.* 2007;298:2289-2295.

26. Eisenhauer EA, Therasse P, Bogaerts J, et al. New response evaluation criteria in solid tumours: revised RECIST guideline (version 1.1). *Eur J Cancer.* 2009;45:228-247.

27. Sohaib SA, Houghton SL, Meroni R, et al. Recurrent endometrial cancer: patterns of recurrent disease and assessment of prognosis. *Clin Radiol.* 2007;62:28-34.

28. Park JY, Kim EN, Kim DY, et al. Comparison of the validity of magnetic resonance imaging and positron emission tomography/computed tomography in the preoperative evaluation of patients with uterine corpus cancer. *Gynecol Oncol.* 2008;108:486-492.

29. Chung HH, Kang WJ, Kim JW, et al. The clinical impact of ((18)F)FDG PET/CT for the management of recurrent endometrial cancer: correlation with clinical and histological findings. *Eur J Nucl Med Mol Imaging.* 2008;35:1018-1088.

30. Par JY, Kim NE, Kim DY, et al. Role of PET or PET/CT in the post-therapy surveillance of uterine sarcoma. *Gynecol Oncol.* 2008;109:255-262.

31. Kirk E, Papageorghiou AT, Condous G, et al. The accuracy of first trimester ultrasound in the diagnosis of hydatidiform mole. *Ultrasound Obstet Gynecol.* 2007;29:70-75.

32. Allen SD, Lim AK, Seckl MJ, Blunt DM, Mitchell AW. Radiology of gestational trophoblastic neoplasia. *Clin Radiol.* 2006; 61:301-313.

33. Van Nagell JR Jr, Depriest PD, Reedy MB, et al. Ovarian cancer screening with annual transvaginal sonography: findings of 25,000 women screened. *Cancer.* 2007;109:1887-1896.

34. Partridge E, Kreimer AR, Greenlee RT, et al. Results from four rounds of ovarian cancer screening in a randomized trial. *Obstet Gynecol.* 2009;113:775-782.

35. Menon U, Gentry-Majaraj A, Hallett R, et al. Sensitivity and specificity of multimodal and ultrasound screening for ovarian cancer, and stage distribution of detected cancers: results of the prevalence screen of the UK Collaborative Trial of Ovarian Cancer Screening (UKCTOCS). *Lancet Oncol.* 2009;10(4):327-340.

36. Axtell AE, Lee MH, Bristow RE, et al. Multi-institutional reciprocal validation study of computed tomography predictors of suboptimal primary cytoreduction in patients with advanced ovarian cancer. *J Clin Oncol.* 2007;25:384-389.

37. Fulham MJ, Carter J, Baldey A, et al. The impact of PET-CT in suspected recurrent ovarian cancer: a prospective multi-centre study as part of the Australian PET Data Collection Project. *Gynecol Oncol.* 2009;112(3):462-468.

38. Risum S, Hogdall C, Loft A, et al. The diagnostic value of PET/CT for primary ovarian cancer: a prospective study. *Gynecol Oncol.* 2007;105:145-149.

39. Nam EJ, Yun MJ, Oh YT, et al. Diagnosis and staging of primary ovarian cancer: correlation between PET/CT, Doppler US, and CT or MRI. *Gynecol Oncol.* 2010;116:389-394.

40. Gu P, Pan LL, Wu SQ, Sun L, Huang G. CA 125, PET alone, PET-CT, CT and MRI in diagnosing recurrent ovarian carcinoma a systematic review and meta-analysis. *Eur J Radiol.* 2009;71:164-174.

41. Kataoka MY, Sala E, Baldwin P, et al. The accuracy of magnetic resonance imaging in staging of vulvar cancer: a retrospective multi-centre study. *Gynecol Oncol.* 2010;117(1): 82-87.

Part II | Disease Sites

Preinvasive Disease of the Lower Genital Tract

Levi S. Downs Jr. and Jori S. Carter

Over the past 3 decades, the work of population scientists, laboratory-based researchers, and clinicians has together promoted the understanding of the pathogenesis of preinvasive disease of the lower genital tract and its associated cancers. Elucidating the progression from preinvasive disease to invasive cancer was the first step in implementing the Pap test as one of the most successful cancer screening program in developed nations and has dramatically lessened the impact of cervical cancer in the United States and other developed countries. Furthermore, with the identification of the human papillomavirus (HPV) as the principal and necessary cause of cervical cancer, the development and application of HPV vaccines will potentially further reduce the burden of cervical cancer and other HPV-induced malignancies.

EPIDEMIOLOGY

Key Points

1. The HPV is the most common sexually transmitted infection and is the necessary cause for cervical dysplasia and cancer. HPV16 and 18 are the most common high-risk types implicated in carcinogenesis.
2. Additional risk factors for genital dysplasia including tobacco smoking, immunosuppression, early age at first intercourse, and multiple sexual partners.

3. The HPV proteins E6 and E7 are critical for malignant transformation; E6 binds and inactives the tumor suppressor gene *p53*, whereas E7 binds and inactivates the tumor supressor gene *pRb*.

Incidence of Cervical Dysplasia

In the United States, 2 to 3 million women are diagnosed with cervical cytologic abnormalities annually. The most common abnormality found by liquid-based cytology is atypical squamous cells of undetermined significance (ASC-US), accounting for 2% to 5% of all Pap test results. In contrast, low-grade squamous intraepithelial lesions (LSIL) account for 2% of Pap test results, and approximately 0.5% of Pap test results are high-grade squamous intraepithelial lesions (HSIL); less than 0.5% are suggestive of invasive cancer. Atypical glandular cells of undetermined significance (AGC) account for an additional 0.2% to 0.8% of Pap test results.

Every year, between 250,000 and 1 million women in the United States are diagnosed with cervical dysplasia. Histologic diagnosis of cervical dysplasia is based on a tissue biopsy and uses the Bethesda nomenclature; this differs from the nomenclature used for cytologic abnormalities diagnosed on Pap testing. Cervical intraepithelial neoplasia (CIN) is the formal histologic diagnosis of cervical dysplasia and is graded as 1, 2, or 3 based on the proportion of atypical cells in the cervical epithelium. CIN can occur at any age; the

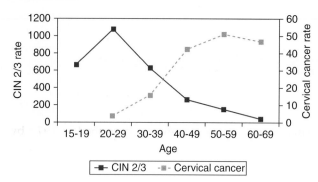

FIGURE 4-1. Incidence of CIN2 and 3 and cervical cancer. Rates shown here are per 100,000 women undergoing routine cytologic screening for CIN2 and 3, and per 100,000 women for cervical cancer. The peak incidence of invasive cervical cancer is observed approximately 25 to 30 years later than for CIN2/3. (Sources: CIN2/3 incidence among screened women [Kaiser Permanente Northwest Health Plan, Portland, Oregon, 1998-2002], Cervical cancer incidence among unscreened women [Connecticut, 1940-1944].)

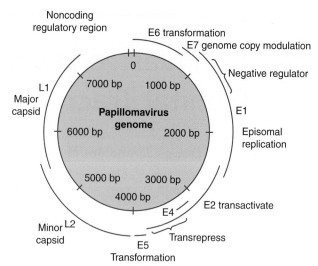

*Bars represent open reading frames.
E = early region; L = late region; bp = base pair

FIGURE 4-2. The 8 open reading frames of the HPV virus. The 6 early proteins (E1-E6) are involved with life cycle and replication; the 2 late proteins (L1 and L2) form the major and minor capsid.

peak incidence is in women between the ages of 25 to 35 years (Figure 4-1).

Human papillomavirus (HPV) is the necessary cause of cervical dysplasia and cervical cancer. HPV is the most common sexually transmitted infection, and is estimated that 6.2 million new infections occur annually in the United States. The overall HPV prevalence in women in the United States is estimated to be 27%. Genital HPV infection has the highest prevalence in young adults under the age of 25 years, with a 25% prevalence in girls aged 14 to 19 years and 45% in women aged 20 to 24 years.[1] More than 100 HPV types have been identified, and more than 40 of these infect the anal/genital area. HPV is a double-stranded DNA virus that encodes 8 open reading frames. The corresponding proteins are described as early proteins, including 6 proteins that are involved with the HPV life cycle and replication. The 2 late proteins, L1 and L2 , are the structural proteins of the virus and form the major and minor capsid, respectively (Figure 4-2).

HPV type is determined by the degree of homology within the region of the DNA that codes for the L1 protein. A new HPV type is identified when the entire genome has been sequenced and there is more than 10% difference from a known L1 sequence. HPV is not only transmitted by sexual intercourse; it is important to recognize that nonpenetrative contact may also lead to new HPV infections. In a 2-year longitudinal study of HPV-negative women, 10% of those having sexual contact, but not sexual intercourse, were positive for HPV at the end of the observation period. It appears that most of these occur within the first few years of initiating sexual activity.

Prospective studies suggest a cumulative incidence of 50% within 3 years of the onset of sexual activity. For most girls/women, genital HPV infections clear within 1 to 2 years of initial detection. The median time to clearance is 8 to 12 months, with more than 90% of infections having cleared within 2 years. It is difficult to determine whether HPV infections become dormant in basal cells and later become reactivated as "latent HPV."[2]

Persistent infection with 1 of the approximately 15 carcinogenic HPV types places women at increased risk for high-grade cervical dysplasia and cervical cancer. There is no consensus on the exact duration of genital HPV infection that constitutes persistent infection; although this has been described differently in many studies, in general it appears to be between 18 and 24 months of detection of the same HPV type. It is believed that persistent infection of 10 to 20 years or more is required for cervical cancer to develop. Although young women under the age of 25 years can be diagnosed with cervical cancer, this is a rare occurrence, and there is little understanding of the circumstances that lead to a more rapid progression of the steps leading to epithelial transformation to malignancy in these rare cases.

HPVs are grouped according to their carcinogenicity. Fifteen high-risk HPV types are found in cervical cancers. These high-risk types may also be found in premalignant lesions of the cervix, but they are much more common in cancer cases than in controls; this provides the epidemiologic evidence of carcinogenicity that is used to classify high-risk and low-risk HPV types. HPV16 is recognized as the most carcinogenic of the high-risk HPV types. HPV type 16 has been identified in 46% of all high-grade premalignant lesions of the cervix and approximately 55% of all cervical cancers. High-risk HPV type 18 can be detected in 16% of all cervical cancers. Other high-risk HPV include types 31, 33, 35, 39, 45, 51, 52, 56, 58, 59, 68, 73, and 82. In contrast, the low-risk HPV types 6 and 11 are the most common types detected in anogenital warts.

Incidence of Vaginal Dysplasia

Vaginal dysplasia is a relatively rare entity and comprises only 0.5% of all female genital tract lesions. The overall incidence in the United States is reported to be between 0.2 and 2 per 100,000 women. It is most commonly diagnosed in women older than 60 years of age who have current or prior diagnoses of cervical or vulvar preinvasive or invasive lesions, as they have many risk factors in common, such as HPV infection and immunosuppression. HPV DNA is present in approximately 80% of vaginal carcinoma in situ. Additional risk factors for vaginal dysplasia include prior pelvic or vaginal radiation and chronic inflammation from pessary use or prolapse. Vaginal dysplasia is usually asymptomatic with absence of a visible lesion. It is often detected by colposcopy during evaluation of an abnormal Pap test, commonly after hysterectomy for cervical dysplasia. When evident, lesions are generally white with sharp borders and are best evaluated after application of dilute acetic acid.

Vaginal intraepithelial neoplasia (VAIN) was first described in 1952 in a woman who had a total hysterectomy for cervical carcinoma in situ several years prior. VAIN was given its nomenclature in 1989 by the International Society for the Study of Vulvar Disease and includes grades 1 through 3 (mild dysplasia, moderate dysplasia, and severe dysplasia/carcinoma in situ) which are defined by the extent of microscopic cellular epithelial abnormalities.

Incidence of Vulvar Dysplasia

In the United States, the incidence of vulvar dysplasia has drastically increased by 411% between 1973 and 2000, with an incidence rate of 0.56 to 2.86 per 100,000 women, and it is becoming more common in younger women aged 20 to 35 years.[3] Approximately 50% of women with vulvar dysplasia have dysplasia at other sites involving the genital tract, most commonly of the cervix.

Vulvar dysplasia was initially described by Bowen in 1912, in which a lesion of the thigh and buttocks was termed *precancerous dermatosis*. These lesions became known as precancerous lesions of the vulva and have adopted several different terminologies over the years, including Bowen disease, erythroplasia of Queyrat, atypical hyperplasia, lichen sclerosis et atrophicus, leukoplakia, leukokeratosis, leukoplakic vulvitis, hyperplastic vulvitis, kraurosis vulvae, neurodermatitis, atypical hyperplasia, dysplasia, atypia, carcinoma in situ, and carcinoma simplex. The original consensus for terminology was described in 1976 by the International Society for the Study of Vulvovaginal Disease, which recommended the adoption of the terms *vulvar dystrophies*, *vulvar atypia*, and *squamous cell carcinoma in situ*. The terminology was further revised in 1989 to include the use of the term *nonneoplastic epithelial disorder* when describing dysplastic conditions such as lichen sclerosis and squamous cell hyperplasia. The 1989 revisions also included the current use of the term *vulvar intraepithelial neoplasia* (VIN), with a grade of 1 to 3 (mild, moderate, and severe/in situ) based on the extent of microscopic cellular epithelial abnormalities, which replaced the terms *atypia* and *carcinoma in situ*. In 2004, the terminology was again revised to include the nomenclature that is currently in use to describe vulvar lesions.

Vulvar lesions are subdivided into 2 major categories: usual type VIN (including warty, basaloid, and mixed warty/basaloid types) which is associated with HPV infection and is generally seen in younger women, and differentiated type VIN, which is not associated with HPV and is generally seen in older women. A third category, unclassified type VIN, was included for rare cases that do not fit either usual or differentiated by histologic criteria.[4]

Risk Factors

Several risk factors for persistent HPV infection, cervical dysplasia, and cervical cancer have been identified. Because these 3 outcomes exist on a continuum, in general, the risk factors are similar for each diagnosis, with duration of exposure being the main differentiating factor. As previously described, persistent genital infection with high-risk HPV types is the most important risk factor for cervical dysplasia, and a history of high-grade cervical dysplasia is the most important risk factor for cervical cancer. When considering the specific high-risk HPV types, it appears that HPV16 infection is more likely to persist beyond 24 months and is more oncogenic than other high-risk HPV types. This is confirmed by epidemiologic data showing that HPV16 is detected in more cervical cancers than any other HPV type. In general, for all HPV infections, the longer that a type-specific infection has persisted, the more likely it is to persist. Additionally, older women with detectable HPV are more likely to have a persistent HPV infection.

Studies have found that tobacco smoking is associated with an increased risk of genital dysplasia.[5] There also appears to be a close association with long-term oral contraceptive use.[6] Coinfection with other sexually transmitted diseases has also been investigated as risk factors for cervical dysplasia. *Chlamydia trachomatis* infection is associated with cervical dysplasia. Studies investigating the role of herpes simplex virus and *Trichomonas vaginalis* have provided inconsistent results. There are not consistent data to support an association with nutritional intake, nutritional supplements, or alcohol use as cofactors for genital dysplasia.

Recent studies have sought to identify the role of host immunity and genetic factors such as human leukocyte antigen class I and II genes and viral factors such as HPV variants or multiple-type HPV infections, viral load, or HPV genome integration sites. More work is needed in this area, and no consistent trends have been identified.

Acquired immunosuppression, specifically human immunodeficiency virus (HIV) infection, and immunosuppressive therapy, specifically in organ transplant recipients, are closely associated with increased risk of genital dysplasia. The prevalence of all cervical cytologic abnormalities is increased in HIV-infected women, with a 3-fold increase in the prevalence of high-grade squamous intraepithelial lesions and cancer. Women receiving lifelong intense immunosuppressive therapy as a strategy to reduce the risk of organ rejection have up to a 2- to 6-fold increased risk of cervical dysplasia, 3-fold increased risk for cervical cancer, and a 50-fold increased risk for vulvar cancer.[7]

Other behavioral factors that are associated with and increased risk of preinvasive disease of the genital tract include early age at first intercourse, multiple sexual partners, and male partners with multiple partners.

HPV and Pathogenesis

Epidemiologic and molecular research has fully defined the relationship between persistent HPV infection and premalignant disease of the lower genital tract. High-risk HPV types 16 and 18 are the types most frequently found in cervical cancer worldwide and therefore are the most well studied. High-risk HPV infection has also been associated with the development of premalignancies and cancers of other sites, such as anal cancer, penile cancer, and malignancies of the head and neck. In contrast to cervical cancer, these cancers are preferentially associated with HPV16. Because the most is known about the molecular biology and pathogenesis at the cervix, this section focuses on specific steps that lead to premalignancy in this organ. It should be recognized, however, that there is increasing evidence that a similar pathogenesis appears to occur in other epithelial tissues where HPV has been implicated as a cause of premalignancy and cancer.

Genital HPV types preferentially infect the cervical transformation zone. Although the majority of HPV infections clear within 1 to 2 years, persistence of infection promotes the development of low-grade and high-grade cytologic and histologic abnormalities. Even after premalignant lesions are identified, some may regress, whereas others progress to an invasive malignancy after what appears to be a period of latency. In HPV-positive cancers, all malignant cells contain at least 1 copy of the viral genome that is actively transcribed. This leads to the overexpression of the viral oncoproteins E6 and E7; the long-term, continuous expression of these oncoproteins in epithelial cells leads to high-grade dysplasia and potentially malignancy.

When host epithelial cells are infected with HPV, it has been shown that the viral genome integrates into the host cell's DNA. This occurs more frequently with high-risk HPV types, and frequency of integration increases with increasing degree of dysplasia/cancer. When integration occurs, the continuous expression of the E6 and E7 genes leads to the transformation of epithelial cells to the malignant phenotype. Both E6 and E7 have specific transforming properties. E6 induces degradation of the tumor suppressor protein p53 via the ubiquitin pathway. p53 is a cellular transcription factor that can trigger cell cycle arrest of apoptosis in response to cellular stress such as hypoxia or DNA damage. The role of p53 is to ensure the integrity of the cellular genome, preventing cell division after DNA damage or delaying it until damage has been repaired. By blocking the function of p53, E6 allows for the accumulation of chromosomal abnormalities, greatly increasing the chance of progression from normal epithelium to high-grade dysplasia and cancer. In a similar manner, E7 binds to the tumor suppressor protein retinoblastoma (pRb1) and its related pocket proteins, p107 and p130. The 3 tumor suppression proteins are critically involved in cell cycle regulation. When these proteins bind to E7, this activates the transcription of a group of genes that encode proteins essential for cell cycle progression. This allows cells to enter into S phase, when, in the absence of E7, they would otherwise undergo cell cycle arrest in G1 phase.[8]

Pathogenesis of Non-HPV Vulvar Dysplasia

Vulvar intraepithelial neoplasia may arise through different mechanisms. HPV-associated vulvar dysplasia is most commonly associated with the HPV16 subtype and is often multifocal and strongly associated with cigarette smoking and has a pathogenesis similar to that of cervical dysplasia. This type of VIN includes the basaloid or warty variants. In contrast, the differentiated VIN variant is not generally associated with HPV infection and is morphologically similar to invasive squamous cell carcinoma in appearance.[9] Non-neoplastic epithelial disorders including lichen sclerosis, lichen simplex chronicus, and squamous cell hyperplasia are often associated with the differentiated type VIN. Although not considered premalignant lesions independently, a well-accepted hypothesis in the pathogenesis of differentiated VIN is that chronic pruritus caused by these disorders, and the resultant inflammation from scratching, plays a role in the progression from lichen sclerosis to lichen simplex chronicus and results in squamous cell hyperplasia, which then progresses to differentiated VIN, and ultimately to invasive carcinoma. Mixed dystrophy refers to lichen sclerosis which is associated with variable degrees of squamous cell hyperplasia and illustrates the progression and spectrum of changes seen in lichen sclerosis.

Lichen sclerosis is a non-neoplastic epithelial disorder of unclear etiology and is most commonly seen in postmenopausal white women. Lesions appear as pale white, flat, plaque-like areas which can resemble thinned parchment paper in advanced cases (Figure 4-3). Histologically, lichen sclerosis shows a thinned epidermis with blunting or loss of rete ridges, a middle layer of homogenous collagenized subepithelial edema, and a lower band of lymphocytic infiltration. When lichen sclerosis is associated with lichen simplex chronicus, it shows epidermal thickening instead of thinning associated with superficial dermal chronic inflammatory infiltrate with vertical collagen streaks in the papillary dermis. Lichen sclerosis with squamous cell hyperplasia has the presence of epidermal hyperplasia without inflammation, atypia, or evidence of a specific dermatosis.

Lichen planus is a dermatosis most commonly seen in women older than 40 years, although it may be present across a wide age range. When symptomatic, women present with burning and pruritus. It is often associated with similar lace-like plaques in the oral or vaginal mucosa. There is a variable appearance histologically, but it is diagnosed by the presence of a bandlike chronic lymphocytic inflammatory infiltrate and the presence of colloid bodies formed as a result of degenerated keratinocytes. Lichen planus can evolve into erosive vulvar disease, which has been associated with invasive vulvar squamous cell carcinoma.[10]

DIAGNOSIS

Key Points

1. The American Cancer Society recommends Pap test screening 3 years after the initiation of sexual intercourse or by 21 years of age. In contrast, the American Congress of Obstetricians/Gynecologists recommends that screening should not begin until 21 years of age.
2. Abnormal Pap tests should trigger subsequent colposcopic examination to obtain directed tissue specimens for histologic evaluation of dysplasia or cancer.
3. The most common presenting symptom of vulvar dysplasia is a pruritic lesion.

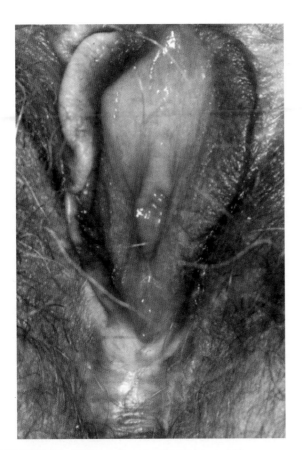

FIGURE 4-3. Lichen sclerosis. White, plaque-like areas can resemble parchment paper.

Cervical Dysplasia

As early as 1932, it was recognized that carcinoma in situ was a precursor to cervical cancer. Papanicolaou and Traut subsequently demonstrated that the exfoliated cells from the ectocervix could be used to detect carcinoma in situ and invasive cancer. In 1969, Richart hypothesized that cervical cancer develops from noninvasive stages, thereby introducing the terminology *cervical intraepithelial neoplasia* (CIN).

Since the 1950s, the Pap smear has been the central component of population-based cervical cancer screening in the United States. Pap-based screening has led to a more than 70% reduction in cervical cancer mortality by making it possible to identify and treat premalignant lesions of the cervix before these lesions develop into cancer. Similarly, the goal of treating vulvar and vaginal dysplasia is primarily to decrease or eliminate the risk of any individual developing cancer of these organs. The Pap smear was originally performed using a wooden or plastic spatula to scrape the ectocervix in a 360-degree circumference. The exfoliated cells were then smeared onto a glass slide, preserved with a spray fixative, processed, and examined by cytopathologists. The degree of cellular atypia and abnormal morphology lead to classifications based on the risk of a histologic abnormality.

The conventional Pap smear is arguably suboptimal due to the frequency of both false-positive and false-negative results, which likely result from the poor quality of sampling and the preparation method. The frequent presence of blood cells or inflammatory cells, poor cell fixation, and inhomogeneous distribution of cells contributes to greater difficulty in detecting epithelial cell abnormalities and impairs the reproducibility of diagnosis. In an attempt to improve test sensitivity, liquid-based cytology may demonstrate superiority to conventional Pap techniques. Exfoliated cells are collected from the ectocervix with a brush designed to match the contour of the cervix, and the cells are rinsed into a vial with a preservative solution. The solution is processed to remove inflammatory and blood cells and debris, and a single-layer slide of epithelial cells is created to facilitate detection of cellular abnormalities. Because only a portion of the preservative is used, the remaining liquid can be used for other purposes, such as HPV detection or other testing. Many prospective studies have suggested that this process improves the sensitivity and positive predictive value for the detection of moderate- or high-grade dysplasia. However, recent studies have challenged these original reports. A large cohort of almost 90,000 women has shown that liquid-based cytology has similar sensitivity and positive predictive value for preinvasive disease of the cervix as that of conventional Pap smears.[11] Despite these recent reports showing similar sensitivities between the 2 methods, the additional benefit of using liquid-based cytology for HPV detection or other testing, faster reading times, and decreased processing costs through automation makes this approach superior to conventional Pap smears. Pap testing with liquid-based cytology has become the primary sampling method used in the United States.

Population-based screening programs have been successful in reducing cervical cancer mortality in developed nations. The optimal screening program has not been defined, and the approach varies throughout the world based on heath system financing and resources allocated to screening programs. For example, screening frequency varies from 5-year intervals in the Netherlands and parts of France to yearly intervals in Germany.

The American Cancer Society (ACS) and the American College of Obstetrics and Gynecology (ACOG) both publish guidelines on cervical cancer screening (Table 4-1). In general, the consensus guidelines of both organizations are supported by the United States Preventative Services Task Force. The 2003 ACS guidelines and the 2009 updated recommendations from ACOG are similar and are presented next. The main area of difference between the 2 organizations is age at which to initiate screening. The ACS recommendations are to begin screening 3 years after the initiation of sexual intercourse or by 21 years of age. In contrast, the updated 2009 ACOG guidelines recommend that screening should not begin until 21 years of age.[12] The recommendation to begin screening at age 21 is based on the very low incidence rate of cervical cancer before age 21 years and the anxiety and harm that diagnosis and treatment of premalignant lesions in this age group may cause. Because the majority of abnormal cytology and premalignant lesions diagnosed in this age group will regress without the need for treatment, the risks of Pap testing may outweigh any benefits. These risks are particularly relevant with the incidence of cervical cancer in women under 21 years of age as low as 1 to 2 per 1,000,000, or only 0.1% of all cervical cancers.

Once cervical cancer screening begins, both ACS and ACOG recommend that screening occurs at a frequency of once every 2 years until age 29 years. Women ≥ 30 years of age with a history of 3 consecutive negative Pap smears may elect to have combination testing with cytology and high-risk HPV detection. With a normal Pap test and absence of high-risk HPV, further screening is deferred for 3 years, at which time the combination screen should be repeated. If HPV testing is not performed along with cytology after age 30 years of age, then testing should be performed every 2 to 3 years. ACS recommendations specify that women who choose to have high-risk HPV testing in this setting should be informed that (1) HPV infection usually is not detectable or harmful; (2) almost everyone who has had sexual intercourse has been exposed to HPV, and infection is very common; (3) a positive HPV test result does not reflect the presence of a sexually transmitted disease, but rather a sexually acquired infection; and (4) a positive HPV test result does not indicate the presence of cancer, and the large majority of women who test positive for an HPV infection will not develop advanced cancer.

Table 4-1 Comparison of ACS and ACOG Guidelines for Screening for Cervical Cancer[12]

Age, Screening Interval, and Test Protocols	ACS 2002	ACOG 2003	ACOG 2009
Age to start	Approximately 3 years after initiation of intercourse or by age 21 years	Approximately 3 years after initiation of intercourse or by age 21 years	Age 21 years
Screening interval in women aged <30 years	Annual with conventional Pap; 2 years with liquid Pap	Annual	Every 2 years
Screening interval in women aged ≥30 years	Every 2-3 years	Every 2-3 years	Every 3 years
Age to stop screening	Age 70 years after 3 negative tests in last 10 years	No upper age limit	Age 65-70 years after 3 negative tests in last 10 years
Women with prior hysterectomy	Discontinue screening if hysterectomy for benign reason	Discontinue screening if hysterectomy for benign reason	Discontinue screening if hysterectomy for benign reason
Screening test options	Conventional Pap test or liquid cytology; option of HPV cotesting starting at age 30 years, repeated no sooner than every 3 years	Conventional Pap test or liquid cytology; option of HPV cotesting starting at age 30 years, repeated no sooner than every 3 years	Conventional Pap test or liquid cytology; option of HPV cotesting starting at age 30 years, repeated no sooner than every 3 years

ACOG, American College of Obstetricians and Gynecologists; ACS, American Cancer Society; HPV, human papillomavirus; Pap, Papanicolaou.

Women who have an intact cervix should continue screening at the 2- to 3-year frequency until age 65 years (per ACOG guidelines) or 70 years (per ACS guidelines). Women may then choose to discontinue routine screening if they have no abnormal cytology or histologic diagnoses of the cervix for the prior 10 years and there is documentation of 3 consecutive normal Pap tests. Screening is recommended to continue, without a maximum age, for women in good health who have not previously undergone screening or if information regarding prior screening is not available. Women who are immunocompromised by organ transplantation, chemotherapy, or chronic corticosteroid treatment or who are HIV positive should be tested twice during the first year after their immunosuppression-related diagnosis and then annually thereafter. There is no recommended age to stop screening in these women. Immunocompromised women should continue screening for as long as they are in good health and are likely to benefit from early detection and treatment of preinvasive disease.

Cytology screening is not recommended for women who have had a hysterectomy for reasons other than gynecologic cancer or cervical dysplasia. If a women has a history of CIN 2 or 3, or if it is not possible to document the absence of CIN 2 or 3 from pathologic reports, cytologic screening should take place for 10 years, and there should be documentation of 3 consecutive normal cytologic screenings at the end of this period.

It is important to recognize that Pap testing is a screening test and indicates women who are at risk for having a histologic diagnosis of cervical dysplasia. When sufficient risk exists that a patient may have cervical dysplasia or cancer, then most often the next step in diagnosis is to perform a colposcopic examination to obtain directed tissue specimens for histologic determination of the presence (or absence) of cervical dysplasia or cancer. The colposcope is a lighted binocular microscope which magnifies the surface of the tissue being examined. It is used to visualize the cervix, vagina, and vulva. Tissue can be magnified between 2× and 25× power. Colposcopes are equipped with various light filters to help better identify vascular patterns that may be associated with varying degrees of dysplasia or cancer. A dilute solution of acetic acid is applied to the cervix during colposcopy. The acetic acid dehydrates cells, thus exaggerating the increased nuclear-to-cytoplasmic ratio found in the cells of dysplastic tissue and cancer. Due to this increased density of DNA, dysplastic cells will reflect the light from the colposcope, and the observer sees a so-called acetowhite lesion. In addition to these acetowhite changes, other colposcopic features suggestive of dysplasia include the margin of the lesion, the presence of vascular patterns referred to punctations or mosaicisms, and size of the lesion relative to the overall size of the cervix. Furthermore, the colposcopist may apply an iodine paint (or Lugol solution) to the cervix to aid in the detection of dysplastic lesions. The iodine solution is thought to stain intracellular glycogen. Normal cells will absorb the iodine and appear brown when viewed through the colposcope. Dysplastic cells, however, absorb less iodine due to their increased nuclear to cytoplasmic ratio and appear yellow or variegated brown/yellow. These features of cervical dysplasia help the colposcopist determine where to biopsy and how many biopsies need to be performed.

The second objective of colposcopy is to exclude a diagnosis of invasive cancer. It is important that the colposcopist be attuned to the visual changes that are predictive of invasive cancer. Fungating lesions or areas of hyperemia and friable areas may be evidence of dysplasia or invasive cancer. In addition, large, complex acetowhite lesions obliterating the cervical os or lesions with irregular and exophytic contour are very concerning for cancer. Lesions that appear to be thick, chalky-white with raised or rolled out margins, or lesions bleeding on touch should be biopsied to evaluate for possible preclinical invasive cancer. An important feature of invasive cancer is the appearance of atypical blood vessels. Atypical vessels occur with blood vessels breaking out from mosaic formations. The atypical vessel patterns are varied and may take the form of hairpins, corkscrews, commas, or have irregular branching patterns with irregular caliber.

Vaginal Dysplasia

As with cervical dysplasia, there are minimal clinical features associated with vaginal dysplasia. The diagnosis of vaginal dysplasia follows the steps described previously for cervical dysplasia. The screening Pap test may result in a diagnosis of a cytologic abnormality; when this occurs after the cervix has been surgically removed, then colposcopy is specifically performed to detect vaginal dysplasia. A detailed examination of the complete vagina is warranted, and it may be necessary to reposition the speculum in this setting so that the lateral and anterior and posterior walls may be fully examined with acetic acid solution. It is often helpful to use Lugol solution during complete colposcopy of the vagina. Abnormal findings should be biopsied and evaluated in a manner similar to that of cervical lesions seen during colposcopic examination.

Vulvar Dysplasia

Most women with vulvar dysplasia are asymptomatic, and the diagnosis is made with a high index of suspicion, colposcopy, and biopsy. When clinically evident, the most common symptom is pruritus. Other symptoms include burning, dyspareunia, erythema, edema, and pain. Lesions have a raised surface and are pigmented in 25% of cases and can also be grey or red (Figure 4-4). Multifocality is a common feature. Lesions are frequently located at the posterior vulva or periclitoral regions and can extend to adjacent structures. Many women have concomitant or previous dysplasia in another location in the genital tract and should be evaluated with colposcopy and liberal biopsies. Half of lesions involved with VIN become acetowhite after the application of 3% to 5% acetic acid, which should be applied for at least 5 minutes before examination. Thorough examination with the colposcope should follow application of acetic acid, and punch biopsies should be taken at each site of a suspicious lesion. These small punch biopsies can be easily performed in the clinic setting after the superficial injection of lidocaine and incorporate the full thickness of the skin for diagnosis.

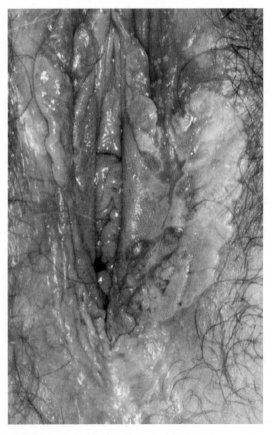

FIGURE 4-4. Vulvar dysplasia. Lesions have a raised surface and may be pigmented.

If needed, hemostasis can be achieved with silver nitrate or a single suture across the area of the biopsy.

PATHOLOGY

Key Points

1. CIN and VIN are reported via a 3-level system, which is based on the proportion of epithelium occupied by abnormal cells measured from the basement membrane.
2. Adenocarcinoma in situ describes cellular atypia involving the glandular epithelium, which may be multicentric (with "skip lesions") and extend to multiple quadrants.

Cervical Cytology

The most frequently used terminology for reporting Pap test results are the Bethesda System criteria, which was last updated in 2001[13] (Table 4-2). Normal squamous and endocervical cells without evidence of HPV infection are considered as "negative for intraepithelial lesion of malignancy." Pap tests with normal endometrial cells may also be placed into this diagnostic category. It is not uncommon that Pap tests of the vagina performed after a hysterectomy show evidence of normal glandular cells. Reasons for this include exfoliated cells from vaginal endometriosis, Bartholin glands, periurethral and perivaginal glands, vaginal adenosis, remnants after surgical or ablative therapies, or prolapsed fallopian tubes. When the glandular cells appear completely benign, they can be considered negative and are included in this diagnostic group.

The category of atypical squamous cells of undetermined significance (ASC-US) is used to describe a finding of equivocal cells. These cells may be atypical secondary to HPV infection, but other reasons include atrophic or reactive processes. Regardless of etiology, the nuclear size of these cells are 2 to 3 times increased over normal cells, with a slight increase in nuclear-to-cytoplasmic ratio. There is mild nuclear hyperchromasia and chromatin irregularity with mild variations in nuclear shape. Atypical parakeratosis may also be seen.

Specimens that are interpreted as atypical squamous cells, favor high grade (ASC-H), contain cells that are suspicious for the presence of high-grade dysplasia but are too limited in volume to permit classification as a high-grade squamous intraepithelial lesion. These specimens typically contain immature cells with atypia and nuclei that are 1.5 to 2.5 times increased over normal. There is an increased nuclear-to-cytoplasmic ratio, similar to high-grade squamous intraepithelial lesion (HSIL), and variations in nuclear size and shape, with nuclear membrane irregularity.

Specimens that are described as low-grade squamous intraepithelial lesions (LSIL) show atypia in mature cells with nuclei that are 3 times normal size. There is a slight increase in nuclear-to-cytoplasmic ratio, with hyperchromasia and coarsely granular chromatin. There are variations is nuclear size and shape, with binucleation and multinucleation. There is irregularity to nuclear membranes, which is variable, and perinuclear cavitation or koilocytosis, sometimes described as a cytoplasmic halo (Figure 4-5).

In contrast to LSIL, Pap tests with HSIL show atypia in immature cells, with variability in cell size, including small cells. There is marked increase in nuclear-to-cytoplasmic ratio, with hyperchromasia with fine to coarse chromatin. There is variation in nuclear size and shape, with marked nuclear membrane irregularity (Figure 4-6).

Cervical Histology

The histologic diagnosis of cervical dysplasia and precancer is referred to as CIN. The standard reporting for histologic diagnoses of CIN involves a 3-level system: CIN1, 2, and 3. The traditional grading of dysplasia is based on the proportion of epithelium occupied by basaloid, undifferentiated cells, with higher grade assigned with the progressive loss of epithelial maturation.

The architectural abnormalities associated with CIN1 are the morphologic manifestations of an active and productive HPV infection. These morphologic changes include pronuclear cytoplasm cavitation with thickening of the cytoplasmic membrane, nuclear atypia, and anisocytosis. Nuclear atypia is present, with nuclear enlargement, hyperchromasia, and irregularity and wrinkling of the nuclear membrane. The loss of maturation is demonstrated by the presence of cells with nuclei near the surface epithelium; these nuclei are somewhat smaller than basal cells. The term *koilocytosis* refers to the combination of the cytoplasmic cavitation (vacuoles) and nuclear atypia. Further, these cells may be binucleated or multinucleated. CIN1 is defined by the limitation of these abnormal, atypical cells to the bottom one-third of the epidermal layer.

An important feature of HPV-induced lesions anywhere in the genital tract is the presence of cellular atypia. In the absence of atypia, these changes are nonspecific, which may be a reflection of atrophy-related vacuolar degeneration or non-HPV infections such as *Gardnerella vaginalis* or candidiasis or squamous epithelium containing abundant amounts of glycogen. These are the most important abnormalities to consider in the

Table 4-2 The 2001 Bethesda System (Abridged)

Specimen Adequacy
Satisfactory for evaluation (*note presence/absence of endocervical/ transformation zone component*)
Unsatisfactory for evaluation . . . (*specify reason*)
  Specimen rejected/not processed (*specify reason*)
  Specimen processed and examined, but unsatisfactory for evaluation of epithelial abnormality because of (*specify reason*)

General Categorization (optional)
Negative for intraepithelial lesion or malignancy
Epithelial cell abnormality
Other

Interpretation/Result
Negative for Intraepithelial Lesion or Malignancy
  Organisms
    T vaginalis
    Fungal organisms morphologically consistent with *Candida* species
    Shift in flora suggestive of bacterial vaginosis
    Bacteria morphologically consistent with *Actinomyces* species
    Cellular changes consistent with herpes simplex virus

  Other non-neoplastic findings (*optional to report; list not comprehensive*)
    Reactive cellular changes associated with
      inflammation (includes typical repair)
      radiation
      intrauterine contraceptive device
    Glandular cells status posthysterectomy
    Atrophy

Epithelial Cell Abnormalities
  Squamous cell
    Atypical squamous cells (ASC)
      of undetermined significance (ASC-US)
      cannot exclude HSIL (ASC-H)
    Low-grade squamous intraepithelial lesion (LSIL)
      encompassing: human papillomavirus/mild dysplasia/cervical intraepithelial neoplasia (CIN) 1
    High-grade squamous intraepithelial lesion (HSIL)
      encompassing: moderate and severe dysplasia, carcinoma in situ; CIN2 and CIN3

  Squamous cell carcinoma
  Glandular cell
    Atypical glandular cells (AGC) (*specify endocervical, endometrial, or not otherwise specified*)
    Atypical glandular cells, favor neoplastic (*specify endocervical or not otherwise specified*)
    Endocervical adenocarcinoma in situ (AIS)
    Adenocarcinoma

Other (*List not comprehensive*)
  Endometrial cells in a woman ≥40 years of age

Automated Review and Ancillary Testing (include as appropriate)

Educational Notes and Suggestions (optional)

differential diagnosis of an LSIL Pap test and represent the diagnostic challenges in correctly identifying CIN1. Specific testing for HPV DNA may help to differentiate these lesions (Figure 4-7).

In CIN2 and CIN3, immature basaloid cells occupy more than the lower one-third of the epithelium. CIN2 is defined as atypical cells confined to the lower two-thirds of the epidermal layer; CIN3 is considered the presence of atypical cells extending more than two-thirds from the basement membrane. Carcinoma in situ is defined as the entire epidermal layer comprising atypical cells, without penetration through the basement membrane. In general, there is nuclear crowding, pleomorphism, and loss of the normal cell polarity. Nuclear enlargement that is more pronounced in the lower portion of the epithelium is present, but it

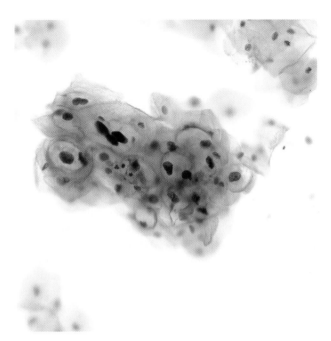

FIGURE 4-5. Low-grade squamous intraepithelial lesions. Cytology shows nuclear atypia, increased nuclear to cytoplasmic ratios, and perinuclear cavitation (koilocytosis).

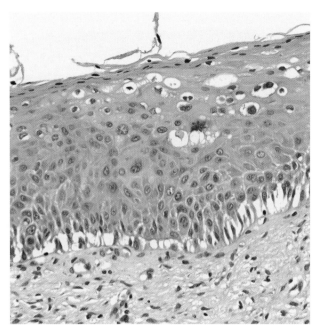

FIGURE 4-7. CIN1. Abnormal, atypical cells are limited to the bottom one-third of the epidermal layer.

occurs throughout the epithelium. This lesion is differentiated from CIN1 in that the nuclear chromatin is more coarsely granular, normal or abnormal mitotic figures are present, and cytoplasm is usually scant. In the superficial layers of the epithelium, individual dyskeratotic cells may be seen (keratinization occurring below the most superficial cells of the epithelium). In

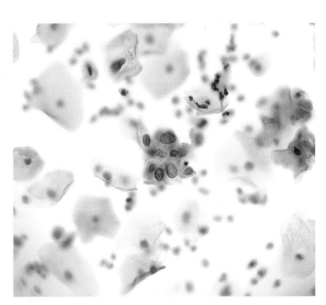

FIGURE 4-6. High-grade squamous intraepithelial lesions. Cytology shows atypia in immature cells, with marked increase in the nuclear to cytoplasmic ratio.

addition, there may be marked variability in nuclear size (anisonucleosis) (Figure 4-8).

Included in the differential diagnosis of CIN2, CIN3 is immature metaplasia and atrophy, the 2 most common lesions mistaken for dysplasia. Although there is a lack of maturity in the epithelium of immature metaplasia and there is a high nuclear-to-cytoplasmic ratio, the absence of nuclear pleomorphism helps to differentiate this lesion from high-grade dysplasia. Immature metaplasia does not contain abnormal mitoses. Additionally there may be mucinous epithelium on the surface of immature metaplastic squamous epithelium, this is rarely seen in high-grade dysplasia. Atrophic epithelium may be mistaken for high-grade dysplasia. Although atrophic epithelium has high nuclear-to-cytoplasmic ratio, atrophic epithelium is thin and shows no nuclear pleomorphism, mitotic activity, atypia, or lack of polarity. Often a repeat biopsy after a trial of vaginal estrogen therapy may help clarify this difference; vaginal estrogen will not alter the histologic appearance of CIN2 or 3.

Adenocarcinoma in situ (ACIS) demonstrates histologic features including preservation of normal glandular architecture and involvement of part or all of the epithelium by enlarged, hyperchromatic, stratified nuclei with coarse chromatin, small nucleoli, mitoses, and apoptosis. The cytoplasm can be depleted or abundant, vacuolated, granular and basophilic, or eosinophilic (Figure 4-9). This histology may frequently coincide with a squamous intraepithelial lesion. It is often difficult to identify these lesions because they

CHAPTER 4

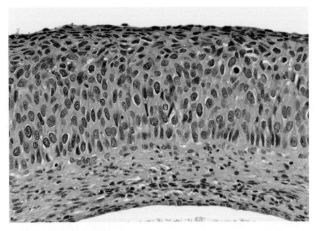

FIGURE 4-8. CIN2 and 3. Abnormal, atypical cells are limited to the lower two-thirds of the epidermal layer for CIN2; for CIN3, atypical cells extend more than two-thirds from the basement membrane.

are located high in the endocervical canal and the cytologic criteria for identifying neoplastic glandular lesions is less clear. An important feature of these glandular lesions is that they may be multicentric. Several foci of ACIS may coexist and be interspersed with normal epithelium within the glandular architecture, leading to histologic findings of "skip lesions."

Vulvar Dysplasia

The histologic diagnosis of premalignant lesions of the vulva is referred to as VIN with a 3-level system: VIN1, 2, and 3. As seen in CIN, VIN is graded into 1 of these 3 levels depending on the level of involvement of the affected epidermis by cellular disarray, atypia, and mitotic activity. In VIN1 (mild dysplasia), the lowest third of the epidermis is involved. In VIN2 (moderate dysplasia), the lower two-thirds are involved, and in VIN3 (severe dysplasia/carcinoma in situ), more than two-thirds of the epithelium are involved. The affected epidermis is apparent when epithelial cells have a high nuclear-to-cytoplasmic ratio and lack cytoplasmic maturation above the basal and parabasal layers. Mitotic figures are present above the basal layer, and multinucleation and dyskeratosis may be seen, often including formation of intraepithelial squamous pearls. The presence of abnormal mitoses is almost always seen in VIN2 and 3 (Figure 4-10).

The grading system for VIN parallels that of cervical dysplasia. However, whereas CIN1 lesions of the cervix are relatively common, VIN1 lesions are rare, as most lesions are diagnosed as VIN2 or 3. Another difference between CIN and VIN is that the origin of atypical

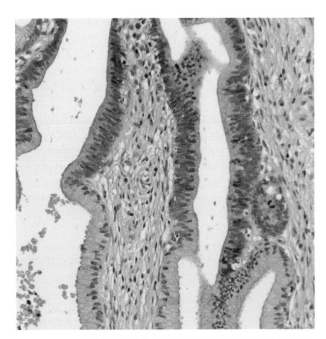

FIGURE 4-9. Adenocarcinoma in situ. Normal glandular architecture is preserved, but atypical cells involve the epithelium. Lesions may be multicentric and interspersed with normal glandular epithelium.

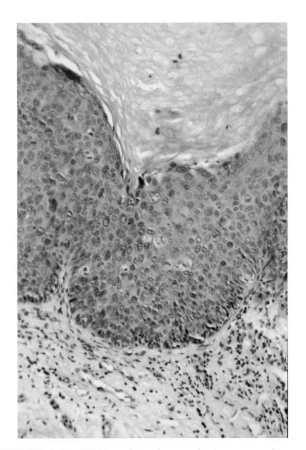

FIGURE 4-10. VIN2 and 3. Abnormal mitoses are characteristic for high-grade vulvar dysplasia.

cells in CIN develops from the endocervical glandular mucosa and the metaplastic squamous epithelium of the transformation zone. VIN originates from mature stratified squamous epithelium of vulvar epidermis or squamous mucosa. In this way there are often more pathologic similarities of VIN to premalignant squamous lesions of the oral cavity and vocal cords.

There are 2 variants of the usual type of VIN, basaloid and warty. The basaloid variant is similar to CIN in its morphology of epithelial changes. There is very little maturation of the keratinocytes, except some keratinization or parakeratosis, which may be seen at the surface. It is associated with uniform, small cells that have hyperchromatic and coarse nuclear chromatin.

The warty variant has larger cells, pleomorphic nuclei, and abnormal mitotic figures. There is often the presence of a prominent granular layer. The nuclear chromatin is clumped and coarse without evidence of nucleoli, despite the presence of mitotic figures. The surface has features similar to condyloma acuminatum with koilocytosis and multinucleation.

The differentiated type of VIN has a thickened epithelium with the presence of parakeratosis. The keratinocytes tend to be large and pleomorphic, with eosinophilic cytoplasm in the cells within the basal and parabasal layer in the base of rete ridges. Within the rete, there is sometimes the presence of keratin pearl formation. Nuclear chromatin is often vesicular with prominent nucleoli, most prominent in the basal and parabasal layers.

Included in the differential diagnosis of VIN are basal cell carcinoma, superficial spreading malignant melanoma, Paget disease, pagetoid urothelial intraepithelial neoplasia, and multinucleated atypia of the vulva. Specifically, differentiated VIN can be mistaken for atypical squamous cell hyperplasia, and the discrimination can be made by evidence of eosinophilic cytoplasm at the base of the rete ridges in differentiated VIN. Immunoperoxidase staining can differentiate the presence of Paget disease or melanoma: Paget disease will stain positive for mucin with mucicarmine stain and stain positive for carcinoembryonic antigen and cytokeratin; melanoma in situ will stain positive for S-100 protein, HMB-45, and Melan-A. An important issue to consider in the evaluation of VIN is that the application of podophyllin on condyloma acuminata on the vulva will cause mitotic arrest, which can easily be misinterpreted as VIN. Therefore, biopsy should be obtained at least after 1 to 2 weeks from the last application of podophyllin.

Squamous histology is the most common histology of premalignant disorders of the vulva. However, glandular histologies are present in vulvar extramammary Paget disease and Bartholin gland tumors (as well as other tumors that arise from other skin appendages,

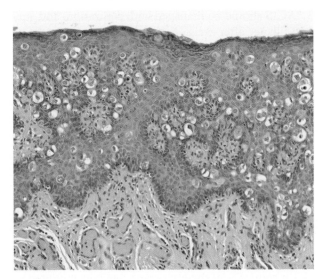

FIGURE 4-11.   Paget disease of the vulva. Paget cells are intraepidermal with abundant pale cytoplasm; they may appear singly, in small clusters, or in large nests.

the urethra, and the Skene gland). Seen primarily in postmenopausal women, Paget disease presents often as multifocal, well-demarcated, scaly, velvet-like, moist, eczematous plaques dotted with small, pale islands. Vulvar Paget disease is primarily an intraepithelial lesion, but has the potential for dermal invasion (4%-26%) and is sometimes associated with an underlying adenocarcinoma (in up to 25% of cases). Frequently, lesions extend beyond the clinically apparent margins and may require extensive surgical resection. Because of this, positive margins are frequent and may account for a high rate of recurrence.

Histologically, Paget cells are large intraepidermal cells with a large nucleus with prominent nucleolus and abundant clear, pale cytoplasm, which stain positive for mucin. These cells may appear singly, in small clusters, or in large nests and may extend into the surrounding hair shafts and skin appendages (Figure 4-11).

TREATMENT

Key Points

1. The mainstay of treatment of high-grade CIN, VIN, and VAIN is surgical excision, although size and number of lesions in VIN and VAIN may influence decisions to treat with topical therapies or CO_2 laser ablation.
2. CIN2 in compliant adolescent and young women may be managed with close surveillance instead of excisional biopsy.

3. ACIS should be managed with conization, and surveillance after excision appears to be safe if margins are negative for disease.

Management of Cervical Cytologic Abnormalities

The American Society for Colposcopy and Cervical Pathology (ASCCP), together with partner organizations and collaborators from the National Institutes of Health, have developed consensus guidelines for the treatment of women with abnormal cervical cancer screening tests, as well as guidelines for the management of CIN or ACIS.[14] The following sections provide a summary of the important concepts included in the most recent full sets of guidelines.

Management of Atypical Squamous Cells

In women older than 20 years of age, the cytologic findings of ASC-US should be managed by DNA testing for high-risk types of HPV. As reported in the ASCUS-LSIL Triage Study (ALTS), women with ASC-US who are high-risk HPV negative can be followed up with repeat cytologic testing in 12 months. In a setting where specific high-risk types are reported, it is recommended to triage women who are positive for types 16 and 18 to colposcopy, whereas women positive for other, less carcinogenic high-risk types, can be followed up with cytologic testing in 12 months (similar to women who are negative for any high-risk type).[15]

Women with ASC-US and who are high-risk type positive (where specific typing is not available) or are specifically HPV16 or 18 positive, as well as women with ASC-H Pap results, should be referred for colposcopic evaluation. Endocervical curettage is preferred for women in whom no lesions are identified or for whom colposcopy is unsatisfactory. When CIN is not identified in these women, acceptable follow-up includes repeat HPV DNA testing at 12 months or cytologic testing at 6 and 12 months, depending on the situation.

An important population in which to discuss the management of Pap test results is adolescent women. Because of the high prevalence of high-risk HPV in this population and the high likelihood for moderate and severe dysplasia to regress, it is recommend that ASC-US be followed with repeat cytology in 12 months. This is the same for ASC-H and LSIL in this population. The guidelines recommend that for adolescents (girls age 20 years and younger), only those with HSIL Pap results be referred for colposcopy.

Management of Low- and High-Grade Squamous Intraepithelial Lesions

In general, women with LSIL and HSIL lesions should be referred for colposcopy. For women with LSIL, if no dysplasia is identified, then surveillance can be performed with testing for high-risk HPV DNA at 12 months or repeat cervical cytology at 6 and 12 months. If the DNA test is negative or if 2 consecutive repeat cytologic tests are negative, then the patient can return to routine cytologic screening. Adolescents with LSIL should not be referred to colposcopy and should be re-screened in 12 months.[16] Postmenopausal women with LSIL can be managed with testing for high-risk HPV with those positive referred for colposcopy and repeat Pap testing at 6 and 12 months. If no abnormalities are found on either of these screens, then return to routine annual screening is safe.

HSIL Pap results are associated with a greater than 50% to 60% risk for high-grade cervical dysplasia. In young women, many of these lesions will spontaneously regress. Nonetheless, in nonadolescents, advanced "see and treat" management options based on cytology results may be appropriate. Options include immediate loop electrosurgical excision (LEEP) or colposcopy with endocervical assessment and directed biopsies. When CIN2 or CIN3 is not identified histologically, then a diagnostic excision procedure or observation with colposcopy and cytology at 6-month intervals for 1 year is acceptable. A diagnostic excisional procedure is recommended in women with HSIL Pap results who also have unsatisfactory colposcopy.

In adolescents with HSIL, immediate referral to colposcopy is the appropriate management. It is not acceptable to perform immediate LEEP on adolescents. When CIN2 or 3 is not identified histologically, then observation for up to 24 months using colposcopy and cytology at 6-month intervals is preferred. If HSIL persists for 24 months, without identification of CIN, then a diagnostic excisional procedure is recommended. After 2 negative cytologic screens, adolescents can return to routine annual screening.

Management of Atypical Glandular Cells

Atypical glandular cells (AGC) is a rare Pap test diagnosis, but it may be associated with an invasive cancer between 3% and 17% of the time.[6] Because this diagnosis can be associated with many different neoplastic entities, the initial evaluation includes multiple tests. Colposcopy with endocervical curettage should be performed for all women with AGC. In women older than 35 years of age, endometrial biopsy should also be performed. In women younger than 35 years with findings that suggest a risk for endometrial cancer, such as irregular vaginal bleeding or chronic anovulation, endometrial biopsy should be performed. HPV testing should be performed at the time of colposcopy in women with atypical endocervical, endometrial, or glandular cells not otherwise specified.

If colposcopy and biopsies are negative after AGC Pap diagnosis, then the recommended follow-up is repeat cytology and HPV DNA testing at 6 months for women who were positive for high-risk HPV and at 12 months for women who were HPV DNA negative. If on subsequent testing they are found to be high-risk HPV positive or have ASC-US or greater abnormality on cytology, then they should be referred for colposcopy. If both tests are negative, then women can be returned to annual cytologic screening.

Management of Cervical Histologic Abnormalities

There are many treatment modalities that are used once a histologic diagnosis of dysplasia has been established. These can be divided into 2 broad categories: ablative techniques and excisional techniques. Ablative techniques destroy the abnormal cells without removing tissue, and such procedures include cryotherapy, laser ablation, and electrofulguration. Excisional techniques include cold-knife conization, LEEP, and laser conization. A recent Cochrane review of these various treatment modalities found similar effectiveness and side effects with ablative procedures of cryotherapy and laser ablation. Risk of residual dysplasia and recurrence appear to be similar. In similar fashion, the excisional procedures are equally effective. The immediate side effects of the procedure—hemorrhage, infection, and vaginal discharge—are similar for each modality.[17]

The most important long-term side effect of excisional procedures is related to pregnancy. These include an increased risk of preterm labor, low-birth-weight infants, and cesarean section. Pregnancy complications have been recognized as a potential outcome of cold-knife cone biopsies for some time. Recent studies have demonstrated a greater frequency of these outcomes than once suspected and that after just 1 procedure, women are at an increased risk for pregnancy complications. There is increasing evidence that LEEP procedures are also associated with an increased risk of pregnancy complications, including an up to 3-fold increase in the risk of preterm delivery.[18]

CIN1

As described earlier, most CIN1 lesions will spontaneously regress without treatment. Progression of CIN1 lesions to CIN2/3 is uncommon. In the ALTS trial, the risk of subsequent diagnosis of CIN2/3 within

2 years of a CIN1 diagnosis was 13%, almost identical the risk of CIN2/3 within 2 years from a normal cervical biopsy (12%).[15] Based on this understanding, the recommendations for management of CIN1 are related to the abnormal Pap test that first led to the colposcopy referral. In cases in which the CIN1 diagnosis was preceded by ASC-US, ASC-H, or LSIL, the recommended management is surveillance with HPV DNA testing every 12 months or repeat cervical cytology every 6 to 12 months. If a patient has persistent CIN1 for 2 years, surveillance or treatment are acceptable options. In this setting either ablation or excisional techniques may be performed. However, if the preceding colposcopic examination is unsatisfactory, the endocervical sample contains CIN, or the patient has been previously treated, then an excisional procedure should be performed.

When a CIN1 diagnosis is preceded by an HSIL or ACG Pap test, either an excisional procedure or observation with colposcopy and cytology at 6-month intervals for 1 year are acceptable options. If colposcopy is unsatisfactory or endocervical curettage is positive for dysplasia, then an excisional procedure is recommended. If during the observation period a repeat Pap test shows HSIL or AGC, then an excisional procedure should be performed. If during the year of observation there are 2 sequential Pap tests that are negative, then the patient can return to routine screening. Hysterectomy should not be considered as the initial treatment for CIN1.

CIN2 or 3

In general, lesions categorized as CIN2 are more likely to regress spontaneously than CIN 3 lesions. However, there is considerable variability in the categorization of the lesions between various pathologists. Based on this, treatment recommendations consider CIN2 as the threshold for recommending treatment, as there is risk for progression to CIN3 and invasive cancer.

Excision or surveillance may be considered in the treatment of CIN2 or 3, depending on the age of the patient. Young women have more robust immune systems, and thus surveillance of CIN2 is acceptable due to the higher rates of regression and risks of pregnancy complications with excisional procedures. These recommendations are supported by a prospective study of young women ages 13 to 24 years with CIN2. In 95 patients, 38% were observed to demonstrate resolution at 1 year, 63% by year 2, and 68% by year 3.[19] Thus, in compliant adolescent patients, CIN2 may be managed with 6-month cytology and colposcopy.[16] For noncompliant or immunosuppressed patients, or in those for whom fertility is not desired, excisional biopsy is recommended.

CIN3 should be managed with excisional biopsy. In these situations, LEEP or conization is both therapeutic and diagnostic. The rationale for excision of CIN3 is underscored by the risks of progression to invasive disease, which is classically described as 12%.[20]

Surveillance after the treatment of CIN2 or 3 can be performed by testing for the presence of high-risk HPV types at 6- to 12-month intervals or cytology alone or cytology with colposcopy at 6-month intervals. If patients are found to have high-risk HPV, or abnormal cytology of ASC-US or greater, colposcopy is then recommended. After 2 consecutive negative screens, patients can return to annual screening and should continue to have screening for the subsequent 20 years. In women found to have positive margins on their excisional biopsy specimen, repeat testing at 4 to 6 months is the preferred management. Immediate re-excision is not necessary, as 50% to 60% of women with positive margins after LEEP or conization will not demonstrate recurrence on subsequent surveillance Pap testing.[21,22]

ACIS

Women with ACIS diagnosed on cervical biopsy should undergo conization to exclude the possibility of invasive adenocarcinoma. In the past, the management of ACIS was somewhat controversial due to the "skip lesions" that can be characteristic of this disease, and subsequent extrafascial hysterectomy was traditionally recommended due to the possibility of residual ACIS, even with negative surgical cone margins. These recommendations were based on studies suggesting up to a 19% incidence of identifying ACIS on hysterectomy specimens after a cone biopsy with negative margins.[23]

More recent data suggest that conservative management is a safe option in women who desire uterine preservation. A large meta-analysis of 671 women followed with surveillance only after a diagnosis of ACIS on cone biopsy identified only a 2.6% rate of recurrence with negative margins and a 19.4% rate of recurrence with positive margins.[24] In this same study, invasive adenocarcinoma was more commonly associated with positive margins (5.2%) compared with negative margins (0.1%). These data support surveillance of women with ACIS and negative margins and consideration of hysterectomy versus re-excision if positive margins are identified at cone biopsy.

Management of Vulvar and Vaginal Dysplasia

Various treatment modalities are used in the management of VIN and VAIN and include topical agents, laser ablation, radiotherapy, and surgical excision. Prospective trials demonstrating the most effective treatment modality for these disease sites are limited, and treatment typically is recommended based on disease and patient factors such as size and number of lesions, as well as performance status of the patient.

Topical agents are noninvasive treatments that can be applied by the patient directly to the dysplastic lesion or to the entire vulvar and/or vaginal mucosal surface. In general, these agents are the recommended therapy for persistent low-grade lesions and multifocal disease, as well as for women who are poor surgical candidates. Five percent imiquimod cream is currently the most commonly used topical agent for the treatment of VIN. It is a topical immune-response modifier that affects local cytokine production and cell-mediated immunity. Two randomized controlled trials have shown that imiquimod is more effective than placebo. Mathiesen and colleagues[25] randomized 32 women with VIN2 or 3 to imiquimod versus placebo and found an 81% complete response rate and 10% partial response rate 2 months after the completion of 16 weeks of treatment. Similarly, van Seters and colleagues[26] demonstrated at least partial response in 81% and a complete response in 35% of 26 women treated with imiquimod. Imiquimod is usually applied on the affected area 2 to 3 times per week, for a total of 16 weeks. Up to two-thirds of patients reduce the frequency or length of treatment due to local side effects of erythema or erosions. Imiquimod has also been examined as a potential topical therapy in the vagina. Use of 1 sachet of 5% cream (0.25 g) once or twice weekly has been shown to induce complete resolution of low-grade VAIN lesions after 1 to 3 treatment cycles. Importantly, vulvar or vestibular excoriation was only reported in 2 of the 56 patients, and none demonstrated vaginal ulceration.[27] For high-grade lesions, a smaller cohort identified an 86% chance of resolution to normal or VAIN1 after use of imiquimod.[28]

Five-fluorouracil (5-FU) cream is another topical agent that induces a chemical degradation of the dysplastic lesion. For VIN, 5-FU is associated with response rates up to 75%; however, local side effects are significantly more severe as compared with imiquimod, with severe inflammation lasting for up to 2 weeks after the completion of a 6- to 10-week course. In the vagina, suppositories of 5% 5-FU may be used once to twice daily for 5 to 14 days or once weekly for 10 weeks. Small cohort studies suggest recurrence rates ranging from 9% to 54%, although completion of therapy has also been limited by the potentially severe side effect of mucosal excoriation.[29,30]

CO_2 laser ablation has shown excellent success for the treatment of both VIN and VAIN. It is well tolerated and results in minimal sexual dysfunction. For VIN, success rates after a single laser treatment are approximately 75%. VIN lesions should be ablated to a depth of 1 mm for non-hairy lesions and 3 mm for hairy lesions. For high-grade VAIN, laser ablation is associated with a curate rate of 69%.[29] Because tissue is not evaluated histologically with laser ablation, biopsies of vulvar and vaginal lesions should be performed preoperatively to exclude invasive disease.

Intracavitary radiation therapy is a modality shown to be effective for the treatment of VAIN. However, radiation is associated with relatively greater morbidity, including vaginal atrophy, stenosis, and shortening. This modality is generally reserved for patients who have failed other therapies, are poor surgical candidates, or have extensive multifocal disease. Small series have examined low-dose-rate vaginal brachytherapy for VAIN3 using personalized vaginal molds with delivery of 60 Gy to 5 mm below the vaginal mucosa. In 28 patients, only 1 recurrence was observed, corresponding to a 5-year local control rate of 93%.[31]

Surgical resection remains the mainstay of the treatment of VIN and VAIN. This modality has several advantages, including removal of diseased tissue while obtaining a histologic diagnosis of the entire lesion of interest. Depending on the extent of disease, surgical excision can be as minimal as a wide local excision or as extensive as a total vulvectomy or vaginectomy. Wide local excision of dysplastic lesions should be performed with a 5-mm margin and is ideal for localized lesions. Primary end-to-end reapproximation of the defect can usually be performed with interrupted dissolvable sutures. Skinning vulvectomy is reserved for large, extensive, or multifocal lesions. This procedure involves the removal of the vulvar skin along the avascular plane beneath the epidermis while preserving the subcutaneous tissue. The defect may require closure with a split-thickness skin graft. For high-grade VAIN lesions, wide local excisions should similarly be performed with a 5-mm margin; curative success with excision of VAIN3 has been reported as 69%.[29]

PREVENTION

In June 2006, the US Food and Drug Administration approved the first vaccine for the prevention of infection from HPV. Today there are 2 commercially available prophylactic HPV vaccines. Both consist of L1 capsid proteins made from recombinant DNA. Each also contains its unique adjuvant to assist in the immune response necessary to induce long-term protection from HPV infection. Gardasil (Merck Corporation) is a quadrivalent vaccine with antigens that mimic the L1 capsid of HPV types 6 and 11, included to decrease the risk of external genital warts, and HPV types 16 and 18, included to decrease the risk of high-grade dysplasia and ultimately cancer. Cervarix (GlaxoSmithKline) is a bivalent vaccine that is made up of the L1 capsid proteins from HPV types 16 and 18.

Both vaccines are effective in preventing HPV16 and 18 infections and the associated high-grade CIN in women ages 15 to 26 years who do not have HPV infection at the time of vaccination.[32,33] Neither shows therapeutic efficacy against current infection. In addition, the quadrivalent vaccine has been shown to prevent VIN and VAIN, as well as genital warts. Although 70% of cervical cancers and 50% of CIN2 and 3 lesions are associated with HPV types 16 and 18, only 35% of LSIL are associated with HPV types 16 and 18. For this reason, it is not anticipated that HPV vaccination will have a major impact on the number of abnormal Pap test results. The full duration of immunity after HPV vaccination is unknown. Phase 2 data provide the longest follow-up data and suggest that immunity persists for at least 5 years for the quadrivalent vaccine and 8.4 years for the bivalent vaccine. In general, HPV vaccination is safe. The only adverse events that were seen in increasing frequency in subjects participating in randomized trials of the vaccines were related to injection site reactions that included erythema, pain, and irritation. An important component of assessing vaccine safety are the post-treatment surveillance registries that specifically monitor any adverse events that occur after vaccination. Uncomplicated syncope has been the most frequently observed adverse event after vaccination. These registries will play a role in identifying any long-term side effects of vaccination. Finally, more recent studies have addressed the efficacy of vaccination in boys and older adult women and will assist in shaping public policy on HPV vaccination recommendations.

PROGNOSIS AND MANAGEMENT OF RECURRENCE

Key Points

1. Surveillance after treatment for CIN, VIN, or VAIN should include routine screening after the post-treatment period.
2. Risk factors for recurrence include positive margins of the excisional biopsy, smoking, immunosuppression, and multifocal disease.

After treatment for cervical, vulvar, or vaginal dysplasia, patients should be monitored closely for evidence of recurrence. There are consensus guidelines for post-treatment surveillance of cervical dysplasia. A recent study of more than 37,000 women treated for CIN1, 2, or 3 has demonstrated that these patients remain at risk for recurrent dysplasia and cervical cancer after treatment. The risk of recurrence is greatest in women treated for CIN2 or 3. The risk of developing recurrent CIN2/3 within the first 6 years after treatment was 9% in women previously treated for CIN3 and 6% in women treated for CIN2. The risk of recurrence was associated with older age at diagnosis and was associated with treatment type, with highest risk in women treated for CIN3 with cryotherapy. The overall incidence of cancer in the cohort of women treated for any dysplasia was 37 cancers per 100,000 woman-years, compared with 6 cancers in a comparison group of women with no history of cervical dysplasia. It is important to strongly encourage women treated for CIN2 and 3 to continue to participate in routine screening programs even after the immediate post-treatment surveillance period.[34]

The clinical course of VIN is varied, and evidence has shown that it may progress, resolve, or become persistent. Differentiated type VIN is more than 5 times more aggressive than usual type VIN, with a rate of 32.8% progression to invasive squamous cell carcinoma in differentiated VIN, as compared with 5.7% progression in usual type after 14 years of follow-up.[35] A meta-analysis showed that untreated VIN3 overall has a 9% rate of progression to invasive vulvar carcinoma in women followed up over 12 to 96 months. In patients who were treated for VIN3, the rate of progression was 3.3%.[36]

At least one-third of patients with VIN will recur regardless of treatment modality, and women should receive long-term follow-up with surveillance of the entire lower genital tract every 6 months for 5 years, and then annually. Risk factors for recurrent disease include cigarette smoking, immunosuppression, multifocal disease, and positive margins on surgical excision. If excisional biopsy has been performed with positive margins, there is 3 times the risk of recurrence as compared with negative margins. For recurrent disease, the recommended treatment takes into consideration the same factors as for primary disease. Surgical excision is preferred, but if this is not feasible because of multiple prior excisions, or if the patient is not an optimal surgical candidate, then topical and laser treatment should be considered after biopsies have excluded invasive carcinoma.

FUTURE DIRECTIONS: HPV AND BIOMARKER DETECTION AS PRIMARY SCREENING

Despite the enormous impact that the Pap test and current management algorithms have had in reducing the burden of cervical cancer in developed countries, the application of this potentially costly and inefficient program is not applicable in poor and underdeveloped parts of the world. A potential approach to addressing this challenge is the development of a cost-effective cervical cancer screening approach that replaces or augments Pap testing. In general, these efforts have focused on HPV detection as a primary tool for cervical cancer screening. HPV testing is presently incorporated into algorithms for triage of women with equivocal cytologic abnormalities, follow-up of women with abnormal screening results, and in determining cervical cancer risk to individualize frequency of Pap testing. Studies also support the use of HPV detection to predict the therapeutic outcome after treatment for CIN. Meta-analyses demonstrate that primary screening for cervical cancer by HPV detection, using various methods of detection, identifies more than 90% of all CIN2, CIN3, or cancer and is 25% more sensitive than cytology alone. However, this approach is also associated with a 6% reduction in specificity, which leads to increased triage to additional testing and affects the cost-effectiveness gained by the improved sensitivity.[37] Recent large studies have attempted to address the reduction in specificity (or positive predictive value) by altering the cutoff for HPV positivity or altering the sequence and components of screening tests and algorithms. In women ages 35 to 60 years, it has been demonstrated that HPV detection (with a cutoff for positive HPV DNA of 2 pg/mL) is 80% more sensitive than conventional Pap testing, and the positive predictive value is essentially unchanged.[38] Another strategy that has improved sensitivity without compromising positive predictive value is primary screening with HPV DNA testing followed by cytologic triage and repeat HPV DNA testing of HPV-positive women whose subsequent cytologic examination was normal. With this algorithm, HPV testing was shown to be 30% more sensitive than conventional Pap testing, with a relatively small decrease in positive predictive value. This approach, however, still resulted in a 12% increase in the number of cytologic tests.[39] Other approaches to molecular testing that are currently being evaluated deal with the decreased sensitivity of HPV DNA detection and include HPV typing for HPV types 16, 18, and 45; testing for markers of proliferative lesions by detection of p16 (a protein that is upregulated downstream of E7 inhibition of pRB activity); and mRNA coding for the viral oncogenes E6 and E7. Several studies have outlined the principles of these screening tests; however, the details and cost-efficacy are still under investigation, and the exact role of these new tests is yet to be defined.

With these advances in HPV testing, the incidence of lower genital tract dysplasias and malignancies may be significantly reduced. Much work is still necessary to target women who do not have access to medical care, both in the United States and in developing nations. Until widespread screening can be implemented, cervical, vulvar, and vaginal dysplasia will still be a significant clinical burden to women worldwide.

REFERENCES

1. Dunne EF, Unger ER, Sternberg M, et al. Prevalence of HPV infection among females in the United States. *JAMA.* 2007;297(8):813-819.

2. Wheeler CM. Natural history of human papillomavirus infections, cytologic and histologic abnormalities, and cancer. *Obstet Gynecol Clin North Am.* 2008;35(4):519-536; vii.

3. Judson PL, Habermann EB, Baxter NN, Durham SB, Virnig BA. Trends in the incidence of invasive and in situ vulvar carcinoma. *Obstet Gynecol.* 2006;107:1018-1022.

4. Heller DS. Report of a new ISSVD classification of VIN. *J Lower Gen Tract Dis.* 2007;11:46-47.

5. Yetimalar H, Kasap B, Cukurova K, Yildiz A, Keklik A, Soylu F. Cofactors in human papillomavirus infection and cervical carcinogenesis. *Arch Gynecol Obstet.* 2011 Aug 10. [Epub ahead of print]

6. Moodley M, Moodley J, Chetty R, Herrington CS. The role of steroid contraceptive hormones in the pathogenesis of invasive cervical cancer: a review. *Int J Gynecol Cancer.* 2003;13(2):103-110.

7. Massad LS, Seaberg EC, Wright RL, et al. Squamous cervical lesions in women with human immunodeficiency virus: long-term follow-up. *Obstet Gynecol.* 2008;111(6):1388-1393.

8. Tjalma WA, Van Waes TR, Van den Eeden LE, Bogers JJ. Role of human papillomavirus in the carcinogenesis of squamous cell carcinoma and adenocarcinoma of the cervix. *Best Pract Res Clin Obstet Gynaecol.* 2005;19(4):469-483.

9. Terlou A, Blok LJ, Helmerhorst TJ, van Beurden M. Premalignant epithelial disorders of the vulva: squamous vulvar intraepithelial neoplasia, vulvar Paget's disease and melanoma in situ. *Acta Obstet Gynecol Scand.* 2010;89(6):741-748.

10. Kennedy CM, Peterson LB, Galask RP. Erosive vulvar lichen planus: a cohort at risk for cancer? *J Repro Med.* 2008;53:781-784.

11. Siebers AG, Klinkhamer PJ, Grefte JM, et al. Comparison of liquid-based cytology with conventional cytology for detection of cervical cancer precursors: a randomized controlled trial. *JAMA.* 2009;302(16):1757-1764.

12. Smith RA, Cokkinides V, Brooks D, Saslow D, Brawley OW. Cancer screening in the United States, 2010: a review of current American Cancer Society guidelines and issues in cancer screening. *CA Cancer J Clin.* 2010;60(2):99-119.

13. Apgar BS, Zoschnick L, Wright TC Jr. The 2001 Bethesda System terminology. *Am Fam Physician.* 2003;68(10):1992-1998.

14. Wright TC Jr, Massad LS, Dunton CJ, et al. 2006 consensus guidelines for the management of women with abnormal cervical cancer screening tests. *Am J Obstet Gynecol.* 2007;197(4):346-355.

15. Solomon D, Schiffman M, Tarone R, ALTS Study Group. Comparison of three management strategies for patients with atypical squamous cells of undetermined significance: baseline results from a randomized trial. *J Natl Cancer Inst.* 2001;93(4):293-299.

16. Moscicki AB. Conservative management of management of adolescents with abnormal cytology and histology. *J Natl Compr Cancer Netw.* 2008;6:101-106.

17. Martin-Hirsch PL, Paraskevaidis E, Kitchener H. Surgery for cervical intraepithelial neoplasia. *Cochrane Database Syst Rev.* 2000(2):CD001318.

18. Jakobsson M, Gissler M, Paavonen J, Tapper AM. Loop electrosurgical excision procedure and the risk for preterm birth. *Obstet Gynecol.* 2009;114(3):504-510.

19. Moscicki AB, Ma Y, Wibbelsman C, et al. Rate of and risks for regression of cervical intraepithelial neoplasia 2 in adolescents and young women. *Obstet Gynecol.* 2010;116:1373-1380.

20. Ostor AG. Natural history of cervical intraepithelial neoplasia: a critical review. *Int J Gynecol Pathol.* 1993;12:186.

21. Livasy CA, Maygarden SJ, Rajaratnam CT, Novotny DB. Predictors of recurrent dysplasia after a cervical loop electrocautery excision procedure for CIN-3: a study of margin, endocervical gland, and quadrant involvement. *Mod Pathol.* 1999;12:233-238.

22. Maluf PJ, Adad SJ, Murta EF. Outcome after conization of cervical intraepithelial neoplasia grade III: relation with surgical margins, extension to the crypts and mitoses. *Tumori.* 2004;90:473-477.

23. McHale MT, Le TD, Burger RA, Gu M, Rutgers JL, Monk BJ. Fertility sparing treatment for in situ and early invasive adenocarcinoma of the cervix. *Obstet Gynecol* 2001;98:726-731.

24. Salani R, Puri I, Bristow RE. Adenocarcinoma in situ of the uterine cervix: a metaanalysis of 1278 patients evaluating the predictive value of conization margin status. *Am J Obstet Gynecol.* 2009;200(2):182.e1-5.

25. Mathiesen O, Buus SK, Cramers M. Topical imiquimod can reverse vulvar intraepithelial neoplasia: a randomised, double-blinded study. *Gynecol Oncol.* 2007;107(2):219-222.

26. van Seters M, van Beurden M, ten Kate FJ, et al. Treatment with vulvar intraepithelial neoplasia with topical imiquimod. *N Engl J Med.* 2008;358:1465-1473.

27. Buck HW, Guth KJ. Treatment of vaginal intraepithelial neoplasia (primarily low grade) with imiquimod 5% cream. *J Low Genit Tract Dis.* 2003;7:290-933.

28. Haidopoulos D, Diakomanolis E, Rodolakis A, Voulgaris Z, Vlachos G, Intsaklis A. Can local application of imiquimod cream be an alternative mode of therapy for patients with high-grade intraepithelial lesions of the vagina? *Int J Gynecol Cancer.* 2005;15:898-902.

29. Rome RM, England PG. Management of vaginal intraepithelial neoplasia: a series of 132 cases with long-term follow-up. *Int J Gynecol Cancer.* 2000;10:382-390.

30. Kirwan P, Naftalin NJ. Topical 5-fluorouracil in the treatment of vaginal intraepithelial neoplasia. *Br J Obstet Gynaecol.* 1985;92:287-291.

31. Blanchard P, Monnier L, Dumas I, et al. Low-dose-rate definitive brachytherapy for high-grade vaginal intraepithelial neoplasia. *Oncologist.* 2011;16:182-188.

32. Garland SM, Hernandez-Avila M, Wheeler CM, et al. Quadrivalent vaccine against human papillomavirus to prevent anogenital diseases. *N Engl J Med.* 2007;356(19):1928-1943.

33. Paavonen J, Naud P, Salmerón J, et al. Efficacy of human papillomavirus (HPV)-16/18 AS04-adjuvanted vaccine against cervical infection and precancer caused by oncogenic HPV types (PATRICIA): final analysis of a double-blind, randomised study in young women. *Lancet.* 2009;374(9686):301-314.

34. Melnikow J, McGahan C, Sawaya GF, Ehlen T, Coldman A. Cervical intraepithelial neoplasia outcomes after treatment: long-term follow-up from the British Columbia Cohort Study. *J Natl Cancer Inst.* 2009;101(10):721-728.

35. van de Nieuwenhof HP, Massuger LF, van der Avoort IA, et al. Vulvar squamous cell carcinoma development after diagnosis of VIN increases with age. *Eur J Cancer.* 2009;45:851-856.

36. van Seters M, van Buerden M, de Craen AJ. Is the assumed natural history of vulvar intraepithelial neoplasia III based on enough evidence? A systematic review of 3322 published patients. *Gynecol Oncol.* 2005;97:645-651.

37. Cuzick J, Arbyn M, Sankaranarayanan R, et al. Overview of human papillomavirus-based and other novel options for cervical cancer screening in developed and developing countries. *Vaccine.* 2008;26(suppl 10):K29-K41.

38. Ronco G, Giorgi-Rossi P, Carozzi F, et al. Results at recruitment from a randomized controlled trial comparing human papillomavirus testing alone with conventional cytology as the primary cervical cancer screening test. *J Natl Cancer Inst.* 2008;100(7):492-501.

39. Naucler P, Ryd W, Törnberg S, et al. Efficacy of HPV DNA testing with cytology triage and/or repeat HPV DNA testing in primary cervical cancer screening. *J Natl Cancer Inst.* 2009;101(2):88-99.

CHAPTER 4

Cervical Cancer

Angela J. Ziebarth, Kenneth H. Kim, and Warner K. Huh

Cervical cancer is one of the most common cancers in women worldwide. Nearly all invasive squamous cell carcinomas are preceded by persistent human papillomavirus (HPV) infection and cervical intraepithelial neoplasia (CIN), and vast improvements in screening over the last 60 years have dramatically lowered the incidence of invasive disease in the developed world. Localized and some advanced cervical cancers in the United States have excellent prognoses, yet in developing countries, this disease remains the most lethal malignancy in women.

EPIDEMIOLOGY

Key Points

1. Minority and low-socioeconomic status patients are still at risk for developing cervical cancer in the United States due to lack of screening and early treatment.
2. The largest risk factor for cervical cancer is persistent HPV infection. Other risk factors include history of sexually transmitted diseases, multiple sexual partners, high parity, immunosuppression, and smoking.
3. The HPV oncoproteins E6 and E7 bind and inactivate the tumor suppressor genes *p53* and *pRB*, respectively, which contributes to cervical carcinogenesis.

Incidence

Cervical cancer is the third most common cancer in women worldwide, with more than 450,000 cases diagnosed annually. Developed countries have demonstrated a decreasing incidence and mortality from squamous cervical cancers over the last 50 years. This is likely due to improved access to screening, decreasing parity, and lower baseline prevalence of HPV. Adenocarcinomas of the cervix account for approximately 15% of cervical cancers in the United States and have risen slightly over the last 20 to 30 years. The recent availability of an HPV vaccine has been shown to decrease the incidence of high-grade CIN and may further reduce the incidence of cervical cancer in years to come.[1]

In 2010, the American Cancer Society estimates 12,200 new cases of cervical cancer in the United States, with 4210 women predicted to die from this disease. The peak incidence for this disease is 45 years. Although the overall incidence of cervical cancer is low in the United States, the incidence in African Americans is nearly 50% higher than in Caucasians, and the incidence in the Hispanic population is more than double that of Caucasians. Furthermore, in comparison with Caucasians. African Americans are more frequently diagnosed with advanced-stage tumors and are less likely to receive treatment.[2]

Risk Factors

Several established risk factors are known to contribute to cervical carcinogenesis. More than 99% of cervical cancers are associated with infection with HPV;

risk factors associated with HPV infection are the same for CIN and cervical cancer. These include multiple sexual partners, history of other sexually transmitted infections, high parity, immunosuppression, and cigarette smoking.[3] Obesity has been associated with a slightly increased risk of adenocarcinoma of the cervix.[4] However, neither parity nor smoking has been associated with increased risk of adenocarcinoma of the cervix.[5] Interestingly, although cervical cancer is not a typical genetically inherited disease, it does tend to aggregate in families.[6]

Women who smoke have a dose-dependent increased risk of having persistent HPV. Cigarette smoking may contribute to the development of high-grade cervical dysplasia in women with underlying HPV infection.[7] This may be due to genotoxicity secondary to the presence of tobacco-derived carcinogens in cervical secretions. Cigarette smoking has also been found to have immunosuppressive effects and may predispose patients to persistent HPV infection.

High parity has been associated with increased rates of cervical cancer and dysplasia, although the mechanism is not clear.[8] Oral contraceptives are a difficult variable to study in regard to HPV infection, because of the difficulty in separating sexual habits and contraceptive use. However, one large multicenter case-control study and several meta-analyses revealed that women taking oral contraceptives may have an elevated risk of invasive cervical cancers.[3,9,10] Parity has also been found to be an independent risk factor, potentially secondary to cervical trauma.[11] Additionally, coinfection with *Chlamydia trachomatis* has also been associated with HPV persistence, cervical neoplasia, and cervical cancer.[12]

Several protective behaviors have been identified as well. Consistent condom use has been associated with a partial protective effect against HPV infection and cervical dysplasia.[13] Additionally, circumcision has been associated with reduced HPV detection in males, and wives of men with multiple sexual partners have been found to have higher rates of cervical cancer.[14]

Patients infected with human immunodeficiency virus (HIV) commonly have concurrent HPV infections. In patients HIV-associated immunosuppression, abnormal cervical cytology rates may be as high as 78%.[15] Increased incidence of abnormal cervical cytology has been correlated with low CD4+ lymphocyte counts, but not with duration of HIV infection, antiretroviral therapy, or viral load.[16]

Pathogenesis

The malignant transformation of cervical cells is intimately related to HPV infection. HPV is an extremely common, double-stranded DNA virus acquired by sexual contact. HPV infects basal keratinocytes and replicates during keratinocyte differentiation. More than 100 types of HPV have been sequenced, and many

more have been partially characterized. Of these, approximately 40 infect the genital tract, and these are responsible for condylomata, some hyperproliferative lesions, and dysplastic lesions of the cervix, vulva, vagina, and anus. In the United States, HPV16 is the most carcinogenic type, and genotypes 16 and 18 have been associated with nearly 70% of cervical cancers worldwide.[17] In particular, HPV18 accounts for approximately 50% of adenocarcinomas, as compared with only 15% of squamous cell carcinoma.[18]

All papillomaviruses have regulatory, early (E), and late (L) genomic regions. Early proteins are required for replication and/or cellular transformation. These include proteins E6 and E7, the major HPV oncoproteins. The E6 protein binds specifically to E6-AP, which associates with the tumor-suppressor protein p53, causing rapid degradation. Loss of p53 results in failure of growth arrest and loss of appropriate apoptotic signaling in response to cell damage. E7 interacts with the retinoblastoma tumor suppressor gene (*pRb*), which normally complexes with E2F transcription factors. Formation of E7-pRb complexes disrupts the pRB-E2F complex, which initiates cell growth. E7 is able to immortalize keratinocytes independently, but the combination of E6 and E7 in transgenic mice have been found to result in aggressive invasive cancers.[19]

HPV genomes initially infect the cell in circular extrachromosomal copies. Over time, however, the HPV viral genome can become inserted into host cell DNA in a process called integration. Integrated HPV has been found to be present in 83% of invasive cervical cancers, as compared with 8% of low-grade squamous epithelial lesions, suggesting that integration may be associated with the transition of low-grade to high-grade lesions.[20] Once integration has occurred, E6 and E7 transcription is not downregulated by the viral regulatory protein E2, and intracellular E6 and E7 oncoprotein levels increase. Keratinocytes that express E6 and E7 are immortalized and may ultimately become tumorigenic.

DIAGNOSIS

Key Points

1. Early-stage cervical cancers are frequently asymptomatic; advanced-stage disease may present with malodorous or bloody vaginal discharge, back pain, hematuria, or rectal bleeding.
2. Cervical cancer staging according to the International Federation of Gynecology and Obstetrics (FIGO) system is performed clinically and may only include such radiographic studies as chest radiograph, intravenous pyelogram, or barium enema.

Clinical Features

The majority of women with early-stage cervical cancers are asymptomatic and are typically diagnosed after evaluation of an abnormal screening Pap smear. For patients with large tumors or advanced-stage disease, the most common presentation is abnormal vaginal bleeding, particularly after intercourse. With tumor growth and necrosis, patients may have additional complaints of malodorous vaginal discharge. In advanced cases, cervical cancer can also cause pelvic pressure and pain or bleeding with urination or defecation. Metastatic disease may cause difficulties with radiating or neuropathic pain, or lower-extremity edema.

On physical examination, the most common finding is a cervical lesion, which should be biopsied. Cervical cancer is clinically staged, and the examination is critical for treatment planning. For this reason, examination should include a detailed description of the size (depth and width) of the primary cervical lesion, as well as documentation of a rectovaginal examination to evaluate for potential parametrial and pelvic sidewall extension. Additionally, regional and distant lymph nodes should be examined for potential metastases; these include the superficial groin and femoral nodes, as well as supraclavicular nodes.

Diagnostic Testing

Diagnostic tests may be included in the clinical staging of cervical cancer; these are limited to standard chest radiography, intravenous pyelogram, and barium enema. Chest radiography may identify metastatic lesions to the lungs, whereas intravenous pyelogram can determine hydronephrosis, suggesting metastatic disease to the pelvic sidewall. Barium enema is useful when patients report rectal bleeding; it can identify metastases to the recto-sigmoid colon.

Although findings from additional imaging tools such as computed tomography (CT), magnetic resonance imaging (MRI), or positron emission tomography (PET) are not formally included in the staging system, they may supplement clinical suspicion of parametrial and sidewall disease and influence treatment planning. Of these techniques, MRI is the most sensitive for detecting locally advanced disease. A prospective collaborative trial sponsored by the American College of Radiology Imaging Network and the Gynecologic Oncology Group (GOG) demonstrated a sensitivity of 53% with MRI compared with 29% for clinical staging and 42% for CT.[21] Furthermore, the negative predictive value of MRI in detecting parametrial invasion is 95%.[22] It is more difficult to determine parametrial invasion based on MRI, and positive predictive value remains significantly lower; this is due to the similarity of the radiographic appearance of parametrial tissue and cervical tumor.[23] In addition, PET imaging may identify lymph nodes suggestive of metastatic disease. PET imaging rapidly evaluates metabolic activity, therefore using physiologic processes rather than the anatomic changes detected by conventional radiography. Fusion of CT and PET images has high sensitivity and specificity in detecting lymph node metastases.[24,25]

Diagnostic Procedures

Several diagnostic procedures are pertinent in the diagnosis of cervical cancer. Small cancers may be identified after cervical conization or loop electrosurgical excision for dysplasia. Because this disease is not staged surgically, operative findings such as lymph node metastases do not influence the staging system. However, examination under anesthesia with cystoscopy and proctoscopy should be considered when office examination is limited due to anatomic distortion from tumor or patient discomfort or when suspicion for bladder or rectal involvement is high.

Role of the General Gynecologist

Primary care providers, including family medicine physicians, internists, obstetrician/gynecologists, as well as physician assistants and nurse practitioners, play a critical role in cervical cancer screening, cervical dysplasia management, and establishing the diagnosis of cervical cancer. The American Cancer Society, American Society for Colposcopy and Cervical Pathology, United States Preventative Services Task force, and the American Congress of Obstetricians and Gynecologists provide regularly updated screening guidelines and recommendations for the general practitioner, which are detailed in Chapter 4. Procedures commonly used by the general obstetrician/gynecologist include colposcopy, cervical biopsy, and cervical conization procedures in the management of cervical dysplasia; once a formal diagnosis of cervical cancer is made, referral should be made to a gynecologic oncologist for definitive treatment planning.

PATHOLOGY

Key Points

1. The majority of cervical cancers are of squamous histology and spread via direct extension.
2. Adenocarcinomas constitute a smaller percentage of cervical cancers, but both the overall incidence and proportion of adenocarcinomas of the cervix appear to be rising.
3. Stage IA1, or microinvasive carcinoma, is defined by a depth of invasion less than 3 mm and a lesion width no greater than 7 mm.

Histopathology

Squamous Cell Carcinoma

The majority of cervical cancers are of squamous cell histology (Table 5-1). Squamous cell cancers develop after an interval of preinvasive disease, as discussed in Chapter 4. Dysplastic cells are characterized by an increased nuclear-to-cytoplasmic ratio and have prominent mitotic figures. CIN can progress to carcinoma in situ, with subsequent invasive disease identified after penetration of dysplastic cells through the basement membrane (Figure 5-1).

Grossly, squamous cell cervical cancers can exhibit a heterogeneous appearance, ranging from small nodular lesions to large, bloody friable tumors with malodorous exudate. Microscopically, cervical cancers demonstrate infiltrative nests of cells with eosinophilic cytoplasm and large, hyperchromatic nuclei. There is frequently a desmoplastic stromal response surrounding the nests of carcinoma. Mitoses are frequently numerous. Lesions may be further characterized as keratinizing or nonkeratinizing, depending on the presence of keratin pearls (Figure 5-2). They are also graded; grade 1 tumors are well differentiated and uncommon. They have mild atypia, large numbers of keratinized cells, and scant mitotic figures. Grade 2 tumors are more common and are largely nonkeratinizing with numerous mitoses, pleomorphic nuclei, and an infiltrative pattern. Grade 3 tumors are poorly differentiated and are pleomorphic with anaplastic nuclei and a tendency to form spindle cells and may be difficult to distinguish from sarcomas without cytokeratin staining.

There are several rare histologic variants of squamous cell carcinomas of the cervix that include verrucous, papillary squamotransitional, warty, and lymphoepithelioma-like carcinomas. Verrucous carcinomas appear grossly as a large, sessile tumor that may be confused for condyloma acuminatum. Clinically, verrucous carcinoma behaves in a slow-growing, locally invasive fashion; however, it rarely involves regional lymph nodes or distant metastases. Histologically, verrucous carcinoma of the cervix is characterized by frond-like papillae, which may be keratinized, without a connective tissue core. In order to make the correct diagnosis, the base of the tumor must be evaluated, as superficial layers frequently lack atypia or frequent mitosis. The basal layer is composed of well-circumscribed invasive nests of epithelium that invade the cervical stroma in a pushing fashion and have a characteristically inflammatory appearance at the base of the epithelium.

Papillary squamotransitional carcinoma may present with a variety of histologic appearances, but often demonstrate superficial papillary architecture with a connective tissue core. They may also have extensive mitoses, nuclear atypia, and keratinization. They may also display the multiple layers and oval-shaped, hyperchromatic nuclei typical of transitional cell carcinomas. Papillary squamotransitional carcinomas typically have immunohistochemistry markers of squamous differentiation. HPV16 has also been found in transitional cell carcinomas.[26]

Warty carcinoma is another rare variant of squamous cell carcinomas with marked condylomatous changes. They are associated with coinfection by several strains of HPV and have deep margins that demonstrate features typical of invasive squamous cell carcinoma.[27] Many warty cell tumors also demonstrate notable cytoplasmic vacuolization. For this reason, they may be confused on cytology as low-grade koilocytosis.

Lymphoepithelioma-like carcinoma of the cervix is more common in Asian women and has been reported to have better prognosis than typical squamous cell carcinomas of the cervix. It has been associated with Epstein-Barr virus.[28] Lymphoepithelioma-like carcinoma of the cervix is histologically similar to nasopharyngeal lymphoepitheliomas: The cells are poorly differentiated, with abundant cytoplasm and enlarged vesicular nuclei. Inflammatory cells including large numbers of T cells are prominent, and therefore, lymphoepithelioma-like carcinomas can be confused for glassy cell carcinoma (Figure 5-3). However, the cells tend to have indistinct cell borders that contrast with the distinctively bordered cells in glassy cell carcinomas.

Adenocarcinoma

Adenocarcinomas are the second most common histologic type of cervical cancer. In contrast to squamous cell

Table 5-1 Histologic Subtypes of Cervical Cancer

Squamous cell carcinoma
Verrucous carcinoma variant
Papillary squamotransitional carcinoma variant
Warty carcinoma variant
Adenocarcinoma
Endocervical-type mucinous adenocarcinoma
Mucinous adenocarcinoma, intestinal-type
Minimal deviation adenocarcinoma (adenoma malignum)
Villoglandular adenocarcinoma
Clear cell adenocarcinoma
Papillary serous carcinoma
Mesonephric adenocarcinoma
Adenosquamous carcinoma
Glassy cell carcinoma
Adenoid cystic carcinoma
Adenoid basal tumors of the cervix
Large-cell neuroendocrine carcinoma
Small-cell carcinoma

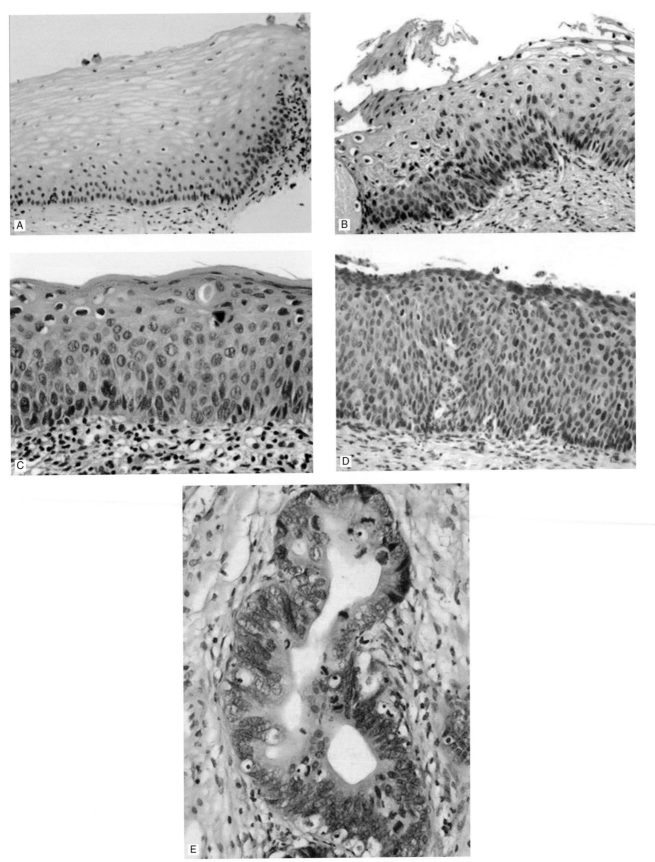

FIGURE 5-1. Demonstration of the progression of cytologic atypia. (A) Normal cervical epithelium; **(B)** cervical intraepithelial neoplasia (CIN) 1; **(C)** CIN2; **(D)** CIN3; **(E)** adenocarcinoma in situ.

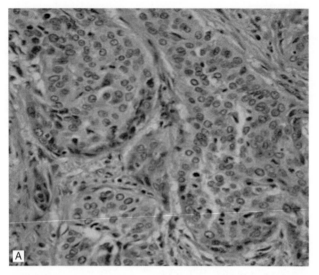
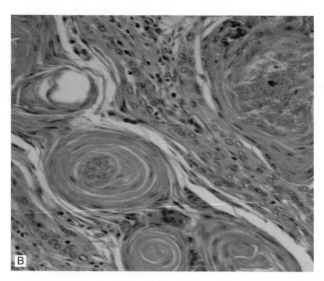

FIGURE 5-2. Invasive squamous cell carcinoma of the cervix. (A) Nonkeratinizing invasive carcinoma; **(B)** keratin pearls.

cancers, adenocarcinomas arise from the endocervical mucus-producing glandular cells. Grossly, the ectocervix may appear benign, but the cervix may be expanded or "barrel-shaped" given the disease in the endocervix. In contrast to squamous cell carcinomas, adenocarcinomas of the cervix may not be confluent and can exhibit so-called skip lesions. Histologically, foci of adenocarcinoma in situ or minimally invasive adenocarcinoma may be interspersed with areas of benign glands.

Endocervical-type mucinous adenocarcinomas are the most common subtype of cervical adenocarcinomas. Their cells resemble columnar cells found in normal endocervical mucosa. They are largely moderately to well-differentiated. The glandular elements may be arranged in a racemose, glandular pattern, appearing similar to the configuration of normal endocervical mucosa. Nuclei are basally located, but appear stratified

with mitotic figures present. Endocervical mucinous adenocarcinomas may have uniform nuclei with minimal stratification. Well differentiated (grade 1) neoplasms demonstrate less than 10% solid components. Moderately differentiated (grade 2) disease displays increased mitotic figures, with solid components comprising up to half of the neoplasm. Poorly differentiated (grade 3) adenocarcinomas have more pleomorphic nuclei, mitoses, and may have a larger solid component, areas of marked desmoplasia, and necrosis (Figure 5-4).

There are also several histologic variants of cervical adenocarcinomas. Mucinous adenocarcinoma may contain goblet cells with intestinal differentiation. They may form glands with papillae or may demonstrate architecture similar to colonic adenocarcinoma. Glands may be lined by pseudostratified, malignant-appearing cells with intracytoplasmic mucinous vacuoles, goblet

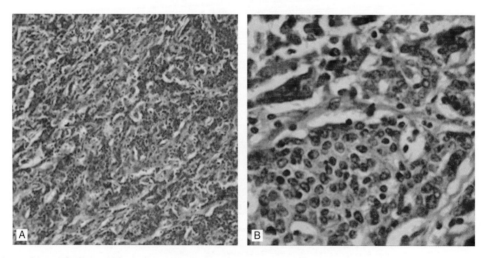

FIGURE 5-3. Lymphoepithelioma-like carcinoma. Note abundant cytoplasm, enlarged vesicular nuclei, and infiltration of inflammatory cells. **A.** Low-power view shows prominent inflammatory cells. **B.** High-power view shows poorly differentiated cells with abundant cytoplasm and enlarged vesicular nuclei.

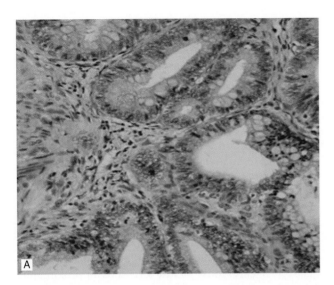 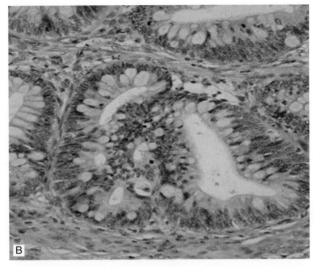

FIGURE 5-4. Invasive adenocarcinoma of the cervix. **(A)** Well differentiated; **(B)** poorly differentiated.

cells, or occasionally Paneth cells. Intestinal subtypes are extremely rare, and care must be taken to rule out metastatic disease from the gastrointestinal tract.

Minimal deviation adenocarcinoma is an uncommon, very well-differentiated form of cervical adenocarcinoma, previously referred to as *adenoma malignum*. Cells do not demonstrate features typical of malignancy. These tumors comprise approximately 1% to 3% of all cervical adenocarcinomas. They may be associated with mucinous adenocarcinomas and sex cord tumors of the ovary.[29] They may occur as a sporadic neoplasm; however, they have also been associated with Peutz-Jeghers syndrome.[30] However, they have not been associated with HPV infection. Clinically, minimal deviation adenocarcinomas may be associated with watery mucinous vaginal discharge or abnormal endocervical cells on cervical cytology. On physical examination, advanced tumors may appear as polypoid lesions and firm yellow neoplasms. Microscopically, glands are more infiltrative in appearance. Nuclei are bland and located at the base of the epithelium. In the endometrioid type, cells lining the glands resemble benign proliferative endometrium. Glands may appear similar to normal endocervical glands; however, they may vary in size or have atypical angular outpouchings surrounded by desmoplasia. Mitotic figures in benign endocervical glands are very rare; however, on high-power magnification, minimal deviation carcinoma can be noted to have mitoses. Therefore, one of the most reliable criteria is the depth of involvement of the cervical stroma. Whereas normal endocervical crypts are rarely deeper than 7 mm, minimal deviation carcinoma may extend through up to two-thirds of the cervical stroma[29] (Figure 5-5). Immunochemistry has revealed that minimal deviation carcinoma may stain focally for carcinoembryonic antigen, and estrogen and progesterone receptors have been found to be uniformly negative in this disease.

Villoglandular adenocarcinomas of the cervix are low-grade carcinomas that may appear similar to intestinal villous adenomas. Villoglandular adenocarcinoma of the cervix is characterized by low-grade atypia and rare mitotic figures. Histologically, these neoplasms have a long, filamentous, often inflammatory-appearing connective tissue core with an overlying layer of well-differentiated cells. They are frequently associated with high-risk HPV. Because these tumors may be associated with more aggressive carcinomas, the formal diagnosis should be made on cone biopsy. Villous adenocarcinomas tend to occur in young women, and unless associated with an underlying adenocarcinoma of poorer prognosis, these tumors have very good prognosis.[31]

Additional cervical adenocarcinomas include clear cell, papillary serous, and mesonephric tumors. Clear cell cancers are associated with intrauterine diethylstilbestrol exposure. Clear cell adenocarcinomas appear histologically as sheets of cells with atypical nuclei, mitotic figures, and abundant clear cytoplasm (Figure 5-6). Papillary serous carcinomas are morphologically similar to the more common papillary serous tumors of the ovary and endometrium and are not associated with HPV infection.[32] Mesonephric neoplasms are a rare glandular subtype derived from wolffian duct remnants. Remnants of the mesonephric ducts are present in the lateral aspects of up to 20% of cervical specimen. They appear as small glandular structures with intraluminal Periodic acid-Schiff (PAS) stain–positive material. They are lined with cuboidal cells. Retiform, tubular, and sex cord patterns have also been described. Patients may develop benign mesonephric hyperplasia of the cervix, and in 2 series of 49 and 14 cases, no consequences of disease were noted.[33,34]

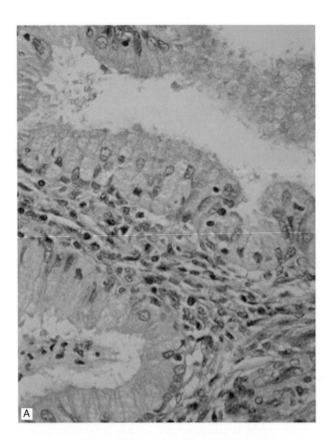

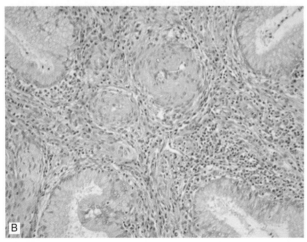

FIGURE 5-5. Minimal deviation adenocarcinoma. A. Mitotic figures in benign endocervical glands are very rare; however, on high-power magnification, minimal deviation carcinoma can be noted to have mitoses. **B.** Deep invasive minimal deviation adenocarcinoma. Therefore, one of the most reliable criteria is the depth of involvement of the cervical stroma.

However, mesonephric hyperplasia may be responsible for cervical cytology revealing atypical glandular cells. Histologically, it may be difficult to differentiate between benign mesonephric hyperplasia in the cervix and mesonephric adenocarcinoma, particularly because mesonephric carcinomas are likely to develop within areas of mesonephric hyperplasia.[33]

Other Epithelial Tumors

In addition to squamous cell and adenocarcinomas, there are several less common types of cervical cancer. For example, adenosquamous carcinomas contain both malignant squamous and glandular cells. Between 5% and 25% of cervical neoplasias are of adenosquamous histology. These tumors tend to behave in a more aggressive fashion. They are more likely to have higher tumor grade, higher incidence of vascular invasion,[35] and higher incidence of lymph node metastasis.[36] Glassy cell carcinomas are a rare, poorly differentiated subtype of adenosquamous carcinoma of the uterine cervix. These behave particularly aggressively and respond poorly to both surgical management and radiotherapy. The mean age of patients affected by glassy cell carcinoma of the cervix is approximately 10 years younger than that of patients with squamous cell and adenocarcinomas of the cervix.[37] Clinically, these may appear on gross examination as a barrel-shaped cervix. Histologically, cells are large, polygonal, with eosinophilic, ground glass–type cytoplasm. Glassy cell carcinomas have abundant mitotic features, well-defined cell borders, and prominent infiltrate of eosinophils and plasma cells (Figure 5-7).

Adenoid cystic carcinoma is a rare neoplasm, comprising 10% to 15% of all salivary neoplasms and 1% to 2% of all head and neck malignancies. Adenoid cystic carcinoma of the cervix is particularly rare and accounts for less than 1% of cervical adenocarcinomas. The tumor is most common in postmenopausal females and is more common in African American patients. It has been associated with high-risk HPV. Clinically, these tumors generally present with a large, palpable lesion that can be ulcerated or friable. Histologically, adenoid cystic carcinoma is characterized by basaloid tumor cells with high nuclear-to-cytoplasmic ratios, numerous mitoses peripheral palisading, and a cribriform appearance, often with areas of necrosis. Lymphatic involvement is common. The cells are cytokeratin positive and also stain positively for MNF-116. This tumor behaves aggressively, with frequent recurrence despite radical surgical management.

Adenoid basal tumors of the cervix may be confused with adenoid cystic carcinoma, but differentiation is important, as adenoid basal tumors rarely exhibit malignant behavior. These tumors may be composed of nests of cells with basaloid, squamous, or glandular differentiation. However, the tumors are typically associated with high-grade squamous intraepithelial lesions and high-risk HPV.[38] Clinically, because these patients may be asymptomatic without grossly visible lesions, these tumors are most commonly detected incidentally. Tumors may be locally aggressive, but rarely metastasize. When the primary tumor is bland in appearance and does not have more atypical features present, it behaves in a benign fashion, and some authors have

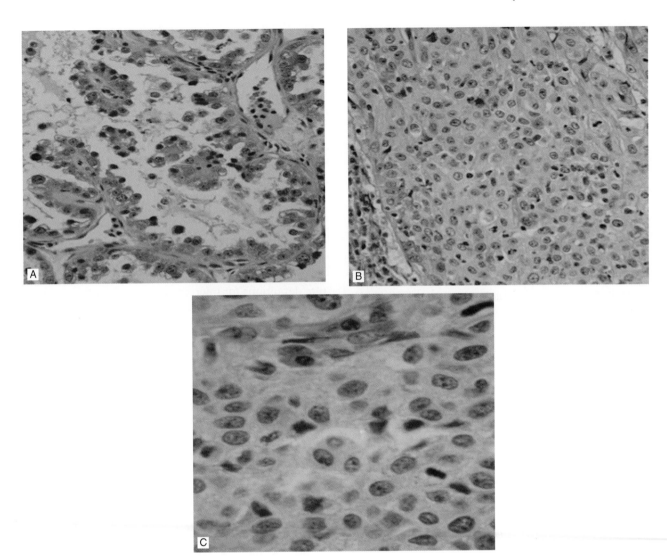

FIGURE 5-6. Glassy cell carcinoma. A. Cells are large and polygonal, with eosinophilic, ground glass–type cytoplasm. **B.** Glassy cell carcinomas have abundant mitotic features, well-defined cell borders, and prominent infiltrate of eosinophils and plasma cells. **C.** High-power view.

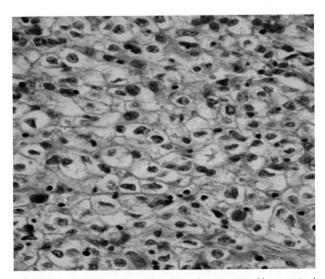

FIGURE 5-7. Clear cell carcinoma, characterized by atypical nuclei, mitotic figures, and abundant clear cytoplasm.

proposed renaming typical adenoid basal tumors of the cervix *adenoid basal epithelioma* to describe their benign course. However, adenoid basal carcinomas are frequently associated with more aggressive histologic subtypes of cervical cancers, which behave more aggressively.

Large-cell neuroendocrine carcinomas are aggressive, rare tumors with a histologic appearance that includes insular, trabecular, glandular, and solid growth patterns. All tumors stain positively for chromogranin, and the majority of the tumors are noted to be argyrophilic, have eosinophilic cytoplasmic granules, and have areas of necrosis (Figure 5-8). Small-cell carcinoma is another rare tumor and is associated with poor outcome, with 5-year survival rates less than 30%. The tumor is composed of sheets and cords of small, anaplastic cells with scant cytoplasm. Lymphatic involvement is common. Immunohistochemistry may

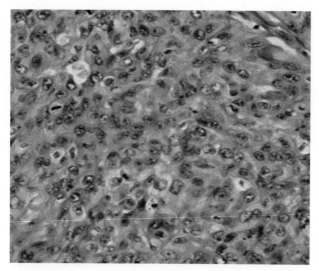

FIGURE 5-8. Large-cell neuroendocrine tumor of the cervix. Such tumors are argyrophilic, have eosinophilic cytoplasmic granules, and have areas of necrosis.

be helpful for diagnosing difficult cases, and these tumors may express chromogranin, synaptophysin, and p53 protein. Approximately 60% of small-cell carcinomas of the cervix are associated with HPV18.

Metastatic Spread Patterns

The most common method of spread of cervical carcinoma is via direct extension to adjacent tissues, including the parametria, the vagina, the pelvic sidewall, and the bladder and rectum. Although less common, cervical cancer may also metastasize to the ovaries. In addition, cervical cancer may spread lymphatically to the parametrial, obturator, and iliac lymph nodes. Hematogenous spread is less common, but may include sites in the lung, bone, liver, and mediastinum and, even less commonly, the spleen, adrenal, and brain.

FIGO Staging

Cervical cancer is clinically staged using a system developed by FIGO and involves bimanual examination with or without anesthesia and limited imaging studies such as chest radiography, intravenous pyelogram, and barium enema. CT, MRI, and PET imaging may be used to assist in case of clinical suspicion of parametrial or sidewall disease; however, identification of lymph nodes suggestive of metastatic disease does not influence the clinically assigned stage.

The FIGO staging system is presented in Table 5-2. Early-stage disease typically refers to FIGO stages I through IIA, and advanced-stage disease describes stages IIB and higher. Identification of hydronephrosis on intravenous pyelogram or CT permits assignation of stage IIIB.

Stage I disease reflects disease limited to the cervix. It is important to note the specific guidelines for stage IA1, or microinvasive squamous cell carcinoma, as this disease may be managed more conservatively. Microinvasive disease is defined by a limited depth of invasion, where only small tongues of malignant cells have penetrated the basement membrane less than 3 mm; the overall width of the lesion can be no larger than 7 mm. This may affect either surface or glandular cervical epithelium. In order for a formal diagnosis of microinvasive squamous carcinoma, the cone or LEEP biopsy must encompass the entire cervical lesion and have negative margins. Microinvasive cells may be larger, with more prominently enlarged, pleomorphic nuclei, more pronounced eosinophilic cytoplasm, and surrounding desmoplastic stromal reaction. Two separate definitions for microinvasive carcinoma have been developed. FIGO has defined microinvasive squamous carcinoma to be stage IA1 lesions. More stringently, the SGO (Society of Gynecologic Oncology) Committee on Nomenclature further defined microinvasive squamous carcinoma as disease that must not exceed a depth of 3 mm and has no lymphovascular space involvement. The application of a microinvasive subtype to adenocarcinomas of the cervix remain controversial, in part due to the presence of skip lesions with this histology.

TREATMENT

Key Points

1. Stage IA1 microinvasive squamous cell carcinoma may be managed conservatively with a cone biopsy or extrafascial hysterectomy.
2. Early-stage disease may be primarily managed surgically with radical hysterectomy and pelvic lymphadenectomy.
3. Chemoradiation is the most effective treatment for advanced-stage disease and may also be employed with great efficacy in patients with early-stage disease who are poor surgical candidates.

Primary Treatment Modalities

Cervical cancer may be treated with several modalities. Early-stage disease is typically managed with surgery, whereas advanced-stage disease is best treated with primary radiation and concurrent low-dose chemotherapy. Treatment options are summarized by stage in Table 5-3.

Early-Stage Disease

Stage IA1, or microinvasive carcinoma, may be managed with either simple hysterectomy or cervical

Table 5-2 Updated FIGO 2009 Staging of Cervical Carcinoma

Stage			Description
I			Carcinoma is strictly confined to the cervix (extension to the uterus is disregarded)
	IA		Invasive carcinoma that can be diagnosed only by microscopy, with deepest invasion ≤5 mm and largest horizontal extension ≤7 mm
		IA1	Stromal invasion ≤3 mm in depth and horizontal extension ≤7 mm
		IA2	Stromal invasion ≤3 mm but ≤5 mm and horizontal extension ≤7 mm
	IB		Clinically visible lesions limited to the cervix, or preclinical/microscopic cancers greater than stage IA
		IB1	Clinically visible lesion ≤4 cm in greatest dimension
		IB2	Clinically visible lesion >4 cm in greatest dimension
II			Cervical carcinoma invading beyond the uterus, but not to the pelvic sidewall or to the lower third of the vagina
	IIA		Without parametrial invasion
		IIA1	Clinically visible lesion ≤4 cm in greatest dimension
		IIA2	Clinically visible lesion >4 cm in greatest dimension
	IIB		With obvious parametrial invasion
III			Cervical carcinoma extending to the pelvic sidewall and/or the lower third of the vagina and/or causes hydronephrosis or nonfunctioning kidney
	IIIA		Extension to the lower third of the vagina with no extension to the pelvic sidewall
	IIIB		Extension to the pelvic sidewall and/or causing hydronephrosis or nonfunctioning kidney
IV			Carcinoma extending beyond the true pelvis or has involved the mucosa of the bladder or rectum.
	IVA		Direct extension to adjacent organs
	IVB		Metastatic spread to distant organs

conization, depending on the patient's desires for future fertility. These guidelines are supported by several studies that have demonstrated that there is minimal risk of nodal involvement in patients with disease

Table 5-3 Treatment Summary for Cervical Cancer by Stage

Stage I
  A1: Extrafascial hysterectomy or cone biopsy
  A2: Radical hysterectomy with pelvic lymphadenectomy
  B1: Radical hysterectomy with pelvic lymphadenectomy
  B2: Radical hysterectomy with pelvic lymphadenectomy

Stage II
  A: Radical hysterectomy with pelvic lymphadenectomy
  B: Chemosensitizing radiation

Stage III
  A: Chemosensitizing radiation
  B: Chemosensitizing radiation

Stage IV
  A: Chemosensitizing radiation
  B: Systemic chemotherapy ± pelvic radiation

less than 3 mm in depth and less than 7 mm in breadth. Takeshima and colleagues analyzed 402 patients with invasive squamous cell carcinoma of the cervix with less than 5 mm of invasion. Only 1 of 82 patients (1.2%) with lesions less than 3 mm in depth demonstrated lymph node metastasis, compared with 5 of 73 (6.8%) in patients with 3 to 5 mm depth of invasion.[39] More recently, Bisseling and colleagues[40] performed a review of the literature reporting on 1565 patients with stage IA1 disease. Eight hundred fourteen patients underwent pelvic lymphadenectomy, of whom 12 had positive nodes. Lymphvascular space invasion (LVSI) was present in 25 patients, none of whom had lymph node metastasis. Because of this low incidence of extra-cervical disease, stage IA1 squamous cell carcinoma of the cervix may thus be managed conservatively with a near-perfect rate of control.[41]

Several tumor characteristics may predict prognosis and recurrence with conservative management of IA1 disease. Roman and colleagues[42] determined that patients with LVSI were more likely to have occult lymph node metastasis, and this finding has been confirmed by others.[43,44] Additionally, Raspagliesi and colleagues[42] showed that patients with LVSI or lateral

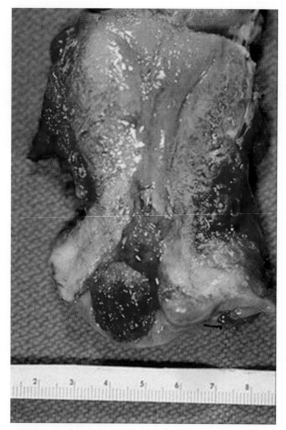

FIGURE 5-9. Standard specimen from type III radical hysterectomy, including parametria, uterosacral ligaments, and upper 2 to 3 cm of the proximal vagina.

negative margins less than 8 mm or apical negative margins less than 10 mm were both associated with recurrence. When fertility is no longer desired, patients with close margins or positive LVSI may be offered completion hysterectomy.

Radical hysterectomy with pelvic lymphadenectomy remains the standard of care for patients with stage IA2, IB, and IIA disease (Figure 5-9). Although some data suggest that patients with stage IA2 disease may be managed with cervical conization or extrafascial hysterectomy without lymphadenectomy, the safety of such a conservative approach has yet to be proven. For example, the risk of lymph node metastases with stage IA2 disease has been shown to be 7.4% in one retrospective review, whereas another study observed a 48% incidence of residual disease in the radical hysterectomy specimen after conization for this stage.[44,45] Radical hysterectomy with pelvic lymphadenectomy should thus be recommended; for patients who are poor surgical candidates, intracavitary brachytherapy may be used with excellent results.

Patients with stage IB to IIA disease may also be managed successfully with either radical hysterectomy and pelvic lymphadenectomy or primary radiotherapy. Landoni and colleagues addressed this issue in

a prospective trial of 469 patients with such disease, randomizing their treatment to either surgery or radiation. In this study, the patients undergoing radical hysterectomy were prescribed subsequent adjuvant radiation in the event of close or positive margins or positive lymph node metastases. They observed a statistically equivalent 5-year overall and disease-specific survival.[46] In this trial, 42 patients (25%) undergoing surgery experienced recurrence, as compared with 44 (26%) in the radiotherapy group. Of note, the surgical patients did demonstrate greater severe morbidity as compared with those who received radiation.

The morbidity of surgery may be minimized with application of a modified approach to the radical hysterectomy. Patients undergoing a type II radical hysterectomy have a less extensive dissection of the parametria and vagina, without impact on survival. This was confirmed in a prospective trial of 243 patients with stage IB and IIA cervical cancer who were randomized to either type II or type III radical hysterectomy. Patients undergoing type II radical hysterectomy had a significantly shorter operative time and late urologic morbidity. Blood loss, need for transfusion, immediate postoperative complications, and postoperative stay were not significantly different. Recurrence and death secondary to disease were not significantly different between the 2 groups of treatment. The authors concluded that both type II and III radical hysterectomies are effective treatment for stage IB and IIA cervical cancer, but that type II hysterectomy was associated with fewer late complications.[47]

The decision to treat with either surgery or radiation depends on several factors, including menopausal status, age, medical comorbidities, tumor histology, and primary tumor diameter. In general, younger and thinner patients without concurrent medical illnesses who desire preservation of ovarian function are better candidates for a surgical approach, although age and obesity are not necessarily contraindications to surgery. Given the radiosensitive nature of the ovaries, women who undergo primary radiotherapy will likely lose ovarian function and can also develop fibrosis of the vagina. A surgical approach allows for preservation of the ovaries and fallopian tubes. The safety of omitting oophorectomy was first established by a prospective GOG trial of 990 patients with stage IB disease; 0.5% of women with squamous cell histologies and 1.7% with adenocarcinomas had ovarian metastases. This was further confirmed in a review of 3471 Japanese patients with early-stage cervical cancers; for women with stage IB to IIA disease, ovarian metastases were observed in less than 1% for patients with squamous cell cancers and less than 5% for those with adenocarcinomas.[48]

Tumor diameter may also influence the decision to treat with surgery or radiation. In general, patients with stage IB2 disease are at higher risk for nodal disease, distant metastasis, and local and distant recurrences.

Patients who undergo radical hysterectomy typically will require postoperative radiotherapy, and the rationale for a primary radiotherapy approach primarily reflects the perceived minimization of morbidity with a single, compared with a multiple, treatment modality. However, several single-institution reviews have reported on the primary management of patients with bulky IB disease with radical hysterectomy, to be followed with adjuvant radiotherapy in patients with particularly high-risk features. Five-year survivals range from 62% to 72%.[49,50] The National Comprehensive Cancer Network (NCCN) panel on cervical cancer's most recent recommendations states that surgery followed by chemoradiation is an acceptable treatment option (category 2); however, they also include pelvic radiotherapy with brachytherapy as a category 1 recommendation.[51]

Occasionally, patients selected for radical hysterectomy are found to have metastatic nodal disease at the time of operation. Options for management intraoperatively remain controversial and include resection of existent adenopathy and performing adjuvant radiation, resection of adenopathy and proceeding with radical hysterectomy and adjuvant radiation, or aborting the procedure entirely and proceeding with curative intent radiation therapy. There are no randomized controlled studies regarding subsequent therapy in this population, and retrospective reviews may be biased because of intraoperative selection. However, Cosin and colleagues[52] identified that patients with macroscopic metastatic lymph nodes who underwent resection had a 50% 5-year survival rate, compared with a 0% 5-year survival rate for those who had bulky adenopathy that was not resected. Although these data are retrospective, they suggest a therapeutic role in resecting grossly metastatic lymph nodes at the time of surgery.

Advanced-Stage Disease

Stage IIIA cervical carcinomas are quite rare and represent a unique therapeutic challenge, owing to the lymphatic drainage of the distal third of the vagina to the inguinal nodes. Although radiotherapy remains primary treatment, there is difficulty in sterilizing inguinal fields without providing inappropriate radiation to the femoral heads. Kavadi and colleagues[53] reviewed cases of stage III disease at the MD Anderson cancer center and found the 5-year survival rate to be 37% and 10-year actuarial survival rate to be 34%. The 5-year survival rate was significantly lower in those patients with parametrial disease (25% vs. 56% [$P = .05$]) and in patients with discontinuous lesions in the lower third of the vagina (15% vs. 48% in patients with contiguous lesions [$P = .05$]).[53] Dittmer et al proposed a unique technique using a posterior field for the pelvis and anterior field for the inguinal nodes; however,

as intensity-modulated techniques improve, this may become a preferred modality for groin irradiation.[54]

For patients with stages IIB, IIIB, and IVA disease, primary radiotherapy, with external beam and intracavitary radiation, is recommended. Several randomized controlled studies examining chemosensitization as an adjunct to radiation confirmed the superior survival when chemotherapy is administered concurrently, and this is now considered the standard of care.[55-57] These findings were recently confirmed by a large-scale population-based study in Ontario.[58] Quantitative meta-analysis by the Cochrane collaborative reveals that there is a 6% improvement in 5-year survival with chemoradiotherapy (hazard ratio [HR] = 0.81; $P < .001$). Radiation with chemosensitization also improved disease-free survival while reducing recurrence and progression. Acute toxicities were increased with chemoradiotherapy; however, there were a limited number of trials with long-term follow-up to comment on long-term toxicity and complications.[59] Weekly single-agent cisplatin is most often administered in this setting, but the NCCN also states that carboplatin or non-platinum chemotherapies may be considered for those patients who may have difficulties with cisplatin-containing options.[60]

Special Situations

Radical Trachelectomy

Radical trachelectomy entails removal of the cervix, the parametrium, and vaginal cuff while leaving the corpus and adnexa intact. This surgery may be approached vaginally, abdominally, or in a laparoscopically assisted manner. This procedure, in combination with a laparoscopic pelvic lymphadenectomy, provides an acceptable fertility-sparing option for patients with early cervical cancer. At case completion, a permanent isthmic cerclage is placed to assist with preventing preterm delivery. Primary cesarean is indicated for patients who have undergone trachelectomy. As of 2008, more than 900 cases had been performed and reported, with nearly 200 subsequent live births. The overall incidence of prematurity before 32 weeks is acceptable (10%), and overall success in curing disease has been high, with 31 recurrences (4%) and 16 deaths (2%).[61] Alternatively, for patients with early-stage operable disease who desire preservation of fertility, radical trachelectomy is a viable option. Multiple studies have shown comparable oncologic outcomes in well-selected patients.[62,63]

Ovarian Transposition

Ovarian transposition or oophoropexy is not in itself a therapeutic procedure; however, in patients who are to undergo primary radiation for cervical disease, ovarian transposition may serve as a way to prevent radiation-induced menopause. In this procedure, the utero-ovarian attachments are ligated, and the infundibulopelvic ligament and ovarian vasculature are mobilized to allow transposition of the ovaries above the pelvic brim. This procedure may be successfully performed abdominally or via laparoscopic approach.[64] Despite transposition, however, up to 50% of patients who subsequently receive postoperative radiotherapy will still develop ovarian failure.

Adjuvant Hysterectomy After Radiation Therapy

In general, adjuvant hysterectomy after primary radiation therapy with chemosensitization should not be offered to patients with bulky cervical cancer. Keys and colleagues[65] examined 256 patients with tumors measuring more than 4 cm who were randomized to either external and intracavitary irradiation or attenuated irradiation with subsequent extrafascial hysterectomy. Hysterectomy was not found to increase grade 3 or 4 toxicity. Although there was a lower incidence of relapse in the hysterectomy cohort at 5 years (27% vs. 14%), there was no impact on overall survival.

Adjuvant Postoperative Pelvic RT

After radical hysterectomy, adjuvant therapy is recommended for patients with intermediate or high risk for recurrence. Intermediate risk is assigned to those patients following an algorithm including large tumor size, deep stromal invasion, and lymphvascular space involvement of tumor. In a randomized study of 277 patients with stage IB disease meeting these criteria, adjuvant radiation was found to significantly improve recurrence-free survival, with a decrease in recurrence from 28% to 15%.[66] Patients at high risk include those with metastatic lymph nodes or obvious extrauterine spread of disease, such as to the adnexae or parametria. Patients with high-risk features should undergo adjuvant radiation with chemosensitization.

Carcinoma of the Cervical Stump

Although the American Congress of Obstetrics and Gynecology states that there is no specific benefit to supracervical hysterectomy, it is not an uncommon procedure in the United States and accounts for a significant portion of hysterectomies performed for benign indications. These patients remain at risk for cervical carcinoma, and their surgical history makes primary treatment more difficult. Radical trachelectomy may be considered in patients with carcinoma of the cervical stump. One large retrospective review of 213 patients with carcinoma of the cervical stump found that although there were no stage-for-stage survival benefits associated with surgical management, there was a significantly higher number of patients

receiving brachytherapy who had improved locoregional control as compared with those undergoing external radiation alone. Complication rates of those patients undergoing primary radiation for cancer of the cervical stump were similar to those of patients undergoing primary radiation for cervical cancer in the intact uterus.[67]

SURVIVAL AND PROGNOSIS

Key Points

1. Early-stage cervical cancer carries an excellent prognosis after appropriate treatment.
2. Lymph node metastasis is the most important prognostic factor in women with cervical cancer.
3. Localized recurrent disease may be successfully treated with pelvic exenteration; extrapelvic recurrence is typically managed with palliative chemotherapy.

Survival Outcomes

With the introduction of chemosensitization to radiotherapy, both in the adjuvant and primary setting, the survival for women with cervical cancer has improved dramatically. In general, patients with stage IA1 and IA2 disease have an overall disease-specific survival of 100%; those with stage IB and IIA disease have long-term survival ranging from 80% to 88%; those with stage IIB to IVA disease have survival of 45% to 65%.[54-56,68]

Prognostic Factors

In addition to the correlation between clinical stage and prognosis, several other elements have been found to affect outcome of patients with cervical cancer; these include primary tumor diameter, lymph node metastasis, lymphatic vascular space invasion, microscopic evidence of parametrial extension, and histology. Although it is not formally part of the FIGO clinical staging for cervical cancer, lymph node involvement is the most important prognostic factor for patients with cervical cancer. Patient 5-year overall survival is dramatically lower in patients with positive lymph node metastasis (50% vs. 85%).[69,70] In addition, tumor size correlates consistently with decreased progression-free and overall survival. The GOG has explored the prognostic factors involved in 1125 patients with stage I squamous cell carcinoma of the cervix who were treated with radical surgery with and without adjuvant radiotherapy. The disease-free interval at 3 years was 94.6% in patients with occult tumors, 85.5% for patients with tumors ~3 cm, and 68.4% in patients with tumors 3 cm or greater.[68] This same study defined several further significant independent prognostic factors. These include capillary or lymphatic involvement of tumor, depth of tumor invasion, and presence of disease at the parametrial margins. All of these factors were associated with decreased disease-free survival and have been confirmed by other investigators.[70,71]

In addition to these surgical-pathologic factors, both anemia and tumor hypoxemia are associated with poorer survival in patients with cervical cancer.[72] The relationship between anemia, tumor oxygen saturation, and prognosis is complex. Although anemia has been associated with poorer outcomes in patients with cervical cancer, it is somewhat unclear whether this is a result of more advanced tumors or whether it is a variable that could influence prognosis if corrected.[73] This complex relationship was observed in a multi-institution retrospective review of 605 Canadian patients that revealed that anemic patients whose hemoglobin levels were corrected to greater than 12 g/dL had similar survival rates as those who had normal hemoglobin without transfusion, noting that correction beyond 13 g/dL was not associated with additional survival improvement.[74] However, other data have suggested that transfusion is associated with increased levels of interleukin-10, diminishing host immunity. In one study designed to study optimal methods of determining intratumoral oxygen tension, only half of patients undergoing transfusion for cervical cancer treatment had increased tumor oxygenation.[75]

Another method that has been proposed to improve tumor oxygenation and hemoglobin is the use of erythropoietins. The Southwest Oncology Group performed a phase 2 trial of women receiving chemoradiation for stage IIB to IVA cervical cancer. They were administered erythropoietin and iron to achieve a hemoglobin level greater than 12.5 g/dL. Although treatment was successful at increasing hemoglobin, there was a 13% incidence of venous thromboembolism during and immediately after treatment. The survival for patients enrolled in this trial was poor when compared with that of prior studies, and although this may have been secondary to baseline patient characteristics, an adverse effect of erythropoietin and iron on survival could not be excluded.[76]

MANAGEMENT OF RECURRENT DISEASE

Key Points

1. A small number of patients with recurrent central cervical cancer may be cured by surgery or radiotherapy.

2. Before proceeding with curative intent salvage, examination and imaging should be used to exclude the possibility of distant metastases.

3. Chemotherapy may assist with improved progression-free survival and palliation of symptoms in the recurrent setting, though it only modestly improves overall survival.

Surveillance

After primary therapy for cervical cancer, women should be followed closely for evidence of recurrence. Typically, women with cervical cancer are followed with office visits, to include directed history and pelvic/rectal examination, with performance of a screening Pap test. Although the utility and cost-effectiveness of Pap testing as a surveillance technique has recently been challenged, abnormal results may indicate early recurrence at the vaginal cuff (after radical hysterectomy) or at the remaining cervix (after primary radiotherapy). In addition, women with cervical cancer are at increased risk for vaginal dysplasia, and Pap testing may be useful to identify such lesions.

Recommended Treatment Options

Despite advances in the management of both early- and advanced-stage cervical cancer, women who develop recurrence of this disease have limited treatment options. The decision to proceed with surgery or chemotherapy depends primarily on the site of recurrence. For those women with small, mobile recurrent tumors limited to the vaginal cuff or cervix, pelvic exenteration is a possibility. This procedure includes radical resection of the pelvic organs, with colostomy and creation of a neo-bladder. Despite the attendant surgical morbidity and mortality, exenteration remains the only modality for long-term survival, as cytotoxic therapy is only palliative.

Pelvic exenteration was first described by Brunschwig as a radical treatment for advanced or recurrent cervical cancer in 1948. This procedure involves complete or partial colpectomy (with hysterectomy if the uterus was not removed at primary therapy) and removal of the bladder and/or rectum with reconstruction of these organs. Exenteration is appropriate to consider in patients with small and central recurrences in the pelvis; furthermore, candidates should not have severe medical comorbidities and must accept the changes in anatomy and self-image inherent with such a radical procedure. When carefully selected, those patients who undergo pelvic exenteration for recurrent cervical cancer previously treated by definitive radiotherapy may have up to a 50% 5-year survival.[77] Despite advances in perioperative management, thromboprophylaxis, antibiotic therapy and surgical technique, exenteration remains a morbid operation, with perioperative mortality that can range from 2% to 14%.

Given the morbidity of this procedure, appropriate patient selection is imperative. Patients with positive nodes at the time of the planned exenteration have a survival of less than 20%. Patients who have positive margins at the time of exenteration have only a 10% 5-year survival rate, with a median overall survival of 4 months. This is in contrast to those with negative margins after exenteration, in whom there is a 55% 5-year survival rate and median overall survival of 22 months.[78] Careful attention must be given to ensuring that the recurrent disease is fully resectable, and preoperative and intraoperative exploration must ensure that there are no sites of metastatic disease outside the pelvis. Preoperative PET is appropriate to help identify metastatic disease and can accurately identify sites of metastasis before planned pelvic exenteration. PET/CT may have improved specificity; however, it may be underutilized as a result of cost considerations. Others propose diagnostic laparoscopy for pre-exenterative evaluation.

In regards to morbidity, Berek and colleagues[77] reported on the University of California, Los Angeles's experience with pelvic exenteration in 75 patients with a median age of 52.5 years. They found that 70.2% of patients had at least 1 major complication, including ileus, ureteral anastomotic insufficiency, abscess, and cardiothrombotic events. Thirty percent developed intestinal fistulae. Goldberg and colleagues reported similar morbidity in 1003 patients undergoing exenteration at Albert Einstein, with complications including ureteral anastomotic leaks (14%) and wound complications (17%).[79] Patients with small central recurrences may be candidates for radical hysterectomy instead of pelvic exenteration. Coleman and colleagues[80] reviewed 50 patients who underwent radical hysterectomy for recurrent or persistent isolated central disease after radiotherapy. One subgroup of 10 patients had normal lesions limited to the cervix less than 2 cm. This subgroup had a 5-year survival rate of 90%. More recently, Maneo et al[81] reported on 34 patients who underwent radical hysterectomy for recurrence after radiotherapy. They confirmed that patients with small tumors had improved outcomes. Both of these studies reported high rates of toxicity, with up to 44% of patients experiencing grade 3 to 4 toxicity and 14% to 28% of patients with fistula.

Alternatively, chemotherapy may be offered to patients with recurrent cervical cancer, especially in patients with extrapelvic sites of disease or who are poor candidates for exenteration. Cisplatin in doses of 50 to 100 mg/m^2 offer response for 4 to 6 months, with overall survival of approximately 7 months. A randomized controlled trial conducted by the GOG compared several regimens of platinum-based chemotherapy for the treatment of recurrent cervical cancer. They found that higher doses of cisplatin (100 mg/m^2 vs. 50 mg/m^2) induced a higher response rate and had greater toxicity, but offered no differences in terms of progression-free or overall survival.[82]

Combination chemotherapies have also been evaluated for recurrent cervical cancer; only until recently, however, has such a regimen been shown to improve survival. In 2005, Long and colleagues[83] reported on a GOG trial designed to determine whether survival is improved with methotrexate, vinblastine, doxorubicin, and cisplatin (MVAC) compared with cisplatin alone, or cisplatin with topotecan. The MVAC arm was closed secondary to treatment-related death. They observed that cisplatin with topotecan offered an improvement in both progression-free survival and overall survival (9.4 vs. 6.5 months) in patients with recurrent cervical cancer. However, this was associated with increased hematologic toxicity,[83] although an ancillary study revealed that overall quality of life was not affected.[84]

FUTURE DIRECTIONS

The treatment of cervical cancer is ever changing, and the standard of care for managing this disease will continue to evolve as new treatment paradigms are explored. There are a vast number of studies currently being conducted regarding cervical cancer therapy. These trials include addition of chemotherapy to chemosensitizing radiotherapy in intermediate-risk patients; the evaluation of preoperative PET and CT imaging to detect lymph node metastases; the use of simple hysterectomy, versus radical, in very early-stage disease; and efficacy of targeted agents such as bevacizumab in addition to cytotoxic chemotherapy in recurrent disease. As surgical management, chemotherapy, and radiotherapy in this disease continue to progress, the survival and morbidities of women undergoing treatment for cervical cancer should continue to improve.

REFERENCES

1. Roden R, Wu TC. How will HPV vaccines affect cervical cancer? *Nat Rev Cancer.* 2006;6(10):753-763.
2. Howell EA, Chen YT, Concato J. Differences in cervical cancer mortality among black and white women. *Obstet Gynecol.* 1999;94(4):509-515.
3. Castellsague X, Munoz N. Chapter 3: cofactors in human papillomavirus carcinogenesis: role of parity, oral contraceptives, and tobacco smoking. *J Natl Cancer Inst Monogr.* 2003(31):20-28.
4. Lacey JV Jr, Swanson CA, Brinton LA, et al. Obesity as a potential risk factor for adenocarcinomas and squamous cell carcinomas of the uterine cervix. *Cancer.* 2003;98(4):814-821.

5. Altekruse SF, Lacey JV Jr, Brinton LA, et al. Comparison of human papillomavirus genotypes, sexual, and reproductive risk factors of cervical adenocarcinoma and squamous cell carcinoma: Northeastern United States. *Am J Obstet Gynecol.* 2003;188(3): 657-663.

6. Lichtenstein P, Holm NV, Verkasalo PK, et al. Environmental and heritable factors in the causation of cancer: analyses of cohorts of twins from Sweden, Denmark, and Finland. *N Engl J Med.* 2000;343(2):78-85.

7. Tolstrup J, Munk C, Thomsen BL, et al. The role of smoking and alcohol intake in the development of high-grade squamous intraepithelial lesions among high-risk HPV-positive women. *Acta Obstet Gynecol Scand.* 2006;85(9):1114-1119.

8. Cervical carcinoma and reproductive factors: collaborative reanalysis of individual data on 16,563 women with cervical carcinoma and 33,542 women without cervical carcinoma from 25 epidemiological studies. *Int J Cancer.* 2006;119(5): 1108-1124.

9. Smith JS, Green J, Berrington de Gonzalez A, et al. Cervical cancer and use of hormonal contraceptives: a systematic review. *Lancet.* 2003;361(9364):1159-1167.

10. Castle PE. Beyond human papillomavirus: the cervix, exogenous secondary factors, and the development of cervical precancer and cancer. *J Low Genit Tract Dis.* 2004;8(3):224-230.

11. Skegg DC. Oral contraceptives, parity, and cervical cancer. *Lancet.* 2002;359(9312):1080-1081.

12. Anttila T, Saikku P, Koskela P, et al. Serotypes of Chlamydia trachomatis and risk for development of cervical squamous cell carcinoma. *JAMA.* 2001;285(1):47-51.

13. Woodman CB, Collins S, Winter H, et al. Natural history of cervical human papillomavirus infection in young women: a longitudinal cohort study. *Lancet.* 2001;357(9271):1831-1836.

14. Castellsague X, Bosch FX, Munoz N, et al. Male circumcision, penile human papillomavirus infection, and cervical cancer in female partners. *N Engl J Med.* 2002;346(15):1105-1112.

15. Duerr A, Paramsothy P, Jamieson DJ, et al. Effect of HIV infection on atypical squamous cells of undetermined significance. *Clin Infect Dis.* 2006;42(6):855-861.

16. Lehtovirta P, Finne P, Nieminen P, et al. Prevalence and risk factors of squamous intraepithelial lesions of the cervix among HIV-infected women: a long-term follow-up study in a low-prevalence population. *Int J STD AIDS.* 2006;17(12): 831-834.

17. Schiffman M, Castle PE, Jeronimo J, Rodriguez AC, Wacholder S. Human papillomavirus and cervical cancer. *Lancet.* 2007;370(9590):890-907.

18. Sherman ME, Wang SS, Carreon J, Devesa SS. Mortality trends for cervical squamous and adenocarcinoma in the United States. Relation to incidence and survival. *Cancer.* 2005;103(6): 1258-1264.

19. Riley RR, Duensing S, Brake T, Munger K, Lambert PF, Arbeit JM. Dissection of human papillomavirus E6 and E7 function in transgenic mouse models of cervical carcinogenesis. *Cancer Res.* 2003;63(16):4862-4871.

20. Hopman AH, Smedts F, Dignef W, et al. Transition of high-grade cervical intraepithelial neoplasia to micro-invasive carcinoma is characterized by integration of HPV 16/18 and numerical chromosome abnormalities. *J Pathol.* 2004;202(1): 23-33.

21. Hricak H, Gatsonis C, Chi DS, et al. Role of imaging in pretreatment evaluation of early invasive cervical cancer: results of the intergroup study American College of Radiology Imaging Network 6651-Gynecologic Oncology Group 183. *J Clin Oncol.* 2005;23(36):9329-9337.

22. Subak LL, Hricak H, Powell CB, Azizi L, Stern JL. Cervical carcinoma: computed tomography and magnetic resonance imaging for preoperative staging. *Obstet Gynecol.* 1995;86(1):43-50.

23. Ascher SM, Takahama J, Jha RC. Staging of gynecologic malignancies. *Top Magn Reson Imaging.* 2001;12(2):105-129.

24. Wright JD, Dehdashti F, Herzog TJ, et al. Preoperative lymph node staging of early-stage cervical carcinoma by [18F]-fluoro-2-deoxy-D-glucose-positron emission tomography. *Cancer.* 2005; 104(11):2484-2491.

25. Grigsby PW, Siegel BA, Dehdashti F. Lymph node staging by positron emission tomography in patients with carcinoma of the cervix. *J Clin Oncol.* 2001;19(17):3745-3749.

26. Lininger RA, Wistuba I, Gazdar A, Koenig C, Tavassoli FA, Albores-Saavedra J. Human papillomavirus type 16 is detected in transitional cell carcinomas and squamotransitional cell carcinomas of the cervix and endometrium. *Cancer.* 1998;83(3): 521-527.

27. Cho NH, Joo HJ, Ahn HJ, Jung WH, Lee KG. Detection of human papillomavirus in warty carcinoma of the uterine cervix: comparison of immunohistochemistry, in situ hybridization and in situ polymerase chain reaction methods. *Pathol Res Pract.* 1998;194(10):713-720.

28. Tseng CJ, Pao CC, Tseng LH, et al. Lymphoepithelioma-like carcinoma of the uterine cervix: association with Epstein-Barr virus and human papillomavirus. *Cancer.* 1997;80(1):91-97.

29. Kaminski PF, Norris HJ. Minimal deviation carcinoma (adenoma malignum) of the cervix. *Int J Gynecol Pathol.* 1983;2(2): 141-152.

30. Young RH, Welch WR, Dickersin GR, Scully RE. Ovarian sex cord tumor with annular tubules: review of 74 cases including 27 with Peutz-Jeghers syndrome and four with adenoma malignum of the cervix. *Cancer.* 1982;50(7):1384-1402.

31. Jones MW, Silverberg SG, Kurman RJ. Well-differentiated villoglandular adenocarcinoma of the uterine cervix: a clinicopathological study of 24 cases. *Int J Gynecol Pathol.* 1993;12(1):1-7.

32. Potter R, Dimopoulos J, Kirisits C, et al. Recommendations for image-based intracavitary brachytherapy of cervix cancer: the GYN GEC ESTRO Working Group point of view: in regard to Nag et al. (Int J Radiat Oncol Biol Phys 2004;60:1160-1172). *Int J Radiat Oncol Biol Phys.* 2005;62(1):293-295; author reply 295-296.

33. Ferry JA, Scully RE. Mesonephric remnants, hyperplasia, and neoplasia in the uterine cervix. A study of 49 cases. *Am J Surg Pathol.* 1990;14(12):1100-1111.

34. Jones MA, Andrews J, Tarraza HM. Mesonephric remnant hyperplasia of the cervix: a clinicopathologic analysis of 14 cases. *Gynecol Oncol.* 1993;49(1):41-47.

35. Wang SS, Sherman ME, Silverberg SG, et al. Pathological characteristics of cervical adenocarcinoma in a multi-center US-based study. *Gynecol Oncol.* 2006;103(2):541-546.

36. Vesterinen E, Forss M, Nieminen U. Increase of cervical adenocarcinoma: a report of 520 cases of cervical carcinoma including 112 tumors with glandular elements. *Gynecol Oncol.* 1989;33(1):49-53.

37. Nasu K, Takai N, Narahara H. Multimodal treatment for glassy cell carcinoma of the uterine cervix. *J Obstet Gynaecol Res.* 2009;35(3):584-587.

38. Parwani AV, Smith Sehdev AE, Kurman RJ, Ronnett BM. Cervical adenoid basal tumors comprised of adenoid basal epithelioma associated with various types of invasive carcinoma: clinicopathologic features, human papillomavirus DNA detection, and P16 expression. *Hum Pathol.* 2005;36(1):82-90.

39. Takeshima N, Yanoh K, Tabata T, Nagai K, Hirai Y, Hasumi K. Assessment of the revised International Federation of Gynecology and Obstetrics staging for early invasive squamous cervical cancer. *Gynecol Oncol.* 1999;74:165-169.

40. Bisseling KC, Bekkers RL, Rome RM, Quinn MA. Treatment of microinvasive adenocarcinoma of the uterine cervix: a retrospective study and review of the literature. *Gynecol Oncol.* 2007;107(3):424-430.

41. Kolstad P. Follow-up study of 232 patients with stage Ia1 and 411 patients with stage Ia2 squamous cell carcinoma of the cervix (microinvasive carcinoma). *Gynecol Oncol*. 1989;33(3): 265-272.

42. Roman LD, Felix JC, Muderspach LI, et al. Influence of quantity of lymph-vascular space invasion on the risk of nodal metastases in women with early-stage squamous cancer of the cervix. *Gynecol Oncol*. 1998;68(3):220-225.

43. Raspagliesi F, Ditto A, Quattrone P, et al. Prognostic factors in microinvasive cervical squamous cell cancer: long-term results. *Int J Gynecol Cancer*. 2005;15(1):88-93.

44. Buckley SL, Tritz DM, Van Le L, et al. Lymph node metastases and prognosis in patients with stage IA2 cervical cancer. *Gynecol Oncol*. 1996;63(1):4-9.

45. Suri A, Frumovitz M, Milam MR, dos Reis R, Ramirez PT. Preoperative pathologic findings associated with residual disease at radical hysterectomy in women with stage IA2 cervical cancer. *Gynecol Oncol*. 2009;112(1):110-113.

46. Landoni F, Maneo A, Colombo A, et al. Randomised study of radical surgery versus radiotherapy for stage Ib-IIa cervical cancer. *Lancet*. 1997;350(9077):535-540.

47. Landoni F, Maneo A, Cormio G, et al. Class II versus class III radical hysterectomy in stage IB-IIA cervical cancer: a prospective randomized study. *Gynecol Oncol*. 2001;80(1):3-12.

48. Shimada M, Kigawa J, Nishimura R, et al. Ovarian metastasis in carcinoma of the uterine cervix. *Gynecol Oncol*. 2006; 101(2):234-7.

49. Havrilesky LJ, Leath CA, Huh W, et al. Radical hysterectomy and pelvic lymphadenectomy for stage IB2 cervical cancer. *Gynecol Oncol*. 2004;93(2):429-434.

50. Kamelle SA, Rutledge TL, Tillmanns TD, et al. Surgical-pathological predictors of disease-free survival and risk groupings for IB2 cervical cancer: do the traditional models still apply? *Gynecol Oncol*. 2004;94(2):249-255.

51. Eifel PJ. Chemoradiotherapy in the treatment of cervical cancer. *Semin Radiat Oncol*. 2006;16(3):177-185.

52. Cosin JA, Fowler JM, Chen MD, Paley PJ, Carson LF, Twiggs LB. Pretreatment surgical staging of patients with cervical carcinoma: the case for lymph node debulking. *Cancer*. 1998; 82(11):2241-8.

53. Kavadi VS, Eifel PJ. FIGO stage IIIA carcinoma of the uterine cervix. *Int J Radiat Oncol Biol Phys*. 1992;24(2):211-215.

54. Dittmer PH, Randall ME. A technique for inguinal node boost using photon fields defined by asymmetric collimator jaws. *Radiother Oncol*. 2001;59:61-64.

55. Stehman FB, Ali S, Keys HM, et al. Radiation therapy with or without weekly cisplatin for bulky stage 1B cervical carcinoma: follow-up of a Gynecologic Oncology Group trial. *Am J Obstet Gynecol*. 2007;197(5):503 e501-506.

56. Eifel PJ, Winter K, Morris M, et al. Pelvic irradiation with concurrent chemotherapy versus pelvic and para-aortic irradiation for high-risk cervical cancer: an update of radiation therapy oncology group trial (RTOG) 90-01. *J Clin Oncol*. 2004;22(5):872-880.

57. Rose PG, Ali S, Watkins E, et al. Long-term follow-up of a randomized trial comparing concurrent single agent cisplatin, cisplatin-based combination chemotherapy, or hydroxyurea during pelvic irradiation for locally advanced cervical cancer: a Gynecologic Oncology Group Study. *J Clin Oncol*. 2007;25(19):2804-2810.

58. Pearcey R, Miao Q, Kong W, Zhang-Salomons J, Mackillop WJ. Impact of adoption of chemoradiotherapy on the outcome of cervical cancer in Ontario: results of a population-based cohort study. *J Clin Oncol*. 2007;25(17):2383-2388.

59. Reducing uncertainties about the effects of chemoradiotherapy for cervical cancer: individual patient data meta-analysis. *Cochrane Database Syst Rev*. 2010(1):CD008285.

60. National Comprehensive Cancer Network. Clinical Practice Guidelines in Oncology v.1.2010. http://www.nccn.org/professionals/physician_gls/f_guidelines.asp. Accessed on 13 January, 2012.

61. Milliken DA, Shepherd JH. Fertility preserving surgery for carcinoma of the cervix. *Curr Opin Oncol*. 2008;20(5):575-580.

62. Plante M. Vaginal radical trachelectomy: an update. *Gynecol Oncol*. 2008;111(2 suppl):S105-S110.

63. Plante M, Renaud MC, Hoskins IA, Roy M. Vaginal radical trachelectomy: a valuable fertility-preserving option in the management of early-stage cervical cancer. A series of 50 pregnancies and review of the literature. *Gynecol Oncol*. 2005;98(1): 3-10.

64. Delotte J, Ferron G, Kuei TL, Mery E, Gladieff L, Querleu D. Laparoscopic management of an isolated ovarian metastasis on a transposed ovary in a patient treated for stage IB1 adenocarcinoma of the cervix. *J Minim Invasive Gynecol*. 2009;16(1):106-108.

65. Keys HM, Bundy BN, Stehman FB, et al. Radiation therapy with and without extrafascial hysterectomy for bulky stage IB cervical carcinoma: a randomized trial of the Gynecologic Oncology Group. *Gynecol Oncol*. 2003;89(3):343-353.

66. Sedlis A, Bundy BN, Rotman MZ, Lentz SS, Muderspach LI, Zaino RJ. a randomized trial of pelvic radiation therapy versus no further therapy in selected patients with stage IB carcinoma of the cervix after radical hysterectomy and pelvic lymphadenectomy: a Gynecologic Oncology Group Study. *Gynecol Oncol*. 1999;73(2):177-183.

67. Barillot I, Horiot JC, Cuisenier J, et al. Carcinoma of the cervical stump: a review of 213 cases. *Eur J Cancer*. 1993;29A(9): 1231-1236.

68. Creasman WT, Zaino RJ, Major FJ, Disaia PJ, Hatch KD, Homesley KD. Early invasive carcinoma of the cervix (3-5 mm invasion): risk factors and prognosis. A Gynecologic Group Study. *Am J Obstet Gynecol*. 1998;178:65-62.

69. Fuller AF Jr, Elliott N, Kosloff C, Hoskins WJ, Lewis JL Jr. Determinants of increased risk for recurrence in patients undergoing radical hysterectomy for stage IB and IIA carcinoma of the cervix. *Gynecol Oncol*. 1989;33(1):34-39.

70. Delgado G, Bundy B, Zaino R, Sevin BU, Creasman WT, Major F. Prospective surgical-pathological study of disease-free interval in patients with stage IB squamous cell carcinoma of the cervix: a Gynecologic Oncology Group study. *Gynecol Oncol*. Sep 1990;38(3):352-357.

71. Rutledge TL, Kamelle SA, Tillmanns TD, et al. A comparison of stages IB1 and IB2 cervical cancers treated with radical hysterectomy. Is size the real difference? *Gynecol Oncol*. 2004;95(1):70-76.

72. Dunst J, Kuhnt T, Strauss HG, et al. Anemia in cervical cancers: impact on survival, patterns of relapse, and association with hypoxia and angiogenesis. *Int J Radiat Oncol Biol Phys*. 2003;56(3):778-787.

73. Fyles AW, Milosevic M, Pintilie M, Syed A, Hill RP. Anemia, hypoxia and transfusion in patients with cervix cancer: a review. *Radiother Oncol*. 2000;57(1):13-19.

74. Grogan M, Thomas GM, Melamed I, et al. The importance of hemoglobin levels during radiotherapy for carcinoma of the cervix. *Cancer*. 1999;86(8):1528-1536.

75. Sundfor K, Lyng H, Kongsgard UL, Trope C, Rofstad EK. Polarographic measurement of pO2 in cervix carcinoma. *Gynecol Oncol*. 1997;64(2):230-236.

76. Lavey RS, Liu PY, Greer BE, et al. Recombinant human erythropoietin as an adjunct to radiation therapy and cisplatin for stage IIB-IVA carcinoma of the cervix: a Southwest Oncology Group study. *Gynecol Oncol*. 2004;95(1):145-151.

77. Berek JS, Howe C, Lagasse LD, Hacker NF. Pelvic exenteration for recurrent gynecologic malignancy: survival and morbidity analysis of the 45-year experience at UCLA. *Gynecol Oncol*. 2005;99(1):153-159.

78. Marnitz S, Kohler C, Muller M, Behrens K, Hasenbein K, Schneider A. Indications for primary and secondary exenterations in patients with cervical cancer. *Gynecol Oncol.* 2006;103(3): 1023-1030.
79. Goldberg GL, Sukumvanich P, Einstein MH, Smith HO, Anderson PS, Fields AL. Total pelvic exenteration: the Albert Einstein College of Medicine/Montefiore Medical Center Experience (1987 to 2003). *Gynecol Oncol.* 2006;101(2): 261-268.
80. Coleman RL, Keeney ED, Freedman RS, Burke TW, Eifel PJ, Rutledge FN. Radical hysterectomy for recurrent carcinoma of the uterine cervix after radiotherapy. *Gynecol Oncol.* 1994;55(1):29-35.
81. Maneo A, Landoni F, Cormio G, Colombo A, Mangioni C. Radical hysterectomy for recurrent or persistent cervical cancer following radiation therapy. *Int J Gynecol Cancer.* 1999;9(4): 295-301.
82. Bonomi P, Blessing JA, Stehman FB, DiSaia PJ, Walton L, Major FJ. Randomized trial of three cisplatin dose schedules in squamous-cell carcinoma of the cervix: a Gynecologic Oncology Group study. *J Clin Oncol.* 1985;3(8):1079-1085.
83. Long HJ 3rd, Bundy BN, Grendys EC Jr, et al. Randomized phase III trial of cisplatin with or without topotecan in carcinoma of the uterine cervix: a Gynecologic Oncology Group Study. *J Clin Oncol.* 20 2005;23(21):4626-4633.
84. Monk BJ, Huang HQ, Cella D, Long HJ 3rd. Quality of life outcomes from a randomized phase III trial of cisplatin with or without topotecan in advanced carcinoma of the cervix: a Gynecologic Oncology Group Study. *J Clin Oncol.* 20 2005;23(21):4617-4625.

CHAPTER 5

6 Endometrial Hyperplasia and Cancer

David A. Iglesias, Marilyn Huang, Pamela T. Soliman,
Bojana Djordjevic, and Karen H. Lu

Endometrial cancer is the most common malignancy of the female genital tract in the United States. Women have an overall lifetime risk of 2.5% of developing endometrial cancer. Fortunately, the majority of endometrial present at early stages with postmenopausal bleeding. Although obesity and estrogen excess remain the strongest risk factors for this disease, Lynch syndrome comprises the majority of inherited endometrial cancer cases; affected women have a 40% to 60% predicted lifetime risk of developing endometrial cancer.

For early-stage disease, standard management includes total abdominal hysterectomy, bilateral salpingo-oophorectomy, and staging. Management for women with advanced-stage disease primarily involves surgical resection and chemotherapy. Radiation therapy may be used for local control or in treating patients with positive lymph nodes, and hormonal therapies have been shown to be effective in a subset of patients. Several novel molecular-targeted therapies have been developed and evaluated for the treatment of endometrial carcinoma. The principal benefit to these drugs, at this time, has been to prolong stable disease.

EPIDEMIOLOGY

Key Points

1. Endometrioid endometrial carcinomas account for approximately 80% of cases and typically occur in perimenopausal or postmenopausal women, are often of lower histologic grade, are often confined to the uterus and have a more favorable prognosis.

2. Risk factors associated with the development of endometrioid endometrial cancer include obesity, tamoxifen use, chronic anovulation, exogenous estrogen administration, nulliparity, early menarche, and/or late menopause.

3. Type 1 and 2 endometrial carcinomas exhibit distinct molecular alterations. The most common molecular alteration associated with type 1 tumors is loss of *PTEN*, whereas in type 2 tumors, it is *p53* mutations.

Incidence

Endometrial cancer is the most common gynecologic malignancy in the United States. An estimated 43,470 women will be diagnosed with uterine cancer in 2010, and it is estimated that 7950 of these women will die of the disease.[1] Endometrial adenocarcinoma typically affects women in their perimenopausal or postmenopausal years and is most frequently diagnosed in women between the ages of 50 and 65 years. However, approximately 5% of cases are diagnosed in women before the age of 40 years, and approximately 10% to 15% of women are diagnosed before the age of 50 years.[2] Women have an overall lifetime risk of 2.53% (1 in 40) of developing endometrial cancer.[1] Approximately 90% of uterine tumors arise within the endometrium and are categorized as endometrial carcinomas. Of the endometrial carcinomas, 80% are endometrioid adenocarcinomas, and 15% to 20% are of more rare subtypes: papillary serous, clear cell, mucinous, or mixed carcinomas. These uncommon subtypes are associated with a poorer prognosis and greater risk of extra-uterine metastases when compared with endometrioid adenocarcinomas.

Risk Factors

Multiple well-defined risk factors are associated with endometrial cancer and vary depending on the histologic subtype (Table 6-1). Type 1 endometrial cancer is associated with estrogenic stimulation; thus conditions that increase a patient's level or duration of exposure to unopposed estrogen, in the absence of progesterone, will increase the risk of developing endometrial hyperplasia and ultimately carcinoma. Risk factors associated with excess or prolonged estrogen exposure include exogenous estrogen administration, chronic anovulation, obesity, tamoxifen use, nulliparity, early menarche, and/or late menopause.

Unopposed estrogen exposure is a well-established risk factor for the development of endometrial hyperplasia and/or carcinoma. Estradiol acts as a mitogen in normal endometrial tissue. During the follicular phase, plasma estradiol levels predominate at normal premenopausal concentrations while progesterone levels are low. Endometrial proliferation rates remain high throughout the follicular phase. Plasma estradiol levels remain elevated until ovulation, when they begin to fall rapidly and the corpus luteum produces and secretes progesterone. During the luteal phase of the menstrual cycle, progesterone predominates and counters the estrogenic effects on the endometrium by promoting the local synthesis of 17β-hydroxysteroid dehydrogenase and estrogen sulfo-transferase, which favor the conversion of estradiol to the less potent estrogen (E1) and into estrogen sulfates that are quickly eliminated from the body.[3] Thus any derangement in the normal balance between estradiol and progesterone will lead to continuous endometrial stimulation and proliferation. Over time, this persistent stimulation may lead to endometrial hyperplasia and/or carcinoma.

Table 6-1 Risk Factors for Endometrial Cancer

Risk Factor	Relative Risk
Unopposed estrogen therapy	10-20
Obesity	2-5
Tamoxifen	2.5
Estrogen-producing ovarian tumors	5
Polycystic ovarian syndrome	3-5
Infertility/nulliparity	2-3
Diabetes	2-3

Tamoxifen is a selective estrogen receptor modulator that demonstrates either estrogenic or antiestrogenic effects in different tissues. In the uterus it functions as an estrogen agonist, whereas in the breast it functions as an estrogen antagonist. Tamoxifen is commonly used in the treatment of estrogen receptor–positive breast cancer, but is also associated with an increased risk of uterine cancer. The National Surgical Adjuvant Breast and Bowel Project (NSABP) B-14 trial compared rates of endometrial cancer in tamoxifen- and non–tamoxifen-treated patients and described the pathologic characteristics of the endometrial cancers.[4] This study demonstrated a 7.5-fold increased risk of endometrial carcinoma in patients treated with tamoxifen relative to placebo controls. The annual hazard rate through all follow-up was 0.2 in 1000 in the placebo group and 1.6 in 1000 in the tamoxifen-treated group. The majority of endometrial cancer cases that developed during this study were of an early stage and low to moderate grade. In the NSABP P-1 chemoprevention trial, 13,388 women at increased risk for breast cancer were randomized to receive either tamoxifen (20 mg/d) or placebo for 5 years.[5] Although tamoxifen reduced the risk of invasive breast cancer by 49% ($P < .00001$), the rate of endometrial cancer was increased in the tamoxifen group (risk ratio, 2.53; 95% confidence interval [CI], 1.35-4.97), particularly in women over the age of 50 years.[5] Current recommendations for management of women treated with tamoxifen include performing an endometrial biopsy for women who develop irregular or postmenopausal vaginal bleeding.

Obesity is an established risk factor for the development of multiple cancer types, cancer-related mortality, and all-cause mortality.[6] Among all cancer types, increasing body mass index (BMI) and obesity is most strongly associated with endometrial cancer incidence and mortality.[6] The development of endometrial cancer in obese women is thought to be a result of the peripheral conversion of androstenedione to estrone by aromatase in adipose tissue. In a recent meta-analysis of 19 reviews and prospective studies, Renehan et al[7] found that each increase in BMI of 5 kg/m^2 significantly increased a woman's risk of developing endometrial cancer (relative risk [RR], 1.59; 95% CI, 1.50-1.68). Endometrial cancer mortality is also adversely affected by obesity, both directly and indirectly. Calle et al,[8] in a prospective study of more than 495,000 women followed for 16 years, examined the relationship between BMI and increased risk of cancer mortality. There was a clear trend associated with increasing BMI; the relative risk of uterine cancer–related death for women considered obese (BMI 30-34.9 kg/m^2) was 2.53, whereas for morbidly obese women (BMI ≥ 40 kg/m^2) it was 6.25.[8] The association between obesity and other medical comorbidities, such as diabetes mellitus and hypertension, adversely affects endometrial cancer–related mortality and all-cause mortality. In a retrospective review of 380 patients with early endometrial cancer, the Gynecologic Oncology Group (GOG) found that morbid obesity was associated with a higher mortality (HR, 2.77; 95% CI, 1.21-6.36) from causes other than endometrial cancer or disease recurrence.[9] Unfortunately, public knowledge of the association between obesity and cancer risk is limited, with a recent survey indicating that up to 58% of women were not aware that obesity increased endometrial cancer risk.[10]

Approximately 5% of endometrial cancer cases are attributed to an inherited predisposition. Hereditary nonpolyposis colorectal cancer (HNPCC), now known as Lynch syndrome, comprises the majority of inherited cases. Affected women have a 40% to 60% predicted lifetime risk of developing endometrial cancer and a 10% to 12% lifetime risk of developing ovarian cancer.[11,12] Lynch syndrome is inherited in an autosomal dominant pattern with incomplete penetrance due to a germline mutation in one of the mismatch repair (MMR) genes. The MMR genes include *MLH1* on chromosome 3, *MSH2* and *MSH6* on chromosome 2, and *PMS2* on chromosome 7. Loss of MMR gene function results in microsatellite instability (MSI), which leads to the accumulation of somatic mutations that are presumed to affect key regulatory genes related to cell growth and/or apoptosis. It is important to note that the incidence of endometrial cancer in female Lynch carriers actually equals or exceeds that of colorectal cancer.[13] Moreover, carriers who develop cancer are also at an increased risk of developing second subsequent metachronous malignancies. In 50% of patients with both colon and endometrial cancers, endometrial cancer is the sentinel event. The risk for women to develop endometrial cancer appears to differ slightly based on the specific germline mutations in MMR genes. The estimated lifetime risk at age 70 years is 26% for *MSH6* mutation carriers and 27% for *MLH1* mutation carriers, whereas it is 40% for *MSH2* mutation carriers.[14-16]

There are 2 primary guidelines used to identify families. The first is the Amsterdam Criteria, originally designed to diagnose Lynch syndrome in certain families based on clinical criteria. However, with the identification of MMR genes and the original criteria not accounting for extra-colonic cancers, the modified Amsterdam Criteria II was revised to be more inclusive (Table 6-2). The Bethesda guidelines were developed as a screening tool to identify which individuals should undergo MSI testing and then genetic testing. These guidelines focus predominantly on colon cancer. The goal of these guidelines was to determine which families should have MSI testing before screening for MMR mutations. The Society of Gynecologic

Table 6-2 Amsterdam II Criteria

Each of the following criteria must be fulfilled:

1. Three or more relatives with an associated cancer (colorectal or endometrial cancer, cancer of the small intestine, ureter, or renal pelvis)

2. Two or more successive generations affected

3. One or more relatives diagnosed before the age of 50 years

4. One should be a first-degree relative of the other two

5. Familial adenomatous polyposis should be excluded in cases of colorectal carcinoma

6. Tumors should be verified by pathologic examination

Oncologists recently published a committee statement with guidelines for identifying women with Lynch syndrome (Table 6-3).[17]

There are limited data on the efficacy of endometrial cancer screening in Lynch syndrome carriers. Current

Table 6-3 Society of Gynecologic Oncologists Statement Guidelines on Risk Assessment for Lynch Syndrome

For patients with 20%-25% risk of Lynch syndrome, genetic risk assessment is strongly recommended. These patients include:

1. Family pedigree meeting Amsterdam Criteria

2. Patients with metachronous or synchronous colorectal and endometrial or ovarian cancers before age 50 years

3. Those with a first- or second-degree relative with a known germline mutation in a MMR gene.

For patients with a 5%-10% risk of having Lynch syndrome, genetic testing was classified as being "helpful." These patients include:

1. Patients with endometrial or colorectal cancer diagnosed before age 50 years

2. Patients with endometrial and/or ovarian cancer and a synchronous or metachronous Lynch-associated malignancy before age 50 years

3. Patients with endometrial or colorectal cancer and a first-degree relative diagnosed with a Lynch-associated malignancy before age 50 years

4. Patients with endometrial or colorectal cancer at any age with ≥2 first- or second-degree relatives diagnosed with a Lynch-associated malignancy at any age

5. A patient with a first- or second-degree relative who meets the above criteria

CHAPTER 6

recommendations advise women to undergo annual endometrial biopsies (EMB) beginning between the ages of 30 and 35 years or 10 years before the first endometrial cancer diagnosis in the family. Several studies have examined the utility of transvaginal ultrasound as a screening modality; however, as the only method, it is ineffective for detecting early endometrial cancer. Prophylactic hysterectomy with bilateral salpingo-oophorectomy has been recommended as a prevention strategy after completing childbearing; however, the specific age remains controversial.[18] Thus counseling for prophylactic surgery in Lynch carriers having completed childbearing is on a case-by-case basis, balancing benefits of ovarian function and reducing cancer risk.

Pathogenesis

Based on epidemiologic, molecular, and prognostic factors, endometrial cancer can be subdivided broadly into 2 types.[19] Type 1 carcinomas, accounting for approximately 80% of cases, are classically of endometrioid histology and are usually preceded by endometrial atypical hyperplasia. These tumors typically occur in perimenopausal or postmenopausal women, are often of lower histologic grade, are often confined to the uterus at presentation, and thus have a more favorable prognosis. Type 1 carcinomas commonly express estrogen and progesterone receptors and are associated with unopposed estrogen exposure. Up to 90% of type 1 endometrial cancer patients are obese.[20]

Type 2 carcinomas are often of nonendometrioid histology and typically arise in a background of atrophic endometrium. These lesions appear to be unrelated to estrogen stimulation and are not typically preceded by endometrial atypical hyperplasia. The precursor lesion of type 2 carcinoma is termed *endometrial intraepithelial neoplasia*. Type 2 lesions include serous and clear cell histologies and have a propensity for early metastatic spread and a poor prognosis. Type 2 tumors are not typically associated with obesity.

Molecular Biology of Endometrial Cancer

Type 1 and type 2 lesions exhibit distinct molecular alterations. The most frequent genetic alteration associated with type 1 lesions is a loss of function of the tumor suppressor *PTEN*. *PTEN* loss of function can be seen in up to 83% of endometrioid carcinomas and 55% of precancerous lesions.[21] Mutations in *PTEN* have been documented in endometrial hyperplasia with and without atypia and thus have been postulated to be an early event in the endometrial tumorigenesis process.[22] PTEN most notably plays a role in the regulation of the phosphotidylinositide 3-kinase (PI3K)-Akt-mammalian target of rapamycin (mTOR) pathway by inhibiting the downstream phosphorylation of AKT,

but its loss of function has also has been shown to result in genomic instability by causing defects in either homologous recombination DNA repair or in cell cycle checkpoints. Mutations on PIK3CA are also relatively common and are seen in up to 36% of endometrioid cancers.[23] These mutations tend to occur in tumors that also have *PTEN* loss.

Other common genetic alterations associated with type 1 endometrial carcinomas include MSI, mutations in K-ras, and mutations in β-catenin. Approximately 20% to 30% of type I lesions exhibit MSI. Microsatellites are repeated sequences of DNA of a set length predominately found in noncoding DNA that are variable from person to person. The propensity of a tumor to develop changes in the number of repeat elements compared with normal tissue due to defects in the DNA mismatch repair process is termed *microsatellite instability*. This leads to replication errors that may inactivate or alter tumor suppressor genes. MSI has also been shown to occur early in the tumorigenesis process and is associated with a higher rate of *PTEN* mutations.[24,25]

K-ras mutations have been found in up to 30% of endometrial cancers.[26] When K-ras is mutated, it functions as an oncogene upregulating signaling through the mitogen-activated protein kinase pathway. As with *PTEN*, mutations in K-ras are more frequent in MSI-positive tumors.[27]

β-catenin plays a role in signal transduction as a transcriptional activator in the Wnt signaling pathway and is a member of the E-cadherin unit of proteins that is essential for maintenance of normal tissue architecture and cell differentiation. Gain of function mutations in β-catenin are seen in 25% to 38% of type 1 lesions.[28] β-catenin mutations have been identified in atypical endometrial hyperplasia, indicating that it also may be an early event in endometrial tumorigenesis.[29] However, whereas MSI and mutations in *PTEN* and K-ras tend to coexist, β-catenin gain of function mutations are usually seen alone.[30]

In contrast, the genetic alterations most commonly seen in type 2 lesions are *p53* mutations, HER-2/*neu* amplification, and *p16* inactivation. The most common of these is a mutation in the tumor suppressor gene, *p53*, which is found in up to 90% of serous carcinomas (compared with 10% of type 1 lesions).[26] Mutations in p53 are also seen in up to 80% of endometrial intraepithelial lesions, the precursor lesions of serous carcinomas.[31] HER-2/*neu* is an oncogene involved in cell signaling. Overexpression and amplification of HER-2/*neu* occurs in 43% and 29% of serous carcinomas, respectively.[32] *p16* is also a tumor suppressor gene involved in cell cycle regulation. Inactivation of *p16* has been identified in 45% of serous carcinomas and less frequently in clear cell carcinomas.[31] These genetic changes are also seen in preneoplastic atrophic endometrium, indicating that they are early events in type 2 endometrial tumorigenesis.[33]

The identification of these genetic alterations has led to the development and implementation of several targeted therapeutic strategies for the management of endometrial cancer, which are reviewed later in this chapter.

DIAGNOSIS

Key Points

1. Postmenopausal bleeding is the most common presenting symptom of endometrial cancer.
2. Endometrial cancer screening strategies are unnecessary for women at general population risk.
4. Transvaginal ultrasound has been evaluated as a diagnostic tool for endometrial cancer in patients with postmenopausal or irregular vaginal bleeding.
5. Dilation and curettage remains the gold standard for diagnosing endometrial cancer; however, in-office endometrial sampling devices have been shown to be highly accurate in women with an endometrial stripe thickness of less than 7 mm.

Clinical Features

Endometrial cancer is classically a disease of perimenopausal and postmenopausal women. The initial endometrial lesion arises in the glandular component of the uterine lining. As it forms a mass, it contains areas of superficial necrosis and becomes more friable (Figure 6-1). As a result, approximately 90% of women with endometrial cancer present with abnormal vaginal

Table 6-4 Differential Diagnosis of Postmenopausal Bleeding

Atrophic endometritis and vaginitis

Benign intracavitary lesions
    Endometrial polyps
    Leiomyomas

Endometrial hyperplasia
Endometrial carcinoma
Cervical carcinoma
Exogenous estrogens
Vaginal or cervical trauma
Bleeding disorders

bleeding. Up to 20% of women with postmenopausal bleeding have an underlying endometrial carcinoma or hyperplasia. Although postmenopausal bleeding is most common, perimenopausal or anovulatory premenopausal women with intermenstrual bleeding or menometrorrhagia should also be evaluated for endometrial cancer. Unfortunately, as there are many potential causes for abnormal bleeding in this patient population, diagnosis may often be delayed (Table 6-4). In some cases, particularly in older women or women who have undergone prior cervical conization or loop electrosurgical excision procedure (LEEP), cervical stenosis may mask the development of postmenopausal bleeding. In this situation, patients may present with hematometra or pyometra. Postmenopausal women experiencing vaginal bleeding, perimenopausal women with heavy or prolonged bleeding, and anovulatory or oligovulatory premenopausal women with abnormal bleeding are considered high risk and warrant endometrial sampling. Furthermore, it is recommended that any woman over the age of 35 years with prolonged or heavy vaginal bleeding undergo endometrial sampling.

On physical examination, finding additional abnormalities is unlikely unless the patient is presenting at an advanced stage of disease with ascites or carcinomatosis. However, it is important to perform a thorough physical examination because a majority of these patients are obese and have other medical comorbidities, including hypertension and diabetes mellitus. On pelvic examination, examination of the vulva, vagina, and cervix is important to exclude metastatic disease. The appearance and patency of the cervical os should be noted, as stenosis may delay the manifestation of postmenopausal bleeding. On bimanual examination, the uterus may feel bulky or tender to palpation, particularly with hematometra, pyometra, or advanced disease. Rectovaginal examination should be performed to palpate the posterior cul-de-sac, adnexa, and parametria.

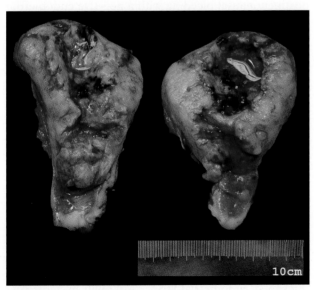

FIGURE 6-1. Endometrial carcinoma (with extension into the cervix).

Screening

Endometrial cancer screening strategies are unnecessary for women at general population risk. Even women who are at increased risk, including those women being treated with tamoxifen, do not benefit from endometrial cancer screening. Pap smear screening for endometrial cancer is unreliable. The finding of atypical glandular cells on Pap smear should warrant further evaluation with endometrial biopsy and endocervical curettage. However, only 50% of patients with endometrial cancer will have an abnormality on Pap smear. Those patients who do are more likely to have more advanced disease. Compared with patients with normal cervical cytology, those with malignant endometrial cells have more than twice the risk of deep myometrial invasion, twice the risk of grade 2 or 3 tumor, and 3 times the risk of positive peritoneal washings.

Transvaginal ultrasonography to evaluate the thickness and contour of the endometrial stripe has been evaluated as a potential endometrial cancer screening technique, especially in women taking tamoxifen. However, Love and colleagues,[34] in an investigation of 357 women treated with tamoxifen and 130 controls who were screened with transvaginal ultrasonography, found that although ultrasound identified a statistically significant ($P < .0001$) positive correlation between length of time on tamoxifen and endometrial thickness, it was a poor screening tool because of the high false-positive rate (46%). Proponents of transvaginal ultrasonography for endometrial screening have argued that it is a relatively noninvasive technique that may help providers determine which patients should undergo endometrial sampling.

Transvaginal ultrasonography has been proposed to identify women with postmenopausal bleeding who are highly unlikely to have endometrial disease so that endometrial sampling may be unnecessary. In a multi-institutional study of more than 1100 women, Karlsson and colleagues[35] established an endometrial stripe thickness cut-off of 5 mm to help triage patients with postmenopausal bleeding toward endometrial biopsy. This yielded a sensitivity of 94%, a specificity of 78%, a positive predictive value (PPV) of 69%, and a negative predictive value (NPV) of 96%. They found that no malignant endometrium was thinner than 5 mm and determined that the risk of finding any endometrial abnormality when the endometrial stripe thickness was ≤4 mm was 5.5%. As a result, they concluded that given the high NPV, it would be reasonable to refrain from endometrial sampling in women with postmenopausal bleeding who cannot undergo endometrial sampling. However, others have argued that the presence of a thin endometrial stripe does not reduce the need for endometrial sampling, because up to 4% of endometrial cancers would be missed

using this strategy, with a false-positive rate as high as 50%.[36] More recently, Timmermans and colleagues[37] conducted a systematic review and meta-analysis of 90 studies reporting on endometrial stripe thickness in women with postmenopausal bleeding and a diagnosis of endometrial carcinoma. The authors concluded that previous studies had likely overestimated the diagnostic accuracy of endometrial stripe thickness in the detection of endometrial cancer and recommended reducing the cut-off to 3 mm.

Diagnostic Testing

Due to the unreliable results associated with Pap screening and the difficulties with conclusively interpreting endometrial stripe thickness, in-office endometrial sampling is a necessary step in the evaluation of women who present with abnormal or postmenopausal vaginal bleeding. Several devices have been developed and are commercially available. These devices are used for direct sampling of the endometrium and allow both cytologic and histologic evaluation of the uterine lining. A meta-analysis reported that the Cornier Pipelle (Prodimed, Neuilly-en-Thelle, France) was the most effective device, with detection rates for endometrial carcinoma in postmenopausal and premenopausal women of 99.6% and 91%, respectively.[38] Use of the Pipelle to detect endometrial carcinoma or hyperplasia has been shown to be effective, with a sensitivity of 84.2%, specificity of 99.1%, accuracy of 96.9%, PPV of 94.1%, and NPV of 93.7%.[39] In addition, the accuracy of in-office endometrial biopsy is comparable to the gold standard of dilation and curettage (D&C) only for an endometrial stripe thickness of less than 7 mm.[40] For an endometrial stripe thickness greater than 7 mm, D&C may be superior. Thus women reporting postmenopausal bleeding with a negative endometrial biopsy warrant further investigation.

The usefulness of combining transvaginal ultrasound with endometrial biopsy has been investigated as a diagnostic schema for the detection of endometrial hyperplasia and carcinoma, with excellent results. In a study of 552 women, Minagawa and colleagues[41] found that the combined method achieved a sensitivity of 100%, a specificity of 99.1%, a PPV of 92.9%, and an NPV of 100% for the detection of endometrial carcinoma. For endometrial hyperplasia, the combined method resulted in a sensitivity of 100%, a specificity of 89.6%, a PPV of 40.0%, and an NPV of 100%.[41]

Diagnostic Procedures

More recently, hysteroscopy has been combined with D&C in the diagnostic evaluation of women with a thickened endometrial stripe. Although hysteroscopy is generally used to identify benign lesions, such as endometrial polyps, it may also be used to examine the uterine lining and specifically biopsy suspicious lesions in the uterine lining under direct visualization.

Role of the General Gynecologist

Because the majority of women with endometrial hyperplasia or carcinoma initially will experience abnormal vaginal bleeding, they often first present to their general gynecologist or primary care provider for evaluation. It is important for the gynecologist to take a thorough history and perform a complete pelvic examination, as described previously. Key aspects of the patient's history that should be considered when establishing a differential diagnosis include menopausal status, age at menarche and menopause, parity, history of infertility, history of hormone therapy use and duration, history of tamoxifen use and duration, and family history of uterine or colon cancers. Women with postmenopausal bleeding should be considered to have endometrial cancer until proven otherwise. The initial evaluation, including a transvaginal ultrasonography and endometrial biopsy as described earlier, is routinely performed by a general gynecologist. Patients with persistent postmenopausal bleeding and a negative endometrial biopsy should consider a definitive diagnostic evaluation with D&C to rule out the presence of malignancy. Referral to a gynecologic oncologist is recommended after a pathologic diagnosis of endometrial carcinoma.

Often women who are diagnosed with endometrial hyperplasia are managed and followed up by their general gynecologist. A discussion on the management considerations for women with endometrial hyperplasia is included later in this chapter.

PATHOLOGY

Key Points

1. Complex atypical hyperplasia is considered a premalignant lesion for endometrioid endometrial cancers.
2. Diagnostic criteria for endometrioid carcinoma include (1) back-to-back proliferation of endometrial glands occupying an area of 2×2 mm; (2) an extensive papillary pattern; and (3) a desmoplastic of fibroblastic stroma infiltrated by irregular glands.
3. Uterine serous carcinoma accounts for approximately 8% to 10% of endometrial cancers and are characterized by early extrauterine metastasis and a worse overall prognosis.
4. Endometrial cancer can spread by direct extension to adjacent structures, lymphatic dissemination, hematogenous dissemination, or transtubal passage of exfoliated cancer cells.

Histopathology

Endometrial Hyperplasia

Endometrial hyperplasia is characterized by the proliferation and crowding of endometrial glands and stroma, resulting in an increased gland-to-stroma ratio. As mentioned previously, endometrial hyperplasia is believed to result from excessive or prolonged exposure to estrogen that is unopposed by the effects of progestin. In 1984, the International Society of Gynecologic Pathologists introduced terminology to classify endometrial hyperplasia that was adopted by the World Health Organization (WHO). According to the WHO definition, endometrial hyperplasia is subdivided into simple and complex on the basis of the architecture of endometrial glands. In simple hyperplasia, the glands maintain round shapes and may be dilated, but there is abundant stroma (Figure 6-2). In contrast, with complex hyperplasia, the glands assume branched and complex outlines and may exhibit back-to-back crowding with little endometrial stroma. In both simple and complex hyperplasia, the cells can have cytologic atypia (Figure 6-3). Cytologic atypia is characterized by a loss of cellular polarity, an increase in the nuclear-to-cytoplasmic ratio, and prominent nucleoli. Thus endometrial hyperplasia can be further divided into 4 subclassifications: (1) simple hyperplasia without atypia, (2) simple atypical hyperplasia, (3) complex hyperplasia without atypia, and (4) complex atypical hyperplasia. Progression to carcinoma varies

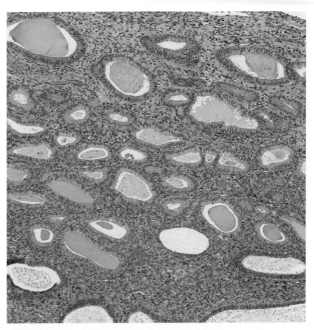

FIGURE 6-2. Simple hyperplasia without atypia. The glands are crowded, but intervening stroma is abundant. The glands maintain round to oval outlines, and there is no cytologic atypia.

CHAPTER 6

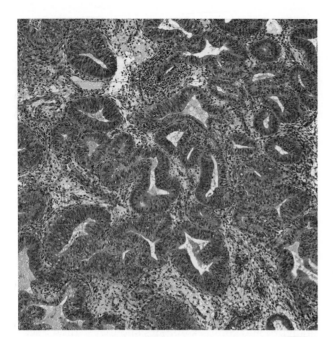

FIGURE 6-3. Complex atypical hyperplasia. The glands are crowded, but intervening stroma is abundant. The glands show complex outlines and cytologic atypia.

based on classification (Table 6-5), but is most prevalent in patients with complex atypical hyperplasia, occurring in up to 26.7% to 29% of cases.[42] Furthermore, these 2 lesions often coexist in the same endometrium. Up to 42.6% of endometrial biopsies with complex atypical endometrial hyperplasia will result in a diagnosis of carcinoma in the subsequent hysterectomy specimen.[43] In addition, a recent study by the GOG showed that the application of WHO criteria for endometrial hyperplasia can be somewhat variable among pathologists, resulting in a relatively low level of reproducibility of the diagnosis of complex atypical endometrial hyperplasia.[44] They concluded that a new classification system, which is both highly reproducible among pathologists and more predictive of lesions on hysterectomy, is needed.

Endometrial Carcinoma

Cancers of the uterine corpus can be divided into epithelial, mesenchymal, mixed epithelial and mesenchymal, and trophoblastic tumors. Mesenchymal uterine tumors and trophoblastic tumors are discussed in Chapter 7 and Chapter 8, respectively. The various histologic subtypes of endometrial carcinoma are listed in Table 6-6.[45]

Endometrioid carcinomas are the most common histologic subtype and comprise approximately 80% to 90% of all endometrial cancers. For a diagnosis of endometrioid endometrial adenocarcinoma, one of the following diagnostic criteria must be met: (1) back-to-back proliferation of endometrial glands occupying an area of 2×2 mm; (2) an extensive papillary pattern; and (3) a desmoplastic of fibroblastic stroma infiltrated by irregular glands.[46] Endometrial tumors are graded based on their degree of differentiation and the amount of solid component present. Grade 1 tumors are well differentiated and have less than 5% of a solid component (Figure 6-4). Grade 2 tumors are of intermediate differentiation and have between 6% and 50% of a solid component (Figure 6-5). Grade 3 tumors are poorly differentiated and have more than 50% of a solid component (Figure 6-6). There are multiple recognized variants within this subtype, including variant with squamous differentiation, villoglandular (or papillary) differentiation, secretory variant, and ciliated-cell variant. These variants all have a similar clinical course and prognosis to that of typical endometrioid adenocarcinoma and as such are grouped together.

Uterine serous carcinomas (USC) are a highly aggressive subtype that histologically resembles high-grade ovarian papillary serous carcinomas (Figure 6-7). USCs, however, are not graded. They account for approximately 8% to 10% of endometrial cancers and are characterized by early extrauterine metastasis and a worse overall prognosis, with a 5-year overall survival rate of approximately 50%.[45,47] Several studies have shown that the depth of myometrial invasion does not correlate with the incidence of extrauterine metastasis. Slomovitz and colleagues[47] found that among patients with no uterine invasion, 37% had extrauterine disease.

Clear cell carcinomas are less common than USCs, accounting for approximately 2% to 3.7% of endometrial cancers.[48] Histologically they resemble clear-cell carcinoma of the ovary and vagina (Figure 6-8). Similar to USCs, uterine clear-cell carcinomas are not

Table 6-5 Comparison of Simple and Complex Hyperplasia With or Without Atypia and Progression to Endometrial Carcinoma

Histology	N	Regressed (%)	Persisted (%)	Progressed to Carcinoma (%)
Simple hyperplasia	93	80	19	1
Complex hyperplasia	29	80	17	3
Simple atypical hyperplasia	13	69	23	8
Complex atypical hyperplasia	35	57	14	29

Adapted from Kurman et al.[70]

Table 6-6 Histologic Subtypes of Endometrial Cancer

Endometrioid adenocarcinoma
  Variant with squamous differentiation
  Variant with villoglandular (or papillary) differentiation
  Secretory variant
  Ciliated cell variant

Uterine papillary serous adenocarcinoma (UPSC)

Clear cell adenocarcinoma

Mucinous adenocarcinoma

Squamous cell carcinoma

Carcinosarcoma

Mixed adenocarcinoma and other rare variants

graded. They also have a higher frequency of extrauterine metastases when compared with endometrioid carcinomas. There is a poor correlation between the depth of myometrial invasion and the presence of extrauterine disease; extrauterine metastases can be found in up to 50% of cases with clear cell carcinoma confined to the inner one-half of the myometrium. McMeekin and colleagues[48] found that clear cell histology was an independent predictor of a worse progression-free survival. The 5-year overall survival rate is 62% for patients with clear cell histology.[45]

Although carcinosarcoma (or malignant müllerian mixed tumor) is not part of the current WHO classification of endometrial carcinoma, clonality and mutational studies have shown that the carcinomatous

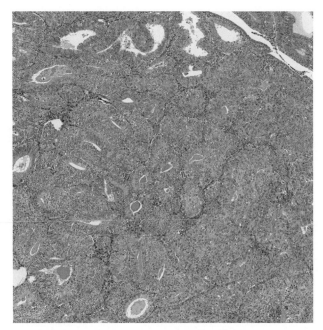

FIGURE 6-5. Grade 2 endometrioid cancer. The tumor is a mixture of back-to-back glands and solid tumor nests.

6-se. solid component

and the sarcomatous components derive from the same precursor.[49-52] In addition, based on patterns of recurrence and metastases, the behavior of this tumor is more akin to that of carcinoma than sarcoma. Tumors designated as carcinosarcoma must contain both a malignant epithelial and a malignant mesenchymal (sarcomatous) component, which can be clearly demarcated from each other on histologic examination (Figure 6-9). When matched for stage, age, patient performance status, and surgical

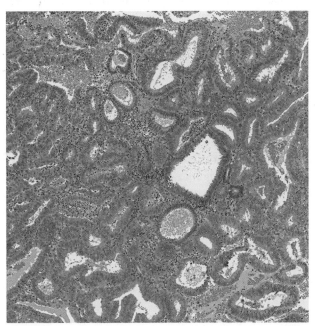

FIGURE 6-4. Grade 1 endometrioid cancer. The majority of the tumor is composed of back-to-back glands, with little to no intervening stroma.

5% solid component

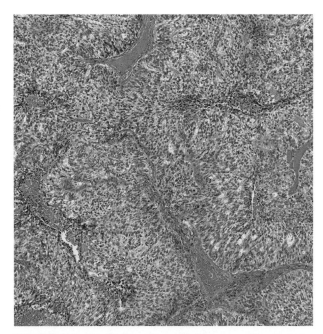

FIGURE 6-6. Grade 3 endometrioid cancer. The majority of the tumor is composed of solid tumor nests.

>50% solid tumor

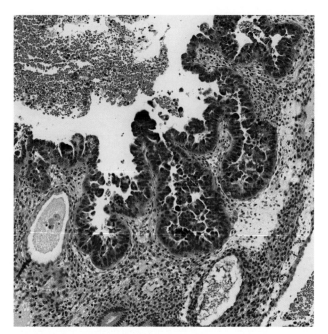

FIGURE 6-7. Uterine serous carcinoma. Tumor cells show high-grade cytologic atypia, loss of intraepithelial polarity, and formation of papillae without fibrovascular cores.

procedure, carcinosarcomas have been found to have a worse outcome than endometrioid, clear cell, and serous carcinomas.[53]

Metastatic Spread Patterns

Endometrial cancer can spread by direct extension to adjacent structures, lymphatic dissemination,

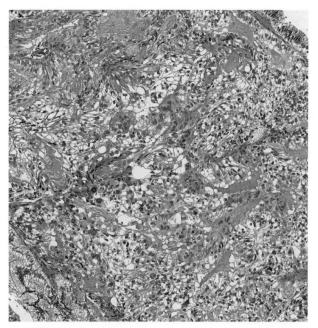

FIGURE 6-8. Clear cell carcinoma. The tumor is composed of sheets of cells with cytoplasmic clearing and high-grade nuclei.

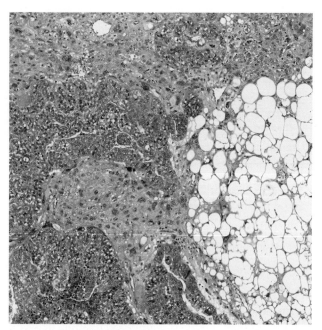

FIGURE 6-9. Carcinosarcoma. The malignant epithelial component (left) is a high-grade endometrioid carcinoma. The malignant stromal component (right) is a high-grade sarcoma with liposarcomatous differentiation. Note the sharp transition between the malignant epithelial and stromal components.

hematogenous dissemination, or passage of exfoliated endometrial cancer cells through the fallopian tubes. The most common route of spread is through direct extension. Initially, the primary endometrial tumor will grow to involve the majority of the endometrial surface and extend into the lower uterine segment. Simultaneously, the tumor invades into the myometrium, extending to eventually involve the uterine serosa and the cervix. On endometrial biopsies, this can represent a diagnostic challenge for the pathologist, because endometrioid endometrial adenocarcinoma and endocervical adenocarcinoma can have overlapping histologic features.

The presence of concurrent complex atypical endometrial hyperplasia in the biopsy favors the diagnosis of endometrial adenocarcinoma, whereas the presence of concurrent adenocarcinoma in situ of the endocervix favors the diagnosis of endocervical carcinoma. In addition, the use of an immunohistochemical staining panel can be helpful to make this distinction. Endometrial adenocarcinoma typically shows diffuse staining for estrogen receptor and vimentin and with patchy staining for *p16*, whereas the carcinoembryonic antigen is negative. In contrast, the endocervical adenocarcinoma usually shows diffuse staining for *p16* and carcinoembryonic antigen, but no staining for estrogen receptor and vimentin.[54]

The location of the primary tumor determines to some degree the timing of cervical involvement. Primary tumors in the uterine fundus often invade and extend to the uterine serosa before involving the cervix. Tumors that originate in the lower uterine segment tend to involve the cervix earlier. The mechanism of spread to the cervix likely involves a combination of surface spread, lymphatic spread, and invasion of deep tissue planes.[55] Once tumors penetrate the uterine serosa, they may directly invade other pelvic structures such as the bladder, rectum, or adnexa, or cells may exfoliate into the peritoneal cavity to form metastatic implants throughout the abdomen.

The uterus has a complex lymphatic network that follows the major blood vessels supplying the uterus. The lymphatic channels that drain the fundal portion of the uterus pass through the infundibulopelvic ligaments and follow the ovarian vessels to the para-aortic lymph nodes. The lymphatic channels that drain the mid and lower portions of the uterus travel through the broad ligament while following the uterine vessels to the pelvic lymph nodes. Small lymphatic channels also travel through the round ligaments to the superficial inguinal lymph nodes. As a result of this complex lymphatic network, nodal metastases can theoretically occur in any combination of nodal basins. Creasman and colleagues[56] have reported on the correlation between tumor histologic grade and depth of myometrial invasion with the incidence of pelvic and para-aortic nodal metastases (Tables 6-7 and 6-8). Studies of endometrial cancer patients from the Mayo Clinic have elucidated the pattern of lymph node spread.[57] The external iliac lymph nodes are the most commonly involved pelvic lymph nodes in tumors confined to the uterus or involving the cervix. However, when compared with tumors confined to the uterine corpus, tumors extending to the uterine cervix have a higher rate of common iliac nodal involvement. Furthermore,

Table 6-8 Frequency of Positive Para-Aortic Nodes in Relationship to Tumor Grade and Depth of Myometrial Invasion

Depth of Invasion	Grade 1 (%)	Grade 2 (%)	Grade 3 (%)
Endometrium only	0	3	0
Inner one-third myometrium	1	4	4
Middle one-third myometrium	5	0	0
Outer one-third myometrium	6	14	23

Adapted from Creasman et al.[64]

although lymphatic channels pass directly from the uterine fundus to the para-aortic lymph nodes, it is rare to find positive para-aortic lymph nodes in the absence of pelvic lymph nodes. In a separate consecutive series of 612 endometrial cancer patients from the Mayo Clinic, Mariani and colleagues[58] identified 2 independent predictive factors of para-aortic nodal metastases: positive pelvic lymph nodes and the presence of lymph vascular space invasion (LVSI). Only 2% of patients with negative pelvic lymph nodes had positive para-aortic lymph nodes, compared with 47% of patients with positive pelvic nodes. Furthermore, when the pelvic lymph nodes and LVSI were both negative, only 0.8% of patients had positive para-aortic lymph nodes, compared with 31% in patients with at least 1 of these variables.

Hematogenous dissemination of endometrial carcinoma does occur, but is less common than lymphatic spread or direct extension. The most common site of hematogenous spread is to the lungs, and liver, brain, and bone are also less common sites of metastasis.

Transtubal migration of exfoliated endometrial cancer cells is a less common route of spread, but may explain the presence of positive peritoneal washings and/or disseminated intraperitoneal metastases in women with otherwise early endometrial cancer. In series of 87 patients who underwent hysterectomy for uterine serous carcinoma, Snyder and colleagues[59] found tumor clusters within the fallopian tube lumen of 16 patients, all of whom had peritoneal spread. Three of these 16 patients had no evidence of myometrial invasion or LVSI. There have also been concerns that hysteroscopy may facilitate transtubal passage of endometrial cancer cells, resulting in peritoneal dissemination. Obermair and colleagues[60] reported on a retrospective analysis of 113 women with stage I endometrial carcinoma confined to the inner half of the myometrium. They noted that 10 patients (9%) had suspicious or positive peritoneal cytology, and this was

Table 6-7 Frequency of Positive Pelvic Nodes in Relationship to Tumor Grade and Depth of Myometrial Invasion

Depth of Invasion	Grade 1 (%)	Grade 2 (%)	Grade 3 (%)
Endometrium only	0	3	0
Inner one-third myometrium	3	5	9
Middle one-third myometrium	0	9	4
Outer one-third myometrium	11	19	34

Adapted from Creasman et al.[64]

significantly associated with a history of hysteroscopy. In general, the prognostic significance of this finding is uncertain. Most recently, positive washings have been removed from surgical staging.

FIGO Staging

Endometrial carcinoma is staged surgically according to the International Federation of Gynecology and Obstetrics (FIGO) staging system. Comprehensive surgical staging includes a hysterectomy, bilateral salpingo-oophorectomy, bilateral pelvic and para-aortic lymphadenectomy, and peritoneal washings. This procedure can be accomplished through either a laparotomy incision or by a laparoscopic or robotically assisted approach.

Before 1988, endometrial cancer was staged clinically based on the depth of the uterine cavity, physical examination findings, and fractional biopsy specimens from the endocervix and endometrium. However, several studies comparing the accuracy of clinical versus surgical staging consistently demonstrated the superiority of surgical staging.[61-63] As a result, clinical staging was abandoned, and in 1988, FIGO approved a surgical staging system for carcinoma of the uterine corpus. This was felt to be inadequate by many, given that uterine sarcomas have a different histologic appearance, clinical behavior, and prognosis than endometrial adenocarcinomas and should, therefore, not be grouped together in the same staging system. In response, FIGO revised the surgical staging system for endometrial carcinomas in 2009 (Table 6-9) and developed a separate staging system for uterine sarcomas (reviewed in Chapter 7).

In 2009, the FIGO staging system was again revised (Table 6-9). The key differences between the 1988 staging system and the revised 2009 staging system include changes in reporting the depth of myometrial invasion, endocervical glandular involvement, and the extent of advanced (stage III) disease. According to the 1988 staging system, tumors confined to the uterine corpus (stage I) were divided into 3 subgroups based on the depth of myometrial invasion. Stage IA was defined as no myometrial invasion, whereas stage IB was defined as the presence of less than 50% myometrial invasion and stage IC as greater than 50% myometrial invasion. However, as data from the FIGO Annual Report showed no significant difference in 5-year survival rates between stage IA grade 1, stage IB grade 1, stage IA grade 2, or stage IB grade 2 (93.4%, 91.6%, 91.3%, and 93.4%, respectively), the previous stage IA and IB were combined into stage IA.[64] Stage IB is now defined by the presence of ≥50% myometrial invasion.

The staging of cervical involvement has also changed for in the FIGO 2009 criteria. Previously, stage II

Table 6-9 FIGO 2009 Surgical Staging for Endometrial Carcinoma

Stage I	Tumor confined to the uterine corpus
IA	<50% myometrial invasion
IB	≥50% myometrial invasion, but does not invade the serosa
Stage II[a]	Invasion of the cervical stroma, but tumor remains confined to uterus
Stage III[b]	Local and/or regional spread of tumor
IIIA	Invasion of the uterine serosa and/or adnexae
IIIB	Involvement of the vagina and/or parametrium
IIIC	Metastases to pelvic and/or para-aortic lymph nodes
IIIC1	Positive pelvic lymph nodes
IIIC2	Positive para-aortic lymph nodes ± pelvic lymph nodes
Stage IV[b]	Tumor invades the mucosa of the bladder or bowel or has metastasized to distant sites
IVA	Tumor invasion of the bladder and/or bowel mucosa
IVB	Distant metastases including intra-abdominal metastases and/or positive inguinal lymph nodes

[a]Endocervical gland involvement only is now considered stage I.
[b]Positive cytology does not affect the stage, but should be reported separately.

endometrial cancer was divided into 2 subgroups based on endocervical glandular involvement (stage IIA) or invasion into the cervical stroma (stage IIB). The revised staging system eliminated these subgroups and classifies only tumors involving the cervical stroma as stage II. Tumors involving the endocervical glands are now classified as stage I and are subdivided based on the presence and depth of myometrial invasion.

The definition of stage III disease has also been refined based on the importance of prognostic features. Positive peritoneal cytology (previously stage IIIA) appears to worsen prognosis when combined with other poor prognostic features, but does not appear to be an independent poor prognostic feature.[65,66] For this reason, it was removed from the revised staging system. It is still an important part of the endometrial cancer staging, but should be reported separately. The presence of parametrial extension was added to stage IIIB. The classification of nodal involvement was also revised. Previously, stage IIIC encompassed the presence of either positive pelvic and/or para-aortic lymph nodes. However, several studies have shown that involvement of para-aortic lymph nodes carry a worse prognosis than involvement of pelvic lymph nodes alone.[67-69] In a recent study of patients with stage IIIC disease, 5-year overall survival and recurrence-free survival with involvement of only the pelvic lymph nodes was 69.7% and 65.6%, respectively, compared with 48.8% and 44.4% when the para-aortic nodes were involved.[68] For this reason, stage IIIC was subdivided into stage IIIC1 (pelvic lymph node involvement) and stage IIIC2 (para-aortic lymph node involvement with or without pelvic lymph node involvement).

In 2009, FIGO also developed a separate staging system for uterine sarcomas (reviewed in Chapter 7). The 1998 FIGO staging system was also felt to be inadequate by many, given that uterine sarcomas have histologic appearance, clinical behavior, and prognosis that are different from those of endometrial adenocarcinomas and should, therefore, not be grouped together in the same staging system.

TREATMENT

Key Points

1. Women with complex atypical hyperplasia have an increased risk of concurrent endometrial cancer, as well as the increased risk of progression to carcinoma. Although hysterectomy is considered standard treatment, progestin therapy may be an option in women who wish to preserve fertility.
2. Early-stage endometrial cancer is often curative with surgical resection alone. Adjuvant radiation therapy has not been shown to improve overall survival in patients with early-stage disease, but may have a role in reducing vaginal cuff recurrence or targeting occult nodal disease in patients at high risk for recurrence.
3. Controversies remain regarding the extent of surgical staging of endometrial cancer, primarily, which patients require lymphadenectomy and what is considered an adequate para-aortic lymph node dissection.
4. Primary radiation therapy is a viable option for patients who are considered to have medically inoperable disease. However, this treatment approach may not be as effective as primary surgery, particularly in stage II and/or high grade tumors.
5. Advanced-stage endometrial cancer is treated primarily with surgical resection (when feasible) and chemotherapy. Radiation therapy has a role in local control and in treating patients with positive lymph nodes. Hormonal therapies have been shown to be effective in patients with grade 1 tumors.

Primary Treatment Modalities

The mainstay of curative therapy for women with endometrial carcinoma is surgical resection, which includes complete hysterectomy, bilateral salpingo-oophorectomy, and comprehensive surgical staging. External pelvic radiotherapy and/or vaginal brachytherapy have not been shown to decrease mortality in early-stage disease. In certain cases, it is used to reduce the risk of vaginal cuff recurrence or to target occult disease in patients at high risk of disease recurrence. In patients who are considered inoperable secondary to significant medical comorbidities, external radiotherapy and/or intracavitary brachytherapy can be used as first-line treatment. The role of chemotherapy has evolved over the last several decades. Historically, chemotherapy was used in the treatment of recurrent disease; however, in the past decade, chemotherapy has played a larger role in the upfront and adjuvant treatment of patients with advanced (stage III and IV) endometrial cancer. Finally, hormonal therapy has also been used in a variety of settings, including in patients with early-stage and low-grade endometrial carcinoma who desire to preserve fertility, in patients with recurrent disease, and in patients with significant comorbidities who are not surgical candidates. Treatment recommendations for endometrial carcinoma by stage and histology are summarized in Tables 6-10 and 6-11.

Treatment of Endometrial Hyperplasia

Treatment of endometrial hyperplasia depends on the patient's age and her desire for future fertility as well as the degree of cytologic atypia. Progression to endometrial carcinoma occurs in 1% and 3% of patients with simple and complex hyperplasia without atypia, respectively.[70] In contrast, up to 29% to 43% of the patients with complex atypical hyperplasia will experience disease progression or already have a concurrent endometrial carcinoma.[43,70] Thus this should be taken into consideration when counseling patients regarding treatment options.

In women diagnosed with simple hyperplasia or complex hyperplasia without atypia, a D&C can be both diagnostic and therapeutic. Also, the use of progestins or combination oral contraceptives may be effective. In a prospective study of 85 postmenopausal women, Ferenczy and colleagues reported that 86% of women with endometrial hyperplasia without atypia responded to oral medroxyprogesterone acetate with only 6% developing a recurrence and none progressing to carcinoma during a mean 7-year follow-up[71].

For complex atypical hyperplasia, the risk of progression to endometrial carcinoma or the presence of a concurrent endometrial carcinoma is sufficiently high that standard therapy for women who have completed childbearing is hysterectomy and bilateral salpingo-oophorectomy. In a study by Kurman and colleagues,[70] 11% of women younger than age 35 years, 12% of women 36 to 54 years, and 28% of women older than 55 years with complex atypical hyperplasia were found to have carcinoma in their uterus after D&C. Younger

Table 6-10 Treatment Summary for Endometrioid Endometrial Carcinoma After Comprehensive Surgical Staging

Stage IA	
Grade 1	
(−) RF	Observe
(+) RF	Observe or VBT
Grade 2-3	
(−) RF	Observe or VBT
(+) RF	Observe or VBT and/or pelvic RT
Stage IB	
Grade 1-2	
(−) RF	Observe or VBT
(+) RF	Observe or VBT and/or pelvic RT
Grade 3	
(−) RF	Observe or VBT and/or Pelvic RT
(+) RF	Observe or pelvic RT and/or VBT ± chemotherapy
Stage II	
Grade 1	VBT and/or pelvic RT
Grade 2	Pelvic RT + VBT
Grade 3	Pelvic RT + VBT ± chemotherapy
Stage IIIA	
Grade 1-3	Chemotherapy ± pelvic RT or Tumor-directed RT ± chemotherapy or Pelvic RT ± VBT
Stage IIIB	Chemotherapy and/or tumor-directed RT
Stage IIIC	Chemotherapy and/or tumor-directed RT
Stage IVA/IVB	Chemotherapy ± RT (optimally debulked)

RF, adverse risk factors (age, positive lymph-vascular space invasion, tumor size, lower uterine [cervical/glandular] involvement); RT, radiation therapy; VBT, vaginal brachytherapy.
Data from the National Comprehensive Cancer Network (NCCN) Guidelines Version 1.2011. http://www.nccn.org/professionals/physician_gls/f_guidelines.asp

women who desire to preserve their fertility are treated with high-dose progestin therapy, usually megestrol acetate 40 mg 3 to 4 times daily. However, patients with complex hyperplasia with atypia respond less to progestin therapy than patients without atypia. In the study described above by Kurman and colleagues,[70] only 50% of patients with complex atypical hyperplasia responded to oral medroxyprogesterone acetate, and of the responders, 50% had recurrence with cytologically atypical disease. Furthermore, 25% developed adenocarcinoma during a mean follow-up of 5.5 years after starting medroxyprogesterone acetate therapy. Furthermore, in a cohort study of 185 women (mean age, 55.9 years) diagnosed with complex hyperplasia with or without atypia and treated with progestin therapy, Reed and colleagues[72] reported that although progestin treatment of women with atypical hyperplasia was associated with an increased likelihood of regression of the lesion during the ensuing 2 to 6 months, persistence or progression was present in 26.9% of treated women. Thus young patients with complex atypical hyperplasia managed conservatively with progestins require close surveillance and long-term follow-up with periodic endometrial sampling, the first at 3 months following initiation of therapy and at least every 6 months thereafter. Although the data suggest that patients with atypical hyperplasia may respond to progestin therapy, even younger patients who fail are at increased risk of progression to endometrial carcinoma and should also be considered for hysterectomy. If the complex atypical hyperplasia is cleared, consideration should be given to periodic progestin treatment or combination oral contraception until the patient chooses to attempt pregnancy because the risk factors that led to the development of endometrial hyperplasia in the first place remain. Younger women diagnosed with polycystic ovarian syndrome and chronic anovulation with hyperplasia who desire

Table 6-11 Treatment Summary for Papillary Serous or Clear Cell Endometrial Carcinoma After Comprehensive Surgical Staging

Stage IA	
No myometrial invasion	Observe or chemotherapy or tumor-directed RT
Myometrial invasion	Chemotherapy ± tumor-directed RT or whole-abdomen RT ± VBT
Stage IB-II	Chemotherapy ± tumor-directed RT or whole-abdomen RT ± VBT
Stage III-IVB	
Optimally debulked	Chemotherapy ± tumor-directed RT or whole-abdomen RT ± VBT
Suboptimally debulked	Chemotherapy

RT, radiation therapy; VBT, vaginal brachytherapy.
Data from the National Comprehensive Cancer Network (NCCN) Guidelines Version 1.2011. http://www.nccn.org/professionals/physician_gls/f_guidelines.asp

children should seek out the opinion of a reproductive endocrinologist and infertility specialist. In morbidly obese women, weight reduction is recommended.

In patients who are inoperable secondary to significant medical comorbidities, long-term high-dose progestin therapy can be used to treat complex atypical hyperplasia (megestrol acetate 80-160 mg/d or its equivalent, depending on the endometrial response). Recent studies have also evaluated the role of the levonorgestrel-containing intrauterine device (IUD).[73] When comparing the levonorgestrel IUD with oral progestin therapy in women aged 30 to 70 years with "low-risk" endometrial hyperplasia, Vereide and colleagues[74] reported that after 3 months, all 26 patients treated with the levonorgestrel IUD showed regression of hyperplasia, whereas 14 of 31 patients in the oral progestin group had persistent disease, suggesting that the levonorgestrel IUD is a superior alternative to oral progestin treatment of endometrial hyperplasia. Also, Gallos and colleagues[75] performed a meta-analysis of 24 studies evaluating the regression rate of endometrial hyperplasia with oral progestins versus the levonorgestrel IUD, which concluded that oral progestins appear to induce a lower disease regression rate than a levonorgestrel-releasing intrauterine system in the treatment of endometrial hyperplasia. In this study, treatment with oral progestins resulted in a lower pooled regression rate compared with the levonorgestrel IUD for complex (66% vs. 92%; $P < .01$) and atypical hyperplasia (69% vs. 90%; $P = .03$). Additional studies will be necessary to fully evaluate the role of the levonorgestrel IUD. Close follow-up is still warranted. Periodic sampling of the endometrium may be performed with the IUD in place.

Treatment of Early-Stage Endometrial Carcinoma

Surgical resection that includes total abdominal hysterectomy, bilateral salpingo-oophorectomy, and staging remains the cornerstone of treatment for early-stage disease. Adjuvant radiation therapy has not been shown to decrease mortality in early-stage patients, but may have a role in reducing the risk of vaginal cuff recurrence and to target occult disease in patients at high risk for recurrence. Recently, the use of hormone therapy for the treatment of early-stage endometrial cancer has been evaluated in younger women who wish to preserve their fertility.

Surgery

Because the majority of women with endometrial cancer present with disease confined to the uterus, surgical resection alone may be curative. As such, surgical resection should be attempted whenever feasible. The goals of surgery should be to provide definitive treatment to those patients whose disease is confined to the uterus, identify women with extrauterine disease who will require adjuvant therapy, and obtain tissue specimens for histopathologic analysis to provide prognostic information. Adequate resection with clear surgical margins can usually be achieved by extrafascial hysterectomy alone; however, in cases in which the tumor involves the cervix, a more extensive radical hysterectomy may be necessary.

Surgical staging of endometrial cancer was traditionally done via a laparotomy; however, with the increasing popularity of minimally invasive surgery, a large proportion of cases are now completed by traditional laparoscopy or by robotic-assisted laparoscopy, including pelvic and para-aortic lymphadenectomy. Descriptions of different uterine surgical procedures are discussed in greater detail in Chapter 25. In a prospective, randomized study of more than 2600 women, the GOG compared laparoscopy with laparotomy for the comprehensive surgical staging of uterine cancer and concluded that minimally invasive surgery was feasible for surgical resection and staging of endometrial cancer. The authors found that compared with women who underwent laparotomy, those patients who underwent laparoscopy had significantly fewer moderate to severe postoperative complications, a shorter length of hospital stay, and equivalent detection rates of advanced-stage disease and had an improved quality of life through 6 weeks after surgery.[76,77] However, a larger percentage of women in the laparoscopy group did not have a complete lymphadenectomy when compared with those who underwent laparotomy (8% vs. 4%). Survival data from this trial are still pending.

The extent of lymphadenectomy for endometrial cancer patients has not been standardized. There is ongoing debate regarding (1) whether all patients with presumed early-stage disease require complete pelvic and/or para-aortic lymphadenectomy, and (2) the extent of a para-aortic lymph node dissection. There can be significant practice pattern variation between institutions and between individual practitioners. There has been a recent movement to identify a group of low-risk patients with minimal risk of lymph node involvement who may not need full lymphadenectomy. In a review of 328 patients with grade 1 or 2 endometrioid endometrial carcinoma, with ≤50% myometrial invasion and no intraoperative evidence of macroscopic extrauterine spread who were treated surgically (57% with lymphadenectomy), Mariani and colleagues[78] found that no patient with tumor diameter ≤2 cm had positive pelvic lymph nodes or died of disease. They concluded that patients who have grade 1 or 2 endometrioid endometrial cancer with greatest tumor surface dimension of ≤2 cm, myometrial invasion

≤50%, and no intraoperative evidence of macroscopic disease are at low risk for nodal metastases and can be treated optimally with hysterectomy alone.

Several recent large, prospective European studies have examined the role of lymphadenectomy. The ASTEC trial (Adjuvant External Beam Radiotherapy in the Treatment of Endometrial Cancer)[79] was a multi-institutional prospective study involving 85 centers in 4 countries that included 1408 women with histologically proven endometrial carcinoma presumed to be confined to the uterus. Patients were randomly assigned to standard surgery, which included hysterectomy, bilateral salpingo-oophorectomy, peritoneal washings, and palpation of para-aortic lymph nodes, or standard surgery plus a systematic bilateral pelvic lymphadenectomy (iliac and obturator nodes). Resection of the para-aortic lymph nodes was left to the discretion of individual practitioners. This study included a second randomization in which 507 patients with intermediate-risk or high-risk (IA or IB with high-grade histology, IC or IIA) early-stage disease, independent of lymphadenectomy, were randomized to pelvic radiotherapy versus observation in order to control for differences in adjuvant therapy dependent on node status. The authors reported a significant difference in 5-year recurrence-free survival (HR, 1.35; 95% CI, 1.06-1.73; $P = .017$) in favor of standard surgery. However, with regard to their primary outcome measure, there was no difference in overall survival or disease- or treatment-related deaths. Furthermore, despite initial randomization, considerable imbalances in baseline characteristics and histology were noted between the arms, with more aggressive tumors (serous, clear cell, grade 3) and more deeply invasive tumors in the lymphadenectomy arm. When adjusting for these differences, recurrence-free survival was no longer significantly different (HR, 1.25; 95% CI, 0.93-1.66; $P = .14$). There were several limitations to this study, including an inadequate sampling of pelvic lymph nodes in the lymphadenectomy group and inclusion of significant number (45%) of patients with low-risk features who would not have undergone or benefited from lymphadenectomy in the first place. The median number of lymph nodes resected was 12, with 35% of patients having fewer than 9 lymph nodes resected. Para-aortic lymphadenectomy was not required or standardized in the ASTEC trial, making it difficult to conclude that lymphadenectomy provides no survival benefit, because patients with isolated para-aortic disease were not captured.

The observations made in the ASTEC trial were supported by a separate prospective, randomized clinical trial from Italy (CONSORT trial) in which 514 patients with stage I endometrial carcinoma were randomly allocated to undergo systematic pelvic lymphadenectomy versus no lymphadenectomy.[80] There

was a higher number of pelvic lymph nodes removed (median = 30) compared with the ASTEC trial. However, only 26% of patients in the lymphadenectomy group underwent para-aortic dissection, because this was left to the discretion of individual practitioners. The authors found that systematic pelvic lymphadenectomy did not improve disease-free or overall survival (81.0% and 85.9% in the lymphadenectomy group and 81.7% and 90.0% in the no-lymphadenectomy group, respectively) in this patient population. Both the ASTEC and CONSORT trials have been limited by failing to standardize the indications for and extent of lymphadenectomy, and therefore definitive data regarding the benefit of lymphadenectomy remain unresolved.

The second main controversy in surgical management of endometrial cancer is the extent of lymphadenectomy. Is a pelvic lymphadenectomy sufficient? Is a para-aortic lymphadenectomy up to the inferior mesenteric artery sufficient, or should a dissection up to the renal vessels be performed? In a prospective evaluation of 422 consecutive patients deemed to be at intermediate or high risk for lymph node metastasis, Mariani and colleagues[81] found that 67% of patients with nodal metastases had para-aortic node involvement, with 16% having isolated para-aortic nodes. In this study, 77% of patients with para-aortic node involvement had positive nodes above the level of the inferior mesenteric artery, arguing for a more extensive para-aortic dissection up to the renal vessels. A study by Soliman et al[82] found that there was significant practice variation among gynecologic oncologists, with approximately 50% using the inferior mesenteric artery as the upper boundary and 11% extending the dissection to the renal vessels.

An additional area of controversy is whether there is a therapeutic benefit and survival advantage to lymphadenectomy.[83-85] A retrospective review of more than 12,300 patients in the Surveillance, Epidemiology, and End Results (SEER) database by Chan and colleagues[86] reported that in intermediate-/high-risk patients (stage IB, grade 3; stage IC and II-IV, all grades), a more extensive lymph node resection (number of nodes retrieved equal to 1, 2-5, 6-10, 11-20, and >20) was associated with improved 5-year disease-specific survival rates across all 5 groups of 75.3%, 81.5%, 84.1%, 85.3%, and 86.8%, respectively ($P < .001$). However, there was no significant benefit of lymphadenectomy in low-risk patients (stage IA, all grades; stage IB, grades 1 and 2; $P = .23$). A retrospective review of 671 patients with high-intermediate risk endometrial cancer in Japan (the SEPAL [Survival Effect of Para-Aortic Lymphadenectomy in Endometrial Cancer] study) who underwent systematic pelvic lymphadenectomy ($n = 325$) or combined pelvic and para-aortic lymphadenectomy to the level of the renal vessels (n = 346) showed a reduction in the risk of death in patients who underwent the combined procedure compared with pelvic lymphadenectomy alone (HR, 0.44; 95% CI, 0.30-0.64; $P < .0001$).[85] Kilgore and colleagues[83] published a single-institution retrospective review of 649 patients with presumed stage I to II endometrial adenocarcinoma who underwent a total abdominal hysterectomy, bilateral salpingo-oophorectomy, and peritoneal washings plus or minus pelvic lymph node dissection. The decision to perform a lymphadenectomy was at the discretion of individual practitioners based on preoperative risk factors. They further subdivided patients who underwent lymphadenectomy into a "multiple-site" pelvic sampling group (nodes sampled from at least 4 different sites: right and left common iliac, external iliac, internal iliac, and obturator nodes) versus a "limited-site" pelvic sampling group (< 4 sites sampled). Of the 649 patients who underwent surgery, 208 did not have a lymphadenectomy, 212 had a multiple-site lymph node sampling, and 205 had a limited-site lymph node sampling. Over a mean follow-up of 3 years, patients who underwent a multiple-site pelvic node sampling had significantly better survival than patients without node sampling ($P = .0002$). Patients were also categorized as low risk (disease confined to the corpus) or as high risk (disease in the cervix, adnexa, uterine serosa, or washings). For both high-risk and low-risk groups, multiple-site pelvic node sampling provided a significant survival advantage compared with patients without node sampling (high risk, $P = .0006$; low risk, $P = .026$). Furthermore, in both the high-risk and low-risk groups, patients who underwent lymphadenectomy and did not receive postoperative pelvic radiotherapy had improved survival compared with similar patients who did not undergo lymphadenectomy but who did receive postoperative pelvic radiotherapy (low risk, $P = .003$; high risk, $P = .041$). These studies are both limited by the inherent biases associated with retrospective studies, and the study by Kilgore et al[83] did not include a para-aortic lymphadenectomy, but they do provide interesting results that must be considered when planning surgical treatment for patients with presumed early-stage endometrial carcinoma. Although these results are promising, a prospective trial evaluating the potential therapeutic benefit of lymphadenectomy is needed.

Moving forward, it is clear that systematic lymphadenectomy may not benefit patients with low-risk endometrioid endometrial carcinoma. Whats remain to be determined are standardized definitions for low-, intermediate-, and high-risk groups, and whether those factors can be determined preoperatively with a high degree of accuracy. Further, whether complete pelvic and para-aortic lymphadenectomy is of benefit in patients who are deemed to be in an intermediate-risk or high-risk group has still not been determined in a prospective study.

Radiation Therapy

Current data show no benefit to adjuvant radiotherapy for overall survival in early-stage disease. Based on 2 prospective randomized trials, the benefit of adjuvant pelvic radiotherapy for early-stage disease is in the reduction of pelvic relapse. As mentioned previously, PORTEC-1 (Post Operative Radiation Therapy in Endometrial Carcinoma 1) and GOG-99 were designed to address the question of whether or not postoperative radiotherapy is of benefit to patients with early-stage, "intermediate-risk" endometrial carcinoma. In the PORTEC-1 trial,[87] 715 patients with stage I endometrial carcinoma (grade 1 with ≥50% myometrial invasion, grade 2 with any invasion, and grade 3 with < 50% invasion) underwent a total abdominal hysterectomy and bilateral salpingo-oophorectomy without lymphadenectomy. Patients were then randomized to receive postoperative pelvic radiotherapy (46 Gy) or no further treatment. Over a median 52-month follow-up period, the 5-year actuarial locoregional recurrence rate was 4% in the radiotherapy group and 14% in the no further treatment group ($P < .001$). However, there was no difference in 5-year overall survival between the 2 groups (81% in radiotherapy group vs. 85% in no further treatment group; $P = .31$). Treatment-related morbidity was higher in the radiotherapy group (25% vs. 6% in the no further treatment group; $P < .0001$). Eight patients experienced grade 3 to 4 toxicities, of whom 7 were in the radiotherapy group. In 2005, specimens of 569 patients (80%) underwent central pathology review, and a significant shift from grade 2 to grade 1 tumors was noted.[88] Of the 569 patients, 134 (24%) were ultimately determined to have grade 1 tumors with superficial myometrial invasion and would have been excluded from the original study. However, when these cases were excluded from the analysis, the results remained essentially the same, with a 10-year recurrence rate of 5% for the radiotherapy group and 17% for the control group ($P < .0001$) and still no difference in 10-year overall survival (65% for the radiotherapy group and 70% for the control group; $P = .23$).

In the GOG-99 trial,[89] 448 women with intermediate-risk, stage IB-II (occult disease) underwent total abdominal hysterectomy and bilateral salpingo-oophorectomy with pelvic and para-aortic lymphadenectomy. Patients were then randomized to receive postoperative pelvic radiotherapy (50.4 Gy) or no further treatment (control). This study was powered to detect a 58% decrease in the recurrence hazard rate and a 56% decrease in the death hazard rate when a minimum of 39 recurrences and 42 deaths were observed. Over a median follow-up time of 69 months,

44 recurrences and 62 deaths were noted. The 2-year cumulative incidence of recurrence was 12% in the control group and 3% in the radiotherapy group ($P = .007$). There was no statistically significant difference in 4-year overall survival (86% in the control group vs. 92% in the radiotherapy group; HR, 0.86; $P = .557$). However, approximately half of the deaths noted during the study were due to causes other than endometrial cancer or related treatment. It should also be pointed out that this study was underpowered to detect a difference in survival, as adjuvant radiotherapy for early-stage endometrial cancer would likely provide a small survival benefit at best. GOG-99 also provided a definition for a new "high-intermediate risk" subgroup based on a patient's age and the presence of various risk factors (Table 6-12). The high-intermediate risk subgroup was defined as patients of (1) any age with the presence of a moderately to poorly differentiated tumor, lymphovascular space invasion, and outer-third myometrial invasion; (2) 50 years of age with any 2 of the preceding risk factors; or (3) 70 years of age with any 1 of the preceding risk factors. Following a subgroup analysis of patients in the high-intermediate risk group, there was an even greater difference in recurrence rates (2-year cumulative incidence of recurrence of 26% in the control group and 6% in the radiotherapy group; HR, 0.42). Therefore, new studies of adjuvant therapy have focused specifically on this group. There were also significant differences in the frequency and severity of hematologic, gastrointestinal, genitourinary, and cutaneous toxicities between the 2 treatment groups ($P < .001$).

These studies both show significant reductions in locoregional recurrence in patients receiving adjuvant pelvic radiotherapy, but no improvement in overall survival. Because there is clearly an increased risk of treatment-related toxicities associated with radiotherapy and no clear benefit in overall survival, the conclusions of these studies have been used to argue against the use of adjuvant external pelvic radiotherapy in patients with early-stage, low-to-intermediate risk endometrial cancer. However, caution should be taken when comparing these 2 studies, as the patient populations and interventions differed. PORTEC-1 excluded

many higher-risk patients (stage IC grade 3 and occult stage II), and patients did not undergo lymphadenectomy, whereas GOG-99, which targeted a higher-risk population, included many lower-risk patients (stage IB grade 1 and 2), and patients did undergo pelvic and para-aortic lymphadenectomy, albeit limited.

Because pelvic radiotherapy did show improved locoregional control, vaginal brachytherapy was then tested, given its improved toxicity profile when compared with external pelvic radiotherapy. To compare the efficacy of vaginal brachytherapy versus pelvic external beam radiotherapy, Nout and colleagues[90] performed an open-label, noninferiority randomized trial (PORTEC-2). In this study, 427 patients with stage I or IIA endometrial carcinoma underwent total abdominal hysterectomy and bilateral salpingo-oophorectomy with pelvic and para-aortic lymph node sampling of suspicious nodes (although no standardized lymphadenectomy was required). Patients were then randomized to postoperative external pelvic radiotherapy (46 Gy) or vaginal brachytherapy (21 Gy high-dose rate in 3 fractions or 30 Gy low-dose rate). After a median follow-up of 45 months, there were no differences between vaginal brachytherapy and external pelvic radiotherapy in 5-year vaginal recurrence rates (1.8% vs. 1.6%; $P = .74$) or 5-year locoregional relapse rates (5.1% vs. 2.1%; $P = .17$). The rates of distant metastases were also similar (8.3% for vaginal brachytherapy and 5.7% for external pelvic radiotherapy; $P = 0.46$). There were also no differences between vaginal brachytherapy and external pelvic radiotherapy in disease-free survival (84.8% vs. 79.6%; $P = .57$) or overall survival (82.7% vs. 78.1%; $P = .74$). However, external pelvic radiotherapy was associated with increased treatment-related acute grade 1 to 2 gastrointestinal toxicity (53.8% vs. 12.6%). A separate quality-of-life assessment of patients in PORTEC-2 showed that patients in the vaginal brachytherapy group reported better social functioning ($P < .002$) and lower symptom scores for diarrhea, fecal incontinence, and limitations in daily activities because of bowel symptoms ($P < .001$).[91] Based on these data, vaginal brachytherapy has been proposed for intermediate-risk early-stage patients, instead of external pelvic radiotherapy, due to

Table 6-12 Gynecologic Oncology Group Criteria for High-Intermediate Risk Group

Risk Factors	High-Intermediate Risk Group
1. Moderately to poorly differentiated tumor grade 2. Presence of LVSI 3. Invasion of the outer third of the myometrium	Any patient that meets the following criteria: 1. >70 years old with 1 risk factor 2. 50-69 years old with 2 risk factors 3. Any age with all 3 risk factors

LVSI, lymphovascular space invasion.
Data from Keys et al.[89]

an improved toxicity profile, improved quality of life, and no difference in locoregional control rates. However, the role of adjuvant radiation therapy in improving mortality is still not resolved.

Combination Chemotherapy and Radiation

Based on previous studies showing similar rates of locoregional control with either pelvic radiotherapy or vaginal brachytherapy, a more favorable toxicity profile associated with vaginal brachytherapy, and a growing understanding of the efficacy of chemotherapy in endometrial cancer, the GOG is currently exploring the effect of vaginal brachytherapy plus combination chemotherapy on recurrence-free survival in high-intermediate risk, early-stage patients. The GOG has an ongoing trial (GOG-249) comparing pelvic radiotherapy versus vaginal cuff brachytherapy plus intravenous carboplatin and paclitaxel. Carboplatin and paclitaxel have been shown to be active in endometrial cancer as well as in other gynecologic malignancies and are generally well tolerated. Eligible patients include those with stage I high-intermediate risk disease (defined as in GOG-99), stage II disease (occult) of any histology with or without risk factors, and stage I-IIB disease of serous or clear cell histology with or without risk factors. When survival data are available from this study, a more refined adjuvant treatment regimen for a subset of high-intermediate risk endometrial cancer patients may be available.

Early-Stage Uterine Serous Carcinoma

Uterine serous carcinoma (USC) is often characterized by extra-uterine spread of disease, even when there is only minimal disease within the uterus. USC also carries a higher risk of distant failure after therapy. Huh and colleagues[92] performed a retrospective study of 60 patients with stage I USC who underwent comprehensive surgical staging. In this study, 40 patients(66%) received no adjuvant therapy, 12 (20%) received adjuvant radiation therapy, 7 (12%) received adjuvant chemotherapy, and 1 (2%) received both radiotherapy and chemotherapy. The investigators found that recurrence rates were lower than previously reported (17% in the no adjuvant therapy group, 16% in the adjuvant radiotherapy group, and no recurrences in patients who received adjuvant chemotherapy). Because USC is of a similar histology and behavior to serous carcinoma of the ovary, the combination regimen of carboplatin and paclitaxel is frequently used. In a multi-institutional retrospective study of early-stage USC, Dietrich and colleagues[93] found that the combination of carboplatin and paclitaxel in the adjuvant setting was effective in improving survival and limiting recurrences. In this study, surgically staged patients with stage I uterine

papillary serous carcinoma (UPSC) who were treated after surgery with 3 to 6 courses of platinum-based chemotherapy and followed up for a minimum of 12 months or until recurrence were included. Twenty-one patients (stage IA-5, IB-13, IC-3) were treated with a combination of carboplatin (AUC [area under the curve] of 6) and paclitaxel (135-175 mg/m^2). Of these 21 patients, only 1 experienced disease recurrence to the vagina after 3 cycles of carboplatin/paclitaxel and was treated with chemoradiation with complete response. At the time of reporting, all 21 patients with stage I UPSC treated after surgical staging with carboplatin/paclitaxel chemotherapy were without evidence of disease over a mean follow-up of 41 months after treatment.

Promising results have been encountered using a combination of systemic chemotherapy with pelvic and/or vaginal radiotherapy. Kelly and colleagues[94] performed a retrospective analysis of 74 patients with stage I USC who underwent comprehensive surgical staging. The authors reported that platinum-based chemotherapy was associated with improved disease-free survival ($P < .01$) and overall survival ($P < .05$). Of the 43 patients who received radiotherapy, none experienced disease recurrence locally at the vaginal cuff, but 6 of the 31 patients (19%) who were not treated with vaginal radiotherapy did recur at the vaginal cuff. Furthermore, in a study by Turner et al,[95] vaginal radiotherapy in combination with chemotherapy in patients with surgical stage I USC was shown to produce a 5-year survival rate of 94%, which is higher than that of most other studies for patients with stage I disease.

Inoperable Patients

Although comprehensive surgical resection and staging is the recommended first-line treatment for the majority of endometrial cancer patients, some patients with endometrial cancer will have sufficiently severe medical comorbidities that render them inoperable due to an unacceptably high surgical risk. In patients who are considered too high risk to undergo upfront surgical management of endometrial cancer due to medical comorbidities, primary treatment with radiation therapy may be a viable option. Several studies have demonstrated the effectiveness and tolerability of primary radiation therapy for early-stage endometrial cancer in medically inoperable patients.[96-98] However, higher-stage and higher-grade lesions are associated with an increased failure rate. Niazi and colleagues[96] treated 38 patients with medically inoperable presumed stage I and II endometrial cancer with radiotherapy as primary treatment and reported on their long-term outcomes. High-dose-rate brachytherapy alone was used in 79% of patients, with the remaining 29% of patients receiving a combination of external pelvic radiotherapy and high-dose-rate brachytherapy. The 15-year disease-specific survival was 78% for all stages, 90% for stage I, and 42% for stage II ($P < .0001$). The 15-year disease-specific survival was 91% for grade 1 and 67% for grade 2 and 3 combined ($P = .0254$).[96] A large number of intercurrent deaths related to medical comorbidities may also affect the survival outcomes. In summary, primary radiation therapy appears to be a feasible alternative to surgery for patients whose medical comorbidities put them at too high a risk to undergo an operation. However, this treatment approach may not be as effective as primary surgery, particularly in stage II and/or high-grade tumors.

Fertility Preservation

Approximately 5% of endometrial carcinoma cases are diagnosed in women before the age of 40 years.[2] The majority of patients diagnosed with endometrial cancer at a young age are nulliparous.[99] As such, occasionally the gynecologic oncologist will be faced with a young patient diagnosed with endometrial carcinoma who has questions regarding fertility preservation. Fortunately, fertility-sparing therapies have been considered feasible in this population, as young women with endometrial cancer tend to have more favorable prognostic factors, tumors that are confined to the inner half of the myometrium, stage I disease, and low-grade endometrioid histology.[100,101] Furthermore, well-differentiated endometrioid lesions are more likely to express progesterone receptors.[102] The GOG has demonstrated that endometrial cancer expressing progesterone receptors are more likely to respond to oral medroxyprogesterone than lesions lacking progesterone receptors (37% vs. 8%; $P < .001$).[103]

Important considerations when counseling patients about conservative, fertility-preserving treatment are tumor histology, grade and receptor status, depth of myometrial invasion, risk of concurrent ovarian involvement due to either metastatic disease or a synchronous primary lesion, and risk of nodal disease. It is recommended to avoid offering conservative management to patients with grade 2 or 3 endometrioid adenocarcinoma and patients with non-endometrioid histologies of any grade due to their increased risk for metastasis.[104] A greater proportion of younger women with endometrial cancer can also have an ovarian malignancy. This can be as a result of direct metastasis from an endometrial primary, which is found in up to 5% of all cases involving grade 1 endometrial adenocarcinoma.[105] However, a significant proportion of younger, premenopausal women actually have a synchronous ovarian primary (11%-29%) when compared with postmenopausal women.[99,106] Thus patients considering fertility-preserving therapy should be

counseled about this risk, and a thorough evaluation of the adnexa is necessary before beginning nonsurgical therapy.

For patients who are considering fertility-preserving therapy, a D&C with or without hysteroscopy is necessary, as this procedure has been shown to be more reliable, with grade 1 lesions upgraded only up to 23% of the time.[107] Often patients present with a diagnosis of endometrial cancer by office endometrial biopsy using a device such as the Pipelle (described earlier). This is insufficient in a patient for whom conservative treatment is being considered, as the rate of upgrading a lesion from grade 1 to grade 2 or 3 is as high as 55%.[108] The depth of myometrial invasion should also be evaluated. In a meta-analysis, Kinkel and colleagues[109] determined that contrast-enhanced MRI was better at detecting myometrial invasion in patient with endometrial cancer than CT, non–contrast-enhanced MRI, or ultrasonography. Contrast-enhanced MRI was particularly effective at excluding deep myometrial invasion. Imaging is also useful in evaluating for extrauterine spread of disease. However, current imaging modalities, including fluorodeoxyglucose positron emission tomography, still lack the sensitivity to reliably exclude nodal metastases.

Fertility-preserving treatments have centered around the use of oral progestins. The most commonly used oral progestins include either medroxyprogesterone acetate (400-800 mg oral daily) or megestrol acetate (160 mg/d divided into 2 or 4 daily doses). Ramirez and colleagues evaluated the use of oral progestins for the conservative treatment of grade 1 endometrioid adenocarcinomas.[110] Of the 81 patients included, the authors reported a complete response rate of 76% with a median time to response of 12 weeks. Of the 62 patients who initially experienced a complete response, 47 (76%) were noted to have a durable response, whereas 15 (24%) experienced disease recurrence at a median time of 19 months. Thus, overall, 58% of patients had a complete and durable response to conservative, fertility-preserving therapy. Progesterone-containing IUDs have more recently been studied to treat grade 1 endometrioid adenocarcinoma. However, in a case series of 4 women with grade 1 endometrioid adenocarcinoma who were treated with the levonorgestrel-containing IUD (the only progesterone-containing IUD currently on the market in the United States), only 1 patient was shown to have a complete response.[111]

Many young patients with endometrial carcinoma have other factors that affect their fertility, including obesity and the polycystic ovarian syndrome. Weight reduction is strongly recommended. Consultation with an infertility specialist may be necessary to achieve pregnancy. Several assisted reproductive technology procedures have been used in endometrial cancer patients after hormonal therapy, including clomiphene citrate with intrauterine insemination and in vitro fertilization.

Treatment of Advanced-Stage or Recurrent Endometrial Cancer

Seven percent of endometrial cancer patients are diagnosed with stage III disease, and 3% are diagnosed with stage IV disease. Management for women with advanced-stage disease has evolved to primarily include surgical resection and chemotherapy. Radiation therapy may have a specific role in local control or in treating patients with positive lymph nodes. In certain cases of advanced or recurrent grade 1 endometrial cancer, hormonal therapies have been shown to be effective. Surgical resection, including comprehensive surgical staging, with the goal to achieve optimal tumor cytoreduction should be performed when feasible. Bristow and colleagues[112] demonstrated that the amount of residual disease after cytoreductive surgery as well as the patient's age and performance status appear to be important determinants of survival in patients with stage IVB endometrial carcinoma. In this study, among patients with optimal surgery, those with only microscopic residual disease survived significantly longer than those with optimal but macroscopic residual tumor. Adjuvant chemotherapy with or without radiation is then recommended after surgical debulking.

Chemotherapy

Several chemotherapeutic agents have shown activity in endometrial cancer. In general, platinum-based combination chemotherapy is used in the treatment of advanced disease. A series of GOG studies have determined the most effective chemotherapeutic regimens for the treatment of endometrial cancer.

Doxorubicin was one of first drugs established as an active agent for endometrial cancer. Doxorubicin is an anthracycline antibiotic that intercalates into DNA, inhibits replication via topoisomerase II stabilization, and generates free radicals that damage DNA. Early GOG studies examined doxorubicin in patients with advanced or recurrent endometrial carcinoma and determined its activity in this setting. Subsequently, the GOG studied cisplatin, an agent that causes intra- and inter-strand DNA cross-links and DNA adducts that disrupt replication. They determined that cisplatin similarly is active in endometrial cancer. The combination of these drugs was prospectively evaluated to assess whether the combination regimen would increase the response rate and prolong progression-free survival or overall survival compared with doxorubicin given as a single agent. Of 281 patients who were randomized and eligible for evaluation, the combination regimen produced an overall response rate that was significantly higher than doxorubicin alone (42% vs. 25%; $P = .004$).[113] The combination regimen also resulted in improved progression-free survival as compared with doxorubicin alone (5.7 months vs. 3.8 months; HR, 0.736; $P = .014$).[113] However, there was no significant difference in overall survival, and increased response rates were at the expense of greater toxicities, including increased grade 3 and 4 hematologic toxicities and nausea/vomiting. Nonetheless, the combination of doxorubicin and cisplatin (AP) became the standard regimen for patients with advanced or recurrent endometrial carcinoma in clinical practice and for future phase 3 chemotherapy trials.

Owing to the sensitivity of early-stage endometrial cancer to radiotherapy and the propensity of advanced-stage disease to relapse within the abdomen, there was interest in evaluating the role of whole-abdomen radiotherapy (WART) in these patients. The GOG performed a phase 3 trial comparing WART (given as 30 Gy in 20 fractions with a 15-Gy boost) versus the combination AP regimen described in the preceding paragraph. In order to be eligible for study entry, patients must have had optimal surgical tumor reduction to less than 2 cm. In this trial, only 50% of patients had endometrioid tumors, whereas 21% had papillary serous tumors. There was improved progression-free survival and overall survival with the AP regimen compared with WART. The HRs for progression and for death adjusted for stage were 0.71 and 0.68, respectively, favoring the AP regimen ($P < .01$).[114] However, acute toxicities were more common with the chemotherapy regimen, including 15% of patients experiencing grade 3 and 4 cardiac toxicities.

Paclitaxel, a mitotic inhibitor, is a commonly used chemotherapeutic in various gynecologic cancers. Paclitaxel produces an overall response rate of 35.7% in advanced or recurrent endometrial carcinoma, suggesting that it is among the most active agents tested in this setting. Although GOG-163[115] showed no benefit of doxorubicin plus paclitaxel compared with AP, the 3-drug regimen of AP plus paclitaxel (TAP) in GOG-177 was shown to significantly improve the objective response rate (57% vs. 35%; $P < .01$), progression-free survival (median 8.3 vs. 5.3 months; $P < .01$), and overall survival (median 15.3 vs. 12.3 months; $P = .037$) when compared with AP in patients with stage III or IV recurrent endometrial cancer.[116] However, the improved response came at the expense of worse grade 3 neurotoxicity in the TAP arm (12% vs. 1%).

Given the excellent response rate with the TAP regimen, it became standard therapy for advanced/recurrent endometrial cancer. However, concern remained about the neurotoxic effects. The combination of a platinum and taxane (dropping doxorubicin from the regimen) was considered a viable alternative with the potential for less neurotoxicity and gastrointestinal upset. Cisplatin and paclitaxel were combined in a phase 2 trial in advanced or recurrent endometrial carcinoma and produced response rates similar to those of the TAP regimen. Of 24 patients treated with cisplatin and paclitaxel, 16 patients (67%) achieved an objective response, including 7 complete responses.[117]

In 2003, carboplatin was established as an active compound for advanced or recurrent endometrial cancer, producing an overall response rate of 24% in a phase 2 trial.[118] A retrospective review demonstrated that the combination of carboplatin and paclitaxel is well tolerated and has significant activity in endometrial adenocarcinoma, with an overall response rate of 87%.[119] Although there have been no published data on the carboplatin and paclitaxel doublet, the GOG recently completed accrual to GOG-209 comparing paclitaxel and carboplatin versus TAP.

Chemotherapy for Advanced or Recurrent Uterine Serous Carcinoma

For advanced-stage USC, much of the available information describing treatment options comes from retrospective, nonrandomized case series or from subset analysis of studies including all types of advanced or recurrent endometrial cancer. Paclitaxel, or the combination of carboplatin and paclitaxel, have shown good activity in several studies. Zanotti and colleagues reported on a retrospective cohort of 24 patients with measurable disease (either progressive disease after initial surgery or recurrent disease) who were treated with platinum-based chemotherapy and paclitaxel. There was an 89% response rate in patients treated after initial surgery and a 64% response rate for patients with recurrent disease, with median progression-free intervals of 13 months and 9 months, respectively.[120] Several agents are under investigation as monotherapy or as part of combination regimens for the treatment of USC.

Hoskins and colleagues also reported on the results of a phase 2 trial for patients with advanced or recurrent endometrial carcinoma.[121] In this study of 63 total patients, 20 patients had advanced serous cancers and 4 had recurrent serous cancers. Patients with radio-encompassable advanced USC received involved-field irradiation (n = 11; 55%). Both groups received carboplatin plus paclitaxel for 3 hours at 4-week intervals. Response rates to chemotherapy were 60% and 50% for advanced and recurrent USC, respectively.[121]

Ramondetta and colleagues[122] performed a phase 2 trial of intravenous paclitaxel for women with advanced or recurrent USC. Twenty patients received from 1 to 11 cycles of therapy, which included paclitaxel 200 mg/m^2 over a 24-hour intravenous infusion every 3 weeks. Among 13 women with measurable tumor receiving ≥2 cycles of therapy, 10 (77%) had an objective response (4 complete responses and 6 partial responses). The median time to progression was 7.3 months (range, 2-21 months). Furthermore, the remaining 3 patients with measurable disease had stable disease for a median of 6 months. The authors concluded that paclitaxel appears to have excellent activity in the treatment of advanced or recurrent USC.

Combination Chemotherapy and Radiation

Adjuvant therapy for advanced-stage endometrial carcinoma most commonly includes chemotherapy; however, when chemotherapy is given alone in this setting, pelvic recurrence rates may be as high as 46.5%.[123] Radiation may play an important role in decreasing pelvic recurrence or in specifically treating patients with node-only disease. In a retrospective analysis of 356 patients with advanced endometrial carcinoma treated with postoperative adjuvant therapy, Secord and colleagues[124] demonstrated that adjuvant chemotherapy and radiation was associated with improved survival when compared with either modality alone. In this study, when only optimally cytoreduced patients were analyzed, the adjusted HR for patients who were treated with either chemotherapy or radiation alone indicated a significantly higher risk for disease progression (HR = 1.84 [P = .038]; HR = 1.80 [P = .020]) and death (HR = 2.33 [P = .024]; HR = 2.64 [P = .004]), respectively, compared with patients who received combination therapy. Thus there has been an interest in exploring the role of radiotherapy in combination with chemotherapy for advanced-stage disease to improve overall response and prevent locoregional recurrence.

The Radiation Therapy Oncology Group performed a phase 2 study to assess the feasibility, safety, toxicity, recurrence rates, and survival with combination chemotherapy and adjuvant radiotherapy for patients with high-risk endometrial cancer.[125] High risk was defined as grade 2 or 3 endometrial adenocarcinoma with either more than 50% myometrial invasion, cervical stromal invasion, or extrauterine disease confined to the pelvis. After standard surgery, radiation included 45 Gy in 25 fractions to the pelvis followed by vaginal brachytherapy. Four cycles of cisplatin and paclitaxel were given at 4-week intervals after completion of radiotherapy. Four-year rates of survival and progression-free survival for stage III patients were 77% and 72%, respectively.[125] There were no recurrences for patients with stage IC, IIA, or IIB disease. Overall, in patients who experienced a recurrence, distant recurrences were the most common (19%). However, this regimen was tolerated well, with excellent pelvic and regional control. As mentioned previously, Hoskins and colleagues[121] also reported on the results of a phase 2 trial for patients with advanced or recurrent endometrial carcinoma. In this study of 63 total patients, 21 patients had advanced, nonserous cancers, and 18 had recurrent, nonserous cancers. Involved-field irradiation was used in patients with advanced, nonserous cancer who had radioencompassable disease (n = 19; 90%), and all groups received carboplatin plus paclitaxel at 4-week intervals. Response rates to chemotherapy for the 4 groups were 78% and 56% for patients with advanced and recurrent nonserous endometrial cancer, respectively.[121] The authors concluded that the combination of carboplatin and paclitaxel is efficacious for managing primarily advanced or recurrent endometrial cancers.

Although chemotherapy is often given concurrent with radiotherapy or after completion of radiotherapy, different administration strategies have been attempted. Most recently, Geller and colleagues[126] completed a phase 2 trial of carboplatin and docetaxel in combination with radiotherapy given in a "sandwich" method for advanced stage or recurrent endometrial carcinoma. Forty-two patients received 3 cycles of docetaxel and carboplatin at 3-week intervals followed by pelvic radiotherapy (45 Gy) with or without brachytherapy and 3 additional cycles of docetaxel and carboplatin. This regimen was noted to be effective, with only 2 patients experiencing disease recurrence in the pelvis or locally (8 had a distant recurrence), with estimated 5-year progression-free and overall survival of 64% and 71%, respectively. However, hematologic toxicities were common, with 30 grade 3 or 4 hematologic events encountered. Klopp et al[127] reported on 71 women who were treated for stage IIIC endometrial adenocarcinoma who had undergone total abdominal hysterectomy, bilateral salpingo-oophorectomy, and lymphadenectomy to evaluate treatment outcomes and patterns of recurrence. Fifty patients received definitive pelvic or extended-field radiotherapy with or without systemic therapy (regional radiotherapy group). Eighteen received adjuvant systemic platinum-based chemotherapy or hormonal therapy without external-beam radiotherapy. The authors noted that 5-year pelvic-relapse-free survival (98% vs. 61%; $P = .001$), disease-specific survival (78% vs. 39%; $P = .01$), and overall survival (73% vs. 40%; $P = .03$) were significantly better for the regional radiotherapy group than the systemic therapy group.[127] The authors concluded that patients with node-positive disease treated without regional radiotherapy had a high rate of locoregional recurrence.

Hormonal Therapy

Progestins are the most widely used form of hormonal therapy in patients with advanced or recurrent endometrial cancer. The GOG randomized 299 women with advanced or recurrent endometrial carcinoma to receive either 200 mg/d or 1000 mg/d of oral medroxyprogesterone acetate (MPA until disease progression or unacceptable toxicity.[103] Of the 145 patients receiving the low-dose (200 mg/d) regimen, there was an overall response rate of 25%, including 25 complete responses (17%) and 11 partial responses (8%). Among the 154 patients receiving the high-dose (1000 mg/d) regimen, the overall response rate was surprisingly lower at 15%, including 14 (9%) complete responses and 10 (6%) partial responses.[103] The median progression-free and overall survival for the low-dose regimen was 3.2 and 11 months, respectively. In contrast, the median progression-free and overall survival for the high-dose regimen was 2.5 and 7 months, respectively. The investigators also found that the response rates were greater for patients with well-differentiated tumors and positive progesterone receptor status; the response rates for patients with grade 3 tumors or progesterone-receptor negative tumors were 9% and 8%, respectively. The GOG concluded that MPA 200 mg/d was a reasonable initial approach in the treatment of patients with advanced or recurrent endometrial carcinoma, particularly in patients with tumors that are well-differentiated and/or progesterone-receptor positive.

Megestrol acetate (MA) has also been evaluated for use in the treatment of patients with advanced or recurrent endometrial carcinoma. Lentz and colleagues[128] enrolled 63 patients with advanced or recurrent endometrial carcinoma who had not been treated with prior cytotoxic or hormonal therapy onto a phase 2 GOG study. Patients were given MA 800 mg/d in divided doses until disease progression or unacceptable toxicity. There were 13 patients (24%) who responded (11% with a complete response and 13% with a partial response), plus an additional 22% with stable disease.[128] The progression-free and overall survival were 2.5 months and 7.6 months, respectively. Although this therapy was generally well tolerated, 5% of patients experienced grade 3 weight gain (> 20% increase in weight) or deaths secondary to cardiovascular events. Furthermore, the response rates achieved with this higher dose were not significantly different when compared with lower-dose regimens. As with the MPA study described previously, it was noted that patients with grade 1 and 2 disease had a significantly improved response rate when compared with patients with poorly differentiated tumors (30% vs. 8%; $P = .02$). Based on these data, the authors concluded that high-dose progestin therapy offers no advantage over low-dose therapy in the treatment of advanced endometrial carcinoma.

Tamoxifen, a selective estrogen receptor antagonist, has estrogenic effects on the endometrium and has been used in the treatment of advanced and recurrent endometrial carcinoma. Several studies have evaluated the use of tamoxifen alone. In a review of the literature, Moore and colleagues[129] reported a pooled response rate of 22% with tamoxifen alone. Perhaps more importantly, tamoxifen has been shown to increase the number of progesterone receptors in human endometrial carcinoma.[130] Given the short response durations seen with MPA and MA alone and the improvement in responses seen in tumors that are progesterone-receptor positive, the GOG sought to evaluate the activity of tamoxifen in combination with either MPA or MA.[131,132] Sixty-one patients with measurable advanced or recurrent endometrial carcinoma were treated with tamoxifen 40 mg oral daily and alternating weekly cycles of MPA 200 mg oral daily. This combination regimen produced an overall response rate of 33%, including 10% complete responses and 23% partial responses.[131] The progression-free and overall survival were 3 months and 13 months, respectively. As the response rate with this combination regimen was better than either drug alone with no significant difference in adverse events, the authors concluded that this combination was active and warranted further investigation in randomized trials.

In a similar study, the GOG treated 61 chemotherapy- or hormonal therapy-naïve patients with measurable advanced or recurrent endometrial carcinoma with MA 80 mg oral twice daily for 3 weeks alternating with tamoxifen 20 mg oral twice daily for 3 weeks. This combination regimen produced an overall response rate of 27%, including 21% complete responses and 7% partial responses.[132] The progression-free and overall survival were 2.7 months and 14 months, respectively. Grade 3 and 4 vascular toxicities were seen in 7% of patients. Similar to the MPA/tamoxifen study, the authors concluded that MA alternating with tamoxifen was active in patients with advanced or recurrent endometrial carcinoma and warranted further investigation.

Recently, another selective estrogen receptor antagonist has been evaluated. In a phase 2 trial, arzoxifene was administered at a dose of 20 mg/d orally to 29 patients and produced responses in 9 (overall response rate, 31%), with a median duration of response of 13.9 months.[133] The progesterone antagonist mifepristone (RU-486) has also been studied to determine its efficacy in women with advanced or recurrent endometrioid adenocarcinoma.[134] In this phase 2 trial, mifepristone (200 mg orally) was given daily to patients with progesterone receptor–positive advanced or recurrent endometrioid adenocarcinoma or low-grade endometrial stromal sarcoma. Of 12 evaluable patients, 3 (25%) were observed to have stable disease (2 with endometrioid endometrial carcinoma and 1 with low-grade endometrial stromal sarcoma). There were no complete or partial responses. The authors concluded that mifepristone as a single agent provided a limited response in women with progesterone receptor–positive uterine tumors.[134]

Aromatase inhibitors are another category of drugs that have been evaluated for their usefulness in the management of advanced or recurrent endometrial carcinoma. Aromatase inhibitors block the peripheral conversion of androgens to estrogens and reduce circulating estrogen levels. The 2 most commonly used aromatase inhibitors are anastrozole and letrozole. A phase 2 trial of anastrozole (1 mg/d orally) in 23 patients with measurable advanced or recurrent endometrial carcinoma demonstrated only minimal activity (9% partial response) with this drug as a single agent.[135] A separate phase 2 trial of letrozole (2.5 mg/d orally) in 32 postmenopausal women with advanced or recurrent endometrial carcinoma refractory to progestins also demonstrated only minimal activity, with a 9.4% overall response rate.[136]

Although their role in the management of advanced or recurrent endometrial cancer has been established and used for several decades, progestins have not been shown to be effective in the adjuvant setting to prolong progression-free and overall survival. A recent Cochrane review, which included 6 randomized controlled trials to assess the effectiveness and safety of hormonal therapy for advanced or recurrent endometrial carcinoma, concluded that, as there has been no demonstrated survival advantage, until more data are available, hormonal therapy should be individualized with the intent to palliate disease rather than being used with curative intent.[137]

Novel Targeted Therapies

With the recent interest in personalizing cancer care and targeting specific aberrations in tumorigenic pathways, several novel therapies have been developed and evaluated for the treatment of endometrial carcinoma (Table 6-13).[138] The PI3K/AKT/mTOR pathway is the most frequently altered pathway in endometrial carcinoma. *PTEN* loss of function and/or PI3K mutations or amplifications are commonly seen, particularly in type 1 tumors. These molecular alterations result in activation of the mTOR signaling pathway, resulting in uncontrolled cell proliferation and survival. After the discovery that the administration of rapamycin produced complete responses in patients who developed Kaposi's sarcoma after kidney transplantation, it was demonstrated that this drug inhibits mTOR signaling. Several rapamycin analogues—everolimus,[139] temsirolimus,[140] and ridaforolimus[141]—have been evaluated as monotherapy in phase 2 trials for endometrial carcinoma (Table 6-13) and are currently being evaluated in combination regimens. The principal benefit to these drugs, at this time, has been to prolong stable disease. The first of these agents evaluated for treatment of endometrial carcinoma was everolimus (RAD001), an orally administered mTOR inhibitor. In a phase 2 study of 28 patients with advanced or recurrent type 1 endometrial carcinoma, the drug produced no complete or partial responses, but did

Table 6-13 Completed Phase 2 Trials of Novel Targeted Agents for Advanced or Recurrent Endometrial Carcinoma

Drug	Target	No. of Patients	Route of Administration	CR (%)	PR (%)	SD (%)
Everolimus[139]	mTOR	28	PO	0	0	42.9
Temsirolimus[140]	mTOR	27	IV	0	7.4	44.4
Ridaforolimus[141]	mTOR	27	IV	0	7.4	25.9
Erlotinib[145]	EGFR	32	PO	0	12.5	46.9
Cetuximab[146]	EGFR	30	IV	0	5	10
Bevacizumab[142]	VEGF	52	IV	1.9	11.5	40.4
Sunitinib[143]	VEGFR	20	PO	0	15	20
Sorafenib[144]	VEGFR	39	PO	0	5	49

CR, complete response; EGFR, epidermal growth factor receptor; IV, intravenous; mTOR, mammalian target of rapamycin; PO, oral; PR, partial response; SD, stable disease; VEGF, vascular endothelial growth factor; VEGFR, vascular endothelial growth factor receptor.
Adapted from Dedes KJ et al.[138]

demonstrate prolonged stable disease in 12 patients (43%) at 8 weeks' evaluation and in 6 patients (21%) at 20 weeks' evaluation.[139] Similarly, in a phase 2 trial of intravenous temsirolimus, 12 of 25 patients (44%) had prolonged stable disease and 2 patients had a partial response (7.4%).[140] These studies have also sought to identify biomarkers that could predict response to mTOR inhibitors. PTEN expression was felt to be a reasonable predictive marker of clinical benefit, but, thus far, has not shown a significant correlation with response. The next generation of rapamycin analogues, which are currently in phase 1 and 2 trials, have been developed to act as dual inhibitors of mTOR and PI3K in an attempt to improve effectiveness.

Angiogenesis is an important and essential characteristic of various cancer types, including endometrial carcinoma. Overexpression of vascular endothelial growth factor (VEGF) results in increased vascular proliferation and delivery of oxygen and nutrients to the tumor; thus VEGF and its receptors have been proposed as therapeutic targets. Bevacizumab is a monoclonal antibody directed against VEGF. In a phase 2 study of 53 women with persistent or recurrent endometrial carcinoma who had received at most 1 to 2 prior cytotoxic regimens, bevacizumab was shown to have modest single-agent activity (13.5% overall response rate, including 1 complete response and 6 partial responses in the 53 participants), but an impressive additional 21 patients(40.4%) had stable disease at 6 months.[142] Table 6-14 shows the list of agents that have been studied by the GOG in women with recurrent endometrial cancer and highlights that although bevacizumab has a similar response rate as other drugs, it is significantly better at maintaining stable disease. Targeting the VEGF receptor (VEGFR)

has also been attempted with modest success. Sorafenib and sunitinib are 2 compounds that block the VEGFR. Sunitinib has been shown to produce a partial response rate of 15%, with an additional 20% of patients with stable disease.[143] In a phase 2 trial of 39 patients, sorafenib demonstrated fewer responses, with a partial response rate of 5%, but almost half of patients (49%) had stable disease.[144] As with many of these novel targeted therapies, the utility of VEGF and VEGFR inhibitors is still being evaluated and may be maximized as part of combination regimens with cytotoxic agents.

Inhibitors of the epidermal growth factor receptor (EGFR)[145,146] and human epidermal growth factor receptor 2 (HER-2) have also been evaluated and completed phase 2 trials for recurrent or metastatic endometrial cancer (Table 6-13).

As the molecular aberrations associated with endometrial carcinoma are further characterized, new targets will be identified and agents that exploit these targets will go into development. Indeed, there are several agents that are currently in phase 1 and 2 trials. Identifying biomarkers that predict response will be essential for the implementation of these therapeutic strategies.

SURVIVAL AND PROGNOSIS

Key Points

1. As the majority of patients with endometrial cancer present at an early stage, overall survival is good.
2. Several factors are associated with a poor prognosis, including increasing age, African American

race, non-endometrioid histology, the presence of lymphovascular space invasion, increasing tumor size, and tumor DNA aneuploidy.

3. Positive peritoneal cytology is not a significant prognostic factor.
4. Estrogen receptor– and progesterone receptor–positive tumors are associated with improved progression-free survival.

Survival Outcomes

Because most endometrial cancer cases are diagnosed at an early stage when often surgery alone is curative, overall survival is good. Long-term survival is related to surgical stage at presentation. The overall 5-year survival rate for endometrial cancer is 83%, with 5-year survival rates for local, regional, and distant metastatic disease of 96%, 67%, and 17%, respectively.[1] In contrast to patients with early-stage disease, patients with advanced or recurrent disease carry a worse prognosis, and therapy can best be characterized as palliative. Although patients with advanced or recurrent disease often respond to cytotoxic chemotherapy and radiotherapy, these responses tend to be of short duration and only provide a limited benefit to progression-free survival.

Prognostic Factors

Prognostic variables that may affect the behavior of endometrial cancer can be broadly divided into demographic factors and pathologic factors. Demographic factors that have been shown to be independent prognostic variables include the patient's age and race. Pathologic factors include the tumor histology, tumor grade, depth of myometrial invasion, the presence of lymphovascular space invasion (LVSI), the hormone receptor status of the tumor, the presence of tumor outside the uterus or in the peritoneal cytology, and the DNA ploidy of the tumor (Table 6-15).

Demographic Factors

Age is an independent prognostic variable. Older patients tend to have tumors of a higher stage and grade as compared with those of younger patients. However, even with early-stage endometrial carcinoma, increased age at time of diagnosis is associated with a worse survival. Zaino and colleagues found that compared with women who are 45 years of age with stage I and II disease, women who are 55, 65, and 75 years of age carry a relative risk of death of 2.3, 4.6, and 7.6, respectively ($P = .0001$).[147] This study also demonstrated that women 40 years of age or younger have a 5-year relative survival rate of 96.3% as compared with 94.4% for women age 41 to 50 years, 87.3% for women age 51 to 60 years, 78% for women 61 to 70 years, 70.7% for women age 71 to 80 years, and 53.6% for women older than 80 years ($P < .001$).[147]

Race also appears to be an independent prognostic variable. White women have a higher survival rate than African American women (Table 6-16). This may be attributed the development of higher-grade tumors and an increased propensity to develop USCs that

Table 6-14 GOG Studies Evaluating Agents for Recurrent Endometrial Cancer

| Protocol | Agent | Evaluable Patients (n) | Probability PFS at 6 Months | | Response | |
			Product Limit Estimate	SE	Patients (n)	%
GOG-129-B	Etoposide	25	0.08	0.05	0	0
GOG-129-C	Paclitaxel	48	0.21	0.06	12	25
GOG-129-E	Dactinomycin	27	0.04	0.04	3	11
GOG-129-H	Liposomal doxorubicin	43	0.23	0.06	4	9
GOG-129-I	Pyrazoloacridine	25	0.16	0.07	1	4
GOG-129-J	Topotecan	28	0.25	0.08	2	7
GOG-129-K	Oxaliplatin	52	0.27	0.06	7	13
GOG-129-L	Irofulven	25	0.28	0.09	1	4
GOG-129-M	Flavopiridol	21	0	0	0	0
GOG-229-B	Thalidomide	24	0.08	0.06	3	12
GOG-229-E	Bevacizumab	52	0.40	0.07	7	13.5

GOG, Gynecologic Oncology Group; PFS, progression-free survival.
Adapted from Aghajanian et al.[142]

Table 6-15 Prognostic Variables for Surgically Staged Endometrial Carcinoma

Prognostic Variable	Relative Risk of Death
Endometrioid	
Grade 1	1.0
Grade 2	1.3
Grade 3	1.8
Serous	4.4
Clear cell	2.5
Endometrioid with squamous differentiation	
Grade 1	1.2
Grade 2	1.0
Grade 3	0.8
Myometrial invasion	
Endometrium only	1.0
Superficial	0.5
Middle	3.3
Deep	4.6
Age, years	
45 (reference)	1.0
55	2.3
65	4.6
74	7.6
Positive LVSI	1.4

LVSI, lymphovascular space involvement.
Adapted from Zaino et al.[144]

Table 6-16 Five-Year Relative Survival Rates Among Patients Diagnosed With Endometrial Cancer by Stage and Race

Stage	5-Year Survival (%)
Localized	
White	96
African American	85
Regional	
White	70
African American	46
Distant	
White	19
African American	11
All stages	
White	85
African American	61

Data from Jemal et al.[1]

present at later stages. Maxwell et al[148] retrospectively reviewed data from 169 African American women and 982 white women with stage III/IV or recurrent endometrial cancer and found that African American women were significantly more likely to have USC ($P < .001$), stage IV disease ($P < .001$), and higher tumor grade ($P < .001$) as compared with white women. Survival was also worse among African American women compared with white women (median survival, 10.6 months vs. 12.2 months, respectively; $P < .001$).

Pathologic Factors

The histologic subtype of the tumor has also been shown to be a strong predictor of survival, with tumors of endometrioid histology with or without squamous differentiation having the most favorable prognosis. Fortunately, most tumors fall into this more favorable category. USC and clear cell carcinoma carry a worse prognosis and when taken together account for up to 10% to 15% of endometrial cancers. In a retrospective analysis of 388 patients, the Mayo Clinic reported that compared with a 92% survival in patients with endometrioid histology, patients who had a lesion with an unfavorable subtype (adenosquamous, serous, clear cell, or undifferentiated) had only a 33% overall survival.[149] This poor survival is likely due to a propensity for extrauterine disease at the time of presentation and a proclivity of recurrence at distant sites. In patients with an unfavorable histologic subtype, 62% had extrauterine spread of disease and 55% had a component of recurrence outside of the abdominal/pelvic cavity.[95] Slomovitz and colleagues[150] reported that the 5-year overall survival for clear cell carcinomas is 53% (stage I/II, 70%; stage III/IV, 39%) and for USC is 49% (stage I/II, 63%; stage III/IV, 33%).

The histologic grade of the tumor is also an important determinant of prognosis. Table 6-16 shows the survival of 895 patients studied by the GOG that relates endometrial carcinoma survival to tumor grade. In summary, Zaino and colleagues[147] found that in patients with stage I or II endometrial carcinoma, those who had grade 3 lesions had a 66.4% 5-year survival rate as compared with 91.1% for those with grade 1 lesions and 82% for those with grade 2 lesions ($P < .001$). Furthermore, in a sentinel article reviewing the surgical and pathologic features of 621 patients with stage I carcinoma of the endometrium, Creasman and colleagues[56] demonstrated that increasing tumor grade and the depth of myometrial invasion are correlated with the risk of tumor spread outside the uterus, specifically to the pelvic and paraaortic lymph nodes (Tables 6-7 and 6-8).

The presence of LVSI has been demonstrated to have a negative effect on survival.[151] The incidence of LVSI increases with greater depth of myometrial invasion and poorer tumor differentiation. However, even in early-stage well-differentiated endometrial

CHAPTER 6

carcinomas, LVSI has been associated with a high risk of death.[152] In a retrospective review of 41 patients with well-differentiated endometrioid adenocarcinoma of the endometrium with more than 50% myometrial invasion, O'Brien and colleagues[153] reported that 60% patients with LVSI died of recurrence.

Schink and colleagues[154] performed a retrospective analysis of 142 women with clinical stage I endometrial carcinoma and reported that tumor size is also prognostic of lymph node involvement and survival. Patients with tumors ≤2 cm in diameter had only a 5.7% incidence of lymphatic metastases. However, when tumors exceeded 2 cm in diameter or involved the entire endometrial surface, metastases were encountered in 15% and 35% of patients, respectively ($P = .01$). The 5-year survival rate was 98% for patients with tumors ≤2 cm, 84% with tumors more than 2 cm, and 64% with tumors involving the whole uterine cavity ($P = .005$).[154]

The importance of positive peritoneal cytology as a prognostic factor is controversial. The GOG reported that the relative risk of death for patients with positive peritoneal washings was 3.0.[147] In contrast, Tebeu and colleagues[155] performed a retrospective analysis of 278 stage I and 53 stage IIIA endometrial cancer patients. They further subdivided patients with stage IIIA disease into "cytological" stage IIIA (ie, stage IIIA by positive peritoneal cytology alone) and "histological" stage IIIA (infiltration of the adnexa or serosa). The authors demonstrated that the 5-year disease-specific survival of cytologic stage IIIA cancer was similar to stage I (91% vs. 92%) and better than histologic stage IIIA cancer (50%; $P < .001$). Reflecting these more recent findings, in the revised FIGO surgical staging (2009), positive cytology is no longer classified as stage IIIA.

DNA ploidy has also been demonstrated to be a significant prognostic variable. Approximately 15% to 30% of patients with endometrial carcinoma have aneuploid tumors.[156,157] In a retrospective study of 217 patients with stage IA, grade 1 to 2 endometrial carcinoma ploidy was demonstrated to be an independent prognostic factor (HR, 4.5; $P = .017$). In these low-risk patients, the recurrence rate was 2.1% for diploid tumors and 12.5% for aneuploid tumors ($P = 0.038$).[156]

Measurement of serum CA-125 is recommended in the preoperative evaluation of endometrial cancer patients and has been proposed as a strategy to predict which patients may have advanced versus early disease in an effort to determine which patients would require lymphadenectomy. Elevated CA-125 levels have been correlated with advanced-stage disease and positive lymph node status.[158] A CA-125 cut-off level of 37 IU/mL has a sensitivity and specificity of 95% and 90%, respectively, with a PPV of 78% and an NPV of 97%.[158] Conversely, a preoperative CA-125 level of less than 20 IU/mL has been associated with only a 3% risk of extrauterine disease with a NPV of 88%, making vaginal hysterectomy a feasible option in patients at high risk for abdominal surgery with low CA-125 levels and low-grade histology.[159] Despite the usefulness of these findings in predicting the presence or absence of extrauterine disease, CA-125 alone is not sufficient to determine which patients will require lymphadenectomy.

Special Management Problems

Approximately 10% to 15% of women with endometrial carcinoma are diagnosed before the age of 50 years.[2] Younger women who present with endometrial carcinoma generally have early-stage disease and a good overall prognosis. As a result, the issue of hormone replacement therapy (HRT) to protect against osteoporosis and manage vasomotor symptoms has been debated. Historically, hormone replacement therapy has been considered contraindicated in patients who have been diagnosed with endometrial carcinoma. However, this notion has been recently challenged. In a small prospective study of 50 endometrial cancer patients who were treated with a continuous daily regimen of 0.625 mg of conjugated equine estrogen plus 2.5 mg of MPA beginning 4 to 8 weeks after surgery and 52 endometrial cancer patients who did not receive HRT (control group), Ayhan and colleagues[160] found that none of the patients who received HRT developed a recurrence over the follow-up period. One patient in the control group developed a recurrence and died of disease. Although the authors concluded that immediate postoperative use of HRT did not increase the recurrence or death rates in endometrial cancer survivors, this study is limited by its small sample size and lack of randomization.

The GOG has performed a prospective, randomized trial of HRT versus placebo in 1236 patients with stage I or II endometrial carcinoma after hysterectomy with or without pelvic and aortic nodal sampling.[161] The investigators planned to administer HRT versus placebo treatment for 3 years, with an additional 2 years of follow-up. The median follow-up time for all 1236 eligible and assessable patients was 35.7 months. Two hundred fifty-one patients (41.1%) were compliant with HRT for the entire treatment period. In patients receiving HRT, 14 (2.3%) experienced disease recurrence, and 5 deaths (0.8%) were attributed endometrial cancer. Eight patients (1.3%) developed a new malignancy. These results did not differ significantly from patients in the placebo treatment group, in which 12 patients (1.9%) experienced disease recurrence, 10 patients (1.6%) developed a new malignancy, and 4 deaths (0.6%) were a result of endometrial cancer.[161] Unfortunately, this study was closed prematurely due to poor accrual after publication of the

Women's Health Initiative in 2002. Although incomplete and incapable of fully supporting or refuting the safety of exogenous HRT with regard to risk of endometrial cancer recurrence, it is reassuring that very few recurrences and cancer-related deaths were noted in the HRT group. This study provides limited information that allows practitioners and patients to discuss options and review the risks and benefits to HRT after an endometrial cancer diagnosis.

FUTURE DIRECTIONS

The incidence of endometrial cancer has continued to rise in the past 2 decades from 34,900 in 1997 to 43,470 in 2010. In addition, despite the introduction and increased use of multimodality therapy and the development of novel targeted agents, yearly deaths related to endometrial cancer have increased by 250% since the mid-1980s—from 2900 to 7950. The central issue surrounding the rising incidence of endometrial cancer is the epidemic of obesity. Controlling the epidemic of obesity, developing effective chemopreventive options, and developing approaches to predict a patient's risk of developing endometrial cancer will be important in decreasing incidence. Continuing to pursue novel targeted therapies will be key to addressing the increased mortality. Finally, refinements in treatment, including further delineating which patients benefit from full lymphadenectomy as well as the role of adjuvant treatment in high-risk, early-stage patients, will assist us in maximizing cures while minimizing treatment side effects.

REFERENCES

1. Jemal A, Siegel R, Xu J, Ward E. Cancer statistics, 2010. *CA Cancer J Clin.* 2010;60(5):277-300.
2. Elwood JM, Cole P, Rothman KJ, Kaplan SD. Epidemiology of endometrial cancer. *J Natl Cancer Inst.* 1977;59(4):1055-1060.
3. Kaaks R, Lukanova A, Kurzer MS. Obesity, endogenous hormones, and endometrial cancer risk: a synthetic review. *Cancer Epidemiol Biomarkers Prev.* 2002;11(12):1531-1543.
4. Fisher B, Costantino JP, Redmond CK, Fisher ER, Wickerham DL, Cronin WM. Endometrial cancer in tamoxifen-treated breast cancer patients: findings from the National Surgical Adjuvant Breast and Bowel Project (NSABP) B-14. *J Natl Cancer Inst.* 1994;86(7):527-537.
5. Fisher B, Costantino JP, Wickerham DL, et al. Tamoxifen for prevention of breast cancer: report of the National Surgical Adjuvant Breast and Bowel Project P-1 Study. *J Natl Cancer Inst.* 1998;90(18):1371-1388.
6. Reeves GK, Pirie K, Beral V, Green J, Spencer E, Bull D. Cancer incidence and mortality in relation to body mass index in the Million Women Study: cohort study. *BMJ.* 2007;335(7630):1134.
7. Renehan AG, Tyson M, Egger M, Heller RF, Zwahlen M. Body-mass index and incidence of cancer: a systematic review and meta-analysis of prospective observational studies. *Lancet.* 2008;371(9612):569-578.
8. Calle EE, Rodriguez C, Walker-Thurmond K, Thun MJ. Overweight, obesity, and mortality from cancer in a prospectively studied cohort of U.S. adults. *N Engl J Med.* 2003;348(17):1625-1638.
9. von Gruenigen VE, Tian C, Frasure H, Waggoner S, Keys H, Barakat RR. Treatment effects, disease recurrence, and survival in obese women with early endometrial carcinoma: a Gynecologic Oncology Group study. *Cancer.* 2006;107(12):2786-2791.
10. Soliman PT, Bassett RL Jr, Wilson EB, et al. Limited public knowledge of obesity and endometrial cancer risk: what women know. *Obstet Gynecol.* 2008;112(4):835-842.
11. Lu KH, Broaddus RR. Gynecologic cancers in Lynch syndrome/HNPCC. *Fam Cancer.* 2005;4(3):249-254.
12. Schmeler KM, Lu KH. Gynecologic cancers associated with Lynch syndrome/HNPCC. *Clin Transl Oncol.* 2008;10(6):313-317.
13. Aarnio M, Sankila R, Pukkala E, et al. Cancer risk in mutation carriers of DNA-mismatch-repair genes. *Int J Cancer.* 1999;81(2):214-218.
14. Hendriks YM, Wagner A, Morreau H, et al. Cancer risk in hereditary nonpolyposis colorectal cancer due to MSH6 mutations: impact on counseling and surveillance. *Gastroenterology.* 2004;127(1):17-25.
15. Aarnio M, Mecklin JP, Aaltonen LA, Nystrom-Lahti M, Jarvinen HJ. Life-time risk of different cancers in hereditary non-polyposis colorectal cancer (HNPCC) syndrome. *Int J Cancer.* 1995;64(6):430-433.
16. Baglietto L, Lindor NM, Dowty JG, et al. Risks of Lynch syndrome cancers for MSH6 mutation carriers. *J Natl Cancer Inst.* 2010;102(3):193-201.
17. Lancaster JM, Powell CB, Kauff ND, et al. Society of Gynecologic Oncologists Education Committee statement on risk assessment for inherited gynecologic cancer predispositions. *Gynecol Oncol.* 2007;107(2):159-162.
18. Schmeler KM, Lynch HT, Chen LM, et al. Prophylactic surgery to reduce the risk of gynecologic cancers in the Lynch syndrome. *N Engl J Med.* 2006;354(3):261-269.
19. Bokhman JV. Two pathogenetic types of endometrial carcinoma. *Gynecol Oncol.* 1983;15(1):10-17.
20. von Gruenigen VE, Gil KM, Frasure HE, Jenison EL, Hopkins MP. The impact of obesity and age on quality of life in gynecologic surgery. *Am J Obstet Gynecol.* 2005;193(4):1369-1375.
21. Mutter GL, Lin MC, Fitzgerald JT, et al. Altered PTEN expression as a diagnostic marker for the earliest endometrial precancers. *J Natl Cancer Inst.* 2000;92(11):924-930.
22. Maxwell GL, Risinger JI, Gumbs C, et al. Mutation of the PTEN tumor suppressor gene in endometrial hyperplasias. *Cancer Res.* 1998;58(12):2500-2503.
23. Oda K, Stokoe D, Taketani Y, McCormick F. High frequency of coexistent mutations of PIK3CA and PTEN genes in endometrial carcinoma. *Cancer Res.* 2005;65(23):10669-10673.
24. Basil JB, Goodfellow PJ, Rader JS, Mutch DG, Herzog TJ. Clinical significance of microsatellite instability in endometrial carcinoma. *Cancer.* 2000;89(8):1758-1764.
25. Bilbao C, Rodriguez G, Ramirez R, et al. The relationship between microsatellite instability and PTEN gene mutations in endometrial cancer. *Int J Cancer.* 2006;119(3):563-570.
26. Lax SF, Kendall B, Tashiro H, Slebos RJ, Hedrick L. The frequency of p53, K-ras mutations, and microsatellite instability differs in uterine endometrioid and serous carcinoma: evidence of distinct molecular genetic pathways. *Cancer.* 2000;88(4):814-824.
27. Caduff RF, Johnston CM, Frank TS. Mutations of the Ki-ras oncogene in carcinoma of the endometrium. *Am J Pathol.* 1995;146(1):182-188.

28. Mirabelli-Primdahl L, Gryfe R, Kim H, et al. Beta-catenin mutations are specific for colorectal carcinomas with microsatellite instability but occur in endometrial carcinomas irrespective of mutator pathway. *Cancer Res.* 1999;59(14):3346-3351.

29. Moreno-Bueno G, Hardisson D, Sanchez C, et al. Abnormalities of the APC/beta-catenin pathway in endometrial cancer. *Oncogene.* 2002;21(52):7981-7990.

30. Saegusa M, Hashimura M, Yoshida T, Okayasu I. beta- Catenin mutations and aberrant nuclear expression during endometrial tumorigenesis. *Br J Cancer.* 2001;84(2):209-217.

31. Bansal N, Yendluri V, Wenham RM. The molecular biology of endometrial cancers and the implications for pathogenesis, classification, and targeted therapies. *Cancer Control.* 2009;16(1):8-13.

32. Morrison C, Zanagnolo V, Ramirez N, et al. HER-2 is an independent prognostic factor in endometrial cancer: association with outcome in a large cohort of surgically staged patients. *J Clin Oncol.* 2006;24(15):2376-2385.

33. Busmanis I, Ho TH, Tan SB, Khoo KS. p53 and bcl-2 expression in invasive and pre-invasive uterine papillary serous carcinoma and atrophic endometrium. *Ann Acad Med Singapore.* 2005;34(7):421-425.

34. Love CD, Muir BB, Scrimgeour JB, Leonard RC, Dillon P, Dixon JM. Investigation of endometrial abnormalities in asymptomatic women treated with tamoxifen and an evaluation of the role of endometrial screening. *J Clin Oncol.* 1999;17(7):2050-2054.

35. Karlsson B, Granberg S, Wikland M, et al. Transvaginal ultrasonography of the endometrium in women with postmenopausal bleeding: a Nordic multicenter study. *Am J Obstet Gynecol.* 1995;172(5):1488-1494.

36. Tabor A, Watt HC, Wald NJ. Endometrial thickness as a test for endometrial cancer in women with postmenopausal vaginal bleeding. *Obstet Gynecol.* 2002;99(4):663-670.

37. Timmermans A, Opmeer BC, Khan KS, et al. Endometrial thickness measurement for detecting endometrial cancer in women with postmenopausal bleeding: a systematic review and meta-analysis. *Obstet Gynecol.* 2010;116(1):160-167.

38. Dijkhuizen FP, Mol BW, Brolmann HA, Heintz AP. The accuracy of endometrial sampling in the diagnosis of patients with endometrial carcinoma and hyperplasia: a meta-analysis. *Cancer.* 2000;89(8):1765-1772.

39. Machado F, Moreno J, Carazo M, Leon J, Fiol G, Serna R. Accuracy of endometrial biopsy with the Cornier Pipelle for diagnosis of endometrial cancer and atypical hyperplasia. *Eur J Gynaecol Oncol.* 2003;24(3-4):279-281.

40. Epstein E, Skoog L, Valentin L. Comparison of Endorette and dilatation and curettage for sampling of the endometrium in women with postmenopausal bleeding. *Acta Obstet Gynecol Scand.* 2001;80(10):959-964.

41. Minagawa Y, Sato S, Ito M, Onohara Y, Nakamoto S, Kigawa J. Transvaginal ultrasonography and endometrial cytology as a diagnostic schema for endometrial cancer. *Gynecol Obstet Invest.* 2005;59(3):149-154.

42. Dunton CJ, Baak JP, Palazzo JP, van Diest PJ, McHugh M, Widra EA. Use of computerized morphometric analyses of endometrial hyperplasias in the prediction of coexistent cancer. *Am J Obstet Gynecol.* 1996;174(5):1518-1521.

43. Trimble CL, Kauderer J, Zaino R, et al. Concurrent endometrial carcinoma in women with a biopsy diagnosis of atypical endometrial hyperplasia: a Gynecologic Oncology Group study. *Cancer.* 2006;106(4):812-819.

44. Zaino RJ, Kauderer J, Trimble CL, et al. Reproducibility of the diagnosis of atypical endometrial hyperplasia: a Gynecologic Oncology Group study. *Cancer.* 2006;106(4):804-811.

45. Creasman WT, Odicino F, Maisonneuve P, et al. Carcinoma of the corpus uteri. FIGO 26th Annual Report on the Results of Treatment in Gynecological Cancer. *Int J Gynaecol Obstet.* 2006;95(suppl 1):S105-S143.

46. Malpica A, Deavers MT, Euscher ED, eds. *Biopsy Interpretation of the Uterine Cervix and Corpus.* Biopsy Interpretation Series. Philadelphia, PA: Lippincott Williams & Wilkins; 2009.

47. Slomovitz BM, Burke TW, Eifel PJ, et al. Uterine papillary serous carcinoma (UPSC): a single institution review of 129 cases. *Gynecol Oncol.* 2003;91(3):463-469.

48. McMeekin DS, Filiaci VL, Thigpen JT, Gallion HH, Fleming GF, Rodgers WH. The relationship between histology and outcome in advanced and recurrent endometrial cancer patients participating in first-line chemotherapy trials: a Gynecologic Oncology Group study. *Gynecol Oncol.* 2007;106(1):16-22.

49. Costa MJ, Vogelsan J, Young LJ. p53 gene mutation in female genital tract carcinosarcomas (malignant mixed mullerian tumors): a clinicopathologic study of 74 cases. *Mod Pathol.* 1994;7(6):619-627.

50. Thompson L, Chang B, Barsky SH. Monoclonal origins of malignant mixed tumors (carcinosarcomas). Evidence for a divergent histogenesis. *Am J Surg Pathol.* 1996;20(3):277-285.

51. Abeln EC, Smit VT, Wessels JW, de Leeuw WJ, Cornelisse CJ, Fleuren GJ. Molecular genetic evidence for the conversion hypothesis of the origin of malignant mixed mullerian tumours. *J Pathol.* 1997;183(4):424-431.

52. Kounelis S, Jones MW, Papadaki H, Bakker A, Swalsky P, Finkelstein SD. Carcinosarcomas (malignant mixed mullerian tumors) of the female genital tract: comparative molecular analysis of epithelial and mesenchymal components. *Hum Pathol.* 1998;29(1):82-87.

53. Vaidya AP, Horowitz NS, Oliva E, Halpern EF, Duska LR. Uterine malignant mixed mullerian tumors should not be included in studies of endometrial carcinoma. *Gynecol Oncol.* 2006;103(2):684-687.

54. McCluggage WG, Sumathi VP, McBride HA, Patterson A. A panel of immunohistochemical stains, including carcinoembryonic antigen, vimentin, and estrogen receptor, aids the distinction between primary endometrial and endocervical adenocarcinomas. *Int J Gynecol Pathol.* 2002;21(1):11-15.

55. Bigelow B, Vekshtein V, Demopoulos RI. Endometrial carcinoma, stage II: route and extent of spread to the cervix. *Obstet Gynecol.* 1983;62(3):363-366.

56. Creasman WT, Morrow CP, Bundy BN, Homesley HD, Graham JE, Heller PB. Surgical pathologic spread patterns of endometrial cancer. A Gynecologic Oncology Group study. *Cancer.* 1987;60(8 suppl):2035-2041.

57. Mariani A, Webb MJ, Keeney GL, Podratz KC. Routes of lymphatic spread: a study of 112 consecutive patients with endometrial cancer. *Gynecol Oncol.* 2001;81(1):100-104.

58. Mariani A, Keeney GL, Aletti G, Webb MJ, Haddock MG, Podratz KC. Endometrial carcinoma: paraaortic dissemination. *Gynecol Oncol.* 2004;92(3):833-838.

59. Snyder MJ, Bentley R, Robboy SJ. Transtubal spread of serous adenocarcinoma of the endometrium: an underrecognized mechanism of metastasis. *Int J Gynecol Pathol.* 2006;25(2):155-160.

60. Obermair A, Geramou M, Gucer F, et al. Does hysteroscopy facilitate tumor cell dissemination? Incidence of peritoneal cytology from patients with early stage endometrial carcinoma following dilatation and curettage (D & C) versus hysteroscopy and D & C. *Cancer.* 2000;88(1):139-143.

61. Cowles TA, Magrina JF, Masterson BJ, Capen CV. Comparison of clinical and surgical-staging in patients with endometrial carcinoma. *Obstet Gynecol.* 1985;66(3):413-416.

62. Ayhan A, Yarali H, Urman B, Yuce K, Gunalp S, Havlioglu S. Comparison of clinical and surgical-pathologic staging in

patients with endometrial carcinoma. *J Surg Oncol.* 1990;43(1): 33-35.

63. Campbell K, Nuss RC, Benrubi GI. An evaluation of the clinical staging of endometrial cancer. *J Reprod Med.* 1988;33(1): 8-10.

64. Creasman W. Revised FIGO staging for carcinoma of the endometrium. *Int J Gynaecol Obstet.* 2009;105(2):109.

65. Takeshima N, Nishida H, Tabata T, Hirai Y, Hasumi K. Positive peritoneal cytology in endometrial cancer: enhancement of other prognostic indicators. *Gynecol Oncol.* 2001;82(3):470-473.

66. Hirai Y, Takeshima N, Kato T, Hasumi K. Malignant potential of positive peritoneal cytology in endometrial cancer. *Obstet Gynecol.* 2001;97(5 Pt 1):725-728.

67. Watari H, Todo Y, Takeda M, Ebina Y, Yamamoto R, Sakuragi N. Lymph-vascular space invasion and number of positive para-aortic node groups predict survival in node-positive patients with endometrial cancer. *Gynecol Oncol.* 2005;96(3):651-657.

68. Hoekstra AV, Kim RJ, Small W Jr, et al. FIGO stage IIIC endometrial carcinoma: prognostic factors and outcomes. *Gynecol Oncol.* 2009;114(2):273-278.

69. Hirahatake K, Hareyama H, Sakuragi N, Nishiya M, Makinoda S, Fujimoto S. A clinical and pathologic study on para-aortic lymph node metastasis in endometrial carcinoma. *J Surg Oncol.* 1997;65(2):82-87.

70. Kurman RJ, Kaminski PF, Norris HJ. The behavior of endometrial hyperplasia. A long-term study of "untreated" hyperplasia in 170 patients. *Cancer.* 1985;56(2):403-412.

71. Ferenczy A, Gelfand M. The biologic significance of cytologic atypia in progestogen-treated endometrial hyperplasia. *Am J Obstet Gynecol.* 1989;160(1):126-131.

72. Reed SD, Voigt LF, Newton KM, et al. Progestin therapy of complex endometrial hyperplasia with and without atypia. *Obstet Gynecol.* 2009;113(3):655-662.

73. Wildemeersch D, Dhont M. Treatment of nonatypical and atypical endometrial hyperplasia with a levonorgestrel-releasing intrauterine system. *Am J Obstet Gynecol.* 2003;188(5): 1297-1298.

74. Vereide AB, Arnes M, Straume B, Maltau JM, Orbo A. Nuclear morphometric changes and therapy monitoring in patients with endometrial hyperplasia: a study comparing effects of intrauterine levonorgestrel and systemic medroxyprogesterone. *Gynecol Oncol.* 2003;91(3):526-533.

75. Gallos ID, Shehmar M, Thangaratinam S, Papapostolou TK, Coomarasamy A, Gupta JK. Oral progestogens vs levonorgestrel-releasing intrauterine system for endometrial hyperplasia: a systematic review and metaanalysis. *Am J Obstet Gynecol.* 203(6):547 e541-e510.

76. Walker JL, Piedmonte MR, Spirtos NM, et al. Laparoscopy compared with laparotomy for comprehensive surgical staging of uterine cancer: Gynecologic Oncology Group Study LAP2. *J Clin Oncol.* 2009;27(32):5331-5336.

77. Kornblith AB, Huang HQ, Walker JL, Spirtos NM, Rotmensch J, Cella D. Quality of life of patients with endometrial cancer undergoing laparoscopic international federation of gynecology and obstetrics staging compared with laparotomy: a Gynecologic Oncology Group study. *J Clin Oncol.* 2009;27(32):5337-5342.

78. Mariani A, Webb MJ, Keeney GL, Haddock MG, Calori G, Podratz KC. Low-risk corpus cancer: is lymphadenectomy or radiotherapy necessary? *Am J Obstet Gynecol.* 2000;182(6): 1506-1519.

79. Kitchener H, Swart AM, Qian Q, Amos C, Parmar MK. Efficacy of systematic pelvic lymphadenectomy in endometrial cancer (MRC ASTEC trial): a randomised study. *Lancet.* 2009;373(9658):125-136.

80. Benedetti Panici P, Basile S, Maneschi F, et al. Systematic pelvic lymphadenectomy vs. no lymphadenectomy in early-stage endometrial carcinoma: randomized clinical trial. *J Natl Cancer Inst.* 2008;100(23):1707-1716.

81. Mariani A, Dowdy SC, Cliby WA, et al. Prospective assessment of lymphatic dissemination in endometrial cancer: a paradigm shift in surgical staging. *Gynecol Oncol.* 2008;109(1):11-18.

82. Soliman PT, Frumovitz M, Spannuth W, et al. Lymphadenectomy during endometrial cancer staging: practice patterns among gynecologic oncologists. *Gynecol Oncol.* 2010;119(2):291-294.

83. Kilgore LC, Partridge EE, Alvarez RD, et al. Adenocarcinoma of the endometrium: survival comparisons of patients with and without pelvic node sampling. *Gynecol Oncol.* 1995;56(1):29-33.

84. Chan JK, Cheung MK, Huh WK, et al. Therapeutic role of lymph node resection in endometrioid corpus cancer: a study of 12,333 patients. *Cancer.* 2006;107(8):1823-1830.

85. Todo Y, Kato H, Kaneuchi M, Watari H, Takeda M, Sakuragi N. Survival effect of para-aortic lymphadenectomy in endometrial cancer (SEPAL study): a retrospective cohort analysis. *Lancet.* 2010;375(9721):1165-1172.

86. Chan JK, Urban R, Cheung MK, et al. Lymphadenectomy in endometrioid uterine cancer staging: how many lymph nodes are enough? A study of 11,443 patients. *Cancer.* 2007;109(12):2454-2460.

87. Creutzberg CL, van Putten WL, Koper PC, et al. Surgery and postoperative radiotherapy versus surgery alone for patients with stage-1 endometrial carcinoma: multicentre randomised trial. PORTEC Study Group. Post Operative Radiation Therapy in Endometrial Carcinoma. *Lancet.* 2000;355(9213): 1404-1411.

88. Scholten AN, van Putten WL, Beerman H, et al. Postoperative radiotherapy for stage 1 endometrial carcinoma: long-term outcome of the randomized PORTEC trial with central pathology review. *Int J Radiat Oncol Biol Phys.* 2005;63(3):834-838.

89. Keys HM, Roberts JA, Brunetto VL, et al. A phase III trial of surgery with or without adjunctive external pelvic radiation therapy in intermediate risk endometrial adenocarcinoma: a Gynecologic Oncology Group study. *Gynecol Oncol.* 2004;92(3):744-751.

90. Nout RA, Smit VT, Putter H, et al. Vaginal brachytherapy versus pelvic external beam radiotherapy for patients with endometrial cancer of high-intermediate risk (PORTEC-2): an open-label, non-inferiority, randomised trial. *Lancet.* 2010;375(9717):816-823.

91. Nout RA, Putter H, Jurgenliemk-Schulz IM, et al. Quality of life after pelvic radiotherapy or vaginal brachytherapy for endometrial cancer: first results of the randomized PORTEC-2 trial. *J Clin Oncol.* 2009;27(21):3547-3556.

92. Huh WK, Powell M, Leath CA 3rd, et al. Uterine papillary serous carcinoma: comparisons of outcomes in surgical Stage I patients with and without adjuvant therapy. *Gynecol Oncol.* 2003;91(3):470-475.

93. Dietrich CS 3rd, Modesitt SC, DePriest PD, et al. The efficacy of adjuvant platinum-based chemotherapy in stage I uterine papillary serous carcinoma (UPSC). *Gynecol Oncol.* 2005;99(3):557-563.

94. Kelly MG, O'Malley DM, Hui P, et al. Improved survival in surgical stage I patients with uterine papillary serous carcinoma (UPSC) treated with adjuvant platinum-based chemotherapy. *Gynecol Oncol.* 2005;98(3):353-359.

95. Turner BC, Knisely JP, Kacinski BM, et al. Effective treatment of stage I uterine papillary serous carcinoma with high dose-rate vaginal apex radiation (192Ir) and chemotherapy. *Int J Radiat Oncol Biol Phys.* 1998;40(1):77-84.

96. Niazi TM, Souhami L, Portelance L, Bahoric B, Gilbert L, Stanimir G. Long-term results of high-dose-rate brachytherapy in the primary treatment of medically inoperable stage I-II endometrial carcinoma. *Int J Radiat Oncol Biol Phys.* 2005;63(4):1108-1113.

97. Shenfield CB, Pearcey RG, Ghosh S, Dundas GS. The management of inoperable stage I endometrial cancer using intracavitary brachytherapy alone: a 20-year institutional review. *Brachytherapy*. 2009;8(3):278-283.

98. Wegner RE, Beriwal S, Heron DE, et al. Definitive radiation therapy for endometrial cancer in medically inoperable elderly patients. *Brachytherapy*. 2010;9(3):260-265.

99. Soliman PT, Oh JC, Schmeler KM, et al. Risk factors for young premenopausal women with endometrial cancer. *Obstet Gynecol*. 2005;105(3):575-580.

100. Yamazawa K, Seki K, Matsui H, Kihara M, Sekiya S. Prognostic factors in young women with endometrial carcinoma: a report of 20 cases and review of literature. *Int J Gynecol Cancer*. 2000;10(3):212-222.

101. Tran BN, Connell PP, Waggoner S, Rotmensch J, Mundt AJ. Characteristics and outcome of endometrial carcinoma patients age 45 years and younger. *Am J Clin Oncol*. 2000;23(5):476-480.

102. Nyholm HC. Estrogen and progesterone receptors in endometrial cancer. Clinicopathological correlations and prognostic significance. *APMIS Suppl*. 1996;65:5-33.

103. Thigpen JT, Brady MF, Alvarez RD, et al. Oral medroxyprogesterone acetate in the treatment of advanced or recurrent endometrial carcinoma: a dose-response study by the Gynecologic Oncology Group. *J Clin Oncol*. 1999;17(6):1736-1744.

104. Frumovitz M, Gershenson DM. Fertility-sparing therapy for young women with endometrial cancer. *Expert Rev Anticancer Ther*. 2006;6(1):27-32.

105. Takeshima N, Hirai Y, Yano K, Tanaka N, Yamauchi K, Hasumi K. Ovarian metastasis in endometrial carcinoma. *Gynecol Oncol*. 1998;70(2):183-187.

106. Gitsch G, Hanzal E, Jensen D, Hacker NF. Endometrial cancer in premenopausal women 45 years and younger. *Obstet Gynecol*. 1995;85(4):504-508.

107. Larson DM, Johnson KK, Broste SK, Krawisz BR, Kresl JJ. Comparison of D&C and office endometrial biopsy in predicting final histopathologic grade in endometrial cancer. *Obstet Gynecol*. 1995;86(1):38-42.

108. Mitchard J, Hirschowitz L. Concordance of FIGO grade of endometrial adenocarcinomas in biopsy and hysterectomy specimens. *Histopathology*. 2003;42(4):372-378.

109. Kinkel K, Kaji Y, Yu KK, et al. Radiologic staging in patients with endometrial cancer: a meta-analysis. *Radiology*. 1999;212(3):711-718.

110. Ramirez PT, Frumovitz M, Bodurka DC, Sun CC, Levenback C. Hormonal therapy for the management of grade 1 endometrial adenocarcinoma: a literature review. *Gynecol Oncol*. 2004;95(1):133-138.

111. Dhar KK, NeedhiRajan T, Koslowski M, Woolas RP. Is levonorgestrel intrauterine system effective for treatment of early endometrial cancer? Report of four cases and review of the literature. *Gynecol Oncol*. 2005;97(3):924-927.

112. Bristow RE, Zerbe MJ, Rosenshein NB, Grumbine FC, Montz FJ. Stage IVB endometrial carcinoma: the role of cytoreductive surgery and determinants of survival. *Gynecol Oncol*. 2000;78(2):85-91.

113. Thigpen JT, Brady MF, Homesley HD, et al. Phase III trial of doxorubicin with or without cisplatin in advanced endometrial carcinoma: a Gynecologic Oncology Group study. *J Clin Oncol*. 2004;22(19):3902-3908.

114. Randall ME, Filiaci VL, Muss H, et al. Randomized phase III trial of whole-abdominal irradiation versus doxorubicin and cisplatin chemotherapy in advanced endometrial carcinoma: a Gynecologic Oncology Group Study. *J Clin Oncol*. 2006;24(1):36-44.

115. Fleming GF, Filiaci VL, Bentley RC, et al. Phase III randomized trial of doxorubicin + cisplatin versus doxorubicin + 24-h paclitaxel + filgrastim in endometrial carcinoma: a Gynecologic Oncology Group study. *Ann Oncol*. 2004;15(8):1173-1178.

116. Fleming GF, Brunetto VL, Cella D, et al. Phase III trial of doxorubicin plus cisplatin with or without paclitaxel plus filgrastim in advanced endometrial carcinoma: a Gynecologic Oncology Group Study. *J Clin Oncol*. 2004;22(11):2159-2166.

117. Dimopoulos MA, Papadimitriou CA, Georgoulias V, et al. Paclitaxel and cisplatin in advanced or recurrent carcinoma of the endometrium: long-term results of a phase II multicenter study. *Gynecol Oncol*. 2000;78(1):52-57.

118. van Wijk FH, Lhomme C, Bolis G, et al. Phase II study of carboplatin in patients with advanced or recurrent endometrial carcinoma. A trial of the EORTC Gynaecological Cancer Group. *Eur J Cancer*. 2003;39(1):78-85.

119. Michener CM, Peterson G, Kulp B, Webster KD, Markman M. Carboplatin plus paclitaxel in the treatment of advanced or recurrent endometrial carcinoma. *J Cancer Res Clin Oncol*. 2005;131(9):581-584.

120. Zanotti KM, Belinson JL, Kennedy AW, Webster KD, Markman M. The use of paclitaxel and platinum-based chemotherapy in uterine papillary serous carcinoma. *Gynecol Oncol*. 1999;74(2):272-277.

121. Hoskins PJ, Swenerton KD, Pike JA, et al. Paclitaxel and carboplatin, alone or with irradiation, in advanced or recurrent endometrial cancer: a phase II study. *J Clin Oncol*. 2001;19(20):4048-4053.

122. Ramondetta L, Burke TW, Levenback C, Bevers M, Bodurka-Bevers D, Gershenson DM. Treatment of uterine papillary serous carcinoma with paclitaxel. *Gynecol Oncol*. 2001;82(1):156-161.

123. Mundt AJ, McBride R, Rotmensch J, Waggoner SE, Yamada SD, Connell PP. Significant pelvic recurrence in high-risk pathologic stage I-IV endometrial carcinoma patients after adjuvant chemotherapy alone: implications for adjuvant radiation therapy. *Int J Radiat Oncol Biol Phys*. 2001;50(5):1145-1153.

124. Alvarez Secord A, Havrilesky LJ, Bae-Jump V, et al. The role of multi-modality adjuvant chemotherapy and radiation in women with advanced stage endometrial cancer. *Gynecol Oncol*. 2007;107(2):285-291.

125. Greven K, Winter K, Underhill K, Fontenesci J, Cooper J, Burke T. Final analysis of RTOG 9708: adjuvant postoperative irradiation combined with cisplatin/paclitaxel chemotherapy following surgery for patients with high-risk endometrial cancer. *Gynecol Oncol*. 2006;103(1):155-159.

126. Geller MA, Ivy JJ, Ghebre R, et al. A phase II trial of carboplatin and docetaxel followed by radiotherapy given in a "Sandwich" method for stage III, IV, and recurrent endometrial cancer. *Gynecol Oncol*. 121(1):112-117.

127. Klopp AH, Jhingran A, Ramondetta L, Lu K, Gershenson DM, Eifel PJ. Node-positive adenocarcinoma of the endometrium: outcome and patterns of recurrence with and without external beam irradiation. *Gynecol Oncol*. 2009;115(1):6-11.

128. Lentz SS, Brady MF, Major FJ, Reid GC, Soper JT. High-dose megestrol acetate in advanced or recurrent endometrial carcinoma: a Gynecologic Oncology Group study. *J Clin Oncol*. 1996;14(2):357-361.

129. Moore TD, Phillips PH, Nerenstone SR, Cheson BD. Systemic treatment of advanced and recurrent endometrial carcinoma: current status and future directions. *J Clin Oncol*. 1991;9(6):1071-1088.

130. Carlson JA Jr, Allegra JC, Day TG Jr, Wittliff JL. Tamoxifen and endometrial carcinoma: alterations in estrogen and progesterone receptors in untreated patients and combination hormonal therapy in advanced neoplasia. *Am J Obstet Gynecol*. 1984;149(2):149-153.

131. Whitney CW, Brunetto VL, Zaino RJ, et al. Phase II study of medroxyprogesterone acetate plus tamoxifen in advanced endometrial carcinoma: a Gynecologic Oncology Group study. *Gynecol Oncol.* 2004;92(1):4-9.

132. Fiorica JV, Brunetto VL, Hanjani P, Lentz SS, Mannel R, Andersen W. Phase II trial of alternating courses of megestrol acetate and tamoxifen in advanced endometrial carcinoma: a Gynecologic Oncology Group study. *Gynecol Oncol.* 2004;92(1):10-14.

133. McMeekin DS, Gordon A, Fowler J, et al. A phase II trial of arzoxifene, a selective estrogen response modulator, in patients with recurrent or advanced endometrial cancer. *Gynecol Oncol.* 2003;90(1):64-69.

134. Ramondetta LM, Johnson AJ, Sun CC, et al. Phase 2 trial of mifepristone (RU-486) in advanced or recurrent endometrioid adenocarcinoma or low-grade endometrial stromal sarcoma. *Cancer.* 2009;115(9):1867-1874.

135. Rose PG, Brunetto VL, VanLe L, Bell J, Walker JL, Lee RB. A phase II trial of anastrozole in advanced recurrent or persistent endometrial carcinoma: a Gynecologic Oncology Group study. *Gynecol Oncol.* 2000;78(2):212-216.

136. Ma BB, Oza A, Eisenhauer E, et al. The activity of letrozole in patients with advanced or recurrent endometrial cancer and correlation with biological markers: a study of the National Cancer Institute of Canada Clinical Trials Group. *Int J Gynecol Cancer.* 2004;14(4):650-658.

137. Kokka F, Brockbank E, Oram D, Gallagher C, Bryant A. Hormonal therapy in advanced or recurrent endometrial cancer. *Cochrane Database Syst Rev.* 2010(12):CD007926.

138. Dedes KJ, Wetterskog D, Ashworth A, Kaye SB, Reis-Filho JS. Emerging therapeutic targets in endometrial cancer. *Nat Rev Clin Oncol.* 2011;8(5):261-271.

139. Slomovitz BM, Lu KH, Johnston T, et al. A phase 2 study of the oral mammalian target of rapamycin inhibitor, everolimus, in patients with recurrent endometrial carcinoma. *Cancer.* 2010;116(23):5415-5419.

140. Oza AM, Elit L, Provencher D. NCIC Clinical Trials Group. A phase II study of temsirolimus (CCI-779) in patients with metastatic and/or locally advanced recurrent endometrial cancer previously treated with chemotherapy: NCIC CTG IND 160b. *J Clin Oncol.* 2008;26:5516.

141. Colombo N, McMeekin DS, Schwartz P. A phase II trial of the mTOR inhibitor AP23573 as a single agent in advanced endometrial cancer. *J Clin Oncol.* 2007;25:5516.

142. Aghajanian C, Sill MW, Darcy KM, et al. Phase II trial of bevacizumab in recurrent or persistent endometrial cancer: a Gynecologic Oncology Group study. *J Clin Oncol.* 2011;29(16):2259-2265.

143. Correa R, Mackay H, Hirte HW, et al. A phase II study of sunitinib in recurrent or metastatic endometrial carcinoma: a trial of the Princess Margaret Hospital, The University of Chicago, and California Cancer Phase II Consortia. *J Clin Oncol.* 2010;28(15s):5038.

144. Nimeiri HS, Oza AM, Morgan RJ, et al. A phase II study of sorafenib in advanced uterine carcinoma/carcinosarcoma: a trial of the Chicago, PMH, and California Phase II Consortia. *Gynecol Oncol.* 2010;117(1):37-40.

145. Oza AM, Eisenhauer EA, Elit L, et al. Phase II study of erlotinib in recurrent or metastatic endometrial cancer: NCIC IND-148. *J Clin Oncol.* 2008;26(26):4319-4325.

146. Slomovitz B *ea.* Phase II study of cetuximab (Erbitux) in patients with progressive or recurrent endometrial cancer [abstract]. *Gynecol Oncol.* 2010;116(Suppl. 1):S13.

147. Zaino RJ, Kurman RJ, Diana KL, Morrow CP. Pathologic models to predict outcome for women with endometrial adenocarcinoma: the importance of the distinction between surgical stage and clinical stage—a Gynecologic Oncology Group study. *Cancer.* 1996;77(6):1115-1121.

148. Maxwell GL, Tian C, Risinger J, et al. Racial disparity in survival among patients with advanced/recurrent endometrial adenocarcinoma: a Gynecologic Oncology Group study. *Cancer.* 2006;107(9):2197-2205.

149. Wilson TO, Podratz KC, Gaffey TA, Malkasian GD Jr, O'Brien PC, Naessens JM. Evaluation of unfavorable histologic subtypes in endometrial adenocarcinoma. *Am J Obstet Gynecol.* 1990;162(2):418-423; discussion 423-416.

150. Slomovitz B, Coleman RL, Soliman PT, et al. Is there a survival difference between clear cell and serous carcinoma of the endometrium? A stage and age-matched cohort study. *J Clin Oncol.* 2005;23(16S):5081.

151. Narayan K, Rejeki V, Herschtal A, et al. Prognostic significance of several histological features in intermediate and high-risk endometrial cancer patients treated with curative intent using surgery and adjuvant radiotherapy. *J Med Imaging Radiat Oncol.* 2009;53(1):107-113.

152. Gemer O, Arie AB, Levy T, et al. Lymphvascular space involvement compromises the survival of patients with stage I endometrial cancer: results of a multicenter study. *Eur J Surg Oncol.* 2007;33(5):644-647.

153. O'Brien DJ, Flannelly G, Mooney EE, Foley M. Lymphovascular space involvement in early stage well-differentiated endometrial cancer is associated with increased mortality. *BJOG.* 2009;116(7):991-994.

154. Schink JC, Rademaker AW, Miller DS, Lurain JR. Tumor size in endometrial cancer. *Cancer.* 1991;67(11):2791-2794.

155. Tebeu PM, Popowski Y, Verkooijen HM, et al. Positive peritoneal cytology in early-stage endometrial cancer does not influence prognosis. *Br J Cancer.* 2004;91(4):720-724.

156. Song T, Lee JW, Kim HJ, et al. Prognostic significance of DNA ploidy in stage I endometrial cancer. *Gynecol Oncol.* 2011;122(1):79-82.

157. Susini T, Amunni G, Molino C, et al. Ten-year results of a prospective study on the prognostic role of ploidy in endometrial carcinoma: DNA aneuploidy identifies high-risk cases among the so-called 'low-risk' patients with well and moderately differentiated tumors. *Cancer.* 2007;109(5):882-890.

158. Jhang H, Chuang L, Visintainer P, Ramaswamy G. CA 125 levels in the preoperative assessment of advanced-stage uterine cancer. *Am J Obstet Gynecol.* 2003;188(5):1195-1197.

159. Sood AK, Buller RE, Burger RA, Dawson JD, Sorosky JI, Berman M. Value of preoperative CA 125 level in the management of uterine cancer and prediction of clinical outcome. *Obstet Gynecol.* 1997;90(3):441-447.

160. Ayhan A, Taskiran C, Simsek S, Sever A. Does immediate hormone replacement therapy affect the oncologic outcome in endometrial cancer survivors? *Int J Gynecol Cancer.* 2006;16(2):805-808.

161. Barakat RR, Bundy BN, Spirtos NM, Bell J, Mannel RS. Randomized double-blind trial of estrogen replacement therapy versus placebo in stage I or II endometrial cancer: a Gynecologic Oncology Group Study. *J Clin Oncol.* 2006;24(4):587-592.

Uterine Sarcomas

Gary S. Leiserowitz

Sarcomas comprise approximately 3% to 7% of uterine corpus malignancies. Although they represent a small proportion of uterine cancers, they disproportionately contribute to mortality. Their biologic behaviors are highly variable, ranging from a locally invasive process with minimal metastatic risk to highly aggressive tumors that are characterized by intra-abdominal or disseminated hematogenous spread. This reflects the complex origin of the malignant tissue components: endometrium, endometrial stroma, and smooth muscle, plus supportive elements of the uterine corpus.

EPIDEMIOLOGY

Key Points

1. Uterine sarcomas represent only 3% to 7% of all uterine malignancies.
2. The median age for patients with uterine sarcomas is 57 years, but patients with carcinosarcoma are approximately 10 years older.
3. African American women have a higher incidence of both leiomyosarcomas and carcinosarcomas.
4. Carcinosarcomas have been associated with a history of previous pelvic radiation and previous tamoxifen use.

Using Surveillance, Epidemiology, and End Results (SEER) data from the National Cancer Institute from 1988 to 2001, there were 48,642 uterine malignancies, of which 3742 were uterine sarcomas (7.7%).[1] The relative proportions of the 4 major uterine sarcoma categories are noted in Table 7-1.[2] Carcinosarcomas are now considered to be an aggressive, dedifferentiated, or metaplastic form of endometrial cancer, and some authors therefore exclude them from the uterine sarcoma classification list.[3] However, the vast majority of previous clinical studies have included carcinosarcomas with other uterine sarcomas, and that convention is followed in this chapter. The World Health Organization (WHO) classification scheme for uterine sarcomas is noted in Table 7-2,[4] and uterine sarcomas are divided into 2 large pathologic categories: mesenchymal and mixed epithelial and mesenchymal tumors. Table 7-2 includes common and uncommon variants, as well as benign tumors (eg, leiomyomas, adenofibromas), malignant tumors (eg, leiomyosarcomas, carcinosarcomas), and those of uncertain malignant behavior (eg, smooth muscle tumor of uncertain malignant potential [STUMP]).

The median age for patients with uterine sarcomas (excluding carcinosarcoma) is 56.6 years, with a range of 20 to 90 years, based on Cancer Registry data from Norway.[5] The median ages for the various histologies are as follows: leiomyosarcoma, 56.6 years; endometrial stromal sarcoma, 50.7 years; adenosarcomas, 65.7 years; and undifferentiated sarcoma, 58.6 years. Only 41% of women with leiomyosarcoma are postmenopausal.[6] The average age of patients with carcinosarcoma tends to be approximately 10 years older than for other sarcomas, with a mean of 65 years.[7] The incidence of carcinosarcoma increases with age.[8]

The incidence of uterine malignancies (endometrial adenocarcinoma and uterine sarcomas) varies significantly by race.[9] Taken from SEER data, Table 7-3

Table 7-1 Percentage of Histologic Categories of Uterine Sarcomas

Leiomyosarcomas	40
Endometrial stroma sarcomas	10-15
Carcinosarcomas	40
Undifferentiated sarcomas	5-10

Table 7-2 World Health Organization Classification System of Uterine Sarcomas[4]

Mesenchymal Tumors
Endometrial stromal and related tumors
Endometrial stromal sarcoma, low grade
Endometrial stromal nodule
Undifferentiated endometrial stromal sarcoma
Smooth muscle tumors
Leiomyosarcomas
Epithelioid variant
Myxoid variant
Smooth muscle tumor of uncertain malignant potential
Leiomyoma, not otherwise specified
Histologic variants
Mitotically active variant
Cellular variant
Hemorrhagic cellular variant
Epithelioid variant
Myxoid
Atypical variant
Lipoleiomyoma variant
Growth pattern variants
Diffuse leiomyomatosis
Dissecting leiomyoma
Intravenous leiomyomatosis
Metastasizing leiomyoma
Miscellaneous mesenchymal tumors
Mixed endometrial stromal and smooth muscle tumor
Perivascular epithelioid cell tumor
Adenomatoid tumor
Other malignant mesenchymal tumor
Other benign mesenchymal tumors
Mixed Epithelial and Mesenchymal Tumors
Carcinosarcoma (malignant mullerian mixed tumor, metaplastic carcinoma)
Adenosarcoma
Carcinofibroma
Adenofibroma
Adenomyoma
Atypical polypoid variant

shows that both carcinosarcomas and leiomyosarcomas are quite infrequent as compared with endometrial adenocarcinomas in all ethnicities. Endometrial adenocarcinomas are approximately half as frequent in Hispanics and blacks. Hispanics have approximately the same incidence of leiomyosarcomas, and a slightly decreased incidence of carcinosarcoma, as compared with whites. Blacks have a significantly higher risk of carcinosarcomas and leiomyosarcomas as compared with whites. Brooks also used SEER data and showed that the age-adjusted incidence of uterine sarcomas in blacks was twice that of whites and other races.[8] They found that even with a racial difference in sarcoma incidence, the survivals of white and black women who received comparable treatment were equivalent.

Several factors may increase the risk of uterine sarcomas. Radiation therapy is commonly noted to be associated with development of carcinosarcomas. Up to 37% of carcinosarcoma patients have a precedent history of pelvic radiation.[2,3] The radiation is more frequently administered for a nongynecologic indication (eg, colon cancer) than for a previous gynecologic malignancy. In contrast, previous radiation is rarely reported with leiomyosarcomas. Giuntoli et al[6] reported only 1 of 208 uterine leiomyosarcoma patients who had previous radiation.

Tamoxifen, a selective estrogen receptor modulator, is associated with an increased risk of endometrial cancer because of its agonistic effects on the genital tract, including the uterus. Several case studies also report a higher than expected rate of high-grade uterine cancers, including sarcomas. An early report from the Yale Tumor Registry appeared to show that tamoxifen-associated endometrial cancers behaved more aggressively and had a worse prognosis.[10] Recent case reports also suggested higher rates of uterine carcinosarcoma.[11,12] Barakat[13] performed a literature review of tamoxifen-related uterine malignancies and concluded that the rate of high-risk uterine malignancies, including carcinosarcoma, was not different from that of non–tamoxifen-related cancers. Clinicians should recognize that some patients with tamoxifen-related cancers may be at risk for uterine carcinosarcoma.

DIAGNOSIS

Key Points

1. Common symptoms include abnormal uterine bleeding, vaginal discharge, pelvic mass, abdominal/pelvic pain, and occasionally constitutional symptoms.
2. Endometrial sampling (with or without hysteroscopy) is typically diagnostic, although leiomyosarcomas may be missed.

3. Imaging tests typically demonstrate a uterine mass, either involving the endometrial cavity of uterine wall. Magnetic resonance imaging may distinguish between benign and malignant tumors, but the diagnostic accuracy is limited.

4. Preoperative imaging tests (eg, chest x-ray, computed tomography or positron emission tomography/computed tomography scans) are valuable to identify patients with uterine sarcomas who have distant metastases, which may influence surgical management.

Patients with uterine sarcomas present with various symptoms depending on the location of the sarcoma. When the endometrium is involved (carcinosarcoma or endometrial stromal sarcoma), abnormal uterine bleeding is usually the first symptom. Even leiomyosarcomas cause abnormal bleeding in 40% of patients. Vaginal discharge (watery or mucous) is commonly seen as well. The malignant tumors can fill the endometrial cavity and the polypoid tumor can protrude through the cervix into the vagina. The uterus is often enlarged, resulting in a palpable pelvic mass. Pain is associated with either an enlarged uterine mass or advanced-stage disease. Locally extensive disease can involve the vagina or parametria or invade the bladder or rectum, resulting in symptoms. Parametrial extension can cause ureteral obstruction, leading to hydronephrosis and flank pain. Advanced-stage disease is often accompanied by constitutional symptoms (fatigue, weight loss, anorexia) and/or medical complications such as venous thromboembolism.

The diagnostic evaluation usually follows from the presenting symptoms. Vaginal bleeding from an endometrial tumor is an indication for endometrial sampling either with an endometrial biopsy or with hysteroscopically directed endometrial sampling. An endometrial biopsy is more than 90% sensitive to detect malignancy when it is present (especially because the lesions often fill the uterine cavity), but sampling error can result in a false-negative result. Persistent abnormal uterine bleeding should always be further investigated, and hysteroscopy is quite effective.

Pelvic ultrasounds are commonly used as an initial diagnostic evaluation for uterine bleeding instead of endometrial sampling because it is very reassuring if normal (ie, it has a high negative predictive value). If a mass is detected in the endometrium on ultrasound, then endometrial sampling is the next step. If a mass is noted in the uterine wall, then the differential diagnosis will include a benign leiomyoma versus a leiomyosarcoma. The evaluation of a uterine wall mass can be problematic. Endometrial sampling may not be effective for diagnosis. Ultrasonic criteria to distinguish between a benign or malignant tumor include a diffuse irregular border, invasion, and a mixed echogenicity (indicative of hemorrhage or necrosis). Color flow Doppler may show irregular vessels with low impedance and high systolic velocities.[14] The detection of a rapidly growing uterine mass is considered a classic presentation for a leiomyosarcoma, but the actual risk is very low, and none of 198 such patients had a sarcoma.[15] The incidence of leiomyosarcoma contained within a leiomyoma is less than 1%, although the rate increases with age.[16]

Magnetic resonance imaging (MRI) is well-suited to delineating tissue planes and has some value in distinguishing between benign and malignant masses.[17] In uterine leiomyosarcoma, the tumors have intermediate-signal intensity on T1- and T2-weighted images, with scattered foci of high-signal intensity on T2 weighting. Classically, leiomyosarcomas have an ill-defined irregular margin and intensely enhance after use of gadolinium contrast. Depending on the location within the uterine wall, it can cause distortion of the endometrial cavity. Endometrial stromal sarcomas usually invade the myometrium and are noted to have an irregular border. They have high-signal intensity on T2 weighting and variable signals on T1 weighting. Diffuse infiltration into adjacent tissues such as the parametrium

Table 7-3 Incidence of Malignant Uterine Corpus Tumors by Histopathologic Category, Race, and Ethnicity: SEER Data (1992-1998)

Histology	White Hispanic		Black		White Non-Hispanic	
	Incidence[a]	Rate Ratio[b]	Incidence	Rate Ratio	Incidence	Rate Ratio
Adenocarcinoma	11.39	0.57	9.2	0.46	20.14	Ref.
Serous and clear cell ACA	0.85	0.72	2.16	1.85	1.17	Ref.
Carcinosarcoma	0.63	0.80	1.82	2.33	0.78	Ref.
Leiomyosarcoma	0.80	1.01	1.24	1.56	0.79	Ref.

Adapted from Sherman et al.[9]
ACA, adenocarcinoma; Ref., referent.
[a]Incidence is defined as the rate per 100,000 woman-years, age-adjusted using the 1979 standard population.
[b]Rate ratio is relative to white non-Hispanics.

and fallopian tube walls can be a distinguishing feature and indicates invasion of blood vessels and lymphatics. Contrast enhancement is commonly seen with endometrial stromal sarcomas. They can be confused with leiomyomas, but the latter are notable for well-defined margins. Carcinosarcomas have a mixed-signal intensity, corresponding to areas of necrosis and hemorrhage. Depending on the degree of invasion, there is a loss of the junctional zone between the endometrium and myometrium. Myometrial invasion can be assessed. Carcinosarcomas usually enhance in the early phase and persist in the delayed phase after use of contrast, which is unusual for endometrial cancers.

In patients with a known uterine sarcoma, various imaging tests can be used for preoperative staging, including a chest x-ray, computed tomography (CT) scan of chest/abdomen/pelvis, and even positron emission tomography (PET) scan. A high proportion of sarcoma patients do have advanced-stage disease, but it is unclear whether imaging tests contribute significantly to the clinical management. In a recent study, imaging tests altered therapy in only 9% of patients and had no effect on survival (when compared with histology, stage, and surgical resection).[18] In the patient who appears to have clinical stage I disease, an imaging test that demonstrate metastases can lead the clinician to avoid unnecessary surgical staging (eg, a patient with lung metastases does not benefit from staging lymphadenectomy) and focus the clinician to consider best palliative care instead of curative intent. There does not appear to be any advantage to the use of a PET scan over a CT scan. Other tests such as bone scans and CT scans of the head should be limited to specific circumstances when bone or brain metastases are clinically suspected.

The gynecologist who sees a patient with abnormal uterine bleeding or a symptomatic uterine mass should consider uterine sarcomas in the differential diagnosis, but endometrial carcinoma and benign leiomyomas will be much more common. Simple diagnostic maneuvers such as an endometrial sampling and/or ultrasound will triage the majority of patients into low- and high-risk categories. If a uterine sarcoma is diagnosed, then the patient will be best managed by those with specialized expertise. However, a certain number of sarcoma patients will not be diagnosed until after hysterectomy, because preoperative testing is never completely predictive.

PATHOLOGY

Key Points

1. Uterine sarcomas can be either mesenchymal or mixed epithelial and mesenchymal tumors.

2. Leiomyosarcomas are characterized by a high mitotic index, hypercellularity, nuclear atypia, and coagulative necrosis.

3. Endometrial stromal sarcomas are typically low-grade, indolent tumors with infiltrating tumor borders, a low mitotic count and mild nuclear atypia. They must be distinguished from endometrial stromal nodules, cellular leiomyomas, and undifferentiated endometrial sarcomas.

4. Carcinosarcomas likely represent undifferentiated metaplastic endometrial carcinomas. These metaplastic tumors have both malignant epithelial and mesenchymal components (the latter of which can be homologous or heterologous). The malignant epithelial component is usually responsible for metastases.

5. International Federation of Gynecology and Obstetrics staging was modified in 2009. Carcinosarcomas are staged as endometrial cancers. Leiomyosarcomas, endometrial stromal sarcomas, and adenosarcomas have new staging criteria derived from the knowledge of soft tissue sarcomas.

Uterine sarcomas are named based on their tissue origin (refer to Table 7-2 for the WHO classification system)—either mesenchymal or mixed epithelial and mesenchymal tumors.

They derive from the endometrium, endometrial stroma, and uterine smooth muscle, plus rare variants derived from other supportive tissue elements such as blood vessels. Several of the sarcomas may have extra-uterine sites as the origin for tumors, such as carcinosarcoma from the ovary or pelvic endometriosis or a leiomyosarcoma of the fallopian tube. The pathologic diagnosis may be problematic at times, with several variants having confusing and subtle tumor characteristics that make distinguishing among the entities challenging. In these cases, review of the pathology slides by an expert gynecologic pathologist will be the key to establishing an accurate diagnosis, because the treatment and prognosis can be dramatically different.

Leiomyosarcoma

These are sarcomas derived from the smooth muscle of the uterus. Leiomyosarcomas typically arise de novo and rarely transition from a benign leiomyomas. Grossly, they are large, solitary, fleshy masses that are greater than 10 cm in diameter and are poorly circumscribed.[19] Intratumoral hemorrhage and necrosis are commonly seen. The mass can be confined to the uterine wall or burst into the abdominal cavity associated with hemoperitoneum. Characteristic pathologic features include a mitotic index >15 mitoses/10 high-power field (hpf), hypercellularity, nuclear atypia, and

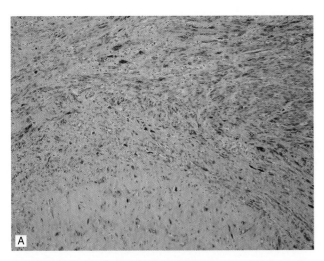 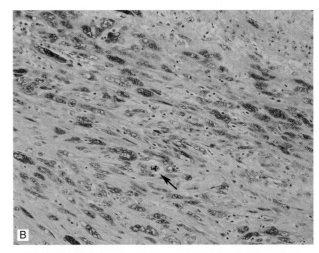

FIGURE 7-1. High-grade leiomyosarcoma. A. There is a sharp demarcation between an area of coagulative necrosis (bottom) and a proliferation of atypical spindle cells (top). ×100 magnification. **B.** Spindle cell proliferation with marked nuclear atypia. An atypical mitotic figure (arrow) is present. ×200 magnification.

coagulative tumor cell necrosis.[3] Examples of a high-grade leiomyosarcoma are seen in Figures 7-1A and 7-1B. The pathologic diagnosis for most leiomyosarcomas is straightforward, because most tumors contain most of these features. There are a number of tumors, though, that do not contain all of these features, and their biologic behavior can be more difficult to predict.[20] Other features that support the diagnosis of leiomyosarcoma include age >51 years, extrauterine disease, tumor size >10 cm, and an infiltrating border.[3] Expression of receptors for estrogen, progesterone, and androgens can be seen in 30% to 40% of leiomyosarcomas, but their presence does not necessarily imply hormonal responsiveness.

Some smooth muscle tumors appear atypical and have some worrisome features; these should be classified as leiomyomas (eg, mitotically active leiomyoma, cellular leiomyoma, leiomyomas with bizarre nuclei; see Table 7-2 for other examples). Smooth muscle tumors of uncertain malignant potential (STUMP) can also be mistaken for leiomyosarcomas. The pathologic criteria for STUMP include (1) tumor cell necrosis in a typical leiomyoma, (2) necrosis of uncertain type with ≥ 10 mitoses/10 hpf or marked diffuse atypia, (3) marked diffuse or focal atypia with borderline mitotic counts, and/or (4) necrosis difficult to classify.[3] These tumors can be mistaken for low-grade leiomyosarcomas, but their behavior is actually bland with few documented recurrences.

The metastatic spread pattern includes local extension, intra-abdominal dissemination, lymphatic, and hematogenous. The lungs are a common source of distant metastases. Lymphatic involvement is variable, ranging from 3.5% to 11%.[6,21] Surgical staging is not considered valuable, because nodal involvement is commonly associated with other extrapelvic metastatic disease[6] and even patients with apparent stage I tumors have a very high relapse rate.

Endometrial Stromal Sarcoma

This is the second most common sarcoma of pure mesenchymal origin, deriving from the endometrial stroma. Endometrial stromal sarcoma is by definition a low-grade malignancy and must be distinguished from an endometrial stromal nodule and an undifferentiated sarcoma (previously referred to as a high-grade endometrial stromal sarcoma). Endometrial stromal sarcoma is an irregularly shaped nodular growth emanating from the endometrium to infiltrate into the myometrium. The mass may include worm-like plugs that may fill the myometrial veins and extend into the broad ligament, pelvic vessels, and even to the right side of the heart.[22] Microscopically, the mitotic count is usually <5 mitoses/hpf, and there is mild nuclear atypia (Figures 7-2A and 7-2B). The cells are round or spindle-shaped and resemble endometrial stroma. There is an infiltrating border of endometrial stromal sarcoma into the myometrium, and vascular invasion is common. Necrosis is unusual.[3] Estrogen receptor (ER) and progesterone receptor (PR) can be identified with immunohistochemistry and may reflect hormonal response to progestational agents.

The pattern of metastatic spread includes local extension, vessel permeation, and nodal spread. Up to 33% of endometrial stromal sarcoma patients have nodal spread. Late recurrences are occasionally seen and are most common in the pelvis and abdomen, but sometimes in the lungs. The indolent nature of endometrial stromal sarcoma, even when recurrent, allows for various salvage treatments, including surgical resection,

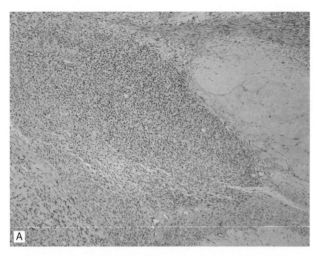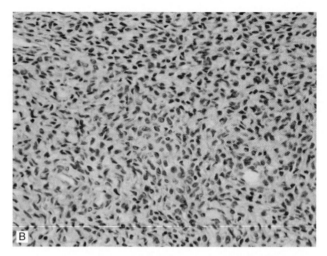

FIGURE 7-2. Endometrial stromal sarcoma. A. Proliferation of endometrial stromal cells. Note the irregular, infiltrating margin. ×100 magnification. **B.** The neoplastic cells resemble endometrial stromal cells with bland, uniform, round to ovoid nuclei and scant cytoplasm. ×200 magnification.

regional radiation, and use of hormonal agents such as progestins or aromatase inhibitors. Endometrial stromal sarcoma can also occur in extrauterine locations in the pelvis (ovary, fallopian tube, parametrium, and retroperitoneum). The distribution may reflect an association with extrauterine endometriosis.[22]

Endometrial Stromal Nodule

This is a rare, benign tumor that superficially resembles endometrial stromal sarcoma. On gross appearance, there is also a tumor mass from the endometrium pushing into the myometrium, with a size ranging from a few centimeters to 22 cm. Endometrial stromal nodules are fleshy and tan-yellow in color. They are circumscribed, but non-encapsulated. Microscopically, they have uniform, small, bland cells that resemble endometrial stromal cells. The distinguishing features of an endometrial stromal nodule are that there are "pushing" borders (instead of infiltrating borders seen with endometrial stromal sarcoma) and no vascular invasion.[23] There may be tongues of tumor extending between muscle fascicles. The diagnosis can be suspected with endometrial curettage, but the distinction between endometrial stromal sarcoma and a stromal nodule is best determined after examining the hysterectomy specimen because the prognosis is quite different between the two. Endometrial stromal nodule can be confused with a cellular leiomyoma, but there are histologic and immunohistochemical differences that will assist with the differential diagnosis.[23]

Undifferentiated Endometrial Sarcoma

These tumors were previously called high-grade endometrial stromal sarcomas, but current classification limits endometrial stromal sarcoma to low-grade tumors.

Undifferentiated endometrial sarcomas are very aggressive malignancies with a high propensity for hematogenous spread, resulting in distant metastases. In contrast to endometrial stromal sarcoma, undifferentiated endometrial sarcoma tumors are often noted to have necrosis and hemorrhage. Microscopically, the cells show marked cellular pleomorphism, nuclear atypia, and a brisk mitotic rate greater than 10 mitoses/10 hpf.[3,23] There is destructive infiltration into the myometrium.

Necrosis is present. Undifferentiated endometrial sarcomas can be confused with some carcinosarcomas, adenosarcomas with sarcomatous overgrowth, or muscle differentiation indicative of a leiomyosarcoma or rhabdomyosarcoma. The differential diagnosis is dependent on extensive tumor sampling and use of immunohistochemistry stains.

The pattern of spread for undifferentiated endometrial sarcomas includes local extension, regional nodal metastases, and distant metastases. In 2 series, 50% to 61% of high-grade endometrial stromal sarcomas were noted to be stage III or IV at presentation in contrast to 23% to 31% for low-grade endometrial stromal sarcoma.[24,25] Involvement of the pelvic and/or para-aortic nodes was noted to range between 12% and 18%.[25,26] Relapse has been documented in the pelvis, abdomen, lymph nodes, and lungs.[24]

Carcinosarcoma

Also known as malignant mixed mullerian tumors (MMMT), carcinosarcomas are biphasic with both malignant epithelial and mesenchymal elements. A number of potential etiologic hypotheses have been proposed for the pathogenesis of carcinosarcomas, including the possibility of a collision tumor, but most authors have now coalesced around the theory that they are metaplastic cancers derived from a monoclonal population of dedifferentiated stem cells.[27] The biologic aggressiveness is driven largely by the carcinomatous component. The behavior and pattern of spread is most similar to that of high-grade endometrial adenocarcinoma and therefore is considered with this group of tumors.

Carcinosarcomas are usually bulky, polypoid masses arising from the endometrium and often prolapsing through the cervical os.[3] Necrosis, hemorrhage, and cystic changes are noted when the uterine specimen is cut open. Gross myometrial invasion is typically seen. The tumors can be confined to an endometrial polyp or involve the entire endometrial cavity, with a size ranging up to 20 cm. Microscopically, the carcinomatous component is usually high grade, with two-thirds being serous and one-third being endometrioid, although other histologies such as clear cell can be seen.[28] The mesenchymal elements can be either homologous (usually spindle cell or pleomorphic, but occasionally leiomyosarcoma) or heterologous (including rhabdomyosarcoma, chondrosarcoma, and osteosarcoma). See Figures 7-3A and 7-3B.

Metastatic spread to the pelvic and para-aortic lymph nodes is the predominant pattern, occurring in 32% of surgically staged patients in one series.[29] Other sites include ovaries, fallopian tubes, omentum, and other intra-abdominal organs.[30] This pattern of spread is similar to what is seen with high-grade endometrial cancers, although with a higher frequency. The risk of metastasis is related to depth of myometrial invasion, but even if the tumor appears confined to an endometrial polyp, there is still significant risk. The metastatic component is usually epithelial, although sarcomatous and mixed components are also seen.[3,22] In a study from MD Anderson Cancer Center, recurrences were noted in 56% of carcinosarcomas seen from 1955 to 1981. The pattern of relapse was locoregional alone (pelvis and vagina) in 10% and distant (abdomen, lungs, supraclavicular nodes) in 49%. The distant recurrences were responsive for 84% of first recurrences and likely reflects that almost all patients received adjuvant whole-pelvic radiation therapy.[31]

Adenosarcoma

This is an unusual tumor of mixed epithelial and mesenchymal histologies. In contrast to carcinosarcomas, adenosarcomas are usually low-grade, indolent tumors. The tumor mass usually emanates from the uterine cavity, but the cervix can also be the origin.[23] A polypoid lesion often fills the cavity and protrudes through the cervix. The tumor margin is usually clear. On microscopic examination, a benign gland is associated with a low-grade sarcomatous element that is typically of the endometrial stromal type. Modest mitotic activity and mild to moderate nuclear atypia are present.[3] The sarcoma is typically homologous, but can be heterologous in uncommon cases. A high percentage of cases express both ER and PR positivity. Adenosarcomas usually act in an indolent fashion and remain confined to the uterine corpus. Relapses can be seen in the vagina, pelvis, and abdomen and can be late occurrences.

An unusual variant is adenosarcomas with sarcomatous overgrowth. In contrast to adenosarcomas, the sarcoma is high grade, and the tumor behavior is aggressive. In a retrospective case series, adenosarcomas with sarcomatous overgrowth were noted to have a higher risk of metastasis to the regional lymph nodes and worse prognosis even when compared with carcinosarcomas from the same period.[32]

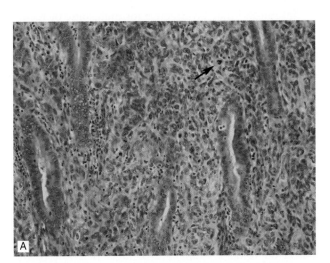
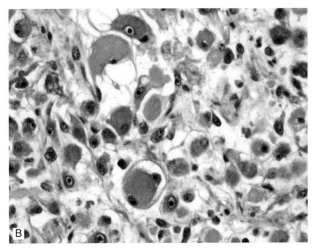

FIGURE 7-3. Carcinosarcoma (malignant mixed mullerian tumor). A. Malignant glands and stroma. Note the stromal mitotic figure (arrow). ×200 magnification. **B.** Heterologous elements are present; malignant cells with abundant eosinophilic cytoplasm show rhabdoid differentiation. ×400 magnification.

FIGO Staging

FIGO made changes in the staging system of uterine sarcomas in 2009. New staging systems were developed for leiomyosarcomas and endometrial stromal sarcomas with adenosarcomas (Table 7-4).[33] Because

Table 7-4   Staging for Uterine Sarcomas (Leiomyosarcomas, Endometrial Stromal Sarcomas, Adenosarcomas, and Carcinosarcomas)[33]

Stage		Definition
Leiomyosarcomas and endometrial stromal sarcomas		
I		Tumor limited to uterus
	IA	<5 cm
	IB	>5 cm
II		Tumor extends to the pelvis
	IIA	Adnexal involvement
	IIB	Tumor extends to extrauterine pelvic tissue
III		Tumor invades abdominal tissues (not just protruding into the abdomen)
	IIIA	1 site
	IIIB	>1 site
	IIIC	Metastatic to pelvic and/or para-aortic lymph nodes
IV	IVA	Tumor invades bladder and/or rectum
	IVB	Distant metastases
Adenosarcomas		
I		Tumor limited to uterus
	IA	Tumor limited to endometrium/endocervix with no myometrial invasion
	IB	≤ Half myometrial invasion
	IC	> Half myometrial invasion
II		Tumor extends beyond the uterus, within the pelvis
	IIA	Adnexal involvement
	IIB	Tumor extends to extrauterine pelvic tissue
III		Tumor invades abdominal tissues (not just protruding into the abdomen)
	IIIA	1 site
	IIIB	> 1 site
	IIIC	Metastatic to pelvic and/or para-aortic lymph nodes
IV	IVA	Tumor invades bladder and/or rectum
	IVB	Distant metastases
Carcinosarcomas		
Carcinosarcomas should be staged as carcinomas of the endometrium.		

Note. Simultaneous tumor of the uterine corpus and ovary/pelvis in association with ovarian/pelvic endometriosis should be classified as independent primary tumors.

carcinosarcoma are considered to be an aggressive form of endometrial cancer, the staging classification is the same [refer to FIGO staging system in Chapter 6]. FIGO noted that the behavior of the uterine sarcomas, other than CS, is qualitatively different from that of endometrial cancer. Somewhat arbitrarily, it was decided that the staging system for soft tissue sarcomas was a better model for these entities, and therefore further refinements in the current system will await the collection of further data. The American Joint Commission on Cancer (AJCC), which uses the TNM system, has adopted the FIGO 2009 modifications in its most recent edition, which maintains concurrence between the two.

TREATMENT

Key Points

1. Standard primary surgical treatment for most uterine sarcomas includes a total hysterectomy and bilateral salpingo-oophorectomy. Surgical staging of the pelvic and para-aortic nodes may be helpful for carcinosarcomas and has less or uncertain value when managing the other uterine sarcoma types. Aggressive tumor debulking may be valuable when there is extrauterine spread.
2. Chemotherapy provides a high response rate in patients of advanced-stage uterine sarcomas, but duration of response is often limited.
3. Most uterine sarcomas are radiosensitive, and therefore, whole pelvic radiation improves pelvic control in the majority of patients. However, improved pelvic regional control does not usually improve overall survival.
4. Hormonal therapies (eg, progestins and aromatase inhibitors) may be effective for metastatic or recurrent uterine sarcomas that express ER and PR (eg, low-grade endometrial stromal sarcomas).

The treatment plans for the various uterine sarcomas are often mired in controversy because (1) these are rare tumors with limited clinical data; (2) the classification of the tumor types has been inconsistent, confusing, and/or lumped together, making assessments of therapeutic response challenging; (3) several of the malignancies are highly aggressive, and many current therapies are ineffective; and (4) there have been few randomized controlled clinical trials, so most of the therapeutic information is derived from case series. The best treatment plans are based on understanding the biologic behavior of the malignancy, the typical pattern of spread and/or relapse, a determination of therapeutic intent (eg, curative, adjuvant, palliative), and assessment of therapeutic efficacy

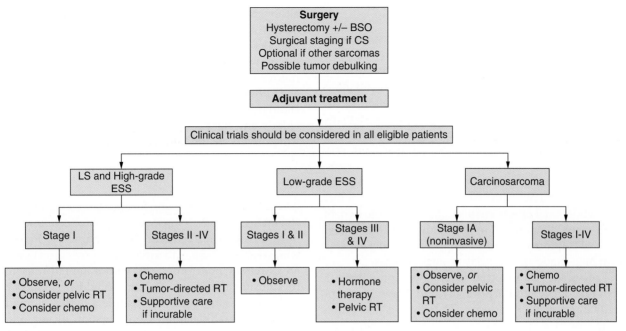

FIGURE 7-4. Treatment summary by stage. Please see the Treatment section for details. Clinical trials should be considered for all patients, when available. Supportive care should be considered for advanced or recurrent disease that is incurable. BSO, bilateral salpingo-oophorectomy; chemo, chemotherapy; CS, carcinosarcoma; ESS, endometrial stromal sarcoma; LS, leiomyosarcoma; RT, radiation therapy. (Adapted from National Comprehensive Cancer Network Guidelines, 2010).[34]

versus treatment toxicity. Assessment of the cancer stage is important to make rational decisions about treatment options. Multimodality treatments are common for uterine sarcomas, but an honest appraisal of benefits and risks should be discussed with the patient and her family when aggressive therapies are offered. A summary of treatment options is noted in Figure 7-4 and includes many aspects from the uterine sarcoma practice guidelines from the National Comprehensive Cancer Network.[34]

Surgery

Primary surgery has several important goals, including primary treatment of the malignancy, surgical staging, and relief of symptoms (eg, uterine bleeding, pelvic pain, bowel obstruction). The components for surgical treatment of uterine sarcomas generally include (1) total hysterectomy, (2) bilateral salpingo-oophorectomy, (3) staging of the pelvic and para-aortic lymph nodes, and (4) cytoreduction of intra-abdominal disease. The therapeutic intent should be thoroughly considered before the patient goes to the operating room, because operations on patients with advanced-stage uterine sarcoma can be fraught with a high risk of morbidity (and occasionally perioperative death). When advanced-stage disease is suspected before surgery, then preoperative imaging is valuable to help with decision making about

the roles of surgical staging, tumor debulking, and symptom relief.

Leiomyosarcoma

Evidence supports a hysterectomy, with or without oophorectomy, and possible cytoreduction to no gross residual disease. There is no evidence that lymphadenectomy is beneficial. Fewer than 50% of patients with leiomyosarcoma have a preoperative biopsy showing leiomyosarcoma, which means that the pathologic diagnosis is usually made after hysterectomy. Lymph node metastases occur infrequently (3.5%-11%)[6,21,35] and usually in the setting of other extrauterine disease.[6,35] Identification of lymph node metastases probably has only prognostic value, because survival with positive nodes is rare, even with adjuvant treatment. Also, lymphadenectomy by itself does not appear to affect survival.[35] Consequently, surgical staging, either at the time of hysterectomy or after hysterectomy, is not justified. There may be some survival advantages to tumor debulking at the time of primary surgery, but only if all gross tumor is resected.[36] Attempts at aggressive cytoreduction should be balanced with the understanding that the morbidity can be high, and current adjuvant chemotherapy has limited efficacy. In rare circumstances with a long disease-free interval, complete resection of recurrent leiomyosarcoma may be beneficial.[37]

Endometrial Stromal Sarcoma

Standard recommendations include a hysterectomy and possibly bilateral salpingo-oophorectomy. Although one-third of endometrial stromal sarcoma patients may have nodal metastases, the value of surgical staging is unclear because the pattern of relapse is often in the abdomen or lungs.[38] Patients who have systematic lymphadenectomy do not experience recurrence in the retroperitoneal nodes,[39] suggesting that there may be benefit to debulking enlarged nodes. Nonetheless, lymphadenectomy itself does not appear to improve survival.[26] Patients with extrauterine disease, whether intra-abdominal or retroperitoneal, do appear to benefit from cytoreduction.[14,39] In the study by Leath et al,[25] optimal cytoreduction appeared to benefit only patients with high-grade endometrial stromal sarcoma.

Low-grade endometrial stromal sarcoma have a high rate of ER and PR positivity, and relapses are typically hormonally responsive. Therefore, conservation of the ovaries is controversial. Still, recurrence and survival are not adversely affected when the ovaries are left in situ,[26,38,40,41] which suggests that ovarian conservation is a reasonable option in young, premenopausal women.

Endometrial Stromal Nodules

Endometrial stromal nodules are best treated by hysterectomy, primarily to endometrial stromal sarcomas, because the final pathologic diagnosis is based on thorough sectioning of the uterine specimen. Because these are not malignancies, neither an oophorectomy nor lymphadenectomy contribute to surgical treatment. In rare cases, where the stromal nodule is diagnosed by endometrial curettings and the tumor is well-defined on a pelvic MRI, then hysterotomy with resection to clear margins would be a consideration for a fertility-sparing procedure.

Carcinosarcoma

Because these are considered a high-grade, metaplastic, biphasic endometrial cancer, then the surgical treatment paradigm is parallel to what is recommended for high-grade endometrial cancers. This includes a hysterectomy, bilateral salpingo-oophorectomy, and staging of pelvic and para-aortic lymph nodes. Surgical staging clearly results in upstaging of patients with clinical stage I and II disease because the risk of nodal involvement is approximately 35%. There is some evidence suggesting that lymphadenectomy improves survival in early-stage carcinosarcoma.[29,42,43] There is limited circumstantial evidence that optimal cytoreduction of intra-abdominal disease is beneficial,[44,45] although it is sometimes performed after the same paradigm of ovarian cancer treatment. A major factor that impedes demonstrating the value of aggressive cytoreduction is the limited response rate to adjuvant chemotherapy and/or radiation therapy. Enthusiasm for aggressive surgery should be tempered with the understanding that many patients with carcinosarcoma are elderly and have a compromised performance status, which limits treatment tolerability.

Adenosarcoma

These tumors act in a similar manner to endometrial stromal sarcomas. Consequently, the recommendations for surgical treatment are comparable.[14] Patients with adenosarcoma with sarcomatous overgrowth have an extremely poor prognosis, with a limited response to adjuvant treatment. Surgery should be guided by symptom relief and should include a hysterectomy to control vaginal bleeding. Consideration of any other surgical maneuvers should be tempered, weighing the limited benefits against potential morbidity.

Chemotherapy

There are a limited number of clinical trials available to assess the efficacy of chemotherapy for uterine sarcomas. Problems in interpreting these data result from a paucity of phase 3 comparative studies, failure to separate the different uterine sarcoma types, use of chemotherapy in patients who have also received radiation therapy, and limited numbers of trial participants. There are 3 indications for use of chemotherapy in the treatment of uterine sarcomas: as adjuvant treatment (after surgery), after recurrence, and for palliation. The majority of the data comes from studies of advanced-stage and recurrent disease, so evidence is lacking that demonstrates the efficacy of adjuvant use in early-stage disease to prevent recurrence. Because the risk of recurrence with leiomyosarcoma, carcinosarcoma, and undifferentiated endometrial stromal sarcoma is at least 50%, even with stage I disease, clinicians may feel compelled to offer adjuvant chemotherapy even in the absence of documented efficacy.

Early clinical trials of chemotherapy did not separate out the different uterine sarcoma categories. One classic study randomized patients with uterine sarcomas (leiomyosarcoma and carcinosarcoma) to use of doxorubicin versus placebo in stages I and II disease.[46] Radiation therapy was given in a nonrandomized fashion. Overall progression-free survival and overall survival were not improved when the groups were combined. Recurrences appeared to be less frequent in the leiomyosarcoma patients who received doxorubicin versus no chemotherapy (44% vs. 61%), but no statistical evaluation was done. Use of radiation therapy did not improve survival, but there were fewer vaginal recurrences in carcinosarcoma patients who received radiation, suggesting some local benefit.

Leiomyosarcoma

Responses to various single and combination chemotherapeutic agents for advanced-stage and recurrent leiomyosarcoma are limited and primarily used for palliation. The response rates (complete plus partial) for the following single agents appear to be the best: doxorubicin (25%),[47] ifosfamide (17%),[48] paclitaxel (9%),[49] gemcitabine (20.5%),[50] and liposomal doxorubicin (16.1%).[51] The current best combination chemotherapy for leiomyosarcoma is gemcitabine and docetaxel. In a phase II Gynecologic Oncology Group (GOG) study evaluating its use as a second-line therapy, gemcitabine and docetaxel provided a 27% response rate; an additional 50% of patients had stable disease.[52] Median survival was greater than 5.6 months. In another phase II GOG study, this time using gemcitabine and docetaxel as first-line agents, the overall response rate was 35.8%, and another 26.2% of patients had stable disease. Median progression-free survival was 4.4 months, and overall survival was greater than 16 months. In both studies, myelosuppression was the most common toxicity, and the rate of grade 3 or 4 toxicity was moderate, with good tolerability. Other chemotherapy combinations show less activity and/or are more toxic.[14]

There are no separate studies that have tested the efficacy of adjuvant chemotherapy for early-stage leiomyosarcoma. The study by Omura, noted earlier, suggested that recurrences were decreased in leiomyosarcoma after adjuvant doxorubicin, but no separate survival data were available.[46] Use of hormonal agents for low-grade leiomyosarcomas that are ER/PR positive is anecdotal and suggests some effectiveness. Several ongoing clinical trials are using targeted agents, such as trabectedin. One anti-angiogenesis agent, sunitinib, has been tested in advanced, recurrent leiomyosarcoma, but was found to be ineffective.[53] A current phase III trial (GOG-250) is investigating whether bevacizumab (an anti-angiogenesis agent) with the current standard of docetaxel and gemcitabine adds additional benefit.

Carcinosarcoma

Response rates to single-agent chemotherapy for advanced-stage and recurrent carcinosarcoma are better than for leiomyosarcomas. The best ones include cisplatin (19%-42%),[54,55] doxorubicin (19%),[56] ifosfamide (18%-36%),[57,58] and paclitaxel (18%).[59] Combination chemotherapy regimens have been shown to have higher response

rates in 2 phase 3 GOG trials. Cisplatin plus ifosfamide was better than ifosfamide alone (response rates, 54% vs. 36%), with improved progression-free survival (6 vs. 4 months), but overall survival was not statistically different.[57] Another combination, ifosfamide plus paclitaxel, was compared with ifosfamide alone in advanced and recurrent carcinosarcoma in a phase 3 trial (GOG-161).[60] The response rates favored the ifosfamide combination (45% vs. 29%). The progression-free survival and overall survival were both statistically better in the combination arm (5.8 vs. 3.6 and 13.5 vs. 8.4 months, respectively). The hazard of death was decreased 31% by the combination arm. The authors noted that the toxicities were predictable and manageable. Thus the GOG considered the combination of ifosfamide and paclitaxel to be the new standard treatment.

Several studies have recently evaluated carboplatin plus paclitaxel for treatment of advanced and recurrent carcinosarcoma. Hoskins et al[61] reported that carboplatin plus paclitaxel showed a response rate of 60% for adjuvant treatment and 55% for recurrent carcinosarcoma, with minimal toxicity. The progression-free survival durations were 16 and 12 months, respectively. A recently reported study, GOG-232, was a phase 2 study of carboplatin and paclitaxel in patients with advanced, persistent, or recurrent carcinosarcoma.[62] The response rate was 54% (13% complete responses, 41% partial responses), and 24% of patients had stable disease. The progression-free survival was 7.6 months, and overall survival was 14.7 months. Toxicity was very manageable, and 59% of patients completed ≥6 cycles, with no deaths attributable to chemotherapy. These results compare very favorably with ifosfamide and paclitaxel. Consequently, GOG has initiated another phase 3 trial to compare ifosfamide plus paclitaxel with carboplatin plus paclitaxel to assess survival and toxicity in carcinosarcoma.

Endometrial Stromal Sarcoma

Adjuvant treatment of endometrial stromal sarcoma is dependent on whether it is low grade or high grade (also known as undifferentiated endometrial sarcoma). Because low-grade endometrial stromal sarcoma often expresses ER and PR, the recommended initial treatment is hormonal.[38] Choices include either a progestational agent such as megestrol or aromatase inhibitors. There are limited data supporting this recommendation, which is based largely on retrospective case series. In a review of uterine sarcomas, Amant et al[14] noted that the reports on endometrial stromal sarcoma showed an overall response rate of 76% for progestational agents and that letrozole (an aromatase inhibitor) provided an 88% response rate. Undifferentiated endometrial sarcoma is typically not responsive to hormones. Some studies suggest that doxorubicin and ifosfamide are active agents with advanced and recurrent endometrial stromal sarcoma.[63,64] A recommended chemotherapy combination is ifosfamide and doxorubicin.[14]

Adenosarcoma

Adenosarcomas typically have a low-grade stromal sarcoma in association with benign epithelium. Their behavior is similar to that endometrial stromal sarcoma, and so the paradigm for treatment is similar. Interestingly, adenosarcomas have a high rate of ER and PR positivity (90% in one immunohistochemistry study).[65] Thus hormonal treatment of advanced and recurrent adenosarcomas should be considered. However, patients with adenosarcoma with sarcomatous overgrowth have far more aggressive disease that is unlikely to respond to hormonal manipulation. Two case reports noted an excellent response to liposomal doxorubicin,[66,67] and in one case, the tumor apparently did not respond to ifosfamide and cisplatin.

Radiation Therapy

Radiation therapy is most commonly used as adjuvant therapy after surgery for uterine sarcomas. There are limited cases in which radiation is used for palliation of local problematic recurrences or as primary therapy when surgery is deemed undesirable (eg, to control bleeding in a patient either with extensive locoregional spread into the pelvis or vagina or a patient with stage IV disease). Uterine sarcomas are radiosensitive as a group, and so radiation therapy is a valuable (and probably underused) tool for palliation of symptoms due to pain or bleeding. However, for the remainder of this discussion, we will limit consideration only to use of adjuvant radiation therapy.

The literature evaluating the efficacy of radiation therapy in the treatment of uterine sarcomas is difficult to interpret. In many cases, radiation therapy is not given alone, but rather is combined with chemotherapy, making it challenging to separate out the relative benefits of this modality. Similar to chemotherapy, studies have commonly combined the results of several categories of uterine sarcomas, so that the responses of the specific sarcoma types are hard to gauge. The vast majority of the studies are retrospective case series, and the limited number of cases diminishes the statistical power to find a difference in benefit. Nonetheless, there are several larger studies from which conclusions can be drawn.

Radiation is a locoregional treatment modality, meaning that cancer control is expected only within the radiation field. Those malignancies that have a significant risk of distant metastases (ie, hematogenous spread) would be unlikely to have an overall benefit with adjuvant radiation. The literature on use of adjuvant radiation therapy for uterine sarcomas consistently reflects this concept. Most studies fail to show an improvement in overall survival when adjuvant radiation is used alone. Studies that do show an improvement in pelvic control and overall survival are an exception.[68,69]

The largest phase 3 randomized controlled trial of adjuvant pelvic radiation versus no further treatment after surgery for stage I or II uterine sarcomas was completed by the European Organisation for Research and Treatment of Cancer.[70] Thirteen years were required to accrue 224 patients, with 219 evaluable patients. Uterine sarcoma subtypes were included, with data on 99 leiomyosarcoma, 92 carcinosarcoma, and 30 endometrial stromal sarcoma patients. Neither disease-free nor overall survival was improved by use of adjuvant radiation. Locoregional control was improved for patients with carcinosarcoma, but not for patients with leiomyosarcoma.

Sampath reported on a nonrandomized, retrospective population-based study of 3650 uterine sarcoma patients, derived from 130 hospital tumor registries in the United States.[71] They evaluated the use of adjuvant radiation using external-beam whole-pelvis radiation (with or without vaginal vault brachytherapy) after surgical treatment for uterine sarcomas. Uterine sarcoma subtypes were separated by type: 1877 carcinosarcomas, 920 leiomyosarcomas, 544 endometrial stromal sarcomas, 130 adenosarcomas, and 179 others. Some patients received chemotherapy, but the report did not note how many received it adjuvantly or for recurrences. Overall survival was not improved with use of radiation or chemotherapy. However, locoregional control was clearly improved for all uterine sarcomas (compared with no adjuvant radiation), and benefit was seen for carcinosarcoma, leiomyosarcoma, and endometrial stromal sarcoma. The benefit was even seen in sarcoma patients with negative lymph nodes (96% vs. 88%).

Several notable earlier GOG studies have also shown decreased rates of pelvic failures associated with adjuvant radiation to the pelvis.[21,46,72] Thus adjuvant radiation does appear to provide improved locoregional control. The benefits of this are difficult to gauge, because recurrences are common outside of the radiation field, and overall survival is not improved.

The issue of multimodality therapy (adjuvant radiation plus chemotherapy) remains unsettled, especially for carcinosarcoma, where there seems to be more support. GOG-150 compared whole abdominal radiation (with a pelvic boost) versus 3 cycles of ifosfamide and cisplatin in patients with stages I to IV carcinosarcoma who were optimally debulked to less than 1 cm.[73] Overall survival was better in the chemotherapy group, but the rate of vaginal failures was higher compared with the radiation therapy group. This suggests that adding radiation to chemotherapy might provide overall benefit. Menczer et al[74] evaluated the outcomes of 49 carcinosarcoma patients who were treated at 3 different hospitals where adjuvant treatment preferences varied (chemotherapy alone, whole pelvic radiation therapy alone, or sequential chemotherapy followed by whole pelvic radiation). This nonrandomized case series found that sequential therapy had superior 5-year survival as compared with chemotherapy alone (75% vs. 22%; $P < .05$), but was not statistically significant when compared with whole pelvic radiation (75% vs. 50.5%; $P = .4$). Cox proportion hazard modeling for survival favored sequential treatment versus either chemotherapy or radiation. A study from the Mayo Clinic reviewed their retrospective experience with 121 patients with stages I to IV carcinosarcoma and compared cancer characteristics and several treatment strategies (surgery alone, chemotherapy alone, pelvic radiation therapy alone, and combined adjuvant radiation and chemotherapy).[75] They found that pelvic adjuvant radiation alone decreased the risk of vaginal recurrences, but had no effect on survival. However, both disease-free and disease-specific survivals were improved with multimodality treatment; however, the number of patients receiving both was small. In combination, these studies suggest that patients with optimally debulked carcinosarcoma may derive the most benefit from combined adjuvant chemotherapy and radiation, although the evidence is very limited.

SURVIVAL AND PROGNOSIS

Key Points

1. Tumor type and stage are the most important prognostic factors in uterine sarcomas.
2. The recurrence rate is greater than 50% in patients with high-grade, stage I uterine sarcomas, making long-term survival very challenging.

Survival in uterine sarcoma patients is highly dependent on the tumor type, and then stage. As noted previously, the various uterine sarcomas have biologic behaviors that range from indolent to highly aggressive with poor survival, even when the tumor is stage I. Figure 7-5 shows the crude survivals of patients with uterine sarcomas (with carcinosarcomas excluded) based on a Norwegian Cancer Registry from 1970 through 2000, which is highly accurate as all cancer cases are reportable by law.[5] Similar data are available in the United States from SEER data from 1988 through 2001 and is stratified by AJCC stage as well as tumor type (carcinosarcoma and mullerian mixed

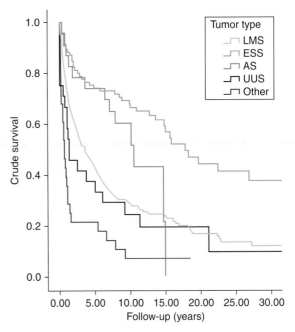

FIGURE 7-5. Crude survival by type of uterine sarcoma. AS, adenosarcoma; ESS, endometrial stromal sarcoma; LMS, leiomyosarcoma; UUS, undifferentiated endometrial or uterine sarcoma. (Reproduced with permission from Abeler et al.[5])

tumors were reported separately; Figure 7-6 and Table 7-5).[1]

The prognostic factors, other than tumor type and stage, are noted in Table 7-6. Not all studies confirm all of the prognostic factors, so various sources are cited.

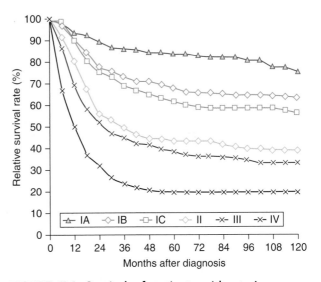

FIGURE 7-6. Survival of patients with uterine sarcomas by American Joint Committee on Cancer stage. Age >20 years, 1988-2001. (Reproduced with permission from Korsary.[1])

Table 7-5 Number, Distribution of Cases, and 5-year Relative Survival Rate by Tumor Types, AJCC Stage, Ages >20 Years, SEER Data, 1988-2001

Histology	AJCC Stage											
	Total		I		II		III		IV		Unknown/Unstaged	
	Cases	5-Year Relative Survival Rate(%)	Cases	5-Year Relative Survival Rate(%)	Cases	5-Year Relative Survival Rate(%)	Cases	5-Year Relative Survival Rate(%)	Cases	5-Year Relative Survival Rate(%)	Cases	5-Year Relative Survival Rate(%)
Total	3742	53.3	2081	70.8	277	43.6	394	38.8	828	19.8	162	39.7
Leiomyosarcoma	939	48.2	623	60.0	28	35.1	64	27.7	185	14.9	39	51.6
Carcinosarcoma[a]	706	53.7	401	73.7	62	43.3	97	26.2	122	13.6	24	~
Endometrial Stromal	610	74.6	372	89.8	27	40.0	85	64.3	106	37.0	20	~
Mullerian[a]	1264	45.3	570	66.7	147	45.7	132	34.8	353	18.2	62	19.4
All other	223	53.6	115	74.3	13	~	16	~	62	21.4	17	~

Adopted from Korsary.[1]
~, Statistic not displayed because there were fewer than 25 cases.
[a]Although carcinosarcoma and mullerian mixed tumors are probably interchangeable terms, they were reported separately in SEER data.

Table 7-6 Adverse Prognostic Factors Associated With Uterine Sarcomas (Other Than Stage)

Tumor Type	Prognostic Factors
Leiomyosarcoma	Tumor size, mitotic index, grade, age, race[5,6,21,35]
Endometrial stromal sarcoma	Mitotic index, tumor cell necrosis, grade[5,24,76]
Carcinosarcoma	Tumor size, grade, type (heterologous worse), nodal metastasis, adnexal involvement, age[21,45,76]
Adenosarcoma	Tumor cell necrosis, deep myometrial invasion, sarcomatous overgrowth[5,32,77]

MANAGEMENT OF RECURRENT DISEASE

Key Points

1. Surveillance for patients with uterine sarcomas is comparable to that of patients with endometrial cancer and includes symptom history, examination, and consideration for serial imaging tests. The efficacy of surveillance is limited by the relatively poor response to salvage therapies, except for patients who have low-grade tumors.
2. Because most patients with recurrent uterine sarcoma have a limited-duration response to salvage treatment, palliation of symptoms is the primary therapeutic goal in most patients.
3. Some patients with low-grade, indolent sarcomas (eg, endometrial stromal sarcomas) can be successfully treated with salvage therapy using a combination of surgery, radiation, and/or hormonal treatments.

Surveillance of patients treated for a uterine sarcoma should follow the same approach as for endometrial cancer. Generally, surveillance includes an interval history, focused physical examination including a pelvic examination, and imaging tests based on symptoms. There is limited value to performing routine imaging tests for surveillance for most asymptomatic patients, although some clinicians recommend annual chest radiographs.

Recurrences are common with all of the uterine sarcomas, with the patterns of relapse noted in the preceding Pathology section. Most recurrences are fatal, unless the patient has an indolent tumor (eg, low-grade endometrial stromal sarcoma). Treatment of recurrent disease is highly dependent on the goals of treatment, the presence of symptoms, and the performance status of the patient. Many of the uterine sarcoma patients are older with a compromised medical status, which limits the options for treatment. In these patients, a frank discussion is appropriate, because responses to chemotherapy are less than 50%, and duration is limited to months. Thus consideration should be given to best supportive care for symptom palliation (which can include targeted radiation therapy) instead of aggressive chemotherapy.

There are several categories of patients who will benefit from treatment of recurrent disease. Patients with a long disease-free interval who experience recurrence with limited-volume disease are the best candidates for aggressive treatment. Classically, these patients have low-grade, indolent sarcomas (eg, endometrial stromal sarcomas). Isolated recurrences, even in the lungs, may be amenable to surgical resection followed by adjuvant treatment including radiation, hormones, and chemotherapy. The majority of patients with recurrent disease are not candidates for repeat surgery, and therefore treatment options include chemotherapy, hormones, and/or radiation. Patients with a good performance status should be offered chemotherapy. Several chemotherapy doublets for carcinosarcoma and leiomyosarcoma are active with very manageable toxicity. The potential agents are listed in the preceding Treatment section by sarcoma type. Patients with recurrent disease should be offered participation in clinical trials.

SPECIAL MANAGEMENT SITUATIONS

Ovarian Conservation

Low-grade leiomyosarcoma often is ER/PR positive (see preceding Pathology section). Therefore, concern has been raised about the deleterious effects of conserving the ovaries when a hysterectomy is done for leiomyosarcoma. Available literature does not show an adverse effect from ovarian conservation.[6,35,36] Also, the risk of ovarian metastases is only approximately 4%, and typically the ovaries are grossly involved.[35] Similarly, ovarian preservation does not appear to adversely affect recurrence or survival in low-grade endometrial stromal sarcoma.[26,40] Consequently, in premenopausal women with leiomyosarcoma or endometrial stromal sarcoma, it is reasonable to conserve normal-appearing ovaries.

Rapidly Enlarging Leiomyomata

It is rare to find leiomyosarcoma in a myomectomy specimen performed as a fertility-sparing procedure.

In their review of 39 studies encompassing 6815 myomectomy patients from 1950 to 1993, Parker et al[15] calculated the risk to be 0.29%. None of their 198 patients with rapidly enlarging fibroids had leiomyosarcoma. Lissoni et al[78] reported on 8 patients who were found to have leiomyosarcoma after a myomectomy who did not have a subsequent hysterectomy. Six of 8 patients had "pushing" tumor borders, and 2 patients had infiltrating borders. None had involvement of the endometrium. Three subsequent pregnancies were reported. One patient was noted to have recurrent leiomyosarcoma in the uterus at the time of cesarean section and later died of disseminated disease. Van Dinh and Woodruff[79] reported on 9 patients found to have leiomyosarcoma associated with a myomectomy. Six patients were managed without hysterectomy, and 1 patient experienced disease recurrence. All appeared to have low-risk leiomyosarcoma (low mitotic count, no necrosis). There were 3 subsequent pregnancies. This suggests that uterine preservation may be an option in young women found to have leiomyosarcoma at myomectomy if given appropriate counseling about their risks.

FUTURE DIRECTIONS

The GOG has coordinated multiple previous cooperative group studies on uterine sarcomas, as noted in the preceding Treatment section. Two phase e studies are ongoing to investigate the best options for leiomyosarcoma and carcinosarcoma. In GOG-250, investigators are evaluating whether the addition of an anti-angiogenesis agent, bevacizumab, to the current standard combination chemotherapy (docetaxel and gemcitabine) improves progression-free survival in patients with recurrent or advanced uterine leiomyosarcoma. GOG-261 is designed to compare the current standard chemotherapy doublet (ifosfamide and paclitaxel, which showed superior results compared with ifosfamide alone in GOG-161[60]) with a commonly used regimen doublet (carboplatin and paclitaxel, which was shown to be effective and well-tolerated in GOG-232B and in a study by Hoskins et al[61]). Both studies will assess the effectiveness and tolerability of the treatment combinations to help clinicians in their choice of chemotherapy for the most common uterine sarcomas.

Investigators are also evaluating the feasibility of molecular targeted agents in the treatment of uterine sarcomas. Leiomyosarcomas express ER and PR in approximately 40% to 80% of patients, especially when tumors are low grade. Objective responses to either progestins or aromatase inhibitors have been noted in case reports. In a retrospective case series, 40 patients with advanced/recurrent leiomyosarcomas were treated with aromatase inhibitors.[80] The 1-year progression-free survival rate was 28% in ER/PR-positive leiomyosarcoma patients, versus 9% for all leiomyosarcoma patients. It is unknown whether the relatively prolonged survival reflected a therapeutic response or simply indolent tumor progression. Other trials using aromatase inhibitors are ongoing.

Use of anti-angiogenesis agents in leiomyosarcomas are also under investigation, examples of which have included thalidomide, sunitinib, and bevacizumab.[53,81,82] The response rates to use of single-agent anti-angiogenesis agents have been limited, despite evidence that the vascular endothelial growth factor pathway activity is associated with poorer outcomes in uterine leiomyosarcoma. The combined use of an anti-angiogenesis agent along with conventional chemotherapy has proven to be more effective than either separately in several other solid tumors, including colon, lung, and breast cancers, and therefore is being tested with other gynecologic cancers such as ovarian cancer. This has been extended to include uterine leiomyosarcoma in GOG-250, as described earlier.

Anti-angiogenesis agents have been investigated in advanced and recurrent endometrial cancer. Bevacizumab has been used as a single agent in recurrent endometrial cancer (GOG-229E) and had 13.5% response rate, and 40.4% of patients were progression-free at 6 months of treatment, suggesting that it acts as a cytostatic agent. Other anti-angiogenesis agents under investigation include: vascular endothelial growth factor-trap, sorafenib, and sunitinib.[83] These agents appear to be candidates to be used in carcinosarcoma as well, given the current belief that carcinosarcoma is a form of poorly differentiated endometrial cancer.

REFERENCES

1. Korsary CL. Chapter 15. Cancer of the Corpus Uteri. In: Ries LAG et al, eds. *SEER Survival Monograph: Cancer Survival Among Adults: US SEER Program, 1988-2001, Patient and Tumor Characteristics.* NIH Pub. No. 07-6215. Bethesda, MD: National Cancer Institute, SEER Program; 2007:123-132.
2. Prat J. FIGO staging for uterine sarcomas. *Int J Gynaecol Obstet.* 2009;104(3):177-118.
3. D'Angelo E, Prat J. Uterine sarcomas: a review. *Gynecol Oncol.* 2010;116(1):131-139.
4. World Health Organization classification of tumours. In: Tavassoli FA, Devilee P, eds. *Pathology and Genetics of Tumours of the Breast and Female Genital Organs.* Lyon, France: IARC Press; 2003.
5. Abeler VM, Royne O, Thoresen S, et al. Uterine sarcomas in Norway. A histopathological and prognostic survey of a total population from 1970 to 2000 including 419 patients. *Histopathology.* 2009;54(3):355-364.
6. Giuntoli RL 2nd, Metzinger DS, DiMarco CS, et al. Retrospective review of 208 patients with leiomyosarcoma of the uterus: prognostic indicators, surgical management, and adjuvant therapy. *Gynecol Oncol.* 2003;89(3):460-469.
7. Doss LL, Llorens AS, Henriquez EM. Carcinosarcoma of the uterus: a 40-year experience from the state of Missouri. *Gynecol Oncol.* 1984;18(1):43-53.

8. Brooks SE, Zhan M, Cote T, et al. Surveillance, epidemiology, and end results analysis of 2677 cases of uterine sarcoma 1989-1999. *Gynecol Oncol.* 2004;93(1):204-208.

9. Sherman ME, Devesa SS. Analysis of racial differences in incidence, survival, and mortality for malignant tumors of the uterine corpus. *Cancer.* 2003;98(1):176-186.

10. Magriples U, Naftolin F, Schwartz PE, et al. High-grade endometrial carcinoma in tamoxifen-treated breast cancer patients. *J Clin Oncol.* 1993; 11(3):485-490.

11. Kloos I, Delaloge S, Pautier P, et al. Tamoxifen-related uterine carcinosarcomas occur under/after prolonged treatment: report of five cases and review of the literature. *Int J Gynecol Cancer.* 2002;12(5):496-500.

12. Bergman L, Beelen MLR, Gallee MPW, et al. Risk and prognosis of endometrial cancer after tamoxifen for breast cancer. Comprehensive Cancer Centres' ALERT Group. Assessment of Liver and Endometrial cancer Risk following Tamoxifen. *Lancet.* 2000;356(9233):881-887.

13. Barakat RR. The effect of tamoxifen on the endometrium. *Oncology (Williston Park).* 1995;9(2):129-134; discussion 139-140, 142.

14. Amant F, Coosemans A, Debiec-Rychter M, et al. Clinical management of uterine sarcomas. *Lancet Oncol.* 2009;10(12): 1188-1198.

15. Parker WH, Fu YS, Berek JS. Uterine sarcoma in patients operated on for presumed leiomyoma and rapidly growing leiomyoma. *Obstet Gynecol.* 1994;83(3):414-418.

16. Leibsohn S, d'Ablaing G, Mishell DR, et al. Leiomyosarcoma in a series of hysterectomies performed for presumed uterine leiomyomas. *Am J Obstet Gynecol.* 1990;162(4):968-974; discussion 974-976.

17. Whitten CR, DeSouza NM. Magnetic resonance imaging of uterine malignancies. *Top Magn Reson Imaging.* 2006;17(6):365-377.

18. Nugent EK, Zighelboim I, Case AS, et al. The value of perioperative imaging in patients with uterine sarcomas. *Gynecol Oncol.* 2009;115(1):37-40.

19. Toledo G, Oliva E. Smooth muscle tumors of the uterus: a practical approach. *Arch Pathol Lab Med.* 2008;132(4):595-605.

20. Bell SW, Kempson RL, Hendrickson MR. Problematic uterine smooth muscle neoplasms. A clinicopathologic study of 213 cases. *Am J Surg Pathol.* 1994;18(6):535-558.

21. Major FJ, Blessing JA, Silverberg SG, et al. Prognostic factors in early-stage uterine sarcoma. A Gynecologic Oncology Group study. *Cancer.* 1993; 71(4 suppl):1702-1709.

22. Brown L. Pathology of uterine malignancies. *Clin Oncol (R Coll Radiol).* 2008;20(6):433-447.

23. Baker P, Oliva E. Endometrial stromal tumours of the uterus: a practical approach using conventional morphology and ancillary techniques. *J Clin Pathol.* 2007;60(3):235-243.

24. Gadducci A, Sartori E, Landoni F, et al. Endometrial stromal sarcoma: analysis of treatment failures and survival. *Gynecol Oncol.* 1996;63(2):247-253.

25. Leath CA 3rd, et al. A multi-institutional review of outcomes of endometrial stromal sarcoma. *Gynecol Oncol.* 2007;105(3):630-634.

26. Chan JK, Kawar NM, Shin JY, et al. Endometrial stromal sarcoma: a population-based analysis. *Br J Cancer.* 2008;99(8): 1210-1215.

27. McCluggage WG. Malignant biphasic uterine tumours: carcinosarcomas or metaplastic carcinomas? *J Clin Pathol.* 2002; 55(5):321-325.

28. D'Angelo E, Spagnoli LG, Prat J. Comparative clinicopathologic and immunohistochemical analysis of uterine sarcomas diagnosed using the World Health Organization classification system. *Hum Pathol.* 2009;40(11):1571-1585.

29. Park JY, Kim DY, Kim JH, et al. The role of pelvic and/or para-aortic lymphadenectomy in surgical management of apparently early carcinosarcoma of uterus. *Ann Surg Oncol.* 2010;17(3): 861-868.

30. Kernochan LE, Garcia RL. Carcinosarcomas (malignant mixed Mullerian tumor) of the uterus: advances in elucidation of biologic and clinical characteristics. *J Natl Compr Canc Netw.* 2009;7(5):550-556; quiz 557.

31. Spanos WJ Jr, Peters LJ, Oswald MJ. Patterns of recurrence in malignant mixed mullerian tumor of the uterus. Cancer. 1986;57(1):155-159.

32. Krivak TC, Seidman JD, McBroom JW, et al. Uterine adenosarcoma with sarcomatous overgrowth versus uterine carcinosarcoma: comparison of treatment and survival. *Gynecol Oncol.* 2001;83(1):89-94.

33. FIGO Committee on Gynecologic Oncology. FIGO staging for uterine sarcomas. *Int J Gynaecol Obstet.* 2009;104:179.

34. National Comprehensive Cancer Network. *NCCN Practice Guidelines in Oncology. Endometrial carcinoma.* 2010. http://www.nccn.org/professionals/physician_gls/f_guidelines.asp. Accessed February 24, 2012.

35. Kapp DS, Shin JY, Chan JK. Prognostic factors and survival in 1396 patients with uterine leiomyosarcomas: emphasis on impact of lymphadenectomy and oophorectomy. *Cancer.* 2008;112(4): 820-830.

36. Dinh TA, Oliva EA, Fuller AF, et al. The treatment of uterine leiomyosarcoma. Results from a 10-year experience (1990-1999) at the Massachusetts General Hospital. *Gynecol Oncol.* 2004;92(2): 648-652.

37. Giuntoli RL 2nd, Metzinger DS, DiMarco CS, et al. Secondary cytoreduction in the management of recurrent uterine leiomyosarcoma. *Gynecol Oncol.* 2007;106(1):82-88.

38. Amant F, De Knijf A, Van Calster B, et al. Clinical study investigating the role of lymphadenectomy, surgical castration and adjuvant hormonal treatment in endometrial stromal sarcoma. *Br J Cancer.* 2007;97(9):1194-1199.

39. Thomas MB, Keeney GL, Podratz KC, et al. Endometrial stromal sarcoma: treatment and patterns of recurrence. *Int J Gynecol Cancer.* 2009;19(2):253-256.

40. Li AJ, Giuntoli RL 2nd, Drake R, et al. Ovarian preservation in stage I low-grade endometrial stromal sarcomas. *Obstet Gynecol.* 2005;106(6):1304-1308.

41. Shah JP, Bryant CS, Kumar S, et al. Lymphadenectomy and ovarian preservation in low-grade endometrial stromal sarcoma. *Obstet Gynecol.* 2008;112(5):1102-1108.

42. Nemani D, Mitra N, Guo M, et al. Assessing the effects of lymphadenectomy and radiation therapy in patients with uterine carcinosarcoma: a SEER analysis. *Gynecol Oncol.* 2008;111(1):82-88.

43. Temkin SM, Hellmann M, Lee YC, et al. Early-stage carcinosarcoma of the uterus: the significance of lymph node count. *Int J Gynecol Cancer.* 2007;17(1):215-219.

44. Arrastia CD, Fruchter RG, Clark M, et al. Uterine carcinosarcomas: incidence and trends in management and survival. *Gynecol Oncol.* 1997;65(1): 158-163.

45. Inthasorn P, Carter J, Valmadre S, et al. Analysis of clinicopathologic factors in malignant mixed Mullerian tumors of the uterine corpus. *Int J Gynecol Cancer.* 2002;12(4):348-353.

46. Omura GA, Blessing JA, Major F, et al. A randomized clinical trial of adjuvant Adriamycin in uterine sarcomas: a Gynecologic Oncology Group Study. *J Clin Oncol.* 1985;3(9):1240-1245.

47. Omura GA, Major FJ, Blessing JA et al. A randomized study of Adriamycin with and without dimethyl triazenoimidazole carboxamide in advanced uterine sarcomas. *Cancer.* 1983;52(4):626-632.

48. Sutton GP, Blessing JA, Barrett RJ, et al. Phase II trial of ifosfamide and mesna in leiomyosarcoma of the uterus: a Gynecologic Oncology Group study. *Am J Obstet Gynecol.* 1992;166(2):556-559.

49. Sutton G, Blessing JA, Ball H. Phase II trial of paclitaxel in leiomyosarcoma of the uterus: a gynecologic oncology group study. *Gynecol Oncol.* 1999;74(3):346-349.

50. Look KY, Sandler A, Blessing JA, et al. Phase II trial of gemcitabine as second-line chemotherapy of uterine leiomyosarcoma: a Gynecologic Oncology Group (GOG) Study. *Gynecol Oncol.* 2004;92(2):644-647.

51. Sutton G, Blessing J, Hanjani P, et al. Phase II evaluation of liposomal doxorubicin (Doxil) in recurrent or advanced leiomyosarcoma of the uterus: a Gynecologic Oncology Group study. *Gynecol Oncol.* 2005;96(3): 749-752.

52. Hensley ML, Blessing J, Mannel R, et al. Fixed-dose rate gemcitabine plus docetaxel as second-line therapy for metastatic uterine leiomyosarcoma: a Gynecologic Oncology Group phase II study. *Gynecol Oncol.* 2008;109(3):323-328.

53. Hensley ML, Sill MW, Scribner DR Jr, et al. Sunitinib malate in the treatment of recurrent or persistent uterine leiomyosarcoma: a Gynecologic Oncology Group phase II study. *Gynecol Oncol.* 2009;115(3):460-465.

54. Gershenson DM, Kavanagh JJ, Copeland LJ, et al. Cisplatin therapy for disseminated mixed mesodermal sarcoma of the uterus. *J Clin Oncol.* 1987;5(4):618-621.

55. Thigpen JT, Blessing JA, Homesley H, et al. Phase II trial of cisplatin as first-line chemotherapy in patients with advanced or recurrent uterine sarcomas: a Gynecologic Oncology Group study. *J Clin Oncol.* 1991;9(11):1962-1966.

56. Muss HB, Bundy B, DiSaia PJ, et al. Treatment of recurrent or advanced uterine sarcoma. A randomized trial of doxorubicin versus doxorubicin and cyclophosphamide (a phase III trial of the Gynecologic Oncology Group). *Cancer.* 1985;55(8):1648-1653.

57. Sutton G, Brunetto VL, Kilgore L, et al. A phase III trial of ifosfamide with or without cisplatin in carcinosarcoma of the uterus: a Gynecologic Oncology Group Study. *Gynecol Oncol.* 2000;79(2):147-153.

58. Sutton GP, Blessing JA, Rosenshein N, et al. A phase II trial of ifosfamide and mesna in patients with advanced or recurrent mixed mesodermal tumors of the ovary previously treated with platinum-based chemotherapy: a Gynecologic Oncology Group study. *Gynecol Oncol.* 1994;53(1):24-26.

59. Curtin JP, Blessing JA, Soper JT, et al. Paclitaxel in the treatment of carcinosarcoma of the uterus: a gynecologic oncology group study. *Gynecol Oncol.* 2001;83(2):268-270.

60. Homesley HD, Filiaci V, Markman M, et al. Phase III trial of ifosfamide with or without paclitaxel in advanced uterine carcinosarcoma: a Gynecologic Oncology Group Study. *J Clin Oncol.* 2007;25(5):526-531.

61. Hoskins PJ, Swenerton KD, Pike JA, et al. Carboplatin plus paclitaxel for advanced or recurrent uterine malignant mixed mullerian tumors. The British Columbia Cancer Agency experience. *Gynecol Oncol.* 2008;108(1):58-62.

62. Powell MA, Filiaci VL, Rose PG, et al. Phase II evaluation of paclitaxel and carboplatin in the treatment of carcinosarcoma of the uterus: a Gynecologic Oncology Group study. *J Clin Oncol.* 2010;28(16):2727-2731.

63. Berchuck A, Rubin SC, Hoskins WJ et al. Treatment of endometrial stromal tumors. *Gynecol Oncol.* 1990;36(1):60-65.

64. Sutton G, Blessing JA, Park R, et al. Ifosfamide treatment of recurrent or metastatic endometrial stromal sarcomas previously unexposed to chemotherapy: a study of the Gynecologic Oncology Group. *Obstet Gynecol.* 1996;87(5 Pt 1):747-750.

65. Amant F, Schurmans K, Steenkiste E, et al. Immunohistochemical determination of estrogen and progesterone receptor positivity in uterine adenosarcoma. *Gynecol Oncol.* 2004;93(3):680-685.

66. del Carmen MG, Lovett D, Goodman A. A case of Mullerian adenosarcoma of the uterus treated with liposomal doxorubicin. *Gynecol Oncol.* 2003;88(3):456-458.

67. Huang GS, Arend RC, Sakaris A, et al. Extragenital adenosarcoma: a case report, review of the literature, and management discussion. *Gynecol Oncol.* 2009;115(3):472-475.

68. Ferrer F, Sabater S, Farrus B, et al. Impact of radiotherapy on local control and survival in uterine sarcomas: a retrospective study from the Grup Oncologic Catala-Occita. *Int J Radiat Oncol Biol Phys.* 1999;44(1):47-52.

69. Smith DC, Macdonald OK, Gaffney DK. The impact of adjuvant radiation therapy on survival in women with uterine carcinosarcoma. *Radiother Oncol.* 2008;88(2):227-232.

70. Reed NS, Mangioni C, Malmstrom H, et al. Phase III randomised study to evaluate the role of adjuvant pelvic radiotherapy in the treatment of uterine sarcomas stages I and II: an European Organisation for Research and Treatment of Cancer Gynaecological Cancer Group Study (protocol 55874). *Eur J Cancer.* 2008;44(6):808-818.

71. Sampath S, Schultheiss TE, Ryu JK, Wong JY. The role of adjuvant radiation in uterine sarcomas. *Int J Radiat Oncol Biol Phys.* 2010;76:728-734.

72. Hornback NB, Omura G, Major FJ. Observations on the use of adjuvant radiation therapy in patients with stage I and II uterine sarcoma. *Int J Radiat Oncol Biol Phys.* 1986;12(12):2127-2130.

73. Wolfson AH, Brady MF, Rocereto T, et al. A Gynecologic Oncology Group randomized phase III trial of whole abdominal irradiation (WAI) vs. cisplatin-ifosfamide and mesna (CIM) as post-surgical therapy in stage I-IV carcinosarcoma (CS) of the uterus. *Gynecol Oncol.* 2007;107(2):177-185.

74. Menczer J, Levy T, Piura B, et al. A comparison between different postoperative treatment modalities of uterine carcinosarcoma. *Gynecol Oncol.* 2005;97(1):166-170.

75. Gonzalez Bosquet J, Terstriep SA, Cliby WA, et al. The impact of multi-modal therapy on survival for uterine carcinosarcomas. *Gynecol Oncol.* 2010; 116(3):419-423.

76. Pautier P, Genestie C, Rey A, et al. Analysis of clinicopathologic prognostic factors for 157 uterine sarcomas and evaluation of a grading score validated for soft tissue sarcoma. *Cancer.* 2000;88(6):1425-1431.

77. McCluggage WG. Mullerian adenosarcoma of the female genital tract. *Adv Anat Pathol.* 2010;17(2):122-129.

78. Lissoni A, Cormio G, Bonazzi C, et al. Fertility-sparing surgery in uterine leiomyosarcoma. *Gynecol Oncol.* 1998;70(3):348-350.

79. Van Dinh T, Woodruff JD. Leiomyosarcoma of the uterus. *Am J Obstet Gynecol.* 1982;144(7):817-823.

80. O'Cearbhaill R, Zhou Q, Iasonos A, et al. Treatment of advanced uterine leiomyosarcoma with aromatase inhibitors. *Gynecol Oncol.* 2010;116(3): 424-429.

81. McMeekin DS, Sill MW, Benbrook D, et al. A phase II trial of thalidomide in patients with refractory leiomyosarcoma of the uterus and correlation with biomarkers of angiogenesis: a Gynecologic Oncology Group study. *Gynecol Oncol.* 2007;106(3):596-603.

82. Wright JD, Viviano D, Powell MA, et al. Bevacizumab therapy in patients with recurrent uterine neoplasms. *Anticancer Res.* 2007;27(5B):3525-3528.

83. Zagouri F, Bozas G, Kafantari E, et al. Endometrial cancer: what is new in adjuvant and molecularly targeted therapy? *Obstet Gynecol Int.* 2010;2010:749579.

8 Gestational Trophoblastic Disease

Diljeet K. Singh

Gestational trophoblastic disease (GTD) represents a spectrum of cellular proliferations arising from the villous trophoblast of the placenta and encompasses 4 clinicopathologic entities: hydatidiform mole (complete and partial), invasive mole, choriocarcinoma (CCA), and placental site trophoblastic tumor (PSTT). The last 3 conditions are associated with more significant clinical sequelae and together comprise the general term *gestational trophoblastic neoplasia* (GTN). In the absence of GTD, a normal pregnancy involves functioning trophoblast that invades the endometrium and recruits a robust vasculature to develop the placenta, which supports intrauterine fetal development. In healthy trophoblastic tissue, these "cancer simulating" behaviors are highly regulated; however, in GTD, normal control mechanisms fail, leading to invasive, vascular tumors with a tendency to metastasize.[1]

Historically, GTD has been associated with significant morbidity and mortality. Hydatidiform moles were typically accompanied by serious bleeding and other medical complications before the development of early detection and effective uterine evacuation in the 1970s. Over the past 50 years, advances in this field have transformed GTN from a high mortality condition to one of the most treatable of all human cancers, with a cure rate exceeding 90%.[2-4] Collaborative global efforts and specialty care centers have promoted the development of highly predictive staging and prognostic scoring systems, which enhance individualization of therapy. Furthermore, several advances in chemotherapy afford ongoing refinement in treatment protocols.[2-6] For women at highest risk of death, the application of multimodal therapy, including chemotherapy, radiation, and surgery, has led to high cure rates while minimizing disease and treatment-related morbidities. In this setting of potentially high cure rates, the onus to identify and appropriately treat GTD falls on the providers entrusted with the primary care of women.

EPIDEMIOLOGY

Key Points

1. The incidence of GTD is approximately 1 per 1000 pregnancies.
2. The most consistently defined risk factors for GTD include extremes of reproductive age and history of prior molar pregnancy. Of all the environmental factors associated with GTD, only low β-carotene and animal fat intake is consistently associated with GTD.
3. Complete hydatidiform molar pregnancy typically results in 1 sperm fertilizing an empty ovum, with subsequent genetic duplication; in contrast, incomplete hydatidiform molar pregnancy typically develops from dispermic fertilization of a normal ovum.

In general, studies conducted in North America, Australia, New Zealand, and Europe indicate the incidence of hydatidiform mole ranges from 0.57 to 1.1 per 1000 pregnancies. In contrast, studies from Southeast Asia and Japan suggest an incidence as high as 2.0 per 1000 pregnancies. As a result of difficulties in obtaining reliable epidemiologic data, it is unclear whether these findings represent a true difference in prevalence or are related to discrepancies between hospital- and population-based data or disparities in the availability of central pathology review.[7] Further complicating the identification of true incidence is the uncommon diagnosis of GTD and the unreliable documentation of early pregnancy loss. Epidemiologic studies do support wide regional variations in the incidence of hydatidiform moles.[7] However, attempts to attribute an increased incidence of hydatidiform mole among American Indians, Eskimos, Hispanics, and African Americans as well as various Asian populations to genetic traits, cultural factors, or differences in reporting have been unsuccessful.[8] Furthermore, some data suggest a decline in the incidence of molar pregnancies, which may be attributed to improved socioeconomic conditions and improvements in diet, which is consistent with studies that show a decreased risk of molar pregnancy with increased consumption of dietary carotene and animal fat.[9,10]

The incidence of CCA and placental-site trophoblastic tumor are even less well known, because these lesions are exceedingly uncommon and because of the difficulty in clinically distinguishing postmolar CCA from invasive mole. In Europe and North America, CCA affects approximately 1 in 40,000 pregnancies, with 1 in 160,000 term pregnancies and 1 in 40 hydatidiform moles. In Southeast Asia and Japan, CCA rates are higher, at 9.2 and 3.3 per 40,000 pregnancies, respectively.[8,11] In the United Kingdom, CCA develops in 1 in 50,000 deliveries, and placental-site trophoblastic tumor accounts for approximately 0.2% of cases of GTD.[12,13] The incidence rates of both hydatidiform mole and CCA have declined over the past 30 years in all populations.[11]

The most consistently documented risk factors for the development of GTD include extremes of reproductive age and history of prior molar pregnancy. Advanced or very young maternal age consistently correlates with higher rates of complete hydatidiform mole. Compared with women aged 21 to 35 years, the risk of complete mole is doubled for those older than 35 years and/or younger than 21 years and is 7.5 times higher for women older than 40 years.[14] A diagnosis of a previous hydatidiform mole confers approximately a 1% risk of repeat molar pregnancy.[15] Although this is 10 times the risk of the general population, most women with history of a molar conception will have normal subsequent pregnancies. If a woman has had more than 2 prior molar pregnancies, the risk for recurrence in latter gestations increases to 15% to 28%, and the risk is not influenced by change of partner.[15-21] Although many possible environmental etiologies for complete mole have been studied, the only consistent association is an inverse relationship between β-carotene and animal fat dietary intake and the incidence of molar pregnancy.[9,10]

Risk factors for CCA include prior complete hydatidiform mole, ethnicity, and advanced maternal age. GTN (invasive mole or CCA) follows a complete molar pregnancy in 15% to 20% of cases.[22-24] CCA is approximately 1000 times more likely after a complete mole than after another pregnancy event. Fewer than 5% of partial moles will develop postmolar GTN; metastases occur rarely, and a histopathologic diagnosis of CCA has never been confirmed after a partial mole.[22,25] The risk of CCA is also increased in women of Asian and American Indian descent and among African Americans. Similar to molar pregnancies, the median age of women with CCA is higher than that for normal pregnancies.[11]

Reproductive factors may play a role in the development of GTD. Women with a history of spontaneous abortion have a 2- to 3-fold increased risk of a molar pregnancy as compared with women without a history of miscarriage.[26] Other studies have suggested that women with menarche after 12 years of age, light menstrual flow, and previous use of oral contraceptives are at increased risk for GTN.[27,28]

Much of the pathogenesis of GTD is well known. In 90% of cases, complete hydatidiform mole occurs when an ovum without maternal chromosomes or with inactive chromosomes is fertilized by 1 sperm that duplicates its DNA, resulting in a 46, XX androgenetic (entirely paternally derived) karyotype.[29] The other 10% of complete moles are 46, XY, or 46, XX, as a result of fertilization of an empty ovum by 2 sperms (dispermy). Although nuclear DNA is entirely paternal, mitochondrial DNA remains maternal in origin.[30] In contrast, partial molar pregnancies demonstrate a triploid karyotype (usually 69, XXY), resulting from the fertilization of an apparently normal ovum by 2 sperms.[22]

Evidence that recurrent molar pregnancies occur even in the setting of different male partners suggests a poorly understood role of maternal factors in the development of molar pregnancy.[31] Some researchers have suggested that ova from older women are more susceptible to abnormal fertilizations than are those from younger women.[1] In addition, there appears to be a relationship between excessive paternal chromosomes and trophoblastic hyperplasia.[24]

DIAGNOSIS

Key Points

1. Classic presenting signs of molar pregnancy include first trimester vaginal bleeding and uterine size greater than expected for gestational dates.

2. Ultrasonography is the imaging modality of choice when GTD is suspected.
3. Markedly elevated human chorionic gonadotropin levels above those of normal pregnancy are a hallmark of hydatidiform moles.

A high index of suspicion on the part of the general obstetrician-gynecologist is essential to the timely diagnosis of GTD and GTN. Clinical features, ultrasound, and serum and urine tests for human chorionic gonadotropin (hCG) aid in the diagnostic process.

In 80% to 90% of cases, complete hydatidiform mole presents with vaginal bleeding, usually at 6 to 16 weeks of gestation (Table 8-1). Other classic clinical signs suggestive of a diagnosis of molar pregnancy include uterine size greater than expected for gestational dates, hyperemesis gravidarum, and pregnancy-induced hypertension. Because the diagnosis of molar disease has shifted earlier in the pregnancy with increasing application of ultrasound technology, these findings are seen much less frequently.[32] To a lesser extent, women with molar disease may also present with pelvic pain due to enlarged theca-lutein cysts and/or clinical signs of hyperthyroidism.

Partial moles present slightly later in pregnancy because they do not grow as rapidly as complete moles. Most (90%) present with symptoms of incomplete or missed abortion, and vaginal bleeding occurs in approximately 75% of patients.[33] The other signs and symptoms seen with complete mole, such as excessive uterine enlargement, hyperemesis, pregnancy-induced hypertension, hyperthyroidism, and theca lutein cysts, are significantly less common.[33]

Presentation of gestational trophoblastic neoplasia depends on the antecedent pregnancy event, extent of disease, and histopathology. Most often postmolar GTN (invasive mole or CCA) presents as irregular bleeding after evacuation of a hydatidiform mole. Clinical signs of postmolar GTN include an enlarged, irregular uterus and persistent bilateral ovarian enlargement. Occasionally, the diagnosis is made at the time of evacuation when a metastatic vaginal lesion is found. Biopsy of suspected vaginal metastases is discouraged because of the risk of substantial bleeding.[34] In patients with postpartum uterine bleeding and subinvolution, the differential should include GTN as well as retained products of conception, endomyometritis, primary or metastatic tumors of other organ systems, or a new pregnancy event (Table 8-1).[35]

Diagnosis of GTN is often made when metastases induce symptoms. The vascular nature of these lesions can lead to bleeding, including intra-abdominal and/or intracerebral hemorrhage, melena, or hemoptysis. Brain metastases and bleeding from these lesions can cause increased intracranial pressure, leading to headaches, seizures, or hemiplegia. Extensive lung metastases can also cause dyspnea, cough, and chest pain. PSTTs and epithelioid trophoblastic tumors almost always cause irregular uterine bleeding, often distant from a preceding nonmolar gestation, and rarely virilization or nephrotic syndrome. The uterus is usually symmetrically enlarged, and serum hCG levels are only slightly elevated.[36,37]

Several diagnostic tests aid in the diagnosis and evaluation of GTD. Ultrasonography has virtually replaced all other means of preoperative diagnosis of both complete and partial mole.[38-40] Characteristic ultrasonographic scans of complete mole show a uterine cavity

Table 8-1 Differential Diagnosis

Signs & Symptoms	Differential Diagnosis
Vaginal bleeding and positive urine pregnancy test	Gestational trophoblastic disease Missed abortion Ectopic pregnancy
Highly elevated hCG	Gestational trophoblastic disease More advanced gestational age than suspected Multiple gestations Erythroblastosis fetalis Intrauterine infections
Molar pregnancy is followed by persistent vaginal bleeding	Postmolar gestational trophoblastic neoplasia New pregnancy event Retained products of conception Endomyometritis Primary metastatic tumors of other organ systems
Molar pregnancy is followed by persistently elevated hCG	Postmolar gestational trophoblastic neoplasia New pregnancy event

hCG, human chorionic gonadotropin.

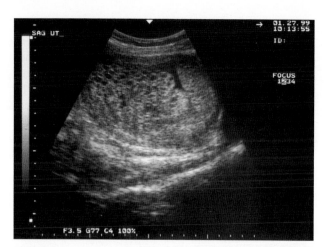

FIGURE 8-1. Pelvic ultrasound of a complete hydatidiform **mole** with the characteristic vesicular pattern of multiple echoes, holes within the placental mass, and no fetus.

filled with a heterogeneous mass (snowstorm pattern), without associated fetal development and with theca lutein ovarian cysts, although these features are not always visible in the first trimester[41] (Figure 8-1). Ultrasonography may also facilitate the early diagnosis of a partial mole by demonstrating focal cystic spaces within the placenta and an increase in the transverse diameter of the gestational sac.[39] Although previous work suggested that ultrasound was diagnostic of complete mole in early pregnancy, larger, more recent studies have shown that only 40% to 60% of cases are detected as molar by sonography in routine clinical practice.[39,40,42,43] In addition, 10% of "molar pregnancies" diagnosed by ultrasound were found to be nonmolar hydropic abortions on histologic review.[42,44] In the United Kingdom, the Royal College of Obstetrics and Gynaecologists recommends that all products of conception from nonviable pregnancies should undergo histologic examination irrespective of ultrasonographic findings, and other authors have recommended routine follow-up of hCG after elective termination.[45,46] The American Congress of Obstetrics and Gynecology suggests pathologic evaluation of tissue after spontaneous and therapeutic abortions, although regulations vary by state.

hCG is a disease-specific tumor marker produced by hydatidiform moles and GTNs. hCG assays are readily available, and levels are easily measured quantitatively in both urine and blood. hCG is made up of an α subunit that is shared with pituitary glycoprotein hormones, including thyroid-stimulating hormone and luteinizing hormone (LH) and a β subunit unique to the placenta that confers specificity. Assays that are designed to detect hCG target the β subunit. In healthy pregnancy, hCG is intact and is hyperglycosylated during the first trimester. However, in GTD, many other subtypes of β-hCG can exist, including free β-hCG, β-core, nicked free β, or c-terminal peptide.[47,48] Because the hCG molecules in

GTD are more heterogenous and degraded than those in normal pregnancy, an assay that detects all forms of hCG and its multiple fragments should be used to follow patients with GTD. Most institutions currently use rapid, automated, radiolabeled monoclonal antibody "sandwich" assays that measure different mixtures of hCG-related molecules. hCG assays are susceptible to false-positive results, usually caused by cross-reacting heterophile antibodies that are found in 3% to 4% of healthy people.[49] These cross-reacting heterophile antibodies are present only in serum and do not pass into the urine. In most cases a negative urine hCG test can confirm that the serum value is a false positive, although referral to a specialty laboratory may be required. These so-called phantom hCG results, with levels reported as high as 800 mIU/mL, have led to treatment of healthy patients with unnecessary surgery and chemotherapy.[50] Additionally, there is some cross-reactivity of hCG with LH, which may lead to falsely elevated low levels of hCG. Measurement of LH to identify this possibility and suppression of LH with oral contraceptive pills prevents this problem.[51]

Markedly elevated hCG levels above those of normal pregnancy are a hallmark of hydatidiform moles, and approximately half of patients with complete mole have pre-evacuation hCG levels greater than 100,000 mIU/mL.[52] However, the differential diagnosis of a significantly elevated hCG level includes the multiple causes of an enlarged placenta, such as misjudged gestational age, multiple gestation, and erythroblastosis fetalis (Table 8-1). Partial molar pregnancies, in contrast, typically do not demonstrate elevated hCG levels; fewer than 10% have hCG levels exceeding 100,000 mIU/mL.[38]

A clinical diagnosis of postmolar GTN is most often made by the finding of rising or plateauing hCG levels after evacuation of a hydatidiform mole. Choriocarcinoma is usually diagnosed by the finding of an elevated hCG level, frequently in conjunction with the discovery of metastases, after other pregnancy events. PSTT is commonly associated with only slightly raised hCG levels; human placental lactogen may be elevated in this variant of trophoblastic disease.

When a diagnosis of GTN is suspected, a metastatic work-up should be conducted. Most patients who develop GTN after a molar pregnancy are detected early by hCG monitoring, so detailed investigation is rarely needed. Diagnostic testing should be guided by findings on complete history and physical examination and laboratory studies including complete blood count, serum chemistries including renal and liver functions panels, blood type and antibody screen, and quantitative serum hCG level. Pulmonary metastases are most common, so chest radiography (CXR) is essential.[2] Chest computed tomography (CT) is not needed when CXR is normal, because discovery of micrometastases, which can be seen in approximately 40% of patients, does not affect outcome.[53] However, if lesions are noted on CXR, CT of the chest, abdomen, and pelvis and brain magnetic resonance imaging (MRI) are obtained to exclude more widespread disease such as the brain or liver metastases, which would substantially change management. Pelvic ultrasound or MRI may also be useful in detecting extensive uterine disease for which hysterectomy may be of benefit.

Several procedures are critical in the diagnosis and management of GTD. A diagnosis of GTD is usually confirmed by cervical dilatation and suction curettage of uterine contents. Some patients who do not desire future fertility may elect to undergo primary hysterectomy for evacuation of the molar gestation, with concurrent sterilization. Due to risks of hemorrhage at the time of evacuation, hysterotomy or induction of labor is not recommended.

Repeat curettage after hydatidiform mole evacuation is not recommended unless there is excessive uterine bleeding and radiologic evidence of substantial intracavitary molar tissue, because repeat curettage does not often induce remission or influence treatment and may result in uterine perforation and hemorrhage.[54-56]

PATHOLOGY

Key Points

1. Complete hydatidiform moles undergo early and uniform hydatid enlargement of villous trophoblast in the absence of a fetus or embryo.
2. Partial, or incomplete, hydatidiform moles demonstrate identifiable fetal tissue and chorionic villi with focal edema that vary in size and shape.
3. Approximately 10% to 17% of hydatidiform moles result in invasive mole, and approximately 15% of these metastasize; the most common site of metastatic spread is to the lungs or vagina.
4. Choriocarcinoma (CCA) is a malignant disease characterized by abnormal trophoblastic hyperplasia and anaplasia, absence of chorionic villi, hemorrhage, and necrosis, with direct invasion into the myometrium and vascular invasion resulting in spread to distant sites.

Molar pregnancies and gestational trophoblastic neoplasia all originate from the placental trophoblast. Hydatidiform moles and CCA arise from villous trophoblast and PSTT from intermediate trophoblast. Normal trophoblast is composed of cytotrophoblast, syncytiotrophoblast, and intermediate trophoblast, all 3 of which may result in GTD when they proliferate.[57] Normal syncytiotrophoblast invades the endometrial

stroma with implantation of the blastocyst and is the cell type that produces hCG. Cytotrophoblast functions to supply the syncytium with cells in addition to forming outpouchings that become the chorionic villi covering the chorionic sac. The villous chorion adjacent to the endometrium and basalis layer of the endometrium together form the functional placenta for maternal-fetal nutrient and waste exchange. Intermediate trophoblast is located in the villi, the implantation site, and the chorionic sac.

Hydatidiform mole is pathologically characterized by varying degrees of trophoblastic proliferation (both cytotrophoblast and syncytiotrophoblast) and vesicular swelling of placental villi associated with an absent or an abnormal fetus/embryo. There are 2 syndromes of hydatidiform mole, which are distinguished by their clinical behavior, morphology, and genetic make-up. Complete hydatidiform moles undergo early and uniform hydatid enlargement of villi in the absence of a fetus or embryo, the trophoblast is consistently hyperplastic with varying degrees of atypia, and villous capillaries are absent (Figure 8-2). Partial, or incomplete, hydatidiform moles demonstrate identifiable fetal or embryonic tissue, chorionic villi with focal edema that vary in size and shape, scalloping and prominent stromal trophoblastic inclusions and a functioning villous circulation, and focal trophoblastic hyperplasia with mild atypia only (Figure 8-3). Invasive mole arises from myometrial invasion of a hydatidiform mole via direct extension through tissue or venous channels (Figure 8-4). Approximately 10% to 17% of hydatidiform moles result in invasive mole, and approximately 15% of these will metastasize; the most common site of metastatic spread is to the lungs or vagina. Invasive moles are most often diagnosed clinically rather than pathologically based on persistent hCG elevation after molar evacuation and are frequently treated with

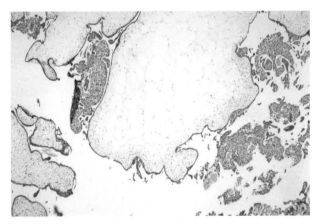

FIGURE 8-2. Complete hydatidiform mole with hydropic villi, absence of villous blood vessels, proliferation of hyperplastic cytotrophoblast, and syncytiotrophoblast.

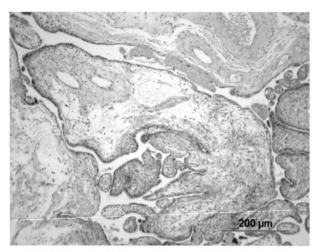

FIGURE 8-3. **Partial hydatidiform mole** with chorionic villi of varying size and shape with focal edema and scalloping, stromal trophoblastic inclusions, and functioning villous circulation, as well as focal trophoblastic hyperplasia.

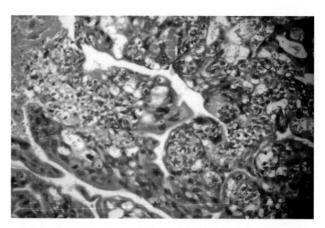

FIGURE 8-5. **Choriocarcinoma** composed of abnormal cytotrophoblast and syncytiotrophoblast with hyperplasia and anaplasia, absence of chorionic villi, hemorrhage, and necrosis.

chemotherapy without a histopathologic diagnosis. CCA is a malignant disease characterized by abnormal trophoblastic hyperplasia and anaplasia, absence of chorionic villi, hemorrhage, and necrosis, with direct invasion into the myometrium and vascular invasion resulting in spread to distant sites, including the lungs, brain, liver, pelvis and vagina, kidney, intestines, and spleen (Figure 8-5). CCA has been reported to occur in association with any pregnancy event. Approximately 25% of cases follow abortion or tubal pregnancy, 25% are associated with term or preterm gestation, and the remaining 50% arise from complete moles. Only 2% to 3% of complete moles progress to CCA. PSTT is an extremely rare disease that arises from the placental implantation site and consists predominantly of mononuclear intermediate trophoblast without chorionic

villi infiltrating in sheets or cords between myometrial fibers (Figure 8-6). PSTT is associated with less vascular invasion, necrosis, and hemorrhage than CCA, and it has a propensity for lymphatic metastasis. Immunohistochemical staining reveals the diffuse presence of cytokeratin and human placental lactogen, whereas hCG is only focal. Cytogenic studies have revealed that PSTTs are more often diploid than aneuploid. Most PSTTs follow nonmolar gestations.[37] Epithelioid trophoblastic tumor (ETT) is a rare variant of PSTT that simulates carcinoma. Based on morphologic and histochemical features, it appears to develop from neoplastic transformation of chorionic-type intermediate trophoblast. Most ETTs present many years after a full-term delivery.[36]

Pathologic diagnosis of complete and partial moles is made by examination of curettage specimens. In the setting of unclear diagnosis, additional testing can be

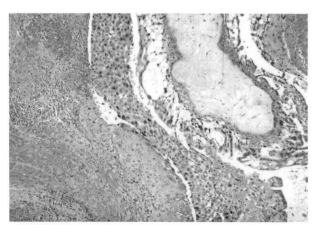

FIGURE 8-4. **Invasive mole** with direct extension of molar tissue, including hydropic villi and covering hyperplastic trophoblast, into the myometrium.

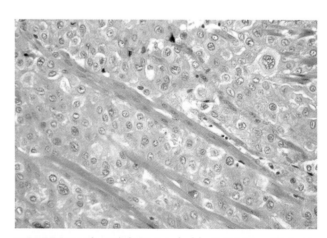

FIGURE 8-6. **Placental-site trophoblastic tumor** with sheets of mononuclear intermediate trophoblast cells without chorionic villi infiltrating between myometrial fibers.

Table 8-2 FIGO Anatomic Staging for Gestational Trophoblastic Neoplasia[1]

FIGO Anatomic Staging	
Stage I	Disease confined to the uterus
Stage II	Disease extends outside the uterus but is limited to the genital structures (adnexa, vagina, broad ligament)
Stage III	Disease extends to the lungs with or without genital tract involvement
Stage IV	Disease involves other metastatic sites

helpful. Immunohistologic staining for *p57* (a paternally imprinted, maternally expressed gene) can differentiate complete moles (absent immunostaining) from hydropic abortuses and partial moles (positively staining), and flow cytometry can distinguish diploid complete moles from triploid partial moles.[58,59] Additionally, pathologic diagnosis of invasive mole, CCA, PSTT, and ETT can sometimes be made by curettage, biopsy of metastatic lesions, or examination of hysterectomy specimens or placentas. Biopsy of a vaginal lesion suggestive of a GTN is dangerous because of the massive bleeding that can occur.[60]

In 2002, the International Federation of Gynecology and Obstetrics (FIGO) defined criteria for the diagnosis of postmolar disease and adopted a combined anatomic staging and modified World Health Organization (WHO) risk-factor scoring system for GTN (Tables 8-2 and 8-3).[61] The components needed to diagnose postmolar GTN include at least 1 of the following:

(1) hCG plateau for 4 consecutive values over 3 weeks, (2) hCG rise of $\geq$10% for 3 values over 2 weeks, (3) hCG persistence 6 months after molar evacuation, (4) histopathologic diagnosis of CCA, or (5) presence of metastatic disease (Figure 8-1). The FIGO stage is designated by a Roman numeral, followed by the modified WHO score designated by an Arabic numeral, separated by a colon. PSTTs and ETTs are classified separately.[5]

Treatment is based on classification into risk groups defined by the stage and scoring system. Patients with nonmetastatic (stage I) and low-risk metastatic (stages II and III, score <7) GTN can be treated with single-agent chemotherapy, with resulting survival rates approaching 100%. Patients classified as having high-risk metastatic disease (stage IV and stages II-III, score $\geq$7) should be treated in a more aggressive manner with multiagent chemotherapy and as needed adjuvant radiation or surgery to achieve cure rates of 80% to 90%. Use of the FIGO staging system is essential for determining initial therapy for patients with GTN to assure the best possible outcomes with the least morbidity.

TREATMENT

Key Points

1. Suction evacuation and curettage is the preferred treatment method for a hydatidiform mole, independent of uterine size, for patients who wish to maintain their fertility.

2. Definitive follow-up requires serial serum quantitative hCG measurements every 1 to 2 weeks until 3 consecutive tests show normal levels, after which hCG

Table 8-3 Modified WHO Prognostic Scoring System as Adapted by FIGO

Risk Factor	Score			
	0	1	2	4
Age	$\leq$39	>39	—	—
Antecedent pregnancy	Mole	Abortion	Term	
Pregnancy event to treatment interval (months)	<4	4-6	7-12	>12
Pretreatment hCG (mIU/mL)	$<10^3$	10^3-10^4	10^4-10^5	$>10^5$
Largest tumor mass, including uterus (cm)	<3	3-4	$\geq$5	—
Site of metastases	—	Spleen, kidney	GI tract	Brain, liver
Number of metastases	—	1-4	5-8	>8
Previous failed chemotherapy	—	—	Single drug	$\geq$2 drugs

Note. The total score for a patient is obtained by adding the individual scores for each prognostic factor: low-risk, <7; high-risk, $\geq$7. To stage and allot a risk factor score, a patient's diagnosis is allocated to a stage as represented by a Roman numeral I, II, III, and IV. This is then separated by a colon from the sum of all the actual risk factor scores expressed in Arabic numerals (eg, stage II:4, stage IV:9). This stage and score will be assigned to the patient. Modified from FIGO Committee on Gynecologic Oncology.[5]

levels should be determined at 3-month intervals for 6 months after the spontaneous return to normal.

3. Patients with nonmetastatic (stage I) and low-risk metastatic (stages II and III, score <7) GTN should be treated with single-agent methotrexate or actinomycin D chemotherapy.

4. Patients with high-risk metastatic GTN (FIGO stage IV and stages II-III score ≥7) should be treated initially with multiagent chemotherapy with or without adjuvant surgery or radiation therapy.

5. Definitive treatment of PSTT and ETT includes hysterectomy with lymphadenectomy.

Once the diagnosis of molar pregnancy is suspected by history, physical examination, hCG levels, and ultrasound findings, the patient should be evaluated for the presence of medical complications (anemia, preeclampsia, hyperthyroidism) and metastases by vital signs and diagnostic tests including complete blood counts, basic chemistry, hepatic and thyroid panels, urinalysis, and CXR. The preoperative evaluation should also include blood type and cross-match, serum hCG level, and electrocardiogram if appropriate.

Suction evacuation and curettage is the preferred treatment method for a hydatidiform mole, independent of uterine size, for patients who wish to maintain their fertility.[51,62] Intraoperative ultrasonography can reduce the risk of uterine perforation. After anesthesia is achieved, the cervix is dilated to allow a 12- to 14-mm suction cannula to pass into the lower uterine segment, which is rotated as the intrauterine contents are removed.[35] An intravenous (IV) oxytocin infusion should be started at the onset of suction curettage and continued for several hours postoperatively to enhance uterine contractility and to minimize blood loss. Suction evacuation should be followed by gentle sharp curettage. Because the risk of bleeding increases with uterine size, at least 2 units of blood should be immediately available when the uterus is greater than 16-week gestational size.

Patient outcomes are improved by use of appropriate equipment, access to blood products, careful intraoperative monitoring, and early anticipation of complications. Patients who are rhesus-negative should receive rhesus immunoglobulin at the time of evacuation because rhesus D factor is expressed on trophoblast.[51,62]

Women who are nulliparous should not be given prostanoids to ripen the cervix because these drugs can induce uterine contractions and might increase the risk of trophoblastic embolization to the pulmonary vasculature.[1] Similarly, medical induction of labor or hysterotomy are not recommended for molar evacuation because they increase trophoblastic dissemination and the development of postmolar GTN requiring chemotherapy.[63] In addition, these methods increase maternal morbidity, such as blood loss, incomplete evacuation ultimately requiring dilation and curettage, and the requirement for cesarean delivery in subsequent pregnancies. Hysterectomy may be considered for women who do not desire further childbearing or have life-threatening hemorrhage.[64] The adnexa may be left intact even in the presence of theca lutein cysts. In addition to evacuating the molar pregnancy, hysterectomy provides permanent sterilization and eliminates the risk of local myometrial invasion as a cause of persistent disease. Hysterectomy does not eliminate the risk of postmolar GTN, which remains at 3% to 5% because of the potential for metastatic disease. hCG surveillance should be continued as after any molar pregnancy (Table 8-4).

Prophylactic administration of either methotrexate or actinomycin D chemotherapy at the time of or immediately after evacuation of a hydatidiform mole is associated with a reduction in incidence of postmolar GTN from approximately 15% to 20% to 3% to 8%. However, the use of prophylactic chemotherapy should be limited to situations in which the risk of postmolar GTN is much greater than normal or in which adequate hCG follow-up is not possible, as essentially all patients who are followed up with serial hCG testing

Table 8-4 Surveillance After Gestational Trophoblastic Disease

Surveillance	After Hydatidiform Mole	After Gestational Trophoblastic Neoplasia
Serum quantitative hCG	Every 1-2 weeks until 3 consecutive normals then every 3 months for 6 months	At 1-month intervals for 12 months
Contraception/delay conception	6-12 months, preferably with oral contraceptives	12 months, preferably with oral contraceptives
Future pregnancies	First-trimester ultrasound Pathologic examination of placenta and other products of conception 6-week postpartum hCG	First-trimester ultrasound Pathologic examination of placenta and other products of conception 6-week postpartum hCG

hCG, human chorionic gonadotropin.

after molar evacuation and found to have persistent GTN can be cured with appropriate chemotherapy.[65]

Follow-up after evacuation of a hydatidiform mole is essential to detect trophoblastic sequelae (invasive mole or CCA), which develop in 15% to 20% of women with complete mole and 1% to 5% of those with partial mole (Figure 8-1 and Table 8-4).[62,66,67] Clinical findings of prompt uterine involution, ovarian cyst regression, and cessation of bleeding are all reassuring signs; however, definitive follow-up requires serial serum quantitative hCG measurements every 1 to 2 weeks until 3 consecutive tests show normal levels, after which hCG levels should be determined at 3-month intervals for 6 months after the spontaneous return to normal. More than half of patients will have complete regression of hCG to normal within 2 months of evacuation. Contraception is recommended for 6 months after the first normal hCG result to distinguish a rising hCG due to persistent or recurrent disease from a rising hCG associated with a subsequent pregnancy. The use of oral contraceptive pills is preferable because they have the advantage of suppressing endogenous LH, which may interfere with the measurement of hCG at low levels, and studies have shown that oral contraceptive pills do not increase the risk of postmolar trophoblastic neoplasia.[68] Pathologic examination of the placenta and other products of conception as well as determination of a 6-week postpartum hCG level is recommended with all future pregnancies. The general obstetrician-gynecologist may be responsible for immediate surveillance after a molar pregnancy and will be essential to ensuring that appropriate studies are carried out after subsequent pregnancy events.

The likelihood of persistent disease developing after evacuation of a complete mole increases with evidence of marked trophoblastic growth, such as a pre-evacuation hCG level greater than 100,000 mIU/mL, excessive uterine growth (>20 weeks size), and theca lutein cysts greater than 6 cm in diameter. Patients with ≥1 of these signs have approximately a 40% incidence of postmolar GTN compared with 4% for those without any of these signs. Patients with age greater than 40 years, a repeat molar pregnancy, an aneuploid mole, and medical complications of molar pregnancy, such as toxemia, hyperthyroidism, and trophoblastic embolization, are also at increased risk for postmolar GTN.[62]

Treatment of Low-Risk Disease

Patients with nonmetastatic (stage I) and low-risk metastatic (stages II and III, score <7) GTN should be treated with single-agent methotrexate or actinomycin D chemotherapy.[69,70] Several outpatient chemotherapy protocols may be used, including weekly intramuscular (IM) or intermittent intravenous (IV) infusion methotrexate, biweekly single-dose actinomycin D, 5-day

methotrexate or actinomycin D, and 8-day methotrexate plus folinic acid. Increased risk of initial chemotherapy resistance is seen with older patient age, higher hCG levels, nonmolar antecedent pregnancy, histopathologic diagnosis of CCA, presence of metastatic disease, and higher FIGO score; these patients may benefit from the 5- or 8-day regimens. Although differences are seen in primary remission rates depending on initial chemotherapy, almost all patients are eventually cured, with most being able to preserve fertility.[71]

Methotrexate 0.4 mg/kg (maximum 25 mg) IM or IV push daily for 5 days every other week appears to be a highly effective treatment protocol. Review of 30 years of experience in treating nonmetastatic GTN at the Brewer Trophoblastic Disease Center (Northwestern University Feinberg School of Medicine, Chicago, IL) with 5-day methotrexate showed that 89% of patients achieved primary remission, 9% were placed into remission with subsequent single-agent actinomycin D, and only 2% required multiagent chemotherapy or hysterectomy for cure. Significant toxicity to methotrexate necessitating a change to another chemotherapeutic agent occurred in 5% of patients, and no life-threatening toxicity occurred. Stomatitis was common, nausea was uncommon, and alopecia did not occur. Factors found to be associated with resistance to initial methotrexate chemotherapy were high pretreatment hCG level, nonmolar antecedent pregnancy, and clinicopathologic diagnosis of CCA. These results of approximately 90% complete response and 100% survival confirm other reports that single-agent methotrexate in a 5-day outpatient course every 2 weeks is a highly effective and well-tolerated treatment.[71]

An alternative methotrexate regimen consists of slightly higher doses of methotrexate (1.0-1.5 mg/kg) IM every other day alternating with folinic acid (0.1-0.15 mg/kg) IM over 8 days with at least a 1-week interval between courses. This methotrexate plus folinic acid protocol demonstrated decreased toxicity, but higher cost and inconvenience, and it more frequently required change in chemotherapy to achieve remission.[72] High-dose methotrexate infusion (100 mg/m² IV push followed by 200 mg/m² IV 12-hour infusion with folinic acid rescue), with interval between doses based on post-treatment hCG trends, is another modified methotrexate dosage schedule used for treatment of low-risk GTN. This regimen also has increased need for second-line therapy and is expensive.[73] Although methotrexate administered in single weekly IM doses of 30 to 50 mg/m² is more convenient, less costly, and less toxic, it has the relatively lowest complete response rate of any regimen and is not appropriate therapy for metastatic disease or CCA.[74]

Actinomycin D (10-12 mg/kg IV daily for 5 days every other week or as a single 1.25 mg/m² IV dose every 2 weeks) is a reasonable alternative to methotrexate, although it has a more toxic side-effect profile (nausea, alopecia) than methotrexate and produces local tissue injury with extravasation. Actinomycin D has mainly been used for methotrexate resistance or as primary therapy for patients with hepatic or renal compromise or effusions contraindicating the use of methotrexate.[75,76]

Several studies have compared different methotrexate and actinomycin D regimens for treatment of low-risk, mostly nonmetastatic GTN. Three randomized clinical trials have compared weekly IM methotrexate with biweekly actinomycin D and demonstrated lower primary remission rates for weekly IM methotrexate (49%-53%) than for pulsed actinomycin D (69%-90%).[77-79] In a randomized trial of patients with non-metastatic GTN, complete remission was achieved in 74% of the women in the methotrexate-folinic acid arm, versus 100% of the women in the actinomycin D arm.[80] In a retrospective analysis of patients with low-risk, mostly nonmetastatic GTN treated with 5-day regimens of methotrexate and actinomycin D or a combination of methotrexate and actinomycin, complete remission rates were not significantly different at 69%, 61%, and 79%, respectively, though adverse side effect rate was much greater with combination therapy (62%) than with single-agent methotrexate (29%) or actinomycin D (19%).[81]

Patients categorized as having low-risk metastatic GTN (FIGO stages II and III, score <7) may be treated successfully with initial single-agent chemotherapy with methotrexate or actinomycin D, as for nonmetastatic disease. The weekly methotrexate or biweekly acti-nomycin D single-dose protocols currently in use for nonmetastatic postmolar disease should not be used for treatment of metastatic disease.[71] The combined experience of 3 specialized trophoblastic disease centers in the United States with single-agent methotrex-ate or actinomycin D treatment of low-risk metastatic GTN revealed excellent outcomes, with 48% to 67% of patients achieving primary remission with the first single-agent chemotherapy regimen.[82-84] Multiagent chemotherapy was used in 1% to 14% of patients after failed sequential single-agent chemotherapy with or without surgery to ultimately cure all of the patients. In low-risk metastatic GTN patients, risk factors for drug resistance to initial single-agent chemotherapy were pretherapy hCG level more than 100,000 mIU/mL, age greater than 35 years, FIGO score greater than 4, and large vaginal metastases.

In all treatment protocols, chemotherapy should be continued until 1 course has been administered past a normal hCG level. Indications to change treatment to an alternative single agent include a plateau in hCG above normal during treatment or toxicity that precludes an adequate dose or frequency of treatment. Multiagent chemotherapy should be initiated if there is a significant elevation in hCG level, development of metastases, or

resistance to sequential single-agent chemotherapy. If fertility preservation is not desired, hysterectomy may be performed as adjuvant treatment at the initiation of che-motherapy to shorten the treatment duration. Hysterec-tomy may also be used to treat hemorrhage or persistent, chemotherapy-resistant disease in the uterus. Hysterec-tomy is the treatment of choice for PSTT and ETT.

In summary, cure rates for both nonmetastatic and low-risk metastatic GTN can approach 100% with the use of initial single-agent methotrexate or acti-nomycin D chemotherapy. Approximately 20% of low-risk patients will develop resistance to the initial chemotherapeutic agent, but more than 90% will be cured by the use of sequential single-agent chemo-therapy. Eventually, approximately 10% of patients will require multiagent chemotherapy with or without surgery to achieve remission.

Treatment of High-Risk Metastatic Disease and Recurrence

Patients with high-risk metastatic GTN (FIGO stage IV and stages II-III score ≥7) should be treated initially with multiagent chemotherapy with or without adjuvant sur-gery or radiation therapy.[70] Several groups have demon-strated the efficacy of the EMA-CO regimen (etoposide, high-dose methotrexate with folinic acid, actinomycin D, cyclophosphamide, and vincristine) as primary ther-apy for high-risk GTN, reporting complete response rates of 71% to 78% and long-term survival rates of 85% to 94%.[85-89] The EMA-CO regimen is currently the initial treatment of choice for high-risk metastatic GTN because of relatively low toxicity, allowing adherence to treatment schedules, high complete response rates, and overall high resultant survival.[1,71] Chemotherapy for high-risk disease is continued for at least 2 to 3 courses after the first normal hCG measurement.[70]

Central nervous system metastases may be treated with whole-brain radiation (3000 cGy in 200-cGy frac-tions) or surgical excision with stereotactic irradiation with simultaneously initiation of systemic chemother-apy. During radiotherapy, the methotrexate infusion dose in the EMA-CO protocol is increased to 1 g/m², and 30 mg of folinic acid is given every 12 hours for 3 days starting 32 hours after the infusion begins. An alternative to brain irradiation is the use of intrathecal as well as high-dose IV methotrexate. Cure rates for brain metastases are 50% to 80%, depending on patient symptoms and size and location of the brain lesions.[90]

Hysterectomy, pulmonary resection, and other adjuvant surgical procedures may be used for chemo-therapy-resistant disease and to control hemorrhage in patients with high-risk GTN. Surgery is used to achieve cure in approximately one-half of high-risk patients.[91-94] Between 1986 and 2005, of 50 patients with high-risk GTN treated with EMA-CO as primary or secondary therapy at the Brewer Center, 24 patients underwent 28 adjuvant surgical procedures, and 21 patients were cured. Surgical procedures that helped to achieve cure included hysterectomy, lung resection, uterine artery embolization, small bowel resection, salpingectomy, and uterine wedge resection.[93]

Approximately 30% of high-risk GTN patients will have an incomplete response to first-line chemotherapy or relapse from remission.[95,96] Multiple metastases to sites other than the lung and vagina and previous inadequate chemotherapy are common in these patients. The majority can be managed with chemotherapy regimens that include etoposide and a platinum agent, which are often combined with surgical excision of persistent tumor. The EMA-EP regimen, substituting etoposide and cisplatin for cyclophosphamide and vincristine in the EMA-CO protocol, is considered the most appropriate therapy for patients who have responded to EMA-CO but have plateauing low hCG levels or who have developed re-elevation of hCG levels after a complete response to EMA-CO.[97,98] Finally, in patients with disease that is resistant to methotrexate-containing protocols, drug combinations containing etoposide and platinum with bleomycin, ifosfamide, or paclitaxel have all been found to be effective.[70,99,100]

In summary, intensive multimodality therapy with EMA-CO chemotherapy and adjuvant radiotherapy or surgery when indicated achieves cure in 80% to 90% of patients with high-risk GTN. Most of the 30% of high-risk patients who fail first-line therapy or relapse from remission can be effectively treated with salvage therapy that includes platinum-containing drug combinations in conjunction with surgical resection of persistent tumor.

Treatment of Placental Site Trophoblastic Tumors and Epithelioid Trophoblastic Tumors

PSTT and ETT differ from invasive mole and CCA in their relative resistance to chemotherapy and their propensity for lymphatic spread. Initial treatment should include hysterectomy with lymph node dissection. Chemotherapy should be used in patients with metastatic disease and in patients with nonmetastatic disease who have adverse prognostic factors, including prolonged interval from last known pregnancy (>2 years), deep myometrial invasion, tumor necrosis and mitotic count greater than 6/10 high-power fields. Although the optimal chemotherapy regimen for PSTT and ETT remains to be defined, the current clinical approach is an etoposide and platinum-containing regimen, such as EMA-EP or a paclitaxel/cisplatin–paclitaxel/etoposide doublet.[71] The survival rate is approximately 100% for nonmetastatic disease and 50% to 60% for metastatic disease.[12,101,102]

Surveillance After GTN

After hCG has returned to normal and chemotherapy has been completed, patients treated for GTN should have serum quantitative hCG levels measured at 1-month intervals for 12 months (Table 8-4). Relapse risk is approximately 3% in the first year after completing therapy and less than 1% after that.[103] Physical examinations are performed every 6 to 12 months, but testing such as x-rays or CT scans are rarely indicated. Contraception, ideally with oral contraceptives, should be used during treatment and for 6 to 12 months after completion of chemotherapy. Because of the 1% to 2% risk of a second gestational trophoblastic disease event in subsequent pregnancies, pelvic ultrasound is recommended in the first trimester of a subsequent pregnancy to confirm a normal gestation, the products of contraception or placentas from future pregnancies should be carefully examined histopathologically, and an hCG level should be obtained 6 weeks after any pregnancy.

SURVIVAL AND PROGNOSIS

Key Points

1. The majority of patients with GTN will be cured with adjuvant therapy.
2. Patients who develop resistance to initial chemotherapy are likely to be cured with subsequent alternative regimens.
3. Future pregnancies should be carefully monitored for the development of a second episode of GTD.

Cure rates for both nonmetastatic and low-risk metastatic GTN approach 100% with the use of initial single-agent methotrexate or actinomycin D chemotherapy. Approximately 20% of low-risk patients will develop resistance to the initial chemotherapeutic agent, but more than 90% will be cured by the use of sequential single-agent chemotherapy. Roughly 10% of patients with low-risk GTN will require multiagent chemotherapy with or without surgery to achieve remission; for high-risk GTN, cure rates are 80% to 90% with intensive multimodality therapy with multiagent chemotherapy, along with adjuvant radiotherapy or surgery when indicated. Approximately 30% of high-risk patients will fail first-line therapy or relapse from remission. Salvage therapy with platinum-containing drug combinations, sometimes in conjunction with surgical resection of sites of persistent tumor, will result in cure of most high-risk patients with resistant disease. Even those patients with metastatic disease to the brain, liver, and gastrointestinal tract now have 75%, 73%, and 50% survival rates, respectively.[3]

Survival rates for PSTT and ETT are highly dependent on the presence of metastatic disease, with cure rates of approximately 100% for nonmetastatic disease and 50% to 60% for metastatic disease.[12,101,102]

Curative treatment of GTN has allowed women to maintain their reproductive potential despite exposure to drugs that have ovarian toxicity and teratogenic potential. Most women resume normal ovarian function after chemotherapy and exhibit no increase in infertility. Many studies have reported successful pregnancies, without an increase in abortions, stillbirths, congenital anomalies, prematurity, or major obstetric complications.[71] Although subsequent pregnancy does not cause "reactivation" of disease, patients who have had 1 episode of GTD are at greater risk for the development of a second episode in a subsequent pregnancy, regardless of whether or not they required chemotherapy. Patients should avoid conception for 6 to 12 months after chemotherapy to allow for disease surveillance via hCG and to theoretically allow for elimination of mature ova that may have been damaged by cytotoxic drugs (Table 8-4).[15,104,105]

The carcinogenic potential of chemotherapy in relatively young patients has led to concern for second malignancies among patients treated for GTN. Although single-agent treatment has not been associated with an increased risk for secondary malignancy, sequential therapy and etoposide-containing drug combinations have been associated with a slight increased risk of secondary malignancies, including acute myelogenous leukemia, colon cancer, melanoma, and breast cancer.[106]

SPECIAL MANAGEMENT PROBLEMS

Quiescent gestational trophoblastic disease is a highly uncommon, presumed inactive form of GTN that is characterized by persistent, unchanging low levels (<200 mIU/mL) of "real" hCG for at least 3 months associated with a past history of GTD or spontaneous abortion but without clinically detectable disease. The hCG levels do not change with treatment, including chemotherapy or surgery. The International Society for the Study of Trophoblastic Disease 2001 provides several recommendations for managing this condition: (1) false-positive hCG level due to heterophile antibodies or LH interference should be excluded, (2) the patient should be thoroughly investigated for evidence of disease, (3) immediate chemotherapy or surgery should be avoided, and (4) the patient should be monitored long term with periodic hCG testing while avoiding pregnancy. Treatment should be undertaken only when there is a sustained rise in hCG or the appearance of overt clinical disease.[107] Subanalysis

of hCG in these patients reveals no hyperglycosylated hCG, which has been associated with cytotrophoblastic invasion. During follow-up of patients with presumed quiescent GTD, approximately one-quarter eventually develop active GTN, which is signaled by an increase in both hyperglycosylated hCG and total hCG.[108,109]

A twin pregnancy consisting of a complete mole and a coexisting normal fetus is estimated to occur once in every 22,000 to 100,000 pregnancies. It must be distinguished from a partial mole (triploid pregnancy with fetus). The diagnosis can usually be established by ultrasound, but cytogenetics may be used to differentiate between chromosomally normal, potentially viable fetuses and triploid nonviable fetuses. Patients with a twin normal fetus/complete mole pregnancy should be cautioned that they may be at increased risk for hemorrhage and medical complications. Suction evacuation and curettage in the operating room is recommended for patients who desire pregnancy termination or develop bleeding or other complications. Evidence from a case series of 77 pregnancies showed that approximately 40% will result in normal viable fetuses if allowed to continue.[110,111]

FUTURE DIRECTIONS

The joint efforts of vigilant primary care providers, obstetricians/gynecologists, and collaborative oncologic specialists have led to excellent short- and long-term outcomes for women with GTD, and the substantial reduction in worldwide mortality from GTN is a triumph of modern global medical efforts. Diagnostic and prognostic tests are still needed to allow earlier identification of GTD patients who will develop postmolar GTN and GTN patients who will require multiagent chemotherapy. These tools could minimize ultimately unnecessary testing and loss to follow-up and ultimately reduce morbidity and mortality by individualizing treatment and decreasing chemotherapy resistance. Finally, a mechanistic understanding of the identified causative gene for repetitive molar pregnancy would not only improve outcomes in the few women affected by this gene, but also would further our comprehension of GTD, making prevention possible.

REFERENCES

1. Seckl MJ, Sebire NJ, Berkowitz RS. Gestational trophoblastic disease. *Lancet.* 2010;376(9742):717-729.
2. Berkowitz RS, Goldstein DP. Current management of gestational trophoblastic diseases. *Gynecol Oncol.* 2009;112(3):654-662.
3. Hoekstra AV, Lurain JR, Rademaker AW, Schink JC. Gestational trophoblastic neoplasia: treatment outcomes. *Obstet Gynecol.* 2008;112(2 pt 1):251-258.

4. Soper JT. Gestational trophoblastic disease. *Obstet Gynecol.* 2006;108(1):176-187.

5. FIGO Committee on Gynecologic Oncology. Current FIGO staging for cancer of the vagina, fallopian tube, ovary, and gestational trophoblastic neoplasia. *Int J Gynaecol Obstet.* 2009;105(1):3-4.

6. Newlands ES. The management of recurrent and drug-resistant gestational trophoblastic neoplasia (GTN). *Best Pract Res Clin Obstet Gynaecol.* 2003;17(6):905-923.

7. Palmer JR. Advances in the epidemiology of gestational trophoblastic disease. *J Reprod Med.* 1994;39(3):155-162.

8. Smith HO. Gestational trophoblastic disease epidemiology and trends. *Clin Obstet Gynecol.* 2003;46(3):541-556.

9. Berkowitz RS, Cramer DW, Bernstein MR, Cassells S, Driscoll SG, Goldstein DP. Risk factors for complete molar pregnancy from a case-control study. *Am J Obstet Gynecol.* 1985;152(8):1016-1020.

10. Parazzini F, La Vecchia C, Mangili G, et al. Dietary factors and risk of trophoblastic disease. *Am J Obstet Gynecol.* 1988;158(1):93-99.

11. Smith HO, Qualls CR, Prairie BA, Padilla LA, Rayburn WF, Key CR. Trends in gestational choriocarcinoma: a 27-year perspective. *Obstet Gynecol.* 2003;102(5 pt 1):978-987.

12. Schmid P, Nagai Y, Agarwal R, et al. Prognostic markers and long-term outcome of placental-site trophoblastic tumours: a retrospective observational study. *Lancet.* 2009;374(9683):48-55.

13. Ngan S, Seckl MJ. Gestational trophoblastic neoplasia management: an update. *Curr Opin Oncol.* 2007;19(5):486-491.

14. Sebire NJ, Foskett M, Fisher RA, Rees H, Seckl M, Newlands E. Risk of partial and complete hydatidiform molar pregnancy in relation to maternal age. *BJOG.* 2002;109(1):99-102.

15. Garrett LA, Garner EI, Feltmate CM, Goldstein DP, Berkowitz RS. Subsequent pregnancy outcomes in patients with molar pregnancy and persistent gestational trophoblastic neoplasia. *J Reprod Med.* 2008;53(7):481-486.

16. Agarwal P, Bagga R, Jain V, Kalra J, Gopalan S. Familial recurrent molar pregnancy: a case report. *Acta Obstet Gynecol Scand.* 2004;83(2):213-214.

17. Al-Hussaini TK, Abd el-Aal DM, Van den Veyver IB. Recurrent pregnancy loss due to familial and non-familial habitual molar pregnancy. *Int J Gynaecol Obstet.* 2003;83(2):179-186.

18. Fisher RA, Hodges MD, Newlands ES. Familial recurrent hydatidiform mole: a review. *J Reprod Med.* 2004;49(8):595-601.

19. Kerkmeijer LG, Wielsma S, Massuger LF, Sweep FC, Thomas CM. Recurrent gestational trophoblastic disease after hCG normalization following hydatidiform mole in The Netherlands. *Gynecol Oncol.* 2007;106(1):142-146.

20. Sebire NJ, Fisher RA, Foskett M, Rees H, Seckl MJ, Newlands ES. Risk of recurrent hydatidiform mole and subsequent pregnancy outcome following complete or partial hydatidiform molar pregnancy. *BJOG.* 2003;110(1):22-26.

21. Williams D, Hodgetts V, Gupta J. Recurrent hydatidiform moles. *Eur J Obstet Gynecol Reprod Biol.* 2010;150(1):3-7.

22. Lage JM, Mark SD, Roberts DJ, Goldstein DP, Bernstein MR, Berkowitz RS. A flow cytometric study of 137 fresh hydropic placentas: correlation between types of hydatidiform moles and nuclear DNA ploidy. *Obstet Gynecol.* 1992;79(3):403-410.

23. Mosher R, Goldstein DP, Berkowitz R, Bernstein M, Genest DR. Complete hydatidiform mole. Comparison of clinicopathologic features, current and past. *J Reprod Med.* 1998;43(1):21-27.

24. Berkowitz RS, Goldstein DP, Bernstein MR. Evolving concepts of molar pregnancy. *J Reprod Med.* 1991;36(1):40-44.

25. Sebire NJ, Makrydimas G, Agnantis NJ, Zagorianakou N, Rees H, Fisher RA. Updated diagnostic criteria for partial and complete hydatidiform moles in early pregnancy. *Anticancer Res.* 2003;23(2C):1723-1728.

26. Parazzini F, Mangili G, La Vecchia C, Negri E, Bocciolone L, Fasoli M. Risk factors for gestational trophoblastic disease: a separate analysis of complete and partial hydatidiform moles. *Obstet Gynecol.* 1991;78(6):1039-1045.

27. Palmer JR, Driscoll SG, Rosenberg L, et al. Oral contraceptive use and risk of gestational trophoblastic tumors. *J Natl Cancer Inst.* 1999;91(7):635-640.

28. Buckley JD, Henderson BE, Morrow CP, Hammond CB, Kohorn EI, Austin DF. Case-control study of gestational choriocarcinoma. *Cancer Res.* 1988;48(4):1004-1010.

29. Fisher RA, Newlands ES. Gestational trophoblastic disease. Molecular and genetic studies. *J Reprod Med.* 1998;43(1):87-97.

30. Azuma C, Saji F, Tokugawa Y, et al. Application of gene amplification by polymerase chain reaction to genetic analysis of molar mitochondrial DNA: the detection of anuclear empty ovum as the cause of complete mole. *Gynecol Oncol.* 1991;40(1):29-33.

31. Tuncer ZS, Bernstein MR, Wang J, Goldstein DP, Berkowitz RS. Repetitive hydatidiform mole with different male partners. *Gynecol Oncol.* 1999;75(2):224-226.

32. Hou JL, Wan XR, Xiang Y, Qi QW, Yang XY. Changes of clinical features in hydatidiform mole: analysis of 113 cases. *J Reprod Med.* 2008;53(8):629-633.

33. Berkowitz RS, Goldstein DP, Bernstein MR. Natural history of partial molar pregnancy. *Obstet Gynecol.* 1985;66(5):677-681.

34. Cagayan MS. Vaginal metastases complicating gestational trophoblastic neoplasia. *J Reprod Med.* 2010;55(5-6):229-235.

35. Lurain JR. Gestational trophoblastic disease I: epidemiology, pathology, clinical presentation and diagnosis of gestational trophoblastic disease, and management of hydatidiform mole. *Am J Obstet Gynecol.* 2010;203(6):531-539.

36. Allison KH, Love JE, Garcia RL. Epithelioid trophoblastic tumor: review of a rare neoplasm of the chorionic-type intermediate trophoblast. *Arch Pathol Lab Med.* 2006;130(12):1875-1877.

37. Baergen RN, Rutgers JL, Young RH, Osann K, Scully RE. Placental site trophoblastic tumor: A study of 55 cases and review of the literature emphasizing factors of prognostic significance. *Gynecol Oncol.* 2006;100(3):511-520.

38. Soto-Wright V, Bernstein M, Goldstein DP, Berkowitz RS. The changing clinical presentation of complete molar pregnancy. *Obstet Gynecol.* 1995;86(5):775-779.

39. Fine C, Bundy AL, Berkowitz RS, Boswell SB, Berezin AF, Doubilet PM. Sonographic diagnosis of partial hydatidiform mole. *Obstet Gynecol.* 1989;73(3 pt 1):414-418.

40. Benson CB, Genest DR, Bernstein MR, Soto-Wright V, Goldstein DP, Berkowitz RS. Sonographic appearance of first trimester complete hydatidiform moles. *Ultrasound Obstet Gynecol.* 2000;16(2):188-191.

41. Reid MH, McGahan JP, Oi R. Sonographic evaluation of hydatidiform mole and its look-alikes. *AJR Am J Roentgenol.* 1983;140(2):307-311.

42. Fowler DJ, Lindsay I, Seckl MJ, Sebire NJ. Routine pre-evacuation ultrasound diagnosis of hydatidiform mole: experience of more than 1000 cases from a regional referral center. *Ultrasound Obstet Gynecol.* 2006;27(1):56-60.

43. Johns J, Greenwold N, Buckley S, Jauniaux E. A prospective study of ultrasound screening for molar pregnancies in missed miscarriages. *Ultrasound Obstet Gynecol.* 2005;25(5):493-497.

44. Fowler DJ, Lindsay I, Seckl MJ, Sebire NJ. Histomorphometric features of hydatidiform moles in early pregnancy: relationship to detectability by ultrasound examination. *Ultrasound Obstet Gynecol.* 2007;29(1):76-80.

45. The management of early pregnancy loss. Green-top guideline. London, England: London Royal College of Obstetricians and Gynaecologists; 2006:1-18.

46. Seckl MJ, Gillmore R, Foskett M, Sebire NJ, Rees H, Newlands ES. Routine terminations of pregnancy—should we screen for gestational trophoblastic neoplasia? *Lancet.* 2004;364(9435):705-707.

47. Cole LA. Human chorionic gonadotropin tests. *Expert Rev Mol Diagn.* 2009;9(7):721-747.

48. Mitchell H, Seckl MJ. Discrepancies between commercially available immunoassays in the detection of tumour-derived hCG. *Mol Cell Endocrinol.* 2007;260-262:310-313.

49. Palmieri C, Dhillon T, Fisher RA, et al. Management and outcome of healthy women with a persistently elevated beta-hCG. *Gynecol Oncol.* 2007;106(1):35-43.

50. Rotmensch S, Cole LA. False diagnosis and needless therapy of presumed malignant disease in women with false-positive human chorionic gonadotropin concentrations. *Lancet.* 2000;355(9205):712-715.

51. Hancock BW, Tidy JA. Current management of molar pregnancy. *J Reprod Med.* 2002;47(5):347-354.

52. Genest DR, Laborde O, Berkowitz RS, Goldstein DP, Bernstein MR, Lage J. A clinicopathologic study of 153 cases of complete hydatidiform mole (1980-1990): histologic grade lacks prognostic significance. *Obstet Gynecol.* 1991;78(3 pt 1):402-409.

53. Darby S, Jolley I, Pennington S, Hancock BW. Does chest CT matter in the staging of GTN? *Gynecol Oncol.* 2009;112(1):155-160.

54. van Trommel NE, Massuger LF, Verheijen RH, Sweep FC, Thomas CM. The curative effect of a second curettage in persistent trophoblastic disease: a retrospective cohort survey. *Gynecol Oncol.* 2005;99(1):6-13.

55. Garner EI, Feltmate CM, Goldstein DP, Berkowitz RS. The curative effect of a second curettage in persistent trophoblastic disease: a retrospective cohort survey. *Gynecol Oncol.* 2005;99(1):3-5.

56. Pezeshki M, Hancock BW, Silcocks P, et al. The role of repeat uterine evacuation in the management of persistent gestational trophoblastic disease. *Gynecol Oncol.* 2004;95(3):423-429.

57. Bentley RC. Pathology of gestational trophoblastic disease. *Clin Obstet Gynecol.* 2003;46(3):513-522.

58. Castrillon DH, Sun D, Weremowicz S, Fisher RA, Crum CP, Genest DR. Discrimination of complete hydatidiform mole from its mimics by immunohistochemistry of the paternally imprinted gene product p57KIP2. *Am J Surg Pathol.* 2001;25(10):1225-1230.

59. Thaker HM, Berlin A, Tycko B, et al. Immunohistochemistry for the imprinted gene product IPL/PHLDA2 for facilitating the differential diagnosis of complete hydatidiform mole. *J Reprod Med.* 2004;49(8):630-636.

60. Berry E, Hagopian GS, Lurain JR. Vaginal metastases in gestational trophoblastic neoplasia. *J Reprod Med.* 2008;53(7):487-492.

61. Ngan HY, Bender H, Benedet JL, Jones H, Montruccoli GC, Pecorelli S. Gestational trophoblastic neoplasia, FIGO 2000 staging and classification. *Int J Gynaecol Obstet.* 2003;83 (suppl 1):175-177.

62. Berkowitz RS, Goldstein DP. Clinical practice. Molar pregnancy. *N Engl J Med.* 2009;360(16):1639-1645.

63. Tidy JA, Gillespie AM, Bright N, Radstone CR, Coleman RE, Hancock BW. Gestational trophoblastic disease: a study of mode of evacuation and subsequent need for treatment with chemotherapy. *Gynecol Oncol.* 2000;78(3 pt 1):309-312.

64. Elias KM, Goldstein DP, Berkowitz RS. Complete hydatidiform mole in women older than age 50. *J Reprod Med.* 2010;55(5-6):208-212.

65. Limpongsanurak S. Prophylactic actinomycin D for high-risk complete hydatidiform mole. *J Reprod Med.* 2001;46(2):110-116.

66. Feltmate CM, Growdon WB, Wolfberg AJ, et al. Clinical characteristics of persistent gestational trophoblastic neoplasia after partial hydatidiform molar pregnancy. *J Reprod Med.* 2006;51(11):902-906.

67. Hancock BW, Nazir K, Everard JE. Persistent gestational trophoblastic neoplasia after partial hydatidiform mole incidence and outcome. *J Reprod Med.* 2006;51(10):764-766.

68. Deicas RE, Miller DS, Rademaker AW, Lurain JR. The role of contraception in the development of postmolar gestational trophoblastic tumor. *Obstet Gynecol.* 1991;78(2):221-226.

69. Lurain JR. Pharmacotherapy of gestational trophoblastic disease. *Expert Opin Pharmacother.* 2003;4(11):2005-2017.

70. Alazzam M, Tidy J, Hancock BW, Osborne R. First line chemotherapy in low risk gestational trophoblastic neoplasia. *Cochrane Database Syst Rev.* 2009(1):CD007102.

71. Lurain JR. Gestational trophoblastic disease II: classification and management of gestational trophoblastic neoplasia. *Am J Obstet Gynecol.* 2011;204(1):11-18.

72. McNeish IA, Strickland S, Holden L, et al. Low-risk persistent gestational trophoblastic disease: outcome after initial treatment with low-dose methotrexate and folinic acid from 1992 to 2000. *J Clin Oncol.* 2002;20(7):1838-1844.

73. Wong LC, Ngan HY, Cheng DK, Ng TY. Methotrexate infusion in low-risk gestational trophoblastic disease. *Am J Obstet Gynecol.* 2000;183(6):1579-1582.

74. Homesley HD, Blessing JA, Rettenmaier M, Capizzi RL, Major FJ, Twiggs LB. Weekly intramuscular methotrexate for nonmetastatic gestational trophoblastic disease. *Obstet Gynecol.* 1988;72(3 pt 1):413-418.

75. Schlaerth JB, Morrow CP, Nalick RH, Gaddis O Jr. Single-dose actinomycin D in the treatment of postmolar trophoblastic disease. *Gynecol Oncol.* 1984;19(1):53-56.

76. Twiggs LB. Pulse actinomycin D scheduling in nonmetastatic gestational trophoblastic neoplasia: cost-effective chemotherapy. *Gynecol Oncol.* 1983;16(2):190-195.

77. Osborne RJ, Filiaci V, Schink JC, et al. Phase III trial of weekly methotrexate or pulsed dactinomycin for low-risk gestational trophoblastic neoplasia: a Gynecologic Oncology Group study. *J Clin Oncol.* 2011;29:825-831.

78. Gilani MM, Yarandi F, Eftekhar Z, Hanjani P. Comparison of pulse methotrexate and pulse dactinomycin in the treatment of low-risk gestational trophoblastic neoplasia. *Aust N Z J Obstet Gynaecol.* 2005;45(2):161-164.

79. Yarandi F, Eftekhar Z, Shojaei H, Kanani S, Sharifi A, Hanjani P. Pulse methotrexate versus pulse actinomycin D in the treatment of low-risk gestational trophoblastic neoplasia. *Int J Gynaecol Obstet.* 2008;103(1):33-37.

80. Lertkhachonsuk AA, Israngura N, Wilailak S, Tangtrakul S. Actinomycin D versus methotrexate-folinic acid as the treatment of stage I, low-risk gestational trophoblastic neoplasia: a randomized controlled trial. *Int J Gynecol Cancer.* 2009; 19(5):985-988.

81. Abrao RA, de Andrade JM, Tiezzi DG, Marana HR, Candido dos Reis FJ, Clagnan WS. Treatment for low-risk gestational trophoblastic disease: comparison of single-agent methotrexate, dactinomycin and combination regimens. *Gynecol Oncol.* 2008;108(1):149-153.

82. Roberts JP, Lurain JR. Treatment of low-risk metastatic gestational trophoblastic tumors with single-agent chemotherapy. *Am J Obstet Gynecol.* 1996;174(6):1917-1923; discussion 1923-1914.

83. Soper JT, Clarke-Pearson DL, Berchuck A, Rodriguez G, Hammond CB. 5-day methotrexate for women with metastatic gestational trophoblastic disease. *Gynecol Oncol.* 1994;54(1):76-79.

84. DuBeshter B, Berkowitz RS, Goldstein DP, Bernstein MR. Management of low-risk metastatic gestational trophoblastic tumors. *J Reprod Med.* 1991;36(1):36-39.

85. Escobar PF, Lurain JR, Singh DK, Bozorgi K, Fishman DA. Treatment of high-risk gestational trophoblastic neoplasia with etoposide, methotrexate, actinomycin D, cyclophosphamide, and vincristine chemotherapy. *Gynecol Oncol.* 2003;91(3):552-557.

86. Lu WG, Ye F, Shen YM, et al. EMA-CO chemotherapy for high-risk gestational trophoblastic neoplasia: a clinical analysis of 54 patients. *Int J Gynecol Cancer.* 2008;18(2):357-362.

87. Lurain JR, Singh DK, Schink JC. Primary treatment of metastatic high-risk gestational trophoblastic neoplasia with EMA-CO chemotherapy. *J Reprod Med.* 2006;51(10):767-772.

88. Matsui H, Suzuka K, Iitsuka Y, Seki K, Sekiya S. Combination chemotherapy with methotrexate, etoposide, and actinomycin D for high-risk gestational trophoblastic tumors. *Gynecol Oncol.* 2000;78(1):28-31.

89. Turan T, Karacay O, Tulunay G, et al. Results with EMA/CO (etoposide, methotrexate, actinomycin D, cyclophosphamide, vincristine) chemotherapy in gestational trophoblastic neoplasia. *Int J Gynecol Cancer.* 2006;16(3):1432-1438.

90. Newlands ES, Holden L, Seckl MJ, McNeish I, Strickland S, Rustin GJ. Management of brain metastases in patients with high-risk gestational trophoblastic tumors. *J Reprod Med.* 2002;47(6):465-471.

91. Alazzam M, Hancock BW, Tidy J. Role of hysterectomy in managing persistent gestational trophoblastic disease. *J Reprod Med.* 2008;53(7):519-524.

92. Fleming EL, Garrett L, Growdon WB, et al. The changing role of thoracotomy in gestational trophoblastic neoplasia at the New England Trophoblastic Disease Center. *J Reprod Med.* 2008;53(7):493-498.

93. Lurain JR, Singh DK, Schink JC. Role of surgery in the management of high-risk gestational trophoblastic neoplasia. *J Reprod Med.* 2006;51(10):773-776.

94. Feng F, Xiang Y. Surgical management of chemotherapy-resistant gestational trophoblastic neoplasia. *Expert Rev Anticancer Ther.* 2010;10(1):71-80.

95. Yang J, Xiang Y, Wan X, Yang X. Recurrent gestational trophoblastic tumor: management and risk factors for recurrence. *Gynecol Oncol.* 2006;103(2):587-590.

96. Powles T, Savage PM, Stebbing J, et al. A comparison of patients with relapsed and chemo-refractory gestational trophoblastic neoplasia. *Br J Cancer.* 2007;96(5):732-737.

97. Newlands ES, Mulholland PJ, Holden L, Seckl MJ, Rustin GJ. Etoposide and cisplatin/etoposide, methotrexate, and actinomycin D (EMA) chemotherapy for patients with high-risk gestational trophoblastic tumors refractory to EMA/cyclophosphamide and vincristine chemotherapy and patients presenting with metastatic placental site trophoblastic tumors. *J Clin Oncol.* 2000;18(4):854-859.

98. Mao Y, Wan X, Lv W, Xie X. Relapsed or refractory gestational trophoblastic neoplasia treated with the etoposide and cisplatin/etoposide, methotrexate, and actinomycin D (EP-EMA) regimen. *Int J Gynaecol Obstet.* 2007;98(1):44-47.

99. Lurain JR, Nejad B. Secondary chemotherapy for high-risk gestational trophoblastic neoplasia. *Gynecol Oncol.* 2005;97(2):618-623.

100. Wang J, Short D, Sebire NJ, et al. Salvage chemotherapy of relapsed or high-risk gestational trophoblastic neoplasia (GTN) with paclitaxel/cisplatin alternating with paclitaxel/etoposide (TP/TE). *Ann Oncol.* 2008;19(9):1578-1583.

101. Hassadia A, Gillespie A, Tidy J, et al. Placental site trophoblastic tumour: clinical features and management. *Gynecol Oncol.* 2005;99(3):603-607.

102. Papadopoulos AJ, Foskett M, Seckl MJ, et al. Twenty-five years' clinical experience with placental site trophoblastic tumors. *J Reprod Med.* 2002;47(6):460-464.

103. Berry E, Lurain, JR. Gestational trophoblastic diseases. In: Raghavan D, Brecher ML, Johnson DH, Meropol NJ, Moots PL, Rose PG, eds. *Textbook of Uncommon Cancer.* 3rd ed. Hoboken, NJ: John Wiley & Sons; 2006.

104. Woolas RP, Bower M, Newlands ES, Seckl M, Short D, Holden L. Influence of chemotherapy for gestational trophoblastic disease on subsequent pregnancy outcome. *Br J Obstet Gynaecol.* 1998;105(9):1032-1035.

105. Matsui H, Iitsuka Y, Suzuka K, et al. Early pregnancy outcomes after chemotherapy for gestational trophoblastic tumor. *J Reprod Med.* 2004;49(7):531-534.

106. Rustin GJ, Newlands ES, Lutz JM, et al. Combination but not single-agent methotrexate chemotherapy for gestational trophoblastic tumors increases the incidence of second tumors. *J Clin Oncol.* 1996;14(10):2769-2773.

107. Hancock BW. hCG measurement in gestational trophoblastic neoplasia: a critical appraisal. *J Reprod Med.* 2006;51(11):859-860.

108. Cole LA, Butler SA, Khanlian SA, et al. Gestational trophoblastic diseases: 2. Hyperglycosylated hCG as a reliable marker of active neoplasia. *Gynecol Oncol.* 2006;102(2):151-159.

109. Khanlian SA, Cole LA. Management of gestational trophoblastic disease and other cases with low serum levels of human chorionic gonadotropin. *J Reprod Med.* 2006;51(10):812-818.

110. Sebire NJ, Foskett M, Paradinas FJ, et al. Outcome of twin pregnancies with complete hydatidiform mole and healthy co-twin. *Lancet.* 2002;359(9324):2165-2166.

111. Matsui H, Sekiya S, Hando T, Wake N, Tomoda Y. Hydatidiform mole coexistent with a twin live fetus: a national collaborative study in Japan. *Hum Reprod.* 2000;15(3):608-611.

9 Vulvar Cancer

Mark Milam and Charles F. Levenback

Vulvar cancers are among the least common gynecologic malignancies. Radical surgery is the primary approach for most patients, and advances in neoadjuvant chemotherapy and radiation may decrease operative morbidity in those patients with locally advanced disease. This chapter focuses on the diagnosis and management of vulvar cancer, with special emphasis on changes in staging and sentinel lymph node biopsy (SLNB). Due to the recent modifications in International Federation of Gynecology and Obstetrics (FIGO) staging, the reported outcomes in this chapter reflect the older staging criteria.

EPIDEMIOLOGY

Key Points

1. Vulvar cancer is the fourth most common gynecologic malignancy, with approximately 3900 diagnoses in 2010.
2. Prevention strategies for cervical dysplasia using the human papillomavirus (HPV) vaccine may decrease the incidence of vulvar dysplasia and vulvar carcinoma.
3. The median age of patients with vulvar cancer is 68 years of age, with approximately 1 in 387 women at risk for a vulvar cancer diagnosis during their lifetime.
4. Risk factors for invasive vulvar cancer depend on age of diagnosis and may include HPV infection, smoking, immunosuppression, and potentially lichen sclerosis.

Vulvar cancer is the fourth most common gynecologic malignancy in the United States, with approximately 3900 diagnoses in 2010.[1] The incidence of this disease increases with age and peaks in the seventh decade of life. The majority of vulvar cancers are of squamous histology, and many develop from progressively worsening dysplastic conditions known as *vulvar intraepithelial neoplasia* (VIN).

In the United States, the demographic characteristics of the 12 areas associated with the Surveillance, Epidemiology, and End Results (SEER) study demonstrate that the median age for patients with a diagnosis of vulvar cancer is 68 years.[2] Only 26.6% of patients have a diagnosis at age younger than 55 years, with most women being in their 60s and 70s at diagnosis.[2] Recently, Kumar and colleagues[3] observed that approximately 19% of women who have a diagnosis of vulvar cancer are younger than 50 years. These women appear to have an overall better prognosis because their tumors are characterized by lower stage and superficial invasion.

Vulvar cancer may arise through 2 distinct pathways, each with its respective risk factors. The first is characterized by nonkeratinizing carcinomas and is more commonly diagnosed in younger women with VIN and concurrent HPV infection. The second pathway results in keratinizing, well-differentiated carcinomas; these are more frequently diagnosed in older women with a background of vulvar dystrophies such as lichen sclerosus. HPV infection is rarely identified in these women.

HPV infection remains a significant risk factor for the development of vulvar dysplasia and subsequent malignant transformation in the first type of invasive vulvar carcinoma.[4] Recent advances in immunization may decrease the incidence of VIN and vulvar cancer through prevention of HPV infection. A recent 4-year trial has demonstrated the benefit of the prophylactic HPV quadrivalent vaccine against low-grade vulvar lesions. These data indicate an efficacy of approximately 100% for vulvar epithelial lesions specifically associated with HPV subtypes 6, 11, 16, and 18 and an efficacy of approximately 75% for vulvar epithelial lesions associated with any HPV type.[5] In the future, the current HPV vaccinations may reduce the overall burden of vulvar cancer. Because there is a prolonged interval between HPV infection and clinical manifestation of vulvar disease, it can potentially be decades before the clinical impact of HPV vaccination is fully appreciated.

Additional risk factors for the development of vulvar cancer include smoking, immunosuppression, and potentially lichen sclerosis. Tobacco smoking in particular promotes carcinogenesis in HPV-associated disease.[6] Immunosuppression is a risk factor likely due to HPV infection and persistence; women with human immunodeficiency virus infection, for example, have an increased incidence of vulvar cancers.[7] Finally, lichen sclerosis is a benign chronic inflammatory vulvar lesion that is associated with vulvar cancer, especially in older women. A causative relationship between lichen sclerosis and invasive vulvar cancer remains controversial, although recent evidence suggests that inactivation of the *p53* tumor suppressor gene in these lesions promotes progression to malignancy.[8]

DIAGNOSIS

Key Points

1. Vulvar cancer often presents with a pruritic or painful lesion.
2. Early biopsy of suspicious vulvar lesions is critical to diagnosis of malignant disease.
3. Clinical features of vulvar cancer are variable, and clinicians should have low thresholds to recommend biopsy of concerning lesions.
4. Physical examination of lymph nodes to determine metastatic disease is unreliable.

Early biopsy of suspicious vulvar lesions is critical to the diagnosis of vulvar cancer. Patients who present with concerns of pruritic or painful vulvar conditions should be evaluated for the possibility of vulvar cancer with a complete pelvic examination and office biopsy. Postmenopausal women who report pruritic vulvar pain that does not resolve with conservative measures

are of special concern, as such symptoms may be an early sign of vulvar cancer. Vulvar cancer is a rare disease; hence patients and clinicians may not be aware of the possibility of development of this tumor, and treatment delay is possible. Reluctance in reporting gynecologic symptoms to clinicians may also make it difficult to articulate concern and lead some women to minimize their symptoms.

The clinician must consider several differential diagnoses when women present with a chief complaint of vulvar pruritus. These are often separated into acute and chronic conditions: Acute conditions may involve infectious processes and possible contact dermatitis; chronic conditions may involve dermatoses, including lichen sclerosis and general atrophy, and also HPV infections.[9] The vulvar manifestation of systemic disease is possible, including but not limited to Crohn disease and other autoimmune conditions[9] (Table 9-1).

It must be underscored that the liberal use of biopsies when evaluating a concerning vulvar lesion will afford definitive pathologic identification of a benign or malignant etiology. Early diagnosis of a small vulvar cancer can result in a less aggressive surgical procedure, with minimal morbidity and decreased risk for potential adjuvant therapy (Figure 9-1). Conversely, a prolonged

Table 9-1 Differential Diagnoses of Pruritic Vulvar Conditions

Acute
Contact dermatitis (allergic or irritant)
Infections
Vulvovaginal candidiasis
Trichomoniasis
Molluscum contagiosum
Scabies and/or pediculosis
Chronic
Dermatoses
Atopic and contact dermatitis
Lichen sclerosis, lichen planus, lichen simplex chronicus
Psoriasis
Genital atrophy
Neoplasia
Vulvar intraepithelial neoplasia or vulvar cancer
Paget disease
Infection
Human papillomavirus infection
Vulvar manifestations of systemic disease
Crohn disease
Diabetes
Human immunodeficiency virus

Modified from ACOG Practice Bulletin No. 93: diagnosis and management of vulvar skin disorders. *Obstet Gynecol.* 2008;111:1243-1253.

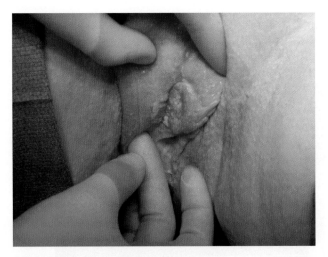

FIGURE 9-1. Early-stage vulvar cancer.

delay in diagnosis may lead to advancing stage of disease, with more extensive and radical surgical intervention and the potential need for adjuvant radiation therapy and potential chemotherapy (Figure 9-2). Rectal or urinary bleeding is suggestive of tumor involvement of the colorectal and/or urinary system, and such metastases will influence the treatment plan and lead to consideration of neoadjuvant chemotherapy and surgery for curative attempts.

The majority of vulvar cancer diagnoses appear to be localized without regional lymph node involvement. SEER data indicate that approximately 61% of all vulvar cancers are confined to the vulva without metastases to the inguinal-femoral lymph node basins.[2] Lymph node metastasis confers worse prognosis, and therefore clear knowledge of nodal metastatic disease is critical for treatment planning. Physical examination of the inguinal/femoral nodes alone is poorly sensitive for the detection of metastases and should not be used

as criteria for evaluation of patients with a known diagnosis of vulvar cancer.[10]

Imaging may assist in the preoperative diagnosis of metastatic disease to the regional lymph nodes and is more sensitive than physical examination and palpation alone. These modalities include computed tomography (CT), magnetic resonance imaging (MRI), positron emission tomography (PET),[11] and lymphoscintigraphy[12] (Figure 9-3). In general, MRI affords superior evaluation of soft tissues, and contrast-enhanced MRI techniques in particular provide improved visualization of lymph node involvement.[13] PET testing, fused with CT images, can also identify potential metastatic lesions in the inguinal-femoral lymph nodes; limitations include potential false-positive findings due to inflammatory processes, with potential inappropriate adjuvant therapy if confirmatory lymphatic dissection is not performed.[11] It is important to note that neither the 1988 nor 2009 FIGO staging criteria for vulvar cancer allow inclusion of preoperative imaging results.

PATHOLOGY

Key Points

1. Squamous cell carcinoma is the most common histology in vulvar cancers, followed by melanoma and adenocarcinoma.
2. Depth of invasion is measured from the epithelial stromal junction of the most superficial dermal papillae to the deepest point of invasion.
3. FIGO staging has changed to reflect metastatic spread patterns that emphasize the prognostic significance of the number and morphology of nodal metastases.

The most common vulvar cancer is squamous cell (approximately 83% of diagnoses), followed by adenocarcinoma (8% of diagnoses), and melanoma (6%).[2,3,14,15] Most vulvar cancers arise from the squamous epithelium of the labia majora and minora, clitoris, or the anterior and posterior fourchette. These areas are characterized by a junction between the keratinized stratified squamous epithelium and the nonkeratinized squamous mucosa of the vagina. Frequently, invasive squamous cell carcinomas of the vulva have adjacent VIN or lichen sclerosis.

Squamous cell carcinomas of the vulva may metastasize via several routes: local expansion, with extension into adjacent tissues; lymphatic spread to the regional nodal tissues; and hematogenous metastases to distant sites. These patterns of metastases are reflected in the 2009 revised FIGO staging for vulvar carcinoma (Table 9-2). Local growth may involve extension of carcinoma to

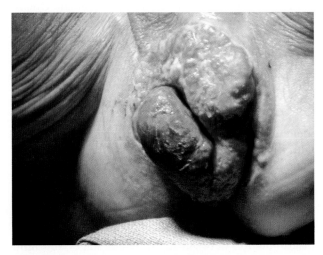

FIGURE 9-2. Late-stage vulvar cancer.

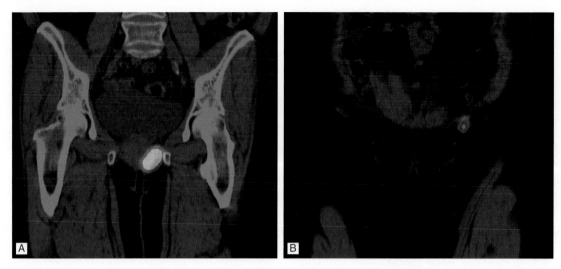

FIGURE 9-3. Metastatic disease demonstrated in preoperative lymphoscintigraphy.

Table 9-2 Revised FIGO Surgical Staging Criteria for Carcinoma of the Vulva[17]

Stage I: Tumor confined to the vulva
IA Lesions ≤2 cm in size, confined to the vulva or perineum and with stromal invasion ≤1.0 mm,[a] no nodal metastasis
IB Lesions >2 cm in size or with stromal invasion >1.0 mm,[a] confined to the vulva or perineum, with negative nodes

Stage II: Tumor of any size with extension to adjacent perineal structures (1/3 lower urethra, 1/3 lower vagina, anus) with negative nodes

Stage III: Tumor of any size with or without extension to adjacent perineal structures (1/3 lower urethra, 1/3 lower vagina, anus) with positive inguinofemoral lymph nodes
IIIA (i) With 1 lymph node metastasis (≥5 mm), or
     (ii) 1-2 lymph node metastasis(es) (<5 mm)
IIIB (i) With ≥2 lymph node metastases (≥5 mm), or
     (ii) ≥3 lymph node metastases (<5 mm)
IIIC With positive nodes with extracapsular spread

Stage IV: Tumor invades other regional (2/3 upper urethra, 2/3 upper vagina), or distant structures
IVA Tumor invades any of the following:
(i) upper urethral and/or vaginal mucosa, bladder mucosa, rectal mucosa, or fixed to pelvic bone, or (ii) fixed or ulcerated inguinofemoral lymph nodes
IVB Any distant metastasis, including pelvic lymph nodes

[a]The depth of invasion is defined as the measurement of the tumor from the epithelial-stromal junction of the adjacent most superficial dermal papilla to the deepest point of invasion.
Reprinted from International Journal of Gynecology & Obstetrics, Vol 105, Iss 2, Pecorelli S, Pecorelli S. Revised FIGO staging for carcinoma of the vulva, cervix, and endometrium. © 2009, with permission from Elsevier.

the urethra, vagina, and anus. Lymphatic embolization occurs first to the regional inguinal-femoral lymph nodes in the groin; further spread to the pelvic and/ or para-aortic lymph nodes is considered as a distant metastasis. Finally, hematogenous dissemination to lung, bone, or liver is uncommon with initial presentation and may be observed with recurrent disease.

The revised staging criteria reflects several modifications over the initial surgical staging system proposed by the FIGO Committee on Gynecologic Oncology in 1988 (Table 9-3). The 1988 criteria changed the staging system from clinical to surgical to better reflect the prognostic significance of metastatic regional lymph nodes. However, this staging system included several heterogeneous populations within stage III. For example, patients were included with small tumors involving the vagina or urethra (but with negative nodes), as were patients with small primary tumors and 1 positive lymph node, and patients with large primary tumors with 2 positive lymph nodes; in a Gynecologic Oncology Group study, survival of these 3 groups ranged from 100%, 95%, and 34%.[16] Furthermore, survival is dramatically worse for patients with increasing number and size of metastatic lymph nodes, as well as for those with extracapsular spread.

To better reflect the prognostic significance of these findings, the 2009 criteria has expanded stage III to include 3 subcategories. Stage IIIA includes patients with 1 lymph node metastasis (≥5 mm) or 1 to 2 lymph node metastases (<5 mm). Stage IIIB includes patients with ≥2 lymph node metastases (≥5 mm) or ≥3 lymph node metastases (<5 mm). Stage IIIC includes those patients with positive nodes with extracapsular spread. The revised criteria should afford improved prognostic discrimination between the different stages and limit the heterogeneity in regards to survival within stages.

Table 9-3 1988 Surgical Staging Criteria for Carcinoma of the Vulva[17]

Stage I: Tumor confined to the vulva
IA Lesions ≤2 cm in size, confined to the vulva or perineum and with stromal invasion ≤1.0 mm,[a] no nodal metastasis
IB Lesions >2 cm in size or with stromal invasion >1.0 mm,[a] confined to the vulva or perineum, with negative nodes

Stage II: Tumor more than 2 cm in greatest dimension confined to the vulva and/or perineum with negative nodes

Stage III: Tumor of any size with or without extension to adjacent perineal structures (1/3 lower urethra, 1/3 lower vagina, anus) or with positive unilateral inguinofemoral lymph nodes

Stage IV: Tumor invades other regional (2/3 upper urethra, 2/3 upper vagina), or distant structures
IVA Tumor invades any of the following:
(i) upper urethral and/or vaginal mucosa, bladder mucosa, rectal mucosa, or fixed to pelvic bone, and/or bilateral regional lymph node involvement
IVB Any distant metastasis including pelvic lymph nodes

[a]The depth of invasion is defined as the measurement of the tumor from the epithelial-stromal junction of the adjacent most superficial dermal papilla to the deepest point of invasion.

Several studies have demonstrated the prognostic significance of the depth of invasion and lymphvascular space invasion in predicting the risk of nodal metastasis. Pathologists must apply strict criteria for assessment of the depth of invasion for all patients diagnosed with vulvar cancer; this includes measurement from the epithelial-stromal junction of the most superficial dermal papilla to the deepest point of invasion.[17]

The prospective Gynecologic Oncology Group (GOG) protocol that evaluated 637 patients with vulvar cancer found on multivariate analysis that factors involved in the risk for lymphatic metastasis in squamous cell vulvar tumors include lymphvascular space invasion (LVSI) and patient age (Table 9-4).[10] They also reported that clinically fixed nodes and utilization of 5-step GOG criteria on grading were associated with nodal metastasis as well. The reproducibility of some of these clinicopathologic risk factors makes tumor depth of invasion and tumor size among the more utilized factors in evaluating the potential risk for nodal metastasis. Grading systems based on 3-tier criteria are not necessarily predictive of nodal metastasis, and LVSI is limited in the tumor beds, with only a small percentage of tumors identified with LVSI.[10,18] This underscores the importance of using pathologists either formally trained or with a background in gynecologic pathology for review of these specimens.

Ultrastaging of lymph node tissue to detect microscopic disease in lymph nodes has demonstrated an increased detection rate for metastatic disease in cervical cancer and may play a role in vulvar cancer.[19] Caution must be advised, however, as some of these identified metastatic lesions may consist of microscopic disease (one report consisted of a single cell in the lymph node), and the clinical outcome may not be clear.[19] Current management of patients identified with this technique is the same as for those with a positive lymph node by conventional techniques until further data are available.

TREATMENT

Key Points

1. Primary treatment of vulvar cancer involves radical surgery to excise the primary lesion with a clinical margin of 1 to 2 cm.
2. Microinvasive, or stage IA, vulvar cancers have a low risk of nodal metastases and may be managed with radical surgical excision alone.

Table 9-4 Risk Factors for Groin Node Metastasis in Squamous Vulvar Carcinoma[10]

Depth of Invasion (mm)	Groin Node Metastasis (%)	Tumor Grade	Groin Node Metastasis (%)	Lymphvascular Space Invasion	Groin Node Metastasis (%)
≤1	2.8	1 (Well)	26.8	Positive	75.0
2	8.9	2 (Moderate)	36.1	Negative	27.4
3	18.6	3 (Poor)	54.8	n/a	-----
4	30.9	n/a	-----	n/a	-----
5	33.3	n/a	-----	n/a	-----
≥5	47.9	n/a	-----	n/a	-----

Modified from Homesley HD, Bundy BN, Sedlis A, et al. Prognostic factors for groin node metastasis in squamous cell carcinoma of the vulva (a Gynecologic Oncology Group study). *Gynecol Oncol.* 1993;49(3):279-283.

3. Ipsilateral inguinal-femoral lymphadenectomy is recommended for all invasive squamous cell vulvar cancers; bilateral inguinal-femoral lymphadenectomy is recommended for patients with lesions less than 2 cm from the midline, with clinically suspicious inguinal lymph nodes, and with positive ipsilateral nodes.

4. Sentinel lymph node biopsies (SLNB) may identify lymph node–positive patients who require additional treatment and lymph node–negative patients who do not require full inguinal-femoral lymphadenectomy.

Treatment of Microinvasive Disease

Stage IA vulvar cancers are characterized by small primary tumors less than 2 cm in size, with clinically negative inguinal/femoral lymph nodes, and with the depth of invasion ≤1.0 mm. Similar to the microinvasive stage IA1 disease of cervical squamous cell cancers, the risk of nodal metastases is minimal, and patients may undergo radical local excision of the primary lesion with 1-cm clinical margins at the time of resection. Inguinal-femoral lymphadenectomy is not indicated for these very low-risk patients.

Treatment of Early-Stage Disease

Surgery is the primary approach for patients with vulvar cancers that do not demonstrate extension to adjacent perineal structures. Depending on the size of the primary tumor, patients may undergo total radical vulvectomy, partial radical vulvectomy, or radical local excision. As opposed to a skinning or simple vulvectomy, the radical nature of this procedure involves excision of the lesion with 1- to 2-cm clinical margins at the time of resection and dissection down to the level of the perineal membrane (previously considered as the deep fascia of the urogenital diaphragm).[20] Resection of the regional inguinal and femoral lymph nodes is also indicated, both for prognostic reasons and adjuvant treatment planning. Patients may undergo ipsilateral inguinal-femoral lymphadenectomy if lesions are of squamous histology; the primary tumor is well lateralized and less than 2 cm in diameter, both groins are clinically negative for metastases, and the ipsilateral groin is pathologically negative for metastases.[21]

Historically, this surgical excision has evolved from a butterfly-shaped resection (removing the vulva, the inguinal and femoral lymph nodes, and the intervening skin and lymphatics in between). Application of 3 incisions has significantly improved morbidity and mortality from this procedure without a cost in survivorship. Attempts to reduce the extent of groin dissection, however, were abandoned when unexpected fatal

recurrences in the groin occurred.[22,23] Historic GOG data suggest that the risk of groin relapse after a radical en bloc dissection of the groin that included skeletonization of the femoral artery and vein and sartorius muscle transposition was less than 1%.[24] In GOG-74, the relapse rate after negative superficial inguinal lymphadenectomy in a very-low-risk patient population was more than 7%. These groin relapses, even when they appear to be detected early, are difficult to treat and are associated with a high mortality rate.

To minimize the morbidity of complete inguinal-femoral lymphadenectomy without a cost in survival, several investigators defined lymphatic drainage patterns with injections of various compounds into the vulva.[25,26] In 1992, the modern sentinel lymph node biopsy (SLNB) technique was described by Morton and colleagues[27] as an alternative to regional lymphadenectomy for patients with cutaneous melanoma. This technique was easily applied to vulvar cancer patients, as the tumor is easy to inject and the lymphatic drainage is predictably to the groin.[28] Multiple single-institution series confirmed the general concept of SLNB in vulvar cancer patients[29] (Table 9-5).

Two recent multi-institution trials suggest that SLNB is an alternative to lymphadenectomy for selected patients with vulvar cancer. The first trial was a collaboration of Dutch investigators led by Van der Zee,[30] who reported the results of the GROinigen International Sentinel Node for Vulvar Cancer trial. This trial had an observational design in which eligible patients with invasive vulvar cancer limited to the vulva and up to 4 cm in diameter were treated with SLNB and resection of the primary tumor. If the sentinel lymph node result was negative, the patients were observed every 2 months for signs of relapse. Of the 403 patients enrolled, 296 were sentinel lymph node negative and were observed. The relapse rate was 3%, within the predetermined statistically acceptable outcome range. Exclusion of patients with multifocal tumors would have reduced the relapse rate to just over 2%. The outcomes for the 8 patients with relapse were poor; however, the overall survival at 3 years was 97% with decreased perioperative morbidity, including lymphedema and wound breakdown, among the SLNB-only patients as compared with the node-positive patients who underwent lymphadenectomy.[30]

The second multi-institutional trial was conducted by the GOG and the study, GOG-173, has been presented in abstract form. This trial enrolled more than 500 patients who had invasive squamous carcinoma 2 to 6 cm in diameter limited to the vulva. The patients underwent SLNB followed by unilateral or bilateral lymphadenectomy depending on the location of the primary tumor. The success of sentinel lymph node identification was improved dramatically by the use of radiocolloid in addition to blue dye. There were 131

Table 9-5 Levenback and GROINS-V Table[30,31]

	GROINS-V	GOG 173
Tumor size	T1 or T2 <4 cm	T2 (2-6 cm)
Mapping technique	Combined	Initially blue dye, combined
Centers	15	47
Skill verification	10 cases	None
Cases/center (median)	21	6
Primary end point	Failure at 2 years (<8%)	SN: ≥88%, false-negative predictive value <5%
Strategy	Only SLN-positive patients undergo inguinal femoral lymph node dissection	All patients undergo SLN, then inguinal femoral lymph node dissection
False-negative rate	8/135 patients (6%)	Tumors <4 cm: 6% (10% overall)[a]
False-negative predictive value	8/276 patients (3%)	Tumors <4 cm: 2.5% (4% overall)[a]

SLN, sentinel lymph node.
[a]Two hundred seventy of the evaluable patients had tumors of less than 4.0 cm in diameter, and the remainder had tumors ≥4.0 cm in size. Thirty-one percent of the patients had lymph node metastases, consistent with the projected rate. The rate of lymph node metastasis was 26% in patients with smaller tumors and 40% in patients with larger tumors.

lymph node–positive patients. The sensitivity and false-negative predictive value in the study group met the predetermined statistical targets, with a sensitivity of approximately 90% and a false-negative predictive value of less than 5%. The false-negative predictive value is the statistical estimate of a false-negative sentinel lymph node when the status of the remaining lymph nodes is not known. Among the patients with tumors less than 4 cm, the false-negative predictive value was less than 3%.[31]

Implementation of SLNB strategy involves teamwork and communication between the gynecologic oncologist, diagnostic radiologist, pathologist, radiation oncologist, and patient. Case selection for best outcome is a patient with a unifocal tumor, less than 4 cm in size, without a history of prior radiotherapy or groin surgery (although prior wide local excision for diagnosis is acceptable). Patients with gross involvement of a lymph node on physical examination or imaging are not considered optimal candidates for SLNB due to alterations in lymphatic drainage. In fact, a solitary grossly involved lymph node is presumed to be the sentinel node, the first site of metastatic disease.

Candidates for SLNB may benefit from preoperative lymphoscintigraphy, which may help guide decisions regarding when to perform unilateral or bilateral groin dissection. Patients with direct tumor involvement of midline structures should have surgical evaluation of both groins, even if a sentinel lymph node is not imaged in one or both of the groins. If the tumor is close to but not involving the midline, and there is ipsilateral unilateral lymphatic drainage on the lymphoscintigram, then unilateral surgical groin evaluation is acceptable. Limitations of this technique include the potential use of painful injections with limited utility in a patient before any surgical intervention; recent data have suggested that use of perioperative Lymphazurin blue dye and technetium-99 during lymphatic mapping negates the need for this imaging technique.[12]

In the operating room, the radioactive tracer is injected intradermally before the patient is prepped, approximately 20 to 30 minutes before groin incision. The blue dye, which is a smaller molecule and travels more rapidly from the injection site to the lymph node than the radiocolloid, is injected after the patient is prepped and draped. It takes approximately 5 minutes for the blue dye to reach the sentinel lymph node. A single groin might have more than 1 sentinel lymph node, and therefore special care must be taken to ensure that all nodes that take up the blue dye or radiocolloid are removed. If a sentinel lymph node is not found, then lymphadenectomy should be performed.

Sentinel lymph nodes are then subjected to pathologic ultrastaging.[32,33] The gross specimen is subjected to serial sectioning and routine hematoxylin and eosin examination. If no metastases are found, then deeper levels are subjected to cytokeratin immunohistochemical staining. Identification of metastatic disease increases

20% to 40% with this analysis.[19,30] A prospective study of 723 sentinel lymph nodes with metastatic disease found that increased size was associated with poorer disease-specific survival (88% for patients with ≤2 mm in size vs. 70% with 2-5 mm in size vs. 69% for >5 mm in size; $P < .01$).[33] Identification of those patients with micrometastatic disease is important for further treatment and also for identifying patients at risk for recurrence. In other disease sites, especially breast cancer, there are patients with micrometastases who may be treated the same as for lymph node–negative patients. With the current fund of knowledge, all patients with micrometastases in a sentinel lymph node should be considered as having metastatic disease and as candidates for further treatment, including lymphadenectomy or possibly radiotherapy.

Treatment of Advanced Disease

Patients with advanced disease with involvement and encroachment of the urethra and rectum may benefit from neoadjuvant chemotherapy and/or radiation. Preoperative radiotherapy may also benefit patients who would otherwise require a pelvic exenteration; shrinkage of the primary tumor may lead to preservation of bowel and bladder functions before more conservative surgical intervention.[34] A combination of chemoradiation in a phase II study by the GOG evaluated this modality in patients with stage III to IV vulvar cancer before surgical intervention; they demonstrated that even in advanced-stage disease, bowel and bladder function can be preserved (2 of 71 patients or 2.8% had residual unresectable disease).[35]

A candid conversation with patients, regardless of age, before surgical intervention should include complete disclosure of unique risks and benefits. It is important to emphasize that besides the usual risks of bleeding, infection, and damage to bowel and bladder, patients must be made aware of the potential impact on sexuality and sexual function. Pretreatment counseling and decision making are critical to patients, especially younger patients who are diagnosed with vulvar cancer, as this dissection and excision may be viewed as a cosmetically mutilating procedure that may change patients' view of self, result in loss of sexual function, and may change the way that they interact with their sexual partner.[36]

Treatment of Metastatic Lymph Nodes

Groin radiation is recommended for those patients with a positive nodal metastasis, with or without a formal full inguinal-femoral node dissection. Patients who undergo this treatment may have issues with vaginal and perivaginal dryness. Hormone replacement therapy for these patients with vaginal dryness with emphasis on quality of life and sexual function is not contraindicated with squamous cell carcinomas treated with surgery and radiation.[37] Certainly, patients who require radiation after surgical resection may undergo early ovarian failure and are candidates for hormone replacement therapy. There is no contraindication for short-term hormone replacement therapy in patients with a history of vulvar cancer.

Treatment of Poor Surgical Candidates

Neoadjuvant chemoradiation may be considered for medically infirm patients, with the potential for decreased morbidity with extensive resection. Patients who have extensive medical issues including diabetes and poor functional status, chronic steroid use with a decrease in functional ability, and concern for bowel and bladder function may need a tailored approach that focuses on treatment cure and on limiting surgical and treatment morbidity.

Further treatment summaries are listed in the treatment box in Figure 9-4, and these underscore the importance of tailored treatment plans based on the patient's clinical presentation. The important point is the potential of decreased lymph node dissection in patients with smaller tumors and with imaging/examination suggesting no lymph node involvement. Patients with positive lymph nodes (either by the traditional lymph node dissection or by SLNB) require further treatment (regardless or tumor size), until further data are available.[33]

SURVIVAL AND PROGNOSIS

Key Points

1. The 5-year median survival of women with vulvar cancer (all histologies included) is approximately 76%.
2. Lymph node metastases remain the most significant prognostic factor in vulvar cancer. Patient age and tumor histology are also predictive of survivorship in vulvar cancer.

In general, survival rates for women with early-stage squamous cell carcinomas of the vulva are excellent, with 5-year survivorship of 80% to 90% for patients with stage I and II disease. Reflecting the significance of nodal metastases as a prognostic factor, patients with stage III disease, categorized by the 1988 FIGO criteria, demonstrate a 55% survival rate at 5 years, and those with stage IV disease are only at 28% (Table 9-6).[15] As discussed previously, the range of survival within stage III disease (per the 1998 criteria) is between 34% and 100%, and prospective application of the 2009 revised

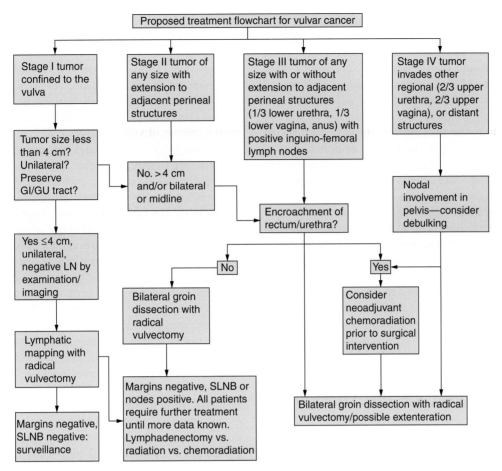

FIGURE 9-4. Flowchart for management (lymphatic mapping with both radioactive tracer and blue dye). T1, ≤1.0 mm, a, without ulceration; T1 b, with ulceration or level IV or V; T2, 1.01 ro 2.0 mm, a, without ulceration; T2 b, with ulceration; T3, 2.01 to 4.0 mm, a, without ulceration; T3 b, with ulceration; T4, >4.0 mm, a, without ulceration; T4 b, with ulceration.

staging criteria should limit the significant heterogeneity observed with the prior system.

In addition to stage, survival in this disease is associated with several additional prognostic features, including patient age and tumor histology. Patients with a diagnosis of vulvar cancer at a younger age have improved survival, with 5-year survival rates of 87.5% for younger women and 52.5% for older women.[3] Older patients have also been demonstrated to have more advanced disease and risk for nodal metastasis; although age is not factored into the staging criteria, it should be considered during patient evaluation.[10,38]

Table 9-6 Five-Year Survival Based on Histology: Modified From SEER Survival Monograph[15]

	Total 5-Year Survival (%)	Stage I (%)	Stage II (%)	Stage III (%)	Stage IV (%)
Squamous (not otherwise specified)	73.7	91.5	77.8	54.7	27.6
Squamous, keratinizing	60.2	82.7	64.4	43.7	23.9
Basal cell	99.4	100.0	97.7	a	a
Melanoma	58.9	83.0	64.3	35.1	a

[a]Percentages are not displayed due to fewer than 25 cases.
Reproduced, with permission, from Kosary CotVilagr C, Young JL, Keel GE, Eisner MP, Lin YD, Horner MJ. SEER Survival Monograph: Cancer Survival Among Adults: US SEER Program 1998-2001, Patient and Tumor Characteristics. Bethesda, MD: National Cancer Institute; 2007.

Tumor histology is also associated with improved survival, with women with vulvar adenocarcinoma having improved 5-year survival rates compared with women with squamous and melanoma vulvar tumors[15] (Table 9-6). As discussed later, vulvar adenocarcinomas are typically indolent in nature and have a decreased risk of advanced lymphatic spread. Melanomas are on the opposite side of the spectrum, with increased risk of metastatic disease despite pathologic evidence of local disease status. This is part of the reason that, based on histology, survival patterns favor adenocarcinoma, followed by squamous tumors, with melanoma having the worst prognosis.[2,3,14,15]

Groin relapse has been demonstrated to have a high mortality rate; patients with a potential for treatment with salvage therapy are often detected early. In the GROINS-V study, patients were followed every 2 months,[30,33] with a reported higher mortality rate in patients with recurrence. At this time, we recommend surveillance every 2 to 3 months with use of imaging modalities based on clinical history, including ultrasound, CT, or MRI.

MANAGEMENT OF RECURRENT DISEASE

Key Points

1. Local recurrence on the vulva may be successfully salvaged surgically with re-excision.
2. Recurrences in the groin are almost uniformly fatal, and chemotherapy remains only palliative.
3. Nonresectable recurrences should include local wound care to address potential erosive disease.

After completion of primary therapy, patients with vulvar cancer should be followed closely, with visits every 3 months for the first 2 to 3 years. These visits should include a detailed history and physical examination, including evaluation of the groin nodes and the vulva, pelvis, and rectum. Visits may be extended to 6-month intervals until 5 years after therapy, when patients may then be seen on an annual basis. If recurrence is suspected on the basis on symptoms or physical findings, biopsy and imaging (using CT, PET, or MRI) should be used. The application of routine imaging in vulvar cancer is not well established, but MRI in particular may have a role in postoperative imaging of this disease.[13]

In the event of recurrence, a detailed evaluation is necessary to characterize the extent of disease. Recurrences may be categorized as local (in the vulva alone), groin (in the inguinal-femoral lymph nodes), or distant (lung, liver, and/or brain). For local recurrences, surgery can be associated with a high morbidity, but can result in cure. Up to 75% of all patients with recurrence limited to the vulva may be successfully treated with salvaged therapy that includes radical wide excision; absence of carcinoma at the margins of resection are predictive of long-term survival. For those patients with groin recurrences, cure is rarely possible. In patients without prior groin radiation, surgical resection with radiation should be considered. In women who experience recurrence in a previously radiated groin or those who present with distant sites of recurrence, palliative treatment is recommended, usually with chemotherapy.

There are few palliative treatment options for women with recurrent disease, and these often involve platinum-based agents that are similar to those used for metastatic cervical cancer. The activity of platinum combination agents and/or taxanes is limited,[39,40] and patients with recurrent disease may best be managed with enrollment in clinical trials. Recent data have demonstrated potential benefit with antagonism of the epidermal growth factor receptor pathway. These studies have shown impressive initial responses in small studies, but durable responses have yet to be seen.[41,42]

Additional palliative care treatment options should be discussed with patients with recurrent vulvar cancer, as this can lead to erosion along the skin surfaces and potentially into the large vessels along the femoral and groin regions. Involvement may also occur along the vaginal periurethral and perirectal areas, limiting the patient's bowel and bladder function; this may require diverting ostomies for palliative benefit.

SPECIAL MANAGEMENT PROBLEMS

Postoperative Complications

There are significant postoperative management considerations in patients who have vulvar cancer and undergo surgery and radiation. Approximately 50% of patients will have complications involving wound breakdown at the groin and/or vulvar incisions, and lymphedema (Figure 9-5).[43] Lymphedema, in particular, results from disruption of the normal lymphatic channels in the groin after inguinal-femoral lymphadenectomy and can be compounded by radiation-induced fibrosis. This complication can be disfiguring, painful, and prone to chronic cellulitides. According to recent data, use of hemostatic agents has not affected the incidence of lymphedema and may worsen perioperative morbidity.[43] In breast cancer, randomized placebo-controlled studies have suggested a potential benefit with α-tocopherol (vitamin E) and pentoxifylline in the reduction of radiation-induced fibrosis and

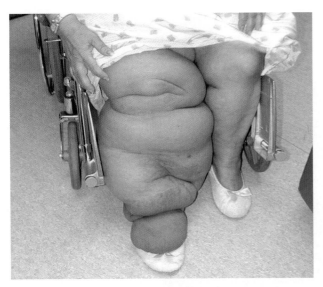

FIGURE 9-5. Severe lymphedema.

arm lymphedema, although other studies failed to replicate any benefit.[44,45] SLNBs can lessen the risks of these complications; in the prospective study by Van der Zee and colleagues,[30] sentinel node dissection was associated with a significant decrease in wound breakdown, cellulitis, and lymphedema.

Vulvar Melanoma

Melanoma is the second most common vulvar cancer and accounts for approximately 10% of all primary malignant neoplasms. This disease occurs predominantly in elderly white women, with the peak frequency between the sixth and seventh decades. Vulvar melanoma can develop on the labia minora, labia majora, or clitoris and can arise from both pigmented lesions and nonpigmented normal-appearing skin. Presenting signs of vulvar melanoma typically include pruritus, bleeding, and an ulcerated lesion. In general, these malignancies are highly aggressive, with a strong propensity for local and distant metastases and recurrences. The 5-year survival rate is 36% and is lower than the survival rate for both cutaneous melanoma and vulvar squamous cell carcinoma.[46]

There are 3 histologic subtypes of vulvar melanoma: superficial spreading melanoma and nodular melanoma are more common, and acral lentiginous melanoma is the rarest. Superficial spreading melanomas demonstrate radial growth of ≥4 retia lateral to the vertical or infiltrative growth. Nodular melanomas, in contrast, have no radial growth. Immununohistochemical staining for the S100 antigen is characteristic for most melanomas and can differentiate this tumor from squamous cell carcinomas.

Vulvar melanomas may be staged via several criteria. The American Joint Committee on Cancer (AJCC) frames its system on the tumor-nodes-metastases (TNM) classification, with tumor thickness (T), regional nodal involvement (N), and the presence or absence of distant metastases (M). The AJCC recently revised these criteria in 2010 to highlight several prognostic factors, including mitotic rate, presence of microtumor burden in lymph nodes, and levels of lactate dehydrogenase in patients with distant metastases.[47] Similarly, the FIGO classification system described for squamous cell carcinomas may also be applied to vulvar melanomas, but criticisms of this staging system include limited assistance in guiding treatment decision making and a weak predictor of survival. As such, vulvar melanoma may be further staged via several microstaging systems for cutaneous melanoma. The Clark system is based on the depth of invasion into the dermis; the Breslow system focuses on tumor thickness (Figure 9-6). Finally, the Chung system is a modification of the Clark criteria specifically for vaginal and vulvar melanoma and reflects the absence of a keratin or granular layer in much of the vulvar vestibule.

Surgery remains the initial treatment modality for most patients with vulvar melanoma. Gynecologic oncologists have traditionally advocated aggressive surgical resection, including radical vulvectomy or radical local excision; however, recent data have shown no differences in survival in patients undergoing radical vulvectomy, simple vulvectomy, partial vulvectomy, or wide local excision.[48] As such, conservative management with less radical procedures, such as wide local excision, is recommended, with the caveat that a 1-cm deep surgical margin should be obtained. For tumors that are less than 1 mm thick, 1-cm lateral surgical margins are appropriate; 2-cm lateral margins are indicated for lesions thicker than 1 mm.

The role of elective inguinal-femoral lymphadenectomy remains controversial in the management of vulvar melanoma. Metastases to the regional groin nodes are rare with thin lesions less than 1 mm (<5%) but significant with lesions greater than 4 mm (>70%). SLNB may be an option for patients with tumors between 1 and 4 mm thick, but this modality remains to be confirmed as standard of care.

Vulvar melanomas carry a poor prognosis and have a high propensity toward hematogenous dissemination to distant sites. Prognostic factors for survival in specifically vulvar melanomas include younger age, localized disease, and negative lymph nodes.[49] In high-risk, resected cutaneous melanomas, adjuvant treatment with high-dose α-interferon demonstrated strong evidence for improved recurrence-free survival and moderate improvement in overall survival in 2 randomized, prospective studies; in a pooled analysis of 4 randomized trials, interferon demonstrated only an improvement in recurrence-free survival.[50]

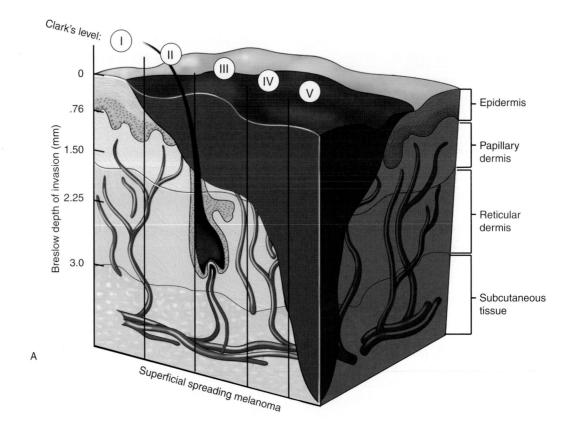

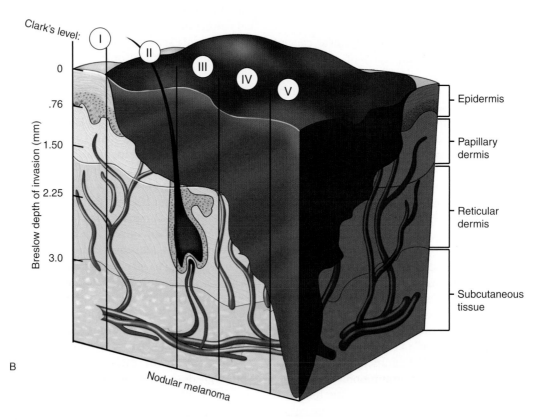

FIGURE 9-6. Microstaging of melanoma according to depth of penetration. A. Superficial spreading melanoma. **B.** Nodular melanoma.

Paget Disease of the Vulva

Paget disease of the vulva is a rare lesion, characterized as a red, velvety, weeping lesion on the labia majora, posterior fourchette, or clitoris. Similar to melanoma, patients with Paget disease tend to be elderly white women. This disease is associated with an underlying invasive adenocarcinoma in 10% to 20% of cases; more recently, a large study of 100 patients with this disease found a 16% incidence of invasive adenocarcinoma or other associated vulvar cancer. In this study, the risk of recurrent Paget disease was reported in 34% of the patients approximately 3 years after primary treatment.[51] Primary management remains surgical and frequently involves wide local excision in the absence of invasive features. Paget disease has a propensity for recurrence, despite negative margins; therefore, 1-cm surgical margins are typically advocated.

FUTURE DIRECTIONS

Significant progress has been made in the surgical management of women with invasive vulvar cancers. As discussed, the potential impact of SLNB may result in dramatically improved quality of life for survivors. Further study is needed in the management of women with groin and distant recurrences, and current treatment strategies remain only palliative in nature. As discussed earlier, the epidermal growth factor receptor pathway may have a role in management of advanced metastatic disease, either alone or in combination with cytotoxic chemotherapy. Similarly, additional study is warranted in patients found to have micrometastatic lymph node disease as a result of ultrastaging techniques. Historically, these patients were considered to have negative nodes; until further data are available, management of these patients should include radiotherapy with potential additive chemotherapy.[52,53]

Future studies should emphasize the transition period that is now underway in vulvar cancer in both staging and the sentinel lymph node technique. Vulvar cancers are rare tumors and require specialized treatment. Owing to the potential local nature of this disease, however, the goal of a cure is attainable at centers that manage this condition. The importance of a focused primary surgical treatment with the idea of curative intent cannot be overemphasized. Further management of metastatic disease may lead to multiple potential biologically plausible treatment pathways.

REFERENCES

1. Jemal A, Siegel R, Xu J, et al. Cancer statistics, 2010. *Ca Cancer J Clin.* 2010;60:277-300.
2. Howlader N, Noone AM, Krapcho M, et al. SEER Cancer Statistics Review, 1975-2008, National Cancer Institute. Bethesda, MD, http://seer.cancer.gov/csr/1975_2008/, based on November 2010 SEER data submission, posted to the SEER web site, 2011. Accessed February 6, 2012.
3. Kumar S, Shah JP, Malone JM Jr, Kumar S, Shah JP, Malone JM Jr. Vulvar cancer in women less than fifty in United States, 1980-2005. *Gynecol Oncol.* 2009;112:283-284; author reply 234.
4. Giuliano AR, Tortolero-Luna G, Ferrer E, et al. Epidemiology of human papillomavirus infection in men, cancers other than cervical and benign conditions. *Vaccine.* 2008;26(suppl 10): K17-K28.
5. Dillner J, Kjaer SK, Wheeler CM, et al. Four year efficacy of prophylactic human papillomavirus quadrivalent vaccine against low grade cervical, vulvar, and vaginal intraepithelial neoplasia and anogenital warts: randomised controlled trial. *BMJ.* 2010;341:c3493.
6. Madsen BS, Jensen HL, van den Brule AJ, Wohlfahrt J, Frisch M. Risk factors for invasive squamous cell carcinoma of the vulva and vagina: population-based case-control study in Denmark. *Int J Cancer.* 2008;122(12):2827-2834.
7. Elit L, Voruganti S, Simunovic M. Invasive vulvar cancer in a woman with human immunodeficiency virus: case report and review of the literature. *Gynecol Oncol.* 2005;98:151.
8. Hantschmann P, Sterzer S, Jeschke U, Friese K. P53 expression in vulvar carcinoma, vulvar intraepithelial neoplasia, squamous cell hyperplasia and lichen sclerosus. *Anticancer Res.* 2005;25(3A):1739-1745.
9. ACOG Practice Bulletin No. 93: diagnosis and management of vulvar skin disorders. *Obstet Gynecol.* 2008;111:1243-1253.
10. Homesley HD, Bundy BN, Sedlis A, et al. Prognostic factors for groin node metastasis in squamous cell carcinoma of the vulva (a Gynecologic Oncology Group study). *Gynecol Oncol.* 1993;49:279-283.
11. Cohn DE, Dehdashti F, Gibb RK, et al. Prospective evaluation of positron emission tomography for the detection of groin node metastases from vulvar cancer. *Gynecol Oncol.* 2002;85: 179-184.
12. Rob L, Robova H, Pluta M. Further data on sentinel lymph node mapping in vulvar cancer by blue dye and radiocolloid Tc99. *Int J Gynecol Cancer.* 2007;17:147-153.
13. Kataoka MY, Sala E, Baldwin P, et al. The accuracy of magnetic resonance imaging in staging of vulvar cancer: a retrospective multi-centre study. *Gynecol Oncol.* 2010;117:82-87.
14. Basta A, Adamek K, Pitynski K. Intraepithelial neoplasia and early stage vulvar cancer. Epidemiological, clinical and virological observations. *Eur J Gynaecol Oncol.* 1999;20:111-114.
15. Kosary CotVilagr C, Young JL, Keel GE, Eisner MP, Lin YD, Horner MJ. SEER Survival Monograph: Cancer Survival Among Adults: US SEER Program 1998-2001, Patient and Tumor Characteristics. Bethesda, MD: National Cancer Institute; 2007.
16. Hacker NF. Revised FIGO staging for carcinoma of the vulva. *Int J Gynaecol Obstet.* 2009;105:105-106.
17. Pecorelli S, Pecorelli S. Revised FIGO staging for carcinoma of the vulva, cervix, and endometrium. *Int J Gynaecol Obstet.* 2009;105:103-104.
18. Sedlis A, Homesley H, Bundy BN, et al. Positive groin lymph nodes in superficial squamous cell vulvar cancer. A Gynecologic Oncology Group study. *Am J Obstet Gynecol.* 1987;156: 1159-1164.
19. Euscher E, Malpica A, Atkinson E, Levenback C, Frumovitz M, Deavers M. Ultrastaging improves detection of metastases in sentinel lymph nodes of uterine cervix squamous cell carinoma. *Am J Surg Pathol.* 2008;32:1336-1343.
20. Morgan MA, Mikuta JJ. Surgical management of vulvar cancer. *Semin Surg Oncol.* 1999;17:168-172.
21. Morrow CP, Curtin JP. Surgery for vulvar neoplasia. In: *Gynecologic Cancer Surgery.* New York, NY: Churchill Livingstone; 1996:381-450.

22. DiSaia PJ, Creasman WT, Rich WM. An alternate approach to early cancer of the vulva. *Am J Obstet Gynecol.* 1979;133:825-832.

23. Stehman FB, Bundy BN, Thomas G, et al. Groin dissection versus groin radiation in carcinoma of the vulva: a Gynecologic Oncology Group study. *Int J Radiat Oncol Biol Phys.* 1992;24:389-396.

24. Stehman FB, Bundy BN, Ball H, Clarke-Pearson DL. Sites of failure and times to failure in carcinoma of the vulva treated conservatively: a Gynecologic Oncology Group study. *Am J Obstet Gynecol.* 1996;174:1128-1132; discussion 1132-1133.

25. Eichner E, Goldberg I, Bove ER. In vivo studies with direct sky blue of the lymphatic drainage of the internal genitals of women. *Am J Obstet Gynecol.* 1954;67:1277-1286.

26. Parry-Jones E. Lymphatics of the vulva. *J Obstet Gynaecol Br Emp.* 1963;70:751-765.

27. Morton DL, Wen DR, Wong JH, et al. Technical details of intraoperative lymphatic mapping for early stage melanoma. *Arch Surg.* 1992;127:392-399.

28. Levenback C, Burke TW, Gershenson DM, Morris M, Malpica A, Ross MI. Intraoperative lymphatic mapping for vulvar cancer. *Obstet Gynecol.* 1994;84:163-167.

29. Frumovitz M, Ramirez P, Levenback C. Lymphatic mapping and sentinel node detection in gynecologic malignancies of the lower genital tract. *Curr Oncol Rep.* 2005;7:435-443.

30. Van der Zee AG, Oonk MH, De Hullu JA, et al. Sentinel node dissection is safe in the treatment of early-stage vulvar cancer. *J Clin Oncol.* 2008;26:884-889.

31. Levenback C, Tian C, Coleman RL, Gold M, Fowler J, Judson P. Sentinel node (SN) biopsy in patients with vulvar cancer: the Gynecologic Oncology Group (GOG) experience. *Ann Surg Oncol.* 2008;15:28.

32. Moore RG, Granai CO, Gajewski W, Gordinier M, Steinhoff MM. Pathologic evaluation of inguinal sentinel lymph nodes in vulvar cancer patients: a comparison of immunohistochemical staining versus ultrastaging with hematoxylin and eosin staining. *Gynecol Oncol.* 2003;91:378-382.

33. Oonk MH, van Hemel BM, Hollema H, et al. Size of sentinel-node metastasis and chances of non-sentinel-node involvement and survival in early stage vulvar cancer: results from GROINSS-V, a multicentre observational study. *Lancet Oncol.* 2010;11:646-652.

34. Hacker NF, Berek JS, Juillard GJ, Lagasse LD. Preoperative radiation therapy for locally advanced vulvar cancer. *Cancer.* 1984;54:2056-2061.

35. Moore DH, Thomas GM, Montana GS, Saxer A, Gallup DG, Olt G. Preoperative chemoradiation for advanced vulvar cancer: a phase II study of the Gynecologic Oncology Group. *Int J Radiat Oncol Biol Phys.* 1998;42:79-85.

36. Likes WM, Stegbauer C, Tillmanns T, et al. Correlates of sexual function following vulvar excision. *Gynecol Oncol.* 2007;105:600-603.

37. Levgur M. Estrogen and combined hormone therapy for women after genital malignancies: a review. *J Reprod Med.* 2004;49:837-848.

38. Kumar S, Shah JP, Bryant CS, et al. A comparison of younger vs older women with vulvar cancer in the United States. *Am J Obstet Gynecol.* 2009;200:e52-e55.

39. Behbakht K, Massad LS, Yordan EL, et al. A bleomycin/ifosfamide/cisplatin regimen exhibits poor activity against persistent or recurrent squamous gynecologic cancers. *Eur J Gynaecol Oncol.* 1996;17:7-12.

40. Witteveen PO, van der Velden J, Vergote I, et al. Phase II study on paclitaxel in patients with recurrent, metastatic or locally advanced vulvar cancer not amenable to surgery or radiotherapy: a study of the EORTC-GCG (European Organisation for Research and Treatment of Cancer—Gynaecological Cancer Group). *Ann Oncol.* 2009;20:1511-1516.

41. Olawaiye A, Lee LM, Krasner C, et al. Treatment of squamous cell vulvar cancer with the anti-EGFR tyrosine kinase inhibitor Tarceva. *Gynecol Oncol.* 2007;106:628-630.

42. Oonk MH, de Bock GH, van der Veen DJ, et al. EGFR expression is associated with groin node metastases in vulvar cancer, but does not improve their prediction. *Gynecol Oncol.* 2007;104:109-113.

43. Carlson JW, Kauderer J, Walker JL, et al. A randomized phase III trial of VH fibrin sealant to reduce lymphedema after inguinal lymph node dissection: a Gynecologic Oncology Group study. *Gynecol Oncol.* 2008;110:76-82.

44. Magnusson M, Höglund P, Johansson K, et al. Pentoxifylline and vitamin E treatment for prevention of radiation-induced side-effects in women with breast cancer: a phase two, double-blind, placebo-controlled randomised clinical trial (Ptx-5). *Eur J Cancer.* 2009;45(14):2488-2495.

45. Gothard L, Cornes P, Earl J, et a. Double-blind placebo-controlled randomised trial of vitamin E and pentoxifylline in patients with chronic arm lymphoedema and fibrosis after surgery and radiotherapy for breast cancer. *Radiother Oncol.* 2004;73(2):133-139.

46. Piura B. Management of primary melanoma of the female urogenital tract. *Lancet.* 2008;9:973-981.

47. Nading MA, Balch CM, Sober AJ. Implications of the 2009 American Joint Committee on Cancer Melanoma Staging and Classification on dermatologists and their patients. *Semin Cutan Med Surg.* 2010;29:142-147.

48. Irvin WP, Legallo RL, Stoler MH, et al. Vulvar melanoma: a retrospective analysis and literature review. *Gynecol Oncol.* 2001;83:457-465.

49. Sugiyama VE, Chan JK, Shin JY, et al. Vulvar melanoma: a multivariable analysis of 644 patients. *Obstet Gynecol.* 2007;110:296-301.

50. Kirkwood JM, Manola J, Ibrahim J, et al. A pooled analysis of Eastern Cooperative Oncology Group and intergroup trials of adjuvant high dose interferon for melanoma. *Clin Cancer Res.* 2004;10:1670-1677.

51. Fanning J, Lambert HC, Hale TM, Morris PC, Schuerch C. Paget's disease of the vulva: prevalence of associated vulvar adenocarcinoma, invasive Paget's disease, and recurrence after surgical excision. *Am J Obstet Gynecol.* 1999;180:24-27.

52. Oonk MH. Prediction of lymph node metastases in vulvar cancer: a review. *Int J Gynecol Cancer.* 2006;16:963-971.

53. Oonk MH, van de Nieuwenhof HP, van der Zee AG, et al. Update on the sentinel lymph node procedure in vulvar cancer. *Exp Rev Anticancer Ther.* 2010;10:61-69.

10 Vaginal Cancer

William J. Lowery, Junzo Chino, and Laura J. Havrilesky

Primary vaginal cancer is an uncommon gynecologic malignancy and constitutes only 1% to 2% of gynecologic malignancies. Because of its rarity, there are specific guidelines for the diagnosis of primary vaginal cancer. A malignancy located in the vagina and not involving any adjacent pelvic organs is considered to be a primary vaginal cancer. If the malignancy extends to the cervix or vulva, it is considered a primary lesion of the nonvaginal site. Based on the observation that 95% of patients with recurrent cervical cancer will experience relapse within 5 years, all squamous cell carcinomas identified in the vagina within this period are defined as recurrences. Only those squamous cell carcinomas found more than 5 years after the diagnosis of cervical cancer are defined as primary vaginal cancers.[1] If there is a history of endometrial cancer, a diagnosis of adenocarcinoma in the vagina is usually considered a recurrence regardless of the time from primary treatment.

Primary vaginal malignancies are most commonly located in the upper third of the vagina and on the posterior wall (Figure 10-1). The most common histologic type is squamous cell carcinoma, which accounts for approximately 80% of all primary vaginal malignancies. Less commonly encountered are adenocarcinomas (10%), melanomas (3%), sarcomas (3%), and other rare tumors. Eighty-four percent of malignancies identified in the vagina are secondary, most commonly originating from the cervix (32%) and endometrium (18%); less common primary sites include the vulva, gastrointestinal tract, and ovary, as well as gestational trophoblastic disease.[2]

Prior to the mid-20th century, vaginal cancer was generally considered to be an incurable disease. Advances in radiation therapy and surgical techniques have been associated with significant improvement in cure rates, even in women with advanced disease.

EPIDEMIOLOGY

Key Points

1. Risk factors for vaginal cancer include human papillomavirus infection, smoking, in utero diethylstilbestrol exposure, and a prior history of cervical cancer.
2. Vaginal intraepithelial neoplasia (VAIN) is a potential precursor lesion to invasive squamous cell carcinoma of the vagina.
3. A history of pelvic radiation is a risk factor for vaginal sarcoma.

Primary vaginal cancer is a rare entity and constitutes only 1% to 2% of gynecologic malignancies. It has an incidence of approximately 1 in 100,000 women per year. The American Cancer Society estimates that there will be 2300 new vaginal cancers diagnosed in 2010 with approximately 780 deaths.[3]

The peak incidence of vaginal cancer is in the sixth and seventh decades. Risk factors for the disease closely mirror those for cervical cancer and include an increased number of lifetime sexual partners, younger

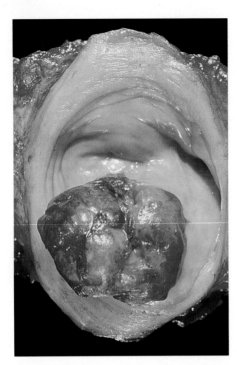

FIGURE 10-1. Squamous cell carcinoma of the vagina. (Reprinted with permission of Robboy SJ and Robboy Associates LLC [Chapel Hill, NC], copyright holder of *Robboy's Pathology of the Female Reproductive Tract*, Elsevier Pub, London.)

age at first intercourse, human papillomavirus (HPV) infection, history of smoking, in utero diethylstilbestrol exposure, and a prior history of cervical cancer.[4,5] There is also an association between vaginal cancer and chronic vaginal irritation, as with long-term pessary use. In a 10-year review of the National Cancer Data Base, Creasman and colleagues[6] observed that survival was related to the stage of disease and the histologic type, with melanoma having the poorest prognosis. In a later review of the Surveillance, Epidemiology, and End Result (SEER) program by Shah and colleagues,[7] stage, tumor size, histology, and treatment modality were the most significant prognostic factors.

Although VAIN is recognized as a premalignant condition, its progression rate to invasive cancer is not well understood. Aho and colleagues[8] followed 23 patients with untreated VAIN in an attempt to define the natural history of the disease and reported a 9% progression rate from high-grade VAIN to vaginal cancer among women who were followed for at least 3 years. A subsequent retrospective study by Schookaert and colleagues[9] examining the incidence of high-grade VAIN after hysterectomy for high-grade cervical intraepithelial neoplasia also suggested progression from VAIN to invasive vaginal cancer. A total of 7.6% of patients developed VAIN 2, VAIN 3, or invasive carcinoma with

a mean interval between hysterectomy and the first vaginal biopsy of 45 months, with 3% of these high-grade vaginal lesions subsequently progressing to invasive vaginal cancer. All of the patients were reported to have had a negative vaginal colposcopy before their hysterectomy for cervical dysplasia, suggesting that the subsequent cancers were of vaginal origin.

One recognized risk factor for the development of vaginal cancer is a history of treatment for an anogenital tumor. In a large, population-based, case control study, Daling and colleagues[5] reported that 30% of women with vaginal cancer had a history of treatment for an anogenital tumor. This is most likely secondary to the shared pathophysiology of HPV infections. Up to 90% of anal cancers in women harbor HPV; previous treatment for a genital cancer confers a 10-fold increased risk of anal cancer.[10] Other risk factors for squamous cell carcinoma of the vagina include pelvic radiation, tobacco abuse, and other factors associated with HPV, such as an increased number of sexual partners and younger age at first intercourse. Finally, 10% to 20% of women with a primary vaginal cancer have a history of pelvic irradiation, most commonly as treatment for cervical cancer. A prior history of pelvic radiotherapy is more frequent in women with vaginal sarcomas than in women with vaginal cancers of other histologic subtypes.

DIAGNOSIS

Key Points

1. Vaginal cancer may present with an abnormal Pap smear or with vaginal bleeding.
2. Biopsy of suspicious vaginal lesions is critical to diagnosis of this disease.

Vaginal cancer is often identified at the time of screening for cervical cancer. Although there is ample literature addressing optimal strategies to screen for cervical cancer, the rarity of vaginal cancer makes it difficult to assess any screening strategy. It is generally accepted that women who have had a hysterectomy for benign disease do not need continued vaginal cytologic screening if there is no evidence of HPV-related cervical lesions on pathology. There is also agreement that it is likely safe for older women to discontinue screening if there is a history of negative cytology and an absence of risk factors. Women who have been treated for cervical cancer should continue to undergo routine surveillance with vaginal cytologic testing. It is also reasonable to continue to screen women who have undergone a hysterectomy and who have a history of cervical dysplasia.[11]

Table 10-1 Differential Diagnosis for Vaginal Lesions

• Anatomic variants
  – Gartner duct cyst
  – Vaginal adenosis
	• Inflammatory/
	  autoimmune
	  – Behcet syndrome
	  – Paget disease

• Malignancy
  – Cervical cancer
  – Metastatic cancer from
    other sites
	• Other
	  – Endometriosis
	  – Vaginal atrophy
	  – Trauma
	  – Foreign body

• Infectious
  – Vaginitis
  – Condyloma
  – Herpes simplex lesion
    and other sexually
    transmitted infections	

The most common presenting symptom of vaginal cancer is abnormal vaginal bleeding. Other presenting symptoms include abnormal discharge and pelvic pain or dysuria, although these often present later in the disease course secondary to tumor spread outside of the vagina. A careful vaginal examination is required in these patients, as a small lesion can be difficult to visualize in the folds of the vagina or can be covered by blades of the speculum. The differential diagnosis for vaginal lesions is broad (Table 10-1), and biopsy should never be delayed when a suspicious lesion is encountered.

The most common symptom at diagnosis of a vaginal melanoma is vaginal bleeding,[12,13] but up to one-third of these lesions present as a mass at the time of routine pelvic examination.[13] The majority of vaginal melanomas are pigmented or ulcerated at diagnosis, but up to one-fourth have been reported as grossly amelanotic.[12,13] The most common location for vaginal melanoma is the lower anterior vaginal wall.

Sarcomas are often bulky lesions that appear most commonly in the upper vagina. Sarcoma botryoides is a subtype of rhabdomyosarcoma and primarily affects children, predominantly arising from the anterior wall of the vagina. The name derives from the Greek word for grapes and grossly has a grapelike cluster appearance.

In general, computed tomography (CT) and, more recently, positron emission tomography (PET) or single-photon emission computed tomography (SPECT) have been shown to be a valuable adjunct in the identification of lymph node metastasis. Although not part of the standard staging criteria, these imaging techniques may have a role in surgical and/or radiation therapy planning.

PATHOLOGY

Key Points

1. Squamous cell carcinomas comprise the majority of vaginal cancers, and up to 70% are associated with infection with high-risk HPV subtypes.
2. Adenocarcinomas of the vagina are commonly of clear cell histology and are attributed to in utero exposure to diethylstilbestrol.
3. Vaginal cancers are clinically staged using International Federation of Gynecology and Obstetrics (FIGO) criteria; this system is limited by the accuracy of determining extension into subvaginal tissues.

Squamous cell carcinomas (Figure 10-2) comprise approximately 80% of primary vaginal malignancies and histologically resemble squamous cell carcinomas of the cervix. There is no established or consistent precursor lesion to vaginal cancer. HPV infection appears to be associated with the development of vaginal cancer, similar to cervical cancer. Daling and colleagues[5] detected HPV in the tissue of more than 80% of patients with carcinoma in situ and more than 60% of patients with invasive squamous cell cancer. More recent studies have suggested that approximately 70% of squamous cell vaginal cancers and greater than 90% of VAIN 2 and VAIN 3 can be attributed to high-risk HPV subtypes.[14,15]

Adenocarcinomas of the vagina (Figure 10-3) account for approximately 10% of primary vaginal carcinomas. The origin of these lesions may include embryonic

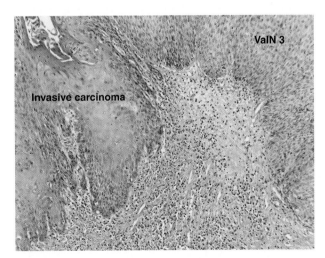

FIGURE 10-2. Squamous cell carcinoma. Hematoxylin and eosin stain of squamous cell carcinoma of the vagina showing malignant invasion of the dermal layer with associated inflammatory reaction. (Image contributed by Dr. Rex Bentley.)

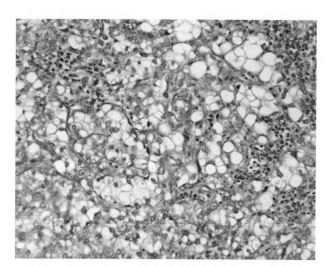

FIGURE 10-3. Clear cell adenocarcinoma. Hematoxylin and eosin stain of clear cell carcinoma of the vagina showing clear cells secondary to a large quantity of glycogen in the cytoplasm. (Image contributed by Dr. Rex Bentley.)

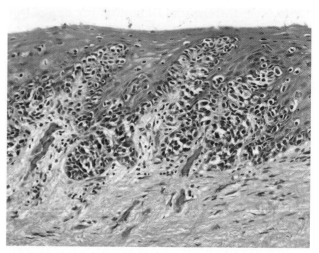

FIGURE 10-4. Melanoma. Hematoxylin and eosin stain of melanoma demonstrating melanocytes proliferating along the dermal/epidermal juction in a continuous band with scattered single melanocytes extending into the upper layers of the dermis. (Image contributed by Dr. Angelica Selim.)

elements and normal glandular tissue residing in the vagina. The majority of reported cases are clear cell adenocarcinomas in individuals exposed in utero to diethylstilbestrol (DES). These DES-associated adenocarcinomas are histologically identical to the clear cell adenocarcinomas of the ovary and endometrium. DES is a synthetic nonsteroidal estrogen that was used from the 1930s until 1971 primarily to prevent spontaneous miscarriage in patients considered as high risk. Herbst and Scully[16] described 7 women aged 15 to 22 years with clear cell adenocarcinoma of the vagina and noted that 6 of these patients had been exposed to DES in utero. DES was subsequently removed from the market in the United States. Herbst and Scully[16] subsequently established a registry to track cases of clear cell adenocarcinoma. As of December 2007, the registry has accessioned approximately 760 cases of clear cell adenocarcinoma of the vagina and cervix, two-thirds of which were associated with DES exposure. Hatch and colleagues[17] examined the cancer risk in daughters exposed to DES and found that the standardized incidence ratio for clear cell adenocarcinoma was 40 times that expected in the general population. The age-incidence curve peaks between the ages of 15 and 25 years, with an estimated risk of development of 1 per 1000 of these individuals exposed, but cases up to the age of 55 have been accessioned to the registry.

The number of DES-associated adenocarcinomas has sharply declined over the last several decades after the removal of DES from the market. Frank and colleagues[18] described a series of patients with primary non–DES-associated adenocarcinoma of the vagina. The patients presented at an older age and, stage for stage, carried a worse prognosis than DES-associated

adenocarcinoma. Local and distant recurrence rates were also higher in non–DES-associated malignancies.[18] The role of HPV in the pathogenesis of non–clear cell adenocarcinomas of the vagina is unclear.

There are several vaginal cancers of less common histology; these include melanomas, sarcomas, verrucous carcinomas, and endodermal sinus tumors. Vaginal melanoma (Figure 10-4) constitutes 3% to 5% of all vaginal malignancies[19,20] and less than 1% of all melanomas[19,21] and occurs at a mean age of 60 to 65 years. Unlike many cutaneous melanomas, exposure to ultraviolet radiation is not a risk factor for mucosal melanomas. Melanoma is thought to arise from melanocytes, which are present as a normal variant in the vaginal epithelium in approximately 3% of women.[22]

Sarcomas account for approximately 3% to 4% of all primary malignancies of the vagina.[6,23] Prior radiotherapy is a risk factor, with 35% of cases having a history of pelvic radiotherapy, usually for cervical cancer, 8 to 26 years prior.[24] Grade is an important prognostic factor; a series of 24 vulvar and vaginal sarcomas demonstrated no deaths in patients with low-grade tumors, whereas the 5-year overall survival rate was approximately 50% for high-grade lesions.[25] There was no survival difference between leiomyosarcomas and other histologic types in this series, although numbers were limited.

Embryonal rhabdomyosarcoma is the most common malignant neoplasm of the vagina in infants and children and accounts for 75% of the vaginal rhabdomyosarcomas. Although a majority of these cases are diagnosed before age 5 years, these malignancies can be found elsewhere in the female genital tract later in life.

Verrucous carcinoma is a rare malignancy of the female genital tract, with only a few cases reported in the vagina. It is primarily found in postmenopausal women. HPV is likely a causative agent or factor in its development, but the pathogenesis is not completely understood. It is a slowly growing tumor that generally "pushes" into adjacent tissue rather than invades it, and accompanying inflammatory enlargement of the regional lymph nodes is encountered as opposed to metastasis.[26]

Endodermal sinus tumors, or yolk sac tumors, are germ cell tumors that are rarely found in the vagina. They are primarily diagnosed before the age of 3 years. The most common presenting symptom is vaginal bleeding. In children, the majority of germ cell tumors are extragonadal, with thoracic and central nervous system being most common. Only a small proportion of these are primary vaginal tumors.[27] The most common presenting symptom is vaginal bleeding. α-Fetoprotein is generally elevated in these patients and can be used as a marker of response to treatment.

Metastatic Spread Patterns

The vagina is bordered laterally by the levator ani muscles, pelvic fascia, and ureters. Deep invasion anteriorly or posteriorly can result in bladder or rectal involvement, which may lead to fistula formation during or after radiotherapy. Disease extending to the sidewall may result in ureteral obstruction and renal failure. The lymphatic drainage of vaginal cancers is complex and depends on the anatomic level of the lesion. Much like cervical cancer, the lymphatic drainage can follow multiple pathways.[28] The upper two-thirds of the vagina drain into the internal and external iliac lymph nodes, whereas the lower one-third drains into the sacral, common iliac, and superficial inguinal lymph nodes.

FIGO Staging

Vaginal cancer is clinically staged using the criteria established by the International Federation of Gynecology and Obstetrics (FIGO) (Table 10-2), which uses history and physical examination, routine laboratory evaluation, bimanual rectovaginal examination, cystoscopy, proctoscopy, intravenous pyelogram, and plain film radiographs if there is a concern for bony metastasis. One of the limitations of this staging system is the inability to accurately determine spread into subvaginal tissues. This is reflected in a wide range of survival data within a given stage. Perez and colleagues[1] have suggested that stage II disease be subdivided into 2 groups: (1) lesions that involve the submucosa but do not extend into the parametria, and (2) lesions that involve the parametria without reaching the pelvic sidewall, but this has not consistently been demonstrated to have prognostic significance.[7,29]

Table 10-2 Staging of Vaginal Cancer Adapted From the International Federation of Gynecology and Obstetrics

FIGO Staging of Vaginal Cancer	
Stage I	Cancer limited to the vaginal wall
Stage II	Cancer with involvement of the subvaginal tissue but no extension to the pelvic sidewall
Stage III	Cancer with extension to the pelvic wall
Stage IV	Cancer with extension beyond the true pelvis or involvement of the mucosa of the bladder or rectum not including bullous edema
IVA	Invasion of the bladder or rectal mucosa and/or direct invasion beyond the true pelvis
IVB	Distant metastasis

Because it does not account for tumor size or regional lymph node status, the FIGO staging system is not generally used for melanomas. Likewise, the Clark and Chung methods are not applicable because of the difference in histologic landmarks between cutaneous structures and the vagina. Vaginal melanomas may best be classified using the Breslow thickness,[30] which describes the tumor thickness, or the American Joint Committee on Cancer (AJCC) staging system (AJCC 2001), which takes into account thickness, presence or absence of ulceration, lymph node metastasis, and other metastatic sites of disease.[19] The size of the lesion is an important prognostic factor as well, with a size of greater than 3 cm generally indicating worse outcomes.[31-33] Similarly, the staging of sarcoma botryoides follows that of pediatric rhabdomyosarcoma.

TREATMENT

Key Points

1. Stage I squamous cell carcinomas of the vagina may be treated primarily with surgical excision or primary radiotherapy. Advanced-stage lesions likely requiring postsurgical radiation are typically managed with primary radiotherapy alone.
2. Lymph node dissection is recommended with surgical excision of early-stage vaginal cancers.
3. Radiotherapy is the treatment of choice for a majority of vaginal cancers because of its effectiveness in achieving long-term survival and preservation of adjacent organs; chemosensitization with platinum regimens may improve disease control.

Surgery

Stage I squamous cell carcinoma of the vagina may be treated either surgically or with primary radiotherapy, and this decision should be tailored not only to the size of the lesion, but also to the patient's desire to maintain optimal sexual function (Figure 10-5). Minimally invasive lesions discovered incidentally at the time of surgical excision of presumed VAIN have been managed with surveillance with acceptable outcomes.[34,35] Women who have small, known invasive lesions and who have previously undergone a hysterectomy are usually treated by partial or total vaginectomy, parametrectomy, and lymph node dissection. For women who have an intact uterus, radical hysterectomy is also indicated.[36-38] A significant portion of patients who undergo primary surgical therapy also receive adjuvant radiotherapy, with lymph node metastasis or surgical margin involvement being the most common indications.[36-39] Those at high risk for requiring postoperative radiation, as when lymph node metastasis is suspected, are generally not also subjected to primary surgical excision, as this combination is associated with higher rates of adverse events.

Adenocarcinoma of the vagina is treated similarly to squamous cell carcinoma. In the past, consideration was given to conservation of ovarian and sexual function, as patients with early-stage DES-associated adenocarcinoma were usually younger, but DES-associated malignancies are now a rare entity. Simple excision is not recommended for adenocarcinomas regardless of size because of their more aggressive nature and propensity for lymphatic spread, and as with squamous cell carcinomas, options include radical surgery or primary radiotherapy with or without chemotherapy.[18]

Although the role of lymph node metastasis is not well defined in the FIGO staging system, it is a poor prognostic indicator. As outlined earlier, the lymphatic drainage of the vagina is somewhat complicated and depends on the level of the lesion. In patients undergoing surgical management of early-stage vaginal cancer, a lymph node dissection is routinely performed.[36,38] Because the majority of patients diagnosed with vaginal cancer undergo radiation therapy, the true incidence of lymph node metastasis is unknown. Identification of sentinel nodes has the potential to aid in radiation treatment planning. Frumovitz and colleagues[40] were able to identify a sentinel node in 79% of the patients with vaginal cancer evaluated with pretreatment lymphoscintigraphy, and van Dam and colleagues[41] were able to detect a sentinel lymph node in 2 of 3 patients with vaginal cancer laparoscopically.

Radiotherapy

Radiotherapy (RT) is an effective, curative treatment modality for vaginal cancer and is often the treatment of choice for many reasons. First, radical surgery to remove large, invasive primary vaginal lesions with negative margins often carries risks of significant morbidity because of the close proximity of the vagina to critical structures; RT affords preservation of adjacent organs. Second, the vagina is an ideal site for brachytherapy (BT) for conformal treatment to curative doses. Finally, given the broad lymph drainage patterns of vaginal cancer, prophylactic nodal treatment is often more appropriately accomplished with whole-pelvic RT than with multiple large dissections.

Combined Chemotherapy and Radiotherapy for Vaginal Cancer

Interest in combining chemotherapy and RT for treatment of vaginal cancer has increased in the last decade as a result of the tremendous success with concurrent

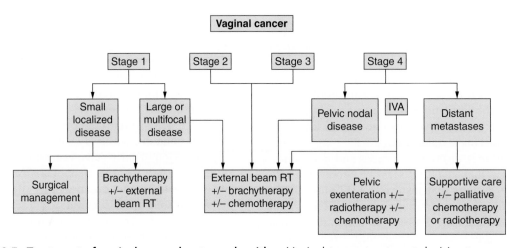

FIGURE 10-5. Treatment of vaginal cancer by stage algorithm. Vaginal cancer treatment decision tree.

cisplatin-based regimens in cervical cancer.[42–45] Because of the small numbers and stage heterogeneity, direct comparison of combined chemotherapy plus RT and RT alone is difficult. Most series include a majority of advanced-stage disease, and in this unfavorable cohort, disease control is achievable using combined chemotherapy and RT in approximately 50% to 60% of patients. Concurrent chemotherapy is generally well tolerated in appropriately selected patients, and there is no evidence of significantly worse late toxicity as compared with RT alone. As such, it has been our approach to include concurrent platinum-based chemotherapy in the treatment of appropriate patients with advanced-stage disease.

Radiation Technique

RT for vaginal cancer is highly individualized and depends on the site and extent of disease, as well as the tolerance of neighboring critical organs. Before initiation of treatment, it is optimal for the radiation oncologist to perform a thorough physical examination to delineate the location of the primary disease and its extent. Often fiducial markers (radio-opaque seeds) are placed during the initial examination so that appropriate boost planning can be performed. If this is not done, in the event of a response to initial external-beam RT, boost planning can only be based on estimates of the initial extent of disease.

The use of brachytherapy alone should be limited to the smallest and most favorable vaginal lesions (low grade, ≤5-mm thick, ≤2 cm in greatest diameter). In these selected cases, the entire vaginal mucosa is treated to between 50 and 60 Gy, with a boost at the primary site to a total dose of 65 to 85 Gy to 5-mm depth. The technique is best established with low-dose rate applicators, although experience with high-dose rate applicators is comparable.[46] Whole vaginal treatment can be accomplished with a single line of intracavitary sources; boost doses can be achieved by loading only the most superior positions in the case of apical lesions, whereas for distal or lateral lesions, using asymmetrically leaded cylinders or differential loading of multicatheter applicators can result in more optimal dose distributions (Figure 10-6). Doses to the normal vaginal mucosa at the apex should be limited to 140 Gy, with the distal mucosa limited to 100 Gy.

Whole-pelvic RT is generally included in unfavorable stage I patients and in all those with stage II or greater disease. For those with disease limited to the proximal third of the vagina, standard pelvic fields are appropriate either via anterior-posterior (AP)/posterior-anterior (PA) field arrangement or a 4-field technique. Care should be taken to extend the field inferiorly to obtain a minimum of a 4-cm margin on the vaginal disease. Doses of 45 to 50 Gy in 1.8- to 2-Gy daily fractions are used. Some investigators advocate the addition of a midline block after 10 to 20 Gy, relying on brachytherapy for treatment of the central disease and thus sparing the bladder and rectum.

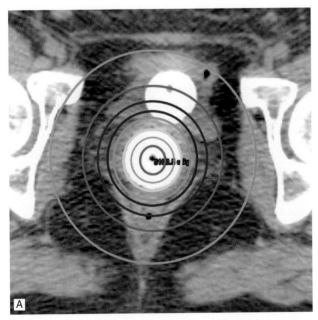
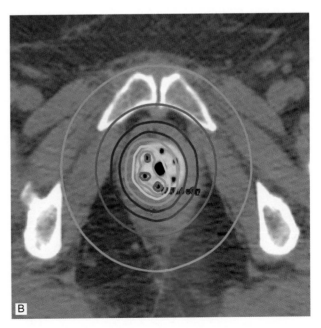

FIGURE 10-6. Intracavitary brachytherapy. A. Single-channel intracavitary brachytherapy for a thin apical lesion. The prescription isodose line is green and is symmetric. **B.** Multichannel intracavitary brachytherapy for a thin lateral wall lesion. The green prescription isodose line is well lateralized.

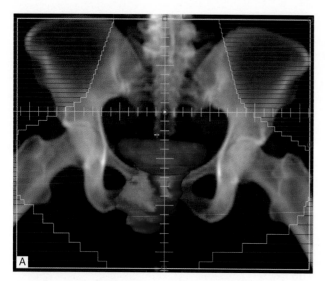
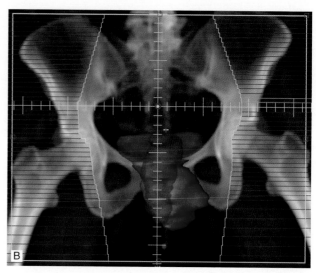

FIGURE 10-7. Wide AP and narrow PA technique for treating inguinofemoral nodes. Wide AP (**A**) and narrow PA (**B**) fields may be used to spare femoral heads; however, the portion of the AP field that is blocked in the PA must be supplemented with additional electrons or low-energy photons to bring dose to prescription.

In situations in which the inguinal nodal basins are at risk (ie, involvement of the distal two-thirds of the vagina), the inguinofemoral nodes must be covered. Opposed AP/PA fields appropriately cover the targets, but lead to a significant dose to the femoral heads. A wide AP (covering the inguinofemoral basins) and narrow PA field (blocking the majority of the femoral heads) may be used, with supplemental anterior electrons or low-energy photons to portions of the AP field blocked in the PA, which can significantly reduce femoral head dose (Figure 10-7).[47] Intensity-modulated radiotherapy (IMRT) has shown promise in reducing dose to the femoral heads, the intergluteal cleft, and nontarget pelvic organs, although special care must be taken to account for both

inter- and intra-fractional organ motion due to the highly conformal nature of the treatment (Figure 10-8).[48-50]

Gross disease should be treated to a total dose 65 to 85 Gy as normal tissue tolerance allows. Generally brachytherapy is the preferred modality for boosting after whole-pelvic RT, as it offers extremely conformal isodose distributions and eliminates the need for organ motion margins. Both intracavitary and interstitial techniques are often used to boost gross disease, as dictated by the extension of the primary and normal tissue tolerance. For thin lesions (≤5 mm) of the vaginal vault, intracavitary techniques previously described are quite sufficient for treatment. For thicker lesions, an interstitial implant is required.

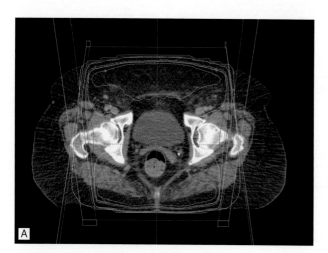
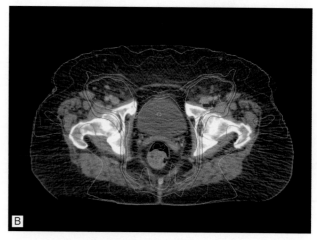

FIGURE 10-8. Opposed AP-PA treatment versus IMRT for treatment of inguinofemoral nodes. A. Opposed AP-PA fields cover targets appropriately but treat the femoral heads to full dose. **B.** IMRT may be used to spare the femoral heads and other neighboring critical structures.

Several techniques exist for interstitial implants, including the Syed-Neblett template, the Martinez Universal Perineal Interstitial Template, and other freehand and custom template techniques (Figure 10-9).[51,52] These techniques all involve the introduction of needles or catheters through the volume, requiring treatment with approximately 1-cm spacing and ideally with a 1- to

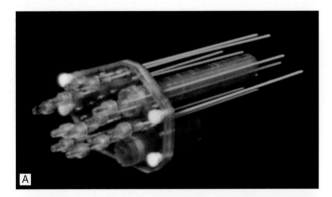

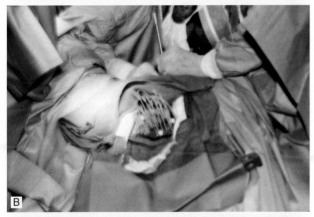

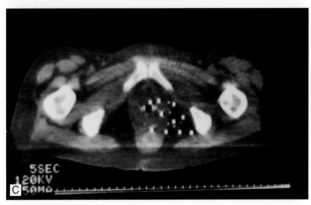

FIGURE 10-9. Customized interstitial template for a deeply invasive lateral lesion. A. A perineal template is fashioned based on clinical examination and imaging, with holes drilled to guide interstitial catheters. **B.** After completing external-beam radiotherapy, the patient is brought to the OR for catheter placement. **C.** CT or MRI 3-dimensional treatment planning is performed, and catheters are loaded with Ir-192 strands in a shielded inpatient room. (Images courtesy of Gustavo Montana, MD.)

2-cm margin around the target. If there is close approximation of the target volume and the peritoneum (such as in a post-hysterectomy apical tumor), laparoscopy is used to ensure that the peritoneal cavity is not entered. Treatment planning can be performed with orthogonal films or with CT and/or magnetic resonance imaging (MRI). Iridium-192 (Ir-192) wires or stranded seeds are then after loaded into the catheters/needles after treatment planning. Interstitial boosts are ideal for thick apical and lateral wall lesions. Discrete distal anterior and posterior lesions can also be treated with interstitial boosts, or combined with an external-beam RT boost.

For large and extensive lesions or for disease extension into areas in which an implant will not cover adequately, 3-dimensional (3D) conformal or IMRT boosts are often required to cover the targets appropriately. Often the dose to the target must be limited to ≤75 Gy due to normal tissue limits. Special care must be taken to ensure that tightly conformal plans are indeed treating the correct volumes, and regular use of real-time confirmation (cone-beam CT and on-board imaging) is extremely useful. Even with the best imaging, however, intra fractional motion must still be accounted for.

An additional application for 3D conformal/IMRT boosts is for node-positive disease. With careful treatment planning and image guidance, boosts to involved lymph nodes can be designed to take these regions of gross disease to 55 to 65 Gy, although this is often limited by approximation to small bowel, particularly in the upper pelvis and para-aortic region. Significant volumes of small bowel should not be taken beyond 50 to 52 Gy due to the risk of obstruction, fistula, and perforation.

Treatment of Melanoma

The primary treatment of vaginal melanoma remains surgical. Although several case series have suggested that radical procedures such as exenteration should be the preferred approach,[33,53] other studies have failed to demonstrate either superior local control or a survival advantage for radical surgery.[32] Given the increased morbidity of radical procedures and the poor 5-year survival of vaginal melanoma regardless of treatment approach, conservative resection procedures are most commonly used. RT has been used for the primary, neoadjuvant, adjuvant, and palliative setting for vaginal melanoma.[19,31,54] Although primary surgical intervention has generally been associated with better outcomes than primary radiotherapy in limited case series of vaginal melanoma, selection of healthier and better-prognosis patients for surgery undoubtedly biases these studies in favor of the surgical approach. In general, primary RT has been reserved for women who refuse surgery or are poor operative candidates.

Primary surgery for vaginal melanoma should consist, at a minimum, of the wide excision of all visible disease.[13] RT has been added after conservative surgery, with several small series suggesting improved locoregional control when radiotherapy is incorporated.[31,55] There are several case reports suggesting satisfactory palliative outcomes with salvage radiotherapy using brachytherapy or external-beam treatment.[56]

Routine inguinal or pelvic lymphadenectomy have no known therapeutic value in the management of vaginal melanoma. Assessment for distant sites of disease is usually made using CT or PET/CT. For patients with vaginal melanoma in whom no distant disease is detected on imaging, consideration may be given to sentinel lymph node assessment; approximately 10 such cases have been reported in the literature.[13,19,57,58] For women with lower vaginal lesions, identification and removal of groin sentinel lymph nodes may be reasonable for prognostic purposes.

Treatment of Sarcoma

Primary surgery is the preferred treatment, with RT reserved for selected postoperative cases, or for definitive management of those who are not appropriate for surgery. There are scant data on chemotherapy for vaginal leiomyosarcoma or carcinosarcoma, and it has not been routinely incorporated into initial treatment for localized disease. Agents chosen to treat recurrent or metastatic vaginal sarcomas are derived from the uterine experience; the preferred agents in leiomyosarcoma are doxorubicin, gemcitabine, and docetaxel, whereas carcinosarcomas are commonly treated with ifosfamide, platinum, and paclitaxel.[59-63]

In children, rhabdomyosarcoma is the dominant histologic type. The prognosis is good in most patients with initial chemotherapy, followed by tailored surgery or RT in those with residual disease. In the National Cancer Data Base study, 30 pediatric patient were identified, the majority with rhabdomyosarcoma.[6] More than 75% of the pediatric cases were treated with chemotherapy, and 80% had surgery.

Treatment of Verrucous Carcinoma

Given the indolent nature of verrucous carcinoma and the fact that spontaneous metastasis is rare, local excision of the tumor is generally accepted as the therapy of choice. The use of RT in the treatment of verrucous carcinoma is controversial. There is concern for anaplastic transformation of verrucous carcinomas of both head and neck sites and the female genital tract,[64,65] but other investigators have used RT with success.[66]

Treatment of Endodermal Sinus Tumor

In the past, the treatment of vaginal endodermal sinus tumors has consisted of chemotherapy in combination with surgery as well as RT. Although effective, this treatment regimen leaves little hope for future fertility. More recently, there have been multiple reports of successful treatment with chemotherapy only, using a regimen of cisplatin, etoposide, and bleomycin.[67,68]

SURVIVAL AND PROGNOSIS

Key Points

1. Stage remains the most important prognostic factor in vaginal cancers.
2. Surgical management may afford improved survival in early-stage vaginal cancers, but data may be biased as a result of patient selection factors.
3. Rhabdomyosarcomas have an excellent prognosis, with 5-year survival rates of 90%.

According to the SEER database, the overall 5-year survival rate after a diagnosis of vaginal cancer is 51.4%. Clinical stage is recognized as the most important prognostic factor. Although vaginal cancer appears to have a shared pathophysiology with cervical and vulvar cancer, it has a worse prognosis at each stage. The 5-year survival rate for each stage is as follows: stage I, 77.6%; stage II, 52.2%; stage III, 42.5%; stage IVA, 20.5%; stage IVB, 12.9%[69] (Figures 10-10 and 10-11).

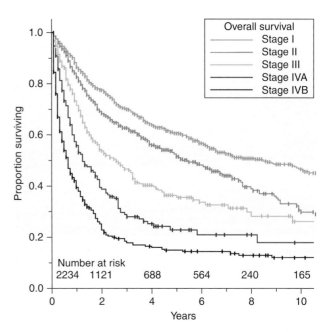

FIGURE 10-10. Vaginal cancer: overall survival by stage. Overall survival by stage for vaginal cancer, adapted from SEER data.

CHAPTER 10

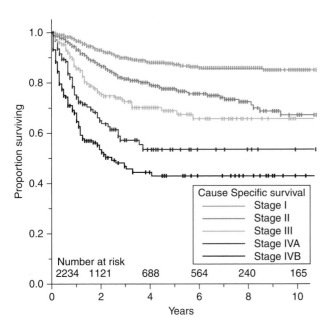

FIGURE 10-11. Vaginal cancer: cause-specific survival by stage. Cause-specific survival by stage for vaginal cancer, adapted from SEER data.

Early Stage-Disease

Selected early-stage disease may be treated with surgery, surgery followed by tailored adjuvant RT, or RT alone (Table 10-3). In retrospective series, women with stage I disease treated with surgery alone, the majority having squamous lesions, have a 5-year survival rate of 85% to 92%.[6,37,38] Those with stage II disease managed surgically have a 49% to 70% 5-year survival rate.[6,38] In these same series, the 5-year survival rates for women with stage I and stage II disease undergoing primary RT are 44% to 63% and 50% to 57%, respectively. Women treated with a combination of surgery and adjuvant RT have comparable outcomes: Tjalma and colleagues[37] reported a 71% 5-year survival rate for women with stage I disease, whereas Davis and colleagues[38] reported a 100% and 69% survival rate for women with stage I and II disease, respectively. Although survival in these series appears to favor the surgical management of early-stage disease, selection bias likely accounts for some of the observed difference in outcomes.

Advanced-Stage Disease

Advanced-stage vaginal lesions are usually treated with concurrent chemotherapy and RT. Historically, prognostic data are based on RT alone, with a 5-year survival rate of approximately 35%,[6] but more recent analyses include patients who received concurrent chemotherapy. The Mallinckrodt Institute[1] reported 212 patients managed with primary RT from 1953 through 1991. The majority of patients with advanced-stage disease received both external-beam RT and brachytherapy; 10-year disease-specific survival was 38% for stage III disease. The MD Anderson Cancer Center reported a series of 301 women, of whom 66% with stage III or IVA disease were treated with external-beam RT alone, whereas 17% of the advanced-stage disease cohort received chemotherapy as well. The 5-year disease-specific survival rate was 58% women with stage III/IVA disease, and 5-year pelvic control was 71%.[70] A series of 153 women from Princess Margaret Hospital (PMH) reported that patients with advanced-stage disease who underwent RT or RT with concurrent chemotherapy had a cause-specific survival of 60% for stage III and 42% for stage IV disease.[71] Vaginal stenosis is commonly encountered after RT, with Kirkbride and colleagues[71] reporting an incidence of 38%. Severe adverse events occur in 10% to 13% of patients undergoing primary RT, most commonly proctitis, vaginal necrosis, intestinal obstruction, or fistula formation.[2,70,71]

For the most part, clinical series include adenocarcinomas. In patients who have clear cell adenocarcinoma as a result of DES exposure in utero, the 5-year survival rate is improved for early-stage disease but worse for late-stage disease. Herbst[72] reported that the 5-year survival rate for women with stage I clear cell adenocarcinoma exceeded 90% but reported no 5-year survivors with stage IV disease.

Rare Tumors/Prognosis

In the National Cancer Data Base study, of 105 adults with vaginal sarcomas, leiomyosarcoma was the dominant histology (46 of 105), with 25 cases of complex, mixed, or stromal tumors.[6] Sixty-seven of 105 were treated surgically, with 29 receiving adjuvant RT and 10 receiving adjuvant chemotherapy. Five-year overall survival rates were 84% in women aged 20 to 49 years and 48% in women aged 50 to 69 years, and 2-year survival was 30% in women ≥70 years. In the largest single series of 17 patients, the 3 long-term survivors had stage I or II disease and had exenteration as primary treatment.[24] The 5-year survival rate for patients with leiomyosarcoma was 36%. It was noted that most recurrences were pelvic; therefore, judicious postoperative RT may be considered when optimal resection is not possible.

Rhabdomyosarcomas typically have a better prognosis. The 5-year survival rate reported in 12 children less than 5 years of ages was 90% in the National Cancer Data Base study. In one series, 38 children with vaginal, vulvar, or uterine rhabdomyosarcoma were enrolled on sequential International Society of Pediatric Oncology trials; the majority were treated with chemotherapy initially, with the most common

Table 10-3 Results for Definitive Radiotherapy With and Without Chemotherapy for Vaginal Cancer by FIGO Stage

| Study | Chemo | N | 5-Year End Points | | | | ≥ G3 Late AE |
			I	II	III	IV	
Surgery alone							
Creasman[6]	No	131	90%[a]	70%[a]	47%[a]		NS
Ball[79]	No	30	84%[a]	75%[a]	50%[a]	0%[a]	23% fistulas
Stock[36]	No	40	56%[b]	68%[b]	—	50%[b]	15%(10 year)
Surgery followed by adjuvant radiation therapy							
Creasman[6]	No	122	79%[a]	58%[a]	60%[a]		NS
Davis[38]	No	14	100%[a]	69%[a]	—		
Stock[36]	No	13	100%[b]	69%[b]	—	0%[b]	
Radiation alone							
Creasman[6]	No	402	63%[a]	57%[a]	35%[a]		NS
Perez[1]	No	192	80%[b] (10 year)	35-55%[b] (10 year)	38%[b] (10 year)		16% crude
Frank[80]	No	193	85%[c]	78%[c]	58%[c]		10% (5 year), 17% (10 year)
de Crevoisier[81]	No	91	65%[a]	62%[a]	42%[a]	2/4 recurred	15% crude
Mock (HDR)[46]	No	86	41%[a]	43%[a]	37%[a]	0%[a]	1-3% crude
Kirkbride[71]	No	118	75%[c]	76%[c]	60%[a]	42%[a]	18% crude
Tran[82]	No	78	92%[c]	68%[c]	44%[c]	13%[c]	16% (5 year)
Ball[79]	No	25	55%[a]	13%[a]	0%[a]	0%[a]	NS
Stock[36]	No	47	80%[b]	31%[b]	0%[b]	0%[b]	11% (10 year)
Chemoradiation							
Creasman[6]	Yes	9	71%[a] (also received surgery)				NS
Frank[80]	Yes	13	4/4 recurred with neoadjuvant drug, 5/9 recurred with concurrent chemo				NS
Kirkbride[71]	Yes	26	50%[c] with 20/26 being stage III or IV				NS
Samant[83]	Yes	12	66%[a], 75%[d] with 6/12 being stage III or IV				2/12 developed fistulas
Nashiro[84]	Yes	6	2/6 recurred, 1/6 died of disease				1/6 developed fistula
Dalrymple[85]	Yes	14	1/14 died of disease, 4/14 died of intercurrent disease				No fistulas
Sinha[86]	Yes	11	55%[d] (7/11 being stage III or IV, 2/11 had surgery)				18% crude

AE, adverse events; FIGO, International Federation of Gynecology and Obstetrics; HDR, high dose-rate; NS, not specified.
[a]Overall survival.
[b]Disease-free survival.
[c]Disease-specific survival.
[d]Freedom from progression.

regimen consisting of ifosfamide, vincristine, and actinomycin D.[73] Seventeen of 38 required additional local treatment, with 10 undergoing RT, 3 undergoing surgery, and 4 undergoing both RT and surgery. The 5-year survival rate was 91%, with a disease-free survival rate of 78%. Additional series from the Intergroup Rhabdomyosarcoma Study support the use of chemotherapy followed by conservative surgery and/or RT for residual disease.[74]

The prognosis of vaginal melanomas is generally poor, with 5-year survival rates ranging from 5% to 25% in various case series.[21,31,55,75]

MANAGEMENT OF RECURRENT DISEASE

Key Points

1. Local recurrences of vaginal cancer may be curable with radiotherapy or pelvic exenteration.
2. Distant recurrences are typically managed with chemotherapy, although prognosis is poor.

Management of recurrent vaginal cancer provides a significant challenge. Factors to consider before determining therapy include previous treatment modalities, extent of recurrent disease, site of recurrence, and the patient's health and performance status. Consideration must also be given to whether the goal of treatment is curative or palliative. Distant metastasis is generally associated with a poor prognosis, but patients with small local recurrences are potentially curable.

The majority of recurrences are pelvic, with a historical 5-year survival rate of 12% after salvage therapy.[70] Improvements in RT and advances in chemotherapy have the potential to increase the survival of this population of women. In patients with central recurrences who underwent surgical management as their primary treatment, the treatment of choice is RT. In patients who have previously received RT with local recurrence, treatment is usually limited to pelvic exenteration. Berek et al[76] noted an approximately 50% 5-year survival rate in patients who underwent pelvic exenterations for recurrent or persistent gynecologic malignancies, including vaginal cancer.

Herbst[4] noted a 23% recurrence rate in patients with a history of clear cell adenocarcinoma of the vagina. Sixty percent of patients had recurrence in the pelvis, 36% in the lungs, and 20% in the supraclavicular lymph nodes. Various treatment strategies were evaluated, including chemotherapy, RT, and radical surgery, with a 3-year survival rate of only 20%. Patients with small central recurrences had an overall better prognosis when treated with surgical management.

SPECIAL MANAGEMENT PROBLEMS

The majority of malignancies identified in the vagina are metastatic in origin. Most cases are secondary to direct invasion or lymphatic spread from the primary tumor, and the diagnosis is easily made. In rare cases, the metastasis is from a distant organ and the diagnosis can prove challenging. Although case reports of metastasis to the vagina are reported from a wide variety of sites, treatment is generally guided by the origin of the primary tumor.

Gestational trophoblastic disease (GTD) often metastasizes to the vagina, which is second only to the lung as the most common site of distant spread. Berry and colleagues[77] reported vaginal metastases from GTD in 4.5% of patients. The World Health Organization does not consider vaginal metastasis as a high-risk prognostic factor, and according to FIGO, GTD with metastasis confined to genital structures is considered stage II disease and is usually treated with single-agent chemotherapy, most commonly methotrexate.[77,78] Although metastatic disease to the vagina has a good prognosis, vaginal tumors are often highly vascular and can cause significant hemorrhage when biopsied.

FUTURE DIRECTIONS

Given the low number of patients diagnosed with primary vaginal cancer, it is unlikely that there will ever be randomized control trials evaluating different treatment regimens. With the shared pathophysiology between squamous cells carcinoma of the vagina and cervix, the results of randomized trials involving cervical cancer may be cautiously applied to the treatment of vaginal cancer. It is likely that widespread acceptance and utilization of the HPV vaccine will further reduce the number of cases of vaginal carcinoma, although the degree of this reduction is a matter of debate.

REFERENCES

1. Perez CA, Grigsby PW, Garipagaoglu M, Mutch DG, Lockett MA. Factors affecting long-term outcome of irradiation in carcinoma of the vagina. *Int J Radiat Oncol Biol Phys.* 1999;44(1):37-45.
2. Fu Y. *Pathology of the Uterine Cervix, Vagina, and Vulva.* 2nd ed. Philadelphia, PA: Saunders; 2002.
3. American Cancer Society. *Vaginal Cancer.* 2010. http://www.cancer.org/Cancer/VaginalCancer/DetailedGuide/vaginal-cancer-key-statistics. Accessed January 10, 2012.
4. Herbst AL, Norusis MJ, Rosenow PJ, Welch WR, Scully RE. An analysis of 346 cases of clear cell adenocarcinoma of the vagina and cervix with emphasis on recurrence and survival. *Gynecol Oncol.* 1979;7(2):111-122.
5. Daling JR, et al. A population-based study of squamous cell vaginal cancer: HPV and cofactors. *Gynecol Oncol.* 2002;84(2):263-270.
6. Creasman WT, Phillips JL, Menck HR. The National Cancer Data Base report on cancer of the vagina. *Cancer.* 1998;83(5):1033-1040.
7. Shah CA, Goff BA, Lowe K, Peters WA. Factors affecting risk of mortality in women with vaginal cancer. *Obstet Gynecol.* 2009;113(5):1038-1045.
8. Aho M, Vesterinen E, Meyer B, Purola E, Paavonen J. Natural history of vaginal intraepithelial neoplasia. *Cancer.* 1991;68(1):195-197.
9. Schockaert S, Poppe W, Arbyn M, Verguts T, Verguts J. Incidence of vaginal intraepithelial neoplasia after hysterectomy for cervical intraepithelial neoplasia: a retrospective study. *Am J Obstet Gynecol.* 2008;199(2):113e1-113e5.

10. Jimenez W, Paszat L, Kupets R, Wilton A, Tinmouth J. Presumed previous human papillomavirus (HPV) related gynecological cancer in women diagnosed with anal cancer in the province of Ontario. *Gynecol Oncol*. 2009;114(3):395-398.

11. ACOG Practice Bulletin no. 109. Cervical cytology screening. *Obstet Gynecol*. 2009;114(6):1409-1420.

12. Gupta D, Malpica A, Deavers MT, Silva EG. Vaginal melanoma: a clinicopathologic and immunohistochemical study of 26 cases. *Am J Surg Pathol*. 2002;26(11):1450-1457.

13. Miner TJ, Delgado R, Zeisler J, et al. Primary vaginal melanoma: a critical analysis of therapy. *Ann Surg Oncol*. 2004;11(1):34-39.

14. Insinga RP, Liaw KL, Johnson LG, Madeleine MM. A systematic review of the prevalence and attribution of human papillomavirus types among cervical, vaginal, and vulvar precancers and cancers in the United States. *Cancer Epidemiol Biomarkers Prev*. 2008;17(7):1611-1622.

15. Smith JS, Backes DM, Hoots BE, Kurman RJ, Pimenta JM. Human papillomavirus type-distribution in vulvar and vaginal cancers and their associated precursors. *Obstet Gynecol*. 2009;113(4):917-924.

16. Herbst AL, Scully RE. Adenocarcinoma of the vagina in adolescence. A report of 7 cases including 6 clear-cell carcinomas (so-called mesonephromas). *Cancer*. 1970;25(4):745-757.

17. Hatch EE, Palmer JR, Titus-Ernstoff L, et al. Cancer risk in women exposed to diethylstilbestrol in utero. *JAMA*. 1998;280(7):630-634.

18. Frank SJ, Deavers MT, Jhingran A, Bodurka DC, Eifel PJ. Primary adenocarcinoma of the vagina not associated with diethylstilbestrol (DES) exposure. *Gynecol Oncol*. 2007;105(2):470-474.

19. Piura B. Management of primary melanoma of the female urogenital tract. *Lancet Oncol*. 2008;9(10):973-981.

20. Sugiyama VE, Chan JK, Kapp DS. Management of melanomas of the female genital tract. *Curr Opin Oncol*. 2008;20(5):565-569.

21. Weinstock MA. Malignant melanoma of the vulva and vagina in the United States: patterns of incidence and population-based estimates of survival. *Am J Obstet Gynecol*. 1994;171(5):1225-1230.

22. Nigogosyan G, Delapava S, Pickren JW. Melanoblasts in vaginal mucosa. Origin for primary malignant melanoma. *Cancer*. 1964;17:912-913.

23. Herbst AL, Green TR Jr, Ulfelder H. Primary carcinoma of the vagina. An analysis of 68 cases. *Am J Obstet Gynecol*. 1970;106(2):210-218.

24. Peters WA 3rd, Kumar NB, Andersen WA, Morley GW. Primary sarcoma of the adult vagina: a clinicopathologic study. *Obstet Gynecol*. 1985;65(5):699-704.

25. Curtin JP, Saigo P, Slucher B, Venkatraman ES, Mychalczak B, Hoskins WJ. Soft-tissue sarcoma of the vagina and vulva: a clinicopathologic study. *Obstet Gynecol*. 1995;86(2):269-272.

26. Powell JL, Franklin EW, 3rd, Nickerson JF, Burrell MO. Verrucous carcinoma of the female genital tract. *Gynecol Oncol*. 1978;6(6):565-573.

27. Handel LN, Scott SM, Giller RH, Greffe BS, Lovell MA, Koyle MA. New perspectives on therapy for vaginal endodermal sinus tumors. *J Urol*. 2002;168(2):687-690.

28. Plentl AA, Friedman EA. Lymphatic system of the female genitalia. The morphologic basis of oncologic diagnosis and therapy. *Major Probl Obstet Gynecol*. 1971;2:1-223.

29. Lian J, Dundas G, Carlone M, Ghosh S, Pearcey R. Twenty-year review of radiotherapy for vaginal cancer: an institutional experience. *Gynecol Oncol*. 2008;111(2):298-306.

30. Breslow A. Thickness, cross-sectional areas and depth of invasion in the prognosis of cutaneous melanoma. *Ann Surg*. 1970;172(5):902-908.

31. Petru E, Nagele F, Czerwenka K, et al. Primary malignant melanoma of the vagina: long-term remission following radiation therapy. *Gynecol Oncol*. 1998;70(1):23-26.

32. Reid GC, Schmidt RW, Roberts JA, Hopkins MP, Barrett RJ, Morley GW. Primary melanoma of the vagina: a clinicopathologic analysis. *Obstet Gynecol*. 1989;74(2):190-199.

33. Van Nostrand KM, Lucci JA, 3rd, Schell M, Berman ML, Manetta A, DiSaia PJ. Primary vaginal melanoma: improved survival with radical pelvic surgery. *Gynecol Oncol*. 1994;55(2):234-237.

34. Hoffman MS, DeCesare SL, Roberts WS, Fiorica JV, Finan MA, Cavanagh D. Upper vaginectomy for in situ and occult, superficially invasive carcinoma of the vagina. *Am J Obstet Gynecol*. 1992;166(1 pt 1):30-33.

35. Peters WA 3rd, Kumar NB, Morley GW. Microinvasive carcinoma of the vagina: a distinct clinical entity? *Am J Obstet Gynecol*. 1985;153(5):505-507.

36. Stock RG, Chen AS, Seski J. A 30-year experience in the management of primary carcinoma of the vagina: analysis of prognostic factors and treatment modalities. *Gynecol Oncol*. 1995;56(1):45-52.

37. Tjalma WA, Monaghan JM, de Barros Lopes A, Naik R, Nordin AJ, Weyler JJ. The role of surgery in invasive squamous carcinoma of the vagina. *Gynecol Oncol*. 2001;81(3):360-365.

38. Davis KP, Stanhope CR, Garton GR, Atkinson EJ, O'Brien PC. Invasive vaginal carcinoma: analysis of early-stage disease. *Gynecol Oncol*. 1991;42(2):131-136.

39. Cutillo G, Cignini P, Pizzi G, et al. Conservative treatment of reproductive and sexual function in young woman with squamous carcinoma of the vagina. *Gynecol Oncol*. 2006;103(1):234-237.

40. Frumovitz M, Gayed IW, Jhingran A, et al. Lymphatic mapping and sentinel lymph node detection in women with vaginal cancer. *Gynecol Oncol*. 2008;108(3):478-481.

41. van Dam P, Sonnemans H, van Dam PJ, Verkinderen L, Dirix LY. Sentinel node detection in patients with vaginal carcinoma. *Gynecol Oncol*. 2004;92(1):89-92.

42. Eifel PJ, Winter K, Morris M, et al. Pelvic irradiation with concurrent chemotherapy versus pelvic and para-aortic irradiation for high-risk cervical cancer: an update of radiation therapy oncology group trial (RTOG) 90-01. *J Clin Oncol*. 2004;22(5):872-880.

43. Rose PG, Ali S, Watkins E, et al. Long-term follow-up of a randomized trial comparing concurrent single agent cisplatin, cisplatin-based combination chemotherapy, or hydroxyurea during pelvic irradiation for locally advanced cervical cancer: a Gynecologic Oncology Group Study. *J Clin Oncol*. 2007;25(19):2804-2810.

44. Whitney CW, Sause W, Bundy BN, et al. Randomized comparison of fluorouracil plus cisplatin versus hydroxyurea as an adjunct to radiation therapy in stage IIB-IVA carcinoma of the cervix with negative para-aortic lymph nodes: a Gynecologic Oncology Group and Southwest Oncology Group study. *J Clin Oncol*. 1999;17(5):1339-1348.

45. Peters WA 3rd, Liu PY, Barrett RJ, 2nd, et al. Concurrent chemotherapy and pelvic radiation therapy compared with pelvic radiation therapy alone as adjuvant therapy after radical surgery in high-risk early-stage cancer of the cervix. *J Clin Oncol*. 2000;18(8):1606-1613.

46. Mock U, Kucera H, Fellner C, Knocke TH, Potter R. High-dose-rate (HDR) brachytherapy with or without external beam radiotherapy in the treatment of primary vaginal carcinoma: long-term results and side effects. *Int J Radiat Oncol Biol Phys*. 2003;56(4):950-957.

47. Gilroy JS, Amdur RJ, Louis DA, Li JG, Mendenhall WM. Irradiating the groin nodes without breaking a leg: a comparison of techniques for groin node irradiation. *Med Dosim*. 2004;29(4):258-264.

48. Taylor A, Powell ME. An assessment of interfractional uterine and cervical motion: implications for radiotherapy target volume definition in gynaecological cancer. *Radiother Oncol*. 2008;88(2):250-257.

49. Beadle BM, Jhingran A, Salehpour M, Sam M, Iyer RB, Eifel PJ. Cervix regression and motion during the course of external beam chemoradiation for cervical cancer. *Int J Radiat Oncol Biol Phys.* 2009;73(1):235-241.

50. Chen YJ, Liu A, Tsai PT, et al. Organ sparing by conformal avoidance intensity-modulated radiation therapy for anal cancer: dosimetric evaluation of coverage of pelvis and inguinal/femoral nodes. *Int J Radiat Oncol Biol Phys.* 2005;63(1):274-281.

51. Fleming P, Nisar Syed AM, Neblett D, Puthawala A, George FW, 3rd, Townsend D. Description of an afterloading 192Ir interstitial-intracavitary technique in the treatment of carcinoma of the vagina. *Obstet Gynecol.* 1980;55(4):525-530.

52. Martinez A, Cox RS, Edmundson GK. A multiple-site perineal applicator (MUPIT) for treatment of prostatic, anorectal, and gynecologic malignancies. *Int J Radiat Oncol Biol Phys.* 1984;10(2):297-305.

53. Geisler JP, Look KY, Moore DA, Sutton GP. Pelvic exenteration for malignant melanomas of the vagina or urethra with over 3 mm of invasion. *Gynecol Oncol.* 1995;59(3):338-341.

54. Bonner JA, Perez-Tamayo C, Reid GC, Roberts JA, Morley GW. The management of vaginal melanoma. *Cancer.* 1988;62(9):2066-2072.

55. Irvin WP Jr, Bliss SA, Rice LW, Taylor PT, Jr., Andersen WA. Malignant melanoma of the vagina and locoregional control: radical surgery revisited. *Gynecol Oncol.* 1998;71(3):476-480.

56. McGuire SE, Frank SJ, Eifel PJ. Treatment of recurrent vaginal melanoma with external beam radiation therapy and palladium-103 brachytherapy. *Brachytherapy.* 2008;7(4):359-363.

57. Abramova L, Parekh J, Irvin WP, Jr., et al. Sentinel node biopsy in vulvar and vaginal melanoma: presentation of six cases and a literature review. *Ann Surg Oncol.* 2002;9(9):840-846.

58. Kobayashi K, Ramirez PT, Kim EE, et al. Sentinel node mapping in vulvovaginal melanoma using SPECT/CT lymphoscintigraphy. *Clin Nucl Med.* 2009;34(12):859-861.

59. Muss HB, Bundy B, DiSaia PJ, et al. Treatment of recurrent or advanced uterine sarcoma. A randomized trial of doxorubicin versus doxorubicin and cyclophosphamide (a phase III trial of the Gynecologic Oncology Group). *Cancer.* 1985;55(8):1648-1653.

60. Sutton G, Blessing JA, Ball H. Phase II trial of paclitaxel in leiomyosarcoma of the uterus: a gynecologic oncology group study. *Gynecol Oncol.* 1999;74(3):346-349.

61. Thigpen JT, Blessing JA, Beecham J, Homesley H, Yordan E. Phase II trial of cisplatin as first-line chemotherapy in patients with advanced or recurrent uterine sarcmas: a Gynecologic Oncology Group study. *J Clin Oncol.* 1991;9(11):1962-1966.

62. Homesley HD, Filiaci V, Markman M, et al. Phase III trial of ifosfamide with or without paclitaxel in advanced uterine carcinosarcoma: a Gynecologic Oncology Group Study. *J Clin Oncol.* 2007;25(5):526-531.

63. Sutton G, Brunetto VL, Kilgore L, et al. A phase III trial of ifosfamide with or without cisplatin in carcinosarcoma of the uterus: a Gynecologic Oncology Group Study. *Gynecol Oncol.* 2000;79(2):147-153.

64. Perez CA, Kraus FT, Evans JC, Powers WE. Anaplastic transformation in verrucous carcinoma of the oral cavity after radiation therapy. *Radiology.* 1966;86(1):108-115.

65. Crowther ME, Lowe DG, Shepherd JH. Verrucous carcinoma of the female genital tract: a review. *Obstet Gynecol Surv.* 1988;43(5):263-280.

66. Huang SH, Lockwood G, Irish J, et al. Truths and myths about radiotherapy for verrucous carcinoma of larynx. *Int J Radiat Oncol Biol Phys.* 2009;73(4):1110-1115.

67. Terenziani M, preafico F, Collini P, Meazza C, Massimino M, Piva L. Endodermal sinus tumor of the vagina. *Pediatr Blood Cancer.* 2007;48(5):577-578.

68. Lacy J, Capra M, Allen L. Endodermal sinus tumor of the infant vagina treated exclusively with chemotherapy. *J Pediatr Hematol Oncol.* 2006;28(11):768-771.

69. Beller U, Benedet JL, Creasman WT, et al. Carcinoma of the vagina. FIGO 6th Annual Report on the Results of Treatment in Gynecological Cancer. *Int J Gynaecol Obstet.* 2006;95 (suppl 1):S29-S42.

70. Chyle V, Zagars GK, Wheeler JA, Wharton JT, Delclos L. Definitive radiotherapy for carcinoma of the vagina: outcome and prognostic factors. *Int J Radiat Oncol Biol Phys.* 1996;35(5):891-905.

71. Kirkbride P, Fyles A, Rawlings GA, et al. Carcinoma of the vagina—experience at the Princess Margaret Hospital (1974-1989). *Gynecol Oncol.* 1995;56(3):435-443.

72. Herbst AL, Anderson D. Clear cell adenocarcinoma of the vagina and cervix secondary to intrauterine exposure to diethylstilbestrol. *Semin Surg Oncol.* 1990;6(6):343-346.

73. Martelli H, Oberlin O, Rey A, et al. Conservative treatment for girls with nonmetastatic rhabdomyosarcoma of the genital tract: a report from the Study Committee of the International Society of Pediatric Oncology. *J Clin Oncol.* 1999;17(7):2117-2122.

74. Andrassy RJ, Hays DM, Raney RB, et al. Conservative surgical management of vaginal and vulvar pediatric rhabdomyosarcoma: a report from the Intergroup Rhabdomyosarcoma Study III. *J Pediatr Surg.* 1995;30(7):1034-1036; discussion 1036-1037.

75. Ragnarsson-Olding B, Johansson H, Rutqvist LE, Ringborg U. Malignant melanoma of the vulva and vagina. Trends in incidence, age distribution, and long-term survival among 245 consecutive cases in Sweden 1960-1984. *Cancer.* 1993;71(5):1893-1897.

76. Berek JS, Howe C, Lagasse LD, Hacker NF. Pelvic exenteration for recurrent gynecologic malignancy: survival and morbidity analysis of the 45-year experience at UCLA. *Gynecol Oncol.* 2005;99(1):153-159.

77. Berry E, Hagopian GS, Lurain JR. Vaginal metastases in gestational trophoblastic neoplasia. *J Reprod Med.* 2008;53(7):487-492.

78. El-Helw LM, Hancock BW. Treatment of metastatic gestational trophoblastic neoplasia. *Lancet Oncol.* 2007;8(8):715-724.

79. Ball HG, Berman ML. Management of primary vaginal carcinoma. *Gynecol Oncol.* 1982;14(2):154-163.

80. Frank SJ, Jhingran A, Levenback C, Eifel PJ. Definitive radiation therapy for squamous cell carcinoma of the vagina. *Int J Radiat Oncol Biol Phys.* 2005;62(1):138-147.

81. de Crevoisier R, Sanfilippo N, Gerbaulet A, et al. Exclusive radiotherapy for primary squamous cell carcinoma of the vagina. *Radiother Oncol.* 2007;85(3):362-370.

82. Tran PT, Su Z, Lee P, et al. Prognostic factors for outcomes and complications for primary squamous cell carcinoma of the vagina treated with radiation. *Gynecol Oncol.* 2007;105(3):641-649.

83. Samant R, Lau B, E C, Le T, Tam T. Primary vaginal cancer treated with concurrent chemoradiation using Cis-platinum. *Int J Radiat Oncol Biol Phys.* 2007;69(3):746-750.

84. Nashiro T, Yagi C, Hirakawa M, et al. Concurrent chemoradiation for locally advanced squamous cell carcinoma of the vagina: case series and literature review. *Int J Clin Oncol.* 2008;13(4):335-339.

85. Dalrymple JL, et al. Chemoradiation for primary invasive squamous carcinoma of the vagina. *Int J Gynecol Cancer.* 2004;14(1):110-117.

86. Sinha B, Stehman F, Schilder J, Clark L, Cardenes H. Indiana University experience in the management of vaginal cancer. *Int J Gynecol Cancer.* 2009;19(4):686-693.

CHAPTER 10

Management of the Adnexal Mass

Ritu Salani and Christa Nagel

Uterine adnexae are defined as the areas adjacent to the uterus that are occupied by the fallopian tubes and ovaries. The embryologic origin of the fallopian tubes and ovaries are 2 distinct events in the development of a female embryo. Development of the ovaries begins before the development of the remainder of the genital tract. The origin of the male and female gonads are similar up until the seventh week of gestation, at which time the primitive sex cords begin to break up in the female embryo. The developing ovary eventually has 3 layers: the surface epithelium, primitive germ cells, and sex cord epithelium. These layers give rise to the 3 main types of ovarian tumors: (1) epithelial tumors, which comprise approximately 70% of all ovarian neoplasms; (2) germ cell tumors, which comprise 15% to 20% of ovarian tumors; and (3) sex cord–stromal tumors, which account for 5% to 10% of ovarian tumors. The remainder of the masses are a result of metastatic or secondary involvement to the ovary.[1]

It is estimated that 289,000 women will undergo surgical intervention for an adnexal mass in the United States every year.[2] This represents one of the most common indications for gynecologic surgery.[3] The determination of whether a mass represents a condition that requires immediate surgical intervention, or is likely to be malignant or benign, is of paramount importance. A patient's demographics, presenting symptoms, physical examination, imaging, laboratory studies, and family history can provide invaluable insights in determining the appropriate treatment plan. Given this information, a physician can form an accurate differential diagnosis and establish an appropriate management plan.

DIAGNOSIS

Key Points

1. Ultrasound characteristics of malignant adnexal masses include presence of complex or solid components, presence of ascites, bilaterality, and size greater than 10 cm.
2. Serum tumor markers useful in the evaluation of adnexal masses include CA125, alpha-fetoprotein, lactate dehydrogenase, human chorionic gonadotropin, and inhibin A and B.
3. Novel markers, including human epididymis 4 protein (HE4), transthyretin, transferrin, β-microglobulin, and apolipoprotein A1 may improve preoperative assessment of the risk of malignancy in adnexal masses.

Symptoms

Not all patients with an adnexal mass initially present with symptoms. Some masses are found incidentally on imaging ordered for the evaluation of unrelated conditions. However, when patients do present with symptoms, detailed evaluation and characterization of the reporting signs can provide insight into the etiology of the mass. Physicians should question patients regarding the duration, intensity, location, and radiation of their pain to determine whether immediate surgical intervention is needed for conditions such as ovarian torsion or ectopic pregnancy. Physicians should also perform a complete review of systems focusing on symptoms that can help elucidate the etiology of an adnexal mass such as the following: fevers, chills, vaginal discharge, vaginal bleeding, weight loss, abdominal bloating, changes in bowel or bladder function, and early satiety.[4]

Abdominal pain is a common presenting symptom for the majority of patients who are diagnosed with an adnexal mass. The first step in treating a patient who presents with abdominal pain is to differentiate those who will ultimately be diagnosed with conditions that require emergent surgical intervention, such as ectopic pregnancy, adnexal torsion, or a ruptured tubo-ovarian abscess (TOA). A pregnancy test should be performed in any woman of reproductive age whose symptoms include abdominal pain and abnormal bleeding. In the case of a ruptured TOA, a patient may have signs and symptoms of an acute abdomen and/or hemodynamic instability, requiring emergent surgical intervention.[5] Similarly, adnexal torsion may be an operative emergency. *Torsion* is defined as the twisting of an ovarian mass around the infundibulo-pelvic ligament, which results in compromise of the arterial and venous blood flow. This is a condition that is often difficult to diagnose and requires a high suspicion from the patient's initial presentation. Findings consistent with adnexal torsion include acute onset of abdominal pain (<8 hours), vomiting, and absence of bleeding or leukorrhea. Thus, particularly in premenopausal women, prompt recognition and treatment is paramount in preserving the involved ovary.[6] Another entity that commonly presents with abdominal pain, a pelvic mass, and fever is a TOA. Leukorrhea combined with a previous diagnosis of pelvic inflammatory disease (PID) or sexually transmitted infection should also raise the suspicion of TOA, as 30% of patients admitted with PID will go on to develop a TOA.[7]

Once emergent situations are excluded, the focus of the evaluation of an adnexal mass turns to determination of its etiology. A patient's presenting symptoms may initially help determine the likelihood that a mass is malignant. In 2000, Goff et al[8] evaluated the symptoms of 1725 women with ovarian cancer and found that 95% had previously presented with symptoms before their diagnosis. The most commonly reported symptoms were related to abdominal and gastrointestinal complaints. They also found that 89% of patients with stage I/II disease had symptomatic complaints before their diagnosis. In supplementary studies, further characterization of symptoms most indicative of malignancy, accounting for duration, intensity, and frequency, was conducted. The Early Ovarian Cancer Detection Study, which comprised a 23-item symptom index in an exploratory group of patients, found that the symptoms that strongly correlated with an ultimate diagnosis of ovarian cancer were pelvic pain, abdominal pain, increased abdominal size or bloating, early satiety, and difficulty eating. Further assessment of a modified symptom index in women with at least 1 symptom for less than a year and occurring greater than 12 times per month had an accuracy of 56.7% in women with early-stage ovarian cancer and in 79.5% in women with advanced-stage disease.[9]

In addition to the symptoms discussed in the preceding paragraph, other presenting complaints, when combined with the finding of an adnexal mass, may point to less common types of ovarian neoplasms. Estrogen-secreting tumors, such as granulosa cell tumors or a thecomas, should be considered in women with an adnexal mass, abnormal uterine bleeding, and breast tenderness, or precocious puberty in prepubertal females.[10-12] In contrast, Sertoli-Leydig tumors, which secrete testosterone, often present with symptoms such as hirsutism and deepening of the voice.[13] Other rare findings may include symptoms of hyperthyroidism in patients with a struma ovarii or symptoms such as flushing, diarrhea, and palpitations in women with a carcinoid tumor of the ovary.

Physical Examination

A thorough physical examination is advocated for the assessment of an adnexal mass, whether detected incidentally in an asymptomatic patient, or for the evaluation of symptoms. The health care provider should note general appearance. This includes assessment for signs of cachexia, such as temporal wasting, which may be found in women with advanced malignancies. Patients with a functional tumor may have signs of virilization, including hirsutism, male pattern balding, clitoromegaly, and acne indicating a hyperandrogenic state, or breast tenderness and vaginal bleeding, possibly suggesting a hyperestrogenic state.

In addition to a general examination, emphasis should be placed on a comprehensive evaluation of supraclavicular, axillary, and inguinal lymph nodes. Abdominal examination is a critical portion of the physical examination, allowing for palpation of large masses and assessment of pain. Tenderness, particularly with fever, may indicate an infectious process, such as a TOA. Presence of a fluid wave or omental caking may be indicative of advanced ovarian cancer.[4,14]

The pelvic examination affords assessment of the uterus and the adnexae. Speculum examination provides evaluation for signs of recent bleeding or displacement of the cervix secondary to the presence of a pelvic mass. Furthermore, characteristics of the mass, such as contour (smooth vs. irregular), firmness (solid, cystic, or mixed), and mobility should be assessed on examination. The rectovaginal examination allows for palpation of the uterosacral ligaments and the cul-de-sac, where nodularity or obliteration may suggest the presence of endometriosis or metastatic cancer. If a primary colonic malignancy is suspected, a stool guaiac should be performed.[4]

Studies have shown that examiners, regardless of experience, tend to underestimate the size of a mass on pelvic examination.[15] In a pooled analysis of studies evaluating the ability of pelvic examination to detect a pelvic mass, sensitivity was 45%.[14] Therefore, one must recognize the limitations of the pelvic examination, which can be further compromised by the presence of a small adnexal mass or in the obese patient.[14,15] Thus a normal examination does not eliminate the need for further evaluation.

Radiographic Imaging

Once an adnexal mass is suspected, the proper imaging modality must be determined. Ultrasound uses high-frequency ultrasonic waves to create a picture of the internal and external structures of a mass (Figure 11-1). Used either transvaginally and/or transabdominally, it is both an inexpensive and accurate way to determine the origin of an adnexal mass and allows further characterization of the mass as benign, malignant, or indeterminate.[16] Table 11-1 provides an overview of

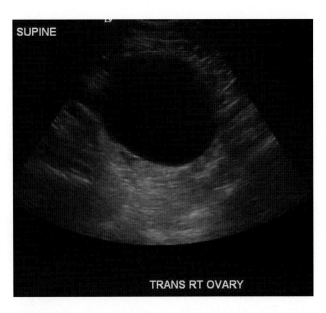

FIGURE 11-1. A simple ovarian cyst on transvaginal ultrasound.

Table 11-1 Ultrasound Characteristics for Common Adnexal Masses

Tumor Type	Ultrasound Appearance
Dermoid cyst	"White ball" appearance secondary to hair and sebaceous fluid Echogenic dots representing free floating hair within the cyst fluid Shadowing secondary to solid/semi-solid components
Endometrioma	Ground glass appearance
Hemorrhagic corpus luteum	"Spider web" secondary to clots of multiple ages No Doppler signal "Jelly-like" movement
Hydro/pyosalpinx	Fluid-filled tubular structure Incomplete septa Visualization of mucosal folds on transverse view
Benign solid lesions (fibromas, fibrothecomas, thecofibromas, thecomas, Brenner tumors)	Well circumscribed Homogenous Solid
Tubo-ovarian abscess	Uni or multilocular "Ground glass" appearance Pain with imaging
Benign cystic lesions (serous cystadenoma, mucinous cystadenoma, adenofibroma)	Uni-bilocular structure Thin walls and septa Homogenous appearance No vegetations
Characteristics concerning for malignancy	Complex or solid mass Ascites Presence of blood flow within a solid papillary projection Diameter >10 cm Irregular internal cyst walls Bilateral tumors Septation >3 mm in width

common characteristic appearances on ultrasound for benign and malignant ovarian masses.[17]

In 2009, Sokalska et al[18] studied the ability of ultrasound to provide a specific diagnosis of an adnexal mass that was compared with final pathology after surgical management. In 800 women with benign processes, the sensitivity of diagnosing dermoid cysts (86%), hydrosalpinges (86%), and endometriomas (77%) were the highest among all ovarian pathologies. In addition to the detection of benign conditions, certain ultrasound findings can also raise the suspicion of a malignant origin. The size, location, locularity, echogenicity, and blood flow of a mass are characteristics used to determine the malignant potential of a pelvic mass. In an evaluation of symptoms in combination with ultrasound findings, the factors that raised the probability of malignancy were a personal history of ovarian cancer, older age, presence of ascites, presence of blood flow within a solid papillary projection, increasing diameter of the solid component of the mass, and irregular internal cyst walls. Factors that decreased the probability of malignancy were the presence of pain during the ultrasound examination, current use of hormonal therapy, and the presence of acoustic shadows. The ultimate sensitivity and specificity of this model were 93% and 76%, respectively.[19] McDonald et al[20] also looked at ultrasound characteristics of adnexal masses that conferred a probability of malignancy. This study confirmed that older age (>55 years), presence of complex or solid components, presence of ascites, bilateral tumors, and a mass greater than 10 cm were all associated with an increased risk of malignancy at the time of surgical intervention.

The use of color flow Doppler, which evaluates the blood flow of a mass, has also been studied for the evaluation of an adnexal mass. However, this technique has been found to be inconsistent in the differentiation between various etiologies and not recommended for routine use at this time.[17] The introduction of 3-dimensional (3D) ultrasound and its utility in the evaluation of a pelvic mass has been less clearly defined. Recent studies have compared the use of 3D ultrasound with conventional ultrasound for the evaluation of a pelvic mass. However, results are premature, and given the limited data, high costs, and availability of 3D ultrasound, its routine use for evaluation of an adnexal mass is not yet recommended.[21]

Though not ideal for initial imaging, the use of magnetic resonance imaging (MRI) may be helpful in further assessing those masses that have an indeterminate malignant potential on ultrasound. The differential diagnosis of an indeterminate adnexal mass on MRI is determined by its dominant signal characteristic. Mature teratomas, hemorrhagic cysts, endometriomas, mucinous cystadenomas, and melanoma metastasis are characterized by a "bright" T1 signal.

The T1 signal helps to further define components of blood, blood clots, fat, and proteinaceous material that suggest a benign lesion, but are not always clearly delineated with ultrasonography. These images are especially helpful in defining heme-filled masses that may appear to be solid in nature on ultrasound. In addition, fat-suppressed T1 images are used to identify small amounts of fat within an adnexal mass that most often signify a mature teratoma.[22] In contrast to this, lesions demonstrating a solid T2 signal may be either malignant or benign. Masses that are homogenously dark, well circumscribed, and smooth are most often leiomyomas or an ovarian fibroma/thecoma. A mixed signal solid mass on T2 imaging should raise an increased suspicion of malignancy. These are usually demonstrated by tumors that express both dark and bright signals. Lastly, tumors that have a predominantly cystic-solid appearance may be aided by further evaluation by MRI. Multilocular benign ovarian cysts, hydrosalpinx, and cystadenomas may appear to have "pseudo-solid" areas on ultrasound that are truly opposed folds of an otherwise cystic mass and that are able to be delineated by MRI. Further characterization of solid-cystic masses can be performed using contrast-enhanced MRI. The addition of contrast helps to more accurately identify solid components, such as mural nodules, areas of necrosis, and vegetations, which are concerning for malignancy.[16,22] Although MRI is expensive, its use to determine the appropriate therapeutic modality in patients with an indeterminate adnexal mass may be warranted. Because the majority of these masses will ultimately be benign in nature, the cost of an MRI may be indicated, as it may prevent patients from undergoing an unnecessary surgical procedure.[22]

In past decades, the use of computed tomography (CT) has been reserved for pre- and postoperative treatment planning for patients with ovarian cancer and not for detailed characterization of adnexal masses. This was mostly secondary to the inadequate characterization of soft tissue densities and the added exposure to radiation.[23] In 1998, the introduction of sub-millimeter spatial resolution and 2- and 3D spatial reconstruction resulted in the ability of CT scans to provide more accurate staging, evaluate disease volume, and determine resectability of metastatic ovarian cancer. In 2008, Tsili et al[23] conducted a prospective study that evaluated the use of CT in the detection and characterization of adnexal masses in patients diagnosed with an adnexal mass on physical exam or ultrasound. Characteristics examined on preoperative CT that were thought to be consistent with a malignant process included a diameter greater than 4 cm, presence of bilateral ovarian masses, cystic and solid components, necrosis present within a solid lesion, and a cystic lesion that contained thick (>3 mm) or irregular walls, septa, or papillary projections, as well

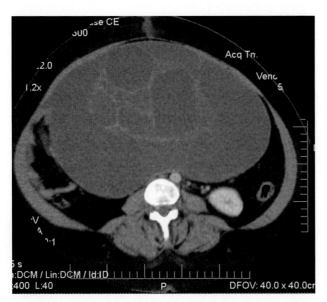

FIGURE 11-2. Large mucinous cystadenoma with multi-loculations (depicted by arrows) on CT scan.

as extra-ovarian disease (Figure 11-2). CT scanning correctly identified the origin of the adnexal mass in 96% of patients, with an overall diagnostic accuracy of 89%,[23] thus concluding that CT scans can provide an accurate characterization of adnexal masses.

The preferred imaging strategy of an adnexal mass is to start with the least expensive and readily available test, which, in most cases, is an ultrasound. For masses that are highly suspicious for malignancy on ultrasound, use of a CT scan may be considered for preoperative staging and determination of disease resectability. If a mass is indeterminate on ultrasound, either an MRI or CT may be used for further evaluation; however, the diagnostic test chosen should take into consideration the availability of resources, costs to the patient, and the implications of radiation exposure.

Tumor Markers

The use of tumor markers may aid in determining the malignant potential and histology of an adnexal mass. Typically elevated in patients who are ultimately diagnosed with cancer, the utility of tumor markers may be helpful in the initial diagnosis, monitoring of response to treatment, and triaging to the appropriate specialist. However, tumor markers should be ordered selectively, and physicians should take into account the patient's age, presentation of symptoms, findings on physical examination, and imaging.

Though currently there are no validated biomarkers for ovarian cancer screening, the use of CA-125 level has been extensively studied. CA-125 is a glycoprotein that is produced by the ovary, peritoneal, and pleural linings.

Although it is frequently elevated in malignant conditions, it can also be increased with benign processes, such as endometriosis and PID. In contrast, patients with early-stage epithelial ovarian carcinoma or borderline tumors may present with a normal CA-125 value.[24] However, when assessing a patient's risk of malignancy, this value may contribute to management decisions.

Germ cell tumors are most commonly associated with secretion of tumor markers. α-Fetoprotein (AFP) is an oncofetal protein that was initially characterized in the fetal liver and yolk sac, and elevation of this protein is often seen in hepatocellular carcinoma, gastric cancer, colon cancer, and pancreatic cancer.[25] Because the fetal liver and yolk sac produce AFP, tumors that resemble these tissues are often associated with increased serum levels. Kawai et al[26] examined at the association of 7 tumor markers with malignant germ cell tumors of the ovary. One hundred percent of patients with endodermal sinus tumors, 61.9% of patients with immature teratomas, and 11.8% of patients with dysgerminomas had elevated serum levels of AFP. More commonly, dysgerminomas, and to a lesser degree other germ cell tumors, are associated with an elevation in lactate dehydrogenase (LDH). Another commonly expressed tumor marker in germ cell tumors is human chorionic gonadotropin (hCG). This glycoprotein hormone, which is produced in pregnancy, is also secreted by germ cell tumors such as choriocarcinoma, embryonal carcinoma, and dysgerminoma (low levels).[26,27]

Inhibin A and B, which belong to heterodimeric glycoproteins of the transforming growth factor β family of growth factors, are the most common tumor markers associated with sex cord–stromal tumors, specifically granulosa cell tumors. In 2007, Mom et al[28] looked at the prevalence of elevations in both inhibin A and B in patients diagnosed with granulosa cell tumors. They found that 89% of patients had an elevated inhibin B level at the time of diagnosis, but only 67% had elevations in inhibin A. More patients were also noted to have an increase in inhibin B at the time of recurrence when compared with inhibin A. The conclusion from this study was that inhibin B levels more accurately reflect disease status in patients with granulosa cell tumors than inhibin A and should be used for diagnosis and monitoring.

Other biomarkers have also been evaluated in the work-up of a pelvic mass. CA 19-9, a monosialoganglioside, is commonly used for mucinous tumors of the gastrointestinal tract, most notably of the pancreas and biliary tract; however, it has also been found to be associated with mucinous tumors of the ovary. Unfortunately, CA 19-9 has not been helpful in separating benign from malignant tumors and is not recommended for use in triaging patients.[29] Another marker is carcinoembryonic antigen (CEA), which is an oncofetal antigen most often found in the colon. In the evaluation of an adnexal mass, CEA has limited potential; however,

Table 11-2 Tumor Marker Recommendations Based on Age

Age	Tumor Markers
≤30 years	AFP, hCG, LDH, inhibin A, inhibin B
30-50 years	Inhibin A, inhibin B, ± CA-125 depending on family history
≥50 years	CA-125, CA 19-9, ± inhibin A and B (if symptoms), ± CEA if suspected colonic primary

AFP, α-fetoprotein; CEA, carcinoembryonic antigen; hCG, human chorionic gonadotropin; LDH, lactate dehydrogenase.

it may be useful for detection of a colonic primary or metastatic disease involving the adnexa.[30]

The routine use of tumor markers in the evaluation of an adnexal mass can be helpful in determining the risk of malignancy, and therefore, the need for surgical intervention or referral. Table 11-2 lists the recommended tumor markers in the initial evaluation of an adnexal mass based on age at presentation. Caution should be used in placing a high degree of emphasis on the results of these laboratory values, and the entire clinical picture should be evaluated when determining a patient's ultimate treatment plan.

Assessing for Risk of Malignancy

When further work-up has confirmed the presence of an adnexal mass, assessment for malignancy is a top priority. Although surgical management may be warranted, the appropriate triage of patients to an oncologist is critical. Studies have shown that women with ovarian malignancies are more likely to undergo optimal cytoreductive surgery and have improved overall survival of more than 1 year when under the care of a gynecologic oncologist rather than a general gynecologist or surgeon.[31,32] Unfortunately, more than 50% of patients diagnosed with ovarian cancer are never seen by a gynecologic oncologist during their care.[31] If suspicious is high or the patient has a strong family history for genetic predisposition for ovarian cancer, referral may reduce the risk of reoperation and increase the rate of optimal cytoreduction, improving survival outcomes.

To help delineate which patients are at higher risk for the presence of an epithelial ovarian malignancy, multiple tests and guidelines have been proposed. In patients with adnexal masses, one of the most widely studied is the use of CA-125 levels. The CA-125 level is elevated in 80% of patients with epithelial cancer; however, this test is often elevated in benign conditions, such as leiomyomas, endometriosis, and diverticulitis. Although it is widely used, more precise

methods exist for discrimination between benign and malignant adnexal masses.[24]

In 2005, the American Congress of Obstetricians and Gynecologists (ACOG), along with the Society of Gynecologic Oncologists (SGO), devised guidelines for referral of the adnexal mass.[33] These guidelines, which are stratified by menopausal status, include assessment of CA-125 levels, presence of extraovarian disease or ascites, and family history. In a retrospective validation study, these guidelines showed that 70% of premenopausal and 94% of postmenopausal women with epithelial ovarian cancer were appropriately identified.[34] These guidelines have been further confirmed by other investigators and provide a simple assessment for referral.[35] It is important to remember that these guidelines assess predominantly for epithelial ovarian cancer. When evaluating a younger patient, in addition to the above assessment, consideration should be given to tumor markers for germ cell tumors, such as AFP, hCG, and LDH.[36]

In 1990, investigators reported on the use of the Risk of Malignancy Index (RMI), incorporating menopausal status, ultrasound characteristics, and CA-125 level, to discriminate between benign and malignant ovarian tumors to triage patients appropriately. Using a simple mathematical formula, an RMI at a value of ≥200 was able to detect women with a more than 40-fold risk of cancer compared with the background risk.[37] Since this time, modifications to the RMI have been studied, such as increasing the cut-off value to ≥450 or incorporating tumor size, which resulted in improvements in referral rates of malignant processes and a reduction in the number of benign tumors.[32,38,39]

Unfortunately, the RMI uses ultrasound as part of the analysis, which is operator dependent. Additionally, many patients are noted to have the presence of an adnexal mass on radiographic imaging such as CT scans, eliminating the need for ultrasonic evaluation. Thus, after a mass has been detected, several studies have examined the use of additional biomarkers. In addition to CA-125 values, the use of human epididymis 4 protein (HE4) has demonstrated potential. In a series of more than 500 women, the use of CA-125 and HE4 in combination successfully classified 94% of patients with epithelial ovarian cancer as high risk.[40] In a study of 65 biomarkers, the combination of CA-125 and HE4 provided the highest level of discrimination between malignant and benign ovarian tumors.[41] When using the Risk of Malignancy Algorithm, which combined the use of HE4 and CA-125 with the presence of an adnexal mass, sensitivity for malignancy was noted to be significantly increased over that of the RMI.[42]

Women with ovarian cancer frequently have a constellation of vague, yet persistent symptoms, including difficulty eating, early satiety, bloating, pain, and gastrointestinal and urinary symptoms. When using a specific symptom index in women with an adnexal mass, the sensitivity of predicting ovarian cancer was 64%. However, when the symptom index was combined with CA-125 and HE4, and 2 of the 3 tests were positive, the rate of detection increased to 84%. When the symptom index was used to triage high-risk patients for further study with CA-125 and HE4 levels, the specificity exceeded 98%.[43] Thus the authors concluded that the symptom index may be used to select for the use of CA-125 and HE4 in high-risk patients.

In early 2010, the US Food and Drug Administration approved the use of the OVA1 test (Vermillion). This test combines 5 immunoassays of CA-125, transthyretin, transferrin, β-microglobulin, and apolipoprotein A1 into a single numerical unit. In an evaluation of 516 women with an adnexal mass, the OVA1 test increased the sensitivity of preoperative assessment from 72.5% to 91.7% for a nongynecologic oncologist and from 77.5% to 98.9% for a gynecologic oncologist. The purpose of this test is to determine which patients should be referred to a gynecologic oncologist and supplements, but does not replace, clinical assessment.[44,45]

Development of the ideal test to distinguish benign from malignant pelvic masses continues to elude practitioners. Currently, using a combination of tumor markers and imaging, along with a thorough review of symptomatology and family history, provides the best assessment. Table 11-3 lists the sensitivity and specificity of the most commonly used tests to assess the risk of malignancy. Health care providers should always assess each patient individually and evaluate the entire clinical picture when determining which patients require referral to a gynecologic oncologists.

Table 11-3 Summary of Studies Assessing for Risk of Malignancy in an Adnexal Mass

Test	Sensitivity (%)	Specificity (%)
CA-125[4,33]	61-90	71-93
Risk of malignancy index[32,37-39]	78-96	70-97
ACOG/SGO guidelines[33-35]	77-94	60-70
HE4 and CA-125[40-42]	77-94	75-85
Symptom index ± HE4, CA-125[43]	58-95	80-88
OVA1[44,45]	92-99	43

PATHOLOGY

Key Points

1. Menopausal status, symptomatology, and risk factors for malignancy influence the differential diagnosis of adnexal masses.
2. The most common epithelial tumor presenting as an adnexal mass is the serous cystadenoma, followed by the mucinous cystadenoma, borderline tumor, mature teratoma, and endometrioma.

Differential Diagnosis

Once the presence of an adnexal mass has been detected, differential diagnoses should consider gynecologic and nongynecologic processes, as well as both benign and malignant entities. The differential for each patient should consider several factors to help tailor the most probable causes. First, identifying the menopausal status of the patient will narrow the possibilities. First, in young women, consideration should be given to pregnancy-related conditions, functional ovarian cysts, germ cell tumors, and entities such as endometriosis. In postmenopausal women, although the risk of malignancy is much higher than for their younger counterparts, the differential should also include cystadenomas and diverticular disease. Second, although many masses are found incidentally, symptomatology should be thoroughly reviewed.[8,9] This includes assessing for the presence of abdominal bloating and pain, as well as abnormal bleeding, suggesting uterine pathology, and evaluation of bowel symptoms, indicating gastrointestinal disease. Third, patient risk factors should be taken into account. Patients with a suspected or known genetic predisposition to ovarian malignancy, such as *BRCA* mutations or Lynch II syndrome, should be assessed appropriately.[33] This may result in favoring surgical management over conservative therapy as well as specific recommendations for surgery, such as a bilateral salpingo-oophorectomy or hysterectomy at the time of intervention. Furthermore, patients with a previous history of malignancy, particularly breast or colorectal cancers, are at risk for metastatic disease to the adnexae, and one should be aware of this possibility.[46] A differential diagnosis of an adnexal mass is provided in Table 11-4.

Benign Epithelial Neoplasms

Epithelial tumors comprise the largest subgroup of ovarian tumors. The most common histology within this subgroup is the serous cystadenoma, which accounts for

Table 11-4 List of Differential Diagnoses of an Adnexal Mass

	Benign	Malignant

Gynecologic causes	Functional cysts
	Benign neoplasms
	  Teratomas
	  Cystadenomas
	Leiomyomas
	Tubal processes
	  Tubo-ovarian abscess
	  Hydrosalpinx
	  Pyosalpinx
	Endometriosis/
	endometrioma
	Pregnancy-related
	conditions
	  Ectopic pregnancy
	  Theca-Lutein cysts
	Embryologic remnants
	  Paratubal cysts
	  Paraovarian cysts
		Epithelial ovarian cancer
		Germ cell tumors
		Sex cord–stromal tumors
		Fallopian tube carcinomas
		Borderline ovarian tumors

Nongynecologic causes	Gastrointestinal conditions
	  Diverticular disease
	  Appendiceal abscess/
	  mucocele
	Retroperitoneal tumors
	Schwannomas
	Urinary tract conditions
	  Ureteral/bladder
	  diverticula
	  Pelvic kidney
		Colorectal cancer
		Small bowel tumors
		Retroperitoneal sarcomas
		Metastatic disease to adnexa
		  Breast cancer
		  Colorectal cancer
		  Lymphoma

almost a quarter of benign ovarian neoplasms. These masses are characterized by a smooth cyst wall and are bilateral in 15% of cases.[47] Loculations may be present, along with the presence of psammoma bodies (calcifications). The second most common histologic subtype is the mucinous cystadenoma. These are often multiloculated and often unilateral. Rarely, these tumors can be associated with the presence of peritoneal implants and gelatinous ascites, known as *pseudomyxoma peritonei*. Less common epithelial tumors may also be encountered. These include Brenner tumors and benign mesotheliomas; the former is characterized by a transitional cell-like epithelium and is a rare ovarian tumor often found incidentally.[47]

Borderline Tumors

Borderline tumors, also known as tumors of low malignant potential, were first described in 1929.[48] These tumors were defined by the presence of proliferative activity, nuclear atypia, and presence or absence of stromal invasion. Histologically, they are classified based on epithelial characteristics, which are also found in their malignant counterparts. Serous and mucinous borderline tumors are the most common subtype encountered, comprising 95% of all borderline tumors.[48,49] These tumors are classically associated with surface papillations and exophytic growth. Less commonly seen subtypes include endometrioid, clear cell, or even Brenner borderline tumors.[48]

Serous borderline tumors are more often bilateral, which occurs in approximately 40% of cases, and more often associated with the findings of extraovarian disease, ranging from 25% to 35% of cases. In comparison, mucinous tumors are bilateral in only 10% of cases and are more often associated with foci of malignancy. Therefore, surgical staging and extensive pathology sampling is warranted.[48]

Recently, more detailed description has been given to the serous subgroup. Kurman et al[49] classified serous borderline tumors into 2 groups based on natural course of the disease process. The first group is defined as the atypical proliferative serous tumors, which behave similarly to benign serous tumors of the ovaries. The second group is the micropapillary serous carcinoma or intraepithelial serous carcinomas. This finding is associated with a poorer outcome and often accompanied by noninvasive implants. If invasive implants are encountered, the tumors may be classified as a low-grade serous carcinoma.[49] Although these terms may not be universally used, careful assessment of the histology will allow for better counseling of these patients.

Mature Teratomas

Although germ cell tumors are discussed in greater detail in Chapter 14, mature teratomas remain one of the most commonly encountered ovarian neoplasm. They account for 20% of all ovarian neoplasms in adults and approximately 50% in the pediatric/adolescent population.[50] These tumors are defined by presence of all 3 pluripotential germ cell layers: (1) ectoderm—such as hair and skin elements; (2) mesoderm—including fat, cartilage, and bone; and (3) endoderm—such as gastrointestinal and thyroid tissue. Rates of bilaterally exceed 10%, and although the mature classification suggests a benign nature, these tumors can, albeit rare, undergo malignant transformation.[50]

Endometriosis/Endometriomas

Endometriosis is an inflammatory condition stimulated by estrogen and is associated with infertility, chronic pelvic pain, and dyspareunia. Although symptoms vary in severity, endometriosis is estimated to affect 5% to 10% of reproductive age women.[51] One of the most common locations is on the ovary, known as an *endometrioma*, which is a cyst wall lined with endometrioid mucosa. Often these tumors have a complex appearance on ultrasound and are associated with an elevated CA-125 level. Additionally, malignant degeneration, typically clear cell or endometrioid carcinoma, is associated with this disease.[51] Thus clinical suspicion and appropriate evaluation will help determine the best management approach.

TREATMENT

Key Points

1. Women with adnexal masses with a high suspicion of malignancy should undergo surgical evaluation either via exploratory laparotomy or laparoscopy with care to avoid intraperitoneal rupture of the mass.
2. Conservative management with close surveillance is appropriate for masses suspected to be benign and are asymptomatic.

The management of an adnexal mass depends highly on the suspicion of malignancy. Presently, the lifetime risk of undergoing surgery for an ovarian neoplasm is 5% to 10%, although it is estimated that less than a quarter of these will be malignant.[4] Clinical decision making regarding a patient with an adnexal mass will result in observation with follow-up or operative management.[52] Patients with adnexal masses can be divided into 3 categories: (1) high suspicion of ovarian cancer, irrespective of symptoms; (2) suspected benign mass with symptoms; and (3) asymptomatic mass with low suspicion of malignancy.

When a patient falls into the first category, surgical intervention is warranted. These patients should be referred to a gynecologic oncologist or have a contingency plan in the event that malignancy is confirmed. Typically, this requires a midline vertical incision to allow for access to pelvic structures as well as the upper abdomen. The use of intraoperative frozen section, which has accuracy rates approaching 95% in the evaluation of ovarian tumors, may help identify a clinically early ovarian cancer and determine the need for surgical staging.[53,54]

Although aspiration of cyst fluid is contraindicated in postmenopausal women secondary to the risk of malignancy, occasionally patients are encountered who have a high likelihood of malignancy but who are not surgical candidates as a result of comorbidities. To establish a diagnosis, biopsy or cytology of an ovarian

mass may be required to confirm diagnosis and allow for commencement of therapy. However, this should be used judiciously, as cytology has poor sensitivity (25%-82%) and is considered a diagnostic tool and not a therapeutic measure.[33]

The management of symptomatic women with a pelvic mass with a low suspicion of malignancy may have an option of management modalities. First, physiologic cysts in women of reproductive age must be excluded. Certain conditions, such as endometriosis and TOAs, may be amenable to medical therapy, such as hormonal manipulation and antibiotics, respectively.[33] However, if symptoms are severe, or the patient declines or is unsuccessfully managed with medical therapy, surgery is often indicated. The extent of surgery should be further tailored by the patient's preference for future fertility and ovarian function. Often patients who are premenopausal may be managed with an ovarian cystectomy or unilateral salpingo-oophorectomy. However, patients should be counseled on the need for performing a bilateral salpingo-oophorectomy, particularly women at high risk for ovarian cancer.[55] Other possibilities for this procedure include bilateral involvement of the ovaries or in women with endometriosis and/or chronic pelvic pain, as rates for repeat operation approach 30%.[55] In patients who have completed child-bearing, the option of undergoing a hysterectomy at the time of surgery to reduce risk of pelvic surgery in the future may be discussed, although benefits of this practice are unclear at this time.

A more complicated scenario is the asymptomatic patient with an adnexal mass that appears to be at low risk for malignancy. In these situations, the risks and costs of surgical intervention often outweigh the benefit of surgery, and often expectant management is the treatment of choice. Several large studies have shown that asymptomatic women with simple, unilocular masses can be managed conservatively, as rates of malignancy are less than 1%.[14,33] Even in the postmenopausal setting, with a normal CA-125 level, expectant management of simple cysts up to 10 cm is recommended. In this scenario, more than two-thirds of these cysts respond without intervention.[56]

In addition to simple cysts of the ovaries, a series evaluating septated tumors, without solid areas or papillary projections, reported a spontaneous resolution rate of almost 40%, and no cases of ovarian cancer were reported with more than 6 years of follow-up.[57] Thus continued surveillance without surgical intervention may be appropriate for this group of patients. However, it is important to conduct follow-up with repeat imaging and CA-125 levels within 6 months to confirm improvement/resolution. If the mass persists, symptoms develop, or CA-125 level becomes abnormal, operative intervention should be considered.[52]

In a woman of reproductive age, findings of an asymptomatic mass often represent functional cysts. These cysts rarely exceed 7 cm, and resolution occurs in more than 70% of cases within 6 weeks.[4] Thus these tumors should be monitored conservatively with repeat imaging after 6 weeks, allowing for potential resolution with the menstrual cycle. Once a cyst is present, the use of oral contraceptives will not result in quicker resolution, but their use may prevent the formation of new cysts.[58] Occasionally, the incidental finding of a small adnexal cyst in the premenopausal woman will be discovered. If the cyst measures ≤2.5 cm, and there are no other concerning signs or symptoms, no further management is warranted.[4] Figures 11-3 and 11-4 provide general management schemas for premenopausal and postmenopausal patients with an adnexal mass.

Once the decision to proceed with surgery has been made, the surgical approach must then be addressed. For any patient with an obvious advanced malignancy, exploratory laparotomy with a vertical midline incision, allowing access to pelvis and upper abdomen, is recommended. In the patient with a suspected benign adnexal mass, laparoscopic management is preferred. Although rates of complications from laparoscopic ovarian procedures are low, ranging from 0% to 30%, and mortality is less than 1%, each decision should be individualized, taking into account the size of the mass, surgeon skill, and other factors, such as surgical and medical history

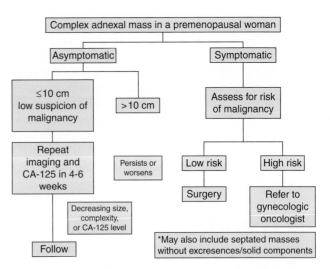

FIGURE 11-4. Schema for the management of a complex adnexal mass in a premenopausal woman.

of the patient.[14] Every effort should be made to avoid rupture, which, if encountered, can result in upstaging of malignancy. Additionally, every patient should be counseled and prepared for a laparotomy, in the event that minimally invasive surgery cannot safely be performed or an unsuspected malignancy is encountered.[52] Regardless of approach, it is important to obtain cytology, assess all peritoneal surfaces, and thoroughly inspect the abdominopelvic cavity.

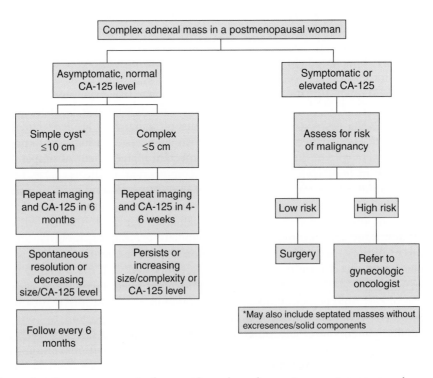

FIGURE 11-3. Schema for the management of a complex adnexal mass in a postmenopausal woman.

SPECIAL MANAGEMENT PROBLEMS

Management of Borderline Tumors

When epithelial ovarian cancer is encountered, surgical staging is recommended; when benign disease is found, either cystectomy or oophorectomy, depending on the patient's age, is warranted. However, when borderline tumors are diagnosed, the management options are varied. If diagnosed on frozen section, complete surgical staging is recommended due to the possibility of identifying invasive cancer on final pathology. For patients desiring fertility-sparing treatment, conservative staging with ovarian cystectomy or unilateral salpingo-oophorectomy with preservation of the contralateral ovary and uterus are acceptable. Patients should be aware that rates of recurrence range from 10% to 30% with this approach.[59] Because frozen section has a notoriously high rate of inaccuracy for the diagnosis of borderline tumors or if not performed, the diagnosis may not be apparent until final pathology.[54] Survival differences were not noted in patients who underwent a restaging operation that resulted in a higher stage of disease.[60] Other studies have supported this finding and reported that complete surgical staging for serous borderline tumors may not be necessary if the intracystic growth pattern has less than a 10% borderline change, as these typically behave like benign serous cystadenomas.[61]

Adnexal Mass in Pregnancy

Due to a delay in child-bearing and improvement in technology, the findings of a pelvic mass at the time of pregnancy are not uncommon, with rates ranging from 2% to 10%.[62] Fortunately, most masses are benign, and spontaneous resolution occurs in a majority of cases, allowing for expectant management. Typically, this includes ultrasound assessment each trimester and repeat assessment in the postpartum period or at the time of caesarean delivery (reserved for obstetrical indications). However, surgical management may be warranted in several clinical situations. First, torsion is reported to occur in 0% to 7% of cases and may require emergent surgery; less common is a mass effect, causing pain or obstructing labor.[62,63] Lastly, clinicians should be aware for the potential of a malignant process, which occurs in approximately 2% to 6%, although some reports indicate the incidence to be as high as 10%.[62] Most often, these malignancies are early-stage epithelial tumors, borderline tumors (51%), or germ cell tumors (39%).[62,63] Because tumor markers are elevated secondary to pregnancy, intervention is based on imaging and clinical suspicion. Although surgery is safe, it should be reserved for surgical emergency or high suspicion of malignancy, as most patients can be managed expectantly.

Adnexal Mass in the Pediatric/Adolescent Population

The finding of an ovarian mass in the pediatric and adolescent population is not uncommonly encountered. An ovarian mass may be discovered as an incidental finding on examination, imaging, or at the time of an operation such as an appendectomy or detected during the evaluation of symptoms, such as abdominal pain or, less commonly, signs of hormone excess such as precocious puberty from a functional tumor. Reports indicate that more than 90% of adnexal tumors are benign in this population, and most patients can be managed with serial evaluation and avoid surgical intervention.[64] However, if a germ cell tumor or other malignancy is suspected, or if surgical emergencies such as torsion occur, surgery may be indicated. As ovarian function is critical to development at this stage, careful evaluation and management are warranted.

FUTURE DIRECTIONS

Over the past several decades, many advances have been made in the assessment of adnexal masses. The improvement in imaging has resulted in the ability to diagnose pelvic masses and evaluate for specific characteristics. Additionally, when appropriate, the use of imaging characteristics may allow for continued surveillance and allow for patients to be conservatively managed, avoiding risks of surgery. Although currently there is no imaging modality that can distinguish benign from malignant lesions perfectly, progress is occurring. This has resulted in improved sensitivity, ultimately allowing for triage of patients with a high suspicion of malignancy to be referred to gynecologic oncologists. Ideally, the ability to distinguish a benign adnexal mass that does not require surgery from a malignant mass should be done with confidence. The use of biomarkers continues to be evaluated for this purpose. Tests such as the use of HE4, OVA1, and combinations have shown potential. Developing algorithms to triage patients appropriately may result in better outcomes for women with pelvic masses.

REFERENCES

1. Barber H. Embryology of the gonad with reference to special tumors of the ovary and testis. *J Ped Surg.* 1988;23:967-972.
2. Timmerman D, Van Calster B, Testa AC, et al. Ovarian cancer prediction in adnexal masses using ultrasound-based logistic regression models: a temporal and external validation study by the IOTA group. *Ultrasound Obstet Gynecol.* 2010;36:226-234.
3. Tsili AC, Tsampoulas C, Argyropoulou M, et al. Comparative evaluation of multidetector CT and MR imaging in the differentiation of adnexal masses. *Eur Radiol.* 2008;18:1049-1057.

4. Stany MP, Maxwell GL, Rose GS. Clinical decision making using ovarian cancer risk assessment. *AJR Am J Roentgenol.* 2010; 194(2):337-342.

5. Nama V, Manyonda I. Tubal ectopic pregnancy: diagnosis and management. *Arch Gynecol Obstet.* 2009;279(4):443-453.

6. Huchon C, Staraci S, Fauconnier A. Adnexal torsion: a predictive score for pre-operative diagnosis. *Hum Reprod.* 2010;25: 2276-2280.

7. Krivak TC, Cooksey C, Propst AM. Tubo-ovarian abscess: diagnosis, medical, and surgical management. *Comp Ther.* 2004; 30:93-100.

8. Goff BA, Mandel L, Muntz HG, et al. Ovarian carcinoma diagnosis results of a national ovarian cancer survey. *Cancer.* 2000; 89:2068-2075.

9. Goff BA, Mandel LS, Drescher CW, et al. Development of an ovarian cancer symptom index. *Cancer.* 2007;109(2):221-227.

10. Malmstrom H, Hogberg T, Risberg B, Simonsen E. Granulosa cell tumors of the ovary: prognostic factors and outcome. *Gynecol Oncol.* 1994;52:50-55.

11. Barrenetxea G, Martin-Mateos M, Barzazan MJ, Montoya F, Matia JC, Rodriguez-Escudero FJ. Serum CA 125, CA 15.3, and CA 19.9 levels and surgical findings in patients undergoing second look operations for ovarian carcinomas. *Eur J Gynaecol Oncol.* 1990;11:369-374.

12. Vassal G, Flamant F, Caillaud JM, et al. Juvenile granulosa cell tumor of the ovary in children: a clinical study of 15 cases. *J Clin Oncol.* 1988;6:990-995.

13. Paraskevas M, Scully RE. Hilus cell tumor of the ovary. A clinicopathological analysis of 12 Reinke crystal-positive and nine crystal-negative cases. *Int J Gynecol Pathol.* 1989;8(4):299-310.

14. Myers ER, Bastian LA, Havrilesky LJ, et al. Management of adnexal mass. *Evid Rep Technol Assess.* 2006;(130):1-145.

15. Padilla LA, Radosevich DM, Milad MP. Limitations of the pelvic examination for evaluation of the female pelvic organs. *Int J Gynaecol Obstet.* 2005;88(1):84-88.

16. Spencer JA, Forstner R, Cunha TM, Kinkel K. ESUR guidelines for MR imaging of the sonographically indeterminate adnexal mass: an algorithmic approach. *Eur Radiol.* 2010;20(1): 25-35.

17. Valentin L. Use of morphology to characterize and manage common adnexal masses. *Best Pract Res Clin Obstet Gynaecol.* 2004;18: 71-89.

18. Sokalska A, Timmerman D, Testa A, et al. Diagnostic accuracy of transvaginal ultrasound examination for assigning a specific diagnosis to adnexal masses. *Ultrasound Obstet Gynecol.* 2009;34:462-470.

19. Timmerman D, Testa A, Bourne T, et al. Logistic regression model to distinguish between the benign and malignant adnexal mass before surgery: a multicenter study by the international ovarian tumor analysis group. *J Clin Oncol.* 2005;23:8794-8801.

20. McDonald J, Doran S, DeSimone C, et al. Predicting risk of malignancy in adnexal masses. *Obstet Gynecol.* 2010;115: 687-694.

21. Geomini P, Coppus S, Kluivers K, et al. Is three-dimensional ultrasonography of additional value in the assessment of adnexal masses? *Gynecol Oncol.* 2007;106:153-159.

22. Spencer JA, Ghattamaneni S. MR Imaging of the sonographically indeterminate adnexal mass. *Radiology.* 2010;256(3):677-694.

23. Tsili AC, Tsampoulas C, Charisiadi A, et al. Adnexal masses: accuracy of detection and differentiation with multidetector computed tomography. *Gynecol Oncol.* 2008;110:22-31.

24. Van Calster B, Timmerman D, Bourne T, et al. Discrimination between benign and malignant adnexal masses by specialist ultrasound examination versus serum CA-125. *J Natl Cancer Inst.* 2007;99:1706-1714.

25. Liu X, Cheng Y, Sheng W, et al. Clinicopathologic features and prognostic factors in alpha-fetoprotein-producing gastric cancers: analysis of 104 cases. *J Surg Oncol.* 2010;102:249-255.

26. Kawai M, Kano T, Kikkawa F, et al. Seven tumor markers in benign and malignant germ cell tumors of the ovary. *Gynecol Oncol.* 1992;45:248-253.

27. Gershenson D. Management of ovarian germ cell tumors. *J Clin Oncol.* 2007;25:2938-2943.

28. Mom CH, Engelen MJ, Willemse PH, et al. Granulosa cell tumors of the ovary: the clinical value of serum inhibin A and B levels in a large single center cohort. *Gynecol Oncol.* 2007;105:365-372.

29. Kelly PJ, Archbold P, Price JH, et al. Serum Ca19.9 levels are commonly elevated in primary ovarian mucinous tumours but cannot be used to predict the histological subtype. *J Clin Pathol.* 2010;63:169-173.

30. Roman LD, Muderspach LI, Burnett AF, Morrow CP. Carcinoembryonic antigen in women with isolated pelvic masses. Clinical utility? *J Reprod Med.* 1998;43:403-407.

31. Gostout BS, Brewer MA. Guidelines for referral of the patient with an adnexal mass. *Clin Obstet Gynecol.* 2006;49(3):448-458.

32. Raza A, Mould T, Wilson M, Burnell M, Bernhardt L. Increasing the effectiveness of referral of ovarian masses from cancer unit to cancer center by using a higher referral value of the risk of malignancy index. *Int J Gynecol Cancer.* 2010;20(4):552-554.

33. ACOG Practice Bulletin. Management of adnexal masses. *Obstet Gynecol.* 2007;110(1):201-214.

34. Im SS, Gordon AN, Buttin BM, et al. Validation of referral guidelines for women with pelvic masses. *Obstet Gynecol.* 2005;105(1):35-41.

35. Dearking AC, Aletti GD, McGree ME, et al. How relevant are ACOG and SGO guidelines for referral of adnexal mass? *Obstet Gynecol.* 2007;110(4):841-848.

36. Guidelines for referral to a gynecologic oncologist: rationale and benefits. The Society of Gynecologic Oncologists. *Gynecol Oncol.* 2000;78:S1-13.

37. Jacobs I, Oram D, Faribanks J, et al. A risk of malignancy index incorporating CA125, ultrasound and menopausal status for the accurate preoperative diagnosis of ovarian cancer. *BJOG.* 1990;97:922-929.

38. Geomini P, Kruitwagen R, Bremer GL, Cnossen J, Mol BWJ. The accuracy of risk scores in predicting ovarian malignancy: a systematic review. *Obstet Gynecol.* 2009;113:384-394.

39. van den Akker PA, Aalders AL, Snijders MP, et al. Evaluation of the Risk of Malignancy Index in daily clinical management of adnexal masses. *Gynecol Oncol.* 2010;116(3):384-388.

40. Moore RG, McMeekin DS, Brown AK, et al. A novel multiple marker bioassay utilizing HE4 and CA125 for the prediction of ovarian cancer in patients with a pelvic mass. *Gynecol Oncol.* 2009;112(1):40-46.

41. Nolen B, Velikokhatnaya L, Marrangoni A, et al. Serum biomarker panels for the discrimination of benign from malignant cases in patients with an adnexal mass. *Gynecol Oncol.* 2010;117:440-445.

42. Moore RG, Jabre-Raughley M, Brown AK, et al. Comparison of a novel multiple marker assay vs the Risk of Malignancy Index for the prediction of epithelial ovarian cancer in patients with a pelvic mass. *Am J Obstet Gynecol.* 2010;203:228.e1-228.e6.

43. Andersen MR, Goff BA, Lowe KA, et al. Use of a symptom index, CA125, and HE4 to predict ovarian cancer. *Gynecol Oncol.* 2010;116:378-383.

44. Ueland F, DeSimone C, Seamon L, et al. The OVA1 test improves the preoperative assessment of ovarian tumors. *Gynecol Oncol.* 2010;116:S23.

45. Muller CY. Doctor, should I get this new ovarian cancer test—OVA1? *Obstet Gynecol.* 2010;116(2):246-247.

46. Simpkins F, Zahurak M, Armstrong D, Grumbine F, Bristow R. Ovarian malignancy in breast cancer patients with an adnexal mass. *Obstet Gynecol.* 2005;105:507-513.

47. Dubeau L. The cell of origin of ovarian epithelial tumours. *Lancet Oncol.* 2008;9(12):1191-1197.

CHAPTER 11

48. Benito V, Lubrano A, Arencibia O, et al. Serous and mucinous borderline ovarian tumors: are there real differences between these two entities? *Eur J Obstet Gynecol Reprod Biol.* 2010;153(2):188-192.

49. Kurman RJ, Seidman JD, Shih IM. Serous borderline tumours of the ovary. *Histopathology.* 2005;47:310-318.

50. Saba L, Guerriero S, Sulcis R, et al. Mature and immature ovarian teratomas: CT, US and MR imaging characteristics. *Eur J Radiol.* 2009;72:454-463.

51. Bulun S. Endometriosis. *N Engl J Med.* 2009;360:268-279.

52. Falcone T. Adnexal masses: when to observe, when to intervene, and when to refer. *Obstet Gynecol.* 2010;115(4):680-661.

53. Yarandi F, Eftekhar Z, Izadi-Mood N, Shojaei H. Accuracy of intraoperative frozen section in the diagnosis of ovarian tumors. *Aust N Z J Obstet Gynaecol.* 2008;48(4):438-441.

54. Medeiros LR, Rosa DD, Edelweiss MI, et al. Accuracy of frozen-section analysis in the diagnosis of ovarian tumors: a systematic quantitative review. *Int J Gynecol Cancer.* 2005;5(2):192-202.

55. Berek JS, Chalas E, Edelson M, et al. Prophylactic and risk-reducing bilateral salpingo-oophorectomy. *Obstet Gynecol.* 2010;116:733-743.

56. Modesitt SC, Pavlik EJ, Ueland FR, et al. Risk of malignancy in unilocular ovarian cystic tumors less than 10 cm in diameter: a long-term follow-up study. *Obstet Gynecol.* 2003;102:594-599.

57. Saunders BA, Podzielinksi I, Ware RA, et al. Risk of malignancy in sonographically confirmed septated cystic tumors. *Gynecol Oncol.* 2010;118:278-282.

58. ACOG Practice Bulletin No. 110: noncontraceptive uses of hormonal contraceptives. *Obstet Gynecol.* 2010;115(1):206-218.

59. Fader AN, Rose PG. Role of surgery in ovarian carcinoma. *J Clin Oncol.* 2007;10;25(20):2873-2883.

60. Zapardiel I, Rosenberg P, Peiretti M, et al. The role of restaging borderline ovarian tumors: single institution experience and review of the literature. *Gynecol Oncol.* 2010;119(2):274-277.

61. Allison KH, Swisher EM, Kerkering KM, Garcia RL. Defining an appropriate threshold for the diagnosis of serous borderline tumor of the ovary: when is a full staging procedure unnecessary? *Int J Gynecol Pathol.* 2008;27(1):10-17.

62. Schwartz N, Timor-Tritsch IE, Wang E. Adnexal masses in pregnancy. *Clin Obstet Gynecol.* 2009;52(4):570-585.

63. Leiserowitz GS, Xing G, Cress R, et al. Adnexal masses in pregnancy: how often are they malignant? *Gynecol Oncol.* 2006;101:315-321.

64. Schultz KA, Ness KK, Nagarajan R, Steiner ME. Adnexal masses in infancy and childhood. *Clin Obstet Gynecol.* 2006;49(3):464-479.

High-Grade Serous Carcinomas of the Ovary, Fallopian Tube, and Peritoneum

David E. Cohn and Ronald D. Alvarez

Epithelial ovarian, fallopian tube, and primary peritoneal cancers remain the most lethal of all the gynecologic malignancies. In 2010, approximately 21,880 women will be diagnosed with ovarian cancer in the United States; of these, 13,850 will be expected to die from this disease.[1] Cancers arising from the fallopian tube and peritoneum are significantly less common that those arising from the ovarian epithelium, but share several similarities in their epidemiology, diagnosis, treatment, and associated outcomes. Because the vast majority of fallopian tube and primary peritoneal cancers exhibit a high-grade papillary serous histology, comparisons to similar disease in primary ovarian cancers suggest common molecular pathways that may promote carcinogenesis within the serous classification of these tumors. Several recent hypotheses also propose a fallopian tube origin for metastatic disease that would traditionally be considered as primary ovarian or peritoneal. Given the recent advances surrounding these diseases, this chapter considers this subset of high-grade serous reproductive cancers as a group, with specific differences highlighted.

EPIDEMIOLOGY

Key Points

1. Women with an inherited ovarian cancer syndrome, particularly those with mutations in the *BRCA1* and *BRCA2* genes, have the highest lifetime risk of developing high-grade, papillary serous epithelial ovarian, primary peritoneal, and fallopian tube cancer.

2. For ovarian cancer, epidemiologic factors that are associated with an increase in lifetime ovulatory cycles confer an increased risk.

3. Bilateral salpingo-oophorectomy, oral contraceptives, tubal ligation, and hysterectomy are all well established risk modifiers of epithelial ovarian, fallopian tube, and primary peritoneal cancer.

Epidemiologic data indicate that ovarian cancer is the ninth most common malignancy affecting women in the United States, with 21,880 cases predicted for 2010; unfortunately, it is the fifth most common cause of cancer-related deaths, with 13,850 women estimated to die of this disease in the same time period.[1] The incidence of ovarian cancer increases with age and is most prevalent in the eighth decade of life, with a rate of 57 per 100,000 women. The median age at diagnosis is 63 years, and 70% of patients present with advanced disease.[2]

The true incidence of fallopian tube and primary peritoneal malignancies is more difficult to quantify. Despite criteria established by the Gynecologic Oncology Group to define primary peritoneal cancers, uniform application by pathologists remains unclear, which clouds identification of the true incidence of this disease. High-grade serous carcinomas of the fallopian tube are rare entities, with 3479 new cases expected to be diagnosed yearly.[3] However, incomplete pathologic sectioning and evaluation of the tubes in women with presumed metastatic ovarian cancer may preclude identification of a true tubal origin. Recent evidence suggests that nearly 60% of all high-grade, non-uterine serous cancers initially classified as primary ovarian or peritoneal in origin demonstrate serous tubal intraepithelial carcinoma (STIC), suggesting that the fallopian tube may be the organ of origin.[4,5]

One of the strongest risk factors for the development of serous gynecologic cancers is the presence of a genetic predisposition to the disease. The majority of patients with a genetic predisposition to ovarian cancer have mutations in the *BRCA1* or *BRCA2* genes. As such, a personal or family history of premenopausal breast cancer or any ovarian cancer suggests that the presence of a *BRCA* gene mutation is more probable and thus increases the risk of these diseases (Table 12-1).

Epithelial ovarian cancer is, however, a disease that occurs most commonly as a result of sporadic (noninherited) acquisition. The median age of patients diagnosed with epithelial ovarian cancer is in the early seventh decade. Epidemiologic studies have established several specific risk modifiers that are associated with an increased risk for the development of ovarian cancer, including increased lifetime exposure to ovulation. These factors include a longer duration of menstruation (early menarche, late menopause), nulliparity, and lack of breast feeding.[6] Although it would intuitively make sense that medications that induce ovulations (such as those used for the treatment of infertility) would increase the risk for ovarian cancer, this has

only been suggested but not proven. Ovarian cancer occurs more frequently in industrialized countries, where obesity and a high-fat diet are more common. The hormonal basis of ovarian cancer is less certain, with some studies associating menopausal estrogen replacement with an increased risk and others with a decreased or no impact on the disease.[7]

Protection against ovarian cancer may be provided through several interventions. Factors that decrease ovulation, such as oral contraceptives, decrease the risk of the disease both in patients with and without a genetic predisposition to developing ovarian cancer. Removal of the ovaries will in large part guarantee the prevention of ovarian cancer, although rare cases of adenocarcinoma of the peritoneal cavity (primary peritoneal cancer) can occur in high-risk women. Likely due to the disruption of the ovarian blood supply, hysterectomy also decreases the risk for developing ovarian cancer. Given the relationship between peritoneal and iatrogenic irritants (possibly such as talc) and ovarian cancer, tubal ligation has been proven to decrease the risk of the disease as well.

High-grade papillary serous epithelial malignancies can arise from numerous anatomic locations in the gynecologic system, including the ovaries, peritoneum, uterus, and cervix. This chapter focuses on the most common sites of epithelial serous malignancies: the ovaries, fallopian tubes, and peritoneum. Epithelial ovarian and peritoneal cancers are predominantly of serous histology (85%) and histologically recapitulate the appearance of the fallopian tubal epithelium. The remaining histologies of epithelial ovarian cancers (endometrioid, mucinous, clear cell, and Brenner tumor) are discussed in Chapter 13.

Serous adenocarcinomas of the ovary, peritoneum, or fallopian tubes can be cytologically low grade or high grade, with high-grade adenocarcinomas comprising more than 80% of all serous cancers. The clinical importance of segregating invasive ovarian neoplasms by cytology relates to the strong influence of grade on the biologic behavior of these. Comparisons of low-grade with high-grade serous ovarian cancers show differences in genetics, response to chemotherapy, and survival. The "2-tier" system has been shown to be both reproducible and biologically relevant. High-grade serous cancers are generally diagnosed at advanced stages and are responsive to taxane and platinum chemotherapy. Low-grade serous cancers are considered to be chemotherapy resistant and may not respond as robustly to the adjuvant chemotherapy generally administered to patients with ovarian cancer.[8] In fact, genetic profiling of low-grade serous cancers demonstrates distinct fingerprints from high-grade tumors, with segregation closer to the profile of borderline cancers.[9] These studies have been invaluable

Table 12-1 Risk Factors for Ovarian Cancer

Increased Risk
Advancing age
Residence in developed world

Nulliparity
    No breast feeding
    Early menarche

Late menopause
Obesity
Menopausal estrogen replacement (variable association)
Perineal talc exposure (variable association)
Infertility medications (variable association)
Personal or family history of premenopausal breast cancer or any ovarian cancer
Decreased Risk
Oral contraceptives
Hysterectomy
Tubal ligation
Oophorectomy

in providing insight into potential molecular targets for the treatment of low-grade serous cancers.

Recently, increasing attention has been paid to the biology and pathogenesis of ovarian cancer. Whereas historically, high-grade serous ovarian cancer was thought to develop from precursor lesions of the ovarian surface epithelium (mesothelium), with metaplastic changes leading to transformation into malignancy, increasing scrutiny has challenged this long-held theory. It is now hypothesized that the majority of epithelial ovarian and primary peritoneal cancers arise from the fallopian tubes, either from high-grade intraepithelial neoplasia of the tubal epithelium or from the ciliated columnar epithelium residing in the para-tubal and para-ovarian tissues.[10] Although this recent shift in the description of the origin of ovarian cancer is conceptually attractive, it is by no means definitive, and substantial research will need to be completed before its universal adoption.

Screening for Ovarian Cancer

Ovarian cancer is a rare disease, with a woman's lifetime risk of being diagnosed approaching 1 in 75 (1.5%) in the general population. The prevalence of the disease is approximately 1 in 2500 in postmenopausal women. This rate, in contrast with a woman's lifetime risk of being diagnosed with breast cancer (1 in 9, or 11%), is responsible for the challenges of ovarian cancer screening in the general population. In women with an increased risk of developing ovarian cancer as a result of a hereditary predisposition, screening becomes more feasible, as the tests required to detect the disease do not require as high a sensitivity and specificity as with detection of a more rare disease. Given that more than 90% of women diagnosed with ovarian cancer have sporadic disease, accurate screening remains a challenge. As such, fewer than 30% of patients with ovarian cancer are diagnosed with stage I disease (when the 5-year survival rates can exceed 90%).

Currently used modalities attempting to identify early-stage ovarian cancer (and thus improve survival) have mainly focused on transvaginal pelvic ultrasonography and serum CA-125 testing. Although novel serum markers and other imaging technologies are in evaluation, previous and current clinical protocols evaluating the role of ovarian cancer screening have tested pelvic ultrasound and CA-125. To date, there has been no evidence in the general population that routine screening for ovarian cancer reduces mortality related to this disease.[11] However, 2 ongoing clinical trials are continuing to gather information to assess the value of screening in the general population. The PLCO (Prostate, Lung, Colorectal, Ovary) screening trial randomized more than 34,000 postmenopausal women without oophorectomy to both annual CA-125 and pelvic ultrasounds for 4 years versus routine care. The most recent results from the screening arm demonstrated that 60 of 89 invasive ovarian or peritoneal cancers were detected by screening, although 72% of the screen-detected cases were diagnosed at an advanced stage.[12] The primary objective of the study, the impact of screening on mortality, has yet to be reported.

In the United Kingdom, the UKCTOCS (Collaborative Trial of Ovarian Cancer Screening) randomized more than 100,000 postmenopausal women to routine care, versus more than 50,000 postmenopausal women to screening with both pelvic ultrasound and CA-125, versus more than 50,000 to pelvic ultrasound alone. Although the data regarding ovarian cancer mortality are not yet mature, preliminary results suggest that the use of multimodality screening with CA-125 and ultrasound is superior to ultrasound alone or routine care in the detection of ovarian cancer.[13] Recently, a single arm multi-institutional study describing the use of the Risk of Ovarian Cancer Algorithm (ROCA) interpretation of the trend of multiple CA-125 levels followed by ultrasound for a positive ROCA screen in a general population cohort of 3251 postmenopausal women over 9 years demonstrated that of the 5 women diagnosed with ovarian cancer, 3 (60%) had early-stage disease, and most had a normal (but increasing by ROCA) level of CA-125 that would have gone without detection by standard CA-125 screening. The ROCA triage strategy was associated with a positive predictive value of 37% and a specificity of 99.9%.[14] Together, these trials suggest that screening of ovarian cancer may be feasible, but data regarding its impact on mortality are imperative for the widespread introduction of this technique into the general population.

DIAGNOSIS

Key Points

1. Women with ovarian cancer often experience symptoms that may include bloating, pelvic or abdominal pain, difficulty eating, early satiety, or urinary symptoms (urgency or frequency).
2. The evaluation of a patient with such symptoms or suspected ovarian cancer should include a thorough abdominal and pelvic examination, selective imaging studies, and selective tumor markers.

Until recently, many providers have described ovarian, fallopian tube, and peritoneal cancers as a "silent" disease, with the thought that there are no classic symptoms until metastases have developed. There is evidence now to suggest that most women with these cancers, including those with early-stage disease, often experience distinct clinical features and symptoms for several months before their initial diagnosis. A national survey of 1500 women, before their diagnosis of ovarian cancer, identified common signs that included abdominal, gastrointestinal, pain, constitutional, urinary, or pelvic symptoms in nature.[15] In a landmark prospective case-control study, Goff et al[16] identified 4 symptoms more likely to occur in women with ovarian cancer than in the general population of women presenting to primary clinics. These symptoms included an increase in abdominal size, bloating, urinary urgency, and pain. Symptoms in women with malignant ovarian masses were likely to be more recent in onset, more frequent, and higher in severity than those experienced by women without an ovarian malignancy. The results of this study and others led to the development of an Ovarian Cancer Symptoms Consensus Statement (Table 12-2).[17]

Fallopian tube cancer may present with similar symptoms. A specific clinical entity, hydrops tubae profluens, is also considered classic for this disease, but is typically not identified in women diagnosed with tubal cancer. This cluster of symptoms includes cramping lower abdominal pain, which resolves after passage of a profuse, watery, and/or yellow vaginal discharge.

The importance of both the patient and the clinician recognizing the symptoms suggestive of epithelial ovarian, fallopian tube, or primary peritoneal cancer cannot be understated. Studies have demonstrated that even 80% to 90% of patients with early-stage disease are symptomatic.[15] Given the lack of effective screening strategies, early recognition of symptoms associated with ovarian cancer may facilitate diagnosis of ovarian cancer at an earlier stage where outcome is improved. Several efforts are underway to develop algorithms that direct the evaluation and management of women who present with symptoms of ovarian cancer that include physical examination by a gynecologist and appropriate imaging and laboratory assessment.

Table 12-2 Symptoms Likely to Occur More Commonly in Women With Ovarian Cancer Than in the General Population

Bloating
Pelvic or abdominal pain
Difficulty eating or feeling full quickly
Urinary symptoms (urgency or frequency)

Patients with symptoms such as those previously described should undergo a thorough physical assessment, which should include an abdominal and pelvic examination. Physical examination findings are often based on the stage of disease. Patients with early-stage disease may be found to have an adnexal mass appreciated on abdominal or pelvic examination.[18] Patients with a malignant ovarian neoplasm may have a mass of various dimensions but typically such masses are solid, irregular, or fixed. However, pelvic examination has limited sensitivity in the detection of adnexal masses; thus many patients with early- or late-stage ovarian cancer have a normal pelvic examination.[19] The adnexal mass may be tender to the patient on palpation, but rarely do patients have significant guarding or rebound tenderness. Patients with more advanced-stage disease are often found to have, along with a pelvic mass, abdominal distension or a fluid wave indicating the presence of ascites. These patients are often noted to have an upper abdominal mass suggestive of omental metastasis.

Physical examination should also include evaluation of the supraclavicular and inguinal lymph nodes to assess for nodal metastasis and evaluation of the breasts and rectum to assess for cancers originating in these organs. Other aspects of the physical examination should focus on evaluation of the other major organ systems to appropriately assess for comorbidities that may affect management decisions.

Various imaging studies can be selectively used to further evaluate a patient with a pelvic mass or with symptoms suggestive of ovarian cancer.[20,21] Pelvic and/or transvaginal ultrasound remains the modality of choice to evaluate a patient with an adnexal mass due to its ease of use and relatively less expense. Pelvic ultrasound can most often distinguish uterine from ovarian pathology, and certain features noted on sonography can raise or lower suspicion for malignant disease. Findings most suggestive of malignancy in the postmenopausal woman with an ovarian mass include the presence of excrescences or papillary structures within a cyst, size greater than 10 cm, a solid or mixed solid and cystic mass, thickened septa, and color or Doppler demonstration of blood flow in the mass.[20,21] Recent studies have confirmed the ability of such ultrasound findings alone and in combination with selective tumor markers (CA-125) to be predictive in discriminating between benign and malignant adnexal masses.[22,23]

Abdominal/pelvic computed tomography (CT) is also a very useful imaging modality, particularly in those patients with nonspecific symptoms suggestive of a malignant ovarian neoplasm or clinical evidence of potential metastatic disease.[20,21] Although not as accurate as ultrasound in characterizing the components of an ovarian mass, abdominal/pelvic CT is able to accurately determine the presence of ascites or metastases to the omentum, peritoneal surfaces, retroperitoneal lymph nodes, or intraparenchymal organs such as the liver and spleen. In addition, valuable information can be ascertained regarding other intraperitoneal organ sites that may be contributing to clinical symptoms and findings or that may be secondarily involved with a malignant ovarian process.

Magnetic resonance imaging (MRI) or positron emission tomography (PET) imaging rarely adds to the assessment of a patient with a pelvic mass or evidence of metastases over that which can be achieved with pelvic ultrasound or abdominal/pelvic CT.[20,21] MRI may be useful in the setting in which there is a sonographically indeterminate or complex pelvic mass and there is uncertainty about the ovary as an origin of the mass. Fluorodeoxyglucose (FDG) PET alone or combined with CT has improved sensitivity over CT in the evaluation of an adnexal mass; however, low specificity and false-positive physiologic signals are not infrequently noted, and rarely does FDG-PET imaging enhance the ability of a clinician to make a management decision over what can be decided with ultrasound or CT imaging.

Serum CA-125 may also be very useful in guiding clinical management decisions in patients with symptoms or physical examination findings suggestive of an ovarian neoplasm, particularly in the postmenopausal woman.[24,25] An elevated CA-125 in the presence of an adnexal mass in a postmenopausal woman is highly predictive of a malignant ovarian neoplasm. Care must be exercised in interpreting a normal serum CA-125 level in a patient with an ovarian mass as an indication that the patient may not harbor a malignant ovarian mass. Serum CA-125 may not be elevated in patients with nonserous (eg, mucinous) ovarian neoplasms and is only elevated in approximately 50% of patients with early-stage ovarian cancer. OVA1 (Vermillion) is a laboratory test recently approved by the US Food and Drug Administration (FDA) that assesses 5 serum biomarkers including CA-125, prealbumin, transferrin, β2 microglobulin, and apolipoprotein A1.[26,27] OVA1 is reported to improve the ability of physicians to predict whether an ovarian mass is malignant when used in combination with clinical and radiographic imaging as compared with when physicians use clinical and radiographic imaging alone. Continued investigation of this multiplex test, as well as others, is needed before its establishment as a routine investigation in women with ovarian cancer or as a screening tool.[28]

The American Congress of Obstetricians/ Gynecologists and the Society of Gynecologic Oncologists have issued guidelines applicable to all primary care physicians that provide recommendations to obstetrician/gynecologists for the evaluation and management of patients with a pelvic or ovarian mass.[29,30]

Table 12-3 Differential Diagnosis of Pelvic Mass

Ovarian
Functional cyst
Benign neoplasm (cystadenoma, cystadenofibroma)
Malignant neoplasm (invasive and borderline cancer)
Fallopian tube
Hydrosalpinx
Tubo-ovarian abscess
Malignant neoplasm
Uterine
Congenital anomaly
Leiomyoma
Other
Colon (diverticular abscess, colon cancer)
Urologic (Bladder obstruction, bladder cancer, pelvic kidney)
Lymphoma
Soft tissue benign or malignant mass

The differential diagnosis in a patient with a pelvic mass should take into consideration problems that can arise from all organ systems located within the pelvis (Table 12-3).

The primary care physician must first have a high index of suspicion for a malignant ovarian neoplasm in patients who present with any of the previously described symptoms or signs commonly experienced in patients with a malignant ovarian mass. A thorough history and physical examination, including an abdominal and pelvic examination, are paramount. Primary care physicians should obtain selective imaging and laboratory studies to evaluate for a possible ovarian neoplasm in women with symptoms or physical examination findings suggestive of an ovarian neoplasm. A pelvic ultrasound can provide useful information about an adnexal mass that can guide clinical management decisions. An abdominal/pelvic CT may be helpful in evaluating whether symptoms may be attributable to other organ systems or, if an adnexal mass is present, whether metastases are present. A serum CA-125 is most useful in determining whether an adnexal mass may be malignant, particularly in the postmenopausal patient. An OVA1 study may also be useful in situations in which a serum CA-125 is normal, characteristics of an adnexal mass are not definitive, and concern persists for the possibility of an ovarian malignancy. It is important that primary care physicians take into consideration all clinical, radiographic, and laboratory findings to guide management decisions, in particular those findings that may determine the need for surgical evaluation or subspecialty referral.

CHAPTER 12

PATHOLOGY

Key Points

1. Metastatic ovarian and primary peritoneal cancer may arise from an abnormal focus in the fallopian tube epithelium.
2. The majority of malignant epithelial ovarian, primary peritoneal, and fallopian tube neoplasms are serous cancers.
3. Staging of gynecologic cancers reflects the distribution of disease, but does not take into consideration other important prognostic factors, such as the volume of disease remaining after surgical resection.

High-grade papillary serous cancers of the ovarian, fallopian tube, and peritoneum share similar histologic characteristics that frequently do not permit determination of the organ of origin. These malignancies are characterized by clusters of atypical cells arranged in papillary patterns with irregular underlying stroma or may appear as sheets of malignant cells with marked atypia without underlying stroma (Figure 12-1). As with all grade 3 malignancies, the nuclear-to-cytoplasmic ratio is high, and observation of atypical mitoses is common. Psammoma bodies are more common in low-grade serous malignancies; they are rarely seen in grade 3 disease.

Spread of serous ovarian, tubal, and peritoneal cancer can be through a number of mechanisms, including direct tumor dissemination into the peritoneal cavity, lymphatic spread, and hematogenous spread

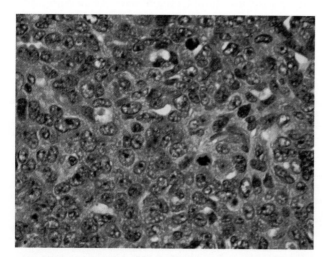

FIGURE 12-1. Photomicrograph of histologic specimen of grade 3 serous adenocarcinoma. (Reproduced, with permission, from Shorge JO, Schaffer JI, Halvorson LM, et al, eds. *Williams' Gynecology.* New York, NY: McGraw-Hill; 2008.)

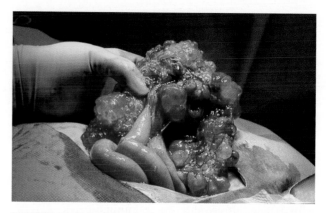

FIGURE 12-2. Omental caking caused by tumor invasion. (Reproduced, with permission, from Shorge JO, Schaffer JI, Halvorson LM, et al, eds. *Williams' Gynecology.* New York, NY: McGraw-Hill; 2008.)

(into solid organs and bone). The vast majority of patients with advanced serous cancers have peritoneal metastases. For epithelial ovarian cancer, disease most commonly spreads to the surface of the peritoneal cavity, the serosa of the large or small intestines, the omentum, and the surface of the liver or diaphragm (Figure 12-2). Although peritoneal spread of advanced ovarian cancer is quite common, it is estimated that at least 50% of these patients have concurrent or isolated retroperitoneal (pelvic, aortic, celiac) lymph node metastasis.[31] The rate of solid organ involvement in newly diagnosed ovarian cancer is quite low,[32] although involvement of solid organs in the context of recurrent disease has been increasing as patients are experiencing increased disease-free survival in the primary and recurrent settings, thus allowing for the manifestations of solid organ metastasis before death from peritoneal spread of ovarian cancer. The pattern of spread of peritoneal cancers is similar to that of ovarian cancers, with common dissemination throughout the peritoneal cavity and spread to the peritoneal surface of the pelvis, intestines, diaphragm, and omentum. Although generally the behavior of these malignancies is similar to those of the ovary and peritoneal cavity, fallopian tube cancers are different in that the rate of disease metastasis to the retroperitoneal lymph nodes exceeds that of the other high-grade serous gynecologic cancers; specifically, in tumors clinically confined to the fallopian tube, more than one-third have pathologic involvement of the retroperitoneal lymph nodes.[33]

The staging system for ovarian cancer was established to provide a common language for the communication of results regarding diagnosis and treatment of the disease. The International Federation of Gynecology and Obstetrics (FIGO) 2009 staging system is shown in Table 12-4. Although stage clearly is an important prognostic factor in patients with ovarian

Table 12-4 FIGO Staging of Ovarian (and Peritoneal) Cancer

Stage I: Limited to 1 or both ovaries
   IA: Involves 1 ovary; capsule intact; no tumor on ovarian surface; no malignant cells in ascites or peritoneal washings
   IB: Involves both ovaries; capsule intact; no tumor on ovarian surface; negative washings
   IC: Tumor limited to ovaries with any of the following: capsule ruptured, tumor on ovarian surface, positive washings

Stage II: Pelvic extension or implants
   IIA: Extension or implants onto uterus or fallopian tube; negative washings
   IIB: Extension or implants onto other pelvic structures; negative washings
   IIC: Pelvic extension or implants with positive peritoneal washings

Stage III: Microscopic peritoneal implants outside of the pelvis; or limited to the pelvis with extension to the small bowel or omentum
   IIIA: Microscopic peritoneal metastases beyond pelvis
   IIIB: Macroscopic peritoneal metastases beyond pelvis <2 cm in size
   IIIC: Peritoneal metastases beyond pelvis >2 cm or lymph node metastases

Stage IV: Distant metastases to the liver or outside the peritoneal cavity

Table 12-5 FIGO Staging of Fallopian Tube Cancer

Stage I: Growth limited to the fallopian tubes
   IA: Growth is limited to 1 tube, with extension into the submucosa and/or muscularis, but not penetrating the serosal surface; no ascites
   IB: Growth is limited to both tubes, with extension into the submucosa and/or muscularis, but not penetrating the serosal surface; no ascites
   IC: Tumor either stage IA or IB, but with tumor extension through or onto the tubal serosa, or with ascites present containing malignant cells, or with positive peritoneal washings

Stage II: Growth involving 1 or both fallopian tubes with pelvic extension
   IIA: Extension and/or metastasis to the uterus and/or ovaries
   IIB: Extension to other pelvic tissues
   IIC: Tumor either stage IIA or IIB and with ascites present containing malignant cells or with positive peritoneal washings

Stage III: Tumor involves 1 or both fallopian tubes, with peritoneal implants outside the pelvis and/or positive retroperitoneal or inguinal nodes; superficial liver metastasis equals stage III; tumor appears limited to the true pelvis, but with histologically proven malignant extension to the small bowel or omentum
   IIIA: Tumor is grossly limited to the true pelvis, with negative nodes, but with histologically confirmed microscopic seeding of abdominal peritoneal surfaces
   IIIB: Tumor involving 1 or both tubes, with histologically confirmed implants of abdominal peritoneal surfaces, none exceeding 2 cm in diameter; lymph nodes are negative
   IIIC: Abdominal implants 2 cm in diameter and/or positive retroperitoneal or inguinal nodes

Stage IV: Growth involving 1 or both fallopian tubes with distant metastases; if pleural effusion is present, there must be positive cytology to be stage IV; parenchymal liver metastases equals stage IV

cancer overall, what is not conveyed in the FIGO staging system is the description of the volume of residual disease after primary cytoreduction in women with advanced ovarian cancer, which has been shown to be the most important prognostic factor in women with metastatic disease. It is important to consider that although distant metastasis (to the upper abdomen or lymph nodes) is generally associated with stage IV disease in most other solid tumors, it is considered stage III in ovarian cancer, with stage IV cases reserved for those with parenchymal liver involvement, cytologically positive pleural effusions, or other extra-abdominal metastasis.

Although the treatment of fallopian tube cancer is identical to that of ovarian cancer, fallopian tube cancers are staged by a separate system (Table 12-5). In order for an adnexal malignancy to be designated a high-grade serous fallopian tube (and not ovarian) cancer, specific pathologic criteria must be met. Specifically, all or most of the adnexal malignancy must arise in the fallopian tube, and a transition from benign to invasive neoplasm must be identified in the fallopian tube.[34,35] In the absence of these criteria, and adnexal malignancy is classified as an ovarian cancer.

Primary peritoneal cancers are staged similarly to epithelial ovarian malignancies. The Gynecologic Oncology Group established pathologic definitions of primary peritoneal cancer in 1993: (1) The ovaries are normal in size or enlarged by a benign process; (2) the involvement in the extraovarian sites must be greater than the involvement on the surface of either ovary; (3) microscopically, the ovaries are not involved with the tumor or exhibited only serosal or cortical implants less than 5 × 5 mm; (4) the histopathologic and cytologic characteristics of the tumor are predominantly of the serous type.[36]

TREATMENT

Key Points

1. Patients with apparently confined or limited ovarian or fallopian tube cancer should undergo comprehensive surgical resection and staging.
2. In patients with metastatic disease, surgical cytoreduction to residual disease less than 1 cm correlates with improved outcome.
3. Combination taxane and platinum-based chemotherapy is the standard of care adjuvant treatment for most patients with newly diagnosed high-risk early-stage or advanced-stage ovarian, fallopian tube, and primary peritoneal cancer.

Treatment of Early-Stage Disease

Surgical Management and Staging

Fewer than 20% of patients with a pelvic mass who are found to harbor an invasive high-grade serous ovarian, tubal, or peritoneal cancer will be diagnosed with disease confined to the ovary, tube, or pelvis at the time of surgical evaluation. When this does occur, it is imperative to surgically resect the affected organ and involved pelvic structures. The decision to remove other involved or uninvolved gynecologic organs may be influenced by the patient's age and her desire for future fertility. It is also important to assess for the presence of occult or microscopic metastasis when disease appears confined to pelvis to provide patients accurate prognostic information and to guide adjuvant therapy decisions. In the classic study of Young et al,[37] 30% of a cohort of 100 patients who were thought to have early-stage ovarian cancer were found to have evidence of metastasis at the time of restaging laparotomy. Despite recent studies that consistently confirm this observation, evaluation of Surveillance, Epidemiology, and End Results data has demonstrated that fewer than 10% of patients with clinically apparent early-stage malignant ovarian neoplasms are comprehensively staged.[38,39]

Procedures involved in the staging of ovarian, tubal, and peritoneal cancers include cytologic evaluation of ascites or abdominopelvic washings, excision or biopsy of suspicious peritoneal implants, omentectomy, and pelvic and para-aortic lymphadenectomy.[40] The contralateral ovary and/or uterus should be removed if there is evidence of metastasis or if future fertility not desired. Although exploratory laparotomy is traditionally the operative modality of choice, recent studies suggest that staging of patients with an ovarian neoplasm can be adequately and safely done using laparoscopic and minimally invasive surgical techniques.[41]

Medical Management

Pathologic assessment of specimens obtained as part of staging in patients with an apparent early-stage high-grade serous cancer provides critical information necessary to assign risk for recurrence and to direct decisions regarding adjuvant therapy. Several prospective randomized clinical trials have provided guidance to clinicians regarding the management of patients with early-stage invasive serous ovarian cancer (Table 12-6). Patients with stage IA/B (grade 1 or 2) invasive serous ovarian cancer have classically been designated as having low risk for recurrence, and studies have demonstrated that the outcome for these patients, particularly when adequately staged, is not improved with the use of adjuvant therapy.[42,43] Those patients with stage IA/B (grade 3), IC, or II invasive serous ovarian cancer are considered as having high risk for recurrence. Although some controversy exists regarding the need for adjuvant therapy in adequately staged patients, most prospective studies have demonstrated improved outcomes in such high-risk early-stage ovarian cancer patients when treated with adjuvant chemotherapy. Specifically, the ACTION (Adjuvant ChemoTherapy In Ovarian Neoplasm)/ICON (International Collaborative Ovarian Neoplasm) studies, which randomized patients with clinically apparent high-risk early-stage ovarian cancer to platinum-based chemotherapy versus observation, did demonstrate superior 5-year survival in chemotherapy-treated patients (82% vs. 74%).[43-45]

In the modern era, a platinum-based regimen, specifically paclitaxel and carboplatin, is currently the most common adjuvant chemotherapy regimen administered to patients with high-risk early-stage invasive serous ovarian or tubal cancers.[46,47] Although there are no randomized trials comparing a paclitaxel and carboplatin regimen with other non–taxane/non–platinum-based regimens, the superior antitumor activity noted with these agents in advanced-staged ovarian cancer justifies adoption of this regimen in patients with early-stage disease. Studies have attempted to identify the optimal number of cycles of chemotherapy for patients with early-stage disease. Specifically, Gynecologic Oncology Group (GOG) 157 randomized patient with high-risk early-stage ovarian cancer to 3 versus 6 cycles of paclitaxel and carboplatin.[46] This study demonstrated that although the risk of recurrence was higher in patients treated with 3 cycles of this regimen compared with 6 cycles (25.4% vs. 20.1%), there was no significant difference in 5-year overall survival (81% vs. 83%). Toxicity, particularly hematologic (neutropenia) and neurologic (sensory neuropathy), was noted to be significantly higher in the patients who received the higher number of cycles. The conclusions rendered by the authors of this study advocated that 3 cycles of paclitaxel and carboplatin should be considered the standard of care in patients with high-risk

Table 12-6 Relevant Randomized Control Trials in Early-Stage Invasive Ovarian Cancer

Trial(s)/Author	Treatment Arms	Overall Survival	Conclusions
Ovarian Cancer Study Group/ GOG (Young, 1990)[42]	Trial 1: Observation vs. melphalan up to 12 cycles	Arm 1: 94% vs. 98%	No adjuvant therapy required in low-risk early-stage ovarian cancer.
	Trial 2: ^{32}P vs. melphalan up to 12 cycles	Arm 2: 78% vs. 81%	^{32}P or melphalans provide similar outcome in high-risk early-stage ovarian cancer.
GOG-95 (Young, 2003)[48]	^{32}P vs. cyclophosphamide/ cisplatin × 3 cycles	78% vs. 83%	Although no difference in survival, lower recurrence and complication rates justify platinum-based chemotherapy as preferred treatment.
ACTION/ICON (Trimbos, 2003)[43]	Observation vs. platinum-based chemotherapy	74% vs. 82%[a]	Platinum-based chemotherapy improved survival in high-risk early-stage ovarian cancer.
GOG-175 (Bell, 2006)[47]	Paclitaxel/carboplatin 3 vs. 6 cycles	81% vs. 83%	Compared with 3 cycles, 6 cycles of paclitaxel and carboplatin did not significantly alter recurrence rate or improve survival and was associated with increased toxicity.
GOG-157 (Mannel, 2010)[48]	Paclitaxel/carboplatin × 3 cycles followed by observation vs. 24 weeks of paclitaxel	85% vs. 86%	The addition of 24 weeks of paclitaxel did not improve survival in patients treated with 3 cycles of paclitaxel and carboplatin.

[a]$P < .05.$

early-stage ovarian cancer. Another recent GOG randomized clinical trial in this same patient population also demonstrated no improvement in outcome with the addition of 24 weeks of paclitaxel after completing 3 cycles of conventional paclitaxel and carboplatin.[47]

Of note, Chan et al,[49] in a post-hoc subset analysis of patients enrolled in GOG-157, suggested that patients with serous cancers (23% of the study population) who underwent 6 cycles of chemotherapy had an improved outcome compared with those with serous cancers receiving 3 cycles. This finding was not noted in high-risk early-stage non-serous ovarian cancers. Specifically, the 5-year recurrence-free survival rate in those patients treated with 6 cycles was 83% in comparison with 60% in those treated with 3 cycles of chemotherapy. Although 3 cycles of paclitaxel and carboplatin should be considered the standard of care in adequately staged high-risk early-stage ovarian cancer patients, up to 6 cycles of chemotherapy should be considered in select patients in whom adequate staging has not been performed or in those patients with higher risk factors such as serous histology or stage II disease. Treatment of early-stage, low- and high-risk serous peritoneal cancer and fallopian tube cancer is identical to that described for ovarian cancer.

Treatment of Advanced-Stage Disease

Surgical Management

More than 70% of patients with ovarian, tubal, and peritoneal cancers present with advanced-stage disease.

The primary approach to the management of such patients has included aggressive surgical cytoreduction followed by the administration of chemotherapy. Griffiths et al,[50] in a landmark article published in 1975, was the first to demonstrate improved outcome in advanced-stage ovarian cancer patients who underwent surgical resection such that there was no residual disease implant greater than 2 cm in diameter (Griffith's definition of an "optimal debulking"). Hoskins et al[51] confirmed these findings in an analysis of patients enrolled on several GOG studies. In a meta-analysis evaluating the effect of cytoreduction on the outcome of 81 advanced ovarian cancer patient cohorts, Bristow et al[52] demonstrated a 10% increase in survival with each 10% increase in the number of patients optimally debulked (Figure 12-3).

The definition of what constitutes "optimal" cytoreduction has evolved and is of continued debate. The modern day definition of optimal debulking is resection of all disease with residual metastatic implants less than 1 cm in diameter. Additional studies suggest that clinical outcome in advanced-stage ovarian, tubal, and peritoneal cancers is significantly improved when there is no macroscopic residual disease; several pundits have advocated that this should be the goal of all attempts at surgical cytoreduction of these patients.[53] In an effort to optimally resect advanced-stage high-grade serous disease, surgeons have traditionally performed bilateral salpingo-oophorectomy, total abdominal hysterectomy, pelvic peritoneal stripping, omentectomy, and selective small and large bowel resection. It is estimated that more

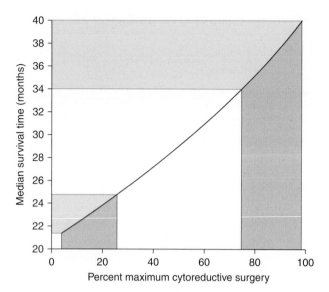

FIGURE 12-3. Simple linear regression analysis displaying de-logged median survival time plotted against the percentage of tumor removed at the time of debulking ("percent maximum cytoreductive surgery").

than a quarter of patients with advanced ovarian cancer undergo an intestinal resection as part of their cytoreductive operation.[54] Increasingly, surgeons are using more advanced upper abdominal debulking surgical techniques such as subdiaphragm peritoneal stripping, splenectomy, and partial pancreatic and hepatic resection to achieve optimal debulking.[55] Several studies have suggested that routine lymphadenectomy in patients with advanced ovarian cancer, particularly in those patients who have all other disease resected, may also be associated with improved outcome.[56,57]

In select patients who are poor surgical candidates or have disease that appears to be unresectable (eg, those with metastases in the liver parenchyma or in the chest), neoadjuvant chemotherapy may be used in lieu of a primary surgical cytoreductive effort. In some of these patients, an "interval" cytoreductive procedure to resect remaining disease may be considered after several cycles of chemotherapy. A randomized clinical trial in European Organization for Research and Treatment of Cancer (EORTC) suggested that an interval cytoreduction in patients with suboptimally resected disease after initial surgery may further render one-third of these patients optimally debulked and improve survival.[58] A similar trial conducted within the GOG did not confirm these findings; the differing conclusions from these studies may be due to the fact that a higher proportion of patients in the GOG study underwent a maximum cytoreductive debulking procedure as compared with those in the EORTC study.[59]

A recent randomized clinical trial conducted within the Gynecologic Cancer Intergroup (GCI) demonstrated that advanced stage IIIC or IV ovarian, tubal, and peritoneal cancer patients managed with neoadjuvant chemotherapy followed by an interval cytoreductive procedure had a similar outcome to those patients managed with primary surgical resection followed by chemotherapy.[60] The percentage of patients rendered optimally resected with disease ≤1 cm in the primary debulking group was 41.6% and in the neoadjuvant chemotherapy group was 80.6%. Postoperative morbidity and mortality tended to be higher after primary debulking. Other studies have concluded that survival in advanced invasive epithelial cancer with neoadjuvant chemotherapy and an interval debulking strategy is associated with an inferior outcome compared with a primary debulking strategy.[61] Additional studies are required to clarify the role of neoadjuvant chemotherapy and interval debulking, but this approach is appropriate in select patients with significant comorbidities or advanced age when all risks versus benefits have been evaluated and discussed.

Medical Management

A combination taxane-platinum chemotherapy regimen is the standard of care for patients with advanced-stage invasive ovarian, tubal, and peritoneal cancers since the results of GOG 111 were published in 1996[62] (Table 12-7). In this study, McGuire et al[62] reported that patients with suboptimally resected ovarian cancers treated with 6 cycles of paclitaxel and cisplatinum had a significantly improved progression-free (18 vs. 13 months) and median overall survival (38 vs. 24 months) compared with those treated with 6 cycles of cyclophosphamide and cisplatin, the standard of care before this study. This study was confirmed by a separate EORTC trial.[63] Given the toxicity associated with the combination of cisplatin and paclitaxel, subsequent studies compared paclitaxel in combination with either cisplatinum or carboplatin (which is associated with decreased long-term toxicity related to neurotoxicity and nephrotoxicity). These results demonstrated that paclitaxel in combination with carboplatin was better tolerated and equally as effective as paclitaxel combined with cisplatin in the management of patients with advanced ovarian cancer.[64,65] Another randomized trial confirmed that the combination of docetaxel and carboplatin was as effective as paclitaxel and carboplatin for patients with newly diagnosed ovarian cancer; although associated with more hematologic toxicity, there was a significant reduction in the rate of neurotoxicity.[66]

Efforts to improve upon the outcome of patients with advanced high-grade, serous cancers have focused on modifying the paclitaxel/platinum combination regimen

Table 12-7 Relevant Randomized Control Trials in Late-Stage Invasive Ovarian Cancer

Trial/Author	Treatment Arms	Overall Survival	Conclusions
Paclitaxel/cisplatin			
GOG-111 (McGuire, 1996)[62]	Cyclophosphamide/cisplatin vs. paclitaxel/cisplatin	PFS: 13 vs. 18 months[a] Median OS: 24 vs. 38 months[a]	Paclitaxel in combination with cisplatin improves PFS and OS over cyclophosphamide and cisplatin.
EORTC (Piccart, 2000)[63]	Cyclophosphamide/cisplatin vs. paclitaxel/cisplatin	PFS: 11.5 vs. 15.5 months[a] Median OS: 25.8 vs. 35.6 months[a]	
Taxanes/carboplatin			
GOG-158 (Ozols, 2003)[64]	Paclitaxel/cisplatin vs. paclitaxel/carboplatin	PFS: 19.4 vs. 20.7 months Median OS: 48.7 vs. 57.4 months	Paclitaxel in combination with carboplatin was equally as effective and better tolerated than paclitaxel and cisplatin.
AGO (du Bois, 2003)[65]	Paclitaxel/cisplatin vs. paclitaxel/carboplatin	PFS: 17.2 vs. 19.1 months Median OS: 43.3 vs. 44.1 months	
SCOTROC (Vasey, 2004)[77]	Paclitaxel/carboplatin vs. docetaxel/carboplatin	PFS: 14.8 vs. 15.0 months 2-year OS: 68.9% vs. 64.2%	Docetaxel/carboplatin appeared to offer similar PFS and OS when compared with paclitaxel/carboplatin.
IP chemotherapy			
GOG-114 (Markman, 2001)[74]	Paclitaxel/cisplatin vs. moderately high dose of IV carboplatin followed by IV paclitaxel and IP cisplatin	PFS: 51 vs. 67 months[a]	An IV/IP taxane/platinum regimen improves outcome over an IV taxane/platinum regimen.
GOG 172 (Armstrong, 2006)[70]	IV paclitaxel and cisplatin vs. IV paclitaxel, IP cisplatin, and IP paclitaxel	PFS: 18.3 vs. 23.8 months[a] Median OS: 49.7 vs. 65.6 months[a]	
Dose-dense paclitaxel			
JGOG (Katsumata, 2009)[75]	Paclitaxel every 3 weeks vs. weekly in combination with carboplatin	PFS: 17.2 vs. 28 months[a] 3-year OS: 65.1% vs. 72.1%[a]	Dose-dense paclitaxel improves outcome.
Bevacizumab			
GOG-218 (Burger, 2010)[76]	Paclitaxel/carboplatin vs. paclitaxel/carboplatin in combination with bevacizumab (cycles 2-6) vs. paclitaxel/carboplatin in combination with bevacizumab followed by maintenance bevacizumab for an additional 15 cycles	PFS: 10.3 vs. 14.1 months[a] CA-125 censored PFS: 12 vs. 18 months	The addition of bevacizumab in combination with paclitaxel and carboplatin improves PFS when compared with chemotherapy alone.
ICON 7			
Maintenance therapy			
GOG 178 (Markman, 2009)[84]	3 vs. 12 cycles of paclitaxel	PFS 14 vs 22 months[a] 5-year OS: 48 vs. 53 months	Maintenance paclitaxel improves PFS but does not appear to improve OS.

AGO, Arbeitsgemeinschaft Gynaekologische Onkologie; EORTC, European Organization for Research and Treatment of Cancer; GOG, Gynecologic Oncology Group; ICON, International Collaborative Ovarian Neoplasm; IP, intraperitoneal; IV, intravenous; JGOG, Japanese Gynecologic Oncology Group; OS, overall survival; PFS, progression-free survival; SCOTROC, Scottish Randomised Trial in Ovarian Cancer.
[a]$p < 0.05$

CHAPTER 12

by adding other active cytotoxic or biologic agents, altering the route of drug delivery, intensifying the dose of paclitaxel, or evaluating various maintenance therapy regimens. Over the past 2 decades, there have been a number of cytotoxic agents that have been demonstrated to have antitumor activity in these diseases. These agents (gemcitabine, topotecan, liposomal doxorubicin) were added to paclitaxel and carboplatin as sequential doublet or triplet regimens in GCI/GOG-182, one of the largest randomized clinical trials in advanced ovarian cancer.[67] This study demonstrated no improvement in outcome in advanced ovarian cancer patients treated with one of the sequential doublet or triplet regimens in comparison with those treated solely with paclitaxel and carboplatin. Recently, a phase 3 comparison of adjuvant intravenous carboplatin with either paclitaxel or gemcitabine demonstrated that the gemcitabine combination provided no additional survival benefit[68] over the standard of carboplatin with paclitaxel.

Altering the route of delivery of chemotherapy has been demonstrated in 3 randomized GOG studies to improve outcome in patients with optimally resected ovarian, tubal, and peritoneal cancer.[69] The results of the latest of these studies, GOG-172, was reported by Armstrong et al[69] and led to the publication of a National Cancer Institute Clinical Alert in 2006.[70] This study randomized patients with optimally resected ovarian cancer to 6 cycles of intravenous paclitaxel and cisplatin versus 6 cycles of intravenous paclitaxel in combination with intraperitoneal cisplatin and intraperitoneal paclitaxel. In this study, patients treated with the intraperitoneal regimen experienced additional complications associated with either the intraperitoneal catheter or the chemotherapy regimen, and only 42% were able to complete all 6 cycles. Nevertheless, the median survival in those treated with the intraperitoneal regimen was significantly improved over that achieved in patients who received traditional intravenous chemotherapy (65.6 vs. 49.7 months). Furthermore, quality of life was similar in both groups of patients 6 months after therapy. Retrospective studies have advocated modification of the intraperitoneal regimen by reducing the dose of cisplatin or using intraperitoneal carboplatin instead of cisplatin.[71,72] Two prior randomized trials conducted within the GOG also demonstrated significant improvement in outcome in optimally debulked advanced-stage ovarian cancer with intraperitoneal chemotherapy regimens compared with those with intravenous chemotherapy alone.[73,74] The decision to use intraperitoneal chemotherapy in this patient population should be individualized and based on a discussion of the risks versus benefits of this approach.

The concept of dose-dense chemotherapy in high-grade serous cancers of the ovary, tube, and peritoneum arises from data in metastatic breast cancer, where studies have demonstrated that intensifying the dose of paclitaxel improves overall survival. In ovarian cancer, a recent randomized Japanese GOG study evaluated the potential of using such an approach.[75] Specifically, 631 eligible patients with stage II to IV ovarian cancer were randomized to receive every-3-weeks paclitaxel (conventional treatment) versus weekly paclitaxel (experimental treatment), both administered in combination with every-3-weeks carboplatin. This study demonstrated a significantly improved median progression-free survival (28.0 vs. 17.2 months) and 3-year overall survival rate (72.1% vs. 65.1%) in patients treated with the dose-dense paclitaxel strategy. Toxicity was similar in both arms with the exception of grade 3 or 4 anemia which was more commonly noted in the dose-dense chemotherapy regimen. The proportion of patients who completed 6 or more cycles of chemotherapy was higher in the conventional treatment arm (73% vs. 62%). Ongoing studies in the GOG are attempting to confirm the findings of this provocative study.

Solid tumors are often dependent on the development of new vessels to facilitate growth and metastasis. Ovarian cancer is no exception, and various studies have linked poor survival in this disease context to increased tumor angiogenesis and increased expression of vascular endothelial growth factor (VEGF), one of the major mediators of tumor angiogenesis.[76] Bevacizumab, a humanized monoclonal antibody to VEGF, has been demonstrated to have significant antitumor activity in a number of solid tumors and has received FDA approval for use in lung and colon cancer. A GOG phase 2 trial demonstrated a 21% response rate and a 40.3% 6-month progression-free survival rate in a cohort of recurrent ovarian cancer patients, 42% of whom were considered to have platinum-resistant disease.[77] Other early-phase and retrospective studies have demonstrated improved responses in patients with recurrent ovarian cancer when various chemotherapy agents were added to bevacizumab.[78,79]

Given the activity of this agent in the recurrent setting, bevacizumab was evaluated in a major GOG phase 3 trial in patients with newly diagnosed advanced-stage ovarian cancer.[80] This study randomized 1873 eligible patients to receive standard paclitaxel and carboplatin alone (control group), chemotherapy in combination with bevacizumab (cycles 2-6), or chemotherapy with bevacizumab (cycles 2-6) followed by an additional 15 cycles of extended bevacizumab maintenance. Bevacizumab was administered at a dose of 15 mg/kg every 3 weeks. This study demonstrated a significant improvement in progression-free survival in the patients who received chemotherapy in combination with both concurrent and maintenance bevacizumab in comparison to the control group of patients (10.3 vs. 14.1 months). There was no difference in progression-free survival between the group of patients treated with chemotherapy and concurrent bevacizumab compared with the control group. Toxicity experienced in the bevacizumab-treated patients included hypertension and gastrointestinal perforation, but the frequency or severity of these toxicities was no more than that encountered in prior ovarian cancer or other solid tumor studies. Overall survival and quality of life analyses are ongoing. The preliminary results of a second trial, ICON 7, also affirm the potential of the anti-angiogenesis agent bevacizumab in this disease context. In this trial, 1528 patients with high-risk early-stage or advanced ovarian, primary peritoneal, or fallopian tube cancer were randomized to receive standard paclitaxel and carboplatin alone or in combination with both concurrent (cycles 2-6) and maintenance bevacizumab (additional 12 cycles). Bevacizumab was administered at a dose of 7.5 mg/kg every 3 weeks.[81] The results of this study demonstrated that the risk of developing progression of disease at 12 months was 15% less in those patients treated with the combination of chemotherapy and bevacizumab when compared with that noted in patients treated with chemotherapy alone. Once mature, the results of GOG-218 and ICON 7 will provide further guidance regarding the role of bevacizumab in newly diagnosed ovarian cancer.

The concept of maintenance chemotherapy is another strategy that has been extensively evaluated as a means to improving outcome in patients with advanced-stage ovarian cancer. The rationale for this approach has been that although more than 70% of patients with advanced-stage ovarian, tubal, and peritoneal cancers will achieve a complete clinical remission with primary surgery and chemotherapy, the majority of these patients will ultimately develop recurrent disease. Investigators have evaluated various maintenance strategies after primary chemotherapy, including the whole abdominal radiation, intraperitoneal radioactive phosphorus (P[32]), and various intravenous and intraperitoneal chemotherapy or biologic agents.[82] The only trial to demonstrate an improvement in outcome (before the results of GOG-218 demonstrating improved outcome in patients with maintenance bevacizumab after carboplatin, paclitaxel, and bevacizumab) was one in which 277 advanced-stage ovarian cancer patients who had achieved a complete clinical response to primary therapy were randomized to monthly paclitaxel for either an additional 3 or 12 months.[83,84] A significant improvement in progression-free survival was noted in the patients who received 12 cycles of monthly paclitaxel (22 vs. 14 months). However, overall survival was noted to be similar in the patients who received 12 cycles of maintenance paclitaxel when compared with those who were treated with 3 cycles (53 vs. 48 months).[84] An ongoing phase 3 trial in the GOG is currently further evaluating the potential of maintenance taxane-based therapies compared with observation in patients with advanced-stage ovarian, peritoneal, and tubal cancers.

In summary, the adjuvant treatment of patients with high-grade serous epithelial ovarian, primary peritoneal, and fallopian tube cancers is directed in large part by the assignment of FIGO stage and by the randomized clinical trials described in this chapter. Table 12-8 provides general recommendations for clinicians managing these patients.

Table 12-8 Treatment for Invasive Serous Epithelial Ovarian Cancer by Stage

Stage	Treatment Options
IA/B, grade 1, 2	Observation
IA/B, grade 3	Clinical trial
IC, II	IV paclitaxel 175 mg/m² and carboplatin AUC 5-7.5 every 21 days × 3-6 cycles
III-IV, optimally debulked	Clinical trial
	IV paclitaxel[a] 175 mg/m² and carboplatin AUC 5-7.5 every 21 days × 6 cycles
	IV paclitaxel[a] 175 mg/m² day 1, IP cisplatin 75-100 mg/m² IP day 2, and IP paclitaxel 80 mg/m² day 8 every 21 days × 6 cycles
	IV paclitaxel 80 mg/m² days 1, 8, 15 and carboplatin AUC 5-7.5 every 21 days × 3-6 cycles
	IV paclitaxel[a] 175 mg/m² and carboplatin AUC 5-7.5 every 21 days × 6 cycles followed by IV paclitaxel 135-175 mg/m² every 28 days × 12 cycles
	IV paclitaxel[a] 175 mg/m², carboplatin AUC 5-7.5 and bevacizumab 15 mg/kg (cycles 2-6) every 21 days × 6 cycles followed by bevacizumab 15 mg/kg every 21 days for 15 cycles

AUC, area under the curve; IP, intraperitoneal; IV, intravenous.
[a]Docetaxel 80 mg/m² may be substituted in appropriate clinical situations.

SURVIVAL AND PROGNOSIS

Key Points

1. Early-stage epithelial ovarian, primary peritoneal, and fallopian tube cancers have a favorable prognosis, with relatively high progression-free and overall survival.
2. Advanced-stage disease is associated with a high likelihood of multiple recurrences, each with increasing chemoresistance.
3. Established prognostic factors for high-grade serous ovarian, peritoneal, and tubal cancers include age at diagnosis, stage of disease, and extent of cytoreduction at primary surgery.

Clinical outcome and survival in women with high-grade serous epithelial ovarian, fallopian tube, and primary peritoneal cancers are influenced by several clinical and pathologic factors. Although large, randomized clinical trials examining women with this disease have included all histologic variants of epithelial ovarian cancer (with many studies including primary peritoneal and fallopian tube malignancies), it is reasonable to extrapolate age at diagnosis, stage of disease, and cytoreductive effort at primary surgery as relevant prognosticators in high-grade, serous disease.

Studies typically report survival as a function of stage (Table 12-9). Again, the majority of data includes all histologic subtypes of epithelial ovarian cancer, and several observational studies confirm similar clinical outcomes for those with fallopian tube and primary peritoneal disease. For stage I and II disease, high-grade serous histology should be considered as high risk for recurrence, and 5-year overall survival rates range from 65% to 89% with adjuvant platinum-based chemotherapy.[43,46] For stage III and IV disease, 5-year survival rates may range from 5% to 75%, depending on therapeutic modality. After an optimal cytoreductive effort, treatment with intravenous platinum and taxane chemotherapy results in a median survival of

Table 12-9 Survival (Overall 5-Year) of Patients With Ovarian Cancer[109]

Stage I	89%
Stage II	65%
Stage III	33%
Stage III (no residual)	75%
Stage III (optimal residual)	25%
Stage III (suboptimal)	5%
Stage IV	18%

50 months, whereas adjuvant therapy with a combined intravenous and intraperitoneal regimen is associated with a 66-month median survival.[70]

Prognostic Factors

Overall, the prognosis of these high-grade serous cancers is predominantly dependent on stage of disease, and the volume of residual cancer after cytoreduction (Table 12-9). Older age is also an established prognosticator, but its clinical impact is relatively limited in comparison with stage and cytoreductive effort. Many women with high-grade serous ovarian, tubal, and peritoneal cancers harbor deleterious mutations in the *BRCA1* and *BRCA2* genes; evidence suggests that tumors associated with *BRCA* mutations are more chemosensitive, with resulting improved overall survival when compared with women with sporadic disease.[85]

MANAGEMENT OF RECURRENT DISEASE

Key Points

1. Patients with recurrent high-grade serous ovarian, tubal, and peritoneal cancers should be classified as having either platinum-sensitive or -refractory disease based on the time interval between end of prior chemotherapy and date of recurrence (treatment-free interval).
2. Secondary cytoreduction should be considered for select patients with recurrent disease; namely, those with long treatment-free intervals and limited sites of recurrent implants.
3. In general, combination platinum-based chemotherapy is the treatment of choice for patients with platinum-sensitive recurrent disease.

Although the majority women with high-grade serous ovarian, tubal, and peritoneal cancers enter remission after surgical resection and advjuant chemotherapy, many will develop recurrence of disease and undergo additional treatment. In general, after completion of primary therapy, women with these diseases are followed at 3-month intervals for the first 2 years, at 4-month intervals for the third year, and then at 6-month intervals thereafter, with discharge at 10 years in the absence of recurrence. During these visits, a focused history and physical examination are performed, including pelvic and rectal evaluation. Traditionally, women have serial serum CA-125 tumor markers drawn, with elevations from their baseline (typically 2 times the nadir value) prompting CT imaging. There is no evidence to support the routine application of CT imaging for surveillance in otherwise asymptomatic patients with normal tumor markers and physical findings.

Several advances have modified this traditional approach to surveillance. Human epididymal secretory protein E4, or HE4, is a novel serum marker that is elevated in women with high-grade serous ovarian cancers, especially compared with those with mucinous or clear cell etiology.[86] HE4 may also provide higher accurancy in differentiating cancer over benign adnexal masses.[87] The FDA has approved HE4 for surveillance and monitoring for recurrent or progressive disease; HE4 has particular utility in following women without prior CA-125 elevations.

In addition, Rustin and colleagues[88] reported on a large randomized trial of women with advanced-stage ovarian cancer and identified no improvement in survival with serial CA-125 monitoring after completion of standard therapy. In this study, women in complete remission underwent CA-125 measurement and clinical examination every 3 months; patients and clinicians were blinded to the CA-125 results. When the CA-125 exceeded twice the upper limit of normal, patients were randomized to either immediate chemotherapy or delay of treatment until relapse became clinical or symptomatic. Investigators could not observe any difference in overall survival and reported decreased quality of life scores in those women randomized to immediate therapy. Although several factors may have influenced these findings (including the very low application of secondary cytoreductive surgery), these findings suggest that serial tumor markers may not influence clinical outcome. CA-125 testing may be omitted except in the event of clinical suspicion of relapse or at the patient's request.

Recommended Treatment Options

Recurrent ovarian, tubal, and peritoneal cancer are diseases unlikely to be cured with the current tools of surgery, chemotherapy, and radiation. As such, the goal of treatment of this disease is palliation of symptoms and extension of disease-free and overall survival. One of the most important factors in predicting outcome related to recurrent ovarian caner is the "platinum-free interval," defined as the time between completion of primary therapy and disease recurrence. The longer this interval, the higher the probability of responding again to platinum-based chemotherapy. For this reason, cancer recurrences that occur greater than 6 months after completion of platinum-based chemotherapy are considered platinum-sensitive, and those occurring less than 6 months from completion of primary treatment are classified as platinum-resistant.

The decision regarding the modality of treatment of recurrent ovarian, tubal, and peritoneal cancer (chemotherapy vs. surgery followed by chemotherapy) is dependent on a variety of factors, not least of which is the judgment of the surgeon. The concept behind performing surgery for recurrent ovarian cancer ("secondary cytoreduction") is based on the principle followed for the primary management of the disease. In primary disease, when there is little or no disease before initiation of chemotherapy, it has been demonstrated that prognosis is better, as delivery of chemotherapy is in theory more effective in the absence of large hypoxic tumors, the probability of sporadic cancer mutation favoring chemotherapy resistance should lessen in the absence of more frequent cellular division in larger tumors, and the total number of cancer cells needed to treat is less. Although these factors should also apply to recurrent ovarian cancer, there are no definitive data suggesting that this intervention improves prognosis in women with recurrent disease. The majority of studies regarding secondary cytoreduction are limited by their varied inclusion criteria, nonrandomized design, long reporting interval, and small sample size. Nonetheless, some general conclusions can be drawn from the literature regarding this intervention. In general, secondary cytoreduction is reserved for patients with platinum-sensitive disease, in that this group of patients has the best prognosis before surgery and the highest likelihood of demonstrating chemosensitive disease after surgery. Furthermore, this procedure is more commonly performed in patients with limited sites of recurrent disease; in those patients with diffuse peritoneal carcinomatosis, it is less likely that optimal resection may be performed.[89] A recent meta-analysis suggested that the survival associated with secondary cytoreduction was significantly associated with complete cytoreduction.[90]

Regardless of whether patients with recurrent disease undergo secondary cytoreduction, patients are generally treated with systemic chemotherapy (unless palliative supportive care is pursued). Patients with platinum-sensitive cancers are treated with either single- or multiagent platinum-containing regimens. To date, 2 randomized clinical trials have reported that treatment of patients with platinum-sensitive recurrent ovarian cancer with combination platinum-paclitaxel or platinum-gemcitabine is associated with improved progression-free survival compared with treatment with platinum alone.[91] Furthermore, the recently reported phase III CALYPSO (CAeLYx in Platinum Sensitive Ovarian) study reported that treatment with liposomal doxorubicin and carboplatin was associated with improved progression-free survival compared with paclitaxel and carboplatin.[92] From these data, most clinicians choose to treat patients with platinum-sensitive recurrent ovarian cancer with platinum-containing doublets. The decision to use one cytotoxic over another (in combination with platinum) often is dictated by the expected toxicity of the combination. As an example, a patient with moderate preexisting peripheral neuropathy would likely be treated with platinum-gemcitabine rather than platinum-paclitaxel for her recurrence. Overall, the expected response rate for platinum-based combinations in the setting of platinum-sensitive recurrent ovarian cancer is approximately 70%.

For patients with persistent disease after primary therapy (platinum-refractory) or platinum-resistant disease, single-agent chemotherapy is often used. Given the poor prognosis associated with recurrent platinum-refractory or -resistant disease, the decision to treat with a specific regimen must be made in the context of maintaining quality of life. Current FDA-approved medications for the treatment of recurrent ovarian cancer include the doublet of carboplatinum and gemcitabine, paclitaxel, liposomal doxorubicin, and topotecan.[93,94] In the setting of platinum-recurrent (or -refractory) disease, these agents are associated with response rates of approximately 15%. During the life of a patient with recurrent ovarian cancer, she will likely be treated with all of these medications; the sequence in which they are given is often based on toxicity and convenience of administration.

Although there is a great deal of enthusiasm regarding the expansion of knowledge related to the human genome and its alterations in cancer, until recently, these scientific discoveries have not translated into substantial improvements in the outcome of patients, recurrent ovarian cancer. Historically, investigation of oncogenic pathways and their inhibitors, such as the epidermal growth factor receptor (EGFR) family of inhibitors (eg, trastuzumab and pertuzumab) have not shown responses much different from those associated with single-agent cytotoxic therapy.[95,96] More recently, investigation of inhibitors of angiogenesis (eg, bevacizumab) in the setting of primary and recurrent ovarian cancer has shown promise. The GOG investigated single-agent bevacizumab and found it to be well tolerated and associated with a greater than 20% response rate (median duration of response, 10 months).[97] This agent has been combined with many other cytotoxic agents and is currently under investigation in patients with platinum-sensitive recurrent ovarian cancer in GOG-213.

More recently, identification of the role of inhibition of the poly (ADP-ribose) polymerase (PARP) pathway in the treatment of ovarian, tubal, and peritoneal cancers has led to enthusiasm in improving outcome in this disease.[98-100] The use of PARP inhibitors in the treatment of cancer represents the first successful clinical exploitation of tumor synthetic lethality (promotion of genomic instability). PARP activity is required for base-excision repair, a DNA-damage repair pathway that recognizes and eliminates the DNA that is commonly damaged during replication. In the absence of PARP activity, these damaged bases accumulate, and replication forks (the location of DNA replication during DNA synthesis) are arrested at sites of the damaged DNA, eventually causing double-strand DNA breaks. Normally, the process of homologous recombination repairs these breaks; in the situation in which this mechanism is unavailable (in the case when *BRCA1* or *BRCA2* is absent), the cell dies. The use of PARP inhibitors exploits this mechanism and causes the accumulation of damaged DNA, limits the repair of double-strand DNA breaks, and inhibits cancer growth. In the absence of 1 copy of the *BRCA* gene (in the case of an inherited *BRCA* defect), the use of PARP inhibitors has been shown to be effective. Patients with hereditary ovarian carcinoma are excellent candidates for treatment with PARP inhibitors, because these patients are heterozygous for mutations in *BRCA1* or *BRCA2* and thus have preserved homologous recombination in their somatic cells, whereas their tumors have lost the remaining wild-type copy of *BRCA1* or *BRCA2* and are therefore deficient in homologous recombination. Because many sporadic ovarian cancers develop somatic acquisition of a *BRCA* mutation, the applicability of PARP inhibitors in the treatment of ovarian cancer extends beyond just treatment of patients with hereditary ovarian cancer syndromes.[101] In a recent phase 2 study of patients with recurrent epithelial ovarian cancer, the overall response rate to the PARP inhibitor olaparib was 33%, much higher than generally reported for this disease when treated with standard chemotherapy.[98] Although encouraging, there is insufficient evidence to date to recommend the routine use of PARP inhibitors in the treatment of recurrent ovarian cancer. Results from ongoing phase 3 trials of PARP inhibitors in ovarian cancer are eagerly awaited.

Palliative Care

Given the usual course of recurrent ovarian cancer (in which patients become refractory to therapy), patients often experience conditions that require specific expertise in palliative care. It is estimated that the majority of patients with recurrent disease will undergo treatment for bowel dysfunction (constipation or obstruction), pain, ascites, pleural effusions, and nausea or emesis. These issues are addressed in general in the following section on Special Management Problems.

SPECIAL MANAGEMENT PROBLEMS

Thoracic Disease

Pleural effusions and intrathoracic metastases are not infrequently noted in patients who present with clinical findings suggestive of an advanced-stage ovarian, tubal, or peritoneal cancer. Eitan et al[102] noted that the outcome in patients with malignant pleural effusions in optimally debulked advanced-stage ovarian cancer was worse than in those patients without an effusion. The optimal management of patients who are noted to have a pleural effusion is not well established, although video-assisted thoracic surgery (VATS) may be used to document intrathoracic disease, to potentially resect macroscopic disease, and to direct therapy in those ovarian cancer patients with moderate to large pleural effusions.[103] For those patients with symptomatic pleural effusions, thoracentesis or VATS-assisted pleurodesis may be considered.

Ascites

Patients with newly diagnosed advanced-stage or recurrent ovarian cancer often experience symptoms related to the accumulation of malignant ascites. A paracentesis may be indicated in instances when patients with ascites experience shortness of breath, significant abdominal bloating, and difficulty with eating. In general, this procedure is accomplished at the bedside with a blind approach or under ultrasound guidance. An indwelling catheter has been demonstrated to be useful in patients with recurrent symptomatic ascites.[104]

Bowel Obstruction

Although uncommonly noted in patients with newly diagnosed ovarian cancer, patients with recurrent disease may often experience bowel dysfunction or obstruction. Clinicians must take into consideration the patient's overall medical and performance status, the burden of disease, and her prior therapy in choosing the appropriate measures to correct or palliate obstructive symptoms. Nonsurgical options include temporary nasogastric suctioning with intravenous fluid supplementation and appropriate electrolyte supplementation. Intravenous octreotide has been reported to be potentially effective in ameliorating obstructive symptoms related to malignancies.[105] A gastrostomy tube placed via endoscopy or by interventional radiology should be considered in those patients who do not respond to conservative measures, who are not good surgical candidates, and who do not have a life expectancy of greater than 3 to 6 months. A colonic stent may be considered in select patients with distal large bowel obstruction, but the reported success rates appear not to exceed 25%.[106]

For select ovarian cancer patients with a bowel obstruction who do not respond to conservative measures, have limited disease, and have a life expectancy of greater than 3 to 6 months, a surgical approach to correct anatomy or palliate their symptoms should be carefully considered. Depending on the nature of the obstruction and intraoperative findings, a surgeon may wish to consider a bowel resection with anastomosis, a bowel bypass, and/or an ileostomy or colostomy. Chi et al[107] reported excellent improvement in symptoms with a surgical approach in a prospectively evaluated cohort of recurrent ovarian cancer patients with a bowel obstruction. However, median survival did not exceed 7 months. Despite only limited data to perform a systematic review, there is a suggestion that surgical management of recurrent ovarian cancer-associated bowel obstruction can improve survival compared with medical management.[108]

FUTURE DIRECTIONS

Substantial progress has been made toward improving the diagnosis and treatment of ovarian cancer, resulting in improved survival. With recent expansion of our understanding of the cancer genome, numerous advances have been made in the diagnosis, prognostication, and treatment of high-grade serous ovarian, peritoneal, and tubal cancers. Although the most encouraging data recently regarding targeted therapies focus on inhibition of angiogenesis with the monoclonal antibody bevacizumab and the exploitation of the PARP pathway, alternative means to inhibit the angiogenesis pathway or investigation of other pathways (eg, those in the EGFR family) have also been described in the treatment of these diseases. Preliminary results using a soluble decoy receptor of VEGF (VEGF trap) and small molecule inhibitors of the VEGF or platelet-derived growth factor pathway (sunitinib, sorafenib) have shown promise in the treatment of recurrent ovarian cancer. Furthermore, inhibition of the EGFR pathway (trastuzumab, cetuximab, pertuzumab, erlotinib) has demonstrated variable response, although at different rates. At this time, these agents remain experimental and are being evaluated in clinical trials in recurrent ovarian cancer. Blockade of other pathways, such as the src kinase inhibitors, antifolates, and insulin-like growth factor 1 receptor inhibitors, also are being studied in clinical trials. Other novel treatment strategies, such as immuno- and gene therapy, are also under development.

REFERENCES

1. Jemal A, Siegel R, Xu J, Ward E. Cancer statistics, 2010. *CA Cancer J Clin.* 2010;60:277-300.

2. Morgan RJ Jr, Alvarez RD, Armstrong DK, et al. Epithelial ovarian cancer. *J Natl Compr Cancer Netw.* 2011;9(1):82-113.

3. Goodman MT, Shvetsov YB. Incidence of ovarian, peritoneal, and fallopian tube carcinomas in the United States, 1995-2004. *Cancer Epidemiol Biomarkers Prev.* 2009;18:132-139.

4. Seidman JD, Zhao P, Yemelyanova A. "Primary peritoneal" high-grade serous carcinoma is very likely metastatic from serous tubal intraepithelial carcinoma. *Gynecol Oncol.* 2011;120(3):470-473.

5. Przybycin CG, Kurman RJ, Ronnett BM, Shih IeM, Vang R. Are all pelvic (nonuterine) serous carcinomas of tubal origin? *Am J Surg Pathol.* 2010;34(10):1407-1416.

6. Schorge JO, Modesitt SC, Coleman RL, et al. SGO White Paper on ovarian cancer: etiology, screening and surveillance. *Gynecol Oncol.* 2010;119:7-17.

7. Santen RJ, Allred DC, Ardoin SP, et al. Postmenopausal hormone therapy: an Endocrine Society scientific statement. *J Clin Endocrinol Metab.* 2010;95:S1-S66.

8. Gershenson DM, Sun CC, Bodurka D, et al. Recurrent low-grade serous ovarian carcinoma is relatively chemoresistant. *Gynecol Oncol.* 2009;114:48-52.

9. Bonome T, Lee JY, Park DC, et al. Expression profiling of serous low malignant potential, low-grade, and high-grade tumors of the ovary. *Cancer Res.* 2005;65:10602-10612.

10. Kurman RJ, Shih IM. The origin and pathogenesis of epithelial ovarian cancer: a proposed unifying theory. *Am J Surg Pathol.* 2010;34(3):433-443.

11. Clarke-Pearson DL. Clinical practice. Screening for ovarian cancer. *N Engl J Med.* 2009;361:170-177.

12. Partridge E, Kreimer AR, Greenlee RT, et al. Results from four rounds of ovarian cancer screening in a randomized trial. *Obstet Gynecol.* 2009;113:775-782.

13. Menon U, Gentry-Maharaj A, Hallett R, et al. Sensitivity and specificity of multimodal and ultrasound screening for ovarian cancer, and stage distribution of detected cancers: results of the prevalence screen of the UK Collaborative Trial of Ovarian Cancer Screening (UKCTOCS). *Lancet Oncol.* 2009;10:327-340.

14. Lu KH, Skates S, Bevers TB, et al. A prospective U.S. ovarian cancer screening study using the risk of ovarian cancer algorithm (ROCA). *J Clin Oncol.* 2010;28(suppl):15S. Abstract 5003.

15. Goff BA, Mandel L, Muntz HG, Melancon CH. Ovarian carcinoma diagnosis—results of a national ovarian cancer survey. *Cancer.* 2000;89:2068-2075.

16. Goff BA, Mandel LS, Melancon CH, Muntz HG. Frequency of symptoms of ovarian cancer in women presenting to primary care clinics. *JAMA.* 2004;291:2705-2712.

17. Women's Cancer Network. Ovarian Cancer Symptoms Consensus Statement. http://www.wcn.org/articles/types_of_cancer/ovarian/symptoms/concensus_statement.html. Accessed January 11, 2012.

18. Ettabbakh GH, Yadav PR, Morgan A. Clinical picture of women with early stage ovarian cancer. *Gynecol Oncol.* 1999:75(3):476-479.

19. Padilla LA, Radosevich DM, Milad MP. Accuracy of the pelvic examination in detecting adnexal masses. *Obstet Gynecol.* 2000;96:593-598.

20. Shaaban A, Rezvani M. Ovarian cancer: detection and radiologic staging. *Clin Obstet Gynecol.* 2009;52:73-93.

21. Iyer VR, Lee SI. MRI, CT, and PET/CT for ovarian cancer detection and adnexal lesion characterization. *AJR Am J Roentgenol.* 2010;194(2):311-321.

22. Van Calster B, Timmerman D, Bourne T, et al. Discrimination between benign and malignant adnexal masses by specialist ultrasound examination versus serum CA-125. *J Natl Cancer Inst.* 2007;99(22):1706-1714.

23. McDonald JM, Doran S, DeSimone CP, et al. Predicting risk of malignancy in adnexal masses. *Obstet Gynecol.* 2010;115(4):687-694.

24. Bast RC, Badgwell D. Lu Z, et al. New tumor markers: CA125 and beyond. *Int J Gynecol Cancer.* 2005:15:274-281.

25. Duffy MJ, Bonfer JM, Kulpa J, et al. CA125 in ovarian cancer: European Group on Tumor Markers guidelines for clinical use. *Int J Gynecol Cancer.* 2005;15(5):679-691.

26. Feng ET. A recipe for proteomics diagnostic test development: the OVA1 test, from biomarker discovery to FDA clearance. *Clin Chem.* 2010;56(2):327-329.

27. Ueland F, DeSimone C, Seamon L, et al. The OVA1 test improves the preoperative assessment of ovarian tumors. *Gynecol Oncol.* 2010;116(suppl):3S. Abstract 54.

28. Muller CY. Doctor, should I get this new ovarian cancer test-OVA1? *Obstet Gynecol.* 2010:116:246-247.

29. American College of Obstetricians and Gynecologists ACOG Committee Opinion: number 280, 2002. The role of the generalist obstetrician-gynecologist in the early detection of ovarian cancer. *Obstet Gynecol.* 2002;100(6):1413-1416.

30. Le T, Glede C, Salem S, et al. Initial evaluation and referral guidelines for management of pelvic/ovarian masses. *J Obstet Gynaecol Can.* 2009;31(7):668-680.

31. Panici PB, Maggioni A, Hacker N, et al. Systematic aortic and pelvic lymphadenectomy versus resection of bulky nodes only in optimally debulked advanced ovarian cancer: a randomized clinical trial. *J Natl Cancer Inst.* 2005;97:560-566.

32. Aletti GD, Podratz KC, Cliby WA, Gostout BS. Stage IV ovarian cancer: disease site-specific rationale for postoperative treatment. *Gynecol Oncol.* 2009;112:22-27.

33. Di Re E, Grosso G, Raspagliesi F, Baiocchi G. Fallopian tube cancer: incidence and role of lymphatic spread. *Gynecol Oncol.* 1996;62:199-202.

34. Hu CY, Taymor ML, Hertig AT. Primary carcinoma of the fallopian tube. *Am J Obstet Gynecol.* 1950;59:58-67.

35. Sedlis A. Carcinoma of the fallopian tube. *Surg Clin North Am.* 1978;58:121-129.

36. Bloss JD, Liao SY, Buller RE, et al. Extraovarian peritoneal serous papillary carcinoma: a case-control retrospective comparison to papillary adenocarcinoma of the ovary. *Gynecol Oncol.* 1993 Sep;50(3):347-351.

37. Young RC, Decker DG, Wharton JT, et al. Staging laparotomy in early ovarian cancer. *JAMA.* 1983;250(22):3072-3076.

38. Le T, Adolph A, Krepart GV, et al. The benefits of comprehensive surgical staging in the management of early-stage epithelial ovarian carcinoma. *Gynecol Oncol.* 2002;85(2):351-355.

39. Trimble EL. Prospects for improving staging of ovarian cancers. *Lancet.* 2001;357(9251):159-160.

40. National Comprehensive Cancer Network. NCCN Ovarian Cancer Guidelines. http://www.nccn.org/professionals/physician_gls/ PDF/ovarian.pdf. Accessed January 11, 2012.

41. Chi DS, Abu-Rustum NR, Sonoda Y, et al. The safety and efficacy of laparoscopic surgical staging of apparent stage I ovarian and fallopian tube cancers. *Am J Obstet Gynecol.* 2005;192(5):1614-1619.

42. Young RC, Walton LA, Ellenberg SS, et al. Adjuvant therapy in stage I and stage II epithelial ovarian cancer. Results of two prospective randomized trials. *N Engl J Med.* 1990;322(15):1021-1027.

43. Trimbos JB, Parmar M, Vergote I, et al. International Collaborative Ovarian Neoplasm trial 1 and Adjuvant ChemoTherapy in Ovarian Neoplasm trial: two parallel randomized phase III trials of adjuvant chemotherapy in patients with early-stage ovarian carcinoma. *J Natl Cancer Inst.* 2003;95(2):105-112.

44. Trimbos JB, Vergote I, Bolis G, et al. Impact of adjuvant chemotherapy and surgical staging in early-stage ovarian carcinoma:

European Organisation for Research and Treatment of Cancer-Adjuvant ChemoTherapy in Ovarian Neoplasm trial. *J Natl Cancer Inst.* 2003;95(2):113-125.

45. Colombo N, Guthrie D, Chiari S, et al. International Collaborative Ovarian Neoplasm trial 1: a randomized trial of adjuvant chemotherapy in women with early-stage ovarian cancer. *J Natl Cancer Inst.* 2003;95(2):125-132.

46. Bell J, Brady MF, Young RC, et al. Randomized phase III trial of three versus six cycles of adjuvant carboplatin and paclitaxel in early stage epithelial ovarian carcinoma: a Gynecologic Oncology Group study. *Gynecol Oncol.* 2006;102(3): 432-439.

47. Mannel R, Brady M, Kohn E, et al. GOG175: a randomized phase III trial of IV carboplatin (AUC 6) and paclitaxel 175 mg/m^2 q 21 days x 3 plus low-dose paclitaxel 40 mg/m^2/wk versus IV carboplatin (AUC 6) and paclitaxel 175 mg/m^2 q 21 days × 3 plus observation in patients with early-stage ovarian cancer. *Gynecol Oncol.* 2010;116:S2. Abstract.

48. Young RC, Brady MF, Nieberg RK, et al. Adjuvant treatment for early ovarian cancer: a randomized phase III trial of intraperitoneal ^{32}P of intravenous cyclophosphamide and cisplatin—a Gynecologic Oncology Group study. *J Clin Oncol.* 2003;21:4350-4355.

49. Chan JK, Tian C, Fleming GF, et al. The potential benefit of 6 vs. 3 cycles of chemotherapy in subsets of women with early-stage high-risk epithelial ovarian cancer: an exploratory analysis of a Gynecologic Oncology Group study. *Gynecol Oncol.* 2010;116(3):301-306.

50. Griffiths CT. Surgical resection of tumor bulk in the primary treatment of ovarian carcinoma. *Natl Cancer Inst Monogr.* 1975;42:101-104.

51. Hoskins WJ, McGuire WP, Brady MF, et al. The effect of diameter of largest residual disease on survival after primary cytoreductive surgery in patients with suboptimal residual epithelial ovarian carcinoma. *Am J Obstet Gynecol.* 1994;170(4):974-979.

52. Bristow RE, Tomacruz RS, Armstrong DK, Trimble EL, Montz FJ. Survival effect of maximal cytoreductive surgery for advanced ovarian carcinoma during the platinum era: a meta-analysis. *J Clin Oncol.* 2002;20(5):1248-1259.

53. Chi DS, Eisenhauer EL, Lang J, et al. What is the optimal goal of primary cytoreductive surgery for bulky stage IIIC epithelial ovarian carcinoma (EOC)? *Gynecol Oncol.* 2006;103(2):559-564.

54. Hoffman MS, Zervos EE. Colon resection for ovarian cancer: intraoperative decisions. *Gynecol Oncol.* 2008;11:56-65.

55. Eisenhauer EL, Abu-Rustum NR, Sonoda Y, et al. The addition of extensive upper abdominal surgery to achieve optimal cytoreduction improves survival in patients with stages IIIC-IV epithelial ovarian cancer. *Gynecol Oncol.* 2006;103(3):1083-1090.

56. Kim HS, Ju W, Jee BC, et al. Systematic lymphadenectomy for survival in epithelial ovarian cancer: a meta-analysis. *Int J Gynecol Cancer.* 2010;20(4):520-528.

57. du Bois A, Reuss A, Harter P, et al. Potential role of lymphadenectomy in advanced ovarian cancer: a combined exploratory analysis of three prospectively randomized phase III multicenter trials. *J Clin Oncol.* 2010;28(10):1733-1739.

58. van der Burg ME, van Lent M, Buyse M, Kobierska A, et al. The effect of debulking surgery after induction chemotherapy on the prognosis in advanced epithelial ovarian cancer. Gynecological Cancer Cooperative Group of the European Organization for Research and Treatment of Cancer. *N Engl J Med.* 1995;332(10):629-634.

59. Rose PG, Nerenstone S, Brady MF, et al. Secondary surgical cytoreduction for advanced ovarian carcinoma. *N Engl J Med.* 2004;351(24):2489-2497.

60. Vergote I, Tropé CG, Amant F, et al. Neoadjuvant chemotherapy or primary surgery in stage IIIC or IV ovarian cancer. *N Engl J Med.* 2010;363(10):943-953.

61. Bristow RE, Eisenhauer EL, Santillan A, Chi DS. Delaying the primary surgical effort for advanced ovarian cancer: a systematic review of neoadjuvant chemotherapy and interval cytoreduction. *Gynecol Oncol.* 2007;104(2):480-490.

62. McGuire WP, Hoskins WJ, Brady MF, et al. Cyclophosphamide and cisplatin compared with paclitaxel and cisplatin in patients with stage III and stage IV ovarian cancer. *N Engl J Med.* 1996;334(1):1-6.

63. Piccart MJ, Bertelsen K, James K, et al. Randomized intergroup trial of cisplatin-paclitaxel versus cisplatin-cyclophosphamide in women with advanced epithelial ovarian cancer: three-year results. *J Natl Cancer Inst.* 2000;92(9):699-708.

64. Ozols RF, Bundy BN, Greer BE, et al. Phase III trial of carboplatin and paclitaxel compared with cisplatin and paclitaxel in patients with optimally resected stage III ovarian cancer: a Gynecologic Oncology Group study. *J Clin Oncol.* 2003;21(17):3194-3200.

65. du Bois A, Lück HJ, Meier W, et al. A randomized clinical trial of cisplatin/paclitaxel versus carboplatin/paclitaxel as first-line treatment of ovarian cancer. *J Natl Cancer Inst.* 2003; 95(17):1320-1329.

66. Vasey PA, Jayson GC, Gordon A, et al. Phase III randomized trial of docetaxel-carboplatin versus paclitaxel-carboplatin as first-line chemotherapy for ovarian carcinoma. *J Natl Cancer Inst.* 2004;96(22):1682-1691.

67. Bookman MA, Brady MF, McGuire WP, et al. Evaluation of new platinum-based treatment regimens in advanced-stage ovarian cancer: a Phase III Trial of the Gynecologic Cancer Intergroup. *J Clin Oncol.* 2009;27(9):1419-1425.

68. Teneriello MG, Gordon AN, Lim P, Janicek M. Phase III trial of induction gemcitabine (G) or paclitaxel (T) plus carboplatin (C) followed by elective T consolidation in advanced ovarian cancer (OC): final safety and efficacy report. *J Clin Oncol.* 2010;28(suppl):18S. Abstract LBA5008.

69. Armstrong DK, Bundy B, Wenzel L, et al. Intraperitoneal cisplatin and paclitaxel in ovarian cancer. *N Engl J Med.* 2006;354(1): 34-43.

70. National Cancer Institute. NCI Clinical Announcement: intraperitoneal chemotherapy for ovarian cancer. http://ctep.cancer.gov/highlights/docs/clin_annc_010506.pdf. Accessed January 11, 2012.

71. Berry E, Matthews KS, Singh DK, et al. An outpatient intraperitoneal chemotherapy regimen for advanced ovarian cancer. *Gynecol Oncol.* 2009;113(1):63-67.

72. Nagao S, Fujiwara K, Ohishi R, et al. Combination chemotherapy of intraperitoneal carboplatin and intravenous paclitaxel in suboptimally debulked epithelial ovarian cancer. *Int J Gynecol Cancer.* 2008;18(6):1210-1214.

73. Alberts DS, Liu PY, Hannigan EV, et al. Intraperitoneal cisplatin plus intravenous cyclophosphamide versus intravenous cisplatin plus intravenous cyclophosphamide for stage III ovarian cancer. *N Engl J Med.* 1996;335(26):1950-1955.

74. Markman M, Bundy BN, Alberts DS, et al. Phase III trial of standard-dose intravenous cisplatin plus paclitaxel versus moderately high-dose carboplatin followed by intravenous paclitaxel and intraperitoneal cisplatin in small-volume stage III ovarian carcinoma: an intergroup study of the Gynecologic Oncology Group, Southwestern Oncology Group, and Eastern Cooperative Oncology Group. *J Clin Oncol.* 2001;19(4):1001-1007.

75. Katsumata N, Yasuda M, Takahashi F, et al. Dose-dense paclitaxel once a week in combination with carboplatin every 3 weeks for advanced ovarian cancer: a phase 3, open-label, randomised controlled trial. *Lancet.* 2009;374(9698):1331-1338.

76. Burger RA. Role of vascular endothelial growth factor inhibitors in the treatment of gynecologic malignancies. *J Gynecol Oncol.* 2010:3-11.

77. Burger RA, Sill MW, Monk BJ, Greer BE, Sorosky JI. Phase II trial of bevacizumab in persistent or recurrent epithelial ovarian

cancer or primary peritoneal cancer: a Gynecologic Oncology Group Study. *J Clin Oncol.* 2007;25(33):5165-5171.

78. Garcia AA, Hirte H, Fleming G, et al. Phase II clinical trial of bevacizumab and low-dose metronomic oral cyclophosphamide in recurrent ovarian cancer: a trial of the California, Chicago, and Princess Margaret Hospital phase II consortia. *J Clin Oncol.* 2008;26(1):76-82.

79. Cheng X, Moroney JW, Levenback CF, et al. What is the benefit of bevacizumab combined with chemotherapy in patients with recurrent ovarian, fallopian tube or primary peritoneal malignancies? *J Chemother.* 2009;21(5):566-572.

80. Burger RA, Brady MF, Bookman MA, et al. Phase III trial of bevacizumab (BEV) in the primary treatment of advanced epithelial ovarian cancer (EOC), primary peritoneal cancer (PPC), or fallopian tube cancer (FTC): a Gynecologic Oncology Group study. *J Clin Oncol.* 2010;28(suppl):18s. Abstract LBA1.

81. Perren TJ, Swart AM, Pfisterer J, et al. A phase 3 trial of bevacizumab in ovarian cancer. *New Engl J Med.* 2011;365:2484-2496.

82. Sabbatini P. Consolidation therapy in ovarian cancer: a clinical update. *Int J Gynecol Cancer.* 2009;19(suppl 2):S35-S39.

83. Markman M, Liu PY, Wilczynski S, et al. Phase III randomized trial of 12 versus 3 months of maintenance paclitaxel in patients with advanced ovarian cancer after complete response to platinum and paclitaxel-based chemotherapy: a Southwest Oncology Group and Gynecologic Oncology Group trial. *J Clin Oncol.* 2003;21(13):2460-2465.

84. Markman M, Liu PY, Moon J, et al. Impact on survival of 12 versus 3 monthly cycles of paclitaxel (175 mg/m2) administered to patients with advanced ovarian cancer who attained a complete response to primary platinum-paclitaxel: follow-up of a Southwest Oncology Group and Gynecologic Oncology Group phase 3 trial. *Gynecol Oncol.* 2009;114:195-198.

85. Cass I, Baldwin RL, Varkey T, et al. Improved survival in women with BRCA-associated ovarian carcinoma. *Cancer.* 2003; 97(9):2187-2195.

86. Köbel M, Kalloger SE, Boyd N, et al. Ovarian carcinoma subtypes are different diseases: implications for biomarker studies. *PLoS Med.* 2008 Dec 2;5(12):e232.

87. Huhtinen K, Suvitie P, Hiissa J, et al. Serum HE4 concentration differentiates malignant ovarian tumours from ovarian endometriotic cysts. *Br J Cancer.* 2009;100(8):1315-1319.

88. Rustin GJ, van der Burg ME, Griffen CL, et al. Early versus delayed treatment of relapsed ovarian cancer (MRC OV05/ EORTC 55955): a randomised trial. *J Clin Oncol.* 2010;376: 1155-1163.

89. Galaal K, Naik R, Bristow RE, et al. Cytoreductive surgery plus chemotherapy versus chemotherapy alone for recurrent epithelial ovarian cancer. *Cochrane Database Syst Rev.* 2010;6: CD007822.

90. Bristow RE, Puri I, Chi DS. Cytoreductive surgery for recurrent ovarian cancer: a meta-analysis. *Gynecol Oncol.* 2009;112: 265-274.

91. Pfisterer J, Plante M, Vergote I, et al. Gemcitabine plus carboplatin compared with carboplatin in patients with platinum-sensitive recurrent ovarian cancer: an intergroup trial of the AGO-OVAR, the NCIC CTG, and the EORTC GCG. *J Clin Oncol.* 2006;24:4699-4707.

92. Pujade-Lauraine E, Mahner S, Kaern J, et al. A randomized, phase III study of carboplatin and pegylated liposomal doxorubicin versus carboplatin and paclitaxel in relapsed platinum-sensitive ovarian cancer (OC): CALYPSO study of the Gynecologic Cancer Intergroup (GCIG). *J Clin Oncol.* 2009;27(suppl):18S. Abstract LBA5509.

93. Sehouli J, Stengel D, Oskay-Oezcelik G, et al. Nonplatinum topotecan combinations versus topotecan alone for recurrent ovarian cancer: results of a phase III study of the North-Eastern German Society of Gynecological Oncology Ovarian Cancer Study Group. *J Clin Oncol.* 2008;26:3176-3182.

94. Mutch DG, Orlando M, Goss T, et al. Randomized phase III trial of gemcitabine compared with pegylated liposomal doxorubicin in patients with platinum-resistant ovarian cancer. *J Clin Oncol.* 2007;25:2811-2818.

95. Bookman MA, Darcy KM, Clarke-Pearson D, Boothby RA, Horowitz IR. Evaluation of monoclonal humanized anti-HER2 antibody, trastuzumab, in patients with recurrent or refractory ovarian or primary peritoneal carcinoma with overexpression of HER2: a phase II trial of the Gynecologic Oncology Group. *J Clin Oncol.* 2003;21:283-290.

96. Makhija S, Amler LC, Glenn D, et al. Clinical activity of gemcitabine plus pertuzumab in platinum-resistant ovarian cancer, fallopian tube cancer, or primary peritoneal cancer. *J Clin Oncol.* 2010;28:1215-1223.

97. Burger RA, Sill MW, Monk BJ, Greer BE, Sorosky JI. Phase II trial of bevacizumab in persistent or recurrent epithelial ovarian cancer or primary peritoneal cancer: a Gynecologic Oncology Group Study. *J Clin Oncol.* 2007;25:5165-5171.

98. Audeh MW, Carmichael J, Penson RT, et al. Oral poly(ADP-ribose) polymerase inhibitor olaparib in patients with BRCA1 or BRCA2 mutations and recurrent ovarian cancer: a proof-of-concept trial. *Lancet.* 2010;376:245-251.

99. Fong PC, Yap TA, Boss DS, et al. Poly(ADP-ribose) polymerase inhibition: frequent durable responses in BRCA carrier ovarian cancer correlating with platinum-free interval. *J Clin Oncol.* 2010;28:2512-2519.

100. Fong PC, Boss DS, Yap TA, et al. Inhibition of poly(ADP-ribose) polymerase in tumors from BRCA mutation carriers. *N Engl J Med.* 2009;361:123-134.

101. Sandhu SK, Wenham RM, Wilding G, et al. First-in-human trial of a poly(ADP-ribose) polymerase (PARP) inhibitor MK-4827 in advanced cancer patients (pts) with antitumor activity in BRCA-deficient and sporadic ovarian cancers. *J Clin Oncol.* 2010;28(suppl):15S. Abstract 3001.

102. Eitan R, Levine DA, Abu-Rustum N, et al. The clinical significance of malignant pleural effusions in patients with optimally debulked ovarian carcinoma. *Cancer.* 2005;103(7):1397-1401.

103. Diaz JP, Abu-Rustum NR, Sonoda Y, et al. Video-assisted thoracic surgery (VATS) evaluation of pleural effusions in patients with newly diagnosed advanced ovarian carcinoma can influence the primary management choice for these patients. *Gynecol Oncol.* 2010;116(3):483-488.

104. Fleming ND, Alvarez-Secord A, Von Gruenigen V, Miller MJ, Abernethy AP. Indwelling catheters for the management of refractory malignant ascites: a systematic literature overview and retrospective chart review. *J Pain Symptom Manage.* 2009; 38(3):341-349.

105. Mystakidou K, Tsilika E, Kalaidopoulou O, et al. Comparison of octreotide administration vs conservative treatment in the management of inoperable bowel obstruction in patients with far advanced cancer: a randomized, double-blind, controlled clinical trial. *Anticancer Res.* 2002;22(2B):1187-1192.

106. Trompetas V, Saunders M, Gossage J, Anderson H. Shortcomings in colonic stenting to palliate large bowel obstruction from extracolonic malignancies. *Int J Colorectal Dis.* 2010; 25(7):851-854.

107. Chi DS, Phaëton R, Miner TJ, et al. A prospective outcomes analysis of palliative procedures performed for malignant intestinal obstruction due to recurrent ovarian cancer. *Oncologist.* 2009;14(8):835-839.

108. Kucukmetin A, Naik R, Galaal K, Bryant A, Dickinson HO. Palliative surgery versus medical management for bowel obstruction in ovarian cancer. *Cochrane Database Syst Rev.* 2010;7:CD007792.

109. Altekruse SF, Kosary CL, Krapcho M, et al, eds. SEER Cancer Statistics Review, 1975-2007, National Cancer Institute. Bethesda, MD, http://seer.cancer.gov/csr/1975_2007/. Accessed January 11, 2012.

13 Epithelial Ovarian Cancers: Low Malignant Potential and Non-Serous Ovarian Histologies

Gregory P. Sfakianos, Angeles Alvarez Secord, and Ie-Ming Shih

Epithelial ovarian cancer is the leading cause of death from gynecologic cancers and the fifth leading cause of all cancer-related deaths among women. The American Cancer Society estimates that 21,880 new cases of ovarian cancer will be diagnosed and 13,850 women will die of the disease in the United States in 2010.[1] Approximately 90% of epithelial ovarian cancers are derived from coelomic epithelium of the ovary, fallopian tube, or peritoneum. Epithelial ovarian cancers are heterogeneous and comprise a group of neoplasms that differ based on their histopathologic and molecular features, as well as their clinical behavior.[2,3] These include low malignancy potential (LMP) tumors and frankly invasive malignant neoplasms. Malignant ovarian cancers can be further subdivided into 2 distinct groups based on their morphologic and molecular genetics features. Type I tumors include low-grade serous, mucinous, low-grade endometrioid, clear cell, and transitional (Brenner) carcinomas. Conversely, type II tumors include high-grade serous carcinoma, high-grade endometrioid carcinoma, malignant mixed mesodermal tumors (carcinosarcomas), and undifferentiated carcinomas.[4] Type II tumors are characterized as highly aggressive, evolving rapidly, and uniformly having poor outcomes. In contrast, LMP and type I tumors tend to be diagnosed at an earlier stage, behave in an indolent fashion, and have a better prognosis.

EPIDEMIOLOGY

Key Points

1. Women with mucinous, endometrioid, clear cell, and low-grade serous ovarian cancers present at a younger age than women with high-grade serous ovarian, tubal, and peritoneal cancers.
2. Mucinous, endometrioid, clear cell, and low-grade serous cancers progress in a stepwise manner from precursor lesions to invasive disease.
3. Type I and type II ovarian cancers may be distinguished by specific and distinct genetic alterations.

Approximately 15% to 20% of all epithelial neoplasms are LMP (also referred to as borderline) tumors, and type I tumors account for 25% of malignant epithelial ovarian cancers (Figure 13-1).[4-6] High-grade serous ovarian, primary peritoneal, and tubal carcinomas are treated in a similar fashion and are discussed in Chapter 12. The histologic subsets of both type I and II tumors comprise 42% serous, including 2% to 10% low-grade serous carcinomas, 7% to 20% endometrioid, 17% undifferentiated, 3% to 12% clear cell carcinoma, and 3.5% to 12% mucinous (Figure 13-2).[6-13] Transitional-cell tumors consist of both Brenner tumors and transitional-cell carcinomas and are exceedingly rare. Only 2% of all epithelial ovarian cancers are Brenner tumors.

Risk factors for type I epithelial ovarian cancers are similar to those with type II disease (see Chapter 12). However, there are differences with regard to certain risk factors between the 2 subtypes. Age is the strongest patient-related risk factor for ovarian cancer and is a prime example of differences between type I and II tumors. In general, epithelial ovarian cancer is a disease of postmenopausal women, with the median age of diagnosis at 63 years. However, women with type I cancers tend to be younger as compared with those women with type II disease.[14-16] Specifically, the mean age in women

CHAPTER 13

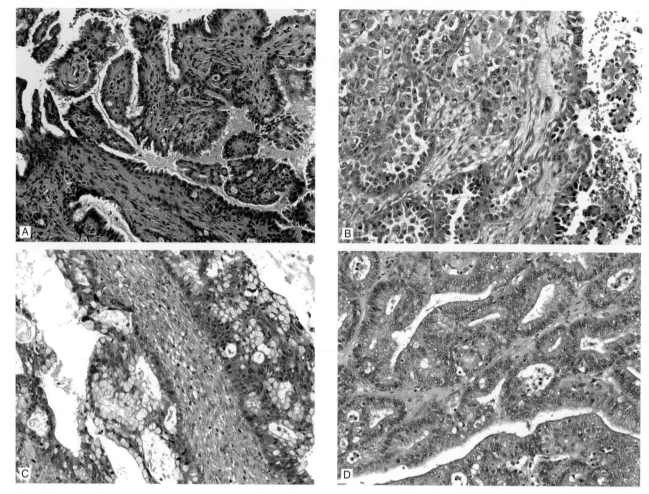

FIGURE 13-1. Representative examples of type I epithelial ovarian tumors. A. Low-grade serous carcinoma. **B.** Clear cell carcinoma. **C.** Mucinous carcinoma. **D.** Low-grade endometrioid carcinoma. (Images contributed by Sonam Loghavi, MD and Denise Barbuto, MD, PhD.)

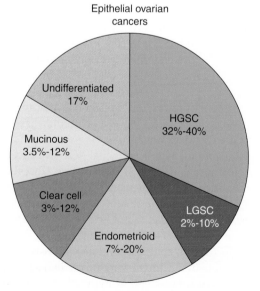

FIGURE 13-2. Histologic subsets for type I and II tumors.[6-13]

with mucinous ovarian cancer is 52 years; endometrioid, 57 to 60 years; clear cell, 53 years; and low-grade serous carcinomas, 55 years.[8,12,15-18] Similarly, patients with LMP tumors are relatively young, with a mean age of 38 years (range, 17-77 years).[19]

Although the differences between LMP tumors and malignant epithelial ovarian cancers are well recognized, the distinction between type I from type II disease is more recent. The stratification of types I and II tumors is based on mounting evidence that demonstrates that the pathogenesis, molecular biology, and clinical behavior of these cancers are not similar.[20] Type I tumors progress in a stepwise manner from well-defined precursor lesions (benign and LMP tumors) to malignant cancer.[21] This stepwise histopathologic progression is often accompanied by an accumulation of genetic mutations that result in the deregulation of critical pathways involved in cellular growth and proliferation and ultimately lead to carcinogenesis. The stepwise sequence from a benign lesion to an LMP tumor to a type I ovarian cancer parallels the widely accepted and recognized sequence seen in colorectal cancers, where an adenomatous lesion can evolve into a carcinoma after a series of genetic alterations.[21] Specifically, low-grade serous carcinomas often arise from cystadenomas and cystadenofibromas, which may transform to serous LMP tumors and micropapillary serous carcinomas. In contrast, although the precursor lesion of high-grade serous carcinomas is largely unknown, recent evidence implicates tubal intraepithelial carcinoma as the originating lesion (Figure 13-3).[22-37] It may be that both low-grade and high-grade serous carcinomas are of tubal origin and the ovary is secondarily involved (Figure 13-4). Kurman and Shih[5] have proposed that tubal epithelium may be directly implanted into the ovary to form an inclusion cyst and can develop into either a low-grade or high-grade serous cancer, depending on the type of genetic alteration incurred.

Endometrioid and clear cell ovarian cancers also develop from a stepwise histopathologic progression from endometriosis to benign endometrioid neoplasm to well-differentiated carcinoma (Figure 13-5).[38] Endometrioid and clear cell cancers most likely originate from endometrial tissue and/or endometriotic implants that via retrograde menstruation become implanted on the ovary or peritoneum (Figure 13-6).[21] The ovarian endometrioid adenoma-carcinoma model of progression may be accompanied by a progressive molecular deregulation of the *Wnt/β-catenin/Tcf* and *PI3KCA/AKT/PTEN* pathways for low-grade tumors (Figure 13-7).

Furthermore, mucinous neoplasms have striking histopathologic and molecular similarities between benign and malignant mucinous tumors, supporting a model of progression from benign to LMP tumors to malignant mucinous ovarian cancer (Figure 13-8). *KRAS* mutations are the most common mutation in mucinous ovarian carcinomas and can also be present in benign-appearing areas of mucinous tumors, adjacent to frank mucinous carcinoma, suggesting that they are an early event during carcinogenesis.[39] In contrast to serous, endometrioid, and clear cell tumors, the origin of mucinous and transitional-cell (Brenner) tumors is perplexing because they do not have mullerian features.[21] These tumors may develop from cortical inclusion cysts or Walthard cell nests that are composed of benign transitional-type epithelium that are frequently found in paraovarian and paratubal locations.[21] In contrast, a precursor lesion for transitional-cell carcinomas has not been as clearly identified.

The histopathologic differences between LMP, type I, and type II tumors are mirrored by differences in their molecular genetic features.[3,38] Although the underlying molecular biology of epithelial ovarian cancers has yet to be completely elucidated, current genomic data

clearly demonstrates that LMP, type I, and type II disease are very distinct entities (See Chapter 2). LMP and type I tumors are genetically more stable than type II tumors and display specific mutations in the different histologic cell types.[40] Mutations that characterize most type I tumors include Kirsten rat sarcoma 2 viral oncogene homolog (*KRAS*), v-raf murine sarcoma viral oncogene homolog (*BRAF*), human epidermal growth factor receptor 2 (HER-2/*neu* [erythroblastic leukemia viral oncogene homolog 2 (*ERBB2*)]), phosphatase and tensin homolog (*PTEN*), beta-catenin (*CTNNB1*), and phosphoinositide-3-kinase, catalytic, alpha polypeptide (*PI3K-CA*) mutations[38] (Tables 13-1 and 13-2). In contrast, high-grade serous carcinoma, the prototypic type II tumor, is characterized by greater genetic instability, tumor protein 53 (*TP53*) mutations, and endcoding cyclin E1 (*CCNE1*) amplification (Table 13-1).[38,41]

Molecular derangements of the mitogen-activated protein kinase (*MAPK*) (*Ras-Raf-MEK-MAPK*) pathway are common in LMP, low-grade serous carcinomas, and mucinous tumors.[42] The *Ras-Raf-MEK-MAPK* pathway plays an important role in cellular proliferation, transformation, and survival (Figure 13-9).[43] Mutations of either *KRAS* or *BRAF* lead to constitutive activation of *MAPK* signaling. Mutations in *KRAS* or *BRAF* mutations are present in more than 50%, 68%, and 80% of serous LMP tumors, low-grade serous cancer, and mucinous LMP tumors, respectively.[38,42,44] In addition, mutations of HER-2/*neu* (*ERBB2*), which activates an upstream regulator of *KRAS*, have also been found in 9% of LMP tumors.[38] Overall, more than 70% to 80% LMP tumors express activated components of the *MAPK* (*Ras-Raf-MEK-MAPK*) pathway.

Other members of the *MAPK* pathway, including *TRAF family-member-associated NF-kappa-B-activator* (*TANK*), poly [ADP-ribose] polymerase 1 (*PARP1*), cell division protein kinase 2 (*CDK2*) and astrocytic phosphoprotein (*PEA15*), have been evaluated in serous LMP, micropapillary serous carcinomas, and low-grade serous tumors. Using real-time quantitative polymerase chain reaction, the differential expression of the 4 genes was not significantly different between these clinical entities, but *TANK*, *PARP1*, and *PEA15* were higher in the low-grade serous tumors. Significantly more intense protein expression was present for TANK and CDK2 in the low-grade serous tumors, whereas PARP1 expression was lowest in the LMP tumors.[37] *KRAS* mutations are also the most common genetic alteration in mucinous carcinomas and are present up to 50% of these malignancies.[45,46] Interestingly, *KRAS* mutations are present in 50% of colorectal cancers.[47] In contrast, *KRAS* or *BRAF* mutations are uncommon in endometrioid (7%) and clear cell cancers (6.3%) and absent in high-grade serous disease.[9,48]

High-grade endometrioid ovarian cancers have a similar gene expression profile to serous carcinomas,

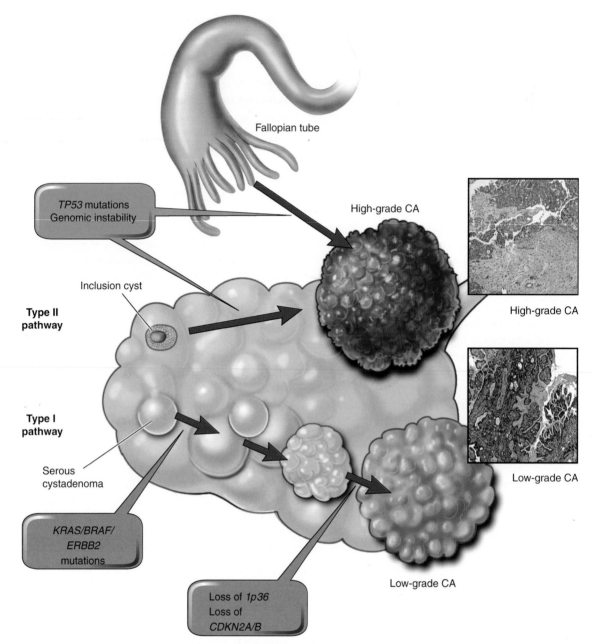

Fallopian tube

High-grade CA

TP53 mutations
Genomic instability

High-grade CA

Inclusion cyst

**Type II
pathway**

Serous
cystadenoma

**Type I
pathway**

Low-grade CA

*KRAS/BRAF/
ERBB2*
mutations

Loss of *1p36*
Loss of
CDKN2A/B

Low-grade CA

FIGURE 13-3. The dualistic pathways in the development of high-grade and low-grade serous carcinoma. Schematic illustration of type I and type II ovarian serous carcinoma pathogenesis. Development of ovarian high-grade (HGSC) and low-grade serous carcinomas (LGSC) involves 2 distinct pathways. LGSCs arise from serous low malignant potential tumors, which in turn develop from serous cystadenomas. This stepwise tumor progression in the low-grade pathway contrasts with the rapid progression pathway of high-grade (type II) carcinomas, for which precursor lesions are not well recognized. APST, atypical proliferative serous tumor; CIN, chromosomal instability; LOH, loss of heterozygosity; MPSC, micropapillary serous carcinoma. (Images contributed by Sonam Loghavi, MD and Denise Barbuto, MD, PhD.)

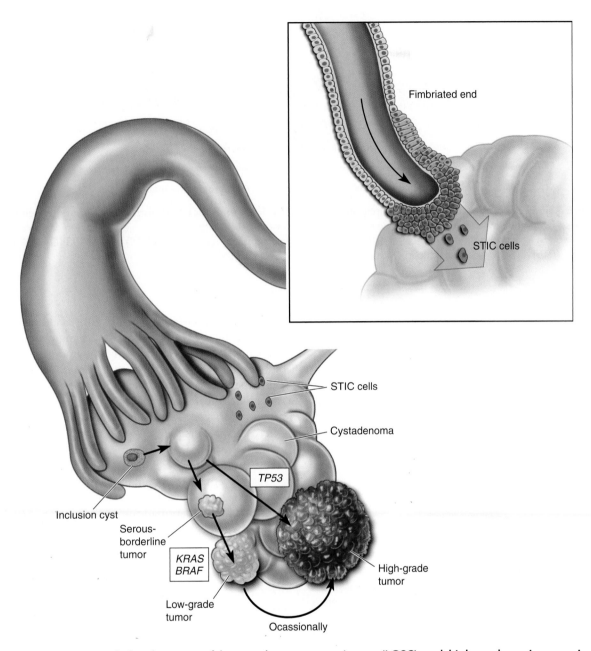

FIGURE 13-4. Proposed development of low-grade serous carcinoma (LGSC) and high-grade serious carcinoma (HGSC). One mechanism involves normal tubal epithelium from the fimbria, which implants on the ovary to form an inclusion cyst. Depending on whether there is a mutation of *KRAS/BRAF/Her2/neu* or *TP53*, an LGSC or HGSC develops, respectively. LGSC often develops from a serous low malignant potential tumors, which in turn arises from a serous cystadenoma. Another mechanism involves exfoliation of malignant cells from a serous tubal intraepithelial carcinoma (STIC) that implants on the ovarian surface, resulting in the development of an HGSC.

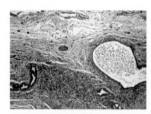

Endometriosis

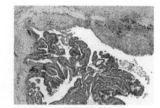

Atypical proliferative
endometrioid tumor
(endometrioid borderline tumor)

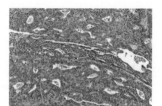

Endometrioid carcinoma

Accumulation of *PTEN*, *CTNNB*1, *PIK*3*CA*, *TP*53, and other mutations

FIGURE 13-5. Low-grade endometrioid carcinomas often arise from endometrioid borderline tumors, which in turn may arise from endometriosis. This stepwise histopathologic progression is often accompanied by accumulation of mutations predicted to deregulate canonical *Wnt/β-catenin/Tcf (Wnt)* signaling (usually *CTNNB1*) and/or *PI3KCA/AKT/PTEN* signaling (*PTEN, PIK3CA*). (Reproduced, with permission, from Cho and Shih.[3])

are more likely to contain *TP53* mutations (>80%),[41,49] and lack alterations of the *Wnt/β-catenin(CTNNB1)/ Tcf* or *PI3K-CA/AKT/PTEN* pathways.[50] In contrast, the low-grade (grade 1) endometrioid tumors typically lack *TP53* mutations and have mutations involving the *Wnt/CTNNB1/Tcf* and *PIK3CA/AKT/PTEN* pathways.[50-53] *CTNNB1* mutations are present in 38% to 58% of cases, *PTEN* mutations in 14% to 21% of

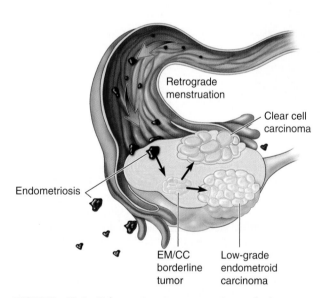

FIGURE 13-6. Schematic representation of the proposed development of clear cell and low-grade endometrioid carcinoma. Endometrial tissue, by a process of retrograde menstruation, implants on the ovarian surface to form an endometriotic cyst, from which a clear cell and low-grade endometrioid carcinoma can develop. CCC, clear cell carcinoma of the ovary; EMC, endometrioid carcinoma of the ovary.

cases, and *PIK3CA* mutations in 20% of endometrioid ovarian cancers. Defects in these 2 signaling pathways appear to be characteristic of low-grade endometrioid disease. Endometrioid carcinomas of the ovary are sometimes associated with hereditary nonpolyposis colon cancer syndrome in patients with germline mutations in a gene encoding a DNA mismatch repair. Microsatellite instability is present in 13% to 20% of endometrioid ovarian cancer and is typically associated with loss of hMLH1 or hMSH2 expression.[3]

Very recent genomic analyses of ovarian clear cell carcinoma have revealed somatic inactivating mutations of a newly identified tumor suppressor, *ARID1A*, in approximately half of the cases, making *ARID1A* mutation the molecular genetic signature in ovarian clear cell carcinoma.[54,55] Similar to low-grade endometrioid carcinoma, mutations involving the *PI3K-CA/ AKT/PTEN* signaling are common in clear cell carcinomas. *PIK3CA* mutations have been found in 20% to 25% to nearly 50% of clear cell tumors,[3,56,57] whereas *PTEN* mutations have been reported in 8% of clear cell lesions.[3] Interestingly, although the gene expression profiles of clear cell ovarian cancers are distinct from other type I cancers, they are remarkably similar to renal clear cell carcinomas.[58] Similar to renal clear cell cancer, 50% of primary and 43% of metastatic clear cell ovarian cancers demonstrated loss of Von Hippel-Lindau (*VHL*) tumor suppressor gene.[59] Loss of *VHL* function results in a marked increase in hypoxia-inducible factor-1α (*HIF-1α*) activity.[60] *HIF-1α* upregulates vascular endothelial growth factor (VEGF) and fms-like tyrosine kinase-1 (*Flt-1*) transcription and induces increased tumor vascularity.

BRCA mutations and *TP53* mutations do not seem to play a significant role in mucinous, low-grade serous, or clear cell cancers.[61-63] *TP53* alterations are present in

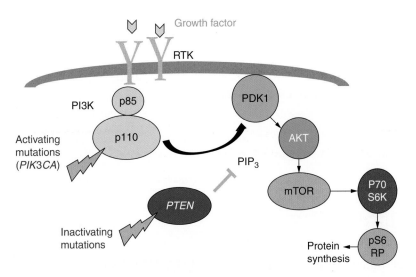

FIGURE 13-7. Activating mutations of *PIK3CA* or inactivating mutations of *PTEN* result in activation of AKT-mediated signaling to downstream effectors that affect protein synthesis. mTOR, mammalian target of rapamycin; PDK1, 3-phosphoinositide-dependent kinase 1; PIP3, phosphatidylinositol (3,4,5)-trisphosphate; PI3K, phosphoinositide-3-kinase; PIK3CA, phosphoinositide-3-kinase (PI3K), catalytic, alpha polypeptide; PTEN, phosphatase and tensin homolog; RTK, receptor tyrosine kinase.

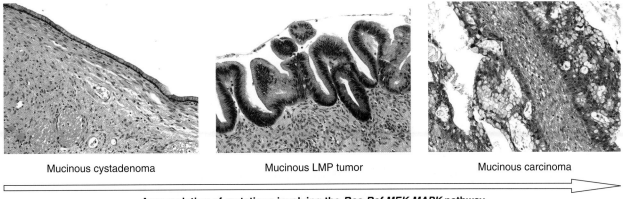

Mucinous cystadenoma   Mucinous LMP tumor   Mucinous carcinoma

Accumulation of mutations involving the *Ras-Raf-MEK-MAPK* pathway

FIGURE 13-8. Mucinous carcinomas often arise from mucinous low malignant potential (LMP) tumors, which in turn may arise from benign mucinous cystadenomas. This stepwise histopathologic progression is accompanied by accumulation of mutations involving *KRAS* and *BRAF*. (Images contributed by Sonam Loghavi, MD and Denise Barbuto, MD, PhD.)

Table 13-1 Genetic Features of Type I and Type II Ovarian Tumors

Genetic Mutation	Type I	Type II
ARID1A mutation	10%-56%	Rare
PI3K/AKT activation	Mutation is common in CCC, LGSC, and EMC	Amplification is common (12%-30%)
TP53 mutation	<10%	>80%
HER-2/*neu* overexpression	Rare	20%-66%
BRAF mutation	Frequent in LGSC	rare
KRAS mutation	Frequent in LGSC and mucinous tumors	rare
PTEN (deletion) mutation or loss of expression	Most common in EMC	5%-10%

LGSC, low-grade serous carcinoma; EMC, endometrioid carcinoma; CCC, clear cell carcinoma.

CHAPTER 13

Table 13-2 Common Precursor Lesions and Molecular Features of Type I Carcinomas

Type I Tumors	Common Precursors	Most Frequent Mutations	CIN[a]
Low-grade serous CA	Serous borderline tumor	*KRAS, BRAF*	Low
Low-grade endometrioid CA	Endometriosis	*CTNNB1, PTEN*	Low
Most clear cell CA[b]	Endometriosis	*PIK3CA*	Low
Mucinous CA	Mucinous borderline tumor	*KRAS*	Low

[a]Low versus high CIN (chromosomal instability) refers to comparison between low-grade and high-grade carcinomas within the same histologic type.
[b]Criteria for classification of clear cell carcinoma (CA) subsets into type I versus type II categories are uncertain. It is thought that most clear cell CAs behave like type I tumors, whereas some clear cell CAs, presumably high grade, may be type II tumors.
Adapted from Cho and Shih.[3]

only 8.3% of clear cell tumors. *BRCA* mutations are not common in endometrioid cancers. Neither clear cell nor low-grade serous disease have significant chromosomal instability.[64] Low-grade serous cancers are usually diploid or near diploid and do not show the complex genetic abnormalities seen in HGSC.[65] Serous ovarian cancers, whether low grade or high grade, have been noted to have higher protein expression of Wilms tumor protein 1 (WT1) as compared with endometrioid, clear cell, and mucinous epithelial ovarian cancer.[3] The molecular changes in transitional-cell carcinomas of the ovary remain largely unknown.

DIAGNOSIS

Key Points

1. The majority of women with LMP and type I ovarian cancers present with earlier-stage disease.
2. The initial evaluation should include a comprehensive history and physical examination, as well as preoperative imaging and serum tumor marker testing.
3. General gynecologists should consider referral to a gynecologic oncologist when malignancy is suspected.

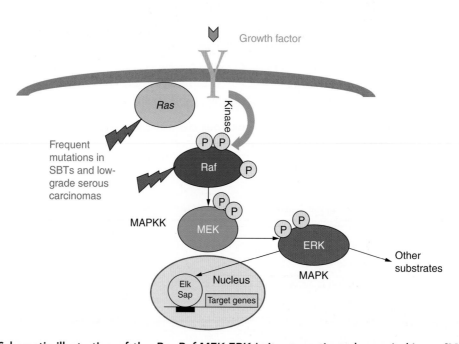

FIGURE 13-9. Schematic illustration of the *Ras-Raf-MEK-ERK* (mitogen-activated protein kinase [MAPK]) signaling pathway. This cell signaling pathway plays a role in cellular proliferation, transformation, and survival in response to a variety of growth and differentiation factors. Aberration of this pathway in low malignant potential tumors and low-grade serous carcinomas is mainly due to activating mutations of *KRAS* and *BRAF*, which result in constitutive activation of MAPK-mediated signaling in these tumors. Activated MAPK signaling alters expression of downstream target genes, including upregulation of cyclin D1. SBT, serous borderline tumors; MAPK, mitogen-activated protein kinase; MAPKK, MAPK kinase; MEK, MAPK/ERK kinase; ERK, extracellular signal-regulated kinase. (Reproduced, with permission, from Cho and Shih.[3])

Approximately 70% to 80% of women with type II epithelial ovarian cancers present with advanced-stage disease at the time of diagnosis, including large-volume intra-abdominal tumor, ascites, and in some cases malignant pleural effusions. Before diagnosis, women with ovarian cancer frequently have vague, nonspecific symptoms. The most common symptoms include abdominal bloating, early satiety, heartburn, constipation, and nausea, as well as genitourinary symptoms including urinary frequency, urgency, or incontinence.[66] In contrast, women with low malignant potential and type I epithelial ovarian cancers are often diagnosed with earlier-stage disease. They may have physical examination findings consistent with a large pelvic-abdominal mass, but typically do not have extensive upper abdominal disease or tense ascites.[67] Nevertheless, symptoms in women with early and advanced disease are strikingly similar. Those with early disease tend to have a decreased frequency of diarrhea and lower use of antidiarrheal medications as compared with those with advanced-stage disease.[68] The general gynecologist and primary care physician should have a heightened awareness regarding ovarian cancer symptoms and conduct a thorough evaluation and refer the patient to a gynecologic oncologist if warranted.

The initial evaluation and differential diagnosis is similar to those with type II epithelial ovarian cancer (see Chapter 12) and include a comprehensive history, physical examination including a pelvic and rectal evaluation, laboratory parameters, and imaging studies if needed. Tumor markers, including CA-125, carcinoembryonic antigen, and CA–19–9 may be useful. Imaging studies such as computed tomography and/or ultrasound imaging can be obtained to determine the extent of the disease and allow preparation for more radical debulking procedures such as hepatic resection and splenectomy. However, preoperative radiographic evaluation is limited in predicting a surgeon's ability to achieve optimal cytoreduction (residual tumor <1 cm) of metastatic ovarian neoplasms. The diagnosis of LMP tumors and type I epithelial ovarian cancer is typically made via surgical exploration. Other options for diagnosis include fine-needle aspiration and core biopsy or cytologic evaluation of pleural or ascitic fluid.

Because these diseases may present with pelvic masses and the absence of obvious metastatic disease, many women with LMP and type I ovarian cancers may be managed initially by a general gynecologist. Surgical staging can be critical in prescribing appropriate adjuvant therapy, and as such referral to a gynecologic oncologist is recommended for those patients with clinical features suggestive of malignant disease. Chapter 11 reviews the management of a pelvic mass.

PATHOLOGY

Key Points

1. LMP tumors are characterized by a degree of cellular proliferation and nuclear atypia in the absence of obvious stromal invasion.
2. Low-grade serous cancers can also be reproducibly distinguished from their high-grade counterparts based primarily on their very uniform nuclei, using low-mitotic rate as a secondary diagnostic criterion.
3. Mucinous ovarian cancers typically present with unilateral, large adnexal masses (up to 30 cm in size).
4. A strong association exists between endometrioid and clear cell ovarian cancers and endometriosis.

The pathologic appearance of type I tumors vary depending on their histologic subtype (Figure 13-1). The histopathologic characteristics are detailed for each tumor type separately in their respective sections. In contrast to type I tumors, type II tumors tend to exhibit papillary, glandular, and solid patterns (Figure 13-10 and 13-11). The metastatic spread patterns for LMP and type I tumors are similar to those of type II

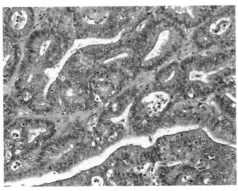
Low-grade

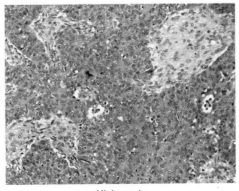
High-grade

FIGURE 13-10. Low- and high-grade endometrioid epithelial ovarian cancer. (Images contributed by Sonam Loghavi, MD and Denise Barbuto, MD, PhD.)

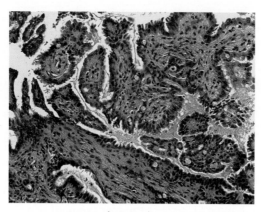
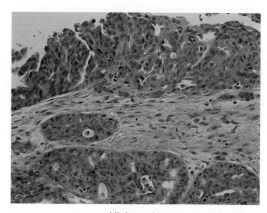

Low-grade

High-grade

FIGURE 13-11. Low- and high-grade serous epithelial ovarian cancer. (Images contributed by Sonam Loghavi, MD and Denise Barbuto, MD, PhD.)

ovarian cancers, and staging is performed using the International Federation of Gynecology and Obstetrics (FIGO) classification (see Chapter 12).

Classically, epithelial ovarian cancers are graded on a 3-tier grading scheme based on architecture (glandular, papillary, or solid), degree of nuclear atypia, and mitotic index.[69] Tumors are graded according to their degree of differentiation. Grade 1 tumors are well-differentiated and maintain their glandular appearance. Grade 2, or moderately differentiated tumors, have both glandular features and sheets of cells. Grade 3, or poorly differentiated tumors, are generally sheets of cells, with little to no architecture. All clear cell carcinomas are considered grade 3. Grade is an important independent predictor of prognosis. In 2004, a 2-tier grading system based on nuclear atypia and mitotic rate was proposed for serous carcinomas, in which tumors are subdivided into low grade and high grade.[70] There is very good correlation between the new 2-tiered system and the established International FIGO and the 3-tiered systems.[71] Furthermore, the distinct epidemiology, biology, and clinical

behavior of low-grade serous and low-grade endometrioid carcinomas compared with high-grade serous and endometrioid carcinomas supports the 2-tiered system.

Low Malignant Potential Tumors

In 1929, Howard Taylor[72] first described LMP tumors as a "semi-malignant" disease with histologic features and biologic behavior between a benign neoplasm and invasive carcinoma. Histologically, LMP tumors are characterized by a degree of cellular proliferation and nuclear atypia in the absence of obvious stromal invasion (Figures 13-5, 13-8, and 13-12). LMP tumors of every surface epithelial cell type (serous, mucinous, endometrioid, clear cell, transitional cell and mixed epithelial cell) have been reported. Serous and mucinous neoplasms constitute the majority of LMP tumors and occur mostly in women of reproductive age (Figure 13-12).[73] According to the 2003 World Health Organization classification schema, LMP ovarian tumors are classified on the basis of histopathology

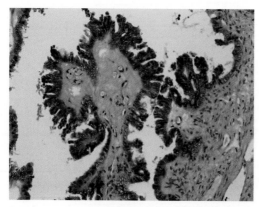
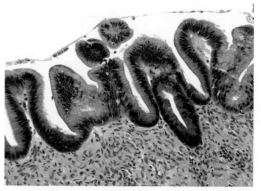

Serous

Mucinous

FIGURE 13-12. Representative sections of serous and mucinous low malignant potential tumors. (Images contributed by Sonam Loghavi, MD and Denise Barbuto, MD, PhD.)

and histogenesis into serous, mucinous, endometrioid, clear cell, and transitional (Brenner) subtypes. The histology of LMP tumors is characterized by the following features: epithelial multilayering of more than 4 cell layers, mitoses ≤4 per 10 high-power field, mild nuclear atypia, increase in nuclear-to-cytoplasmic ratio, slight-to-complex branching of epithelial papillae and pseudopapillae, epithelial budding and cell detachment into the lumen, architecturally complex glands, and no destructive stromal invasion.

Low-Grade Serous Carcinoma

The separation of serous carcinomas into low-grade and high-grade types is a recent development and was first described by Singer et al[9] followed by other investigators.[2,10] Similar to high-grade serous cancers, most women with low-grade serous disease present with advanced-stage disease and have bilateral tumors. These tumors are characterized by micropapillae and small, round nests of cells that infiltrate the stroma and are frequently surrounded by a clear space (Figures 13-1 and 13-13). They are often associated with a serous adenofibroma, atypical proliferative serous tumor, or noninvasive micropapillary serous carcinoma. Psammoma bodies are common. The nuclei are uniform, small, and round to oval. The chromatin is even, and mitotic features are infrequent. The nuclear-to-cytoplasmic ratio may be high. However, only mild variation in size and shape of nuclei are allowed for a diagnosis of low-grade serous carcinoma. Serous tumors with cells showing ≥3:1 variation in nuclear size and shape are classified as high-grade disease.[74] Low-grade serous cancers can also be reproducibly distinguished from their high-grade counterparts, based primarily on their very uniform nuclei, using low-mitotic rate as a secondary diagnostic criterion.[10,17] Low-grade serous tumors are also almost invariably positive for hormone receptor expression (estrogen and/or progesterone receptors).[65] Only rarely do these tumors progress to higher-grade tumors.[75]

Mucinous Carcinoma

Mucinous cancers of the ovary comprise approximately 15% of all ovarian epithelial tumors. The majority of mucinous ovarian tumors are benign, with 15% being LMP and only 3.5% being malignant.[7] Clinically, mucinous tumors may grow quite large, reaching 30 cm in size and weighing as much as 40 kg.[76] Although malignant mucinous tumors may be bilateral in 10% to 20% of cases,[7] benign tumors are rarely bilateral. Eighty-three percent of mucinous ovarian carcinomas but only 4% of serous ovarian carcinomas are stage I at diagnosis.[77]

Microscopically, mucinous tumors are often compared with mucinous cells of the endocervix or colon.[77] However, the mucinous epithelium that characterizes type I epithelial ovarian cancer more closely resembles gastrointestinal mucosa than the endocervix.[21] Mucinous adenocarcinomas also demonstrate gland formation, similar to endometrioid ovarian cancers, but the tumor cell cytoplasm is mucin rich (Figure 13-1). Microscopic features that favor the diagnosis of primary ovarian mucinous carcinoma include the coexistence of LMP and benign mucinous components, an expansile (confluent) pattern of invasion, and a coexisting ovarian teratoma, Brenner tumor, or mural nodule. Mucinous adenocarcinomas often contain areas indistinguishable from mucinous cystadenomas and mucinous LMP tumors. To be classified as an LMP mucinous tumor, the epithelium lining the papillae should generally not exceed 3 cell layers in thickness and lack the following: a marked overgrowth of atypical cells; solid, cellular masses devoid of connective tissue support; severely anaplastic nuclear features; and destructive stromal invasion (Figures 13-6 and 13-11).[77] In contrast, the following microscopic features favor the diagnosis of metastatic adenocarcinoma to the ovary: prominent desmoplastic response, nodular pattern of invasion (ie, tumor nodules among structures indigenous to the ovarian parenchyma), small clusters of tumor cells within corpora lutea or albicantia, numerous pools of mucin dissecting the ovarian stroma (ie, pseudomyxoma ovarii) in the absence of a coexistent ovarian teratoma, an extensive signet-ring cell pattern, ovarian surface involvement, vascular invasion, hilar involvement, and an extensive infiltrative pattern of invasion (Figure 13-10).[78,79] Pseudomyxoma peritonei is a rare condition that is characterized by copious mucin and clusters of well-differentiated mucinous cells throughout the abdomen.[76] Mucinous tumors can be associated with appendiceal tumors, and appendiceal involvement is frequently observed when pseudomyxoma peritonei is encountered.[44,80]

Of significant concern is the finding that only 23% of invasive mucinous carcinomas of the ovary are actually primary ovarian cancers.[81] Making the distinction between primary and metastatic gastrointestinal cancers to the ovary can be difficult. Immunohistochemistry may assist in determining the primary site of a mucinous carcinoma. Primary ovarian mucinous carcinomas tend to be positive for CK7 and CK20 with a predominance of CK7 expression, whereas colorectal primaries tend to express CK20 only.[82,83]

Endometrioid Carcinoma

Endometrioid ovarian cancer has morphologic features similar to the endometrioid endometrial cancers and has varying amounts of gland formation, sometimes accompanied by squamous differentiation. It appears that endometrioid ovarian cancer, similar to serous cancer, may be stratified into 2 distinct entities based on grade (Figures 13-1 and 13-11). These cancers are frequently associated with endometriosis,[84] benign endometrioid neoplasms such as endometrioid adenofibroma, endometrioid LMP tumors, and well-differentiated endometrioid carcinoma. On gross examination these tumors vary in size from 12 to 25 cm.[63,85] They are often fleshy in character and more cystic than serous tumors.[76] Microscopically they resemble endometrioid adenocarcinomas of the endometrium. A concomitant endometrial primary may occur in 10% to 25% of cases.[86-89]

In 1985, Ulbright and Roth[90] developed pathologic criteria to help distinguish metastatic disease from synchronous primary tumors. More recently, Scully et al[91] described a similar but more extensive list of clinicopathologic features used to differentiate endometrial disease with metastasis to the ovary, ovarian disease with metastasis to the endometrium, and independent primary cancers.

Clear Cell Carcinoma

Similar to endometrioid ovarian cancers, a strong association exists between clear cell carcinoma and endometriosis in more than 50% of cases.[12,92] Clear cell cancers present predominantly as a large pelvic mass measuring 3 to 20 cm[12] and are bilateral in 12% of cases.[93] Grossly, clear cell carcinomas resemble endometrioid tumors and cannot be distinguished from serous disease. They may be predominantly solid or cystic and contain white, yellow, or pale brown polypoid masses protruding into the lumen of cysts.[94] Nearly one-third of clear cell ovarian cancers are stage I at diagnosis.[7]

Clear cell carcinoma of the ovary is morphologically similar to the clear cell carcinoma of the endometrium and the clear cell vaginal and cervical cancers seen in young women exposed to diethylstilbestrol.[95] Microscopically, the tumors are composed of clear cells and hobnail cells. The clear cell appearance is due to the presence of copious cytoplasmic glycogen (Figure 13-1). The hobnail cells are when the nuclei, instead of being basal, appear to stand on a narrow stalk of cytoplasm, resembling a large-headed hobnail, and protrude into the lumen. The tumor cell may be arranged in solid, tubulocystic, or papillary patterns. Clear cell carcinomas have relatively low-mitotic rates, and it is therefore not surprising that responses to agents targeting dividing cells are poor.[64,96]

It is uncertain whether clear cell epithelial ovarian cancer should be classified into type I and type II subsets, similar to serous and endometrioid tumors. Clear cell carcinomas are typically considered high grade by definition.[97] Currently, most clear cell epithelial ovarian cancers are thought to behave similar to other type I tumors. However, it is obvious that some clear cell cancers behave in a more aggressive fashion, as manifested by an increased risk of recurrence and worse survival.

Transitional-Cell Tumors

Brenner tumors are almost always benign, and rarely are these tumors of LMP or frankly malignant. There are 2 variants of malignant tumors: malignant Brenner tumors and transitional-cell carcinomas. Benign Brenner tumors are predominantly small (<5 cm), solid, and often associated with mucinous tumors. In contrast, Brenner LMP tumors usually are large cysts, and the malignant tumors contain both solid and cystic areas. Both benign and malignant Brenner tumors have areas of stromal calcification. Brenner tumors have 2 important distinguishing features: epithelial cords with coffee-bean shaped cells and a dense, fibrous, and abundant stroma. Transitional-cell carcinomas have a urothelial-like appearance but, unlike bladder, epithelium will demonstrate cytokeratin-7–positive staining.

The transitional-cell carcinomas tend to present at higher stages and be associated with a greater risk for recurrence compared with malignant Brenner tumors. However, DNA content studies on Brenner tumors have shown that diploid tumors tend to be benign and nonaggressive, whereas those with aneuploid features are typically aggressive and have a worse prognosis.[98,99]

TREATMENT

Key Points

1. LMP tumors diagnosed by frozen section at the time of surgery should undergo staging, as invasive ovarian cancer may be found on final pathologic analysis. Adjuvant therapy may be considered for advanced disease or invasive implants, but remains controversial.
2. Women with stage IA or IB disease with grade 1 or 2 histology are unlikely to benefit from chemotherapy and may undergo close surveillance.
3. Women with advanced-stage type I ovarian cancers should be treated with platinum- and taxane-based regimens until further evidence confirms the use of alternative chemotherapeutic agents in non–high-grade serous disease.

Low Malignant Potential Tumors

Intraoperative management of LMP is similar to that for invasive ovarian cancers and may include systematic staging and abdominal exploration. The primary treatment modality is surgical resection of gross disease. There is considerable debate regarding the extent of surgery as well as the role of lymphadenectomy. Patients with advanced-stage disease who have completed childbearing should undergo a hysterectomy, bilateral salpingo-oophorectomy, omentectomy, complete peritoneal resection of macroscopic lesions, multiple peritoneal biopsies if indicated, and peritoneal washings and may also undergo pelvic and para-aortic lymphadenectomy. For premenopausal women with early-stage disease and/or those who strongly desire future fertility, conservative fertility-sparing surgery with unilateral salpingo-oophorectomy or ovarian cystectomy combined with surgical staging can be performed.[100] Although the conservative approach is associated with a higher recurrence rate, overall survival is likely not compromised.[100]

The role of lymphadenectomy is controversial and has not been shown to confer a reduction in recurrence or a survival benefit.[100,101] However, these tumors can be large, and a definitive diagnosis excluding invasive ovarian cancer based on intraoperative frozen section evaluation is limited. Specifically, 11% to 28% of invasive carcinomas were underdiagnosed in LMP tumors at the time of frozen section.[102-104] In a meta-analysis, Tempfer et al[104] found that intraoperative frozen section analysis had an overall sensitivity of 71.1% and an overall positive predictive value of 84.3%. Thus, given the inaccuracy of frozen sections and risk of nodal recurrence, it is reasonable to perform a pelvic and para-aortic lymphadenectomy in patients with LMP tumors identified on frozen section at the time of surgery.

Treatment recommendations for women with LMP tumors are determined based on the presence or absence of invasive implants. For patients who have no microscopically demonstrable invasive implants, adjuvant chemotherapy has not been shown to be beneficial. The use of chemotherapy even in those women with advanced-stage disease and invasive implants is controversial, with many studies showing no benefit, most likely due to the relative chemoresistant nature of these tumors.[73,100,101] Thus, in women with invasive implants, treatment options may include observation or treatment with adjuvant chemotherapy regimens similar to those used in epithelial ovarian cancer.[99]

Type I Tumors

In general, women with type I and type II epithelial ovarian cancers are treated in a similar fashion with regard to surgical management, adjuvant therapy, and surveillance. Mucinous LMP tumors and epithelial ovarian cancer are frequently associated with appendiceal neoplasms, especially when pseudomyxoma peritonei is encountered. Therefore, appendectomy is recommended at the time of surgical resection of mucinous ovarian tumors. Although high-grade serous cancers tend to be chemo-responsive, mucinous, clear cell, and low-grade serous disease do not have as high as a response rate to the traditional platinum- and taxane-based chemotherapy regimens.

Women with stage IA or 1B, grade 1 or 2 disease are unlikely to benefit from adjuvant chemotherapy and may undergo close surveillance. Women with 1B, grade 2 disease may also be offered chemotherapy with intravenous (IV) taxane and carboplatin chemotherapy for 3 to 6 cycles. For those with stage 1A, 1B clear cell or grade 3 disease or 1C, grade 1, 2, or 3 disease, intravenous taxane and carboplatin chemotherapy for 3 to 6 cycles is recommended. Patients with stage II, III, and IV disease should be counseled regarding combination intraperitoneal/intravenous chemotherapy versus intravenous chemotherapy alone for a total of 6 to 8 cycles.[99] Neoadjuvant chemotherapy followed by interval debulking is an option for select patients and does not appear to negatively impact survival compared with primary debulking surgery in a large European study.[99,105] Typically, neoadjuvant therapy is reserved for individuals who have significant malnutrition, a poor performance status, and tense ascites, or extensive disease that would not be amendable to optimal resection (mediastinal adenopathy, unresectable liver disease). Neoadjuvant therapy may be less beneficial in women with certain type I tumors, as they are less likely to respond to taxane and platinum-based chemotherapy compared with high-grade serous cancers.[106-110] Participation in clinical trials, if they are available, should be encouraged.

Many of the landmark studies that have guided the management of epithelial ovarian cancers have included mostly women with high-grade serous disease. Patients with mucinous, endometrioid, clear cell, and low-grade serous cancer typically comprise only a fraction, if any, of these patient populations. A retrospective analysis of a large Gynecologic Oncology Group (GOG) trial in women with early-stage disease was conducted to explore histologic subsets of patients who may benefit from 6 versus 3 cycles of chemotherapy. Thirty percent of the patient population had clear cell carcinoma, whereas 25% had endometrioid, 23% had serous, 7% had mucinous, and 15% had other cell types. The risk of recurrent disease was significantly lower in women with serous cancers who were treated with 6 versus 3 cycles of chemotherapy (hazard ratio [HR] = 0.33; confidence interval [CI] = 0.14-0.77; P = .04). In contrast, there was no difference in recurrence risk between the 2 chemotherapy groups in women with non-serous cancers (HR = 0.94; CI = 0.60-1.49).[111] This study did not distinguish between low-grade and high-grade serous disease, and most women in the trial had grade 3 tumors. However, the authors did conduct additional subgroup analyses and did not detect any differences with regard to grade in women with serous cancers.[111]

Alternative chemotherapeutic regimens are under evaluation in women with type I ovarian cancers.

Collaborative groups in the United States, Europe, and Japan are currently undertaking prospective studies with chemotherapy and biologically targeted therapies in patients with advanced or recurrent mucinous ovarian cancer. Given the morphologic and molecular similarities between mucinous ovarian cancer and colorectal cancers, it is reasonable to treat these diseases with a similar chemotherapeutic regimen. The GOG has developed a phase 3 clinical trial comparing paclitaxel and carboplatin to capecitabine and oxaliplatin (a regimen commonly used in colorectal cancers) with and without bevacizumab. Given the frequent alterations involving components of the *Ras-Raf-MEK-MAPK* pathway, agents that inhibit this cascade are of interest in the treatment of mucinous epithelial ovarian cancer.

SURVIVAL AND PROGNOSIS

Key Points

1. Type I ovarian cancers have improved survival in comparison with type II disease, in part due to the earlier stage at presentation and lower grade.
2. Clear cell and mucinous ovarian cancers have worse prognosis than low-grade serous and endometrioid disease, potentially resulting from relative chemoresistance.

The survival and prognosis for LMP tumors are significantly better compared with those of type I and II epithelial ovarian cancers. LMP tumors are usually confined to the ovary, occur predominantly in premenopausal women, and are associated with good outcomes. Approximately 75% of LMP tumors are stage I at the time of diagnosis. The majority of patients presents at an early stage and have excellent 5-year survival rates approaching 100%.[112] The recurrence and the overall survival rates of LMP tumors with noninvasive implants is time dependent,[113] but for patients with peritoneal implants, the 10-year survival rate is between 70% and 95%, caused by late recurrence.[114,115] However, a lower 5-year survival rate of 69.3% was reported for mucinous LMP in one study. The 5-year survival for stage I and stage II/ III disease was 93% and 15%, respectively. The lower than expected survival rate may have been secondary to the inclusion of women with pseudomyxoma peritonei, which tends to have a worse prognosis.[116]

There has been considerable controversy regarding serous LMP tumors and the "noninvasive" variant, micropapillary serous carcinomas. Some studies have indicated that the latter are more likely to have invasive implants, advanced disease, increased risk of tumor recurrence, and worse clinical outcome than serous LMP. In 2010, May and colleagues[37] reported their results regarding gene expression profiling in serous LMP, serous LMP-micropapillary serous carcinoma, and invasive low-grade serous cancers. The gene expression profile of micropapillary serous carcinomas was similar to low-grade malignancies and distinct from serous LMP tumors.[37] Given these findings, micropapillary serous carcinomas may require more extensive surgical staging and cytoreductive surgery as well as more frequent surveillance.

Type I ovarian cancers for the most part are considered to be indolent cancers, and the survival for women with type I tumors is overall better than that for type II disease (see Chapter 12). The improved survival probably is in part a reflection of stage and grade, as most of the type I cancers are diagnosed at earlier stages compared with their more aggressive counterpart and are well-differentiated tumors. Women with stage I disease, with appropriate surgical staging, have a 5-year survival rate of 90% when treated with surgery alone. Those with stage II, III, and IV disease have 5-year survival rates of 74%, 15% to 37%, and 5% to 25%, respectively.[98,99] Similar to type II tumors, survival is also associated with the amount of residual tumor (see Chapter 12).

There is also evidence that the clinical behavior of type I histologic subtypes are distinct even from each other with regard to prognosis and survival. For example, women with clear cell carcinoma of the ovary have a worse prognosis than those with serous and endometrioid ovarian cancers.[117,118] The 5-year survival for women with stage I clear cell cancers was 60%, compared with 12% for other stages.[98] Similarly, most women with mucinous carcinomas are diagnosed with early-stage disease, and the overall prognosis for women with primary mucinous ovarian cancer is better than for those with high-grade serous disease. However, those with advanced-stage mucinous carcinomas of the ovary have a worse prognosis, as manifested by a worse progression-free and overall survival than those with advanced-stage serous, endometrioid, and clear cell carcinomas (Figure 13-13).[117] The relative risk of death for women with mucinous cancers was increased 4.1-fold compared with those with serous cancer ($P < .001$).[117] The worse prognosis noted for advanced clear cell and mucinous type I tumors may be due to resistance to traditional chemotherapy regimens often used for type II tumors.[5] Another explanation for the poor prognosis and lack of response for advanced mucinous ovarian cancers is that some of these malignancies represent metastatic disease rather than primary ovarian cancers.

Conversely, women with endometrioid cancer are more likely to undergo optimal cytoreduction, have a better prognosis, and have longer progression-free and overall survival compared with those with serous, mucinous, or clear cell cancer.[16,117] Patients with concurrent

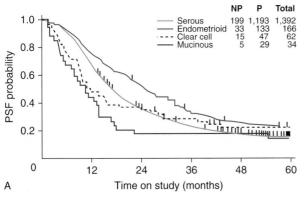
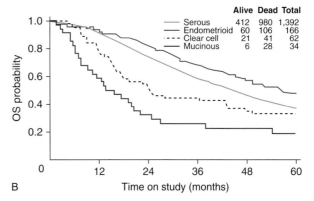

FIGURE 13-13. Progression-free and overall survival in epithelial ovarian cancer. A retrospective review was conducted on 1895 patients with stage III epithelial ovarian cancer (EOC) who had undergone primary surgery followed by 6 cycles of intravenous platinum/paclitaxel on Gynecologic Oncology Group protocols. **A.** The estimated progression-free survival (PFS) in 4 subtypes of EOC revealed that women with endometrioid cancers had a decreased risk of progression of 0.76 (95% CI, 0.64-0.92; P = .004) compared with those with serous cancers. Those with clear cell and mucinous cell type had a significantly increased risk of disease progression (1.37 [95% CI, 1.01-1.85; P = .04] and 2.18 [95% CI, 1.48-3.22; P <.001], respectively) compared with women with serous cancers. Women with the mucinous cell type had a marginally increased risk for disease progression compared with those with clear cell type (1.59 [95% CI, 0.98-2.59; P = .06]). **B.** Similar findings were noted for overall survival (OS). The OS probability adjusted relative risk of death for endometrioid, clear cell, and mucinous cell type as compared with serous cell type was 0.79 (95% CI, 0.65-0.97; P = .02), 1.74 (95% CI, 1.26-2.41; P <.001), and 4.14 (95% CI, 2.77-6.19; P <.001), respectively. Women with mucinous versus clear cell type cancer had a 2.4-fold increased risk of death (2.38 [95% CI, 1.43-3.95; P <.001]). (Reproduced, with permission, from Winter et al.[117])

endometrioid ovarian and endometrial malignancies had a survival advantage compared with those with ovarian carcinoma alone.[16] Soliman et al[89] reported a median survival approaching 10 years for women with concurrent endometrioid tumors of the endometrium and ovary.

Women with low-grade serous cancers have a better prognosis than those with high-grade disease and were found to have a longer median survival (median not reached) compared with those with high-grade disease (median, 39 months).[17] Although low-grade serous cancers typically have a relatively indolent course, they tend to be chemoresistant, and treatment can be challenging.[14,119]

MANAGEMENT OF RECURRENT DISEASE

Key Points

1. Surgical resection of recurrent disease remains the cornerstone for women with LMP tumors; chemotherapy may be considered with the presence of invasive metastases.
2. Secondary cytoreductive surgery may be considered for women with recurrent low-grade serous, endometrioid, or mucinous cancers, but attention to the treatment-free interval is critical given the relative chemoresistance of these malignancies.

3. Chemotherapeutic agents active in type II ovarian, tubal, and peritoneal disease may also be effective in recurrent type I ovarian cancer.

Patients with LMP tumors should be monitored with a careful review of symptoms and clinical examinations every 3 to 6 months for up to 5 years and then annually. Ultrasounds are indicated for women who underwent fertility-sparing surgery. After completion of child-bearing, patients who underwent fertility-sparing surgery should be counseled regarding completion surgery.[99] CA-125 tumor marker assessment can be performed at the discretion of the treating physician. Radiographic studies may be obtained as needed to investigate new symptoms or findings on examination.

The treatment of recurrent disease for women with LMP tumors is typically surgery, but depends on the patient's comorbidities and disease characteristics. The use of adjuvant therapy in the recurrent setting is based on the presence of invasive disease. Those with noninvasive disease can be observed, whereas those with invasive disease may be considered for treatment with chemotherapy.[99] Given the relative chemoresistance of LMP tumors,[114] alternative therapies are needed. Agents targeting the *Ras-Raf-MEK-MAPK* pathway would be of interest given the high frequency of aberrations in LMP tumors.

Currently the surveillance, management of recurrent disease, and palliative care for type I epithelial ovarian cancers is the same as type II cancers (see Chapter 12). The role of secondary cytoreductive surgery, which is considered in women who have at least a treatment-free interval of 6 months before relapse, may have an even more prominent part in the management of type I ovarian cancers given their relative chemoresistant nature as compared with type II cancers. There are several chemotherapy options available, and current US Food and Drug Administration–approved drugs for the treatment of ovarian cancer include carboplatin, cisplatin, paclitaxel, liposomal doxorubicin, topotecan, and gemcitabine in combination with carboplatin. The type of relapse therapy used depends of the treatment-free interval, prior toxicities, the patient's comorbidities, convenience, quality of life, and the goals of therapy. The treatment-free interval is an important prognostic factor, and women are treated differently based on whether they have platinum-resistant or sensitive disease (see Chapter 12).

The preferred chemotherapy regimens for women for platinum-sensitive disease include platinum monotherapy or platinum doublets combined with either paclitaxel, docetaxel, gemcitabine, or liposomal doxorubicin.[99] For women with platinum-resistant disease, single-agent non-platinum therapy is preferred with the following agents; docetaxel, etoposide, gemcitabine, liposomal doxorubicin, weekly paclitaxel, or topotecan. Additional therapies include altretamine, capecitabine, cyclophosphamide, ifosfamide, irinotecan, melphalan, oxaliplatin, conventional dose paclitaxel, nab-paclitaxel, pemetrexed, and vinorelbine.[99] Biologic therapies are also being used in the recurrent setting. Bevacizumab, a monoclonal antibody that binds to VEGF has been shown to have activity in ovarian cancer. Antitumor activity has also been demonstrated for other antiangiogenic therapies, as well as mammalian target of rapamycin (mTOR) and PARP1 inhibitors.

A specific concern for type I ovarian cancers is their chemoresistant nature,[120] and there is an acute need for effective systemic therapy. Given the poor responses of low-grade serous carcinomas to traditional chemotherapy and strong association with alterations of the *MAPK* pathway, the GOG evaluated AZD6244, a biologic agent that inhibits the MAPK, MEK-1/2, in women with recurrent ovarian and peritoneal low-grade serous disease. The trial is closed to enrollment, and data are not yet available but are eagerly awaited. The GOG has also activated a phase 2 trial of sunitinib, a tyrosine kinase inhibitor that inhibits VEGF and platelet-derived growth factor receptors in women with persistent and recurrent clear cell epithelial ovarian cancer. Clear cell cancers have poor response rates ranging from 15% to 45%. Given the molecular similarities between clear cell epithelial ovarian cancer and renal carcinomas, there is interest in evaluating biologic therapies, such as sunitinib, that are active in renal cell cancers in women with clear cell ovarian cancer.

Other agents to consider include mTOR, PIK3, and AKT inhibitors in clear cell and mucinous cancers, as they have frequent alterations in the *PIK3-CA/AKT/PTEN* pathway. This pathway is very complex, activated by numerous factors, and plays a pivotal role in cellular transformation (Figure 13-7). AKT is the major known effector of the *PI3K-CA/AKT/PTEN* pathway and phosphorylates multiple downstream proteins, including mTOR. mTOR is involved in protein synthesis and regulates cellular proliferation, growth, and survival. A strategy of combining multiple agents that inhibit different pathways such as *PARP1* and *MAPK* may be of particular interest in select cancers such as low-grade serous disease that exhibit aberrations in both these pathways.

Hormonal therapies in ovarian cancer have a response rate of approximately 10% in previously treated patients. A correlation may exist between the presence of hormone receptors and a response to therapy. A variety of agents have been used, including progestational agents such as megestrol acetate, gonadotropic-releasing analogs (leuprolide acetate), selective estrogen receptor modulators (tamoxifen), anti-androgen agents, and aromatase inhibitors (anastrozole and letrozole).[98,99] Given the presence of hormone receptors on low-grade serous and endometrioid cancers, hormonal agents should also be evaluated.

FUTURE DIRECTIONS

As we continue to recognize the varying clinical behavior and molecular biology of patients with LMP tumors and type I epithelial ovarian cancers, the management of these distinct histologic subtypes may change dramatically in the future. Paradigms for screening, recommended prophylactic procedures, surgery, treatment, and surveillance may all be altered. Biologic therapies that target the underlying molecular biology of these ovarian cancer subtypes may be exceedingly important, as most of these tumors are resistant to traditional chemotherapeutic regimens used in type II disease. Translational research objectives should be incorporated in the design of clinical trials to correlate specific mutational status or pathway activation to clinical response and survival outcomes. This will enhance the ability to identify patients who are most likely benefit from these therapies and provide guidance regarding future implementation of adjuvant and relapse therapy. These unique tumors represent an exceptional and exciting opportunity to develop individually tailored cancer therapy based on molecular alterations and potentially improve outcome for women with type I ovarian cancer.

REFERENCES

1. Jemal A, Siegel R, Xu J, et al. Cancer statistics, 2010. *CA Cancer J Clin.* 2010;60(5):277-300.

2. Shih IeM, Kurman RJ. Ovarian tumorigenesis: a proposed model based on morphological and molecular genetic analysis. *Am J Pathol.* 2004;164(5):1511-1518.

3. Cho KR, Shih IeM. Ovarian cancer. *Annu Rev Pathol.* 2009; 4:287-313.

4. Chu CS, Rubin SC. Epidemiology, staging, and clinical characteristics. In: RE Bristow, BY Karlan, eds. *Surgery for Ovarian Cancer: Principles and Practices.* Boca Raton, FL: Taylor and Francis; 2007:13-15.

5. Kurman RJ, Shih IeM. The origin and pathogenesis of epithelial ovarian cancer: a proposed unifying theory. *Am J Surg Pathol.* 2010;34(3):433-443.

6. Kuo KT, Guan B, Feng Y, et al. Analysis of DNA copy number alterations in ovarian serous tumors identifies new molecular genetic changes in low-grade and high-grade carcinomas [Erratum in: *Cancer Res.* 2009;69(12):5267]. *Cancer Res.* 2009; 69(9):4036-4042.

7. Robboy SJ, Duggan M, Kurman RJ. The female reproductive system. In: Rubin E, Farber J, eds. *Pathology.* 2nd ed. Philadelphia, PA: JB Lippincott; 1988.

8. Gilks CB. Molecular abnormalities in ovarian cancer subtypes other than high-grade serous carcinoma. *J Oncol.* 2010;2010: 740968.

9. Singer G, Kurman RJ, Chang HW, et al. Diverse tumorigenic pathways in ovarian serous carcinoma. *Am J Pathol.* 2002; 160(4):1223-1228.

10. Seidman JD, Horkayne-Szakaly I, Cosin JA, et al. Testing of two binary grading systems for FIGO stage III serous carcinoma of the ovary and peritoneum. *Gynecol Oncol.* 2006;103(2): 703-708.

11. Stern RC, Dash R, Bentley RC, et al. Malignancy in endometriosis: frequency and comparison of ovarian and extraovarian types. *Int J Gynecol Pathol.* 2001;20(2):133-139.

12. Behbakht K, Randall TC, Benjamin I, et al. Clinical characteristics of clear cell carcinoma of the ovary. *Gynecol Oncol.* 1998;70(2):255-258.

13. Disaia PJ, Creasman WT. Germ cell, stromal and other ovarian tumors. In: DiSaia PJ, Creasman WT, eds. *Clinical Gynecologic Oncology.* 5th ed. St Louis, MO: Mosby Year Book; 1997, Chapter 11.

14. Gershenson DM, Sun CC, Lu KH, et al. Clinical behavior of stage II-IV low-grade serous carcinoma of the ovary. *Obstet Gynecol.* 2006;108(2):361-368.

15. Schmeler KM, Gershenson DM. Low-grade serous ovarian cancer: a unique disease. *Curr Oncol Rep.* 2008;10(6):519-523.

16. Storey DJ, Rush R, Stewart M, et al. Endometrioid epithelial ovarian cancer: 20 years of prospectively collected data from a single center. *Cancer.* 2008;112(10):2211-2220.

17. Plaxe SC. Epidemiology of low-grade serous ovarian cancer. *Am J Obstet Gynecol.* 2008;198(4):459.e1-e8; discussion 459.e8-e9.

18. Kennedy AW, Hart WR. Ovarian papillary serous tumors of low malignant potential (serous borderline tumors). A long-term follow-up study, including patients with microinvasion, lymph node metastasis, and transformation to invasive serous carcinoma. *Cancer.* 1996;78(2):278-286.

19. Kaern J, Tropé CG, Kristensen GB, et al. DNA ploidy; the most important prognostic factor in patients with borderline tumors of the ovary. *Int J Gynecol Cancer.* 1993;3(6):349-358.

20. Riman T, Dickman PW, Nilsson S, et al. Risk factors for invasive epithelial ovarian cancer: results from a Swedish case-control study. *Am J Epidemiol.* 2002;156(4):363-373.

21. Heintz AP, Odicino F, Maisonneuve P, et al. Carcinoma of the ovary. FIGO 6th Annual Report on the Results of Treatment in Gynecological Cancer. *Int J Gynaecol Obstet.* 2006; 95(suppl 1): S161-S192.

22. Callahan MJ, Crum CP, Medeiros F, et al. Primary fallopian tube malignancies in BRCA-positive women undergoing surgery for ovarian cancer risk reduction. *J Clin Oncol.* 2007; 25(25):3985-3990.

23. Carcangiu ML, Radice P, Manoukian S, et al. Atypical epithelial proliferation in fallopian tubes in prophylactic salpingo-oophorectomy specimens from BRCA1 and BRCA2 germline mutation carriers. *Int J Gynecol Pathol.* 2004;23(1):35-40.

24. Carlson JW, Jarboe EA, Kindelberger D, et al. Serous tubal intraepithelial carcinoma: diagnostic reproducibility and its implications. *Int J Gynecol Pathol.* 2010;29(4):310-314.

25. Finch A, Shaw P, Rosen B, et al. Clinical and pathologic findings of prophylactic salpingo-oophorectomies in 159 BRCA1 and BRCA2 carriers. *Gynecol Oncol.* 2006;100(1):58-64.

26. Folkins AK, Jarboe EA, Roh MH, et al. Precursors to pelvic serous carcinoma and their clinical implications. *Gynecol Oncol.* 2009;113(3):391-396.

27. Folkins AK, Jarboe EA, Saleemuddin A, et al. A candidate precursor to pelvic serous cancer (p53 signature) and its prevalence in ovaries and fallopian tubes from women with BRCA mutations. *Gynecol Oncol.* 2008;109(2):168-173.

28. Kuhn E, Meeker A, Wang TL, et al. Shortened telomeres in serous tubal intraepithelial carcinoma: an early event in ovarian high-grade serous carcinogenesis. *Am J Surg Pathol.* 2010;34(6):829-836.

29. Paley PJ, Swisher EM, Garcia RL, et al. Occult cancer of the fallopian tube in BRCA-1 germline mutation carriers at prophylactic oophorectomy: a case for recommending hysterectomy at surgical prophylaxis. *Gynecol Oncol.* 2001;80(2):176-180.

30. Piek JM, van Diest PJ, Zweemer RP, et al. Dysplastic changes in prophylactically removed Fallopian tubes of women predisposed to developing ovarian cancer. *J Pathol.* 2001;195(4): 451-456.

31. Piek JM, van Diest PJ, Zweemer RP, et al. Tubal ligation and risk of ovarian cancer. *Lancet.* 2001;358(9284):844.

32. Piek JM, Verheijen RH, Kenemans P, et al. BRCA1/2-related ovarian cancers are of tubal origin: a hypothesis. *Gynecol Oncol.* 2003;90(2):491.

33. Przybycin CG, Kurman RJ, Ronnett BM, et al. Are all pelvic (nonuterine) serous carcinomas of tubal origin? *Am J Surg Pathol.* 2010;34(10):1407-1416.

34. Sehdev AS, Kurman RJ, Kuhn E, et al. Serous tubal intraepithelial carcinoma upregulates markers associated with high-grade serous carcinomas including Rsf-1 (HBXAP), cyclin E and fatty acid synthase. *Mod Pathol.* 2010;23(6):844-855.

35. Shaw TJ, Senterman MK, Dawson K, et al. Characterization of intraperitoneal, orthotopic, and metastatic xenograft models of human ovarian cancer. *Mol Ther.* 2004;10(6):1032-1042.

36. Shih IeM. Ovarian serous low malignant potential (borderline) tumor—does "micropapillary" matter? *Gynecol Oncol.* 2010; 117(1):1-3.

37. May T, Virtanen C, Sharma M, et al. Low malignant potential tumors with micropapillary features are molecularly similar to low-grade serous carcinoma of the ovary. *Gynecol Oncol.* 2010;117(1):9-17.

38. Modugno F, Ness RB, Allen GO, et al. Oral contraceptive use, reproductive history, and risk of epithelial ovarian cancer in women with and without endometriosis. *Am J Obstet Gynecol.* 2004;191(3):733-740.

39. Cuatrecasas M, Villanueva A, Matias-Guiu X, et al. K-ras mutations in mucinous ovarian tumors: a clinicopathologic and molecular study of 95 cases. *Cancer.* 1997;79(8):1581-1586.

40. Hankinson SE, Colditz GA, Hunter DJ, et al. A quantitative assessment of oral contraceptive use and risk of ovarian cancer. *Obstet Gynecol.* 1992;80(4):708-714.

CHAPTER 13

41. Ahmed AA, Etemadmoghadam D, Temple J, et al. Driver mutations in TP53 are ubiquitous in high grade serous carcinoma of the ovary. *J Pathol.* 2010;221(1):49-56.

42. Malpica A, Deavers MT, Tornos C, et al. Interobserver and intraobserver variability of a two-tier system for grading ovarian serous carcinoma. *Am J Surg Pathol.* 2007;31(8):1168-1174.

43. Bonni A, Brunet A, West AE, et al. Cell survival promoted by the Ras-MAPK signaling pathway by transcription-dependent and -independent mechanisms. *Science.* 1999;286(5443):1358-1362.

44. Ronnett BM, Zahn CM, Kurman RJ, et al. Disseminated peritoneal adenomucinosis and peritoneal mucinous carcinomatosis. A clinicopathologic analysis of 109 cases with emphasis on distinguishing pathologic features, site of origin, prognosis, and relationship to "pseudomyxoma peritonei". *Am J Surg Pathol.* 1995;19(12):1390-1408.

45. Gemignani ML, Schlaerth AC, Bogomolniy F, et al. Role of KRAS and BRAF gene mutations in mucinous ovarian carcinoma. *Gynecol Oncol.* 2003;90(2):378-381.

46. Mok SC, Bell DA, Knapp RC, et al. Mutation of K-ras protooncogene in human ovarian epithelial tumors of borderline malignancy. *Cancer Res.* 1993;53(7):1489-1492.

47. Williams AC, Browne SJ, Yeudal WA, et al. Molecular events including p53 and k-ras alterations in the in vitro progression of a human colorectal adenoma cell line to an adenocarcinoma. *Oncogene.* 1993;8(11):3063-3072.

48. Singer G, Oldt R 3rd, Cohen Y, et al. Mutations in BRAF and KRAS characterize the development of low-grade ovarian serous carcinoma. *J Natl Cancer Inst.* 2003;95(6):484-486.

49. Salani R, Kurman RJ, Giuntoli R 2nd, et al. Assessment of TP53 mutation using purified tissue samples of ovarian serous carcinomas reveals a higher mutation rate than previously reported and does not correlate with drug resistance. *Int J Gynecol Cancer.* 2008;18(3):487-491.

50. Wu R, Hendrix-Lucas N, Kuick R, et al. Mouse model of human ovarian endometrioid adenocarcinoma based on somatic defects in the Wnt/beta-catenin and PI3K/Pten signaling pathways. *Cancer Cell.* 2007;11(4):321-333.

51. Obata K, Morland SJ, Watson RH, et al. Frequent PTEN/MMAC mutations in endometrioid but not serous or mucinous epithelial ovarian tumors. *Cancer Res.* 1998;58(10):2095-2097.

52. Palacios J, Gamallo C. Mutations in the beta-catenin gene (CTNNB1) in endometrioid ovarian carcinomas. *Cancer Res.* 1998;58(7):1344-1347.

53. Catasús L, Bussaglia E, Rodrguez I, et al. Molecular genetic alterations in endometrioid carcinomas of the ovary: similar frequency of beta-catenin abnormalities but lower rate of microsatellite instability and PTEN alterations than in uterine endometrioid carcinomas. *Hum Pathol.* 2004;35(11):1360-1368.

54. Jones S, Wang TL, Shih IeM, et al. Frequent mutations of chromatin remodeling gene ARID1A in ovarian clear cell carcinoma. *Science.* 2010;330(6001):228-231.

55. Wiegand KC, Shah SP, Al-Agha OM, et al. ARID1A mutations in endometriosis-associated ovarian carcinomas. *N Engl J Med.* 2010;363(16):1532-1543.

56. Nakayama K, Nakayama N, Kurman RJ, et al. Sequence mutations and amplification of PIK3CA and AKT2 genes in purified ovarian serous neoplasms. *Cancer Biol Ther.* 2006;5(7):779-785.

57. Kuo KT, Mao TL, Jones S, et al. Frequent activating mutations of PIK3CA in ovarian clear cell carcinoma. *Am J Pathol.* 2009;174(5):1597-1601.

58. Zorn KK, Bonome T, Gangi L, et al. Gene expression profiles of serous, endometrioid, and clear cell subtypes of ovarian and endometrial cancer. *Clin Cancer Res.* 2005;11(18):6422-6430.

59. Simsir A, Palacios D, Linehan WM, et al. Detection of loss of heterozygosity at chromosome 3p25-26 in primary and metastatic ovarian clear-cell carcinoma: utilization of microdissection and polymerase chain reaction in archival tissues. *Diagn Cytopathol.* 2001;24(5):328-332.

60. Semenza GL. Targeting HIF-1 for cancer therapy. *Nat Rev Cancer.* 2003t;3(10):721-732.

61. Evans DG, Young K, Bulman M, Shenton A, Wallace A, Lalloo F. Probability of BRCA1/2 mutation varies with ovarian histology: results from screening 442 ovarian cancer families. *Clin Genet.* 2008;73(4):338-345.

62. Schuijer M, Berns EM. TP53 and ovarian cancer. *Hum Mutat.* 2003;21(3):285-291.

63. Schueller EF, Kirol PM. Prognosis in endometrioid carcinoma of the ovary. *Obstet Gynecol.* 1966;27(6):850-858.

64. Press JZ, De Luca A, Boyd N, et al. Ovarian carcinomas with genetic and epigenetic BRCA1 loss have distinct molecular abnormalities. *BMC Cancer.* 2008;8:17.

65. Pradhan M, Davidson B, Tropé CG, et al. Gross genomic alterations differ between serous borderline tumors and serous adenocarcinomas—an image cytometric DNA ploidy analysis of 307 cases with histogenetic implications. *Virchows Arch.* 2009;454(6):677-683.

66. Goff BA, Mandel L, Muntz HG, Melancon CH. Ovarian carcinoma diagnosis. *Cancer.* 2000;89(10):2068-2075.

67. Goff BA, Mandel LS, Drescher CW, et al. Development of an ovarian cancer symptom index: possibilities for earlier detection. *Cancer.* 2007;109(2):221-227.

68. Olson SH, Mignone L, Nakraseive C, et al. Symptoms of ovarian cancer. *Obstet Gynecol.* 2001;98(2):212-217.

69. Shimizu Y, Kamoi S, Amada S, et al. Toward the development of a universal grading system for ovarian epithelial carcinoma: testing of a proposed system in a series of 461 patients with uniform treatment and follow-up. *Cancer.* 1998;82(5):893-901.

70. Malpica A, Deavers MT, Lu K, et al. Grading ovarian serous carcinoma using a two-tier system. *Am J Surg Pathol.* 2004; 28(4):496-504.

71. Shimizu Y, Kamoi S, Amada S, et al. Toward the development of a universal grading system for ovarian epithelial carcinoma. I. Prognostic significance of histopathologic features—problems involved in the architectural grading system. *Gynecol Oncol.* 1998;70(1):2-12.

72. Taylor HC Jr. Malignant and semi-malignant tumors of the ovary. *Surg Gynecol Obstet.* 1929;48:204-230.

73. Acs G. Serous and mucinous borderline (low malignant potential) tumors of the ovary. *Am J Clin Pathol.* 2005; 123 (suppl): S13-S57.

74. Vang R, Shih IeM, Kurman RJ. Ovarian low-grade and high-grade serous carcinoma: pathogenesis, clinicopathologic and molecular biologic features, and diagnostic problems. *Adv Anat Pathol.* 2009;16(5):267-282.

75. Dehari R, Kurman RJ, Logani S, Shih IeM. The development of high-grade serous carcinoma from atypical proliferative (borderline) serous tumors and low-grade micropapillary serous carcinoma: a morphologic and molecular genetic analysis. *Am J Surg Pathol.* 2007;31(7):1007-1012.

76. Ozols RF, Rubin SC, Thomas GM, et al. Epithelial ovarian cancer. In: Hoskins WJ, Perez CA, Young RC, Barakat RR, Markman M, Randall ME, eds. *Principles and Practice of Gynecologic Oncology.* 4th ed. Philadelphia, PA: Lippincott Williams & Wilkins; 2005:910-911.

77. Seidman JD, Horkayne-Szakaly I, Haiba M, et al. The histologic type and stage distribution of ovarian carcinomas of surface epithelial origin. *Int J Gynecol Pathol.* 2004;23(1):41-44.

78. Hart WR. Mucinous tumors of the ovary: a review. *Int J Gynecol Pathol.* 2005;24(1):4-25.

79. Lee KR, Young RH. The distinction between primary and metastatic mucinous carcinomas of the ovary: gross and histologic findings in 50 cases. *Am J Surg Pathol.* 2003;27(3):281-292.

80. Prayson RA, Hart WR, Petras RE. Pseudomyxoma peritonei. A clinicopathologic study of 19 cases with emphasis on site of origin and nature of associated ovarian tumors. *Am J Surg Pathol.* 1994;18(6):591-603.

81. Seidman JD, Kurman RJ, Ronnett BM. Primary and metastatic mucinous adenocarcinomas in the ovaries: incidence in routine practice with a new approach to improve intraoperative diagnosis. *Am J Surg Pathol.* 2003; 27(7):985-993.

82. Frumovitz M, Schmeler KM, Malpica A, Sood AK, Gershenson DM. Unmasking the complexities of mucinous ovarian carcinoma. *Gynecol Oncol.* 2010;117(3):491-496.

83. Rekhi B, George S, Madur B, Chinoy RF, Dikshit R, Maheshwari A. Clinicopathological features and the value of differential Cytokeratin 7 and 20 expression in resolving diagnostic dilemmas of ovarian involvement by colorectal adenocarcinoma and vice-versa. *Diagn Pathol.* 2008;3:39.

84. Stern RC, Dash R, Bentley RC, Snyder MJ, Haney AF, Robboy SJ. Malignancy in endometriosis: frequency and comparison of ovarian and extraovarian types. *Int J Gynecol Pathol.* 2001;20(2):133-139.

85. Long ME, Taylor HC Jr. Endometrioid carcinoma of the ovary. *Am J Obstet Gynecol.* 1964;90:936-950.

86. Kline RC, Wharton JT, Atkinson EN, Burke TW, Gershenson DM, Edwards CL. Endometrioid carcinoma of the ovary: retrospective review of 145 cases. *Gynecol Oncol.* 1990;39(3): 337-346.

87. Czernobilsky B, Silverman BB, Mikuta JJ. Endometrioid carcinoma of the ovary. A clinicopathologic study of 75 cases. *Cancer.* 1970;26(5):1141-1152.

88. Tidy J, Mason WP. Endometrioid carcinoma of the ovary: a retrospective study. *Br J Obstet Gynaecol.* 1988;95(11):1165-1169.

89. Soliman PT, Slomovitz BM, Broaddus RR, et al. Synchronous primary cancers of the endometrium and ovary: a single institution review of 84 cases. *Gynecol Oncol.* 2004;94(2):456-462.

90. Ulbright TM, Roth LM. Metastatic and independent cancers of the endometrium and ovary: a clinicopathologic study of 34 cases. *Hum Pathol.* 1985;16(1):28-34.

91. Scully RE, Young RH, Clement PB. Tumors of the ovary, maldeveloped gonads, fallopian tube, and broad ligament. In: *Atlas of Tumor Pathology.* Bethesda, MD: Armed Forces Institute of Pathology; 1998.

92. Brescia RJ, Dubin N, Demopoulos RI. Endometrioid and clear cell carcinoma of the ovary. Factors affecting survival. *Int J Gynecol Pathol.* 1989;8(2):132-138.

93. Scully RE, Young RH, Clement PB. Tumors of the ovary, maldeveloped gonads, fallopian tube, and broad ligament. In: *Atlas of Tumor Pathology.* Third series, Fascicle 23. Washington, DC: Armed Forces Institute of Pathology; 1999.

94. Eastwood J. Mesonephroid (clear cell) carcinoma of the ovary and endometrium: a comparative prospective clinico-pathological study and review of literature. *Cancer.* 1978;41(5):1911-1928.

95. Toki T, Fujii S, Silverberg S. A clinicopathologic study on the association of endometriosis and carcinoma of the ovary using a scoring system. *Int J Gynecol Cancer.* 1996;6:68-75.

96. Köbel M, Kalloger SE, Boyd N, et al. Ovarian carcinoma subtypes are different diseases: implications for biomarker studies. *PLoS Med.* 2008;5(12):e232.

97. Tavassoli FA, Devilee P, eds. *World Health Organization Classification of Tumors: Pathology and Genetics. Tumours of the Breast and Female Genital Organs.* Lyon, France: IARC Press; 2003.

98. Ozols RF, Rubin SC, Thomas GM, et al. Epithelial ovarian cancer. In: Hoskins WJ, Perez CA, Young RC, Barakat RR, Markman M, Randall ME, eds. *Principles and Practice of Gynecologic Oncology.* 4th ed. Philadelphia, PA: Lippincott Williams & Wilkins; 2005.

99. National Comprehensive Cancer Network (NCCN). NCCN Clinical Practice Guidelines in Oncology: Ovarian Cancer. V.1.2008. http://www.nccn.org/. Accessed March 13, 2008.

100. Cadron I, Leunen K, Van Gorp T, et al. Management of borderline ovarian neoplasms. *J Clin Oncol.* 2007;25(20):2928-2937.

101. Leake JF, Rader JS, Woodruff JD, et al. Retroperitoneal lymphatic involvement with epithelial ovarian tumors of low malignant potential. *Gynecol Oncol.* 1991;42(2):124-130.

102. Houck K, Nikrui N, Duska L, et al. Borderline tumors of the ovary: correlation of frozen and permanent histopathologic diagnosis. *Obstet Gynecol.* 2000;95(6 pt 1):839-843.

103. Menzin AW, Rubin SC, Noumoff JS, et al. The accuracy of a frozen section diagnosis of borderline ovarian malignancy. *Gynecol Oncol.* 1995;59(2):183-185.

104. Tempfer CB, Polterauer S, Bentz EK, et al. Accuracy of intraoperative frozen section analysis in borderline tumors of the ovary: a retrospective analysis of 96 cases and review of the literature. *Gynecol Oncol.* 2007;107(2):248-252.

105. Vergote I, Tropé CG, Amant F, et al. Neoadjuvant chemotherapy or primary surgery in stage IIIC or IV ovarian cancer. *N Engl J Med.* 2010;363(10):943-953.

106. Goff BA, Sainz de la Cuesta R, Muntz HG, et al. Clear cell carcinoma of the ovary: a distinct histologic type with poor prognosis and resistance to platinum-based chemotherapy in stage III disease. *Gynecol Oncol.* 1996;60(3):412-417.

107. Pectasides D, Fountzilas G, Aravantinos G, et al. Advanced stage clear-cell epithelial ovarian cancer: the Hellenic Cooperative Oncology Group experience. *Gynecol Oncol.* 2006;102(2): 285-291.

108. Itamochi H, Kigawa J, Sugiyama T, et al. Low proliferation activity may be associated with chemoresistance in clear cell carcinoma of the ovary. *Obstet Gynecol.* 2002;100(2): 281-287.

109. Sugiyama T, Kamura T, Kigawa J, et al. Clinical characteristics of clear cell carcinoma of the ovary: a distinct histologic type with poor prognosis and resistance to platinum-based chemotherapy. *Cancer.* 2000;88(11):2584-2589.

110. Crotzer DR, Sun CC, Coleman RL, Wolf JK, Levenback CF, Gershenson DM. Lack of effective systemic therapy for recurrent clear cell carcinoma of the ovary. *Gynecol Oncol.* 2007;105(2):404-408.

111. Chan JK, Tian C, Fleming GF, et al. The potential benefit of 6 vs. 3 cycles of chemotherapy in subsets of women with early-stage high-risk epithelial ovarian cancer: an exploratory analysis of a Gynecologic Oncology Group study. *Gynecol Oncol.* 2010;116(3):301-306.

112. Barnhill DR, Kurman RJ, Brady MF, et al. Preliminary analysis of the behavior of stage I ovarian serous tumors of low malignant potential: a Gynecologic Oncology Group study. *J Clin Oncol.* 1995;13(11):2752-2756.

113. Silva EG, Gershenson DM, Malpica A, et al. The recurrence and the overall survival rates of ovarian serous borderline neoplasms with noninvasive implants is time dependent. *Am J Surg Pathol.* 2006;30(11):1367-1371.

114. Kane A, Uzan C, Rey A, et al. Prognostic factors in patients with ovarian serous low malignant potential (borderline) tumors with peritoneal implants. *Oncologist.* 2009;14(6): 591-600.

115. Tropé C, Davidson B, Paulsen T, et al. Diagnosis and treatment of borderline ovarian neoplasms "the state of the art". *Eur J Gynaecol Oncol.* 2009;30(5):471-482.

116. Nakashima N, Nagasaka T, Oiwa N, et al. Ovarian epithelial tumors of borderline malignancy in Japan. *Gynecol Oncol.* 1990;38(1):90-98.

117. Winter WE 3rd, Maxwell GL, Tian C, et al. Prognostic factors for stage III epithelial ovarian cancer: a Gynecologic Oncology Group Study. *J Clin Oncol.* 2007;25(24):3621-3627.

118. Montag AG, Jenison EL, Griffiths CT, et al. Ovarian clear cell carcinoma. A clinicopathologic analysis of 44 cases. *Int J Gynecol Pathol.* 1989;8(2):85-96.

119. Schmeler KM, Sun CC, Bodurka DC, et al. Neoadjuvant chemotherapy for low-grade serous carcinoma of the ovary or peritoneum. *Gynecol Oncol.* 2008;108(3):510-514.

120. Gershenson DM, Sun CC, Bodurka D, et al. Recurrent low-grade serous ovarian carcinoma is relatively chemoresistant. *Gynecol Oncol.* 2009;114(1):48-52.

Germ Cell and Sex Cord-Stromal Ovarian Cancers

Susan C. Modesitt and Jubilee Brown

Germ Cell Tumors

Germ cell tumors of the ovary comprise fewer than 5% of all malignant ovarian tumors. Germ cell tumors arise from the primordial germ cells and sex cord-stromal derivatives; they are exceedingly common in that they account for approximately one-quarter of all ovarian tumors, yet only 1% to 5% of germ cell tumors are malignant.[1-5] This disease is characterized by a young age at diagnosis. Survival is excellent due to the typically early stage at diagnosis and the relative chemosensitivity of even advanced disease, especially in comparison with epithelial ovarian, tubal, and peritoneal cancers.

EPIDEMIOLOGY

Key Points

1. The peak incidence of these tumors occurs in the 15- to 19-year-old age range.
2. Germ cell tumors may occur in setting of dysgenetic gonads, so karyotype testing may be warranted.

Within the United States, the incidence (age-adjusted) of malignant germ cell tumors is estimated at between 0.34 to 0.41 per 100,000, and rates appear to have declined over the last 30 years.[1,2] Risk factors are not well understood, but include younger age; the 15- to 19-year-old age group has by far the highest incidence rates. Studies have not consistently confirmed other specific demographic characteristics, such as in utero exposures (hormones, pesticides, smoking, or alcohol), maternal reproductive history, parental occupation, or congenital abnormalities as associated risk factors for germ cell tumors.[6-8] Racial differences exist in that dysgerminoma occurs twice as often in whites and other nonwhites as compared with blacks, and teratoma incidence is increased for blacks and other nonwhites as compared with whites; there appear to be no significant differences for the remainder of types.[2,9]

As opposed to some epithelial and stromal ovarian malignancies, germ cell tumors in females do not appear to be related to any yet-identified inherited cancer susceptibility syndromes (eg, *BRCA* mutations for epithelial ovarian, tubal, and peritoneal cancers and Peutz-Jegher syndrome for certain ovarian stromal tumors).[10] Surprisingly, in a recent review of pediatric germ cell tumors, a family history of testicular cancer was correlated with an increased risk of male germ cell tumors; however, a family history of ovarian or uterine cancer was inversely correlated with female germ cell tumors.[10] In contrast, there have been several case reports of familial clustering of germ cell tumors, and authors have hypothesized that a fraction of ovarian germ cell tumors could be a rare manifestation of a familial gonadal tumor syndrome.[11]

Of particular note, however, is that women with gonadal dysgenesis are at very high risk for the development of germ cell tumors. *Gonadal dysgenesis* is defined as a defect in development that causes abnormal sex steroid production and subsequent clinical manifestations such as delayed puberty or primary amenorrhea. In general, Turner syndrome (normally 45 X, or rarely a mosaic form of 45 X with a partial Y fragment) accounts for approximately two-thirds of diagnosed dysgenetic gonads. The majority of patients with Turner syndrome who develop tumors have the mosaic karyotype. Gonadal dysgenesis may also occur in 46 XX or 46 XY individuals. The greatest risk for germ cell tumors, especially dysgerminomas, is found in patients with Swyer syndrome (complete gonadal dysgenesis with 46 XY, but a female phenotype) and may affect more than 30% of patients[12]; prophylactic removal of both gonads should be strongly considered as soon as one of these syndromes is diagnosed.[13]

DIAGNOSIS

Key Points

1. Pelvic pain or mass is the most common presenting symptom of women with germ cell tumors.
2. The majority of germ cell tumors are stage IA at diagnosis.
3. Malignant germ cell tumors characteristically appear solid on imaging ultrasonography.

Most women with germ cell tumors present during the reproductive years, with a mean age in the early 20s. The most frequent symptoms are pelvic pain and/or mass (up to 85% of patients) followed by abdominal distension (30%), fever (10%), vaginal bleeding (10%), or ovarian torsion.[1,3,5] Of note, in ovarian torsion cases, up to 10% of adult cases but fewer than 2% of pediatric cases are ultimately proven to be caused by a malignant process.[5,14,15]

As part of the initial work-up for a pelvic mass in a young woman, ultrasound is the preferred radiographic modality due to the information gleaned regarding ovarian morphology and the lack of radiation. The majority of germ cell tumors are also unilateral. Only dysgerminomas are observed to be bilateral in 10% to 15% of cases.[3,5]

In addition, the majority of the malignant germ cell tumors will be predominantly solid (Figure 14-1).[16,17] Ultrasound alone may be able to raise the suspicion for an immature teratoma (or other malignant germ cell tumor) as opposed to its far more common benign

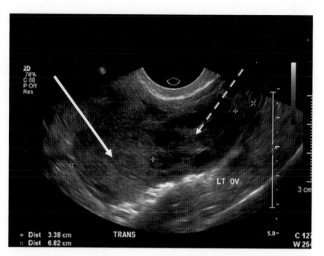

FIGURE 14-1. Ultrasound demonstrating a dysgerminoma of the ovary (white solid arrow) with the adjacent normal ovarian tissue with follicles (white dashed arrow).

counterpart, a mature cystic teratoma. A recent study from Canada evaluating ultrasound characteristics in teratomas found that benign cystic teratomas were more commonly predominantly cystic (77% vs. 18%), and the entirely solid tumors were all immature teratomas.[17] Another recent study in the pediatric population also observed that the benign ovarian germ cell tumors were smaller (7.65 cm vs. 16.9 cm; $P < .001$) and more often cystic compared with their malignant counterparts.[16] For evaluation of extraovarian disease, magnetic resonance imaging (MRI), computed tomography (CT), and positron emission tomography (PET) may be used, but due to the relatively low likelihood of malignancy and incidence of extraovarian metastases in germ cell tumors, this is often omitted during the initial mass evaluation.

Diagnostic testing should include preoperative evaluation of tumor markers and should include quantitative human chorionic gonadotropin (hCG), lactate dehydrogenase, α-fetoprotein (AFP), CA-125, and baseline blood work for surgery.[1,3,5,18,19] The most commonly abnormal tumor markers are hCG and AFP, and elevations are virtually diagnostic of a malignant germ cell tumor; specific patterns of tumor markers vary by tumor types (Table 14-1). Newer tumor markers may help differentiate malignant from benign masses; for example, the newly US Food and Drug Administration–approved OVA1 test (representing a combination of 5 immunoassays, including CA-125, transthyretin, apolipoprotein A1, β-2 microglobulin, and transferrin) demonstrated a 78% sensitivity for malignant nonepithelial ovarian cancers. Further research is needed, however, before applying the OVA1 test to these rare tumor types.[20] For patients with suspected gonadal dysgenesis, a karyotype should be

Table 14-1 Tumor Markers in Germ Cell Tumors

Tumor	Tumor Marker	
	AFP	β-hCG
Dysgerminoma	Usually normal	May be elevated
Immature teratoma	May be elevated	Normal
Endodermal sinus tumor	Elevated	Normal
Embryonal carcinoma	Elevated	Elevated
Choriocarcinoma	Normal	Elevated

Note. Lactate dehydrogenase and CA-125 may be more useful for documenting recurrence because they are unreliable for initial diagnosis in young women.
AFP, α-fetoprotein; β-hCG, β human chorionic gonadotropin.

Table 14-2 Categories of Germ Cell Tumors

I. Primitive germ cell tumors
  Dysgerminoma
  Endodermal sinus tumor (yolk sac tumor)
  Embryonal carcinoma
  Polyembryoma
  Nongestational choriocarcinoma
  Mixed germ cell tumor

II. Biphasic or triphasic teratoma
  Immature teratoma
  Mature teratoma
    Solid
    Cystic (dermoid)
    Fetiform teratoma (homunculus)

III. Monodermal teratoma and somatic-type tumors associated with group II (above)
  Thyroid (struma ovarii)
  Carcinoid
  Neuroectodermal
  Carcinoma
  Melanocytic
  Sarcoma
  Sebaceous
  Pituitary-type
  Other

Adapted from World Health Organization classification of tumors: Tavassoli FA, Deville P. *Pathology and Genetics of Tumors of the Breast and Female Genital Organs.* Lyon, France: International Agency for Research on Cancer; 2003.

performed before surgery, if possible, to ensure both ovaries are removed if indicated.

Definitive diagnosis is via surgical removal using a method that allows full surgical staging if necessary and can be done via laparotomy or laparoscopy, depending on patient and mass characteristics, as well as surgeon preference. The ovary should be removed intact (ie, no intra-abdominal morcellation). Frozen section can confirm the diagnosis and further surgical management undertaken as appropriate (see Treatment section).

PATHOLOGY

Key Points

1. Dysgerminoma and immature teratoma are most common malignant types of germ cell tumors.
2. Immature teratomas are defined by the presence of immature neural elements.
3. The hallmark histopathologic feature of endodermal sinus tumors is the Schiller-Duval body.

In the latest World Health Organization (WHO) classification, germ cell tumors are categorized into 3 broad categories (Table 14-2) that include (1) primitive germ cell tumors, (2) biphasic or triphasic teratoma, and (3) monodermal teratomas (including somatic tumors arising within teratomas). Malignant germ cell tumors include immature teratomas, dysgerminomas, and endodermal sinus tumors, along with the less common types. A recent Surveillance, Epidemiology, and End Results (SEER) data review of malignant germ cell tumors found that the most frequently diagnosed subtypes were immature teratoma (36%), dysgerminoma (33%), endodermal sinus tumor (15%), mixed non-dysgerminoma types (5%), embryonal (4%), mature teratoma with malignant degeneration (3%), and choriocarcinoma (2%).[2]

Grossly and histologically, several tumor types have distinctive appearances. Dysgerminomas are primarily solid tumors with a gray/white appearance and microscopically have sheets of vesicular cells with large nuclei with a fibrous stroma separating them (Figure 14-2). Immature teratomas are usually more solid than cystic and may contain hair or sebaceous material in a similar manner to mature teratomas; there is often extensive necrosis and hemorrhage. The immature components are comprised of neural tissue (required for diagnosis; Figure 14-3); they may also include glands, bone, or muscle.[20] Endodermal sinus tumors may be both solid and cystic with soft, friable tissue that may often be either hemorrhagic or necrotic (Figure 14-4). The hallmark histologic feature associated with endodermal sinus tumors is the Schiller-Duval body, which most closely resembles a renal glomerulus. Embryonal carcinomas maybe histologically solid (with diffuse sheets of anaplastic cells), tubular, or papillary; frequently there is a combination of these patterns (Figure 14-5). There is commonly foci of coagulative necrosis, and spindle cell stroma around tumor nests.

solid w/ gray/white appearance

sheets of vesicular cells w/ lg nuclei + fibrous stroma separating them

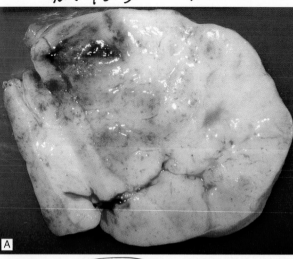

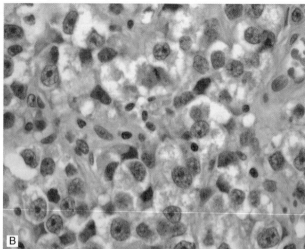

FIGURE 14-2. Dysgerminoma. A. Gross picture of dysgerminoma. **B.** Micrograph of dysgerminoma. (Image contributed by Dr. Kristen Atkins, Department of Pathology, University of Virginia Health System.)

TREATMENT

Key Points

1. Complete surgical resection is critical in the management of germ cell tumors.
2. Controversy exists regarding the need for comprehensive surgical staging in the pediatric population.
3. Adjuvant platinum-based chemotherapy has been recommended for treatment of all malignant germ cell tumors except stage I dysgerminoma and stage I, grade 1 immature teratomas.   *BEP*
4. In general, germ cell tumors are both chemo- and radiosensitive, even in advanced or recurrent disease.

radiation as good cure rates w/ chemo

Surgery

The mainstay of treatment for malignant germ cell tumors is surgery, as approximately 60% of all germ cell tumors will be confined to the ovary, and most (except dysgerminomas) are unilateral.[3,5] Although ovarian cystectomy is not recommended if the diagnosis is known intraoperatively, excellent survival rates after cystectomy for immature teratoma have been reported, but notably, most patients received adjuvant chemotherapy.[21] Few dispute the necessity of removal of the involved ovary, but there are divergent opinions regarding the extent (or necessity) of comprehensive surgical staging. In the gynecologic

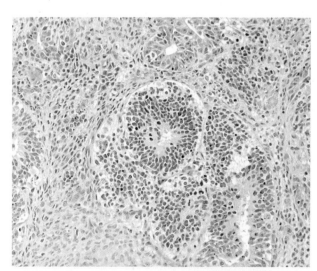

FIGURE 14-3. Micrograph of immature teratoma. (Image contributed by Dr. Kristen Atkins, Department of Pathology, University of Virginia Health System.)

cystic + solid components w/ hemorrhage + necrosis. comprised of neural tissue

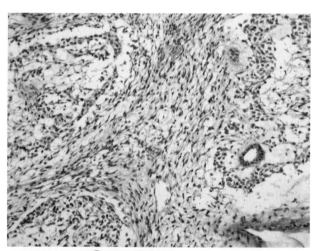

FIGURE 14-4. Endodermal sinus tumor. A. Micrograph of endodermal sinus tumor with typical vitelline growth pattern. (Image contributed by Dr. Kristen Atkins, Department of Pathology, University of Virginia Health System.) **B.** Micrograph of endodermal sinus tumor with associated Schiller-Duval body. *solid + cystic w/ soft friable tissue that is necrotic or hemorrhagic*

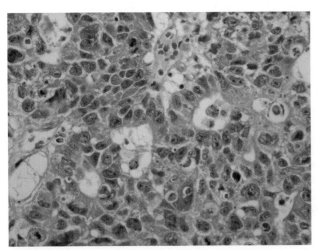

FIGURE 14-5. Micrograph of embryonal carcinoma.

oncology community, the standard recommended surgery has included a unilateral salpingo-oophorectomy (and bilateral salpingo-oophorectomy with hysterectomy if future fertility is not desired), peritoneal cytology, peritoneal biopsies, omentectomy, and retroperitoneal lymphadenectomy, including removal of bilateral pelvic and para-aortic nodes and any abnormal tissue. Because of the extremely chemosensitive nature of the disease, extensive and aggressive surgical resection procedures may not be advised if they increase morbidity or would delay chemotherapy.

In one of the largest reviews of lymph node metastasis, Kumar et al[4] found that approximately half of all patients with germ cell tumor in the SEER database diagnosed between 1988 and 2004 did not have lymph node dissection done as part of their surgery. Of the patients who did undergo lymph node dissection, overall 18% had positive nodes, and women with dysgerminoma had the highest rate of node metastases at 28%. Positive lymph nodes, not surprisingly, were an independent negative predictor of survival. Another study by Palenzuela et al[22] noted that only approximately half of the malignant germ cell tumors underwent comprehensive staging; none of the stage IA patients who underwent complete surgical staging experienced recurrence during observation without adjuvant chemotherapy, and none of the stage I patients who received adjuvant chemotherapy experienced recurrence, whereas approximately 40% of the patients with presumed (but not fully staged) stage I disease had recurrence.

In the pediatric oncology and surgery community, there has been a potential shift toward even more minimal surgery (unilateral salpingo-oophorectomy, washings, directed peritoneal biopsies, and careful abdominal inspection without retroperitoneal lymphadenectomy or omentectomy unless abnormalities are detected/palpated).[23] This change has occurred, in large part, from a study by Billmire et al[24] that reviewed the role and

outcomes of surgical staging in germ cell tumors in children and adolescents enrolled in 2 large intergroup trials that involved postoperative chemotherapy treatment (bleomycin, etoposide, and cisplatin [BEP] or high-dose cisplatin with etoposide and bleomycin). They found that deviations from standard surgical guidelines were the norm (most often the omission of lymphadenectomy), but that survival was excellent regardless of the extent of staging. They concluded that surgery should include washings, excision of any abnormal peritoneal surfaces, biopsy of any abnormal nodes or an abnormal contralateral ovary, and removal of the tumor-containing ovary. [23,24] However, all of the participants in this study received adjuvant platinum-based chemotherapy, which may have minimized any benefit of surgical staging in this very chemosensitive group of tumors.[24,25]

Most recently, a large Children's Oncology Group (COG) study examining surveillance of patients with stage I germ cell tumors who did not undergo chemotherapy closed to accrual in 2010; however, these data are not yet available. Of note, the COG uses a modified staging system (not the standard International Federation of Gynecology and Obstetrics [FIGO] staging[26]) in which lymphadenectomy and omentectomy are not routinely performed, tumor markers and radiographic imaging are employed as part of the staging assignment process, and patients who have positive washings/cytology/ascites are classified as having a stage III tumor[25] (Table 14-3, COG staging; Table 14-4, FIGO staging).

In summary, in adult women, full staging including lymphadenectomy allows better counseling regarding

Table 14-3 Children's Oncology Group Staging for Ovarian Germ Cell Tumor

Stage I	Limited to the ovary Peritoneal evaluation negative No clinical, radiographic, or histologic evidence of disease beyond the ovary
Stage II	Microscopic residual disease Peritoneal evaluation negative Failure of tumor markers to normalize or decrease with an appropriate half-life
Stage III	Lymph node involvement Gross residual disease or diagnosis by biopsy only Contiguous visceral involvement (omentum, intestine, bladder) Peritoneal evaluation positive
Stage IV	Distant metastases (including liver)

Note. Recommended surgical evaluation includes peritoneal washings, excision of any abnormal peritoneal surfaces, biopsy of any abnormal nodes or an abnormal contralateral ovary, and removal of the tumor containing ovary.

Table 14-4 FIGO Staging for Ovarian Tumors

Stage I	Tumor limited to ovaries
	Stage IA: Growth limited to 1 ovary, negative peritoneal cytology, capsule intact, and no tumor on external surface
	Stage IB: Growth limited to both ovaries, negative peritoneal cytology, capsule intact, and no tumor on external surface
	Stage IC: Tumor either stage IA or B but with positive cytology, rupture, or surface involvement
Stage II	Pelvic extension
	Stage IIA: Involvement of uterus and/or fallopian tubes
	Stage IIB: Extension to other pelvic structures
	Stage IIC: Either IIA or B but with positive cytology, rupture, or surface involvement
Stage III	Regional extension
	Stage IIIA: Tumor limited to pelvis but with microscopic involvement of abdominal peritoneum, small bowel, or omentum
	Stage IIIB: Visible tumor (<2 cm) in locations of IIIA
	Stage IIIC: Peritoneal metastases >2 cm or positive retroperitoneal nodes
Stage IV	Distant metastases with positive pleural cytology or intraparenchymal liver metastases

Note. Recommended surgical staging includes unilateral salpingo-oophorectomy (possible bilateral salpingo-oophorectomy /hysterectomy) with peritoneal cytology, biopsies, omentectomy, retroperitoneal lymphadenectomy. Adapted from the FIGO staging.[26]

the need for postoperative adjuvant therapy; however, gynecologic oncologists need to be aware that this may not be the standard practice in pediatric patients who undergo surgery with other specialists.

Chemotherapy

Postoperative chemotherapy has been generally recommended for all malignant germ cell tumors with the exception of stage I dysgerminomas and stage I immature teratomas (low grade). There has been a recent trend toward the consideration of surveillance in all stage I germ cell tumors, as many contend that recurrences are almost always successfully treated with salvage therapy; this would obviate the need for initial adjuvant chemotherapy and eliminate chemotherapy-associated short- and long-term adverse sequelae.[1,3,27] Given the rarity of this disease and the overall excellent prognosis of patients with stage I disease, no randomized trial comparing surveillance with adjuvant therapy in adults will likely ever be undertaken, although a surveillance study has been completed (but not reported) in the COG for all stage I malignant germ cell tumors.

To evaluate the strategy of surveillance after surgery for all stage IA germ cell patients, Patterson et al[27] reported a recurrence rate of 22% in dysgerminomas and a 36% recurrence rate for the other types. Additionally, they reported a salvage/cure rate of 90% in patients with recurrent disease. The authors concluded that all patients with stage I disease may be safely observed; however, their recurrence rates are much higher than those reported for stage I patients receiving adjuvant treatment, and not all recurrences were cured. Further, this was a small study with 37 patients (some previously

reported), and this limits the conclusions.[27] In other studies reported in the late 1990s and early 2000s, 3 groups evaluated surveillance alone in stage I germ cell tumors (83 patients), with an overall survival rate of 97%; 92% (12 of 13) of those patients who experienced disease recurrence were subsequently cured with chemotherapy.[3,28-31] A recent study by Vicus et al[32] of pure dysgerminomas found that the recurrence rate for stage IA patients without adjuvant therapy was 22% compared with 0 for those who received adjuvant treatment; again, all patients who experienced recurrence were cured. Of note, only 4 patients of the entire 65 patients in that study underwent full surgical staging (including lymphadenectomy and omentectomy).

Ultimately, the choice of adjuvant chemotherapy for stage I germ cell malignancy remains controversial and is influenced by both patient and physician preferences. Chemotherapy may be overtreatment for many women, whereas surveillance may represent undertreatment for others who might not be cured at the time of recurrence. Especially, in the absence of full surgical staging, the recurrence rates for presumed stage I malignant germ cell tumors will be approximately 20% to 40%.

Historically, the cure rate for malignant germ cell tumors has been exceedingly poor, as all women with advanced-stage disease died, and a minority of even patients with presumed stage I disease survived before the advent of chemotherapy.[3] Initially, vincristine, actinomycin D, and cyclophosphamide (VAC) was used, and cure rates improved. With the advent of platinum agents, cure for this disease, even in advanced stages, is the rule rather than the exception. The mainstay of platinum-based regimens for this disease is currently BEP, and this is the recommended primary adjuvant therapy according to several large Gynecologic Oncology Group studies as well as the National Comprehensive Cancer Network guidelines.[1,3,5,18,25] A common adult regimen is bleomycin 30 units/wk, etoposide 100 mg/m^2/d for 5 days, and cisplatin 20 mg/m^2/d for 5 days on a 4-week schedule, but multiple other dosing schemes are reported. For other patients for whom toxicity concerns are a priority, an alternate regimen is etoposide (120 mg/m^2/d for 3 days) and carboplatin (400 mg/m^2 on day 1) for 3 cycles on a 4-week schedule or EP (BEP regimen without the bleomycin). Other active regimens that have been used include cisplatin, vincristine, methotrexate, and bleomycin (POMB); vinblastine, bleomycin, and cisplatin; actinomycin D, cyclophosphamide, and etoposide (ACE); or vincristine, ifosfamide, and cisplatin (VIP).

Most women who present with advanced-stage disease at diagnosis still undergo surgical staging and/or debulking followed by chemotherapy. Given the extremely chemosensitive nature of the disease, however, there have been recent reports advocating the possible use of neoadjuvant chemotherapy (where chemotherapy is given before surgical resection) and fertility preservation. Raveendran et al[33] reported 2 patients with advanced germ cell tumors who underwent neoadjuvant chemotherapy (BEP) and had no viable tumor at interval surgery with excellent survival.

Radiation

Germ cell tumors are also very radiosensitive, with excellent responses after radiation therapy. Since the advent of effective chemotherapy, however, the use of radiation in the adjuvant setting for germ cell tumors has been largely abandoned due to the detrimental effects on future fertility and the potential for late side effects. In the past, women with dysgerminomas were treated with either pelvic and para-aortic radiation or whole abdominal radiation with cure rates approaching 100% for early stage and approximately 60% for advanced disease.[5,32]

SURVIVAL AND PROGNOSIS

Key Points

1. In general, survival for germ cell tumors is excellent, and most women are cured with surgery and chemotherapy.
2. Advanced stage remains the most important negative prognostic factor.
3. Elevated initial tumor markers may portend worse prognosis.

The overall survival for malignant ovarian germ cell tumors remains excellent, and the reported 5-year survival rates range from 80% to 97% and vary according to well-established prognostic factors, particularly stage.[2,4,9,14,24,27,34-36] Since the advent of platinum-based chemotherapy, cure rates for stage I disease are almost 100%, and even in advanced disease, cure rates approach 75%.[3]

Stage remains the most important prognostic factor in determining both recurrence risk and overall survival.[1,3,5,35-37] Almost all stage I/II cancers are cured, but patients with advanced-stage disease are more likely to experience recurrence. For example, Chan et al[36] reported a significant survival difference (97.6% for stage I/II vs. 85.5% for stage III/IV); $P < .0001$) for all germ cell tumors in a recent SEER analysis. All advanced-stage tumors were treated with adjuvant chemotherapy as described previously. Similarly, the presence of lymph node involvement (denoting advanced stage) in a recent SEER analysis conferred a 3-fold increase risk of death compared with women without lymph node involvement.[4]

Tumor marker elevation (primarily hCG and AFP) at diagnosis has been relatively consistently linked to increased recurrence rates (3- to 4-fold relative risk), but although this finding has been consistent, it is not necessarily universal.[5,37,38] Failure to normalize tumor markers indicates persistent disease and mandates further treatment.

Histologic type has also been found to be indicative of recurrence. Dysgerminomas have a better prognosis than the other types and have less recurrence risk.[3,5,35,36] In a comparison of the impact of the 3 main histologic types, dysgerminomas appear to have the best 5-year survival rates, followed by immature teratomas and then endodermal sinus tumors (99.5% vs. 94.3% vs. 85.5%; $P < .0001$).[36] Lai et al[35] found a 100% 5-year overall survival rate for the dysgerminoma and immature teratoma patients compared with 80% other types combined ($P = .0004$). Data on endodermal sinus tumors are limited to case series from single institutions or SEER data but indicate a 5-year survival rate of 72% to 90%.[36,39-41] Of note, these tumors may more often be late stage; in one series, 31% of patients with endodermal sinus tumors experienced recurrence (all within 8 months), and only 1 patient was cured.[39]

Racial disparities have also been documented, with black and white women having lower survival rates compared with other nonwhites; it has been hypothesized that this discrepancy for black women may represent diminished access to treatment.[2] Another study found a difference in survival for white compared with blacks (92% vs. 86%; $P = .02$) . However, on multivariate analysis that controlled for complete surgical staging, stage, and histologic type, this difference was no longer significant.[9]

MANAGEMENT OF RECURRENT DISEASE

Key Points

1. The majority of women with recurrent disease naïve to chemotherapy can be treated and cured.
2. Most recurrences are diagnosed within a year and very rarely after 2 years. Options for platinum-resistant disease are limited.

Most recurrences of germ cell tumors occur within the first year, and almost none is ever reported after 2 years of follow-up.[1,3,5,35,37,38] Recurrences are most often detected by tumor markers but also are detected on physical or radiographic imaging. For those patients who did not receive initial chemotherapy and then experience recurrence during surveillance, BEP remains the drug regimen of choice, with an almost 100% cure rate. When including all patients with recurrent germ cell tumors, the overall salvage rate for recurrence, however, is approximately 50%.[3] The optimal treatment of recurrent cancer in those women previously treated with BEP is less clear, in part due to the paucity of patients, and regimens have been adopted based on the testicular germ cell trials. Some small studies suggest a role for high-dose salvage chemotherapy with stem cell transplant, with successful long-term cures documented, but most data on this modality are from the testicular germ cell tumors.[35,42] Other options that have been reported with varying success include all the previously mentioned chemotherapeutic combinations in upfront therapy (eg, BEP, VIP, PVB, POMB, ACE) as well as some new regimens undergoing evaluation, including paclitaxel/carboplatin/ifosfamide, gemcitabine, oxaliplatin/paclitaxel, and targeted therapies including bevacizumab, sunitinib, and flavopiridol.

Data supporting a role for surgical resection for chemotherapy-refractory recurrent disease are limited. In one of the only case series reported, Munkarah et al[43] demonstrated limited efficacy and suggested that the role of secondary cytoreductive surgery might be limited to immature teratoma.

SPECIAL MANAGEMENT ISSUES

Fertility Preservation

Because most women with germ cell tumors are of reproductive age, fertility-sparing surgery has become the standard of care and does not adversely affect clinical outcomes.[1,3,5,14,18,22-24,27,36,37,44] Fertility-sparing surgery is defined as preserving the uterus at a minimum and usually preserving the normal contralateral ovary

as well. A recent SEER database review found that the median age of patients with germ cell tumors in the United States was 23 years, and the vast majority of patients had stage I or II disease. In this review, 41% received fertility-preserving surgery; this percentage increased over the time period studied, with almost half (48.4%) having fertility preservation for the most recent time period examined (1998-2001).[36] There were no significant survival differences observed between women treated with fertility-preserving surgery compared with those undergoing hysterectomy and bilateral salpingo-oophorectomy.

For those young women who undergo fertility preservation, several studies have documented that most will return or attain normal menstrual function, even after chemotherapy administration.[14,44,45] Yoo et al[45] found that 89% of prepubertal girls and 94% of adolescents treated with chemotherapy (primarily BEP), subsequently experienced normal menses; similarly, Biswajit[14] reported 100% resumption of normal menses after treatment with chemotherapy. Gershenson et al[44] surveyed 132 women who had undergone treatment for germ cell malignancies and found that approximately 54% had fertility preservation and 87% of those still reported normal menstrual function; successful pregnancies were reported in approximately a third of the fertile women (of note, almost 40% were using birth control at the time of the survey). Several other authors have also reported that women can achieve pregnancy after treatment for germ cell tumors: Tangir et al[46] reported 76%, Zanetta et al[47] reported 86%, and de La Motte Rouge[40] reported that 75% of women who attempted pregnancy were able to conceive.

Long-Term Sequelae of Treatment

Given the young age at diagnosis, women undergoing treatment for germ cell tumors also can develop late effects relating to therapy (primarily chemotherapy). In addition to the hormonal and reproductive factors addressed previously, women can develop from delayed puberty, irregular menses, and premature menopause. Of note, germ cell cancer survivors who were younger at diagnosis and report fewer gynecologic symptoms have associated better physical functioning.[48] Additionally, women may develop neurotoxicity due to chemotherapy, and this finding is the most highly predictable for decreased physical quality of life.[48] In comparing germ cell survivors with controls, survivors were more likely to report high blood pressure, high cholesterol, and chronic functional problems, including numbness, tinnitus, or nausea, but were less likely to report joint pain or muscle cramps.[49] Most survivors have a quality of life comparable to that of controls with these minimal exceptions.

One of the most devastating potential late toxicities is the development of a secondary malignancy; this is most commonly attributed to etoposide and/or cisplatin and may approach 1% of all patients.[5]

FUTURE DIRECTIONS

Young women with malignant germ cell tumors have generally excellent cancer-specific outcomes and can return to almost normal life after treatment. Further research needs to confirm whether surveillance can replace adjuvant chemotherapy in all presumed stage I cancers, even if comprehensive surgical staging has not been performed. Additional therapies are needed for the rare platinum-refractory recurrences, and this may be anti-angiogenesis agents or other targeted therapies.

Sex Cord-Stromal Ovarian Tumors

Sex cord-stromal ovarian tumors are considered rare ovarian tumors and comprise between 3% and 10% of all ovarian malignancies. Because of their relative rarity, treatment guidelines are based on limited data that combine histologic subtypes. In general, most ovarian stromal tumors are clinically indolent and are reported to have excellent long-term prognoses. However, many occur in adolescent and reproductive-aged women, and therefore, individualized treatment with consideration for fertility preservation is of great importance. Appropriate treatment guidelines are based on individual factors and consist of surgical staging, tumor reduction, and systemic therapy. Stromal tumors of the ovary represent a small portion of ovarian cancers, but are important to distinguish from other types of ovarian neoplasms, because their histologic origin, natural history, and treatment recommendations are distinct from other ovarian cancer histologies.

EPIDEMIOLOGY

Key Points

1. The majority of sex cord-stromal cell tumors occur in women of reproductive age.
2. Sex cord-stromal tumors account for 10% to 15% of all childhood ovarian malignancies.
3. Adult granulosa cell tumors represent the most common histologic subtype.

Ninety percent of ovarian malignancies are epithelial in origin, with the remaining 10% comprising sex cord-stromal tumors, germ cell tumors, soft tissue tumors not specific to the ovary, unclassified tumors, and metastatic tumors.[50] The histologic classification of ovarian stromal tumors is presented in Table 14-5.[50] Estimates from the SEER database between 1975 and 1998 suggest that for each 5-year interval between ages 15 and 40 years, the incidence of non–germ cell ovarian malignancy increases from 8 per million to 79 per million women per year.[51] However, these data are not specific for stromal ovarian tumors. In general, it has been estimated that malignant stromal tumors of the ovary account for between 3% and 10% of all ovarian malignancies.[52-54]

Granulosa cell tumors, the most common histologic subtype, comprise between 2% and 5% of all ovarian cancers and represent 90% of stromal ovarian tumors, yielding an incidence of 0.58 to 1.6 cases per 100,000 women.[55-57] Both adult- and juvenile granulosa cell tumors occur, with the adult subtype representing

Table 14-5 World Health Organization for Classification of Stromal Tumors of the Ovary

I. Granulosa stromal cell tumors
Granulosa cell tumors
Juvenile
Adult
Thecomas/fibromas
Thecoma
Fibroma
Cellular fibroma
Fibrosarcoma
Stromal tumor with minor sex cord elements
Sclerosing luteoma
Unclassified (fibrothecoma)
II. Sertoli-stromal cell tumors; androblastomas
Well differentiated
Sertoli Cell tumor; androblastoma
Sertoli-Leydig cell tumor
Leydig cell tumor
Intermediate differentiation
Variant, with heterologous elements
Poorly differentiated (sarcomatoid)
Variant, with heterologous elements
Retiform
Mixed
III. Sex cord stromal with annular tubules (SCTAT)
IV. Gynandroblastoma
V. Steroid (lipid) cell tumor
Stromal luteoma
Leydig cell tumor
VI. Unclassified

95% of all granulosa cell tumors. Most adult granulosa cell tumors occur during the reproductive or perimenopausal years, whereas most juvenile types occur during childhood and adolescence. The designation of juvenile versus adult granulosa cell tumors is not based on age alone, as they are distinct in natural history and pathologic characteristics.

Many of these tumors occur in adolescent and young women and require special consideration with regard to fertility preservation. Although most adolescents and young adults with ovarian malignancies do have ovarian germ cell tumors, 10% to 15% of childhood ovarian tumors are sex cord-stromal,[58] with juvenile granulosa cell tumors most often occurring in childhood and Sertoli-Leydig cell tumors and unclassified sex cord-stromal tumors occurring during puberty.[59] One study identified 38 cases of pediatric ovarian tumors, and 15% were stromal ovarian tumors, all of which were juvenile granulosa cell tumors.[60] Neonatal presentations of juvenile granulosa cell tumors also occur.[11]

Thecomas, fibromas, and fibrothecomas usually occur in postmenopausal women. The mean age at diagnosis is 48 years, and only 10% of patients are less than 30 years of age.[61,62] These tumors are most often benign and are not usually considered to be malignant. However, ovarian fibromas are the most common type of ovarian stromal tumor, and when combined, these tumors account for 1% of all ovarian neoplasms.

Sertoli-Leydig cell tumors may contain only Sertoli cells, only Leydig cells, or both. These rare tumors represent fewer than 1% of all ovarian tumors. They are classified into 5 groups: well differentiated, intermediately differentiated, poorly differentiated, retiform, and mixed. Sertoli-Leydig cell tumors tend to occur in young adult women with a mean age of 25 years. Intermediate and poorly differentiated tumors tend to be more aggressive and occur approximately 10 years earlier than intermediate or poorly differentiated tumors. The retiform type is usually diagnosed at an even younger age than intermediate or poorly differentiated types.[63,64] Both isolated Sertoli tumors and Sertoli-Leydig tumors usually occur in women in their teens and 20s. Thus fertility preservation is an important consideration in many of these patients, and this is usually appropriate, as more than 95% of all tumors are unilateral with a normal uterus.[65-67]

Sex cord tumor with annular tubules (SCTAT), first described by Scully[68] in 1970, was identified in association with Peutz-Jeghers syndrome. Approximately 15% of these tumors are associated with adenoma malignum of the cervix.[69] These tumors are uncommon in adolescents, but have been reported to present with isosexual precocity.[70]

Gynandroblastomas are a separate, rare type of stromal tumor, which occur most often during the third to fifth decades of life and account for fewer than 1% of all ovarian stromal tumors.[71]

Steroid (lipid) cell tumors consist of stromal luteomas, Leydig cell tumors, and steroid cell tumors not otherwise specified. In combination, these 3 neoplasms represent fewer than 0.1% of all ovarian tumors. Stromal luteomas are benign lesions that represent approximately one-fourth of steroid cell tumors. These may occur during pregnancy but are most common during the postmenopausal years. Leydig cell tumors represent 15% to 20% of all steroid cell tumors of the ovary and usually occur in postmenopausal women. Steroid cell tumors not otherwise specified are the most common type of steroid cell tumor and can be malignant and quite aggressive. Steroid cell tumors not otherwise specified present at a mean age of 43 years.

Sclerosing stromal tumor of the ovary is an extremely rare benign ovarian neoplasm that occurs primarily in women under 30 years of age and is usually unilateral.[72]

DIAGNOSIS

Key Points

1. Women with sex cord-stromal tumors typically present with signs and symptoms of a pelvic mass.
2. Women with granulosa cell tumors may present with hemoperitoneum.
3. Elevations in inhibin A, inhibin B, and/or CA-125 serum levels may suggest a sex cord-stromal tumor preoperatively.

The definitive diagnosis of an ovarian sex cord-stromal tumor is based on histologic evaluation of the removed tumor specimen. However, the history and physical examination, radiographic imaging, and laboratory testing may suggest the diagnosis preoperatively.

In a woman with a pelvic mass, a detailed patient history may offer suggestions regarding the tumor histology. The patient is often in her adolescent or young adult years, as noted previously. She may present with symptoms of a pelvic mass, including bloating, pelvic pressure or pain, increase in abdominal girth, and gastrointestinal or urinary symptoms. Abdominal pain may be a presenting complaint, especially in patients with hemoperitoneum resulting from a granulosa cell tumor. The physical examination usually suggests a pelvic mass. In the case of a ruptured granulosa cell tumor, signs of hemoperitoneum can include abdominal tenderness, peritoneal signs, a fluid wave, and even hemodynamic instability.

Because stromal tumors of the ovary arise from steroid-producing cells, these tumors are often hormonally active, producing estrogen, progesterone, and androgens. Therefore, hirsutism, virilism, and/or isosexual precocious puberty may be present.[73] During the reproductive years, patients may present with menorrhagia, irregular menstrual bleeding, and amenorrhea. Postmenopausal patients may report vaginal bleeding, breast enlargement or tenderness, and vaginal cornification.[74]

Patients with adult granulosa cell tumors can frequently present with abnormal vaginal bleeding, abdominal distention and/or pain, and occasionally signs of virilism and usually present with a unilateral pelvic mass.[74,75] The potential for a hereditary component has been suggested in a report regarding 2 first-degree relatives, but this observation is isolated. Therefore, family history should not be assumed to be a risk factor or suggest a diagnosis.[76]

Patients with a juvenile granulosa cell tumor typically present with a palpable mass on pelvic or rectal examination, and more than 95% are unilateral.[77,78] An association has been described between juvenile granulosa cell tumors and Ollier disease (enchondromatosis) and Maffucci syndrome (enchondromatosis and hemangiomatosis). An increased risk for the development of breast cancer has also been reported.[79]

Thecomas are often hormonally active and may cause abnormal vaginal bleeding as the most common presenting symptom. Endometrial hyperplasia occurs in 37% to 50% of patients with thecomas, and up to 27% have an associated endometrial carcinoma.[61,62,80] Therefore, any patient presenting with abnormal bleeding should always have the endometrium sampled preoperatively. Thecomas may also be luteinized, which may cause androgen production and virilization.[81]

In contrast, fibromas are usually benign, unilateral, and hormonally inactive tumors, and therefore, patients may present with pelvic pressure or pain and a mass. Approximately 30% of patients with tumors more than 6 cm in size have ascites. This can lead to hydrothorax in 1% of patients with fibromas; the constellation of hydrothorax, ascites, and ovarian fibroma is known as Meigs syndrome.[82]

Sertoli-Leydig cell tumors cause virilization in approximately 50% of patients. This finding is independent of tumor size.[63] Patients with SCTAT usually present with abnormal vaginal bleeding, and abdominal pain and intussusception have been reported. Gynandroblastomas present with symptoms and signs related to estrogen and androgen overproduction in 60% of patients. These patients may have virilization in the setting of endometrial hyperplasia.[83] Also, most gynandroblastomas are appreciated on the pelvic examination because of their size. Approximately 50% of patients with steroid cell tumors demonstrate androgenic changes.[84]

During the diagnostic and/or preoperative evaluation, abnormal uterine bleeding should prompt consideration for an endometrial biopsy. In women of reproductive age, pregnancy must first be excluded. Because endometrial hyperplasia can result from excess estrogen production by the ovarian stromal tumor, the endometrium must be evaluated, either preoperatively or intraoperatively upon the diagnosis of an ovarian stromal tumor.[85]

Imaging tests, including transvaginal ultrasound, CT, and MRI, may prove useful in the diagnosis of the adnexal mass but are nonspecific for ovarian sex cord-stromal tumors. The findings may also identify hemoperitoneum or ascites. Adult granulosa cell tumors have variable amounts of solid, cystic, hemorrhagic, and necrotic components, so they may appear as solid masses, multilocular cystic lesions, or completely cystic tumors.[86] Ultrasound often shows increased vascularity by color flow Doppler.[87]

In contrast, Sertoli-Leydig cell tumors often appear as well-defined solid enhancing mass with cysts within the tumor on CT and appear hypointense with multiple variable-sized cystic areas on MRI. The amount of fibrous stroma determines the low-signal intensity on T2-weighted MRI.[86] Radiographically, 79% of thecomas are solid on CT and show delayed accumulation of contrast material.[88] Fibromas appear as hypointense on T1-weighted MRI with very low-signal intensity on T2-weighted imaging, often with dense calcifications.[86]

Preoperative laboratory tests that may be helpful include inhibin A, inhibin B, and, less often, CA-125, in addition to routine preoperative laboratory testing. These levels may act as tumor markers, facilitating preoperative diagnosis but more importantly serving as a baseline by which to judge efficacy of therapy.[89,90]

PATHOLOGY

Key Points

---

1. Adult-type granulosa cells demonstrate grooved "coffee-bean" nuclei, and frequently exhibit Call-Exner bodies.
2. Leydig cell tumors may exhibit crystals of Reinke.

Specialized gonadal stromal cells and their precursors can give rise to sex cord-stromal tumors of the ovary, originating within one or both ovaries, either as an isolated histologic subtype or in combination. The WHO classification is presented in Table 14-5.[50] Specifically, granulosa cells and Sertoli cells arise from sex cord cells, whereas theca cells, Leydig cells, lipid cells, and fibroblasts arise from stromal cells and their pluripotential mesenchymal precursors.

Adult granulosa cell tumors represent 95% of granulosa cell tumors, whereas juvenile granulosa cell

Meigs Synd: ovarian fibroma, hydrothorax, ascites.

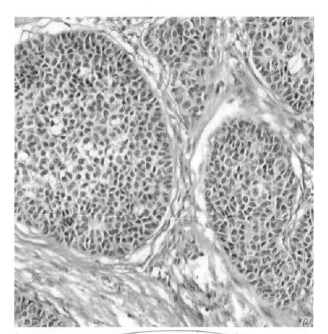

FIGURE 14-6. Adult granulosa cell tumor. Hematoxylin and eosin stain, ×100. Insulae of uniformly staining cells are seen with Call-Exner bodies throughout.

& grooved coffee bean nuclei

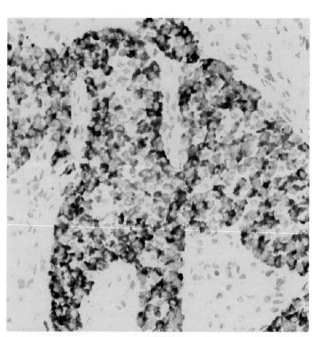

FIGURE 14-7. Juvenile granulosa cell tumor immunostained for inhibin A. Hematoxylin and eosin stain, ×100. Uniform cells are seen amid an edematous, loose stroma. Cytoplasmic staining for inhibin A is present in the majority of cells.

tumors represent 5% of granulosa cell tumors. The gross appearance of both subtypes is similar, most commonly presenting with a tumor with cystic and solid components. Microscopic examination reveals 2 characteristics that distinguish juvenile from adult granulosa cell tumors: the nuclei of juvenile granulosa cell tumors are rounded and hyperchromatic with moderate to abundant eosinophilic or vacuolated cytoplasm, and the theca cell component is luteinized in juvenile granulosa cell tumors (Figures 14-6 and 14-7).[91] Adult type tumors demonstrate granulosa cells with grooved "coffee bean" nuclei; furthermore, they may exhibit Call-Exner bodies, a histologic finding characterized by a rosette arrangement of cells around a central eosinophilic fluid space.

Thecomas and fibromas have significant overlap. Often, these tumors cannot be assigned to either the distinct thecoma or fibroma category based on the clinical or microscopic examination.[91] Thecomas are composed of lipid-laden stromal cells that may or may not demonstrate luteinization. When these tumors exhibit nuclear atypia and mitoses, they may represent low-grade stromal sarcomas or fibrosarcomas and may have a malignant course.[92] Fibromas are usually solid and white, with an average size of 6 cm.[93] Approximately 10% of fibromas show light microscope evidence of hypercellularity, as well as pleomorphism and mitoses. Tumors of low malignant potential (cellular fibromas) are designated as those with an increased cellular density, mild nuclear atypia, and fewer than 3 mitotic figures per high-power field. Fully malignant fibrosarcomas

have greater cellular density, marked pleomorphism, and more than 10 mitoses per high-power field. These tumors are highly aggressive and are usually large, unilateral, and highly vascular, with rupture, adhesions, hemorrhage, and necrosis often seen at the time of surgery.[94]

Sertoli-stromal cell tumors, or androblastomas, represent a group of tumors that differentiate toward testicular structures. These tumors were originally named arrhenoblastomas in 1931 by Meyer, but were renamed Sertoli-Leydig cell tumors in 1958 by Morris and Scully.[95] On gross examination, Sertoli-Leydig cell tumors are solid or mixed cystic and solid (Figure 14-8). There are no features pathognomonic for Sertoli-Leydig cell tumors grossly. The size ranges from microscopic to 25 cm.[63] Well-differentiated tumors tend to be smaller than poorly differentiated tumors.[64] Well-differentiated tumors, which account for 11% of cases, have a predominantly tubular pattern on light microscopy. The Sertoli cells are cuboidal or columnar with round nuclei, but with no prominent nucleoli. Atypical nuclei are absent or rare, and few mitotic figures are seen. The stroma consists of nest of Leydig cells. As seen in Table 14-1, the most common variants are intermediate differentiation (54%) and poor differentiation (13%). These subgroups are characterized by a continuum of different patterns and combinations of cell types, with both Sertoli and Leydig components exhibiting various degrees of maturity.

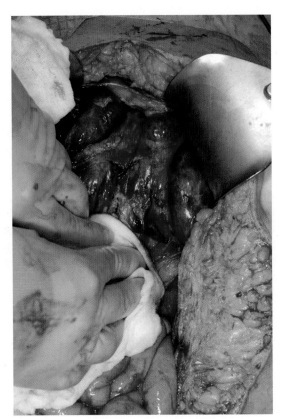

FIGURE 14-8. Gross photograph of Sertoli-Leydig cell tumor. Recurrent tumor filled the abdomen and pelvis, invading small bowel, diaphragm, and liver. Tumor appears as dark maroon, hemorrhagic, fleshy, and solid.

A retiform component is present in 15% of tumors, demonstrating tubules and cysts arranged in a pattern that resembles the rete testis (Figure 14-9).

SCTATs are characterized by either simple or complex ring-shaped tubules. It is controversial whether

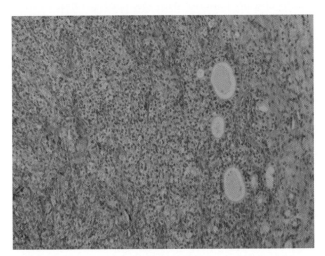

FIGURE 14-9. Sertoli-Leydig cell tumor demonstrates both Sertoli and Leydig cells in trabeculae. Hematoxylin and eosin stain, ×100.

these tumors are more closely related to granulosa cell tumors or Sertoli-Leydig cell tumors, as the cellular elements appear to be somewhat intermediate in nature, but they do seem to represent a distinct entity.[91]

Gynandroblastomas comprise granulosa cell elements, tubules, and Leydig cells. The specific cell of origin remains debated, but it may arise from undifferentiated mesenchyme.[71] Most of these tumors are solid and large, measuring between 7 and 10 cm in size, with yellow-white cystic areas present. Microscopically, these tumors show unequivocal granulosa/theca cell elements, must be well differentiated, and must demonstrate intimate mixing of all the constituent cell types.[71]

Steroid cell tumors consist of stromal luteomas, Leydig cell tumors, and steroid cell tumors not otherwise specified. Stromal luteomas are often small; half measure less than 5 cm.[96] Microscopically, they consist of large, rounded or polyhedral cell resembling Leydig cells, luteinized ovarian stromal cells, and adrenocortical cells. Leydig cell tumors are subdivided into tumors of hilar and non-hilar type, and both are benign. Inspection reveals small, unilateral tumors with a median size less than 3 cm.[97] Histologically, they consist solely of Leydig cells, and crystals of Reinke are seen. These crystals are intracytoplasmic rectangular structures seen in up to 40% of Leydig tumors. Steroid cell tumors not otherwise specified are larger than the other steroid cell tumors with an average size of 8.5 cm and are often bilateral. These lipid cell tumors lack the specific characteristics of stromal luteomas or Leydig cell tumors. The strongest prognostic factor other than stage is the number of mitotic figures, because more than 90% of tumors with more than 2 mitoses per 10 high-power fields are malignant.[96]

Vascular endothelial growth factor is overexpressed in a majority of stromal ovarian tumors, which may account for the vascularity, angiogenesis, and response to anti-angiogenic agents.[98] Inhibin and calretinin may also be helpful immunohistochemical stains to aid in the pathologic diagnosis of sex cord-stromal ovarian tumors.[99,100] SF-1 is a diagnostically useful immunohistochemical marker that aids in the differential diagnosis of Sertoli cell tumors.[101]

Of interest, a single recurrent somatic mutation (402 C to G) in the *FOXL2* gene has been identified as occurring in adult granulosa cell tumors.[102] Validation and confirmation as a driver mutation have yet to be published.

TREATMENT

Key Points

1. Staging and tumor cytoreductive surgery (with metastatic disease) is essential at the time of diagnosis of a sex cord-stromal tumor.

2. Routine lymphadenectomy is not required for a complete staging procedure, as lymphatic metastases are exceedingly rare.
3. Adjuvant chemotherapy consists of bleomycin, etoposide, and cisplatin versus paclitaxel and a platinum agent; these regimens are currently being compared in a randomized trial.

Surgical Therapy and Staging

The appropriate treatment of stromal ovarian tumors is determined by patient age, parity, desire for future fertility, extent of disease, and comorbid conditions. The goals of surgical therapy are accurate diagnosis, removal of the mass, comprehensive staging, tumor cytoreduction when disseminated disease is present, and preservation of fertility when desired and feasible in patients of reproductive age.

Intraoperative pathologic diagnosis is often difficult, and intraoperative determination of the precise histology may be impossible. Therefore, general guidelines should be applied for nonepithelial ovarian tumors during the initial operative management, and the need for adjuvant or additional therapy should be determined based on the final pathology results. With close attention to detail, the need for reoperation and more extensive surgery can be minimized. Alternatively, the frozen section diagnosis may be rendered in the intraoperative setting, in which case guidelines for specific stromal ovarian tumors can be followed.

In general, a preoperative discussion should be held with any woman of childbearing age who has an adnexal mass regarding her wishes for future fertility depending on operative findings. This conversation, although difficult, is better discussed preoperatively with the patient than intraoperatively with the next of kin when a malignancy is encountered.[67]

Minimally invasive surgery (laparoscopy with or without robotic assistance) is appropriate in the occasional patient with a small solid adnexal mass or complex ovarian cyst.[103,104] However, any patient with a large, solid adnexal mass or evidence of hemodynamic instability should undergo laparotomy through a vertical skin incision to remove the mass without morcellation and allow for appropriate surgical staging or tumor reductive surgery.[56]

The surgical procedure consists of pelvic washings and evacuation of hemoperitoneum, if present. The site of hemorrhage is most commonly the mass itself, and therefore surgical removal may stop the bleeding. A unilateral mass in a patient of any age should be removed by unilateral salpingo-oophorectomy and sent for immediate intraoperative histologic evaluation.[56,67] Cystectomy, rupture, and morcellation of suspicious masses should be avoided.[105] Intraoperative rupture of granulosa cell tumors during laparoscopic management can result in subsequent peritoneal seeding and convert an early-stage malignancy to one with disseminated disease.[105] When laparoscopy is the initial approach, a bag with an extended incision should be used or the procedure should be converted to a laparotomy to avoid morcellation. If a cystectomy is initially performed and the frozen section returns as a stromal ovarian tumor, the remainder of the adnexa should immediately be removed, as cystectomy is not adequate therapy.[67, 106] It should be noted that "conservative management" of these tumors invariably describes unilateral salpingo-oophorectomy with conservation of the uterus and normal-appearing contralateral ovary in the setting of limited disease. Therefore, unilateral salpingo-oophorectomy is the initial step in the treatment of patients with disease apparently confined to 1 ovary.[67,106]

Once an ovarian sex cord-stromal tumor is diagnosed, exploration of the abdominopelvic cavity should be performed, inspecting all peritoneal surfaces and abdominopelvic organs. A complete staging procedure should be performed, including cytologic evaluation of each hemidiaphragm, infracolic omentectomy, and peritoneal biopsies from each paracolic gutter, the vesicouterine fold, and the pouch of Douglas. Additionally, biopsies of any suspicious areas should be performed. The bowel should be inspected from the ileocecal valve to the ligament of Treitz, with specific evaluation for tumor implants and sites of obstruction. Maximal tumor cytoreductive surgery should be performed in patients with advanced disease, preferably leaving the patient with no macroscopic disease.[67,106]

Historically, pelvic and para-aortic lymphadenectomy were performed as a component of surgical staging. However, lymph node metastasis in stromal ovarian tumors is extremely rare.[107,108] In one report examining 58 patients with sex cord-stromal ovarian tumors who had lymph nodes sampled during primary surgery, none had positive nodes.[108] Therefore, lymphadenectomy may be omitted in the staging of patients with this disease.

Patients who have completed childbearing should undergo total abdominal hysterectomy and bilateral salpingo-oophorectomy, regardless of the stage of disease. However, preservation of fertility should always be attempted in young patients seeking future fertility.[67] If the contralateral ovary and/or uterine serosa are grossly involved by tumor, the uterus and both adnexae should be removed. If the contralateral ovary and uterine serosa appear normal, conservative management with preservation of the uterus and contralateral adnexa is safe and appropriate, as 95% of sex cord-stromal tumors are unilateral.[66,67,74,106] Staging should still be performed. Fertility-sparing surgery does not obviate the need for staging and refers to the safe preservation of a normal-appearing contralateral ovary and uterus in the setting of apparent limited disease.

Some sex cord-stromal tumors may present with abnormal uterine bleeding. In this case, a preoperative endometrial biopsy or intraoperative endometrial curettage should be performed to exclude endometrial hyperplasia or malignancy. If a uterine malignancy is encountered, the uterus should be removed regardless of patient age.[85]

When juvenile granulosa cell tumors are diagnosed intraoperatively, most are diagnosed as stage IA tumors.[77,78] It is essential to stage each of these patients, because platinum-based chemotherapy is recommended for any patient with disease over stage IA.

Conversely, thecomas, fibromas, and fibrothecomas are uniformly benign, so surgical resection alone without staging or adjuvant treatment is the appropriate therapy. Because many of these patients are diagnosed after their reproductive years, fertility preservation is rarely appropriate.[74]

The management of patients with Sertoli-Leydig cell tumors follows the preceding guidelines, and fertility preservation is important for many of these patients. In patients of reproductive age, a unilateral salpingo-oophorectomy and staging is usually appropriate, as 95% of lesions are unilateral.[66,67] In patients finished with childbearing, a total hysterectomy and bilateral salpingo-oophorectomy with staging procedure is indicated.[74]

Ovarian SCTATs occur in 2 clinical subgroups. The first is associated with Peutz-Jeghers syndrome and is typically multifocal, bilateral, small, and almost always benign. Such patients should be carefully assessed for adenoma malignum of the cervix, as 15% of patients have an occult lesion,[69] and hysterectomy should be strongly considered. The second subgroup of ovarian SCTATs is unrelated to Peutz-Jeghers syndrome and presents with larger tumors with a significant potential for malignant behavior. The basis of treatment remains surgical resection.

Patients with gynandroblastomas require surgical staging, and metastatic tumor should be resected. However, stromal luteomas and Leydig cell tumors are benign and do not require staging or postoperative therapy. Childbearing potential should be maintained in the occasional young patient with this diagnosis. Conversely, steroid cell tumors not otherwise specified can be malignant and aggressive, and therefore, when a steroid cell tumor is diagnosed intraoperatively, staging and aggressive surgical resection of metastases should be performed.

Adjuvant Therapy

Because sex cord-stromal tumors are rare ovarian neoplasms, clinical trials designed to determine which treatment regimens are best for specific histologic subtypes of this disease are not feasible. Most published studies combine most or all subtypes of stromal ovarian tumors, and therefore treatment recommendations are based on limited data. Most data have been gathered from patients with adult granulosa cell tumors, but occasionally other tumor types are encountered, and treatment is generalized to these types as well.[67,75]

Adjuvant therapy is not indicated for patients with surgically staged stage I disease.[109] Patients with stage IC disease may benefit from some adjuvant therapy, either using platinum-based chemotherapy or hormonal therapy with leuprolide acetate.[62]

Patients with more advanced disease are typically treated with combination chemotherapy. The data regarding platinum-based therapy originated in the 1970s and 1980s. Several investigators published anecdotal reports of several complete and partial responses to platinum-containing regimens, including VAC, doxorubicin/cisplatin, cyclophosphamide/doxorubicin/cisplatin, and altretamine/cisplatin.[110-112] Colombo[113] subsequently investigated bleomycin, vinblastine, and cisplatin in patients with newly diagnosed advanced disease and found that 9 of 11 patients responded but with severe toxicity. Later trials used etoposide in place of vinblastine, and in 1996, Gershenson[114] reported an 83% response rate in 9 patients with advanced stromal tumors of the ovary. In 1999, Homesley[115] reported the utility of bleomycin, etoposide, and cisplatin (BEP) in 57 evaluable patients with stage II to IV disease. Sixty-one percent of patients experienced grade 4 myelotoxicity, and several cases of pulmonary toxicity occurred, but 69% of patients with advanced-stage primary and 51% of patients with recurrent disease remained progression free. The progression-free interval was 24 months. As a result, many patients have been treated with 3 to 4 courses of BEP, and this has become a commonly used treatment for patients with stromal ovarian tumors. Most recently, paclitaxel and carboplatin combination therapy have been reported to be effective in stromal tumors with fewer toxic effects compared with BEP.[116,117] Of 22 newly diagnosed patients, 11 treated with BEP and 11 treated with a taxane/platinum regimen, 9 patients in each group were without evidence of disease at the completion of chemotherapy. No differences were detected in response rate, progression-free survival, or overall survival.[117] Confirmation of equivalent outcomes between these 2 regimens awaits performance of a larger prospective randomized trial, which is currently underway.

More than 90% of patients with Sertoli-Leydig cell tumors have stage IA disease. This is largely dependent on grade, with well-differentiated tumors tending to be of limited stage. Only one death from disease has been reported in a patient with a well-differentiated tumor. However, 10% of intermediate, 60% of poorly differentiated, and 20% of retiform and heterologous subtypes show malignant behavior. Therefore, patients with Sertoli-Leydig cell tumors staged IC disease or greater, with poorly differentiated tumors of any stage, or with heterologous elements should receive adjuvant therapy with either BEP or paclitaxel and carboplatin.[118] Radiation and hormone therapy have been described,[64] but there is very limited information on which to base treatment.

Patients with steroid cell tumors not otherwise specified who have tumors that are pleomorphic, have an increased mitotic count, are large, or are at an advanced stage should be treated with additional postoperative platinum-based chemotherapy.[119]

No prospective randomized studies showing the value of radiotherapy in stromal ovarian tumors exist, but several retrospective studies have demonstrated the utility of radiation therapy in select patients with advanced disease.[120,121]

SURVIVAL AND PROGNOSIS

Key Points

1. In general, ovarian sex cord-stromal tumors follow an indolent clinical course.
2. These tumors may recur on multiple occasions with long disease-free intervals.
3. Juvenile granulosa cell tumors, Sertoli-Leydig cell tumors with poor prognostic factors, and steroid cell tumors not otherwise specified can be aggressive.
4. Stromal luteomas, fibromas, and thecomas follow a benign course.

Several large series have reported on survival and prognostic factors of ovarian sex cord-stromal tumors.[55,62] The overall 20-year survival rate of women with this disease approximates 40%. The strongest prognostic factor is the stage at presentation, with the 5- to 10-year survival rate being more than 90% for stage I, 55% for stage II, and 25% for stage III tumors. The natural history of adult granulosa cell tumors is characterized by late recurrence, sometimes over a decade after the initial diagnosis. The average time to recurrence is 5 to 10 years. Poor prognostic factors include tumor size, rupture, and bilaterality. In patients with stage I disease, the recurrence rate is rare in tumors less than 5 cm, 20% in tumors 5 to 15 cm in size, and more than 30% in tumors greater than 15 cm.[122]

Overall, the prognosis for patients with juvenile granulosa cell tumor is favorable but is related to stage. The 5-year survival rate for patients with stage IA disease is 99%, but this declines to 60% for patients with advanced disease.[71]

The prognosis of patients with Sertoli-Leydig cell tumors is related to grade, stage, and histologic subtype. Patients with well-differentiated tumors tend to be of early stage. Such patients have an excellent prognosis, with no reports of advanced stage or recurrence, and only 1 death from disease has been reported in a patient with a well-differentiated tumor. However, 10% of intermediate, 60% of poorly differentiated, and 20% of retiform and heterologous subtypes show malignant behavior.[118]

Unfortunately, eventual prognosis is poor for recurrent stromal ovarian tumors, and the overall mortality rate is 70% in the recurrent setting despite treatment.[62]

MANAGEMENT OF RECURRENT DISEASE

Key Points

1. Multiple tumor cytoreductive surgeries may be employed in the treatment of recurrent sex cord-stromal tumors.
2. Chemotherapy, radiation therapy, and hormonal therapy may be useful in treating recurrent disease.
3. Anti-angiogenic therapy has a biologic basis and may be an option for treating recurrent disease refractory to traditional chemotherapy regimens.

Patients with recurrent disease may achieve long-term survival through secondary cytoreductive surgery, sometimes on multiple occasions after long treatment-free intervals.[116] In cases of widespread disease or disease refractory to surgery, chemotherapy and hormonal therapy are options for treatment. The most effective chemotherapeutic regimens appear to be platinum-based, with either BEP or a taxane-platinum combination most commonly used, yielding similar response rates of 54% and 72%, respectively.[117]

Other chemotherapeutic agents with demonstrated response include carboplatin; cisplatin, doxorubicin, and cyclophosphamide; etoposide and cisplatin; VAC; oral etoposide; topotecan; liposomal doxorubicin; paclitaxel; and ifosfamide and etoposide. Paclitaxel and carboplatin remain the most commonly used single agents at first and second relapse.[116]

Likely due to the expression of steroid receptors, responses have been reported after treatment with gonadotropin-releasing hormone antagonists, progestins, and aromatase inhibitors.[123,124]

The use of radiation for the treatment of recurrent disease has also been reported, with some responses noted in patients with localized or symptomatic disease. However, based on the small numbers of patients, the data are anecdotal, the response rates are short, and the impact on survival remains unknown.[125]

Antiangiogenic agents have also been investigated in patients with recurrent adult granulosa cell tumor, due to the overexpression of vascular endothelial growth factor and vascularity of these tumors. Promising results have been noted, and a cooperative group trial investigating bevacizumab is currently underway.[98]

SPECIAL MANAGEMENT PROBLEMS

Key Points

1. Consideration of fertility preservation is key in patients with limited disease.
2. Inadequate staging at the initial surgery may require consideration of repeat surgery for staging versus careful observation.

Fertility preservation has been discussed under Surgical Considerations. This is an important issue in many patients with ovarian sex cord-stromal tumors, as the age distribution is often among women of reproductive age. Because the majority of tumors are unilateral and disease is often grossly confined, unilateral salpingo-oophorectomy can safely be performed with preservation of a normal-appearing contralateral adnexa and uterus. In the unlikely event of bilateral ovarian involvement with a normal-appearing uterus, both adnexae should be removed and the uterus can be preserved for consideration of donor egg–assisted reproduction post-treatment. A key feature of such conservative management is a preoperative discussion with any patient in whom a stromal ovarian tumor is suspected.[67]

The treatment of patients who have had inadequate staging is a difficult issue. Limited information exists regarding the best course of action for these patients. If the patient has documented large amounts of residual disease after a limited initial attempt at tumor reduction, repeat surgical exploration with staging and tumor-reductive surgery would be reasonable. If the patient has had an inadequate exploration, such as through a small Pfannenstiel incision or through a limited laparoscopy, more information needs to be collected before making a decision about postsurgical treatment. Several options may be considered, including repeat laparoscopic or open exploration with full surgical staging or, in some circumstances, a physical examination, CT, and measurement of serum inhibin and serum CA-125 levels. If the results of all of these are negative, the decision may be made to observe the patient clinically, with or without hormonal suppression

therapy using leuprolide acetate. Lack of lymphadenectomy during staging, however, should not warrant reoperation, as the risk of nodal involvement approaches zero.[108]

FUTURE DIRECTIONS

Research in rare tumors is a difficult issue and is best performed in a cooperative group setting. Currently, the Gynecologic Oncology Group is partnering internationally in a randomized phase II trial to determine the most effective therapy—BEP versus paclitaxel and carboplatin—for patients with newly diagnosed advanced and recurrent chemotherapy-naive patients with ovarian sex cord-stromal tumors. Additionally, bevacizumab is being investigated for use in patients with recurrent ovarian sex cord-stromal tumors in a phase II trial of the Gynecologic Oncology Group. The results of these trials will provide solid recommendations for treatment in patients with newly diagnosed and recurrent disease.

One of the most interesting facets of recent research has been the elucidation of the *FOXL2* gene mutation as a suspected driver mutation for the development of adult granulosa cell tumors.[102] Further research into the mechanism of this mutation and targeted therapy directed against this gene may provide new avenues of understanding and novel therapy for patients with ovarian stromal tumors.

REFERENCES

1. Patterson DM, Rustin GJ. Controversies in the management of germ cell tumours of the ovary. *Curr Opin Oncol.* 2006;18(5):500-506.
2. Smith HO, Berwick M, Verschraegen CF, et al. Incidence and survival rates for female malignant germ cell tumors. *Obstet Gynecol.* 2006;107(5):1075-1085.
3. Gershenson DM. Management of ovarian germ cell tumors. *J Clin Oncol.* 2007;25(20):2938-2943.
4. Kumar S, Shah JP, Bryant CS, et al. The prevalence and prognostic impact of lymph node metastasis in malignant germ cell tumors of the ovary. *Gynecol Oncol.* 2008;110(2):125-132.
5. Pectasides D, Pectasides E, Kassanos D. Germ cell tumors of the ovary. *Cancer Treat Rev.* 2008;34(5):427-441.
6. Chen Z, Robison L, Giller R, et al. Environmental exposure to residential pesticides, chemicals, dusts, fumes, and metals, and risk of childhood germ cell tumors. *Int J Hyg Environ Health.* 2006;209(1):31-40.
7. Chen Z, Robison L, Giller R, et al. Risk of childhood germ cell tumors in association with parental smoking and drinking. *Cancer.* 2005;103(5):1064-1071.
8. Chen Z, Stewart PA, Davies S, et al. Parental occupational exposure to pesticides and childhood germ-cell tumors. *Am J Epidemiol.* 2005;162(9):858-867.
9. Bryant CS, Kumar S, Shah JP, et al. Racial disparities in survival among patients with germ cell tumors of the ovary—United States. *Gynecol Oncol.* 2009;114(3):437-441.

10. Poynter JN, Radzom AH, Spector LG, et al. Family history of cancer and malignant germ cell tumors in children: a report from the Children's Oncology Group. *Cancer Causes Control.* 2010;21(2):181-189.

11. Giambartolomei C, Mueller CM, Greene MH, Korde LA. A mini-review of familial ovarian germ cell tumors: an additional manifestation of the familial testicular germ cell tumor syndrome. *Cancer Epidemiology.* 2009;33(1):31-36.

12. Michala L, Goswami D, Creighton S, Conway G. Swyer syndrome: presentation and outcomes. *BJOG.* 2008;115(6): 737-741.

13. Jonson AL, Geller MA, Dickson EL. Gonadal dysgenesis and gynecologic cancer. *Obstet Gynecol.* 2010;116(suppl 2):550-552.

14. Biswajit D, Patil CN, Sagar TG. Clinical presentation and outcome of pediatric ovarian germ cell tumor: a study of 40 patients. *J Pediatr Hematol Oncol.* 2010;32(2):e54-e56.

15. Oltmann SC, Fischer A, Barber R, Huang R, Hicks B, Garcia N. Pediatric ovarian malignancy presenting as ovarian torsion: incidence and relevance. *J Pediatr Surg.* 2010;45(1):135-139.

16. Vaysse C, Delsol M, Carfagna L, et al. Ovarian germ cell tumors in children. Management, survival and ovarian prognosis. A report of 75 cases. *Journal of Pediatric Surgery.* 2010;45(7): 1484-1490.

17. Alotaibi MOS, Navarro OM. Imaging of ovarian teratomas in children: a 9-year review. *Can Assoc Radiol J.* 2010;61(1): 23-28.

18. National Comprehensive Cancer Network. NCCN Clinical Practice Guidelines in Oncology: Ovarian Cancer, Vol 2010. http://www.nccn.org. Accessed February 24, 2010.

19. Sturgeon CM, Duffy MJ, Stenman U-H, et al. National Academy of Clinical Biochemistry Laboratory Medicine Practice Guidelines for Use of Tumor Markers in Testicular, Prostate, Colorectal, Breast, and Ovarian Cancers. *Clin Chem.* 2008;54(12):e11-e79.

20. Crum C. The female genital tract. In: Kumar V, AbbasAK, Fausto N, eds. *Robbins and Cotran Pathologic Basis of Disease.* 4th ed. Philadelphia, PA: Elsevier; 2005.

21. Beiner ME, Gotlieb WH, Korach Y, et al. Cystectomy for immature teratoma of the ovary. *Gynecol Oncol.* 2004;93(2):381-384.

22. Palenzuela G, Martin E, Meunier A, et al. Comprehensive staging allows for excellent outcome in patients with localized malignant germ cell tumor of the ovary. *Ann Surg.* 2008;248(5):836-841.

23. Billmire DF. Germ cell tumors. *Surg Clin North Am.* 2006;86(2): 489-503, xi.

24. Billmire D, Vinocur C, Rescorla F, et al. Outcome and staging evaluation in malignant germ cell tumors of the ovary in children and adolescents: an intergroup study. *J Pediatr Surg.* 2004;39(3):424-429; discussion 424-429.

25. Rogers PC, Olson TA, Cullen JW, et al. Treatment of children and adolescents with stage II testicular and stages I and II ovarian malignant germ cell tumors: A Pediatric Intergroup Study—Pediatric Oncology Group 9048 and Children's Cancer Group 8891. *J Clin Oncol.* 2004;22(17):3563-3569.

26. Current FIGO staging for cancer of the vagina, fallopian tube, ovary, and gestational trophoblastic neoplasia. *Int J Gynecol Obstet.* 2009;105(1):3-4.

27. Patterson DM, Murugaesu N, Holden L, Seckl MJ, Rustin GJ. A review of the close surveillance policy for stage I female germ cell tumors of the ovary and other sites. *Int J Gynecol Cancer.* 2008;18(1):43-50.

28. Cushing B, Giller R, Ablin A, et al. Surgical resection alone is effective treatment for ovarian immature teratoma in children and adolescents: a report of the pediatric oncology group and the children's cancer group. *Am J Obstet Gynecol.* 1999;181(2):353-358.

29. Marina NM, Cushing B, Giller R, et al. Complete surgical excision is effective treatment for children with immature teratomas with or without malignant elements: A Pediatric

Oncology Group/Children's Cancer Group Intergroup Study. *J Clin Oncol.* 1999;17(7):2137-2143.

30. Gobel U, Schneider DT, Calaminus G, Haas RJ, Schmidt P, Harms D. Germ-cell tumors in childhood and adolescence. GPOH MAKEI and the MAHO study groups. *Ann Oncol.* 2000;11(3):263-271.

31. Baranzelli MC, Bouffet E, Quintana E, Portas M, Thyss A, Patte C. Non-seminomatous ovarian germ cell tumours in children. *Eur J Cancer.* 2000;36(3):376-383.

32. Vicus D, Beiner ME, Klachook S, Le LW, Laframboise S, Mackay H. Pure dysgerminoma of the ovary 35 years on: a single institutional experience. *Gynecol Oncol.* 2010;117(1):23-26.

33. Raveendran A, Gupta S, Bagga R, et al. Advanced germ cell malignancies of the ovary: should neo-adjuvant chemotherapy be the first line of treatment? *J Obstet Gynaecol.* 2010;30(1):53-55.

34. Billmire DF. Malignant germ cell tumors in childhood. *Semin Pediatr Surg.* 2006;15(1):30-36.

35. Lai CH, Chang TC, Hsueh S, et al. Outcome and prognostic factors in ovarian germ cell malignancies. *Gynecol Oncol.* 2005;96(3):784-791.

36. Chan JK, Tewari KS, Waller S, et al. The influence of conservative surgical practices for malignant ovarian germ cell tumors. *J Surg Oncol.* 2008;98(2):111-116.

37. Murugaesu N, Schmid P, Dancey G, et al. Malignant ovarian germ cell tumors: identification of novel prognostic markers and long-term outcome after multimodality treatment. *J Clin Oncol.* 2006;24(30):4862-4866.

38. Tangjitgamol S, Hanprasertpong J, Manusirivithaya S, Wootipoom V, Thavaramara T, Buhachat R. Malignant ovarian germ cell tumors: clinico-pathological presentation and survival outcomes. *Acta Obstet Gynecol Scand.* 2010;89(2):182-189.

39. Cicin I, Saip P, Guney N, et al. Yolk sac tumours of the ovary: evaluation of clinicopathological features and prognostic factors. *Eur J Obstet Gynecol Reprod Biol.* 2009;146(2):210-214.

40. de La Motte Rouge T, Pautier P, Duvillard P, et al. Survival and reproductive function of 52 women treated with surgery and bleomycin, etoposide, cisplatin (BEP) chemotherapy for ovarian yolk sac tumor. *Ann Oncol.* 2008;19(8):1435-1441.

41. Shah JP, Kumar S, Bryant CS, et al. A population-based analysis of 788 cases of yolk sac tumors: a comparison of males and females. *Int J Cancer.* 2008;123(11):2671-2675.

42. Muller AM, Ihorst G, Waller CF, Dolken G, Finke J, Engelhardt M. Intensive chemotherapy with autologous peripheral blood stem cell transplantation during a 10-year period in 64 patients with germ cell tumor. *Biol Blood Marrow Transplant.* 2006;12(3):355-365.

43. Munkarah A, Gershenson DM, Levenback C, et al. Salvage surgery for chemorefractory ovarian germ cell tumors. *Gynecol Oncol.* 1994;55(2):217-223.

44. Gershenson DM, Miller AM, Champion VL, et al. Reproductive and sexual function after platinum-based chemotherapy in long-term ovarian germ cell tumor survivors: a Gynecologic Oncology Group Study. *J Clin Oncol.* 2007;25(19):2792-2797.

45. Yoo S-C, Kim WY, Yoon J-H, Chang S-J, Chang K-H, Ryu H-S. Young girls with malignant ovarian germ cell tumors can undergo normal menarche and menstruation after fertility-preserving surgery and adjuvant chemotherapy. *Acta Obstet Gynecol Scand.* 2010;89(1):126-130.

46. Tangir J, Zelterman D, Ma W, Schwartz PE. Reproductive function after conservative surgery and chemotherapy for malignant germ cell tumors of the ovary. *Obstet Gynecol.* 2003; 101(2):251-257.

47. Zanetta G, Bonazzi C, Cantu M, et al. Survival and reproductive function after treatment of malignant germ cell ovarian tumors. *J Clin Oncol.* 2001;19(4):1015-1020.

48. Champion V, Williams SD, Miller A, et al. Quality of life in long-term survivors of ovarian germ cell tumors: A Gynecologic Oncology Group Study. *Gynecol Oncol.* 2007;105(3):687-694.

49. Matei D, Miller AM, Monahan P, et al. Chronic physical effects and health care utilization in long-term ovarian germ cell tumor survivors: a Gynecologic Oncology Group study. *J Clin Oncol.* 2009;27(25):4142-4149.

50. World Health Organization. *International Histologic Classification of Tumors, No. 9.* Geneva, Switzerland: World Health Organization; 1973.

51. Brown J. Female genital tract cancer. In: Bleyer A, O'Leary M, Barr R, Ries LAG, eds. Cancer Epidemiology in Older Adolescents and Young Adults 15-29 Years of Age, Including SEER Incidence and Survival: 1975-2000. NIH Pub No. 06-5767. Bethesda, MD: National Cancer Institute; 2006

52. Gershenson DM, Copeland LJ, Kavanagh JJ, et al. Treatment of metastatic stromal tumors of the ovary with cisplatin, doxorubicin, and cyclophosphamide. *Obstet Gynecol.* 1987;70:765-769.

53. Jacobs AJ, Deppe G, Cohen CJ. Combination chemotherapy of ovarian granulosa cell tumor with cis-platinum and doxorubicin. *Gynecol Oncol* 1982;14:294-297.

54. Koonings PP, Campbell K, Mishell DR Jr, et al. Relative frequency of primary ovarian neoplasms: a 10-year review. *Obstet Gynecol* 1989;74:921-926.

55. Bjorkholm E, Silfversward C. Granulosa and theca cell tumors: incidence and occurrence of second primary tumors. *Acta Radiol Oncol.* 1980;19:161.

56. Schumer ST, Cannistra SA. Granulosa cell tumor of the ovary. *J Clin Oncol.* 2003;21:1180-1189.

57. Stenwig JT, Hazekamp JT, Beecham JB. Granulosa cell tumors of the ovary: a clinicopathologic study in 118 cases with long term follow-up. *Gynecol Oncol.* 1979;7:136.

58. Schultz KA, Sencer SF, Messinger Y, et al. Pediatric ovarian tumors: a review of 67 cases. *Pediatr Blood Cancer.* 2005;44:167-173.

59. Schneider DR, Calaminus G, Harms D, et al. Ovarian sex cord-stromal tumors in children and adolescents. *J Reprod Med* 2005;50:439-446.

60. Gribbon M, Ein SH, Mancer K. Pediatric malignant ovarian tumors: a 43-year review. *J Pediatr Surg* 1992;27:480.

61. Bjorkholm E, Silfverswand C. Theca cell tumors: clinical features and prognosis. *Acta Radiol.* 1980;19:241.

62. Evans AT, Gaffey TA, Malkasian GD, et al. Clinicopathological review of 118 granulosa and 82 thecal cell tumors. *Obstet Gynecol.* 1980;55:231.

63. Roth LM, Anderson MC, Govan DT, et al. Sertoli-Leydig cell tumors: a *clinicopathologic* study of 34 cases. *Cancer.* 1981;48:187.

64. Zaloudek C, Norris HJ. Sertoli-Leydig tumors of the ovary: a clinicopathologic study of 64 intermediate and poorly differentiated neoplasms. *Am J Surg Pathol.* 1984;8:405.

65. Alam K, Maheshwari V, Rashid S. Bilateral Sertoli-Leydig cell tumor of the ovary: a rare case report. *Indian J Pathol Microbiol.* 2009;52:97-99.

66. Gershenson DM. Management of early ovarian cancer: germ cell and sex cord stromal tumors. *Gynecol Oncol.* 1994;55(suppl):S62-S72.

67. Gershenson DM. Fertility-sparing surgery for malignancies in women. *J Natl Cancer Inst Monographs.* 2005;34:43-47.

68. Scully RE. Sex cord tumor with annular tubules: a distinctive ovarian tumor of the Peutz-Jeghers syndrome. *Cancer.* 1970;25:1107.

69. Srivasta PJ, Keeney GL, Podratz KC. Disseminated cervical adenoma malignum and bilateral ovarian sex cord tumors with annular tubules associated with Peutz-Jeghers syndrome. *Gynecol Oncol.* 1994;53:256.

70. Nosov V, Park S, Rao J, et al. Non-Peutz-Jeghers syndrome associated ovarian sex cord tumor with annular tubules: a case report. *Fert Ster.* 2009;92:1497.

71. Anderson MC, Rees DA. Gynandroblastoma of the ovary. *Br J Obstet Gynecol.* 1975;82:68.

72. Chang W, Oiseth SJ, Orentlicher R, et al. Bilateral sclerosing stromal tumor of the ovaries in a premenarchal girl. *Gynecol Oncol.* 2006;101:342-345.

73. Young RH, Scully RE. Endocrine tumors of the ovary. *Curr Topics Pathol.* 1992;85:113-164.

74. Gershenson DM, Hartmann LC, Young RH. Ovarian sex cord-stromal tumors. In: Hoskins WJ, Perez CA, Young RC, eds. *Principles and Practice of Gynecologic Oncology*, 4th ed. Philadelphia, PA: Lippincott Williams & Wilkins; 2004.

75. Nakashima N, Young RH, Scully RE. Androgenic granulosa cell tumors of the ovary. *Arch Pathol Lab Med.* 1984;108:786.

76. Stevens TA, Brown J, Zander DS, et al. Adult granulosa cell tumors of the ovary in two first-degree relatives. *Gynecol Oncol.* 2005;98:502-525.

77. Lack EE, Perez-Atayde AR, Murthy ASK, et al. Granulosa theca cell tumors in premenarchal girls: a clinical and pathological study of ten cases. *Cancer.* 1981;48:1846.

78. Young RH, Dickersin GR, Scully RE. Juvenile granulosa cell tumor of the ovary. *Am J Surg Pathol.* 1984;8:575.

79. Schoefield DE, Fletcher JA. Trisomy 12 in pediatric granulosa-stromal cell tumors. *Am J Pathol.* 1992;141:1265.

80. Stage AH, Grafton WD. Thecomas and granulosa-theca cell tumors of the ovary: an analysis of 51 tumors. *Obstet Gynecol.* 1977;50:21.

81. Zhang J, Young RH, Arseneau J, et al. Ovarian stromal tumors containing lutein or Leydig cells—a clinicopathologic analysis of fifty cases. *Int J Gynecol Pathol.* 1982;1:270.

82. Meigs JV. Fibroma of the ovary with ascites and hydrothorax—Meigs syndrome. *Am J Obstet Gynecol.* 1954;67:962.

83. Novak ER. Gynandroblastoma of the ovary: review of 8 cases from the Ovarian Tumor Registry. *Obstet Gynecol.* 1967;30:709.

84. Powell JL, Dulaney DP, Shiro BC. Androgen-secreting steroid cell tumor of the ovary. *Southern Med J.* 2000;93:1201-1204.

85. Unkila-Kallio L, Tiitinen A, Wahlstrom T, et al. Reproductive features in women developing ovarian granulosa cell tumour at a fertile age. *Hum Reprod.* 2000;15:589-593.

86. Jung SE, Rha SE, Lee JM, et al. CT and MRI findings of sex cord-stromal tumor of the ovary. *Am J Roentgen.* 2005;185:207-215.

87. Van Holsbeke C, Domali E, Holland TK. Imaging of gynecological disease: clinical and ultrasound characteristics of granulosa cell tumors of the ovary. *Ultrasound Obstet Gynecol.* 2008;31:450-456.

88. Bazot M, Ghossain MA, Buy JN, et al. Fibrothecomas of the ovary: CT and US findings. *J Comput Assist Tomogr.* 1993;17:754.

89. Choi YL, Kim HS, Ahn G. Immunoexpression of inhibin alpha subunit, inhibin/activin beta subunit, and CD 99 in ovarian tumors. *Arch Pathol Lab Med.* 2000;124:563-569.

90. Robertson DM, McNeilage J. Inhibins as biomarkers for reproductive cancer. *Semin Reprod Med.* 2004;22:219-225.

91. Brown J, Jhingran A, Deavers M, et al. Stromal tumors of the ovary. In: Raghaven D, Brecher ML, Johnson DH, et al, eds. *Textbook of Uncommon Cancer.* West Sussex, UK: John Wiley and Sons; 2006

92. Waxman M, Vultein JC, Urcuyo R, et al. Ovarian low grade stromal sarcoma with thecomatous features. *Cancer.* 1979;44:2206.

93. Dockherty MB, Masson JC. Ovarian fibromas: a clinical and pathologic study of two hundred and eighty three cases. *Am J Obstet Gynecol.* 1944;47:741.

94. Prat J, Scully RE. Cellular fibromas and fibrosarcomas of the ovary. *Cancer.* 1981;47:2663.

95. Morris JM, Scully RE. *Endocrine Pathology of the Ovary.* St. Louis, MO: Mosby; 1958.

96. Hayes MC, Scully RE. Stromal luteoma of the ovary: a clinicopathologic analysis of 25 cases. *Int J Gynecol Pathol.* 1987;6:313.

CHAPTER 14

97. Roth LM, Sternberg WH. Ovarian stromal tumors containing Leydig-cells. II. Pure Leydig-cell tumor, non-hilar type. *Cancer.* 1973;32:952.

98. Tao X, Sood AK, Deavers MT, et al. Anti-angiogenesis therapy with bevacizumab for patients with ovarian granulosa cell tumors. *Gynecol Oncol.* 2009;114:431-436.

99. McCluggage WG, Maxwell P, Sloan JM. Immunohistochemical staining of ovarian granulosa cell tumors with monoclonal antibody against inhibin. *Hum Pathol.* 1997;28:1034-1038.

100. Rishi M, Howard LN, Brathauer GL, et al. Use of monoclonal antibody against human inhibin as a marker for sex cord-stromal tumors of the ovary. *Am J Surg Pathol.* 1997;21:583-589.

101. Zhao C, Barner R, Vinh TN, et al. SF-1 is a diagnostically useful immunohistochemical marker and comparable to other sex cord-stromal tumor markers for the differential diagnosis of ovarian sertoli cell tumor. *Int J Gynecol Pathol.* 2008;27:507-514.

102. Shah SP, Kobel M, Senz J, et al. Mutation of FOXL2 in granulosa-cell tumors of the ovary. *N Engl J Med.* 2009;360:2719-2729.

103. Canis M, Mage G, Pouly JL, et al. A 12 year experience with long term follow-up. *Obstet Gynecol.* 1994;83:707-712.

104. Mettler L, Semm K, Shive K. Endoscopic management of adnexal masses. *J Soc Laparosc Surg.* 1997;2:103-112.

105. Salani R, Goodrich K, Song C, et al. Three case reports of laparoscopic management of granulosa cell tumor with intraoperative rupture and subsequent upstaging. *J Min Invasive Gynecol.* 2008;15:511-513.

106. Schumer ST, Cannistra SA. Granulosa cell tumor of the ovary. *J Clin Oncol.* 2003;21:1180-1189.

107. Abu-Rustum NR, Restivo A, Ivy J, et al. Retroperitoneal nodal metastasis in primary and recurrent granulosa cell tumors of the ovary. *Gynecol Oncol.* 2006;103:31-34.

108. Brown J, Sood AK, Deavers MT, et al. Patterns of metastasis in sex cord-stromal tumors of the ovary: can routine staging lymphadenectomy be omitted? *Gynecol Oncol.* 2009;113:86-90.

109. Herbst AL. Neoplastic diseases of the ovary. In: Mishell DR, Stenchever MA, Droegemueller W, Herbst AL, eds. *Comprehensive Gynecology.* 3rd ed. New York, NY: Mosby-Year Book; 1997.

110. Camlibel FT, Caputo TA. Chemotherapy of granulosa cell tumors. *Am J Obstet Gynecol.* 1983;145:763-765.

111. Jacobs AJ, Deppe G, Cohen CJ. Combination chemotherapy of ovarian granulosa cell tumor with cis-platinum and doxorubicin. *Gynecol Oncol.* 1982;14:294-297.

112. Neville AJ, Gilchrist KW, Davis TE. The chemotherapy of granulosa cell tumors of the ovary: experience of the Wisconsin Clinical Cancer Center. *Med Pediatric Oncol.* 1984;12:397-400.

113. Colombo N, Sessa C, Landoni F, et al. Cisplatin, vinblastine, and bleomycin combination chemotherapy in metastatic granulosa cell tumor of the ovary. *Obstet Gynecol.* 1986;37:265-268.

114. Gershenson DM, Morris M, Burke TW, et al. Treatment of poor-prognosis sex cord-stromal tumors of the ovary with the combination of bleomycin, etoposide, and cisplatin. *Obstet Gynecol.* 1996;87:527-531.

115. Homesley HD, Bundy BN, Hurteau JA, et al. Bleomycin, etoposide, and cisplatin combination chemotherapy of ovarian granulosa cell tumors and other stromal malignancies: a Gynecologic Oncology Group study. *Gynecol Oncol.* 1999;72:131-137.

116. Brown J, Shvartsman HS, Deavers MT, et al. The activity of taxanes in the treatment of sex cord-stromal ovarian tumors. *J Clin Oncol.* 2004;22:3517-3523.

117. Brown J, Shvartsman HS, Deavers MT, et al. The activity of taxanes compared with bleomycin, etoposide, and cisplatin in the treatment of sex cord-stromal ovarian tumors. *Gynecol Oncol.* 2005;97:489-496.

118. Brown J, Gershenson DM. Treatment for rare ovarian malignancies. In: Eifel PJ, Gershenson DM, Kavanagh JJ, Silva EG, eds. *M.D. Anderson Cancer Care Series Gynecologic Cancer.* New York, NY: Springer-Verlag; 2006.

119. Khoo SK, Buntine D. Malignant stromal tumor of the ovary with virilizing effects in an XXX female with streak ovaries. *Aust N Z J Obstet Gynecol.* 1980;20:123.

120. Savage P, Constenla D, Fisher C, et al. Granulosa cell tumors of the ovary: demographics, survival, and the management of advanced disease. *Clin Oncol (R Coll Radiol).* 1998;10:242-245.

121. Wessalowski R, Spaar HJ, Pape H, et al. Successful liver treatment of a juvenile granulosa cell tumor in a 4-year-old chile by regional deep hyperthermia, systemic chemotherapy, and irradiation. *Gynecol Oncol.* 1995;57:417-422.

122. Bjorkholm E, Silfversward C. Prognostic factors in granulosa-cell tumors. *Gynecol Oncol.* 1981;11:261-274.

123. Martikainen H, Penttinen J, Huhtaniemi I, et al. Gonadotropin-releasing hormone agonist analog therapy effective in ovarian granulosa cell malignancy. *Gynecol Oncol.* 1989;35:406.

124. Tresukosol D, Kudelka AP, Edwards CL, et al. Recurrent ovarian granulosa cell tumor: a case report of a dramatic response to Taxol. *Int J Gynecol Cancer.* 1995;5:156-159.

125. Wolf JK, Mullen J, Eifel PJ, et al. Radiation treatment of advanced or recurrent granulosa cell tumor of the ovary. *Gynecol Oncol.* 1999;73:35-41.

Breast Cancer and Related Diseases

Catherine M. Dang and M. William Audeh

Breast cancer is the most common malignancy in women throughout the world, and particularly in Westernized, developed countries. The relative roles of genetic, environmental, and lifestyle factors in explaining the high incidence of breast cancer in the modern world is a subject of much debate. However, it is clear that the complex biology of the human breast and its involvement in the reproductive cycle is also the basis for the increased susceptibility of this organ to malignant transformation.[1]

EPIDEMIOLOGY

Key Points

1. The most significant risk factors for breast cancer include increasing age and deleterious mutations in the *BRCA1* and *BRCA2* genes.
2. Reproductive factors that contribute to breast cancer risk are related to the length of estrogen and progesterone exposure.
3. The total number of ovulatory cycles promotes an increased estrogenic exposure that can modulate breast cancer risk.

Breast cancer remains the most common cancer diagnosed in women worldwide. In the United States, more than 209,060 new cases of breast cancer are expected in 2011.[2] Despite the preponderance of epidemiologic studies examining risk factors and causes of breast cancer, only very few highly significant risk factors, such as increasing age and deleterious mutations in the *BRCA* genes, have been identified.[3] Epidemiologic factors reproducibly associated with increased risk of breast cancer are shown in Table 15-1.[4-6] Although increasing age is recognized as a universal risk factor for many cancers, including that of the breast, reproductive factors play a significant role in modulating breast cancer risk. The common thread appears to be the timing and length of exposure to estrogen and progesterone, and the age at which a pregnancy is first carried to term, leading to differentiation of the breast epithelium, lactation, and eventual involution. Furthermore, breast density, as measured on mammography, appears to be an anatomical surrogate for the glandular and potentially proliferative cellular content of the breast and is increasingly recognized as an additional marker of risk.[7] In addition, a growing body of evidence supports the cancer-promoting effect of increasing length of exposure of the breast tissue to estrogen and progestin as a result of the use of postmenopausal hormone replacement therapy (HRT).[8] The use of as little as 2 years of postmenopausal HRT yields an increased risk.[9]

Beyond purposeful exposure to postmenopausal HRT, however, there are the underlying changes in the lifestyle of women in Westernized, developed countries and societies that also affect hormonal factors.[8,10] Women in such societies have on average earlier onset of menses, later and fewer full-term pregnancies, and a lesser likelihood of breast feeding than women in less developed societies, where the rates of breast cancer are much lower. The overall result of these factors

Table 15-1 Risk Factors for Breast Cancer

Risk Factor	Relative Risk (at extremes)
General	
Age (20-70 years)	30
Body mass index	2
Exposure	
Alcohol intake	1.2
Passive smoking	1.2
Hormone replacement therapy	2
Chest irradiation during adolescence	30
Reproductive/hormonal	
Age of menarche	2
Age of first live birth	3
Age of menopause	4
Breast density	6
Family history	
First-degree relative with breast cancer	3
Second-degree relative with breast cancer	1.5

Modified from Gail,[18] Li and Rosen,[21] and Mack et al.[22]

Table 15-2 Germ-line Genes Associated With Increased Risk of Breast Cancer

BRCA1
BRCA2
p53
PTEN
CHEK2
ATM
NBS1
RAD50
BRIP1
PALB2

is to dramatically increase the total number of ovulatory cycles a woman may undergo in her lifetime. Although this increased estrogen effect has been primarily attributed to lifestyle and reproductive history, worldwide environmental exposure to estrogenic compounds is of increasing concern, with potential sources being dietary phytoestrogens, xenobiotic pesticides, and plastic-related exposures to estrogenic substances such as dioxin and bisphenol-A.[11,12]

Efforts to identify genetic factors associated with breast cancer risk have succeeded in identifying very likely all highly penetrant, but relatively rare genes, which are associated with positive family history of cancer[13] (Table 15-2). These genes are all involved in DNA damage detection and repair and, when mutated, confer extremely high lifetime risks of breast (and other) cancers. Of all the identified high-penetrance genes associated with breast cancer, the *BRCA1* and *BRCA2* genes account for as much as 5% or 10% of all breast cancers, with the lifetime risk of breast cancer in mutation carriers ranging from 55% to 87%.[14,15]

The search for genetic factors which may affect the risk of breast cancer in women without a family history has involved genome-wide association studies, seeking genetic markers and polymorphisms.[16] These studies have yielded a growing list of common genetic variants and polymorphisms that exert their effect by modest functional changes, rather than loss of function

through mutation. The strongest candidate for a "universal" breast cancer risk factor is fibroblast growth factor receptor 2 (*FGFR2*),[16,17] in which single nucleotide polymorphisms (SNPs) have been associated with risk of breast cancer. However, as this and the 6 other major risk-associated SNPs were identified from unselected populations in genome-wide searches, no gene–environment or gene–gene interactions have been defined, and no functional biologic associations have been proposed. Therefore, attempts to combine these 7 SNPs with traditional epidemiologic risk factors, as developed in the Gail model, have failed to show any additional predictive power with the addition of this level of genetic information.[18]

The pathogenesis of breast cancer is complex. The evolutionary function of the breast in all mammals is primarily to provide nourishment to newly born offspring. Therefore, breast development and differentiation to provide this function in the female is limited to the reproductive years; it is not required to begin until puberty and is no longer required after menopause. As a result, the breast tissue is minimally formed during embryogenesis, with a single epithelial ectodermal bud, and grows postnatally but without differentiation in keeping with body size. Breast tissue then enters a phase of rapid proliferation and ductal branching with puberty.[1] The development of the breasts under the influence of pituitary and ovarian hormones at the onset of puberty is a so-called invasive process, in which branching morphogenesis by the epithelial ductal tree spreads through the mammary fat pad. The tips of the branching structure are the terminal end buds (TEBs), in which highly proliferative cells drive growth and expansion through the stroma. This process is driven by molecular pathways involved in the so-called epithelial-mesenchymal transition, similar to those seen in embryogenesis, as well as those frequently identified in aggressive invasive malignancies[19] (Figure 15-1). Molecular pathways

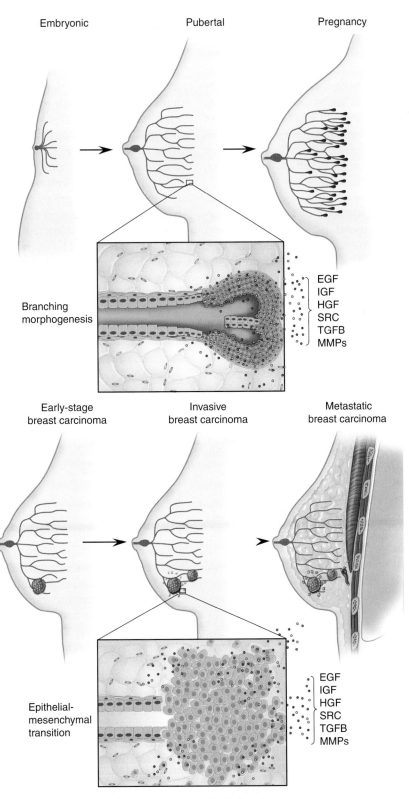

FIGURE 15-1. Similarities between breast development and invasive breast cancer.

involving epidermal growth factor, insulin-like growth factor, src kinase, hepatocyte growth factor/scatter factor, Wnt, transforming growth factor β, and matrix metalloproteinases, among others, are integral to the biology of the developing breast and may explain why they are often upregulated in breast cancers and provide active targets for cancer therapy.[20] In addition, many of the cells of the breast TEB possess stem-cell properties and may represent the vehicle by which mammary stem cells, thought by many to be the origin of breast cancer, spread and populate the breast tissue.[21,22]

From puberty until first pregnancy, the breast epithelial ductal structure is made up of 15 to 20 lactiferous ducts ending in a terminal duct containing from 6 to 11 ductules, forming the terminal duct lobular unit (TDLU)[23] (Figure 15-2). This initial lobular unit is the least differentiated in postpubertal, nulliparous women; has the highest proliferative rate as measured by Ki-67; and has been termed Lob 1.[24] Nearly all epithelial malignancies of the breast are thought to arise from the Lob 1 TDLU. In order to perform the function for which the breast has evolved, namely to produce milk after a full-term pregnancy, the lobular units must remain poised to rapidly proliferate in response to the hormones of pregnancy, first from the pituitary and ovaries, and later from the placenta and fetus itself. Until this occurs, the cells of the breast epithelium must remain in a state of undifferentiated plasticity, which carries with it the risk of malignant transformation.

In animal models, these undifferentiated lobules have been found to be most susceptible to carcinogenesis, with susceptibility diminishing and DNA-repair proficiency increasing, with the differentiated state induced by pregnancy. With pregnancy, the Lob 1 structure is induced to differentiate and branch to a

level of approximately 65 to 90 ductules per TDLU, known as Lob 3, and during lactation, Lob 4. The majority of TDLUs in the breasts of women who have undergone full-term pregnancy before age 30 years are Lob 3, whereas those of nulliparous or late pregnancy women remain primarily Lob 1. Although the classification of lobules as Lob 1 or 3 is based on histology and morphology, the genomic signature underlying these phenotypes has recently been studied and may provide insights into the differing susceptibility to malignant transformation and the observed protective effects of early pregnancy.[25,26] The genomic signature induced by the first full-term pregnancy remains detectable in the breast epithelium after menopause and is characterized by more than 200 genes that have either been up- or downregulated and involve functions of DNA repair, carcinogen metabolism, and regulation of apoptosis, among others. The analysis of the genomic pathways that may affect breast cancer development could allow the identification of factors that may be used to identify women at increased risk, interventions to reduce risk, and new targets for therapy of established cancer. Indeed, the management of breast cancer, perhaps more than any other solid tumor, has been dramatically changed by the introduction of genomic and molecular information into the clinic.[27]

DIAGNOSIS

Key Points

1. The Gail model can predict breast cancer risk in women older than 35 years and includes reproductive history, history of prior breast biopsies, history of hormone use, and family history.
2. Abnormal mammogram findings that are often associated with malignancy include masses, clustered calcifications, architectural distortion, asymmetric density, skin thickening, and abnormal axillary lymph nodes.
3. The American Congress of Obstetrics and Gynecology recommends screening mammography every 1 to 2 years in women between the ages of 40 and 49 years and annually for women 50 years of age and older.
4. Breast imaging for screening and diagnosis may include mammography, ultrasound, and/or magnetic resonance imaging (MRI).

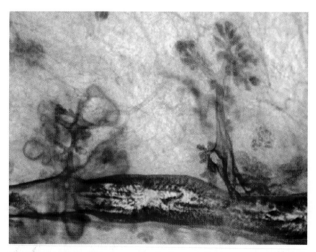

FIGURE 15-2. The terminal duct lobular unit. (Reproduced, with permission, from World Cancer Research Fund and American Institute for Cancer Research.[10])

Traditionally, the diagnosis of breast cancer and related diseases was based primarily on history and physical examination. A detailed reproductive history (age at menarche, childbearing, breastfeeding, age at menopause); history of previous breast surgeries or biopsies, particularly biopsies showing atypia or lobular carcinoma in situ (LCIS); history of medication and hormone use; and family history of breast and ovarian cancer are particularly important components of the initial history. These factors form the basis of the Gail model, which may be used to predict breast cancer risk in women older than 35 years.[28] Additionally, the patient should be asked about breast symptoms, including pain, tenderness, mass, nipple discharge and retraction, changes in size or contour of the breast, and changes in the skin of the breasts. In patients in whom a cancer diagnosis has been confirmed or is suspected, systemic complaints of weight loss, fatigue, abdominal pain, bone pain, and neurologic symptoms should also be elicited.

Physical examination usually begins with visual inspection with the patient sitting upright. Asymmetries; skin changes such as erythema, edema, ulceration, or thickening; nipple retraction or excoriation (a sign of Paget disease); and skin dimpling should be noted. Having the patient raise the arms overhead may exaggerate subtle skin dimpling or nipple retraction. Next, examination of the regional lymph node basins (supraclavicular, infraclavicular, cervical, and axillary) is performed to detect enlarged and/or firm lymph nodes. Finally, the breasts are systematically examined with the patient supine and the ipsilateral arm raised above the head. Aside from distinct masses, more vague asymmetrically dense areas and any nipple discharge should be noted and characterized by color and whether it is emanating from a single or multiple ductal orifices. Nipple fluid that is bloody, spontaneous, and arises from a single ductal orifice is more likely to be related to underlying malignancy than nipple discharge that is bilateral, nonspontaneous, and nonbloody. Although malignancy must be excluded, intraductal papillomas, which are generally benign, are the most common cause of spontaneous, bloody nipple discharge. Milky nipple discharge, or galactorrhea, in a nonpregnant or nonlactating woman may be sign of a pituitary prolactinoma or hypothyroidism. Thyroid function tests and prolactin levels should be evaluated in this instance. Hemoccult testing can be performed on nipple fluid if it seems bloody, although this is not strictly necessary. Of potentially greater value is preparation of smears of nipple fluid for cytologic analysis, which can identify atypical or even malignant epithelial cells in nipple fluid.[29]

Breast imaging is preferably performed before biopsy of any physical exam finding and for screening purposes in asymptomatic women. Since its introduction in the 1930s, mammography, in which the breast is compressed and x-ray images are obtained, has become the standard modality for breast imaging. Screening mammography, which images each breast in 2 views, is performed in asymptomatic women.[30] Diagnostic mammography, in which magnification and/or additional views of the breast are obtained, is usually performed in patients with breast symptoms, physical examination findings, lesions detected by screening mammography, and for short-interval follow-up of probably benign findings detected on prior mammograms.[31] Mammography is effective as a screening tool because cancers are often denser radiographically than the surrounding normal glandular breast tissue, which in turn is denser than fatty breast tissue. Premenopausal women, especially women younger than 30 years, may have very dense glandular breast tissue, which severely limits the sensitivity of mammography. Generally, the glandular breast tissue atrophies and is replaced by fatty tissue as a woman ages, especially after menopause. Consequently, the breasts become less dense mammographically and the sensitivity of mammography for cancer detection increases with age.

Mammogram reports generally specify whether the breasts are fatty, heterogeneously dense, dense, or extremely dense. Abnormal mammogram findings that are often associated with malignancy include masses, clustered calcifications (≥ 5 calcifications in a <2 cm^3 area), architectural distortion, asymmetric density, skin thickening, and abnormal axillary lymph nodes. Specifically, masses are noted to be suspicious for malignancy if the margins are obscured, ill-defined, or spiculated (irregular) (Figure 15-3), and calcifications are noted to be indeterminate or more likely to be malignant if they are amorphous or pleomorphic (heterogeneous) in shape and linear or branching in orientation (Figure 15-4). To standardize the reporting of mammograms and other breast imaging modalities, radiologic findings in the breast are rated using the Breast Imaging Reporting and Data System (BI-RADS) developed by the American College of Radiology (Table 15-3). The positive predictive value of a lesion identified as being suspicious on mammography is estimated to be between 10% and 40%. Thus the vast majority of mammographically detected lesions are benign. Breastfeeding and pregnancy are relative contraindications to the use of mammography.[32]

Current recommendations for annual screening mammography are controversial. Screening mammography is performed in asymptomatic women because, theoretically, screen-detected cancers will be smaller, associated with better prognosis, and require less radical treatment than cancers detected by physical examination. The Health Insurance Plan (HIP) of Greater New York study was the first randomized controlled trial to demonstrate a survival benefit with the use of screening mammography. The trial followed a cohort of women aged 40 to 64 years who were randomly

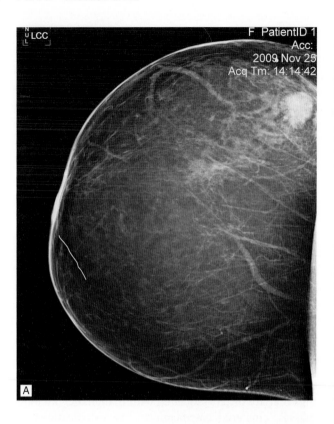

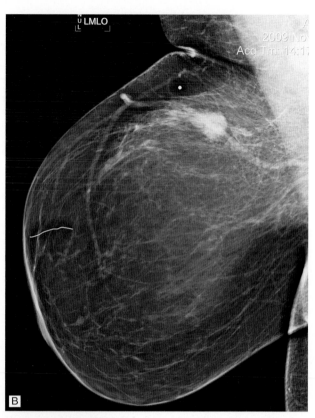

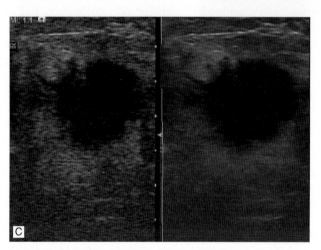

FIGURE 15-3. Mammogram images **(A, B)** indicate an irregular mass in the upper outer left breast. Ultrasound of the left breast **(C)** shows this to be a solid, hypoechoic mass with very irregular borders and confirms its suspicious nature. The mass was subsequently biopsied and demonstrated to be an invasive ductal carcinoma.

assigned to either undergo 3 annual screening mammograms versus no mammography. After 18 years of follow-up, women ages 40 to 49 and 50 to 59 years at enrollment who had undergone screening mammography had a 25% reduction in breast cancer-related mortality.[33] Subsequently, 7 other prospective, randomized trials worldwide have demonstrated that screening mammography decreases the risk of death from breast cancer.[32] However, the age of mammogram

screening, screening interval, and method varied in these trials, and the benefit of mammogram screening in average-risk women between the ages of 40 and 49 years is highly debated. Proponents for mammogram screening in women 40 to 49 years argue that breast cancer is the leading cause of death in this population; this population accounts for 20% of all breast cancer–related deaths and 34% of years of life lost to breast cancer; and breast cancers in younger women

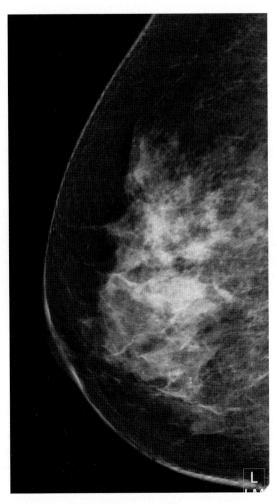

FIGURE 15-4. Mammogram images indicate a suspicious cluster of microcalcifications, which were subsequently biopsied and demonstrated to be associated with ductal carcinoma in situ.

tend to be more aggressive. Arguments against routine annual screening mammograms in this younger age group include the following: only 16% of breast cancers occur in women under the age of 50 years, there is a decreased sensitivity of screening mammography in this age group, and there are significant psychological and physical harms associated with the relatively high false-positive rate of biopsies and unnecessary imaging tests associated with screen-detected lesions.[32,34] Furthermore, in 2009, the US Preventative Services Task Force (USPSTF) dramatically changed their recommendation for screening mammography to biennially (every 2 years) for women between the ages of 50 and 74 years. They recommended *against* screening mammography for all women ages 40 to 49 years, with the disclaimer that the decision to begin screening mammography before the age of 50 years should be made on an individualized basis. The USPSTF acknowledged that the relative risk reduction of screening mammography was similar in the 40 to 49 and 50 to 59 year age groups (15% and 14%, respectively). However, they argued that the absolute benefit is less in women 40 to 49 years of age because of the lower incidence of breast cancer in this age group. The USPSTF also noted that there are insufficient data to recommend for or against mammogram screening in women 75 years of age and older. However, The American Cancer Society, with support from the American College of Surgeons, continues to recommend annual screening mammography in addition to clinical breast examination in women aged 40 years and older and note that women ages 20 to 39 years of age should undergo clinical breast examination every 3 years.[35,36] The American Congress of Obstetrics and Gynecology, meanwhile,

Table 15-3 Breast Imaging Reporting and Data System (BI-RADS) Categories and Recommendations

Category	Assessment	Recommendation	Examples
0	Incomplete	Additional imaging is required	Negative mammogram, but palpable mass
1	Negative	Routine screening	Normal
2	Benign	Routine screening	Simple cyst
3	Probably benign	Short-term follow-up (usually 3-6 months) is recommended to establish stability	Fibroadenoma, complex cyst
4	Suspicious abnormality	Biopsy should be considered	Spiculated mass, pleomorphic calcifications
5	Highly suggestive of malignancy	Biopsy should be considered and appropriate action to be taken	
6	Known breast malignancy	Appropriate action to be taken	

recommends screening mammography every 1 to 2 years in women between the ages of 40 and 49 years and annually for women 50 years of age and older.[37] Women with family history of premenopausal breast cancer in first-degree relatives (ie, mother, sister) may choose to begin annual mammogram screening 10 years before the age at diagnosis of the affected relative, but no later than age 40 years.[35]

Advances in mammographic technology including digital mammography and computer-aided diagnosis (CAD) systems may improve the efficacy of screening mammography. Full-field digital mammography captures digital images of the breasts that can be manipulated and processed to optimize image quality while minimizing radiation exposure. The average radiation dose to the breast with digital mammography is approximately 22% less than with film screen mammography.[38] The Digital Mammographic Imaging Screening Trial, a retrospective, multicenter trial conducted at 33 academic medical centers by the American College of Radiology Imaging Network (ACRIN) demonstrated that the sensitivity of digital mammography for cancer detection (59%) is greater than that of film mammography (27%) in pre- or perimenopausal women younger than 50 years with dense breasts, although this did not apply to other subgroups, particularly older women with fatty breasts.[39] With CAD, digital or digitized mammogram images are subjected to computer analysis after initial radiologist interpretation of the films. The computer software may highlight additional lesions for the radiologist to review and make the final determination regarding whether the lesion is real or artifact and the nature of the lesion. No prospective randomized, controlled trials of CAD exist, although multiple retrospective and cohort studies have demonstrated some improvement in sensitivity (range, 1.7%-19.5% increased sensitivity) along with decreased specificity and increased recall rate for additional imaging with the use of CAD.[40]

Ultrasound is an important adjunct to mammography in evaluation of the breasts. It can help distinguish cystic from solid lesions and further characterize solid lesions as being probably benign or suspicious in nature (Figure 15-3). Unlike mammography, ultrasound is usually performed in a targeted fashion for diagnostic purposes rather than for breast cancer screening. Breast ultrasound is commonly used to evaluate palpable masses or lesions, mammographic abnormalities, and nipple discharge and is also used to guide percutaneous needle biopsies and cyst aspirations and localize nonpalpable lesions for surgical excision; it is also used for intraoperative assessment of margins at surgery.[41] Advantages of ultrasound include no exposure to ionizing radiation, patient comfort, and anatomic evaluation of the breast. Ultrasound, however, is operator dependent and can be time-consuming. Because of the limited sensitivity of

mammography in women with denser breasts, screening whole-breast ultrasound in conjunction with screening mammography is currently being investigated in the prospective, multicenter ACRIN 6666 trial of a high-risk cohort of 2637 women. Initial results of the first round of screening with both mammography and ultrasound indicate that the addition of ultrasound screening detected an additional 4.2 (95% confidence interval, 1.1-7.2) cancers per 1000 women at high risk for breast cancer, but also increased the false-positive biopsy rate.[42]

MRI is now also commonly used to evaluate the breasts. Dynamic contrast-enhanced MRI to evaluate the breast parenchyma employs intravenous gadolinium, which is contraindicated in patients with renal insufficiency and during pregnancy. MRI relies on angiogenesis and the abnormal microvasculature surrounding tumors to detect cancers. Both the degree of contrast enhancement and the perfusion pattern or kinetics of a lesion, along with lesion morphology, are taken into consideration to distinguish between suspicious and benign lesions[43] (Figure 15-5). Although it does not replace mammography, MRI has a number of advantages over mammography: no exposure to ionizing radiation, no limitations due to breast density, better spatial localization, and assessment of the extent of lesions.[32] Furthermore, the sensitivity of MRI for detection of invasive breast cancer, ranging from 91% to 100% in the literature, is far greater than that of mammography and ultrasound, although the specificity of MRI is certainly no better and perhaps worse (as low as 30%) than that of mammography and ultrasound. The sensitivity of MRI for detection of ductal carcinoma in situ (DCIS) is especially low and is

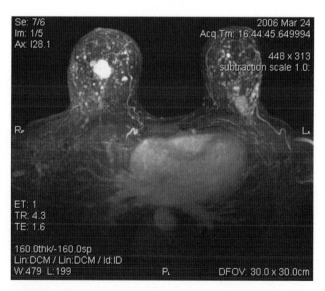

FIGURE 15-5. Dynamic contrast-enhanced MRI of an enhancing, irregular mass that has a "washout" perfusion pattern of enhancement, indicative of malignancy.

also lower for intermediate-grade DCIS.[43] Diagnostic breast MRI is frequently performed for the following reasons: to define the extent of the index lesion, to identify of otherwise occult ipsilateral or contralateral breast lesions, and to evaluate response to neoadjuvant chemotherapy.[44] In women diagnosed with breast cancer, meta-analysis of observational studies indicates that preoperative MRI identifies otherwise occult (not detected by physical examination, mammography, or ultrasound) cancer foci in the ipsilateral breast in 16% of cases and in the contralateral breast in 4% of cases. Accordingly, preoperative MRI changes surgical management in 11.3% of cases, generally resulting in more extensive surgical resection than originally planned, and has been linked to increased rates of mastectomy in women with early-stage breast cancer.[45] However, use of MRI preoperatively has not been shown to decrease rates of reoperation after lumpectomy to achieve adequate surgical margins in the randomized, prospective Comparative Effectiveness of MRI in Breast Cancer (COMICE) trial.[46] Furthermore, to date, there are no randomized prospective trials that demonstrate that preoperative MRI use improves breast cancer survival or reduces recurrence.[45] In summary, routine use of preoperative MRI in women newly diagnosed with breast cancer remains controversial.

Screening breast MRI in high-risk, asymptomatic populations, by contrast, is routinely performed. The American Cancer Society and American College of Surgeons recommends annual screening breast MRI be performed in the following populations at high risk for developing breast cancer: (1) women with deleterious *BRCA1* or *BRCA2* gene mutations and first-degree relatives of *BRCA* carriers who themselves have not undergone genetic testing; (2) women estimated to have at least 20% lifetime risk of breast cancer; (3) women who have undergone chest wall radiation therapy (eg, Hodgkin disease treatment) between the ages of 10 and 30 years; and (4) women with *p53* gene mutations (Li-Fraumeni syndrome, Cowden syndrome, Bannayan-Riley-Ruvalcaba syndrome) and their first-degree relatives. Currently, there is insufficient evidence to support the use of routine screening MRI in women who are at moderately increased risk for breast cancer (15%-20% lifetime risk), including those with a personal history of breast cancer, history of biopsy showing atypia or lobular carcinoma in situ (LCIS), or extremely dense breasts.[35]

After breast imaging, tissue diagnosis is obtained either with an open surgical biopsy or preferably via minimally invasive, percutaneous needle biopsy. Surgical biopsy, both excisional and incisional, is generally performed in the outpatient setting. Surgical biopsy of nonpalpable lesions detected by mammography, ultrasound, or MRI requires preoperative placement of a wire (or needle) by radiology under local anesthesia to guide surgical excision. Intraoperative specimen radiograph or ultrasound should be performed to confirm complete excision of these nonpalpable lesions. Because 70% to 80% of all biopsies yield benign results, surgical incisions should be made as cosmetically as possible, generally along the Langer lines of skin tension, which are oriented concentric with the nipple. Incisions in the cleavage area (upper inner quadrants) should be avoided if possible.[47] Surgical biopsy, however, is more costly and has the potential for greater disfigurement, morbidity, and loss of productivity for the patient. Additionally, patients whose cancer diagnosis is made by surgical biopsy will frequently need at least one other surgery for definitive treatment of their cancer.[48]

A number of options for percutaneous biopsy exist. Fine-needle aspiration (FNA) biopsy is inexpensive and easy to perform in the office setting with a 10- or 20-mL syringe and 22- or 25-gauge needle. Local anesthetic can be used to anesthetize the skin if desired. While pulling back on the syringe to generate suction, the needle is moved back and forth at different angles within the lesion of interest to dislodge cells, which are then aspirated into the syringe. Slides can then be made with the aspirated material, which are sent in fixative for review by a qualified cytopathologist. The accuracy of FNA approaches 80%, but false-negative rates remain as high as 15%-20%, and in some cases, there is insufficient material for analysis. FNA can identify malignant cells but cannot distinguish between in situ and invasive carcinoma. FNA can also be used to completely aspirate cystic lesions. Core (cutting) needle biopsy can be performed on any palpable lesion and on nonpalpable lesions with ultrasound, MRI, and mammogram (stereotactic core needle biopsy) guidance. Because core needle devices are larger (18 to 7 gauge), the skin and surrounding tissue should be well anesthetized with local anesthetic before making the small skin incision required to accommodate introduction of the biopsy needle into the breast.[47] Using a larger-gauge needle and vacuum assistance decreases the potential for sampling error. A radiopaque tissue marker (clip) is generally placed at the time of biopsy to facilitate subsequent lesion identification and confirm sampling of benign lesions on follow-up imaging. Core needle biopsy provides an accurate tissue diagnosis in approximately 98% of cases. The potential for sampling error, however, exists with any needle biopsy technique, and surgical excision is still recommended after benign core needle biopsy results if the pathology findings are discordant with the imaging impression, atypical ductal or lobular hyperplasia (discussed later), LCIS, papillary lesion, or radial scar. When surgical excision is performed subsequent to core needle biopsy showing atypical ductal hyperplasia, for example, 10% to 20% of cases will be found to have DCIS or invasive cancer. Also as a result of sampling error, surgery performed for DCIS may occasionally yield invasive cancer.[44,48]

PATHOLOGY

Key Points

1. The majority of breast cancers are classified as invasive ductal carcinoma and invasive lobular carcinoma.
2. The critical proteins resulting from underlying genomic abnormalities in breast cancer include Ki67, estrogen receptor (ER), progesterone receptor (PR), and HER2; presence or absence of these proteins correlates with clinical outcome and affects adjuvant therapy.
3. Lobular carcinoma in situ (LCIS) is associated with increased risk of both ipsilateral and contralateral breast cancer.

Breast cancer is a clinically heterogeneous and diverse disease, and morphology-based histopathology has attempted to classify breast cancer into categories that would predict clinical and biologic behavior, with limited success.[49] The true basis of the pathology that produces the clinically recognizable entity of "breast cancer" is to be found at the level of the genome: genetic changes inherited and acquired in the course of carcinogenesis, passed on through cell division to daughter cells, involving multiple molecular networks and pathways that have promoted the survival of the malignant clone and produce the phenotype of breast cancer.[50]

Traditional histopathology identifies the phenotypic effects of the underlying molecular and genetic lesions. Immunohistochemistry (IHC) and fluorescent in situ hybridization (FISH) identify the presence and amount of specific proteins expressed as a result of the underlying genomic abnormalities associated with malignancy of the breast. The critical proteins include Ki67, a general marker of proliferation[51]; nuclear and cytoplasmic receptors for estrogen and progesterone, ER and PR[52]; and the cell surface signaling molecule HER2.[53] This gene expression profiling of breast cancers yields the beginnings of a molecular "taxonomy" of breast cancer that has added considerable insight to the previously identified but clinically heterogeneous histopathologically defined subtypes. Standard management guidelines for breast cancer at the present time are based on traditional histopathology and IHC—the tissue, cellular, and protein level of analysis.[49]

The current morphologic classification of invasive epithelial cancers of the breast cancer recognizes at least 18 distinct histologic types (Table 15-4), although the majority of all breast cancers (50%-80%) are

Table 15-4 Histopathologic Subtypes of Epithelial Breast Cancer

Invasive ductal carcinomas (not otherwise specified)
Carcinoma with osteoclast-like giant cells
Invasive lobular carcinomas
Pure tubular carcinoma
Invasive cribriform carcinoma
Medullary carcinomas
Mucinous carcinoma
Neuroendocrine tumors
Invasive papillary carcinoma
Invasive micropapillary carcinoma
Apocrine carcinoma
Metaplastic carcinoma
Lipid-rich carcinoma
Secretory carcinoma
Oncocytic carcinoma
Adenoid cystic carcinoma
Acinic-cell carcinoma
Glycogen-rich clear-cell carcinoma
Sebaceous carcinoma

classified in this system as invasive ductal carcinoma, not otherwise specified (IDC-NOS).[49] This places the burden of identifying clinically meaningful subtypes at the molecular level, by IHC and genomic measures. Therefore, within invasive ductal (Figure 15-6) and invasive lobular (Figure 15-7), an additional 5% to 15%, subsets are more usefully defined by ER, PR, and HER2 expression through IHC. HER2-positive

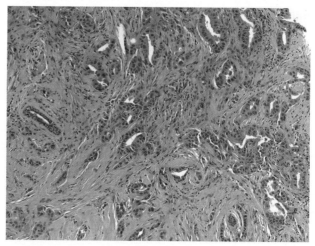

FIGURE 15-6. Invasive ductal carcinoma. (Image contributed by Dr. Shika Bose, Cedars-Sinai Department of Pathology.)

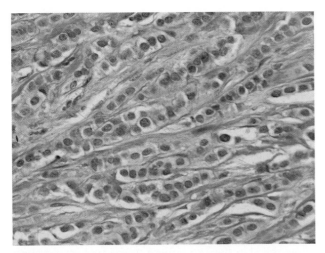

FIGURE 15-7. Invasive lobular carcinoma. (Image contributed by Dr. Shika Bose, Cedars-Sinai Department of Pathology.)

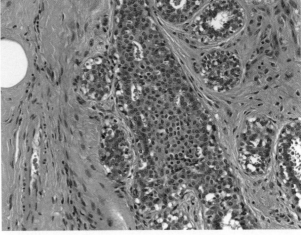

FIGURE 15-8. Atypical ductal hyperplasia. (Image contributed by Dr. Shika Bose, Cedars-Sinai Department of Pathology.)

cancers represent approximately 20% of all breast cancers, ER negative/PR negative/HER2 negative (triple negative) cancers approximately 15%, with the remaining being ER positive/PR positive and ER positive/PR negative.

Histopathology also assigns the tumor grade though morphologic features, which correlate with the degree of differentiation of the tumor. This is subject to considerable interobserver variation; although efforts have been made to diminish this variability, with the introduction of descriptive morphology assigning numerical weights to specific features (eg, the Nottingham and Bloom-Richardson grading systems), analysis of grade at the genomic level again suggests the superiority of molecular analysis to light microscopy.[54,55] A Genomic Grade Index (GGI), based on 97 genes representing several genomic pathways, including cell cycle and proliferation, proved capable of predicting response to therapy more accurately than traditional grading, with a high degree of reproducibility.

Noninvasive but malignant disease of the breast (so-called premalignant states) has been increasingly detected with improvements in breast imaging.[56,57] Proliferative breast disease involves a continuum of increasing genomic and histologic pathology, with enhanced proliferation and/or diminished apoptosis being among the earliest of biologic changes.[58] In addition, the associated risk of subsequent invasive cancer also increases along this continuum.[59,60] Currently, data suggest that noninvasive breast cancer may be a marker as well as a non-obligate precursor to invasive disease.[61]

Intraductal proliferative lesions are categorized into 3 groups: usual ductal hyperplasia (UDH), atypical ductal hyperplasia (ADH) (Figure 15-8), and ductal carcinoma in situ (DCIS) (Figure 15-9). The risk of subsequent invasive cancer associated with these lesions is approximately 1.5-fold with UDH, 4- to 5-fold with ADH, and 8- to 10-fold with DCIS.[58] Lobular intraepithelial neoplasia (LIN) provides the lobular counterpart, with a similar continuum of pathology from atypical lobular hyperplasia to LCIS (Figure 15-10). The subsequent risk of invasive breast cancer, either ductal or lobular, is approximately 8.7%. Unique to LIN is the increased risk of both ipsilateral and contralateral breast cancer, with each breast carrying a risk of more than 4%, supporting the concept of such pathology as a marker of increased susceptibility to lobular neoplasia throughout the breast epithelium.

Two additional pathologic entities warrant further mention. Paget disease of the breast is not considered a distinct histopathologic subtype, but is rather an in situ neoplasm in the squamous epithelium of the nipple and is clinically identified as an eczematoid or crusting

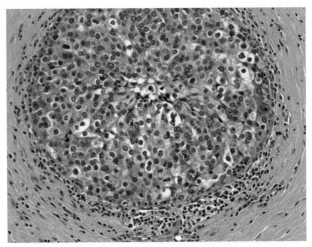

FIGURE 15-9. Ductal carcinoma in situ. (Image contributed by Dr. Shika Bose, Cedars-Sinai Department of Pathology.)

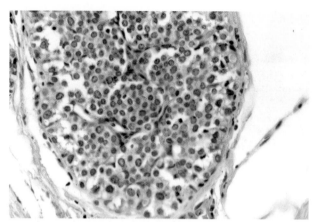

FIGURE 15-10. Lobular carcinoma in situ. (Image contributed by Dr. Shika Bose, Cedars-Sinai Department of Pathology.)

lesion.[62] Although treated as a noninvasive form of breast cancer with local surgical excision, its true significance is as a marker of malignancy elsewhere in the breast. Paget disease may be associated with underlying DCIS or invasive cancer, with the majority of these invasive cancers being ER negative and of high grade. Phyllodes tumor of the breast[63] is another rare entity, less than 1% of all breast neoplasms, and is thought to be of fibroepithelial origin and mimics the shape of leaves, hence the term *phylloides* from the Greek word for "leaf." The challenge with such tumors is to recognize the benign versus the malignant form, for which no specific molecular biomarkers have been established. It is most often seen in young women as a rapidly enlarging lesion and is also treated with wide local excision.[63]

Breast cancers are staged using the American Joint Committee on Cancer (AJCC) TNM staging classification (Table 15-5).

TREATMENT

Key Points

1. Modified radical mastectomy with axillary lymphadenectomy is the surgical treatment of choice for women who have large cancers with clinically apparent axillary lymph node involvement at the time of diagnosis.
2. Smaller cancers with clinically negative lymph node involvement may be treated conservatively with lumpectomy and sentinel lymph node dissection followed by radiation.
3. Expression of ER, PR, and HER2 in breast cancers allows for administration of targeted anti-estrogen and anti-HER2 therapy.

Surgery/Radiation Therapy

Breast cancer treatment is based on the clinical and pathologic stage of the cancer at the time of diagnosis. Treatment usually involves multiple modalities, including surgery, radiation therapy, chemotherapy, and endocrine therapy.

Surgical treatment of breast cancer continues to evolve. In the 1890s, William Halsted propagated the idea of the radical mastectomy in which the breast and overlying teardrop-shaped skin paddle was resected en bloc with the pectoralis major and minor muscles and axillary and supraclavicular lymph nodes. Skin grafts were routinely used to cover the large skin defect. Drains were placed temporarily after mastectomy to allow the skin flaps to adhere to the underlying chest wall. The radical mastectomy quickly achieved widespread acceptance because it conferred significantly improved survival and lower local recurrence rates when compared with the lesser operations being performed at the time. Most breast cancers in this era were also large and locally advanced at diagnosis. A number of developments in the latter half of the 20th century led to the adoption of less radical operations for breast cancer, including modified radical mastectomy and simple mastectomy. Introduced in the 1960s, mammography allowed identification of smaller, earlier-stage breast cancers. Cobalt beam radiation therapy became available in the 1960s, only to be replaced in the 1970s by linear accelerators, which are primarily used to deliver radiation therapy today. Finally, the fact that breast cancer is potentially a systemic disease and the development of adjuvant chemotherapy led to the demise of the radical mastectomy, which is now generally performed only for locally advanced cancers.[64]

Modified radical mastectomy, in which a skin ellipse encompassing the nipple-areola complex is resected in continuity with the underlying breast tissue and level I and II axillary lymph nodes (nodes lateral to the lateral border of the pectoralis minor muscle and nodes located beneath the pectoralis minor, respectively), became the standard surgical treatment for breast cancer beginning in the 1970s. As opposed to a radical mastectomy, the pectoralis muscles and level III nodes (medial to pectoralis minor muscle) are left intact, and skin flaps are reapproximated primarily in a modified radical mastectomy. Two randomized, prospective trials conducted in the 1970s compared overall survival and locoregional recurrence rates in women treated with radical mastectomy versus modified radical mastectomy. Both trials demonstrated no difference in overall survival or locoregional recurrence rates for women with stage I and II disease.[65,66] Currently, modified radical mastectomy is the surgical treatment of choice for women who have large cancers with clinically apparent axillary lymph node involvement at the time of diagnosis.

Table 15-5 AJCC TNM Staging Classification for Breast Cancer

Primary Tumor (T)	
Tx	Cannot be assessed
T0	No evidence of primary tumor
Tis	Carcinoma in situ
Tis (DCIS)	Ductal carcinoma in situ
Tis (LCIS)	Lobular carcinoma in situ
Tis (Paget)	Paget disease of nipple not associated with invasive *or* in situ carcinoma elsewhere in the breast parenchyma
T1	Tumor ≤20 mm in greatest dimension
T1mi	Tumor ≤1 mm in greatest dimension
T1a	Tumor >1 mm but ≤5 mm in greatest dimension
T1b	Tumor >5 mm but ≤10 mm in greatest dimension
T1c	Tumor >10 mm but ≤20 mm in greatest dimension
T2	Tumor >20 mm but ≤50 mm in greatest dimension
T3	Tumor >50 mm in greatest dimension
T4	Tumor of any size with direct extension to chest wall and/or skin (ulceration or skin nodules)
T4a	Tumor extends to chest wall, not including only pectoralis muscle adherence/invasion
T4b	Ulceration and/or ipsilateral satellite nodules, and/or skin edema (including peau d'orange)
T4c	Both T4a and T4b
T4d	Inflammatory carcinoma
Regional Lymph Nodes	
Nx	Regional lymph nodes cannot be assessed (eg, previously removed)
N0	No regional lymph node metastasis
N0(i−)	No regional lymph node metastasis, negative immunohistochemistry
N0(mol−)	No regional lymph node metastasis, negative molecular findings (RT-PCR)
N0(i+)	Malignant cells ≤0.2 mm in regional lymph node(s)
N0(mol+)	Positive molecular findings (RT-PCR) but histologically negative regional lymph nodes
N1mi	Micrometastases >0.2 mm but ≤2 mm
N1	Metastases to 1 to 3 regional lymph nodes
N1a	Metastases to 1 to 3 axillary lymph nodes
N1b	Metastases to 1 to 3 internal mammary lymph nodes detected by sentinel node biopsy only
N1c	Metastases to 1 to 3 axillary and internal mammary nodes detected by sentinel node biopsy only
N2	Metastases to 4 to 9 axillary lymph nodes or in any clinically detected internal mammary lymph nodes
N2a	Metastases >2 mm in size in 4 to 9 axillary lymph nodes
N2b	Metastases in clinically detected internal mammary lymph nodes in the absence of axillary lymph node metastases
N3	Metastases in ≥10 axillary lymph nodes, clinically detected internal mammary nodes *and* axillary lymph nodes, level 3 (infraclavicular) lymph nodes, or ipsilateral supraclavicular lymph nodes
N3a	Metastases in ≥10 axillary lymph nodes or level 3 (infraclavicular) lymph nodes
N3b	Metastases in clinically detected internal mammary nodes *and* axillary lymph nodes *or* metastases in >3 axillary lymph nodes and internal mammary nodes detected by sentinel node biopsy
N3c	Metastases in ipsilateral supraclavicular lymph nodes

(Continued)

Table 15-5 AJCC TNM Staging Classification for Breast Cancer (Continued)

Distant Metastases (M)	
M0	No distant metastases
cM0(+)	No clinical or radiographic evidence or symptoms of distant metastases in a patient with molecularly or microscopically detected tumor cells (≤0.2 mm) in circulating blood, bone marrow, or nonregional nodal tissue
M1	Distant metastases >0.2 mm in size

Stage	T	N	M
0	Tis	N0	M0
IA	T1	N0	M0
IB	T0	N1mi	M0
	T1	N1mi	M0
IIA	T0	N1	M0
	T1	N1	M0
	T2	N0	M0
IIB	T2	N1	M0
	T3	N0	M0
IIIA	T0	N2	M0
	T1	N2	M0
	T2	N2	M0
	T3	N1	M0
	T3	N2	M0
IIIB	T4	N0	M0
	T4	N1	M0
	T4	N2	M0
IIIC	Any T	N3	M0
IV	Any T	Any N	M1

AJCC, American Joint Committee on Cancer; DCIS, ductal carcinoma in situ; LCIS, lobular carcinoma in situ; RT-PCR, reverse transcriptase polymerase chain reaction.
Reproduced with permission from AJCC. Breast. In: Edge SB, Byrd DR, Compton CC, et al, eds. *AJCC Cancer Staging Manual.* 7th ed. New York, NY: Springer; 2010:347-376.

Taking the trend toward less aggressive surgery further, breast conservation was demonstrated to be a viable alternative to modified radical mastectomy in women with early-stage breast cancer in the late 1970s and early 1980s. The National Surgical Adjuvant Breast and Bowel Project (NSABP) B-06 trial randomized women with tumors less than 4 cm in size and clinically negative lymph nodes (stages I and II) to one of 3 treatment arms: modified radical mastectomy, lumpectomy with axillary lymph node dissection (levels I and II), and lumpectomy with axillary lymph node dissection plus adjuvant whole-breast external-beam radiation therapy (50 Gy). After more than 20 years of follow-up, NSABP B-06 demonstrated that overall survival and disease-free survival were equivalent in each of the treatment arms. Although local and regional (axillary) recurrence was lowest in the group who underwent modified radical mastectomy, the addition of radiation therapy decreased the local recurrence rate from 39.2% for those who underwent lumpectomy and axillary node dissection alone to 14.3% in those treated with lumpectomy, axillary node dissection, and radiation therapy.[67] Five other randomized, prospective trials, including the Milan I trial, Institute Gustave-Roussy trial, National Cancer Institute trial, European Organization for Research and Treatment of Cancer (EORTC) 10801 trial, and Danish Breast Cancer Group trial, also confirmed the lack of a survival benefit for mastectomy over breast-conserving surgery.[68-72] In summary, most women with early-stage breast cancers are candidates for breast-conserving therapy. Absolute contraindications to breast conservation include pregnancy, multicentric (cancer in ≥2 quadrants of the breast) disease, history of prior radiation therapy to the breasts or inability to tolerate radiation therapy, and persistently positive surgical margins. Furthermore, relative contraindications to breast conservation include tumor volume to breast volume ratio that would preclude acceptable cosmesis, large area of multifocal (cancers all in same quadrant of the breast) disease, and history of collagen vascular disorder.[73]

The surgical approach to the axilla has also become less radical because standard axillary lymph node dissection places the patient at risk for significant morbidity, including lymphedema (15%-20% incidence), neurovascular injury such as a winged scapula deformity, limited range of shoulder motion, acute pain and discomfort (drains are usually placed after standard axillary dissection), and chronic pain syndromes.[74] The NSABP B-04 trial randomized women with clinically negative lymph nodes to 1 of 3 treatments: radical mastectomy, total (simple) mastectomy in which only skin and breast tissue are removed alone, or total mastectomy plus radiation (50 Gy) to the chest wall and axilla. Women with clinically positive lymph nodes at enrollment were randomized to either radical mastectomy or total mastectomy with axillary radiation. Adjuvant chemotherapy was not given, and women who initially were treated with total mastectomy alone and later developed clinical evidence of axillary lymph node involvement underwent delayed axillary lymph node dissection. After 25 years of follow-up, in the node-negative group, there was no statistically significant difference in overall survival or disease-free survival in the 3 treatment groups. Although overall survival was lower in the clinically node-positive patients, there was also no difference between the 2 treatment subgroups with positive nodes: radical mastectomy versus total mastectomy with radiation.[75]

With the knowledge that the timing and mode of treatment of the axillary lymph nodes does not affect survival, the NSABP B-32 trial was conducted to compare standard axillary lymph node dissection with sentinel lymph node dissection in women with invasive breast cancers and clinically negative axillae. Sentinel lymph node dissection, which is based on the premise that tumors have specific lymphatic drainage patterns, was first demonstrated to be effective in the staging and treatment of malignant melanoma. To identify the sentinel lymph node(s), vital blue dye (methylene blue or isosulfan blue) and/or technetium-radiolabeled sulfur colloid is injected either into the breast at the site of the tumor or into the subareolar Sappey plexus of lymphatics or intradermally. Either through a separate axillary incision or mastectomy incision, the clavipectoral fascia is then divided and the axilla carefully inspected, and lymph nodes that are blue and/or radioactive, as measured with a hand-held gamma probe, are resected. If no sentinel nodes can be identified, standard axillary lymph node dissection should be performed. Intraoperative frozen section analysis of the sentinel lymph node(s) can be performed, but this adds additional time and cost to the operation. Lymphoscintigraphy can also be performed preoperatively to facilitate identification of the sentinel lymph node. At most institutions, sentinel lymph nodes are subjected to histologic analysis with both conventional hematoxylin and eosin staining and immunohistochemical staining. A number of studies have shown that the combined use of blue dye and radioisotope may yield a slightly lower false-negative rate than blue dye alone, although both techniques confer equivalent rates of sentinel lymph node identification.[76] Completion axillary lymph node dissection is then performed only in the event that lymph node metastases are identified in the sentinel lymph node(s).

In the NSABP B-32 trial, women with clinically node-negative, invasive breast cancer were randomly assigned to either sentinel lymph node dissection followed by immediate completion axillary lymph node dissection or sentinel lymph node dissection alone. Patients in the latter group underwent delayed completion axillary dissection only if histologic analysis identified metastases in the sentinel lymph nodes. Both blue dye and radioisotope were used to identify sentinel nodes. Sentinel lymph nodes were successfully identified in 97.2%, and the overall accuracy was 97.1% with a false-negative rate of 9.8%.[77] Overall morbidity, including lymphedema (14% standard axillary dissection vs. 8% sentinel lymph node dissection), was lower in the group who underwent sentinel lymph node dissection alone.[78] Since the study completed enrollment in 1994, the primary end points of survival and recurrence have yet to be reported, although sentinel lymph node dissection is now the preferred method of axillary staging in women with invasive breast cancer and clinically negative lymph nodes.[44]

Consistent with the concern for improved cosmesis in women undergoing prophylactic surgery and breast cancer treatment, skin-sparing and nipple-sparing mastectomy are also being performed in many centers nationwide. In a skin-sparing mastectomy, the nipple and areola are resected along with the breast, but as much of the native skin envelope as possible is preserved to facilitate immediate breast reconstruction. Initially, the oncologic safety of this approach was questioned. A recent meta-analysis of 9 retrospective, observational studies demonstrated that that there appears to be no significant difference in local recurrence rates between women who underwent skin-sparing mastectomies for cancer (range, 3.8%-10%) and those who had non–skin-sparing mastectomies (range, 1.7%-11.5%). Complication rates, including flap necrosis, were similar between the 2 groups.[79] Nipple-sparing mastectomy preserves the entire skin envelope, including the dermis and epidermis of the nipple, and can be performed via circumareolar, transareolar, transnipple, or inframammary incisions. To minimize residual breast tissue, the major ducts leading to the nipple should be excised and sent for biopsy separately to confirm the abscess of malignancy. Among the small number of published retrospective studies, local recurrence rates after nipple-sparing mastectomy range from 1% to 28%, although it was noted that recurrences most frequently occurred in the skin flap overlying the site of the primary tumor rather than in the retained nipple. Because the major blood supply to the nipple normally courses through the breast parenchyma deep to the nipple, viability of the nipple is a concern with nipple-sparing mastectomy. Necrosis of the retained nipple reportedly occurs in 2% to 20% of cases.[80] Optimal patient selection for nipple-sparing mastectomy is critical to the success of the operation, and generally nipple-sparing mastectomy should be reserved for women with small to moderate breast volume and mild to moderate breast ptosis who are undergoing prophylactic surgery or surgery for cancers that are smaller, peripherally located, and not multicentric.

Breast reconstruction after mastectomy can be performed either immediately after mastectomy or in a delayed fashion. Reconstruction is an important part of breast cancer treatment because it can restore the patient's body image and improve quality of life. Most women who undergo mastectomy can be safely offered breast reconstruction. For the vast majority of women who do not undergo nipple-sparing mastectomy, reconstruction initially involves creation of a new breast mound followed by creation of a new nipple and areola. Approximately 70% of reconstructive breast surgery involves implant-based reconstruction, in which a breast implant is placed posterior to the skin and pectoralis major and serratus anterior muscles (Figure 15-11). This is most frequently achieved initially by placing a tissue expander at the time of the mastectomy, followed by serial addition of saline to the tissue expander over a period of weeks to months, and finally exchange of the tissue expander for a breast implant (silicone or saline). Less frequently, a submuscular implant is placed at the time of mastectomy, although radiated cadaveric human skin is often incorporated to create an adequate muscular pocket for the implant.

Alternatively, a number of autogenous tissue-based options for reconstruction exist. The most commonly used autogenous reconstruction is the transverse rectus abdominis muscle (TRAM) flap, in which excess skin, fat, and a portion of the rectus abdominis muscle are resected and either rotated or transposed freely on a superior epigastric vascular pedicle into the mastectomy defect. A low transverse abdominal incision is left at the donor site. Patients who undergo TRAM reconstructions may be prone to develop abdominal

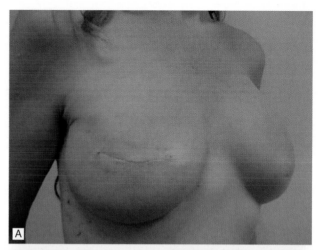

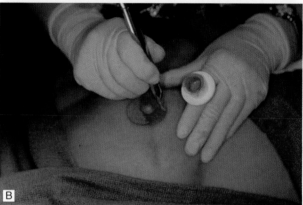

FIGURE 15-11. A. Reconstructed breast with implants after bilateral skin-sparing mastectomy. **B.** Tattoo of the reconstructed nipple and areola after skin-sparing mastectomy and implant reconstruction. (Image contributed by Dr. R. Kendrick Slate.)

wall hernias. The deep inferior epigastric perforator (DIEP) flap is similar to the TRAM flap in that excess skin and fat from the infraumbilical abdominal wall is harvested, although the rectus abdominis muscles are preserved in a DIEP flap. DIEP flaps rely on microvascular anastomosis and are technically more difficult to perform. A hybrid option for breast reconstruction is the latissimus dorsi myocutaneous flap, in which skin, fat, and a portion of the back muscle is rotated on the thoracodorsal vascular pedicle anteriorly to fill the mastectomy defect. Frequently an implant is also placed posterior to the flap to provide more volume to the reconstruction.[81]

Radiation therapy is an integral part of breast cancer treatment, especially in women who desire breast conservation. The NSABP-06 trial demonstrated the importance of adjuvant radiation therapy in decreasing local and regional recurrences in women undergoing lumpectomy for early-stage breast cancer. Most commonly, external-beam whole-breast radiation therapy using tangential photon fields generated by a linear accelerator (to limit exposure to the underlying heart and lungs) is used. Typically in the United States, a total dose of 50 Gy is delivered in 25 to 28 daily fractions, 5 days per week, for a total of 5 to 7 weeks, to the entire breast or chest wall. The boundaries of the radiation field include the inferior clavicular head superiorly, midline medially, 2 cm below the inframammary fold inferiorly, and mid- to posterior axillary line laterally. In women who opt for breast conservation with lumpectomy, an additional 10- to 15-Gy "boost" dose is generally delivered to the lumpectomy cavity to further reduce the risk of local failure. Radiation fields may be expanded to include the entire axilla, intramammary, and/or supraclavicular lymph node basins in women who are deemed to be at high risk for regional recurrence in these areas due to the extent of regional lymph node involvement.[82] Hypofractionated whole-breast radiation therapy in which larger treatment fractions are delivered over a shorter period of time (3 weeks) is also being used more commonly as concerns about the potential adverse effects on cosmesis and local recurrence in select patient populations have been disproved.[83] External-beam radiation therapy to the chest wall after mastectomy and chemotherapy is also recommended for women with T3 or T4 lesions, tumor invading skin or chest wall, and ≥4 axillary lymph nodes with metastatic cancer.[84]

Chemotherapy/Endocrine Therapy/ Targeted Therapy

In stages I to III breast cancers, where cure is achievable, systemic therapy is used to eradicate micrometastatic disease; in the case of neoadjuvant therapy, it is used to reduce the tumor burden before surgery. The efficacy of adjuvant chemotherapy of breast cancer has been established for more than 25 years, whereas hormonal therapy, in the form of surgically or medically induced menopause, has been recognized as early as the 19th century. Depending on the type of breast cancer, modern adjuvant systemic therapy now includes cytotoxic chemotherapy and targeted therapy directed against estrogen (estrogen production or the ER) and against the human epidermal growth factor receptor 2 (HER2). The routine molecular profiling of breast cancer allowing stratification into biologically and therapeutically distinct subsets has improved the therapeutic index of systemic therapy, allowing for increased survival rates with fewer patients receiving toxic therapy when predicted to be ineffective.[85,86] Regimens for therapy are also determined by stage of disease and level of risk of micrometastatic disease, allowing for shorter courses and fewer drugs in stage I, low-risk disease versus aggressive, dose-dense, and extended regimens for high-risk patients, particularly those with multiple axillary nodes involved (stage IIB and III).[87]

Chemotherapy

Systemic adjuvant chemotherapy for breast cancer is accomplished with a variety of regimens, with first-, second-, and third-generation regimens increasing in aggressiveness and effectiveness.[87] All regimens use some combination of an alkylating agent (usually cyclophosphamide), a taxane (either paclitaxel or docetaxel), and/or an anthracycline (either doxorubicin or epirubicin). For ER-positive disease, anti-estrogen therapy is given after chemotherapy, usually for a total of 5 years, whereas for HER2-positive breast cancer, therapy with a monoclonal antibody, trastuzumab, directed at the HER2 receptor is given concurrently with chemotherapy, as well as after chemotherapy, usually for a total of 12 months.

First-generation chemotherapy regimens include modestly toxic combinations such as cyclophosphamide, methotrexate, and fluorouracil for 6 cycles and doxorubicin plus cyclophosphamide (AC) or docetaxel plus cyclophosphamide (TC) for 4 cycles and are appropriate for patients with stage I and low-risk stage II disease. Second-generation regimens include fluorouracil, epirubicin, and cyclophosphamide for 6 cycles; cyclophosphamide, doxorubicin, and fluorouracil for 6 cycles; and standard AC/T: AC for 4 cycles followed by a taxane for 4 cycles, given every 21 days, or weekly paclitaxel for 12 weeks. Second-generation regimens are thought to have somewhat superior efficacy to first-generation regimens, with an approximately 20% improvement in survival, but with longer duration of therapy and increased toxicity. Third-generation regimens include TAC (with all 3 agents given concurrently rather than in sequence as in AC/T), and AC/T given at 2-week intervals rather than 3 (so-called dose-dense AC/T) and are thought to provide an additional 20% improvement in survival over second-generation regimens for high-risk subsets, but with considerable increase in toxicity and a requirement for active growth factor support. The decision regarding which regimen to select is based on stage of disease, prognostic factors such as grade, and the ability of the patient to tolerate therapy as a result of comorbidities such as underlying cardiac, hepatic, and renal function. In addition, the incremental benefit of chemotherapy in prolonging overall survival is contingent on the expected actuarial survival of the individual, such that 2 women with breast cancer similar in stage and prognostic features may receive different therapies if one has no comorbidities and the other has significant health issues other than breast cancer that are expected to affect her overall survival.

The rapid increase in the molecular understanding of breast cancer, and the observation of molecularly defined subsets with distinct biologic behavior, has revealed differing cellular pathways that are up- or downregulated depending on tumor type. This body of information, however, has not been fully integrated into standard clinical decision making for breast cancer chemotherapy; it may serve to guide, in some cases, the decision regarding whether chemotherapy should be used at all.[88] The commercially available 70-gene and 21-gene profiles use differing sets of genes, whose expression levels predict the likelihood of metastases and/or the likelihood of response to anti-estrogen therapy and chemotherapy.

Targeted Therapy: Anti-Estrogen

All breast cancers expressing ER in greater than 1% of tumor cells are expected to benefit from the use of anti-estrogen therapy.[89] The role of the PR in predicting the degree of benefit remains controversial, and it is thought that the absence of PR predicts less benefit; it is also possible that the rare tumors classified as ER negative but PR positive may represent technical errors in processing, rather than a true subset.[52] The degree of benefit of anti-estrogen therapy may be predicted in breast cancer by examining the expression levels of 16 genes,[88] with 5 additional reference genes making up a 21-gene profile. Three levels of benefit are identified based on gene expression: a low-risk profile indicating extreme sensitivity to anti-estrogen therapy and no incremental benefit predicted from the addition of standard chemotherapy; a high-risk profile indicating significantly less sensitivity to anti-estrogen therapy than anticipated despite the presence of ER, but with a commensurately increased sensitivity and benefit from cytotoxic chemotherapy; and an intermediate-risk group, in which the reciprocal trends of sensitivity to anti-estrogen and chemotherapy vary as a continuous variable. A large cooperative group trial designed to determine the optimal therapy for patients in the intermediate category is currently underway.[90]

Targeted therapy directed against estrogen in the premenopausal woman with intact ovarian function is limited to blockade of estrogen binding to the ER by the drug tamoxifen. The pituitary-ovarian axis is often disrupted by tamoxifen, with estrogen "deficiency" sensed by the pituitary, resulting in an increase in luteinizing hormone and follicle-stimulating hormone, which in turn induces increased ovarian production of estrogen. Estrogen levels in women taking tamoxifen may be extremely elevated as result of this feedback mechanism. Tamoxifen acts as an antagonist to estrogen in the breast, but may have agonist effects in the uterus and elsewhere, such that not all women experience menopausal sequelae or become amenorrheic on the drug.

In the postmenopausal woman with no ovarian function, the preferred anti-estrogen therapy is the reduction of non-ovarian estrogen production through the use of inhibitors of the enzyme aromatase, found throughout the body in various tissues, including the breast itself. Aromatase inhibitors (AI) such as anastrozole, letrozole, and exemestane have been proven superior to tamoxifen in several large clinical trials, and, like tamoxifen, are given for a period of 5 years.[89] Longer use of AIs has not been documented as yet to be of benefit, although the use of 5 years of AI after an initial 5 years of tamoxifen does add a small incremental benefit to disease-free survival. Due to the profound reduction in estrogen caused by inhibition of aromatase, menopausal symptoms may be exacerbated, and accelerated loss of bone density may occur. This latter effect warrants the yearly assessment of bone mineral density, calcium, and vitamin D supplementation and often therapy to prevent or treat osteoporosis.

Targeted Therapy: Anti-HER2 Therapy

Overexpression of the HER2 receptor and excessive signaling through this pathway is an important driver of growth and angiogenesis in breast cancer cells. Until the advent of HER2-directed therapy, HER2 positivity identified the worst prognosis subset of breast cancer. However, a monoclonal antibody binding to HER2, trastuzumab, has proven effective in the metastatic setting, in combination with chemotherapy, and in the adjuvant setting; in some cases, use of trastuzumab doubled the survival seen with chemotherapy alone.[91] The addition of trastuzumab to adjuvant chemotherapy for HER2-positive breast cancer is now the standard of care. Additional methods of targeting HER2 function, as with the small molecule tyrosine kinase inhibitor lapatinib, are undergoing testing in clinical trials at this time.

Special Situations

Ductal carcinoma in situ (DCIS), which accounts for approximately 20% to 25% of all newly diagnosed breast cancers, is treated slightly differently than invasive breast cancer. Overall prognosis for DCIS is good: 10-year overall survival for women with DCIS is 96%-98%. DCIS is most frequently asymptomatic at presentation and detected mammographically as suspicious microcalcifications. In some cases, DCIS may be a precursor lesion to invasive breast cancer. Consequently, treatment of DCIS is geared to preventing progression to invasive breast cancer. After mastectomy for DCIS, the risk of local recurrence is 1%.[60] With lumpectomy for DCIS, the risk of local recurrence was 26.8% in the NSABP B-17 trial. The addition of external-beam whole-breast radiation therapy to lumpectomy decreased this local recurrence risk to 12.1%. Furthermore, half of the local recurrences were invasive breast cancers. Although radiation therapy may play an important role in decreasing local recurrence in women undergoing lumpectomy for DCIS, there may be some patients treated with lumpectomy for DCIS in whom radiation therapy can be safely omitted. Specifically, it may be plausible to omit radiation therapy in older women with smaller areas of low-grade DCIS and wide surgical margins, as summarized by the University of Southern California/Van Nuys Prognostic Index.[92] In most cases of DCIS, sentinel lymph node biopsy/axillary staging is not necessary because the risk of lymph node metastasis associated with surgically excised DCIS is only approximately 5%. However, when mastectomy is performed for DCIS, sentinel node biopsy should be considered due to the possibility of subsequent identification of invasive cancer in the mastectomy specimen. Tamoxifen is also recommended for women with DCIS that is positive immunohistochemically for ER.[60]

SURVIVAL AND PROGNOSIS

Key Points

1. The majority of early-stage breast cancers are curable, and prognosis is related to ER, PR, and HER2 status.
2. Breast cancers that do not express ER, PR, or HER2 (triple-negative disease) have a greater risk of relapse, usually within 5 years.
3. Breast cancers that are positive for ER may recur as late as 10 to 25 years after primary diagnosis.

Breast cancer is detected at earlier stages then ever before in the United States, due to heightened public awareness and generally widespread access to mammography[34]; the majority of patients are now diagnosed with highly curable stage 0 to stage II disease. The ability to reliably document the "cure" of breast cancer in an affected individual with early-stage disease varies by the type of breast cancer due to the observation that the likelihood of relapse varies over time by ER, PR, and HER2 status.[89] Basal or triple-negative and HER2-positive breast cancers are characterized by rapid proliferative rates and early risk of relapse, primarily within the first 5 years of diagnosis. ER-positive breast cancer, on the other hand, may relapse as late as 10 to 25 years after diagnosis,[93] with clear proof of genetic relatedness of the relapsing cancer to the original primary tumor.[94] Breast cancer is also a highly chemo-responsive tumor relative to other solid tumors, such that the average 5-year survival rate of patients with metastatic disease is at least 20%[95] and may extend for a decade or more in the case of breast cancer metastatic to bone only. In addition to the heterogeneous clinical behavior of breast cancer subtypes, the collection of survival statistics lags well behind the incorporation of new therapies into the standard of care, causing widely cited summaries

Table 15-6 Five-Year Survival by Stage of Breast Cancer

Stage	5-Year Survival Rate (%)
0	100
I	100
II	86
III	57
IV	20

From reference 95 based on data from 1988 to 2001.

of survival by stage, as in Table 15-6,[95] to be of limited value in assessing the prognosis of an individual patient. Specific predictions through computer-based clinical subset data or genomic profiling[96] appear to be far more accurate.

MANAGEMENT OF RECURRENT DISEASE

Key Points

1. Recurrent breast cancer is managed primarily with chemotherapy and agents targeting known expression of ER and HER2.
2. Novel targeted agents, such as trastuzumab and olaparib, have demonstrated significant activity in certain subsets of recurrent breast cancer.

The management of recurrent breast cancer is dictated by the molecular biomarkers known to drive breast tumor growth. Therefore, estrogen-driven tumors expressing ER and PR are preferentially treated with anti-estrogen therapy typically involving tamoxifen and aromatase inhibitors, as well as the selective down-modulator of ER, fulvestrant.[97] For HER2-positive disease, the anti-HER2 antibody trastuzumab is combined with chemotherapy such as taxanes, and on progression, alternative HER2 targeting with the tyrosine kinase inhibitor lapatinib, in combination with the fluorouracil pro-drug capecitabine, is employed.[98] More recently, however, dual targeted therapy of molecular targets has been studied, for example, by combining lapatinib and trastuzumab (dual HER2 targeting)[99] and lapatinib and an aromatase inhibitor (HER2 and ER targeting).[100]

Recognition of the role of DNA repair proficiency in response to chemotherapy in recurrent disease has led to the use of therapy directed at specific subsets of breast cancer in which DNA repair deficiency is suspected, as in the triple-negative breast cancer, or confirmed, as in *BRCA*-mutated breast cancer. In triple-negative breast cancer, the high rate of genomic instability suggested a potential sensitivity to agents that would further disable DNA repair, such as inhibitors of poly (ADP ribose) polymerase (PARP), an essential component of single-strand, base excision repair.[101] When combined with carboplatin and gemcitabine in a phase II study, the PARP inhibitor iniparib achieved a tripling of response rate and prolongation of survival in metastatic triple-negative breast cancer over chemotherapy alone. In an even more compelling proof of the concept of targeting DNA repair deficiency, in BRCA-mutated breast cancer known to be deficient in homologous double-strand repair, the use of the PARP inhibitor olaparib alone, without chemotherapy, produced a greater than 40% response rate in heavily pretreated BRCA-mutated cancers.[102] This approach, using a genetically targeted therapy that takes advantage of the presence of an intrinsic sensitivity within the cancer cell, has been dubbed "synthetic lethality" and has been applied with similar success to BRCA-mutated ovarian cancer as well.[103]

For the vast majority of patients with recurrent breast cancer, the choice of therapy is limited to the use of single-agent chemotherapy, with the goal being to maintain control of disease while striving to maintain quality of life. With the advent of targeted therapies with generally lesser toxicity, appearing to show synergy with chemotherapy and in some cases superiority, this goal is increasingly achievable with the additional promise of prolonged survival. As in all cases of advanced cancer, the best therapeutic choice is likely to be a clinical trial.

SPECIAL MANAGEMENT PROBLEMS

Approximately 5% of breast cancers in the United states occur in carriers of BRCA gene mutations. For BRCA gene mutation carriers, the lifetime breast cancer risk is estimated to be between 26% and 85%. Breast cancers in women with BRCA1 gene mutations are more likely to occur at younger ages and be higher grade and ER negative. Although commonly used screening protocols have not been prospectively validated, heightened surveillance is generally recommended for this high-risk population. The National Comprehensive Cancer Network recommends annual screening mammography, annual screening breast MRI, and clinical breast examination every 6 months beginning at the age of 25 years. Prophylactic bilateral salpingo-oophorectomy in BRCA carriers not only reduces the risk of gynecologic malignancies, but also significantly reduces the BRCA-associated breast cancer risk. Prophylactic mastectomy furthermore reduces breast cancer risk by more than 90%.[104] The prognosis in terms of survival and local recurrence of BRCA-associated breast cancers,

however, remains the same, stage for stage, as that of similar cancers in women who are not BRCA carriers. BRCA carriers who develop breast cancer, however, are more likely to develop contralateral and new primary ipsilateral breast cancers at a rate of approximately 3% per year.[105] Consequently, bilateral mastectomy is often recommended for BRCA carriers who develop breast cancer.

Breast cancer diagnosed during pregnancy also provides special challenges in terms of diagnosis, staging, and treatment. Although traditionally a diagnosis of breast cancer during pregnancy was associated with worse prognosis, it now appears that this is largely due to the more advanced stage at the time of diagnosis of cancer in women who are pregnant. Expeditious and appropriate therapy, therefore, may result in survival comparable to that of nonpregnant women with breast cancer. In pregnant women, clinical breast examination is less sensitive as a result of glandular hyperplasia and increased density of the breasts. Mammography and other forms of ionizing radiation, furthermore, should generally be avoided in pregnancy. Although MRI itself is safe in pregnancy, gadolinium, the contrast agent used for breast MRIs, does cross the placenta and has not yet been studied in pregnancy. Breast ultrasound is the only safe imaging modality in pregnant women. Breast cancer treatment during pregnancy largely depends the gestational age of the fetus when the cancer is diagnosed. In the first trimester, most pregnant women with breast cancer will be recommended to undergo modified radical mastectomy because adjuvant radiation therapy, which should ideally be started within 8 weeks of successful lumpectomy, cannot be safely given until at least the second trimester. Axillary lymph node dissection, rather than sentinel node biopsy, is performed in pregnancy because the blue dyes and radioactive isotopes used to identify the sentinel lymph nodes have not been demonstrated to be safe for the developing fetus. Chemotherapy should be avoided in the first trimester and stopped at least 3 weeks before anticipated delivery of the baby to allow time for recovery of immune function. Tamoxifen and other estrogen receptor modulators may have teratogenic effects and should not be given during pregnancy. For women diagnosed with stage III or IV breast cancer during the first trimester of pregnancy, termination of the pregnancy should be considered.[106]

Unlike the far more common epithelial breast cancers, treatment of phyllodes tumors, regardless of whether they are classified as being benign or malignant, is wide local excision to at least 1-cm margins because of the propensity for even benign phyllodes tumors to recur locally. At times, mastectomy may be required to achieve the desired surgical margins. Axillary lymph node dissection is not routinely performed because lymph node metastases with phyllodes tumors are rare, and the role of chemotherapy and radiation therapy has not been established in the management of phyllodes tumors.[107]

FUTURE DIRECTIONS

The therapy of breast cancer has evolved dramatically in the past 30 years. For the management of local disease, this era has been marked by the steadily diminishing extent of surgery on the breast, with lumpectomy replacing mastectomy in many cases, and in the axilla, with sentinel lymph node sampling replacing full axillary dissection for many women. In radiation oncology, new technology has allowed a reduction in the extent of radiation therapy both to the breast and surrounding normal tissues, with a resulting decrease in toxicity to normal structures. In the use of systemic adjuvant therapy to control the risk of micrometastatic disease, in combination with definitive local therapy, molecular analysis and genomic profiling of breast cancers have allowed the avoidance of unnecessary chemotherapy and the identification of patients for whom specific chemotherapies may be remarkably effective. The use of less toxic, targeted therapy directed against the intrinsic biology of breast cancer has led to large, incremental increases in rates of cure and diminished reliance on chemotherapy. In the metastatic setting, the growing understanding of the unique and heterogeneous biology of breast cancer, characterized at the level of the genome, transcriptome, and proteome, has created an explosion of new molecular targets and potential therapies directed against these targets. The future of breast cancer is at the molecular and genomic level; a new generation of clinical trials has incorporated this level of definition of breast cancer into the design of studies involving the rational combination of targeted agents to enhance efficacy and reduce resistance. This approach relies on the biologic knowledge derived from the laboratory and applied to the clinic. For example, the knowledge that resistance to HER2-directed therapy with trastuzumab occurs through the activation of the PI3-kinase/AKT survival pathway leads to trials with trastuzumab and inhibitors of the PI3-kinase pathway[108]; knowledge that therapy-resistant ER-positive breast cancer increasingly acquires an epithelial to mesenchymal transition (EMT)-like profile leads to the combination of src-inhibitors with ER blockade[109,110]; knowledge that fibroblast growth factor receptor polymorphisms increase risk of breast cancer and that fibroblast growth factor receptor genes are amplified in subsets of breast cancer leads to trials of agents targeting this pathway.[111] Adding to this expanding molecular world is the discovery of microRNA; this represents untranslated regulatory genetic material with diagnostic, prognostic, and ultimately therapeutic potential in breast cancer.[112] By examining, understanding, and now defining breast cancer by the disease-causing pathology at the level of the genome, new insights are gained and opportunities revealed for both improvements in cancer therapy and the advancement of cancer biology.

REFERENCES

1. Russo JR, Russo I. *Molecular Basis of Breast Cancer: Prevention and Treatment*. New York, NY: Springer; 2004.
2. Jemal A, Siegel R, Xu U, Ward E. Cancer statistics, 2010. *CA Cancer J Clin*. 2010;60;277-300.
3. Weinberg RA. *The Biology of Cancer*. New York, NY: Garland Science; 2007.
4. Evans DG, Howell A. Breast cancer risk-assessment models. *Breast Cancer Res*. 2007;9(5):213.
5. Reynolds P, Goldberg D, Hurley S, et al. Passive smoking and risk of breast cancer in the California Teachers Study. *Cancer Epidemiol Biomarkers Prev*. 2009;18(12):3389-3398.
6. Henderson TO, Amsterdam A, Bhatia S, et al. Systematic review: surveillance for breast cancer in women treated with chest radiation for childhood, adolescent, or young adult cancer. *Ann Intern Med*. 2010;152(7):444-455.
7. McCormack VA, Perry NM, Vinnicombe SJ, dos Santos Silva I. Changes and tracking of mammographic density in relation to Pike's model of breast tissue aging: a UK longitudinal study. *Int J Cancer*. 2010;127(2):452-461.
8. Henderson BP, Ponder B, Ross RK, eds. *Hormones, Genes, and Cancer*. New York, NY: Oxford University Press; 2003.
9. Chlebowski RT, Kuller LH, Prentice RL, et al. Breast cancer after use of estrogen plus progestin in postmenopausal women. *N Engl J Med*. 2009;360(6):573-587.
10. World Cancer Research Fund, American Institute for Cancer Research. *Food, Nutrition, Physical Activity, and the Prevention of Cancer: a Global Perspective*. 2nd ed. Washington, DC: American Institute for Cancer Research; 2007.
11. Roy JR, Chakraborty S, Chakraborty TR. Estrogen-like endocrine disrupting chemicals affecting puberty in humans—a review. *Med Sci Monit*. 2009;15(6):137-145.
12. Groff T. Bisphenol A: invisible pollution. *Curr Opin Pediatr*. 2010;22(4):524-529.
13. Walsh T, King M-C. Ten genes for inherited breast cancer. *Cancer Cell*. 2007;11(2):103-105.
14. Domchek SM, Friebel TM, Singer CF, et al. Association of risk-reducing surgery in BRCA1 or BRCA2 mutation carriers with cancer risk and mortality. *JAMA*. 2010;304(9):967-975.
15. Linger RJ, Kruk PA. BRCA1 16 years later: risk-associated BRCA1 mutations and their functional implications. *FEBS J*. 2010;277(15):3086-3096.
16. Easton DF, Pooley KA, Dunning AM, et al. Genome-wide association study identifies novel breast cancer susceptibility loci. *Nature*. 2007;447(7148):1087-1093.
17. Prentice RL, Huang Y, Hinds DA, et al. Variation in the FGFR2 gene and the effects of postmenopausal hormone therapy on invasive breast cancer. *Cancer Epidemiol Biomarkers Prev*. 2009;18(11):3079-3085.
18. Gail MH. Discriminatory accuracy from single-nucleotide polymorphisms in models to predict breast cancer risk. *J Natl Cancer Inst*. 2008;100(14):1037-1041.
19. Micalizzi D, Farabaugh S, Ford H. Epithelial-mesenchymal transition in cancer: parallels between normal development and tumor progression. *J Mammary Gland Biol Neoplasia*. 2010;15(2):117-134.
20. Thiery JP, Acloque H, Huang RYJ, Nieto MA. Epithelial-mesenchymal transitions in development and disease. *Cell*. 2009;139(5):871-890.

21. Li Y, Rosen JM. Stem/progenitor cells in mouse mammary gland development and breast cancer. *J Mammary Gland Biol Neoplasia.* 2005;10(1):17-24.

22. Mack DL, Smith Gilbert H, Booth Brian W. Mammary glands, stem cells, and breast cancer. In: Giordano A, Normanno N, eds. *Breast Cancer in the Post-Genomic Era.* New York, NY: Humana Press; 2009:19-38.

23. Tot T. DCIS, cytokeratins, and the theory of the sick lobe. *Virchows Archiv.* 2005;447(1):1-8.

24. Russo JR, I. The genomic basis of breast development and differentiation. In: Giordano A, Normanno N, eds. *Breast Cancer in the Post-Genomic Era.* New York, NY: Humana Press; 2009:1-18.

25. Balogh GA, Heulings R, Mailo DA, et al. Genomic signature induced by pregnancy in the human breast. *Int J Oncol.* 2006;28(2):399-410.

26. Russo J, Balogh GA, Russo IH. Full-term pregnancy induces a specific genomic signature in the human breast. *Cancer Epidemiol Biomarkers Prev.* 2008;17(1):51-66.

27. Giordano A, Normanno N, eds. *Breast Cancer in the Post-Genomic Era.* New York, NY: Humana Press; 2009.

28. National Cancer Institute. Breast Cancer Risk Asessment Tool. http://www.cancer.gov/bcrisktool/. Accessed January 18, 2012.

29. Goodson WH, King EB. Discharges and secretions of the nipple. In: Bland K, Copeland EM, eds. *The Breast: Comprehensive Management of Benign and Malignant Disorders.* St. Louis, MO: Saunders; 2004:65-90.

30. Birdwell RL, Wang SC. Mammography: screening. In: Berg A, Birdwell RL, eds. *Diagnostic Imaging: Breast.* Salt Lake City, UT: Amirsys; 2006:6-11.

31. Wang SC. Mammography. In: Berg A, Birdwell RL, eds. *Diagnostic Imaging: Breast.* Salt Lake City, UT: Amirsys; 2006:12-17.

32. Bassett LS. Breast imaging. In: Berg A, Birdwell RL, eds. *Diagnostic Imaging: Breast.* Salt Lake City, UT: Amirsys; 2006:611-665.

33. Shapiro S. Periodic screening for breast cancer: the HIP randomized controlled trial. Health Insurance Plan. *J Natl Cancer Inst Monograph.* 1997;22:27-30.

34. U.S. Preventive Services Task Force. Screening for Breast Cancer: U.S. Preventive Services Task Force Recommendation Statement. *Ann Intern Med.* 2009;151(10):716-726.

35. Smith RA, Cokkinides V, Brooks D, Saslow D, Brawley OW. Cancer screening in the United States, 2010: a review of current American Cancer Society Guidelines and issues in cancer screening. *CA Cancer J Clin.* 2010;60(2):99-119.

36. American College of Surgeons. American College of Surgeons voices strong support for American Cancer Society screening mammography guidelines. 2009. http://www.facs.org/news/mammography1109.html. Accessed February 24, 2012.

37. ACOG. American College of Obstetrics and Gynecology: ACOG statement on revised US Preventative Services Task Force recommendations on breast cancer screening. 2009. http://www.acog.org/from_home/publications/press_releases/nr11-16-09.cfm. Accessed January 18, 2012.

38. Hendrick RE, Pisano ED, Averbukh A, et al. Comparison of acquisition parameters and breast dose in digital mammography and screen-film mammography in the American College of Radiology Imaging Network Digital Mammographic Imaging Screening Trial. *Am J Roentgenol.* 2010;194(2):362-369.

39. Pisano ED, Hendrick RE, Yaffe MJ, et al. DMIST Investigators Group Diagnostic accuracy of digital versus film mammography: exploratory analysis of selected population subgroups in DMIST. *Radiology.* 2008;246(2):376-383.

40. Helvie M. Improving mammographic interpretation: double reading and computer-aided diagnosis. *Radiol Clin North Am.* 2007;45(5):801-811.

41. Kennedy A, Berg WA. Ultrasound. In: Berg A, Birdwell RL, eds. *Diagnostic Imaging: Breast.* Salt Lake City, UT: Amirsys; 2006:32-35.

42. Berg WA, Blume JD, Cormack JB, et al. Combined screening with ultrasound and mammography vs mammography alone in women at elevated risk of breast cancer. *JAMA.* 2008;299(18):2151-2163.

43. Kuhl C. The current status of breast MR imaging, part I. Choice of technique, image interpretation, diagnostic accuracy, and transfer to clinical practice. *Radiology.* 2007;244(2):356-378.

44. Silverstein MJ, Recht A, Lagios MD, et al. Image-detected breast cancer: state-of-the-art diagnosis and treatment. *J Am Coll Surg.* 2009;209(4):504-520.

45. Houssami N, Hayes DF. Review of preoperative magnetic resonance imaging (MRI) in breast cancer: should MRI be performed on all women with newly diagnosed, early stage breast cancer? *CA Cancer J Clin.* 2009;59(5):290-302.

46. Turnbull L, Brown S, Harvey I, et al. Comparative effectiveness of MRI in breast cancer (COMICE) trial: a randomised controlled trial. *Lancet.* 2010;375(9714):563-571.

47. Urisst MB, Bland KI. Indications and techniques for biopsy. In: Bland K, Copeland, EM, ed. *The Breast: Comprehensive Management of Benign and Malignant Disorders.* St Louis, MO: Saunders; 2004:787-801.

48. Bruening W, Fontanarosa J, Tipton K, Treadwell JR, Launders J, Schoelles K. Systematic review: comparative effectiveness of core-needle and open surgical biopsy to diagnose breast lesions. *Ann Intern Med.* 2010;152(4):238-246.

49. Weigelt B, Reis-Filho JS. Histological and molecular types of breast cancer: is there a unifying taxonomy? *Nat Rev Clin Oncol.* 2009;6(12):718-730.

50. Stratton MR, Campbell PJ, Futreal PA. The cancer genome. *Nature.* 2009;458(7239):719-724.

51. Schnitt SJ. Classification and prognosis of invasive breast cancer: from morphology to molecular taxonomy. *Mod Pathol.* 2010;23(S2):S60-S64.

52. Hammond MEH, Hayes DF, Dowsett M, et al. American Society of Clinical Oncology/College of American Pathologists guideline recommendations for immunohistochemical testing of estrogen and progesterone receptors in breast cancer (unabridged version). *Arch Pathol Lab Med.* 2010;134(7):e48-e72.

53. Sauter G, Lee J, Bartlett JMS, Slamon DJ, Press MF. Guidelines for human epidermal growth factor receptor 2 testing: biologic and methodologic considerations. *J Clin Oncol.* 2009;27(8):1323-1333.

54. Liedtke C, Hatzis C, Symmans WF, et al. Genomic grade index is associated with response to chemotherapy in patients with breast cancer. *J Clin Oncol.* 2009;27(19):3185-3191.

55. Filho OM, Ignatiadis M, Sotiriou C. Genomic grade index: an important tool for assessing breast cancer tumor grade and prognosis. *Crit Rev Oncol Hematol.* 2011;77(1):20-29.

56. Pinder SE. Ductal carcinoma in situ (DCIS): pathological features, differential diagnosis, prognostic factors and specimen evaluation. *Mod Pathol.* 2010;23(S2):S8-S13.

57. Berman HK, Gauthier ML, Tlsty TD. Premalignant breast neoplasia: a paradigm of interlesional and intralesional molecular heterogeneity and its biological and clinical ramifications. *Cancer Prev Res.* 2010;3(5):579-587.

58. Ellis IO. Intraductal proliferative lesions of the breast: morphology, associated risk and molecular biology. *Mod Pathol.* 2010;23(S2):S1-S7.

59. Ansquer Y, Delaney S, Santulli P, Salomon L, Carbonne B, Salmon R. Risk of invasive breast cancer after lobular intraepithelial neoplasia: review of the literature. *Eur J Surg Oncol.* 2010;36(7):604-609.

60. Allegra CJ, Aberle DR, Ganschow P, et al. National Institutes of Health State-of-the-Science Conference Statement: Diagnosis and Management of Ductal Carcinoma In Situ September 22–24, 2009. *J Natl Cancer Inst.* 2010;102(3):161-169.

61. Venkitaraman R. Lobular neoplasia of the breast. *Breast Jl.* 2010;16(5):519-528.

62. Chen CY, Sun LM, Anderson BO. Paget disease of the breast: changing patterns of incidence, clinical presentation, and treatment in the U.S. *Cancer.* 2006;107(7):1448-1458.

63. Stamatakos M, Tsaknaki S, Kontzoglou K, Gogas J, Kostakis A, Safioleas M. Phylloides tumor of the breast: a rare neoplasm, though not that innocent. *Int Semin Surg Oncol.* 2009;6(1):6.

64. Frykberg EB, Bland KI. Evolution of surgical prinicples and techniques for the management of breast cancer. In: Bland K, Copeland EM, eds. *The Breast: Comprehensive Management of Benign and Malignant Disorders.* St Louis, MO: Saunders; 2004:759-785.

65. Maddox WA, Carpenter JT Jr, Laws HL, et al. A randomized prospective trial of radical (Halstead) mastectomy versus modified radical mastectomy in 311 breast cancer patients. *Ann Surg.* 1983;198(2):207-212.

66. Turner L, Swindell R, Bell WG, et al. Radical versus modified radical mastectomy for breast cancer. *Ann R Coll Surg Engl.* 1981; 63(4):239-243.

67. Fisher B, Anderson S, Bryant J, et al. Twenty-year follow-up of a randomized trial comparing total mastectomy, lumpectomy, and lumpectomy plus irradiation for the treatment of invasive breast cancer. *N Engl J Med.* 2002;347(16):1233-1241.

68. Veronesi U, Cascinelli N, Mariani L, et al. Twenty-year follow-up of a randomized study comparing breast-conserving surgery with radical mastectomy for early breast cancer. *N Engl J Med.* 2002;347(16):1227-1232.

69. Arriagada R, Le M, Rochard F, Contesso G. Conservative treatment versus mastectomy in early breast cancer: patterns of failure with 15 years of follow-up data. Institut Gustave-Roussy Breast Cancer Group. *J Clin Oncol.* 1996;14(5):1558-1564.

70. Jacobson JA, Danforth DN, Cowan KH, et al. Ten-year results of a comparison of conservation with mastectomy in the treatment of stage I and II breast cancer. *N Engl J Med.* 1995;332(14):907-911.

71. van Dongen JA, Voogd AC, Fentiman IS, et al. Long-term results of a randomized trial comparing breast-conserving therapy with mastectomy: European Organization for Research and Treatment of Cancer 10801 Trial. *J Natl Cancer Inst.* 2000;92(14):1143-1150.

72. Blichert-Toft M, Rose C, Anderson J, et al. Danish randomized trial comparing breast conservation therapy with mastectomy: six years of life-table analysis. Danish Breast Cancer Cooperative Group. *J Natl Cancer Inst Monogr.* 1992;11:19-25.

73. Kontiras HD, De Los Santos JF, Bland KI. Breast conservation in invasive breast cancer. In: Bland K, Copeland EM, eds. *The Breast: Comprehensive Management of Benign and Malignant Disorders.* St. Louis, MO: Saunders; 2004:885-898.

74. Gaskin T. Rehabilitation. In: Bland K, Copeland EM, eds. *The Breast: Comprehensive Management of Benign and Malignant Disorders.* St. Louis, MO: Saunders; 2004:1545-1555.

75. Fisher B, Jeong J-H, Anderson S, Bryant J, Fisher ER, Wolmark N. Twenty-five-year follow-up of a randomized trial comparing radical mastectomy, total mastectomy, and total mastectomy followed by irradiation. *N Engl J Med.* 2002;347(8):567-575.

76. Grube BG, Giuliano AE. Lymphatic mapping and sentinel lymphadenectomy for breast cancer. In: Bland K, Copeland EM, eds. *The Breast: Comprehensive Management of Benign and Malignant Disorders.* St. Louis, MO: Saunders; 2004:1041-1079.

77. Krag DN, Anderson SJ, Julian TB, et al. Technical outcomes of sentinel-lymph-node resection and conventional axillary-lymph-node dissection in patients with clinically node-negative breast cancer: results from the NSABP B-32 randomised phase III trial. *Lancet Oncol.* 2007;8(10):881-888.

78. Ashikaga T, Krag DN, Land SR, et al. Morbidity results from the NSABP B-32 trial comparing sentinel lymph node dissection versus axillary dissection. *J Surg Oncol.* 2010;102(2):111-118.

79. Lanitis S, Tekkis PP, Sgourakis G, Dimopoulos N, Al Mufti R, Hadjiminas DJ. Comparison of skin-sparing mastectomy versus non-skin-sparing mastectomy for breast cancer: a meta-analysis of observational studies. *Ann Surg.* 2010;251(4):632-639.

80. Chung AP, Sacchini V. Nipple-sparing mastectomy: where are we now? *Surg Oncol.* 2008;17(4):261-266.

81. Cordeiro PG. Breast reconstruction after surgery for breast cancer. *N Engl J Med.* 2008;359(15):1590-1601.

82. Marks L. Radiotherapy techniques. In: Bland K, Copeland EM, eds. *The Breast: Comprehensive Management of Benign and Malignant Disorders.* St. Louis, MO: Saunders; 2004:1139-1144.

83. Whelan TJ, Pignol JP, Levine MN, et al. Long-term results of hypofractionated radiation therapy for breast cancer. *N Engl J Med.* 2010;362(6):513-520.

84. Pierce L. Postmastectomy radiotherapy. In: Bland K, Copeland EM, eds. *The Breast: Comprehensive Management of Benign and Malignant Disorders.* St. Louis, MO: Saunders; 2004: 1165-1172.

85. Kelly CM, Warner E, Tsoi DT, Verma S, Pritchard KI. Review of the clinical studies using the 21-gene assay. *Oncologist.* 2010;15(5):447-456.

86. Mook S, Knauer M, Bueno-de-Mesquita J, et al. Metastatic potential of T1 breast cancer can be predicted by the 70-gene mammaprint signature. *Ann Surg Oncol.* 2010;17(5):1406-1413.

87. Adjuvant Online. http://www.adjuvantonline.com. Accessed January 18, 2012.

88. Albain KS, Barlow WE, Shak S, et al. Prognostic and predictive value of the 21-gene recurrence score assay in postmenopausal women with node-positive, oestrogen-receptor-positive breast cancer on chemotherapy: a retrospective analysis of a randomised trial. *Lancet Oncol.* 2010;11(1):55-65.

89. Burstein HJ, Prestrud AA, Seidenfeld J, et al. American Society of Clinical Oncology Clinical Practice Guideline: update on adjuvant endocrine therapy for women with hormone receptor–positive breast cancer. *J Clin Oncol.* 2010;28(23):3784-3796.

90. Sparano JA, Paik S. Development of the 21-gene assay and its application in clinical practice and clinical trials. *J Clin Oncol.* 2008;26(5):721-728.

91. Brufsky A. Trastuzumab-based therapy for patients with HER2-positive breast cancer: from early scientific development to foundation of care. *Am J Clin Oncol.* 2010;33(2):186-195.

92. Silverstein MJ, Woo C. Ductal carcinoma in situ: diagnostic and therapeutic controversies. In: Bland K, Copeland EM, eds. *The Breast: Comprehensive Management of Benign and Malignant Disorders.* St. Louis, MO: Saunders; 2004:985-1018.

93. Willis L, Alarcón T, Elia G, et al. Breast cancer dormancy can be maintained by small numbers of micrometastases. *Cancer Res.* 2010;70(11):4310-4317.

94. Shah SP, Morin RD, Khattra J, et al. Mutational evolution in a lobular breast tumour profiled at single nucleotide resolution. *Nature.* 2009;461(7265):809-813.

95. American Cancer Society. Breast cancer survival by stage. http://www.cancer.org/Cancer/BreastCancer/DetailedGuide/breast-cancer-staging. Accessed January 18, 2012.

96. Park JY, Lee SY, Jeon H-S, et al. Polymorphism of the DNA repair gene XRCC1 and risk of primary lung cancer. *Cancer Epidemiol Biomarkers Prev.* 2002;11(1):23-27.

97. Pritchard K, Rolski J, Papai Z, et al. Results of a phase II study comparing three dosing regimens of fulvestrant in postmenopausal women with advanced breast cancer (FINDER2). *Breast Cancer Res Treat.* 2010;123(2):453-461.

CHAPTER 15

98. Cameron D, Casey M, Oliva C, Newstat B, Imwalle B, Geyer CE. Lapatinib plus capecitabine in women with HER-2-positive advanced breast cancer: final survival analysis of a phase III randomized trial. *Oncologist.* 2010;15(9):924-934.

99. Campone M, Juin P, André F, Bachelot T. Resistance to HER2 inhibitors: is addition better than substitution? Rationale for the hypothetical concept of drug sedimentation. *Crit Rev Oncol Hematol.* 2011;78(3):195-205.

100. Sherrill B, Amonkar MM, Sherif B, Maltzman J, O'Rourke L, Johnston S. Quality of life in hormone receptor-positive HER-2+ metastatic breast cancer patients during treatment with letrozole alone or in combination with lapatinib. *Oncologist.* 2010;15(9):944-953.

101. Annunziata CM, O'Shaughnessy J. Poly (ADP-ribose) polymerase as a novel therapeutic target in cancer. *Clin Cancer Res.* 2010;16(18):4517-4526.

102. Tutt A, Robson M, Garber JE, et al. Oral poly(ADP-ribose) polymerase inhibitor olaparib in patients with BRCA1 or BRCA2 mutations and advanced breast cancer: a proof-of-concept trial. *Lancet.* 2010;376(9737):235-244.

103. Audeh MW, Carmichael J, Penson RT, et al. Oral poly(ADP-ribose) polymerase inhibitor olaparib in patients with BRCA1 or BRCA2 mutations and recurrent ovarian cancer: a proof-of-concept trial. *Lancet.* 2010;376(9737):245-251.

104. Jatoi I, Anderson WF. Management of women who have a genetic predisposition for breast cancer. *Surg Clin North Am.* 2008;88(4):845-861.

105. Bordeleau L, Panchal S, Goodwin P. Prognosis of BRCA-associated breast cancer: a summary of evidence. *Breast Cancer Res Treat.* 2010;119(1):13-24.

106. Navrozoglou I, Vrekoussis T, Kontostolis E, et al. Breast cancer during pregnancy: a mini-review. *Eur J Surg Oncol.* 2008;34(8):837-843.

107. Mies C. Mammary sarcoma and lymphoma. In: Bland K, Copeland EM, eds. *The Breast: Comprehensive Management of Benign and Malignant Disorders.* St. Louis, MO: Saunders; 2004:305-323.

108. O'Brien NA, Browne BC, Chow L, et al. Activated phosphoinositide 3-kinase/AKT signaling confers resistance to trastuzumab but not lapatinib. *Mol Cancer Ther.* 2010;9(6):1489-1502.

109. Chen Y, Alvarez E, Azzam D, et al. Combined Src and ER blockade impairs human breast cancer proliferation in vitro and in vivo. *Breast Cancer Res Treat.* 2010:1-10.

110. Mayer EL, Krop IE. Advances in targeting Src in the treatment of breast cancer and other solid malignancies. *Clin Cancer Res.* 2010;16(14):3526-3532.

111. Hynes NE, Dey JH. Potential for targeting the fibroblast growth factor receptors in breast cancer. *Cancer Res.* 2010;70(13):5199-5202.

112. Janssen EAM, Slewa A, Gudlaugsson E, et al. Biologic profiling of lymph node negative breast cancers by means of microRNA expression. *Mod Pathol.* 2010;23(12):1567-1576.

16 Cancer in Pregnancy

Malaika Amneus and Christine H. Holschneider

The diagnosis of cancer complicates approximately 1 in 1000 pregnancies. Once diagnosed, emotional, ethical, diagnostic, and treatment dilemmas confront both the patient and the treating physicians, posing unique challenges. Questions regarding whether or not to terminate the pregnancy, potential maternal risk of delays in cancer treatment, fetal risks of early delivery, and maternal and fetal effects of cancer treatments during gestation are complex and competing factors that make decision making both medically and emotionally challenging. Limited data on the treatment of malignancies during pregnancy and absence of randomized controlled studies in this population contribute to the lack of generalized treatment algorithms. Individualization of treatment planning with a multidisciplinary team is essential. Considerations not only include the risk/benefit assessment of treatment modalities such as chemotherapy, radiation therapy, and surgery during pregnancy, but also include the potential maternal and fetal consequences of diagnostic procedures.

The most common malignancies during pregnancy include those that are most commonly found in women of reproductive age and include cervical and ovarian cancer. The most common nongynecologic malignancies are breast cancer, malignant melanoma, thyroid cancer, and hematologic malignancies.[1-3] Given that the incidence of malignancies increases with increasing age, as more women choose to delay childbearing, it is expected that the incidence of cancer during pregnancy will increase.

RADIATION IN PREGNANCY

Key Points

1. The developmental effects of radiation exposure on pregnancy is related both to the dose of radiation as well as the gestational age.
2. Computed tomography and magnetic resonance imaging, including scans of the pelvis, are associated with negligible fetal risk.

Ionizing radiation is used routinely during imaging for cancer staging or disease surveillance, and radiation therapy is a common component of the treatment of many cancers in the nonpregnant patient. In pregnancy, consideration has to be given not only to the radiation exposure of the mother, but also that of the developing fetus. Much of what we know about the effects of radiation on pregnancy is based on animal studies, accidental or incidental human exposures to diagnostic and therapeutic radiation, and data gathered from victims of radiation exposure after the atomic bombings of Hiroshima and Nagasaki. There are many confounding factors that limit our interpretation of these data, including species differences, potential differential effects of various types of ionizing radiation, lack of certainty regarding the doses of radiation received, potential differential effects of single versus multiple exposures, and the baseline rate of human malformations and other negative outcomes. Given the lack of controlled studies on the issue, patient counseling regarding radiation exposure in pregnancy may be challenging, even as it relates to imaging procedures. The growing importance of this issue is evidenced by a recent review that noted a 107% increase over the past decade in the use of imaging studies using ionizing radiation during pregnancy.[4]

The developmental effects of radiation exposure on a pregnancy are related not only to the dose of radiation, but also to the gestational age of the pregnancy. Gestation can be generally divided into 3 periods: preimplantation (0-2 weeks after conception), organogenesis (2-8 weeks after conception), and the fetal period (>8 weeks after conception). Radiation exposure has different potential developmental effects during each of these periods (Table 16-1).[5,6] In addition, radiation exposure can lead to genetic cell injury and an increased malignancy risk at any gestational age.

During the preimplantation period, radiation exposure is thought to have an "all or none" effect; that is, the embryo dies, or there is no consequence.[7] This may be explained by the fact that at this early stage of development, the embryo is composed of totipotent cells. If the radiation causes the death of a sufficient number of these cells, the embryo will not survive. Otherwise, the remaining cells will continue to divide and the insult will be overcome without further sequelae. Exposure to 10 cGy (10 rads) or more is generally thought to result in pregnancy loss during the preimplantation period.[8]

During the period of organogenesis, the fetus is most susceptible to the teratogenic effects of radiation exposure. Notable effects include microcephaly, microphthalmia, eye anomalies, mental retardation, genital malformations, and growth restriction.[6,9] It is the current consensus that exposure to <5 cGy (<5 rads) of radiation is not related to an increased risk of fetal malformation,[8] and it is important to note that no single common diagnostic imaging procedure in use today results in exposures at this level (Table 16-2). However, such levels can be quickly reached with multiple imaging studies, therapeutic radiation, and fluoroscopic procedures. Although concerns about exposure in the range of 5 to 10 cGy (5-10 rads) have been raised, significantly increased developmental risk to the embryo and fetus is not known until the absorbed dose reaches at least 10 cGy (10 rads).

During the fetal period, the effects of radiation exposure seem to be limited to growth retardation,

Table 16-1 Developmental Effects of Ionizing Radiation at Different Gestational Ages[7,8]

Developmental Period	EGA	Age of Conceptus	Estimated Threshold Dose	Main Effect
Any	Any	Any	5 cGy (5 rads)	Noncancer health effects not detected below threshold
Developmental Effects				
Preconception	1-2 weeks	n/a	n/a	Mother has not yet ovulated
Preimplantation period	3-4 weeks	<2 weeks	10 cGy (10 rads)	Main risk: Pregnancy loss (baseline population risk below threshold)
Organogenesis	4-10 weeks	2-8 weeks	10-20 cGy (10-20 rads)	Greatest risk for major malformations; lesser risk for growth restriction (baseline population risk below threshold)
Fetal period	8-17 weeks[a]	6 (8)-15 weeks[a]	For severe mental retardation: 10 cGy (10 rads)[b]	Greatest risk for growth restriction, microcephaly, and mental retardation (baseline population risk below threshold)
	18-27 weeks	16-25 weeks	For reduction in IQ :10 cGy (10 rads)[c]	Main risk: Cognitive impairment, growth restriction, death (baseline population risk below threshold)
	28 weeks to term	26 weeks to term	50 cGy (50 rads)	Main risk: Cognitive impairment, growth restriction, death (baseline population risk below threshold)

Note. Gray (Gy) is the International System unit for the radiation absorbed dose rad, which is the old but still frequently used unit (1 Gy = 100 rads; 1 cGy = 1 rad). Radiographic exposure from a single diagnostic procedure to less than 5 cGy (5 rads) has not been associated with an increase in fetal abnormalities or pregnancy loss. Although concerns about exposure in the range from 5 to 10 cGy (5-10 rads) have been raised, serious developmental risk to the fetus is not known until the absorbed dose reaches 10 cGy (10 rads).
[a]Overlap observed in main effects during late organogenesis/early fetogenesis.
[b]Available data suggest that the risk of severe mental retardation is approximately 40% per 100 cGy (100 rads) of exposure above 10 cGy (10 rads).
[c]Available data suggest that the risk of severe mental retardation is approximately 9% per 100 cGy (100 rads) of exposure above 10 cGy (10 rads). Risk of reduction in IQ is estimated at 13 to 21 points per 100 cGy (100 rads) of exposure.

Table 16-2 Estimated Fetal Radiation Exposure From Common Diagnostic Radiologic Procedures[10,11]

Procedure	Fetal Exposure cGy (rad)
Chest x-ray (2 views)	$2\text{-}7 \times 10^{-5}$
Mammogram (4 views)	0.01-0.04
Abdominal x-ray (1 view)	0.1-0.3
Pelvic x-ray (1 view)	0.2-0.35
Ventilation–perfusion scan	0.01-0.04
Helical CT chest	$1\text{-}10 \times 10^{-3}$
CT abdomen	1.7-3.5
CT pelvis	1.0-4.6

microcephaly, and central nervous system (CNS) defects (decreased IQ and mental retardation).[5,6] The period from the 8th to 15th weeks appears to be the period of greatest vulnerability of the CNS, and it is estimated that the probability of mental retardation is approximately 40% for every 100 cGy (100 rads) exposure above 10 cGy (10 rads).[12] The sensitivity of the CNS to radiation is less during the 16th to 25th weeks, and studies have estimated a 13- to 21-point reduction in IQ for every 100 cGy (100 rads) of radiation exposure above 10 cGy (10 rads).[5] The radiation sensitivity of the CNS is even further reduced after 25 weeks.

In addition to the potential developmental effects of radiation exposure, there is also concern for an increased risk of childhood cancers (both leukemias as well as solid tumors) in children exposed to radiation in utero. The relative risk for childhood cancer associated with in utero radiation exposure, as found in the large Oxford Survey of Childhood Cancers as well as in a 1993 meta-analysis, is approximately 1.4.[13] The excess childhood cancer risk attributable to in utero radiation exposure is estimated to be 6% per 100 cGy, with an increase in risk starting to become appreciable at doses as low as 1 cGy.[13] Although it may sound alarming that a standard pelvic CT scan may potentially double the risk of fatal childhood cancer, this must be viewed in context of the low baseline risk (approximately 1 in 2000)[9] and the potential benefit to the management of mother and pregnancy of the information gained by the imaging study. One significant difficulty in interpreting this literature is due to the fact that much of the data stem from case-control studies collected over many decades, during and after which radiation exposure with diagnostic imaging has been greatly reduced. In fact, recent population-based data from Ontario using 1.8 million maternal-child pairs from 1991 to 2008 found no increase in childhood cancers in the

offspring of 5590 mothers exposed to major radiodiagnostic testing in pregnancy (crude hazard ratio of 0.69; 95% confidence interval, 0.26-1.82).[14]

Computed Tomography in Pregnancy

It is generally agreed that imaging modalities that do not involve ionizing radiation, such as ultrasound and magnetic resonance imaging (MRI), are preferred in pregnancy as long as they adequately provide the desired diagnostic information. However, as demonstrated in Table 16-1, the radiation dose to the fetus from a computed tomography (CT) scan, even of the pelvis, is below a dose expected to be associated with considerable fetal risk. It is thus unacceptable to delay diagnostic work-up of a pregnant patient with suspected cancer if the information gained from the imaging study is expected to affect management. In addition, such exposure per se should not alter the management of the pregnancy. Despite this, a survey of physicians published in 2004 indicated that up to 6% would recommend pregnancy termination after an abdominal CT scan in early pregnancy,[15] highlighting the need for provider education. In addition to the potential effects of exposure to ionizing radiation during a CT scan discussed previously, there may also be concerns about the safety of intravenous (IV) contrast administration during pregnancy. Iodinated contrast media do not appear to be teratogenic in animals. Human data are lacking, and thus they are considered US Food and Drug Administration (FDA) category B drugs. The use of iodinated contrast agents is considered acceptable in human pregnancy when it is necessary for appropriate diagnosis and after informed consent.[16] There is a theoretical risk of depression of neonatal thyroid function with in utero exposure to iodinated agents. However, there are no clear data that demonstrate any considerable increased risk associated with contrast exposure for CT scan during pregnancy. The thyroid function of neonates is routinely assessed in the United States, regardless of any in utero exposure to iodinated agents.

Magnetic Resonance Imaging in Pregnancy

MRI during pregnancy has been used for both maternal and fetal indications, and there is no evidence that human fetal exposure to MRI with 1.5 Tesla magnets has resulted in any negative fetal effects. The 2007 American College of Radiology Guidance Document for Safe MR Practices states that it is acceptable to perform magnetic resonance scans at any time point during pregnancy when the radiologist and referring physician believe that the risk-benefit ratio warrants performance of the study.[17] Some theoretical concerns involve potential teratogenicity and acoustic damage. However, thus far, studies have failed to substantiate these concerns. A study of 35 children who were exposed to 1.5-Tesla MRI during the third trimester of pregnancy found no harmful effects attributable to MRI, in particular no negative effects on vision or hearing.[18] Normal pediatric assessment and developmental outcomes were found in a study of 20 9-month-old infants who were exposed in utero to 4 series of echoplanar imaging MRI between 20 weeks and term.[19]

The use of gadolinium-based contrast is controversial. Animal studies have shown potential teratogenic effects at high doses.[6] Studies show that the contrast agents cross the placenta, are filtered by fetal kidneys, and appear in fetal urine. Because they are excreted into the amniotic fluid, there are concerns regarding potential long-term exposure of the fetus due to recirculation and delayed elimination. The American College of Radiology recommends that before administration of gadolinium-based contrast agents in pregnancy, "a well-documented and thoughtful risk-benefit analysis…" be performed that substantiates an "overwhelming potential benefit to the patient or fetus…",.[17] However, the US FDA classifies gadolinium as a class C drug, and the European Society of Radiology states that based on available evidence, the use of gadolinium in pregnancy appears to be safe.[20] Thus, even though current radiology practices and recommendations in the United States discourage the use of gadolinium-based contrast agents during pregnancy because their safety for the fetus has not yet been proven, gadolinium use should be considered when the diagnostic study is important for the health of the mother.

Therapeutic Radiation in Pregnancy

Although the dose of fetal radiation for most diagnostic procedures is low, administration of therapeutic radiation during pregnancy can result in significant fetal doses. Therapeutic radiation to sites remote from the uterus may be indicated during pregnancy for some cancers and can be administered to a well-informed patient. The dose of radiation administered to the fetus depends on several factors, including the target dose of radiation, the size of the radiation field, the type of teletherapy machine used, the distance of the fetus from the edge of the radiation field, and the use of wedges, blocks, and other objects that cause scatter.[21] In addition to the scatter from the teletherapy machine and from beam modifiers, internal scatter within the patient also affects the dose received by the fetus. The use of proper shielding of the uterus can reduce the fetal dose by up to a factor of 4.[22,23] Cobalt-60 irradiation is associated with a higher fetal dose compared with high-energy photons. Additionally, the use of high-energy photon beams >10 MV

produce a photoneutron contribution to the radiation dose, and it is generally recommended that photons <10 MV be used whenever possible.

Woo et al[24] reported on 16 patients with Hodgkin lymphoma who were treated with radiation during pregnancy. Eleven patients received mantle radiation, 3 received radiation to the neck and mediastinum, and in 2 patients, radiation was limited to the neck. The dose to the mid-fetus was estimated in 9 cases and ranged from 1.4 to 5.5 cGy with 6-MV photons and from 10 to 13.6 cGy for cobalt-60. All patients went on to delivery healthy infants. Antypas et al[25] performed in vivo as well as phantom measurements of the fetal dose of radiation in a patient irradiated for breast cancer from the second to sixth week of gestation. There was no shielding used. The total tumor dose was 46 Gy, and the fetal dose was estimated at 3.9 cGy. The importance of gestational age and uterine size for the fetal dose of radiation is exemplified when these measurements are compared with those obtained by Ngu et al[26]; breast irradiation to 50 Gy in late pregnancy resulted in an estimated 21-cGy unshielded dose, which reduced to 14 to 18 cGy with shielding.

If a patient presents with an unplanned pregnancy during radiation therapy for cancer, the risk of poor fetal outcome after fetal radiation exposure is dependent on the fetal dose received. The radiation oncologist and physicist involved in the patient's radiotherapy should be asked to estimate fetal radiation exposure. The results of such evaluation should be discussed with the patient and her family to allow her to make an informed decision regarding her pregnancy in the context of her underlying disease and other concurrent therapy received or planned.

CHEMOTHERAPY IN PREGNANCY

Key Points

1. Chemotherapy exposure in the first trimester is associated with a 20% incidence of fetal malformations, which exceeds the 3% to 4% rate of fetal malformations in the general population.
2. In the second and third trimester, the most significant potential negative effects of chemotherapy during pregnancy are growth restriction and preterm birth.

To patients, the prospect of undergoing chemotherapy is often accompanied by apprehension and fear, both in relation to the anticipated physical and emotional effects of treatment, as well as in regard to whether or not the treatment will be effective. When a pregnant patient faces chemotherapy, these concerns are compounded by concerns about the effect of the treatment on the pregnancy and the developing fetus. Several factors, including the chemotherapeutic agent, placental transfer, timing of treatment, dose, and frequency of exposure, influence the effects of chemotherapy on the fetus. Again, there is a lack of controlled data in humans, and thus our knowledge of the effects of chemotherapy during pregnancy are limited to animal studies and human case series and case reports. Depending on the type of malignancy, the stage of disease, and the gestational age of the pregnancy, there are times when appropriate therapy can be delayed until after delivery, or other modalities of treatment, such as surgery, can be used during the pregnancy with adjuvant therapy delayed until after delivery. However, when chemotherapy is likely to improve maternal outcome, it can be administered during pregnancy to an appropriately informed patient.

The concepts regarding the importance of gestational age on the effects of chemotherapy on a developing pregnancy are similar to those in radiation. Chemotherapy within the first 2 weeks after conception appears to have an "all or none" effect, resulting in either spontaneous abortion or no effect. The most sensitive time for potential teratogenesis is during organogenesis. The organs that continue to develop throughout gestation, such as the nervous system, eyes, and bone marrow, remain at risk even after this window. In general, chemotherapy exposure in the first trimester is associated with a 20% incidence of fetal malformations, which exceeds the 3% to 4% rate of fetal malformations in the general population.

In the second and third trimester, the most significant potential negative effects of chemotherapy during pregnancy are growth restriction and preterm birth. A review of published cases of in utero exposure to chemotherapy identified a less than 4% incidence of malformations, a 7% incidence of intrauterine growth restriction, and a 5% incidence of spontaneous preterm delivery. Of the 11 cases of malformation, 9 were associated with first trimester exposure.[27] The most recent large report comes from the Cancer and Pregnancy Registry and includes data from 231 women diagnosed with a variety of cancers during pregnancy who were voluntarily reported to the registry. Of these patients, 13 terminated their pregnancy and 157 received chemotherapy during pregnancy. Of the infants exposed to chemotherapy in utero, 3.8% had a malformation. Fewer than 8% of infants had a birthweight less than the 10th percentile, and 6% spontaneously delivered prematurely (iatrogenic preterm delivery excluded).[28] The rates of malformation, intrauterine growth restriction and spontaneous preterm delivery in these studies do not exceed those seen in the general population. Although these data are encouraging and can be used for the counseling of patients, some uncertainty

continues as a result of the lack of long-term follow-up. The incidence of clear cell carcinoma of the cervix and vagina in women exposed to diethylstilbestrol in utero is a reminder of the importance of continued long-term follow-up.

Although the timing of delivery is not always predictable for obstetrical reasons, it is generally recommended to avoid delivery during the peak of the hematologic toxicity of chemotherapy treatment in the mother. An additional consideration is the potential for neonatal myelosuppression. For example, in a study on the treatment of leukemia during pregnancy, one-third of the infants exposed to chemotherapy within 1 month before delivery were cytopenic at birth.[29] Due to this potential complication and the resultant potential risk for neonatal sepsis or bleeding, it is typically recommended that administration of chemotherapy be avoided within 3 weeks of anticipated delivery. This also allows for fetal drug excretion via the placenta, as drug metabolism in the neonate may be impaired, leading to potential increased toxicity.

In addition to the concerns regarding potential consequences of chemotherapy exposure for the fetus, careful consideration must be given to the physiologic changes that accompany the pregnant state and how those may affect the dosing and toxicity of chemotherapy. Such physiologic changes include an increased plasma volume, an increased glomerular filtration rate, decreased serum albumin, delayed gastric emptying and reduced intestinal motility, alterations in hepatic metabolism, and the creation of a physiologic third space (amniotic fluid). These changes may significantly affect the pharmacokinetics of drugs due to increased volume of distribution, altered protein binding, increased renal clearance, altered drug absorption, enterohepatic circulation, and hepatic clearance, with subsequent effects on peak drug concentration, drug half-life, and area under the curve (Table 16-3). Due to the paucity of data, chemotherapy during pregnancy is usually administered without dose modification compared with nonpregnant patients. Toxicities, response to treatment, and fetal well-being must be carefully followed throughout treatment and adjustments to treatment regimens and supportive care made when clinically indicated.

Chemotherapeutic Agents in Pregnancy

Information regarding the use of specific chemotherapeutic agents during pregnancy is limited largely to case reports, small case series, and some registry reports of single-agent or combination therapy use. In addition to the FDA classification of drugs in pregnancy (Table 16-4), several resources can provide information to guide clinicians in the administration of chemotherapy in this setting. These include textbooks

Table 16-3 Pharmacokinetic Consideration Regarding Chemotherapeutic Drugs in Pregnancy[30,31]

Physiologic Changes in Pregnancy	
Volume of distribution	↑
Protein binding	↑
Renal clearance	↑
Enterohepatic circulation	↑ or ↓
Hepatic clearance	↑ or ↓
Pharmacokinetic Effects	
Peak drug concentration	↓
Area under the curve	↓ (or ↑)
Drug clearance	↑ (or ↓)
Drug absorption	↑ or ↓

such as *Drugs in Pregnancy and Lactation: A Reference Guide to Fetal and Neonatal Risk* (Briggs, Freeman, and Yaffe, now in the 9th edition), as well as internet-based resources such as Reprotox (www.reprotox. org), TERIS (depts.washington.edu/terisweb), and the Cancer and Pregnancy Registry (www.cooperhealth. org/content/pregnancyandcancer.htm).

Antimetabolites

Antimetabolites, especially folic acid antagonists, are the agents most commonly associated with fetal malformations. First-trimester exposure to aminopterin is associated with a series of abnormalities that includes cranial dysostosis, hypertelorism, abnormalities of the external ear, and micrognathia, as well as potential limb deformities and neurologic abnormalities. Methotrexate exposure in the first trimester has resulted in similar anomalies, and methotrexate is considered one of the most teratogenic medications and is classified as a class X drug by the FDA. These findings have been termed *aminopterin-methotrexate syndrome*. Of 6 first-trimester exposures to cytarabine (alone or in combination with other chemotherapeutic agents), there were 2 congenital abnormalities.[32] Mercaptopurine appears to be associated with a low rate of congenital malformations, with 1 abnormality noted of 34 cases of first-trimester exposure.[33] A recent series of breast cancer patients treated with chemotherapy during pregnancy included 9 patients who received combination therapy with cyclophosphamide, methotrexate, and fluorouracil (none in the first trimester), with no adverse outcomes noted.[34]

Alkylating Agents

A review of use of alkylating agents during pregnancy found a 14% incidence of malformation with administration in the first trimester, but when treatment was limited to the second and third trimester, the rate of malformations was not above that of the general population.[35] Reported malformations after administration of cyclophosphamide during the first trimester of pregnancy have included absent or hypoplastic

Table 16-4 United States Food and Drug Administration (FDA) Classification of Fetal Risks due to Pharmaceuticals[36]

Pregnancy Category	Evidence
A	Adequate and well-controlled human studies have failed to demonstrate a risk to the fetus in the first trimester of pregnancy (and there is no evidence of risk in later trimesters).
B	Animal reproduction studies have failed to demonstrate a risk to the fetus, and there are no adequate and well-controlled studies in pregnant women OR animal studies have shown an adverse effect, but adequate and well-controlled studies in pregnant women have failed to demonstrate a risk to the fetus in any trimester.
C	Animal reproduction studies have shown an adverse effect on the fetus and there are no adequate and well-controlled studies in humans, but potential benefits may warrant use of the drug in pregnant women despite potential risks.
D	There is positive evidence of human fetal risk based on adverse reaction data from investigational or marketing experience or studies in humans, but potential benefits may warrant use of the drug in pregnant women despite potential risks.
X	Studies in animals or humans have demonstrated fetal abnormalities and/or there is positive evidence of human fetal risk based on adverse reaction data from investigational or marketing experience, and the risks involved in use of the drug in pregnant women clearly outweigh potential benefits.

digits, eye abnormalities, cleft palate, flat nasal bridge, and many other abnormalities.[27,33] An interesting case report involves a diamniotic-dichorionic twin pregnancy treated with cyclophosphamide throughout pregnancy for acute lymphocytic leukemia. One twin (female) was without abnormalities, whereas the other (male) had multiple abnormalities including but not limited to esophageal atresia, an upper extremity deformity, and a renal abnormality. He also went on to develop thyroid cancer at 11 years of age and neuroblastoma at 14 years of age.[37] Chlorambucil administration during the first trimester is associated with renal agenesis in both animals and humans.[33] Dacarbazine is used in the treatment of Hodgkin lymphoma and has been administered during pregnancy as part of the doxorubicin, bleomycin, vinblastine, and dacarbazine (ABVD) regimen. In one review, no malformations were noted in 15 pregnancies (some included first-trimester use).[38]

Antibiotics

Anthracyclines incompletely cross the placenta, and their use in pregnancy has not been associated with an increase in fetal malformations. A recent review of the literature analyzed outcomes in 160 pregnancies exposed to anthracyclines (90% in combination regimens). This included 31 patients exposed in the first trimester. They noted a malformation in 3% and fetal death in 9%. Eighty percent of the malformations were associated with first-trimester exposure. Fetal death was in conjunction with maternal death in 40% of the cases. Of the fetal deaths, 87% were in patients with acute leukemia, and 73% were associated with daunorubicin exposure, leading many to now avoid this agent in pregnancy in favor of doxorubicin.[39] An additional concern with the use of anthracyclines in pregnancy is the potential for cardiac toxicity in children exposed to the agents in utero. A recent report with long-term outcomes (mean, 17 years) of cardiac function of such children was encouraging, finding no evidence of late cardiac toxicity.[40] Bleomycin use in pregnancy is somewhat more controversial. At least 9 cases of bleomycin, etoposide, and cisplatin (BEP) use in pregnancy have been reported; in 2 of those poor neonatal outcomes that were noted, 1 included ventriculomegaly and cerebral atrophy.[41]

Vinca Alkaloids

Vinca alkaloids are embryocidal and teratogenic in animal studies, and scattered reports suggest potential malformations after administration of these drugs.[30,33,38] However, several case reports also suggest the relative safety of these agents in human pregnancy.[30] For example, in a review of 6 cases of vinorelbine exposure during pregnancy (none in the first trimester), there

were no malformations noted, and short-term outcomes of the infants were positive.[42] The use of vinblastine and vincristine (including during the first trimester) has also been reported, and there is no clear evidence of an increased risk of fetal malformations.[33]

Platinum Agents

Although platinums are the most commonly used chemotherapeutic agents in pregnancy, data regarding the use of these agents during pregnancy is still limited. There are several case reports on the use of cisplatin or carboplatin alone or in combination with other agents after the first trimester without resultant congenital abnormalities.[10,43-46] A recent review by Mir et al[47] identified 43 patients in the literature who had been treated with cisplatin (36 patients), carboplatin (6 patients), or both (1 patient), with more than 80% of the cases receiving combination therapy. In the 36 cases of cisplatin exposure, they noted 3 cases of intrauterine growth restriction (IUGR), 2 cases of oligohydramnios, 1 case of polyhydramnios, 1 case of microphthalmos, and 1 case of ventriculomegaly. The association of these malformations with cisplatin remains speculative due to concomitant exposure to other potentially teratogenic drugs. Unremarkable neonatal examination and pediatric development were reported in 34 of 36 children after in utero exposure to cisplatin. In the small number of carboplatin exposure cases described, there were no noted malformations or fetal toxicities noted. A recent study of 7 women who received cisplatin monotherapy for cervical cancer in the second and third trimester of pregnancy reports the concentration of cisplatin in the maternal blood, umbilical cord blood, and amniotic fluid measured at the time of delivery. Maternal serum cisplatin concentrations ranged widely, depending on the number of prior cycles and time interval to last treatment. Amniotic fluid cisplatin concentrations were 13% to 42% and umbilical artery levels 31% to 65% of the maternal serum concentration. Eight healthy infants were born with no anomalies and normal short-term development.[48]

Taxanes

The large molecular weight and high degree of protein binding of paclitaxel likely limit transfer of the drug across the placenta.[33] Human data remain very limited. There are case reports of paclitaxel administration along with a platinum agent for the treatment of ovarian cancer during pregnancy[10,49] without evidence of fetal malformation or developmental abnormalities. Additional cases of taxane administration during pregnancy are reported through the Cancer and Pregnancy Registry[28] without fetal malformations.

Topoisomerase Inhibitors

Data regarding the use of etoposide, topotecan, and irinotecan during pregnancy are scant to nonexistent. Use of etoposide has been reported during the second and third trimester, and pancytopenia and IUGR have been noted,[50,51] but there are no reports of fetal malformations.

Supportive Medications

Recombinant erythropoietin does not appear to cross the placenta and does not seem to pose a risk to the fetus. Given the increased risk of thromboembolic disease associated with the use of recombinant erythropoietin and darbepoetin in cancer patients[52] and the already increased risk of thromboembolic disease associated with pregnancy,[53] caution may be warranted.

Granulocyte colony-stimulating factor administration is not teratogenic in animals.[33] It does cross the placenta,[54] but administration during pregnancy appears to be safe. For example, a study from the Severe Chronic Neutropenia International Registry included 20 pregnancies exposed to treatment, with no adverse outcomes noted.[55]

The antiemetics metoclopramide and ondansetron are pregnancy class B and considered safe in pregnancy. Although malformations have been described in children exposed to prochlorperazine in utero, a large study including 2023 total exposures and 877 exposures during the first trimester found no increase in malformations and no other negative impact.[56]

Large studies have noted an association between the use of systemic corticosteroids in the first trimester and orofacial clefts. For example, a case-control study noted an odds ratio (OR) of 4.3 for isolated cleft lip with or without cleft palate and an OR of 5.3 for isolated cleft palate with first trimester exposure.[57]

The antihistamines ranitidine, cimetidine, and diphenhydramine are all class B agents and are considered safe in pregnancy. Due to concerns about antiandrogenic activity of cimetidine, some recommend that ranitidine is preferred over cimetidine.[58]

For pain control, acetaminophen is the first-line choice for mild pain and is not teratogenic. Nonsteroidal anti-inflammatory drugs (NSAIDs) have been associated with an increased rate of spontaneous abortion with first trimester use. Additionally, in the third trimester, NSAIDs have been linked to decreased amniotic fluid volume and constriction of the ductus arteriosus.[59] Additionally, a large nested case-control study with more than 36,000 pregnant women noted that the OR for congenital anomalies for women who filled prescriptions for NSAIDs during the first trimester was 2.21 (95% confidence interval [CI], 1.72-2.85) and for anomalies related to cardiac septal closure

the OR was 3.34 (95% CI, 1.87-5.98).[60] Opioids are not teratogenic, but do cross the placenta and pose the risk of fetal or neonatal withdrawal. Acute opioid withdrawal should be avoided during pregnancy, as it can be life-threatening to the fetus. Infants born to mothers who chronically take opioids should be carefully monitored for neonatal abstinence syndrome, characterized by apnea, autonomic dysfunction, diarrhea, diaphoresis, lacrimation, irritability, respiratory distress, seizures, tachypnea, and wakefulness, and treated with careful weaning of opioids.

CERVICAL CANCER

Key Points

1. The mechanisms to diagnose cervical cancer during pregnancy are the same as those used in nonpregnant patients and include cytology, colposcopy, cervical biopsy, and, in carefully selected cases, cervical conization.
2. There is a high rate of postpartum regression of abnormal cervical cytology and cervical dysplasia diagnosed in pregnancy.
3. Management of invasive cervical cancer diagnosed in pregnancy must include consideration of gestational age, fetal viability, disease stage, and patient preferences regarding pregnancy and treatment.

Epidemiology

The incidence of cervical cancer in pregnancy varies from 0.12 to 1.06 per 1000 pregnancies. It is the most common gynecologic malignancy diagnosed during pregnancy as well as the most common malignancy in pregnancy worldwide. Three percent of cervical cancers are diagnosed during pregnancy. For many women, especially those of lower socioeconomic status, pregnancy may be the only time they receive medical attention. Cervical cancer screening guidelines recommend to start cervical cytology screening at 21 years of age regardless of pregnancy status. The use of Pap tests and gynecologic examination as a component of routine prenatal care likely contributes to the high rate of cervical cancer diagnosis during pregnancy.

Risk factors for the development of cervical cancer in nonpregnant and pregnant populations appear to be similar, with human papilloma virus (HPV) infection, multiple sexual partners, early coitarche, smoking, immunosuppression, human immunodeficiency (HIV) infection, low socioeconomic status, and nonwhite race associated with higher incidence. Cervical cancers diagnosed during pregnancy tend to be of lower stage, with one study finding a 3.1 relative risk of having stage I disease.[61] The histologic spectrum is similar in pregnant and nonpregnant populations, with squamous cell histology predominating.

Diagnosis

The mechanisms to diagnose cervical cancer during pregnancy are the same as those used in nonpregnant patients and include cytology, colposcopy, cervical biopsy, and, in carefully selected cases, cervical conization. The incidence of abnormal cervical cytology in pregnancy is similar to that seen in nonpregnant cohorts, with rates of approximately 5% to 8%. The performance characteristics of cervical cytology do not appear to differ in pregnant and nonpregnant patients. Pregnancy is associated with increased vascularity and altered appearance of the cervix, leading to exaggerated colposcopic findings, which are more difficult to interpret. Thus, if colposcopy is performed during pregnancy, it should be done by a provider with specific expertise in that area. The reliability of expert colposcopic-directed biopsies during pregnancy appears similar to that of the nonpregnant patient, with 83.7% and 89.4% concordance, respectively, with the final diagnosis.[62]

Cervical biopsies are safe to perform in pregnancy. Despite the increased vascularity of the pregnant cervix, significant hemorrhage rarely occurs. When bleeding does occur, it can usually be controlled by the application of pressure. If necessary, use of Monsel solution to the biopsy site is another alternative for obtaining hemostasis. Suture ligature is rarely required. Use of an endocervical brush to obtain a cytologic specimen is a safe practice,[63,64] but endocervical curettage is omitted during pregnancy due to concerns for possible disruption of the pregnancy. Theoretical complications, such as rupture of membranes, are of concern, despite a lack of definitive evidence for this concern. As in nonpregnant patients, any suspicious cervical mass in pregnancy should be biopsied to exclude potential malignancy.

Cervical conization during pregnancy carries considerable risks, including bleeding, miscarriage, preterm labor, preterm delivery, and infection. The incidence of hemorrhage (>500 cc) with cold knife conization of the cervix is correlated with the trimester during which the procedure is performed; there is minimal risk during the first trimester, 5% in the second trimester, and 10% in the third trimester.[65,66] Fetal loss rates are on the order of 4.5%.[65,67] Given these risks, cervical conization during pregnancy should only be used when there is strong suspicion for an invasive malignancy based on cytology, cervical biopsy, or colposcopic appearance, and when the diagnosis of invasive malignancy would significantly alter the management of the pregnancy and the timing or route of delivery. In these situations, consideration should be given to performing a cerclage during the conization procedure in pregnancy, whether performed as cold knife conization or loop electrosurgical excision procedure cone.[68]

Treatment

Abnormal Cervical Cytology and Cervical Dysplasia

Studies indicate a high rate of postpartum regression of abnormal cervical cytology and cervical dysplasia diagnosed in pregnancy. A recent study of 1079 patients who underwent colposcopy during pregnancy, mostly without biopsy (93%), found postpartum regression to normal for 64% of patients referred with atypical squamous cells of undetermined significance (ASCUS) or low-grade squamous intraepithelial lesion (LSIL) Paps, and 53% for those with high-grade squamous intraepithelial lesion (HSIL) Paps.[69] In a study of 153 cases of biopsy-proven cervical intraepithelial neoplasia (CIN) II and CIN III in pregnancy, no cases of progression to invasive or microinvasive disease were found. This study also noted high resolution rates, with 39% of CIN II and 37% of CIN III regressing to normal postpartum.[70] In line with these high rates of regression and low rates of progression to invasive disease during pregnancy, the 2006 Bethesda consensus guidelines for the management of abnormal cervical cancer screening tests and CIN favor a conservative approach in the absence of suspected malignancy and aim to avoid treatment during pregnancy.[71,72]

The management of abnormal Pap tests in pregnancy is summarized in Figure 16-1. ASCUS cytology in pregnancy can be managed the same as in a nonpregnant patient, but colposcopy may be deferred until at least 6 weeks postpartum. For LSIL cytology in pregnancy, the American Society for Colposcopy and Cervical Pathology (ASCCP) guidelines state a preference for performing colposcopy during pregnancy, but it is acceptable to defer this until postpartum. For HSIL, atypical squamous cells, cannot rule out a high-grade lesion (ASC-H), and atypical glandular cells (AGC) cytology during pregnancy, colposcopy is recommended. During colposcopy, biopsies should be taken of any lesions suspicious for CIN II/III or cancer. For histologic abnormalities, the ASCCP guidelines recommend follow-up without treatment in CIN I, with re-evaluation with cytology and colposcopy postpartum. For CIN II and CIN III, repeat colposcopy and cytology at 12-week intervals during pregnancy is reasonable, or repeat cytology and colposcopy may be deferred to the postpartum period, depending on the index of suspicion and the gestational age. Treatment of CIN during pregnancy is not indicated. The only indication for treatment of cervical neoplasia during pregnancy is invasive cancer.

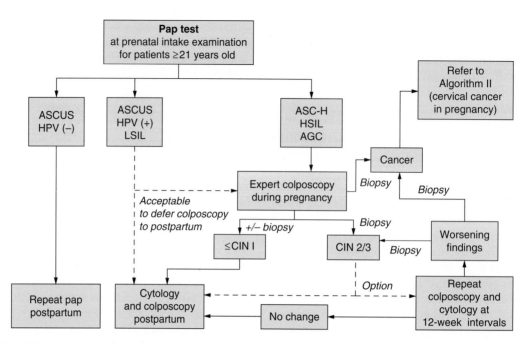

FIGURE 16-1. Management of an abnormal pap test and cervical intraepithelial neoplasia in pregnancy. Based on the 2006 American Society for Colposcopy and Cervical Pathology/Bethesda Consensus Guidelines.[65,66] AGC, atypical glandular cells; ASC-H, atypical squamous cells, cannot rule out a high-grade lesion; ASCUS, atypical squamous cells of undetermined significance; CIN, cervical intraepithelial neoplasia; LSIL, low-grade squamous intraepithelial lesion; HPV, human papillomavirus; HSIL, high-grade squamous intraepithelial lesion.

Invasive Cervical Cancer

Once invasive cervical cancer is confirmed by biopsy, a careful staging examination and MRI are indicated to assess for size of disease, sites of disease involvement, and evidence of metastatic disease. If cervical cancer is diagnosed in a pregnant woman at an advanced gestational age with expected fetal lung maturity, expedited delivery and initiation of definitive treatment should be undertaken. A cervical cancer diagnosis made in a pre-viable undesired pregnancy should be managed with immediate initiation of appropriate definitive therapy and resultant termination. For all other patients, decisions regarding the treatment of cervical cancer diagnosed during pregnancy are more challenging and should involve a multidisciplinary approach and careful consideration of disease stage, the gestational age of the pregnancy, the patient's wishes regarding the pregnancy, and the patient's preferences for therapy.

Figure 16-2 provides an overview of management options for patients diagnosed with invasive cervical cancer during pregnancy. When the decision for definitive treatment has been made for a patient who does not desire to continue a previable pregnancy, recommendations and treatment options are generally the same as those in nonpregnant patients. For patients who wish to continue a previable pregnancy and those who have a potentially viable but premature pregnancy, careful individualized balancing of maternal treatment needs and the desire to allow for fetal maturation must

be done. In general, immediate treatment is appropriate in cases of locally advanced disease, documented lymph node metastasis, progression of disease during pregnancy, and when desired by the patient. In some cases, neoadjuvant chemotherapy may provide an opportunity to treat the mother while allowing for further fetal maturation and deferring definitive therapy to the immediate postpartum period.

Stage IA1

Patients with stage IA1 disease diagnosed on cone biopsy with negative margins can be followed for the remainder of the pregnancy and anticipate vaginal delivery. This approach is supported by data in nonpregnant patients and reports of excellent outcomes in women treated with conization in pregnancy for both stage IA1 squamous cell and IA1 adenocarcinoma of the cervix. In a study of 8 women with squamous cell carcinoma treated with conization and managed expectantly throughout pregnancy, no invasive disease was found at the time of postpartum hysterectomy.[73] Similarly, in a small study of 4 pregnant women with stage IA1 adenocarcinoma, no residual invasive cancer was found in postdelivery treatment specimens.[74] Because there is no convincing evidence suggesting that vaginal delivery in patients with stage IA1 cervical cancer after conization with negative margins compromises outcomes, cesarean section should be reserved for obstetrical indications. In patients requiring

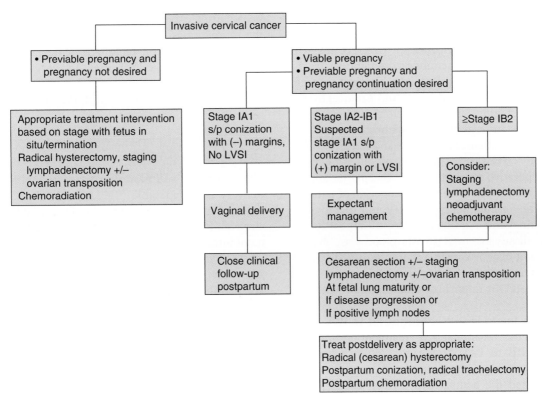

FIGURE 16-2. Possible management options of invasive cervical cancer in pregnancy. LVSI, lymphovascular space invasion.

cesarean section who do not desire future fertility, consideration may be given to cesarean hysterectomy, bearing in mind the higher morbidity of hysterectomy at the time of cesarean section.

Extrapolating from data in nonpregnant patients, it can be expected that the risk of residual microinvasive disease after conization for apparent stage IA1 disease with a conization margin positive for CIN III is approximately 22%, and the risk of more than microinvasive disease approximates 10%.[75] Therefore, it is imperative that pregnant patients with positive cone margins be followed closely during pregnancy and thoroughly evaluated postpartum. Given these risks, we recommend monthly clinical examinations and colposcopy every 3 months during pregnancy. A detailed discussion regarding route of delivery follows. Subsequent treatment for a patient who had been followed through pregnancy after conization for apparent stage IA1 disease with a conization margin positive for CIN III will depend on the patient's wishes for future fertility and should at a minimum entail repeat conization. If the patient wishes for more definitive therapy, a frozen cone-hysterectomy[76] postpartum is a reasonable management option.

Early-Stage Disease: Stages IA2 to IIA

In early-stage patients (stages IA2-IIA) who desire termination of a previable pregnancy and immediate definitive therapy, radical hysterectomy and lymphadenectomy with the fetus in situ is generally recommended. In this typically young patient population,

surgical management as opposed to radiation therapy may be preferable because it may allow for preservation of ovarian function and avoidance of radiation complications such as vaginal stricture and long-term gastrointestinal toxicity. Some authors recommend evacuation of the uterus before radical hysterectomy when the procedure will be performed at greater than 20 weeks.[77] This may be accomplished via hysterotomy during the same procedure. Primary radiation treatment with concomitant chemotherapy may be an alternative option for patients with early-stage disease, especially those who are poor surgical candidates. Consideration should be given to the pretreatment injection of a feticidal agent for second-trimester patients to honor possible patient preferences, avoid the possibility of a live birth during the procedure, and reduce the risk of violating legislation surrounding late previable pregnancy termination.[78]

The operative morbidity and outcomes of radical hysterectomy appear to be similar in pregnant and nonpregnant populations. In a case-control study of 26 patients who underwent radical hysterectomy for the treatment of cervical cancer during pregnancy, there was no difference in operative time, hospital stay, postoperative bladder function, or postoperative complications compared with nonpregnant matched controls. Blood loss was significantly more in the pregnant group, but blood transfusion was no more frequent. There was also no difference in disease status at last contact, with only 1 patient in the pregnant group dead of disease after an average follow-up period of more than 12 years.[79]

CHAPTER 16

For early-stage patients diagnosed near term and those who choose to delay definitive therapy until after a viable delivery, radical cesarean hysterectomy with lymphadenectomy is generally recommended. In this approach, the patient undergoes a classical cesarean section, the hysterotomy is closed, and a radical hysterectomy and staging lymphadenectomy is performed. Radical cesarean hysterectomy has been shown to be associated with a higher blood loss and need for blood transfusion.[80] However, the rates of other operative and postoperative morbidities are acceptable and on par with radical hysterectomy in nonpregnant patients. The benefits of completing delivery and therapy in a timely manner and in a single procedure appear to outweigh the disadvantage of greater blood loss. Ovarian transposition may be considered if intraoperative findings and tumor characteristics place a young patient at high likelihood for requiring radiation treatment.

Locally Advanced Disease: Stages IIB to IVA

In general, the recommended treatment for patients with stage IIB to IVA disease is radiation with concomitant sensitizing chemotherapy. Very few studies have evaluated the management of cervical cancer in pregnancy with radiotherapy or chemoradiation.[81-83] In early pregnancy, chemoradiation treatment can commence without prior evacuation of the uterus. In the majority of cases, fetal death is expected to occur within 2 to 3 weeks and abortion by 20 to 45 days after the beginning of radiotherapy.[84,85] Data suggest that pregnancy loss during radiation is delayed and occurs less reliably later in gestation. In a series of 14 patients who underwent radiation therapy for cervical cancer during pregnancy, pregnancy loss occurred an average of 33 days after the initiation of treatment in the first trimester and 44 days after initiation of treatment in the second trimester.[86] Because of this, some recommended uterine evacuation before initiation of radiotherapy in previable gestations greater than 20 weeks. If hysterotomy is planned for uterine evacuation, lymphadenectomy may be performed during the same surgical procedure. Medical abortion is another alternative for uterine evacuation and has been successfully used to induce uterine evacuation in cases where radiation therapy resulted in fetal death, but not spontaneous abortion.[87] Injection of a selective feticidal agent should be considered not only before pregnancy evacuation procedures, but also before the initiation of chemoradiation for patients in the second trimester, given the potential psychological impact on patient, family, and providers of performing radiotherapy with a live fetus in utero.

For patients with locally advanced disease with a viable premature or a strongly desired previable pregnancy, management decisions are complex and need to take into consideration the impact of delaying definitive therapy for the mother, the role of staging lymphadenectomy and neoadjuvant chemotherapy during the pregnancy, and the morbidity associated with a premature delivery for the child, all discussed in more detail next.

Fortunately, stage IVB disease is very rare in pregnancy. As in nonpregnant patients, a systemic approach to treatment is usually used, with local therapy focused on palliation of symptoms.

Delaying Treatment

The morbidity and mortality associated with preterm delivery is considerable (Table 16-5). Short delays in delivery may have a significant impact on neonatal survival. For example, in infants admitted to the neonatal intensive care unit without congenital abnormalities, the mortality rate is approximately 30% at 25 to 26 weeks, compared with less than 10% at 28 week and less than 2% at 34 to 35 weeks. Although neonatal survival rates have been improving remarkably at US referral centers, neurodevelopmentally intact survival is still problematic for very prematurely born babies.[88] Given the risks associated with prematurity, an effort must be made to balance the desire to optimize fetal outcome with the potential risks of delaying treatment for the mother. Data from many case reports, case series, and case-control studies indicate that there is likely minimal maternal risk associated with delaying treatment of cervical cancer when early-stage disease (stages IA-IB1) is diagnosed during the late second or early third trimester of pregnancy. In a review of 129 pregnancies during which cervical cancer therapy was deliberately delayed for 3 to 4 weeks, excellent outcomes were achieved. More than 95% of patients were alive and without evidence of disease at last follow-up (Table 16-6). Given these data, delaying treatment

Table 16-5 Neonatal Outcomes of Extremely Preterm Infants[88]

Gestational Age at Birth (weeks)	Birthweight (mean, g)	Survival (%)	Survival Without Major Morbidity[a]
22	511	6	0
23	581	26	8
24	651	55	9
25	744	72	20
26	854	84	34
27	960	88	44
28	1082	92	57

[a]Proportion among infants who survived. Major morbidity defined as severe intraventricular hemorrhage, periventricular leukomalacia, bronchopulmonary dysplasia, necrotizing enterocolitis, infections, and retinopathy of prematurity stage ≥3.

Table 16-6 Reported Experience With Deliberate Delay of Therapy in Patients With Invasive Cervical Cancer to Allow for Fetal Maturation[44]

Author/Year	N	Stage	EGA at Diagnosis	EGA at Delivery	Delay in Treatment (weeks)	Disease Progression	Follow-Up (month; mean/range)	Maternal Outcome
Prem et al, 1966[86]	4	I	28	35-36	6 (average)	—	All >60 months	All NED
Prem et al, 1966[86]	5	I	20-34	34-38	11-17	—	34-64	All NED
Boutselis, 1972[189]	5	IA1	8-24	3rd trimester	—	—	72-180	All NED
Dudan et al, 1973[190]	2	IB	—	—	8-24	2	—	1 DOD
Thompson et al, 1975[191]	7	IA	—	3rd trimester	5-28	—	50 (3-120)	All NED
Lee et al, 1981[81]	9	IA-II	24	3rd trimester	<12	No	—	All NED
Nisker and Shoubat, 1983[192]	1	IB	—	3rd trimester	24	1	—	DOD
Greer et al, 1989[193]	5	IB	20-24	28-37	6-17	No	23 (13-35)	4 NED 1 DOD
Monk and Montz, 1992[80]	4	IA2-IB	10-23	3rd trimester	10-23	No	40 (2-228)	All NED
Duggan et al, 1993[194]	8	IA1-IB1	11-31	31-40	8-30	No	33 (3-124)	All NED
Sorosky et al, 1995[195]	8	IB1	0-34[a]	33-38	3-40	No	33 (13-68)	All NED
Sorosky et al, 1996[196]	4[b]	IB1-IB2	18-32	35-36	4-15	—	51 (12-120)	3 NED 1 DOD
Sood et al, 1996[79]	11	IA1-IB1	—	3rd trimester	3-32	—	118 (12-360)	All NED
van Vliet et al, 1998[197]	4	IB	23-32	32-35	3-10	—	67 (16-106)	All NED
Trakushi et al, 2002[73]	12	IA1-IB2	12-27	30-term	6-25	No	70-156	All NED
Taen et al, 2006[198]	1	IB1	14	31	17	No	17	NED
Germann et al, 2005[199]	9	IB1	1st and 2nd trimester	3rd trimester	4-24 (16)	No	63 (2-168)	All NED
Lee et al, 2008[200]	12	IA1-IIIB	6-32	—	3-34	—	~40	10 NED 2 DOD
Gonzalez-Bosquet et al, 2008[201]	1	IB	25	33	8	No	12	NED
Yahata et al, 2008[74]	4	IA1[c]	16-23	37-41	>16-25	No	24-155	All NED
Ishioka et al, 2009[202]	4	IB1-IIB	11-25	29-34	2-19	—	10-111	4 NED
Favero, 2010[203]	9	IA1-IB1	6-23	32-36	9-28	—	38 (5-128)	All NED
Total	129	IA1-IIIB	0-34	3rd trimester	3-40	3	2-360	122 NED 7 DOD

Note. In some cases treatment delay was greater than the time difference of diagnosis to delivery as postdelivery irradiation may not have started for several weeks postpartum.
EGA, estimated gestational age; NED, no evidence of disease; DOD, dead of disease.
[a]One patient was diagnosed in the cycle before conception and followed through pregnancy.
[b]Excluded 3 cases that were doubly reported in Sorosky's 1995 and 1996 series.
[c]All adenocarcinomas
Modified with permission from Karam et al.[46]

for early-stage cervical cancer until fetal lung maturity is obtained may be a reasonable treatment option for patients who desire to continue their pregnancy. It is unlikely that this carries considerable risk of inferior cancer outcome for the mother. When choosing to delay therapy, close surveillance is imperative. Progression of disease during this period has been observed, portends a poor prognosis, and warrants immediate initiation of treatment. Given these risks, we recommend monthly clinical examinations and colposcopy every 3 months during pregnancy. One of the greatest challenges lies in determining an individual patient's risk in delaying therapy.

Several authors have advocated operative (laparoscopic or open) lymphadenectomy during pregnancy to gain accurate knowledge regarding lymph node status, which is the most important negative prognostic factor for the mother.[89,90] If nodal metastases are found, the recommendation is for pregnancy termination or delivery, with immediate definitive therapy for the mother.

Neoadjuvant Chemotherapy

The administration of neoadjuvant chemotherapy during pregnancy followed by definitive treatment after delivery is another potential treatment option. Theoretically, it can be used to reduce or stabilize tumor size and to control micrometastatic disease while delaying definitive management until after delivery. A meta-analysis that included 2078 nonpregnant patients showed a survival advantage for neoadjuvant chemotherapy using cycles of 14 days or less or cisplatin dose intensities of at least 25 mg/m²/wk.[91] There are several case reports in the literature on the use of neoadjuvant chemotherapy with cisplatin alone or in combination regimens for the treatment of cervical cancer in pregnant patients. Maternal outcomes have been variable, but all infants were normal, without congenital abnormalities (Table 16-7).

Delivery Route

There are no randomized studies evaluating the mode of delivery and maternal outcomes for patients with cervical cancer in pregnancy. Retrospective and case-control studies have suggested that vaginal delivery through a cervix with microscopic cervical cancer generally does not alter maternal prognosis. For patients with greater than microinvasive cervical cancer, it is generally recommended that delivery should be by cesarean section, as there is concern for infection, hemorrhage, obstructed labor, dissemination of tumor cells caused by dilation of the cervix, and poorer maternal survival. In a matched case-control study of 56 women diagnosed with cervical cancer during pregnancy and 27 diagnosed within 6 months postpartum, 14% experienced recurrence if delivered by cesarean section, compared with 59% who delivered vaginally.[92] Although other studies of similar design suggest that route of delivery may have no impact on maternal survival outcome,[61,93] there are reports of at least 13 cases of cervical cancer metastasis and recurrence in the episiotomy site after vaginal delivery with a significant associated morbidity and approximately 50% mortality,[94] supporting the recommendation for delivery by cesarean section for patients with frankly invasive cervical cancer.

Survival and Prognosis

Survival for women diagnosed with cervical cancer during pregnancy does not appear to be worse than for nonpregnant women. In a study of 40 cervical cancer cases during pregnancy by Zemlickis et al,[61] in which pregnant cervical cancer patients were matched by age, stage, and years of diagnosis with nonpregnant cases, 30-year survival rates were similar. Likewise, a case-control study by Van der Vange et al[93] involving 44 pregnancy-associated cervical cancers did not show an adverse prognosis for pregnancy-associated cases, with 5-year survival rates of 80% and 82% in pregnant and nonpregnant patients, respectively. The largest reported experience comes from Sweden.[95] These authors reported on a total of 18,474 cases of cervical cancer over a 90-year period of time, which included 219 cases occurring in pregnancy. They noted that over the study period the incidence of cervical cancer diagnosed in pregnancy declined, and cases were diagnosed at an earlier stage. Actuarial 10-year survival rates were not different for those diagnosed in pregnancy compared with age-matched controls. In addition, these authors showed that the incidence of second primary cancers did not differ between the groups (5.5% vs. 5.4%).

OVARIAN CANCER

Key Points

1. The majority of malignant ovarian tumors diagnosed in pregnancy are of epithelial histology (and mainly comprise low malignant potential tumors) followed by germ cell tumors.
2. Adjuvant chemotherapy is not commonly indicated with malignant tumors diagnosed during pregnancy, but should be delayed after the first trimester.
3. Pregnancy does not adversely affect the clinical outcome of ovarian cancer.

Table 16-7 Experience With Neoadjuvant Chemotherapy in Pregnancy for Cervical Cancer[44]

Author/Year	N	Path	Stage	EGA at Diagnosis (weeks)	EGA at Delivery (weeks)	Delay in Delivery (weeks)	Chemotherapy	F/U (months)	Maternal Outcome	Neonatal Outcome
Giacalone, 1996[45]	1	SCCA	IB1	17	32	15	P 75 mg/m² × 3	12	NED	Normal
Lai, 1997[204]	2	n/a	IB2 or IIA	12 weeks and n/a	n/a	n/a	P 50 mg/m² plus V 1 mg/m² plus B 25 mg/m² (max 30 mg) × 3	52 and 59	DOD DOD	Normal
Tewari, 1998[205]	2	SCCA	IB2-IIA	16-21	32-34	11-18	P 50 mg/m2 plus V 1 mg/m² × 4-6	5-24	NED (IB2) DOD (IIA)	Normal
Marana, 2001[206]	1	SCCA	IIB	14	38	24	B 30 mg plus P 50 mg/m² × 2	13 (mother), 36 (child)	DOD[a]	Normal
Caluwaerts, 2006[207]	1	SCCA	IB1	15	32	17	P 75 mg/m² × 6	10	NED	Normal
Benhaim, 2008[208]	1	SCCA	IIIB	22	28	6	P 50 mg/m² × 2	10	DOD	Normal
Karam, 2007[46]	1	SCCA	IB2	23	33	10	P 40 mg/m² × 7	9	NED	Normal
Bader, 2007[209]	1	SCCA	IIA	19	33	14	P 50 mg/m² plus V 1 mg/m² × 4	80	NED	Normal
Palaia, 2007[210]	1	SCCA	IIB	19	35	16	T 175 mg/m² × 1 P 75 ng/m² × 5	10	NED	Normal
Seamon, 2009[211]	1	glassy cell	IIIB	23	31	8	P 30-40 mg/m² plus V 1.5 mg/m²	49	NED	Normal
Rabaiotti, 2010[212]	1	SCCA	IB2	15	32	17	P 75 mg/m²	48	DOD	Normal
Favero, 2010[203]	5	SCCA (3) Adeno (2)	IB1	14-22	32-36	14-19	P monotherapy	5-12	NED	Normal

Path, pathology; SCCA, squamous cell carcinoma; Adeno, adenocarcinoma; EGA, estimated gestational age; P, cisplatin; V, vincristine; B, bleomycin; T, paclitaxel; F/U, follow-up; NED, no evidence of disease; DOD, dead of disease.
[a]Refused treatment.
Modified with permission from Karam et al.[46]

Epidemiology

An adnexal mass is diagnosed in up to 6% of pregnancies. In a study of 3000 consecutive pregnant patients who underwent ultrasound before 14 weeks' gestation with visualization of both ovaries, 161 women were found to have simple cysts greater than 2.5 cm in size or complex cysts.[96] More than 71% resolved spontaneously; only 4% required intervention, and 3% underwent torsion. Similarly, in a study of 79 pregnant patients found to have adnexal masses greater than 3 cm (out of a prospectively analyzed group of more than 6000 patients), 51% spontaneously resolved, and less than 4% required intervention.[97] Data such as these indicate that the majority of adnexal masses in pregnancy are benign, with many cysts being functional and resolving spontaneously by the mid-second trimester and few requiring intervention during pregnancy. Conversely, malignant ovarian tumors during pregnancy are rare, explaining the paucity of reports in the literature. Despite this, ovarian cancer is the second most common gynecologic cancer diagnosed during pregnancy. The incidence of ovarian cancer during pregnancy is estimated at 0.018 to 0.11 per 1000 pregnancies.[98]

Not surprisingly, the distribution of histology in malignant ovarian tumors in pregnancy is more similar to the distribution of malignant ovarian tumors in young, reproductive-age women than it is to the ovarian cancer population as a whole. A recent population-based study of adnexal masses in pregnancy found that in the 206 malignant and low malignant potential ovarian tumors identified, 79% were epithelial, whereas 16% were germ cell tumors. Of the epithelial tumors, 72% were of low malignant potential. More than 83% of the invasive cancers were stage I, as were 95% of the low malignant potential tumors.[99,100] This is in stark contrast to the greater than 50% incidence of advanced-stage disease in the general ovarian cancer population. Additionally, pregnant patients with ovarian cancer tended to be older and were more likely to be non-Hispanic white when compared with pregnant patients without a diagnosis of ovarian cancer.[99]

Diagnosis

A review of pregnancy-associated ovarian cancer cases noted that 50% of malignant adnexal masses were found on routine ultrasound examination, whereas 31% presented with pain, 15% presented with distention or a mass, and 4% were found incidentally at the time of cesarean section.[98] Definitive diagnosis of ovarian cancer requires surgical removal of the mass and pathologic analysis. Great care should be taken when making the decision of observation or surveillance, as undergoing adnexal surgery during pregnancy is not without potential complications. For example, in the first trimester, disruption of the corpus luteum without subsequent pharmacologic supplementation can result in pregnancy loss. Additionally, Leiserowitz et al[99] noted an increased risk of prematurity, very low birthweight infants, and an increased length of neonatal hospitalization in patients who underwent surgery for benign ovarian masses in pregnancy. There is also concern that adnexal masses are at risk for torsion during pregnancy or the immediate postpartum period, which could lead to the need for emergent surgery and therefore pose a potential risk to the pregnancy. Estimates on the risk of torsion of an adnexal mass during pregnancy vary widely (1%-15%), but masses 6 to 10 cm in size seem to be at the highest risk for torsion.[101,102] In general, many believe that small, asymptomatic adnexal masses with features suggesting a low risk of malignancy can be safely followed during pregnancy.

Care should also be taken not to delay potentially life-saving surgery for a woman based on her pregnancy. In many women with ovarian cancer diagnosed during pregnancy, surgery alone will be the only treatment intervention required during the pregnancy. Masses with ultrasonographic features that are highly suspicious for malignancy (eg, those with solid, mural nodules, thick septations, papillations, or excrescences), a size greater than 8 to 10 cm, rapid growth (>3.5 cm/wk), and those that persist into the second trimester carry a higher risk of malignancy, and surgical management should be considered.[99-102] When possible, it is preferred to perform surgery in the second trimester when organogenesis is complete, the placenta has taken over as the source of progesterone, and the risk of pregnancy loss after surgery is small.[103]

Treatment

Surgical management of an adnexal mass suspicious for malignancy during pregnancy usually proceeds through laparotomy. This allows for adequate visualization with minimal need to manipulate the uterus. The use of laparoscopy for the surgical management of adnexal pathology during pregnancy is widely reported and usually well tolerated[104,105] and may be considered. Abdominopelvic washings should be obtained, just as in nonpregnant cases. In the setting of a mass suspicious for malignancy, salpingo-oophorectomy is recommended as opposed to cystectomy. A frozen-section analysis by pathology should be obtained. The contralateral adnexa and peritoneal surfaces should be carefully inspected and sampled if suspicious lesions are noted. If malignancy is confirmed by pathology, a complete surgical staging procedure should be performed, especially in patients who appear to have stage I disease. If metastatic epithelial ovarian cancer is encountered, complete cytoreduction to no visible residual disease should generally be attempted. In the setting of metastatic germ cell tumors, which are generally highly chemosensitive, the degree of cytoreduction should be carefully considered while weighing the potential risks and benefits for the mother and the fetus of an extensive cytoreductive effort. Even in the setting of advanced-stage disease, surgical tumor debulking rarely requires uterine removal or disruption of the pregnancy. However, especially in women diagnosed in the first trimester of pregnancy and those with advanced-stage disease, termination of pregnancy should be discussed.

Given the favorable histology and stage distribution of ovarian cancer during pregnancy, adjuvant therapy is not commonly required. As previously discussed, the majority of ovarian cancers diagnosed during pregnancy are of low malignant potential and do not require adjuvant chemotherapy. However, in advanced-stage epithelial ovarian cancer, high-risk early-stage epithelial ovarian cancer, and germ cell tumors (with the exception of stage IA dysgerminomas and stage I, grade 1 immature teratomas), adjuvant treatment with chemotherapy is generally recommended.

If adjuvant chemotherapy is required, initiation of treatment should generally be avoided during the first trimester of pregnancy given the risks of pregnancy loss and fetal malformations. Chemotherapy can be administered during the second and third trimesters of pregnancy, and care should be taken to avoid chemotherapy within 3 weeks of anticipated delivery. In patients with early-stage, completely resected disease, delaying chemotherapy until after delivery, especially when a diagnosis has been made in the late second or third trimester, is a reasonable option that allows avoidance of fetal exposure to chemotherapy and is unlikely to be associated with a significant effect on outcome. However, in the setting of advanced-stage disease or the presence of residual disease, we would not recommend delaying the initiation of chemotherapy more than would be considered reasonable in a nonpregnant patient.

The standard first-line adjuvant treatment for epithelial ovarian cancer is a combination regimen of a platinum and a taxane. The use of single-agent platinum may also be considered.[106] Studies on chemotherapy during pregnancy for the treatment of epithelial ovarian cancer are rare. A recent review found only 13 reported cases in the literature.[98] Although platinum derivatives are the most commonly used chemotherapeutic agents in pregnancy, as discussed earlier in the section on chemotherapy, data on the use of platinum plus taxane regimens for ovarian cancer during pregnancy remain very limited.[107] Data from pregnant cancer patients treated with chemotherapeutic regimens containing taxanes attest to the feasibility of administration of taxanes during the second and third trimester, and no fetal malformations were noted.[39] However, given the more limited data on the use of taxanes during pregnancy, many clinicians prefer to administer single-agent platinum chemotherapy during

pregnancy and complete adjuvant therapy with a platinum/taxane regimen after delivery to minimize fetal exposure while maximizing maternal outcomes.

For germ cell tumors, the standard chemotherapy regimen used in nonpregnant patients is BEP. There are several case reports of the use of this regimen for ovarian germ cell tumors during pregnancy, including 1 report of a fetal anomaly (ventriculomegaly and cerebral atrophy).[108]

Given the limited data on the possible long-term fetal effects of exposure to the various chemotherapy regimens during pregnancy, patients must be appropriately counseled in regard to the uncertainty. However, the reports that exist on these regimens in the treatment of ovarian cancer during pregnancy are overall reassuring and support their indicated use in the second and third trimesters.

Survival and Prognosis

There is no evidence that pregnancy adversely affects outcomes in ovarian cancer. To the contrary, the favorable histology and stage distribution of disease are likely responsible for the overall more favorable outcomes for ovarian cancer patients diagnosed during pregnancy compared with that of the general ovarian cancer population. In a population-based study, ovarian cancer–related mortality for those diagnosed in pregnancy was less than 5%.[99] A literature review including only epithelial ovarian cancer cases in pregnancy noted a 28% ovarian cancer–related mortality rate.[98] For the infants born to women with ovarian cancer during pregnancy, the outlook is also encouraging. A recent single-institution retrospective analysis of patients with ovarian cancer during pregnancy noted that of the 26 intrauterine pregnancies, all delivered healthy full-term infants.[109] There were no congenital malformations and no evidence of metastases to the placenta or fetus.

BREAST CANCER

Key Points

1. Similar to nonpregnant young women diagnosed with breast cancer, the majority are infiltrating ductal adenocarcinomas with larger tumor size, higher rates of lymph node metastases, higher tumor grade and stage, and higher rates of estrogen and progesterone receptor (ER and PR) negativity.
2. Mastectomy is generally preferred over lumpectomy to avoid the need for breast radiation.
3. Future pregnancies after a diagnosis of breast cancer appear to be safe in successfully treated women.

Epidemiology

Breast cancer is the most common invasive malignancy diagnosed in pregnancy and complicates approximately 1 in 3000 pregnancies. In women younger than 30 years, up to 20% of breast cancer diagnoses occur during pregnancy or during the first postpartum year.[110] As in nonpregnant women, the most common histology of breast cancer in pregnancy is infiltrating ductal adenocarcinoma (approximately 85%). Patients with pregnancy-associated breast cancers tend to have worse clinicopathologic characteristics than the general breast cancer population, including larger tumor size, higher rates of lymph node metastasis and lymphovascular space invasion, higher tumor grade and stage, and higher rates of ER and PR negativity.[111] These clinicopathologic findings are similar to those found in nonpregnant, young breast cancer patients, such that the biology of these tumors is more likely related to the age at diagnosis and not the state of pregnancy.[112]

Evidence also suggests that despite the long-term protective effects of pregnancy and lactation on breast cancer risk, there is a transient increased risk for breast cancer after pregnancy. Albrektsen et al[113] reported a transient increase in risk that peaked 3 to 4 years after delivery, followed by a long-term decrease in risk. Wohlfahrt et al[114] similarly noted a transient increased risk of breast cancer after delivery in uniparous and biparous women and additionally noted an increased risk of diagnosis at a more advanced stage.

Diagnosis

Diagnosing breast cancer during pregnancy, as well as in lactating women, can be difficult, and delays in diagnosis are unfortunately common. In part, delays may be due to the physical changes of the breast during pregnancy and lactation causing difficulty with physical examination or difficulty with interpretation of diagnostic studies. Additionally, patients themselves may note a change, but may fail to report it to a physician, believing that the change is physiologic, not pathologic. Finally, physicians may not maintain a high enough index of suspicion and may fail to recognize an abnormality. Delays in diagnosis and treatment may at least partially account for some of the adverse features of pregnancy-associated breast cancer, such as larger tumor size and increased nodal involvement.

Although in older studies, delays of 6 months or more were noted, in more contemporary reports, delays are more on the order of 1 to 2 months.[111] However, the impact of even a short delay in diagnosis can be very significant. Nettleton et al[115] constructed a mathematical model to estimate the increased risk in nodal metastasis (the most important prognostic factor in breast cancer) attributable to treatment delay. They estimated that for a tumor with a 130-day doubling time (considered a moderately growing tumor), a 1-month delay in the treatment of early-stage breast cancer would increase the risk of axillary lymph node involvement by 0.9%. This risk increases to 2.6% for a 3-month delay and to 5.1% for a 6-month delay. Taken in the context of the estimated 4500 cases of pregnancy-associated breast cancer annually in the United States, a 2-month delay in treatment would correspond to an additional 76 cases of lymph node metastases.

The most common presentation for breast cancer in pregnancy is a breast mass. Despite the fact that approximately 80% of breast mass biopsies performed in pregnant women are benign, a high index of suspicion should be maintained, and any mass that persists for 2 to 4 weeks should be further investigated.[112,117] Ultrasound is a commonly used initial imaging study for breast masses during pregnancy; it is inexpensive and does not expose the mother or fetus to potentially dangerous radiation. It has demonstrated an excellent ability to distinguish normal breast tissue from a mass in an area of palpable abnormality and can distinguish a cystic versus a solid lesion in the majority of cases.[111,117] Mammography during pregnancy is considered safe, with a standard 4-view mammogram of both breasts with abdominal shielding exposing the fetus to only 0.01 to 0.04 cGy.[118] However, mammography has been reported to have a higher false-negative rate during pregnancy, largely due to the increased density of breast tissue in pregnancy. Series have shown pregnancy-associated breast cancers to be mammographically visible in as few as 62.5% of cases.[119] A more recent large series reported mammographically visible breast cancers in 90% of cases imaged during pregnancy.[117] These authors also point to the importance of the complimentary role of ultrasound and mammography, as in those cases where mammography was unable to identify a lesion, ultrasound revealed a suspicious mass. Data on the use of breast MRI during pregnancy is extremely limited.

Masses that are suspicious based on physical examination or imaging findings should be biopsied to establish a definitive diagnosis. Fine-needle aspiration biopsy, core biopsy, incisional biopsy, and excisional biopsy are all techniques than can be performed safely during pregnancy.

Treatment

Treatment of breast cancer during pregnancy largely parallels treatment offered to nonpregnant patients, with surgery, chemotherapy, and radiotherapy all having a potential role in the treatment algorithm. Locoregional treatment is generally accomplished by surgery. Mastectomy has traditionally been preferred to breast-conserving surgery during pregnancy to avoid the need for breast radiation. However, depending on the timing of diagnosis and the patient's desires, breast-conserving surgery can be performed and radiation can sometimes be deferred until after delivery. Significantly delaying radiation therapy should be carefully considered, as treatment delays are related to worse outcomes. One study has shown worse local control, overall survival, and disease-free survival in patients in whom radiation was delayed greater than 6 months from diagnosis.[120]

The regional lymph nodes must also be addressed, as their status is critical in treatment planning. In nonpregnant patients, sentinel lymph node biopsy, as opposed to full axillary lymph node dissection, is often performed in patients with early-stage breast cancer with clinically negative axillary lymph nodes. Vital dyes should not be administered to pregnant women; however, radiolabeled colloids are felt to be safe, and recent data demonstrate that the dose of radiation to the fetus is minimal. The use of this technique for breast cancer in pregnancy has not been fully evaluated in clinical trials, and the American Society of Clinical Oncology does not recommend the use of sentinel lymph node biopsy for breast cancer in pregnancy.[121] However, a recent series of 12 patients who underwent sentinel lymph node biopsy for breast cancer during pregnancy reported identification of sentinel lymph nodes in all patients. There have been no axillary recurrences in patients with negative sentinel lymph nodes with a median follow-up of 32 months, and there were no fetal malformations attributable to the procedure.[122] Similarly, in another small series of 9 pregnant patients (6 with melanoma and 3 with breast cancer) who underwent sentinel lymph node biopsy, there were no adverse reactions and no adverse fetal effects.[123] Given such data, as well as the minimal radiation exposure to the fetus for such a procedure,[124] the use of sentinel lymph node biopsy in breast cancer during pregnancy may be gaining favor for appropriately selected and informed patients. The recommendations from an international consensus meeting in 2010 include sentinel lymph node biopsy as a treatment option and state "sentinel lymph node biopsy (SLNB) for staging of the regional lymph nodes can be performed safely during pregnancy."[125]

The majority of patients with breast cancer in pregnancy meet criteria for adjuvant chemotherapy treatment. Additionally, in patients with advanced disease, the use of neoadjuvant chemotherapy can be considered before surgery, which may also have the added benefit of allowing for timing of surgery and radiation until after delivery. The 3 largest series on the use of chemotherapy for breast cancer during pregnancy come from MD Anderson Cancer Center, a French National Survey, and the pooled experience of 5 London teaching hospitals. In the MD Anderson series, 57 patients were treated prospectively with 5-fluorouracil, doxorubicin, and cyclophosphamide in the adjuvant or neoadjuvant setting. There were no perinatal mortalities. Three children had congenital or chromosomal abnormalities (Down syndrome, club foot, and congenital bilateral ureteral reflux).[126] In the French national survey, 20 patients who were treated with various chemotherapy regimens during pregnancy for breast cancer were retrospectively identified and completed questionnaires. The 2 pregnancies where chemotherapy was initiated in the first trimester ended in miscarriage. One of the remaining 18 pregnancies resulted in stillbirth, and there was one perinatal death of the 17 pregnancies that resulted in live births. There were no reports of congenital abnormalities.[127] Similarly, the series from London reported no serious neonatal consequences in the 23 pregnancies where chemotherapy was administered after the first trimester.[34]

Data on the use of biologic agents during pregnancy are minimal. There are reports on the use of trastuzumab, which has shown benefit in HER2-overexpressing breast cancer, during pregnancy; however, oligohydramnios and anhydramnios are common occurrences (>50% of reported cases).[128] Lapatinib has also been reported in a single pregnancy, with no adverse consequences noted.[129] The use of selective estrogen receptor modulators such as tamoxifen during pregnancy has been associated with teratogenic effects in mice, and birth defects have been reported in the offspring of women taking tamoxifen during pregnancy. Their use is not recommended during pregnancy.[125]

Survival and Prognosis

Studies in which pregnancy-associated breast cancer patients are matched for age and stage with non–pregnancy-associated breast cancer patients indicate that those diagnosed in pregnancy do not have an inferior prognosis.[130,131] A recent large report that included 652 breast cancer patients diagnosed at less than 35 years of age found that the patients with pregnancy-associated breast cancer did not have an inferior locoregional recurrence-free survival, distant metastasis-free survival, or overall survival compared with patients with breast cancers that were not associated with pregnancy, despite having a higher T classification, N classification, and stage at diagnosis.[110] Outcomes for pregnancy-associated breast cancer patients are poor in comparison with those of the general breast cancer population, but this is likely due to tumor factors related to the young age at diagnosis and not pregnancy itself. Termination of pregnancy does not appear to improve outcomes in breast cancer diagnosed during pregnancy.

Although there is a lack of prospective studies on the effects of additional pregnancies on survival outcomes in breast cancer patients, it is the general consensus that future pregnancies are safe for women who have been successfully treated for breast cancer. Many retrospective studies have found that women who become pregnant after treatment for breast cancer do not have worse outcomes.[132,133] Some studies, including a recent large meta-analysis, indicate that women who become pregnant after treatment may have improved outcomes.[134-136] Many clinicians recommend that patients avoid pregnancy for 2 years after treatment. The risk of recurrent disease is greatest during the first 2 years after treatment. The recommendation to delay future pregnancies stems more from the concern that a coincident pregnancy could complicate treatment options for recurrent disease than from concerns that the pregnancy will negatively impact the woman's outcome.

MELANOMA

Key Points

1. Malignant melanoma is the most common malignancy found in metastases to the placenta or fetus.
2. Excisional, rather than shave, biopsy should be performed in pregnant women with lesions suspicious for melanoma.
3. Pregnancy does not appear to independently influence clinical outcome in women diagnosed with melanoma.

Epidemiology

The incidence of melanoma is rising. Approximately 30% to 35% of women with melanoma are of childbearing age, and approximately 1% of female melanoma patients are pregnant. Melanoma represents approximately 8% of cancers diagnosed during pregnancy, with an estimated incidence of 0.1 to 0.28 per 1000 pregnancies.[137] In a recent population-based study from Norway, melanoma represented 31% of all malignancies diagnosed during pregnancy,[2] highlighting the importance of population-specific awareness of cancer risks.

Malignant melanoma is the most common malignancy found in metastases to the placenta or fetus. A recent review described malignant melanoma as the involved cancer in 24 of 77 cases (31%) of placental metastasis and in 6 of 15 cases (40%) of fetal metastasis.[137] Accurate assessment of the incidence of placental or fetal metastases in pregnant patients with melanoma is not available. Given the risk exists and its potential implications for diagnosis and treatment of the baby, it is recommended that the placentas of all pregnancies complicated by a diagnosis of maternal cancer,

especially malignant melanoma, be sent to pathology for full evaluation for possible metastatic disease.

Although malignant melanoma is not considered a hormonally dependent tumor, much research has been conducted evaluating the potential impact of hormones on malignant melanoma. The common occurrence of increased pigmentation associated with pregnancy and, less commonly, with exogenous estrogen use (eg, melasma, darkening of the linea nigra) is likely partially responsible for concerns regarding the potential impact of pregnancy, oral contraceptives, and hormone therapy on the development, prognosis, and recurrence risk of melanoma. The impact of pregnancy on the prognosis of melanoma will be addressed in the discussion of survival and prognosis of melanoma in pregnancy. As for oral contraceptives and hormone replacement, there are no conclusive data indicating either an increased risk for developing melanoma or a worsened prognosis.[138]

Diagnosis

Often, melanoma presents with a change in the size, shape, color, or feel of an existing nevus. During pregnancy, many women note changes in the appearance of nevi. The majority of these lesions are not melanomas, and the changes often disappear after childbirth. However, a high index of suspicion must be maintained to prevent delays in diagnosis during pregnancy. Patients and physicians alike should be aware of the "ABCD" findings suggestive of melanoma and evaluate all suspicious changes: *Asymmetry*, irregular or blurred *Borders*, changes in or unevenness of *Color*, and/or an increase in *Diameter* of nevi should heighten suspicion. When technically feasible and cosmetically acceptable, an excisional biopsy with a 1- to 2-mm margin of normal skin should be performed and extended into the subcutaneous fat. Shave biopsies should be avoided.[139] Incisional or punch biopsy may lead to underestimation of tumor thickness if the thickest portion of the melanoma is not biopsied.

Treatment

After a diagnosis of malignant melanoma is made on biopsy, complete surgical excision with a margin is the standard initial treatment. Guidelines regarding the width of the margin of normal tissue vary based on the thickness of the melanoma. Because of a lack of clear data regarding the ideal surgical margin for tumors of varying thickness, the guidelines between different organizations remain inconsistent.[140] In general, for in situ lesions, a 5-mm margin is considered adequate. For tumors of less than 1 mm in thickness, a 1-cm margin is recommended. For tumors of 1- to 4-mm thickness, a 1- to 2-cm margin is recommended. For tumor greater than 4-mm thickness, a 2- to 3-cm margin is recommended.

Sentinel lymph node biopsy is generally recommended for all patients with clinically negative lymph nodes and T2, T3, and T4 disease and select high-risk T1b disease (see Table 16-8 for the melanoma staging system), with full lymph node dissection reserved for patients with clinically positive nodes or positive sentinel lymph node(s). The incidence of positive sentinel lymph nodes varies with the primary tumor thickness and is approximately 4%, 12%, 28%, and 44% for tumor of less than 1 mm, 1.01 to 2 mm, 2.01 to 4 mm, and more than 4 mm.[141] The presence of positive lymph nodes is the most important predictor of prognosis. Many believe that pregnancy should not influence the decision to perform sentinel lymph node biopsy with radiolabeled colloids, where recent data demonstrate that the dose of radiation to the fetus is minimal.[142] Because it is theoretically possible to have higher fetal exposures when the lesion is located very close to the uterus, some experts recommend decreasing the activity of the tracer and collecting imaging for twice the usual duration as well as minimizing the time interval from injection to operation to further minimize the fetal exposure.[142] Complete regional lymphadenectomy is an alternative to sentinel lymph node biopsy.

For stage I to IIA disease ($\leq$ T3a, N0, M0), surgical therapy alone is highly curative and adjuvant therapy is not recommended outside of clinical trials. However, for patients with localized stage IIB and above tumors, where the risk of recurrence ranges from 30% to 80%, adjuvant therapy should generally be considered. For nonpregnant patients, treatment with high-dose interferon α is the adjuvant therapy with the most evidence-based support. Despite an initial analysis of the Eastern Cooperative Oncology Group (ECOG) 1684 trial that reported both an improved relapse-free (9-month prolongation) and overall survival (1-year prolongation)

Table 16-8 TNM Staging of Melanoma

Classification		
T	**Tumor Thickness (mm)**	**Ulceration Status/Mitoses**
Tis		
T1	N/A	N/A
T2	$\leq$1.00	a: without ulceration and mitosis <1/mm²
T3		b: with ulceration or mitoses $\geq$1/mm²
T4	1.01-2.00	a: without ulceration
		b: with ulceration
	2.01-4.00	a: without ulceration
		b: with ulceration
	>4.00	a: without ulceration
		b: with ulceration
N	**Number of Metastatic Nodes**	**Nodal Metastatic Burden**
N0	0	N/A
N1	1	a: micrometastasis (diagnosed after sentinel lymph node biopsy)
		b: macrometastasis (clinically detectable nodes confirmed positive by pathology)
N2	2-3	a: micrometastasis
		b: macrometastasis
		c: in-transit metastases/satellites without metastatic nodes
N3	4+ positive nodes or matted nodes or in-transit metastases/satellites with metastatic nodes	
M	**Site of Metastasis**	**Serum LDH**
M0	No distant metastases	N/A
M1a	Distant skin, subcutaneous, or nodal metastases	Normal
M1b	Lung metastases	Normal
M1c	All other visceral metastases	Normal
	Any distant metastases	Elevated

LDH, lactate dehydrogenase.
Modified with permission from Balch et al.[139]

for patients who were randomized to receive high-dose interferon α as adjuvant therapy for 1 year,[143] a subsequent updated reanalysis of pooled ECOG trials failed to demonstrate an improvement in overall survival, and only the improvement in relapse-free survival remained significant.[144] Trials using lower doses of interferon α generally show less or no benefit.[145-147] A report from Germany outlines the disease course of a patient who was diagnosed with malignant melanoma during pregnancy and was treated with interferon α from the 8th through 36th weeks of pregnancy.[148] She was diagnosed with metastatic disease in the 36th week of pregnancy, underwent induction of labor, and delivered healthy twins. She died 1 year later as a result of her disease. Interferon α has not been shown to cross the placenta and is not teratogenic in animal studies. There is some concern for a possible increased incidence of IUGR in fetus exposed interferon α; however, no causative link has been established. There also does not appear to be an increase in fetal malformations.[149] Administration of interferon α in pregnant melanoma patients may be warranted in some circumstances after careful consideration and counseling of the patient regarding the potential risks and benefits. In select situations, adjuvant radiation therapy either to the primary site or to an involved nodal basin may be recommended.[150] In a pregnant patient, such a recommendation should take into consideration the distance of the site from the uterus, the gestational age, and the ability to adequately shield and reduce scatter of radiation to the fetus.

In the setting of distant metastasis, prognosis is extremely poor. In nonpregnant patients, dacarbazine is a standard chemotherapy agent for metastatic melanoma and has a response rate of 15% to 25%.[151] A randomized trial has shown equivalent activity for dacarbazine and temozolomide, and the later has the advantage of being orally administered.[152] Another option for the treatment of metastatic disease is interleukin-2 therapy, either alone or in combination with other chemotherapy agents (biochemotherapy). The toxicity of such regimens is significant, and there are no reports of their use during pregnancy.

Survival and Prognosis

Analysis of the American Joint Committee on Cancer Melanoma Staging Database indicates that the most important pathologic prognostic factors in malignant melanoma are tumor thickness, presence or absence of ulceration, mitotic rate, and presence of lymph node metastasis. For a tumor thickness of less than 1 mm, 1.01 to 2 mm, 2.01 to 4 mm, and more than 4 mm, the associated 10-year survival rates are 92%, 80%, 63%, and 50%, respectively. Mitotic rate was the second most powerful pathologic predictor of

survival, with the most significant threshold being 1 mitosis/mm^2.[139] Although some evidence suggests that melanomas diagnosed during pregnancy tend to have a greater thickness, other recent studies do not show such a trend.[153,154]

Clinical prognostic factors, including older age, male sex, and axial location of the lesion, are associated with a worse prognosis. Beginning in the 1950s, uncontrolled case series indicating worse outcomes in women diagnosed with melanoma during pregnancy caused concern among many clinicians and even led some to recommend surgical sterilization of female melanoma patients. However, more recent controlled studies do not support a negative impact of pregnancy on outcomes in melanoma. O'Meara et al[153] performed an analysis of California databases and identified 412 women with melanoma diagnosed during pregnancy ($n = 149$) or within 1 year after pregnancy ($n = 263$) and compared them with a group of age-matched nonpregnant controls. There was no statistically significant impact of pregnancy on survival. In a Swedish database study by Lens et al,[154] 185 women with melanoma during pregnancy were compared with 5348 women with melanoma who were of childbearing age but were not pregnant. Pregnancy status was not found to be a predictor of survival (hazard ratio, 1.08; 95% CI, 0.60-1.93). In this study, pregnancy after diagnosis was also found to not be a predictor of survival. Other small studies provide additional support that melanoma patients who later become pregnant do not suffer a worse prognosis.[155]

Most available data regarding the impact of pregnancy on melanoma outcomes deals with patients with localized disease. Data regarding a potential impact of pregnancy on advanced disease is very limited, possibly in part due to many such patients deciding to terminate the pregnancy in the face of advanced, poor-prognosis disease.

THYROID CANCER

Key Points

1. Prior radiation exposure, family history of thyroid cancer or thyroid disease, and irregular menses are risk factors for thyroid cancers diagnosed during pregnancy.
2. Radioactive iodine scanning is contraindicated in pregnancy, and diagnosis should be made with fine-needle aspiration biopsy.
3. Adjuvant postoperative radioiodine ablation should be delayed until after delivery, and lactation is contraindicated.

EPIDEMIOLOGY

Thyroid cancer is the most common endocrine malignancy and is 3 times more common in women than men. It is especially common among women of childbearing age. Approximately 10% of thyroid cancers in this group are diagnosed during pregnancy or within 1 year after a birth. A recent population-based review noted an incidence of thyroid cancer during pregnancy of 0.14 per 1000 live births.[1] Greater than 90% of thyroid cancers belong to the category of differentiated thyroid cancer, which includes papillary and follicular cancers.[156] Other less common histologies include anaplastic cancer (thought to arise from differentiated cancers), medullary thyroid cancer, Hürthle cell tumors, and primary thyroid lymphoma.

Exposure to ionizing radiation is a well-established risk factor for the development of thyroid cancer. A population-based case-control study evaluating risk factors for the development of thyroid cancer in pregnancy also noted a family history of thyroid cancer or thyroid disease and irregular menses to be associated with increased risk, but not age of menarche, pregnancy history, or use of oral contraceptive pills.[157]

Diagnosis

Thyroid cancer most commonly presents with a palpable thyroid mass that is either noted by the patient or found by a physician. It is estimated that approximately 5% of women have a palpable thyroid nodule.[156] The incidence of malignancy in a solitary nodule is approximately 8% to 17% in the general population.[158] However, reports of thyroid nodules in pregnancy indicate that in the pregnant population this figure may be as high as 39% to 43%.[159] Thyroid cancer discovered during pregnancy may be more likely to be asymptomatic and found by a physician on routine examination, highlighting the importance of a careful and thorough physical examination during prenatal care.

The work-up of a thyroid mass in pregnancy should proceed along the same lines as in nonpregnant patients, with the exception that radioactive iodine scanning is contraindicated. Ultrasound is a safe and inexpensive tool that can elucidate the size, number, and characteristics of thyroid masses, but cannot rule in or rule out malignancy. It can also be used in the evaluation of the regional lymph nodes.

Fine-needle aspiration biopsy is the diagnostic procedure of choice for the evaluation of thyroid nodules. This can be done either with or without ultrasound guidance, depending on the clinical situation. A recent study indicates that the diagnostic performance of fine-needle aspiration biopsy may be improved by use of ultrasound guidance.[160]

Treatment

Surgery is generally the primary treatment of choice for thyroid cancer, but at what point the operation should occur when the diagnosis is made during pregnancy is debated. Some advocate for surgery in the second trimester when possible, especially when biopsy indicates an aggressive histology. Most agree that the majority of cancers diagnosed in the third trimester can be observed until after delivery.[161] Some even advocate for delaying diagnostic procedures until after delivery in certain clinical situations.[162]

In a study that included 61 women with thyroid cancer diagnosed during pregnancy, Moosa and Mazzaferri[160] found that the tumor size, incidence of nodal metastasis, and risk of recurrence did not differ between patients who underwent surgery during pregnancy compared with those in whom surgery was delayed until after delivery. However, delay in therapy may negatively affect survival. In a study of a group of more than 1300 thyroid cancer patients (men and women), it was noted that the time from diagnosis to initiation of therapy had an independent effect on outcome. Cancer-related mortality was 4% in patients who began therapy within 1 year of diagnosis and 10% in those who began therapy more than a year after diagnosis. Patients who died from their disease had a median delay of 18 months, as opposed to 4 months among cancer survivors.[163] In general, the timing of surgery for thyroid cancer in pregnancy should be determined after thoughtful discussion with the patient and should take into account the lesion size, rate of growth, histology, evidence of metastatic disease, gestational age at diagnosis, and the patient's desires.

Postoperative radioiodine ablation is a commonly used adjuvant treatment for papillary thyroid cancer and has been shown to improve outcomes in many populations of thyroid cancer patients, and it is recommended in a variety of clinical scenarios.[156] Because of radiation risks to the fetus or breast-feeding infant, this therapy is reserved until after delivery, and lactation is contraindicated. Papillary cancers express the thyroid-stimulating hormone (TSH) receptor and respond to TSH stimulation with an increase in growth rate. For patients with papillary thyroid cancer with intermediate or high-risk features, suppression of TSH with levothyroxine is recommended,[156] as it has been shown to improve clinical outcomes.[164] It is also recommended for low-risk patients who have not undergone thyroid remnant ablation.[156] When surgical management of papillary thyroid cancer is deferred until after delivery, levothyroxine suppression is recommended during pregnancy.[165,166] Dosing should be carefully monitored and adjusted during pregnancy to maintain adequate levels of suppression.

Survival and Prognosis

Although the survival outcomes for thyroid cancer in general are excellent, approximately 20% of patients will have a recurrence. Young age at diagnosis and female sex are associated with good prognosis.[164] Several studies indicate that women diagnosed with thyroid cancer during pregnancy have a similar prognosis as that of age-matched controls.[167-169] However, the potential stimulatory effects of human chorionic gonadotropin and estrogen on the thyroid gland lead to concerns that the hormonal changes associated with pregnancy may have a negative impact on thyroid cancer prognosis. A recent study indicated a worse prognosis for women diagnosed in pregnancy and also demonstrated increased ERα expression in tumors diagnosed during pregnancy or within 1 year after delivery.[170]

Pregnancy after successful treatment for thyroid cancer does not seem to be associated with recurrence. In a recent study of 63 women with a history of thyroid cancer, there was no evidence of disease progression during pregnancy in any of the patients who had no evidence of disease before pregnancy. However, there was a strong correlation between the presence of persistent disease before pregnancy and progression during pregnancy. Nearly half of the patients in the study who had evidence of disease before pregnancy had evidence of disease progression during pregnancy.[171] Similar findings that pregnancy was unlikely to lead to recurrence, but was associated with progression in patients with known disease before pregnancy, has also been noted by others.[172]

HEMATOLOGIC MALIGNANCIES

Key Points

1. Hodgkin lymphoma is the most common hematologic malignancy in pregnancy.
2. Treatment with chemotherapy should not be delayed in pregnant women with acute myelogenous leukemia.

Epidemiology

Hematologic malignancies account for approximately one-quarter of all malignancies during pregnancy.[3] Of the hematologic malignancies, Hodgkin lymphoma (HL) is by far the most common, accounting for more than half of all hematologic malignancies in pregnancy.[173] Its incidence in pregnancy is estimated at 1:1000 to 1:6000.[3] As in nonpregnant patients, the most common histologic subtype of HL in pregnancy is nodular sclerosis. The etiology of HL is likely multifactorial, involving genetic, immunologic, and environmental factors. Epstein-Barr virus is believed to play a significant role in many cases of HL. Non-Hodgkin lymphoma (NHL) is much less common in pregnancy than HL. When NHL occurs in pregnancy, there may be an association with more aggressive subtypes.[174] Outcomes in NHL are worse than those in HL.[175]

Leukemias occur more rarely in pregnancy, with an estimated incidence of 1 in 75,000-100,000 pregnancies.[3] Approximately 90% of leukemias in pregnancy are acute; two-thirds are acute myelogenous leukemia (AML), and one-third are acute lymphocytic leukemia (ALL).[173,176] As in HL, a single cause for development of leukemia has not been identified. However, several genetic disorders (eg, Down syndrome, Fanconi anemia), exposure to certain chemotherapeutic agents (eg, alkylating agents), ionizing radiation, and some viruses (eg, HTLV-I, Epstein-Barr virus) have been linked to the development of leukemia.

Diagnosis

HL, in pregnant and nonpregnant patients alike, usually presents with painless lymphadenopathy. Diagnosis is made via lymph node biopsy. Additional work-up includes laboratory studies, bone marrow biopsy, and imaging for staging. In nonpregnant patients, staging imaging with CT scan is generally used. In pregnant patients, a chest x-ray with abdominal shielding and either abdominal ultrasound or MRI to evaluate the liver and spleen and assess for lymphadenopathy are often the imaging studies of choice.

The symptoms of leukemia are nonspecific and overlap with some of the common complaints during pregnancy: fatigue, weakness, dyspnea. Other findings may include easy bruising and epistaxis. Lymphadenopathy, hepatomegaly, and splenomegaly are rare in acute leukemias. Abnormalities in the peripheral blood smear may raise suspicion for leukemia, but the diagnosis is made based on morphologic, immunophenotypic, and cytogenetic studies of a bone marrow sample.[173]

Treatment

For nonpregnant patients with early-stage HD, combined-modality therapy consisting of epirubicin, bleomycin, vinblastine, and dacarbazine or doxorubicin, bleomycin, vinblastine, and dacarbazine (ABVD) followed by low-dose involved-field radiation therapy has gained strong acceptance given the excellent overall survival rate of 93% reported with this treatment strategy.[177] In pregnant patients, several management options exist, and the risks and benefits of each should be carefully considered with the patient and multidisciplinary team. Some advocate that treatment of HD can safely be deferred until after delivery in the majority of cases.[178] In 17 cases managed at the BC Cancer Agency, 11 patients received no treatment during pregnancy. Six patients were given single-agent vinblastine to control their disease until term. All reportedly delivered normal babies, and 13 of the 17 are alive at a median of 15 years from delivery.[179] Consideration can also be given in select, well-counseled patients to treatment with single-agent chemotherapy during the first trimester with a transition to ABVD in the second trimester or to initial treatment with ABVD starting in the second trimester.[180] Radiation therapy for supradiaphragmatic early-stage disease in pregnancy has also been described with acceptable fetal radiation estimates and no reported abnormalities in the offspring.[22] Depending on the timing of treatment initiation and response, patients could also be treated with ABVD during the second and third trimester and complete involved-field radiation therapy after delivery.

For patients with advanced-stage HD, multiagent chemotherapy is the preferred treatment, with consideration given to consolidation radiation in some situations. As in early-stage disease, ABVD is generally the preferred multiagent regimen in pregnancy. Mustargen, vincristine, procarbazine, and prednisone (MOPP) is an alternative regimen that has also been used in pregnant patients. If the diagnosis is made in the first trimester, some recommend termination of pregnancy before treatment.[180] However, there are reports of successful term deliveries with no congenital malformations in pregnant patients who initiated treatment with the ABVD or MOPP regimens in the first trimester,[181] and some patients may reasonably elect to continue the pregnancy and initiate treatment in the first trimester. When consolidation radiation is recommended, it is usually deferred until after delivery, especially when targeting infradiaphragmatic disease.

AML is extremely aggressive, and it seems clear that maternal outcomes are significantly compromised when initiation of treatment is delayed. In a recent series, 75% of patients who elected to delay treatment until after delivery died of disease within days of initiating chemotherapy.[182] Immediate induction chemotherapy is almost always indicated, with one exception being when diagnosis is made in the late third trimester when immediate delivery before initiation of treatment is an alternative. When diagnosis is made in the first trimester, it is generally recommended that the patient terminate the pregnancy before treatment.

Induction chemotherapy for AML typically includes cytarabine and an anthracycline. Cytarabine is an antimetabolite and may be teratogenic. Fetal malformations have been reported.[38,183] Anthracyclines cross the placenta incompletely, and studies have indicated that only relatively small quantities can be detected in the fetus (100- to 1000-fold less that that seen in adult tissues).[39] Doxorubicin is the preferred anthracycline in pregnancy and is not associated with an increased risk for severe congenital malformations.[176] Given the cardiotoxicity of anthracyclines, it is reasonable to be concerned about potential long-term cardiac dysfunction in children exposed to anthracyclines in utero. However, a recent study that followed the cardiac function of 81 such children did not show any evidence of late cardiac toxicity.[40]

Induction chemotherapy is generally followed by consolidation chemotherapy in patients who achieve a complete remission (approximately 30% of young adults) and, in pregnancy, usually includes the same drugs as used for induction. Allogenic hematopoietic stem-cell transplant is an option in those who fail to achieve a complete remission, although there is no reported experience in pregnancy.[176]

Leukemia and lymphoma have both been found to be metastatic to the placenta and fetus.[184] The placenta from pregnancies complicated by hematologic malignancy should be sent for histologic evaluation.

Survival and Prognosis

The modified Ann Arbor disease stage and patient age are the most important prognostic factors in HL. Young patients with early-stage disease have long-term survival rates of more than 90%.[173,177] Pregnancy does not appear to adversely affect prognosis. An analysis of pregnancy-associated lymphomas that included 17 cases of HL (stage IIA-IVB) also noted a 5-year survival rate of more than 90%.[175] Additionally, a study of 48 patients with HL in pregnancy in which cases were matched for age, stage, and year of treatment revealed no difference in survival for patients with HL in pregnancy. There was also no difference in the stage distribution for patients with HL in pregnancy when compared with the distribution in nonpregnant reproductive-age patients treated for HL at the same institution. Fetal outcomes were also reassuring in this study, with no increased risk for stillbirth, prematurity, IUGR, or fetal malformation noted. There was 1 malformation noted in the group of HL patients: a case of hydrocephaly resulting in neonatal death in a patient exposed to MOPP in the first trimester of pregnancy.[185] Birth outcomes for patients with a history of previously treated HL also appear to be excellent. A recent large study that included 192 women who gave birth with a history of HL showed no increased risk of preterm birth, low birthweight at term, stillbirth, or congenital abnormalities.[186]

In AML, long-term disease-free survival is expected in fewer than 25% of adult cases.[187] Pregnancy itself does not appear to adversely affect outcomes in acute leukemia.[32,182,188] A recent single-institution series reports an 86% complete response rate for patients newly diagnosed with AML during pregnancy who initiated chemotherapy during the pregnancy. Of these, more than half were long-term survivors.[182] Overall, pregnancy outcomes appear to be compromised with premature birth rates greater than 50% and stillbirth in up to 17%.[173] The series by Greenlund et al[182] reports that in 14 patients who were diagnosed with acute leukemia in pregnancy and elected to continue with the pregnancy, there were 9 live births (5 preterm), 1 spontaneous abortion (4 weeks after diagnosis and before initiation of treatment), 3 IUFDs, and 1 fetal death in association with maternal death. It is difficult to separate effects of the malignancy itself on pregnancy outcomes from the potential effects of treatment.

CONCLUSIONS

A cancer diagnosis during pregnancy remains a relatively rare finding, but in general pregnancy itself does not influence the overall clinical outcome of these women. Individualization of care, with respect to patient wishes, gestational age and viability of the fetus, and stage and grade of the malignancy, remains a critical aspect in the management of malignancy identified during pregnancy. A multidisciplinary approach is often critical to successfully treat these patients to afford excellent outcomes for both mother and infant.

REFERENCES

1. Smith LH, Danielsen B, Allen ME, Cress R. Cancer associated with obstetric delivery: results of linkage with the California cancer registry. *Am J Obstet Gynecol*. 2003;189(4):1128-1135.
2. Stensheim H, Moller B, van Dijk T, Fossa SD. Cause-specific survival for women diagnosed with cancer during pregnancy or lactation: a registry-based cohort study. *J Clin Oncol*. 2009; 27(1):45-51.
3. Pavlidis NA. Coexistence of pregnancy and malignancy. *Oncologist*. 2002;7(4):279-287.
4. Lazarus E, Debenedectis C, North D, Spencer PK, Mayo-Smith WW. Utilization of imaging in pregnant patients: 10-year review of 5270 examinations in 3285 patients—1997-2006. *Radiology*. 2009;251(2):517-524.
5. De Santis M, Di Gianantonio E, Straface G, et al. Ionizing radiations in pregnancy and teratogenesis: a review of literature. *Reprod Toxicol*. 2005;20(3):323-329.
6. Patel SJ, Reede DL, Katz DS, Subramaniam R, Amorosa JK. Imaging the pregnant patient for nonobstetric conditions: algorithms and radiation dose considerations. *Radiographics*. 2007;27(6):1705-1722.
7. Brent RL. Saving lives and changing family histories: appropriate counseling of pregnant women and men and women of reproductive age, concerning the risk of diagnostic radiation exposures during and before pregnancy. *Am J Obstet Gynecol*. 2009;200(1):4-24.
8. De Santis M, Cesari E, Nobili E, Straface G, Cavaliere AF, Caruso A. Radiation effects on development. *Birth Defects Res C Embryo Today*. 2007;81(3):177-182.
9. Chen MM, Coakley FV, Kaimal A, Laros RK Jr. Guidelines for computed tomography and magnetic resonance imaging use during pregnancy and lactation. *Obstet Gynecol*. 2008;112 (2 Pt 1):333-340.
10. Mendez LE, Mueller A, Salom E, Gonzalez-Quintero VH. Paclitaxel and carboplatin chemotherapy administered during pregnancy for advanced epithelial ovarian cancer. *Obstet Gynecol*. 2003;102(5 Pt 2):1200-1202.
11. Holschneider CH. Surgical diseases and disorders in pregnancy. In: De Cherney AH, Nathan L, Goodwin TM, Laufer L, eds. *Current Obstetric and Gynecological Diagnosis and Treatment*. 10th ed. New York, NY: Lange Medical Books/McGraw-Hill; 2006:418.
12. Otake M, Schull WJ. In utero exposure to A-bomb radiation and mental retardation; a reassessment. *Br J Radiol*. 1984; 57(677):409-414.
13. Doll R, Wakeford R. Risk of childhood cancer from fetal irradiation. *Br J Radiol*. 1997;70:130-139.
14. Ray JG, Schull MJ, Urquia ML, You JJ, Guttmann A, Vermeulen MJ. Major radiodiagnostic imaging in pregnancy and the risk of childhood malignancy: a population-based cohort study in Ontario. *PLoS Med*. 2010;7(9):e1000337.
15. Ratnapalan S, Bona N, Chandra K, Koren G. Physicians' perceptions of teratogenic risk associated with radiography and CT during early pregnancy. *AJR Am J Roentgenol*. 2004;182(5): 1107-1109.
16. American College of Radiology. ACR manual on contrast media, version 7. Administration of contrast medium to pregnany of potentially pregnant patients, 2010. http://www.acr.org/SecondaryMainMenuCategories/quality_safety/contrast_manual.aspx. Accessed June 12, 2011.
17. Kanal E, Barkovich AJ, Bell C, et al. ACR guidance document for safe MR practices: 2007. *AJR Am J Roentgenol*. 2007;188(6):1447-1474.
18. Kok RD, de Vries MM, Heerschap A, van den Berg PP. Absence of harmful effects of magnetic resonance exposure at 1.5 T in utero during the third trimester of pregnancy: a follow-up study. *Magn Reson Imaging*. 2004;22(6):851-854.
19. Clements H, Duncan KR, Fielding K, Gowland PA, Johnson IR, Baker PN. Infants exposed to MRI in utero have a normal paediatric assessment at 9 months of age. *Br J Radiol*. 2000;73(866):190-194.
20. Webb JA, Thomsen HS, Morcos SK. The use of iodinated and gadolinium contrast media during pregnancy and lactation. *Eur Radiol*. 2005;15(6):1234-1240.
21. Fenig E, Mishaeli M, Kalish Y, Lishner M. Pregnancy and radiation. *Cancer Treat Rev*. 2001;27(1):1-7.
22. Kal HB, Struikmans H. Radiotherapy during pregnancy: fact and fiction. *Lancet Oncol*. 2005;6(5):328-333.
23. Han B, Bednarz B, Xu XG. A study of the shielding used to reduce leakage and scattered radiation to the fetus in a pregnant patient treated with a 6-MV external X-ray beam. *Health Phys*. 2009;97(6):581-589.
24. Woo SY, Fuller LM, Cundiff JH, et al. Radiotherapy during pregnancy for clinical stages IA-IIA Hodgkin's disease. *Int J Radiat Oncol Biol Phys*. 1992;23(2):407-412.
25. Antypas C, Sandilos P, Kouvaris J, et al. Fetal dose evaluation during breast cancer radiotherapy. *Int J Radiat Oncol Biol Phys*. 1998;40(4):995-999.
26. Ngu SL, Duval P, Collins C. Foetal radiation dose in radiotherapy for breast cancer. *Australas Radiol*. 1992;36(4):321-322.
27. Cardonick E, Iacobucci A. Use of chemotherapy during human pregnancy. *Lancet Oncol*. 2004;5(5):283-291.
28. Cardonick E, Usmani A, Ghaffar S. Perinatal outcomes of a pregnancy complicated by cancer, including neonatal follow-up after in utero exposure to chemotherapy: results of an international registry. *Am J Clin Oncol*. 2010;33(3):221-228.

29. Reynoso EE, Shepherd FA, Messner HA, Farquharson HA, Garvey MB, Baker MA. Acute leukemia during pregnancy: the Toronto Leukemia Study Group experience with long-term follow-up of children exposed in utero to chemotherapeutic agents. *J Clin Oncol.* 1987;5(7):1098-1106.

30. Wiebe VJ, Sipila PE. Pharmacology of antineoplastic agents in pregnancy. *Crit Rev Oncol Hematol.* 1994;16(2):75-112.

31. Van Calsteren K, Verbesselt R, Ottevanger N, et al. Pharmacokinetics of chemotherapeutic agents in pregnancy: a preclinical and clinical study. *Acta Obstet Gynecol Scand.* 2010;89(10): 1338-1345.

32. Caligiuri MA, Mayer RJ. Pregnancy and leukemia. *Semin Oncol.* 1989;16(5):388-396.

33. Briggs GG, Freeman RK, Yaffe SJ. *Drugs in Pregnancy and Lactation.* 7th ed. Philadelphia, PA: Lippincott Williams & Wilkins; 2005.

34. Ring AE, Smith IE, Jones A, Shannon C, Galani E, Ellis PA. Chemotherapy for breast cancer during pregnancy: an 18-year experience from five London teaching hospitals. *J Clin Oncol.* 2005;23(18):4192-4197.

35. Doll DC, Ringenberg QS, Yarbro JW. Antineoplastic agents and pregnancy. *Semin Oncol.* 1989;16(5):337-346.

36. Meddows M. Pregnancy and the drug dilemma. FDA Consumer magazine. 2001. http://www.perinatology.com/Archive/ FDA%20CAT.htm. Accessed June 14, 2011.

37. Zemlickis D, Lishner M, Erlich R, Koren G. Teratogenicity and carcinogenicity in a twin pregnancy exposed in utero to cyclophosphamide. *Teratog Carcinog Mutagen.* 1993;13(3):139-143.

38. Ebert U, Loffler H, Kirch W. Cytotoxic therapy and pregnancy. *Pharmacol Ther.* 1997;74(2):207-220.

39. Germann N, Goffinet F, Goldwasser F. Anthracyclines during pregnancy: embryo-fetal outcome in 160 patients. *Ann Oncol.* 2004;15(1):146-150.

40. Aviles A, Neri N, Nambo MJ. Long-term evaluation of cardiac function in children who received anthracyclines during pregnancy. *Ann Oncol.* 2006;17(2):286-288.

41. Amant F, Van Calsteren K, Halaska MJ, et al. Gynecologic cancers in pregnancy: guidelines of an international consensus meeting. *Int J Gynecol Cancer.* 2009;19(suppl 1):S1-S12.

42. Mir O, Berveiller P, Ropert S, et al. Emerging therapeutic options for breast cancer chemotherapy during pregnancy. *Ann Oncol.* 2008;19(4):607-613.

43. Tabata T, Nishiura K, Tanida K, Kondo E, Okugawa T, Sagawa N. Carboplatin chemotherapy in a pregnant patient with undifferentiated ovarian carcinoma: case report and review of the literature. *Int J Gynecol Cancer.* 2008;18(1):181-184.

44. Han JY, Nava-Ocampo AA, Kim TJ, Shim JU, Park CT. Pregnancy outcome after prenatal exposure to bleomycin, etoposide and cisplatin for malignant ovarian germ cell tumors: report of 2 cases. *Reprod Toxicol.* 2005;19(4): 557-561.

45. Giacalone PL, Laffargue F, Benos P, Rousseau O, Hedon B. Cis-platinum neoadjuvant chemotherapy in a pregnant woman with invasive carcinoma of the uterine cervix. *Br J Obstet Gynaecol.* 1996;103(9):932-934.

46. Karam A, Feldman N, Holschneider CH. Neoadjuvant cisplatin and radical cesarean hysterectomy for cervical cancer in pregnancy. *Nat Clin Pract Oncol.* 2007;4(6):375-380.

47. Mir O, Berveiller P, Ropert S, Goffinet F, Goldwasser F. Use of platinum derivatives during pregnancy. *Cancer.* 2008;113(11): 3069-3074.

48. Marnitz S, Kohler C, Oppelt P, et al. Cisplatin application in pregnancy: first in vivo analysis of 7 patients. *Oncology.* 2010; 79(1-2):72-77.

49. Sood AK, Shahin MS, Sorosky JI. Paclitaxel and platinum chemotherapy for ovarian carcinoma during pregnancy. *Gynecol Oncol.* 2001;83(3):599-600.

50. Buller RE, Darrow V, Manetta A, Porto M, DiSaia PJ. Conservative surgical management of dysgerminoma concomitant with pregnancy. *Obstet Gynecol.* 1992;79(5 Pt 2):887-890.

51. Murray NA, Acolet D, Deane M, Price J, Roberts IA. Fetal marrow suppression after maternal chemotherapy for leukaemia. *Arch Dis Child Fetal Neonatal Ed.* 1994;71(3):F209-210.

52. Bennett CL, Silver SM, Djulbegovic B, et al. Venous thromboembolism and mortality associated with recombinant erythropoietin and darbepoetin administration for the treatment of cancer-associated anemia. *JAMA.* 2008;299(8): 914-924.

53. Marik PE. Venous thromboembolism in pregnancy. *Clin Chest Med.* 2010;31(4):731-740.

54. Calhoun DA, Rosa C, Christensen RD. Transplacental passage of recombinant human granulocyte colony-stimulating factor in women with an imminent preterm delivery. *Am J Obstet Gynecol.* 1996;174(4):1306-1311.

55. Dale DC, Cottle TE, Fier CJ, et al. Severe chronic neutropenia: treatment and follow-up of patients in the Severe Chronic Neutropenia International Registry. *Am J Hematol.* 2003;72(2):82-93.

56. Slone D, Siskind V, Heinonen OP, Monson RR, Kaufman DW, Shapiro S. Antenatal exposure to the phenothiazines in relation to congenital malformations, perinatal mortality rate, birth weight, and intelligence quotient score. *Am J Obstet Gynecol.* 1977;128(5):486-488.

57. Carmichael SL, Shaw GM. Maternal corticosteroid use and risk of selected congenital anomalies. *Am J Med Genet.* 1999;86(3):242-244.

58. Smallwood RA, Berlin RG, Castagnoli N, et al. Safety of acid-suppressing drugs. *Dig Dis Sci.* 1995;40(suppl 2):S63-S80.

59. Briggs GG, Freeman RK, Yaffe SJ. *Drugs in Pregnancy and Lactation.* 8th ed. Philadelphia, PA: Lippincott Williams & Wilkins; 2008.

60. Ofori B, Oraichi D, Blais L, Rey E, Berard A. Risk of congenital anomalies in pregnant users of non-steroidal anti-inflammatory drugs: a nested case-control study. *Birth Defects Res B Dev Reprod Toxicol.* 2006;77(4):268-279.

61. Zemlickis D, Lishner M, Degendorfer P, Panzarella T, Sutcliffe SB, Koren G. Maternal and fetal outcome after invasive cervical cancer in pregnancy. *J Clin Oncol.* 1991;9(11):1956-1961.

62. Baldauf JJ, Dreyfus M, Ritter J, Philippe E. Colposcopy and directed biopsy reliability during pregnancy: a cohort study. *Eur J Obstet Gynecol Reprod Biol.* 1995;62(1):31-36.

63. Paraiso MF, Brady K, Helmchen R, Roat TW. Evaluation of the endocervical Cytobrush and Cervex-Brush in pregnant women. *Obstet Gynecol.* 1994;84(4):539-543.

64. McCord ML, Stovall TG, Meric JL, Summitt RL Jr, Coleman SA. Cervical cytology: a randomized comparison of four sampling methods. *Am J Obstet Gynecol.* 1992;166(6 Pt 1): 1772-1777; discussion 1777-1779.

65. Averette HE, Nasser N, Yankow SL, Little WA. Cervical conization in pregnancy. Analysis of 180 operations. *Am J Obstet Gynecol.* 1970;106(4):543-549.

66. Douvier S, Filipuzzi L, Sagot P. [Management of cervical intra-epithelial neoplasm during pregnancy]. *Gynecol Obstet Fertil.* 2003;31(10):851-855.

67. Hannigan EV, Whitehouse HH 3rd, Atkinson WD, Becker SN. Cone biopsy during pregnancy. *Obstet Gynecol.* Oct 1982; 60(4):450-455.

68. Goldberg GL, Altaras MM, Block B. Cone cerclage in pregnancy. *Obstet Gynecol.* 1991;77(2):315-317.

69. Fader AN, Alward EK, Niederhauser A, et al. Cervical dysplasia in pregnancy: a multi-institutional evaluation. *Am J Obstet Gynecol.* 2010;203(2):113 e111-116.

70. Yost NP, Santoso JT, McIntire DD, Iliya FA. Postpartum regression rates of antepartum cervical intraepithelial neoplasia II and III lesions. *Obstet Gynecol.* 1999;93(3):359-362.

CHAPTER 16

71. Wright TC Jr, Massad LS, Dunton CJ, Spitzer M, Wilkinson EJ, Solomon D. 2006 consensus guidelines for the management of women with abnormal cervical cancer screening tests. *Am J Obstet Gynecol.* 2007;197(4):346-355.

72. Wright TC Jr, Massad LS, Dunton CJ, Spitzer M, Wilkinson EJ, Solomon D. 2006 consensus guidelines for the management of women with cervical intraepithelial neoplasia or adenocarcinoma in situ. *Am J Obstet Gynecol.* 2007;197(4):340-345.

73. Takushi M, Moromizato H, Sakumoto K, Kanazawa K. Management of invasive carcinoma of the uterine cervix associated with pregnancy: outcome of intentional delay in treatment. *Gynecol Oncol.* 2002;87(2):185-189.

74. Yahata T, Numata M, Kashima K, et al. Conservative treatment of stage IA1 adenocarcinoma of the cervix during pregnancy. *Gynecol Oncol.* 2008;109(1):49-52.

75. Roman LD, Felix JC, Muderspach LI, Agahjanian A, Qian D, Morrow CP. Risk of residual invasive disease in women with microinvasive squamous cancer in a conization specimen. *Obstet Gynecol.* 1997;90(5):759-764.

76. Giuntoli RL 2nd, Winburn KA, Silverman MB, Keeney GL, Cliby WA. Frozen section evaluation of cervical cold knife cone specimens is accurate in the diagnosis of microinvasive squamous cell carcinoma. *Gynecol Oncol.* 2003;91(2):280-284.

77. Nguyen C, Montz FJ, Bristow RE. Management of stage I cervical cancer in pregnancy. *Obstet Gynecol Surv.* 2000;55(10):633-643.

78. Nucatola D, Roth N, Gatter M. A randomized pilot study on the effectiveness and side-effect profiles of two doses of digoxin as fetocide when administered intraamniotically or intrafetally prior to second-trimester surgical abortion. *Contraception.* 2010;81(1):67-74.

79. Sood AK, Sorosky JI, Krogman S, Anderson B, Benda J, Buller RE. Surgical management of cervical cancer complicating pregnancy: a case-control study. *Gynecol Oncol.* 1996;63(3):294-298.

80. Monk BJ, Montz FJ. Invasive cervical cancer complicating intrauterine pregnancy: treatment with radical hysterectomy. *Obstet Gynecol.* 1992;80(2):199-203.

81. Lee RB, Neglia W, Park RC. Cervical carcinoma in pregnancy. *Obstet Gynecol.* 1981;58(5):584-589.

82. Sood AK, Sorosky JI, Mayr N, et al. Radiotherapeutic management of cervical carcinoma that complicates pregnancy. *Cancer.* 1997;80(6):1073-1078.

83. Benhaim Y, Haie-Meder C, Lhomme C, et al. Chemoradiation therapy in pregnant patients treated for advanced-stage cervical carcinoma during the first trimester of pregnancy: report of two cases. *Int J Gynecol Cancer.* 2007;17(1):270-274.

84. Creasman WT. Cancer and pregnancy. *Ann N Y Acad Sci.* 2001;943:281-286.

85. Creasman WT, Rutledge FN, Fletcher GH. Carcinoma of the cervix associated with pregnancy. *Obstet Gynecol.* 1970;36(4):495-501.

86. Prem KA, Makowski EL, McKelvey JL. Carcinoma of the cervix associated with pregnancy. *Am J Obstet Gynecol.* 1966;95(1):99-108.

87. Ostrom K, Ben-Arie A, Edwards C, Gregg A, Chiu JK, Kaplan AL. Uterine evacuation with misoprostol during radiotherapy for cervical cancer in pregnancy. *Int J Gynecol Cancer.* 2003;13(3):340-343.

88. Stoll BJ, Hansen NI, Bell EF, et al. Neonatal outcomes of extremely preterm infants from the NICHD Neonatal Research Network. *Pediatrics.* 2010;126(3):443-456.

89. Alouini S, Rida K, Mathevet P. Cervical cancer complicating pregnancy: implications of laparoscopic lymphadenectomy. *Gynecol Oncol.* 2008;108(3):472-477.

90. Favero G, Lanowska M, Schneider A, Marnitz S, Kohler C. Laparoscopic pelvic lymphadenectomy in a patient with cervical cancer stage Ib1 complicated by a twin pregnancy. *J Minim Invasive Gynecol.* 2010;17(1):118-120.

91. Neoadjuvant chemotherapy for locally advanced cervical cancer: a systematic review and meta-analysis of individual patient data from 21 randomised trials. *Eur J Cancer.* 2003;39(17):2470-2486.

92. Sood AK, Sorosky JI, Mayr N, Anderson B, Buller RE, Niebyl J. Cervical cancer diagnosed shortly after pregnancy: prognostic variables and delivery routes. *Obstet Gynecol.* 2000;95(6 Pt 1):832-838.

93. van der Vange N, Weverling GJ, Ketting BW, Ankum WM, Samlal R, Lammes FB. The prognosis of cervical cancer associated with pregnancy: a matched cohort study. *Obstet Gynecol.* 1995;85(6):1022-1026.

94. Baloglu A, Uysal D, Aslan N, Yigit S. Advanced stage of cervical carcinoma undiagnosed during antenatal period in term pregnancy and concomitant metastasis on episiotomy scar during delivery: a case report and review of the literature. *Int J Gynecol Cancer.* 2007;17(5):1155-1159.

95. Pettersson BF, Andersson S, Hellman K, Hellstrom AC. Invasive carcinoma of the uterine cervix associated with pregnancy: 90 years of experience. *Cancer.* 2010;116(10):2343-2349.

96. Condous G, Khalid A, Okaro E, Bourne T. Should we be examining the ovaries in pregnancy? Prevalence and natural history of adnexal pathology detected at first-trimester sonography. *Ultrasound Obstet Gynecol.* 2004;24(1):62-66.

97. Zanetta G, Mariani E, Lissoni A, et al. A prospective study of the role of ultrasound in the management of adnexal masses in pregnancy. *BJOG.* 2003;110(6):578-583.

98. Palmer J, Vatish M, Tidy J. Epithelial ovarian cancer in pregnancy: a review of the literature. *BJOG.* 2009;116(4):480-491.

99. Leiserowitz GS, Xing G, Cress R, Brahmbhatt B, Dalrymple JL, Smith LH. Adnexal masses in pregnancy: how often are they malignant? *Gynecol Oncol.* 2006;101(2):315-321.

100. Leiserowitz GS. Managing ovarian masses during pregnancy. *Obstet Gynecol Surv.* 2006;61(7):463-470.

101. Yen CF, Lin SL, Murk W, et al. Risk analysis of torsion and malignancy for adnexal masses during pregnancy. *Fertil Steril.* 2009;91(5):1895-1902.

102. Lee GS, Hur SY, Shin JC, Kim SP, Kim SJ. Elective vs. conservative management of ovarian tumors in pregnancy. *Int J Gynaecol Obstet.* 2004;85(3):250-254.

103. Giuntoli RL, 2nd, Vang RS, Bristow RE. Evaluation and management of adnexal masses during pregnancy. *Clin Obstet Gynecol.* 2006;49(3):492-505.

104. Mathevet P, Nessah K, Dargent D, Mellier G. Laparoscopic management of adnexal masses in pregnancy: a case series. *Eur J Obstet Gynecol Reprod Biol.* 2003;108(2):217-222.

105. Stepp KJ, Tulikangas PK, Goldberg JM, Attaran M, Falcone T. Laparoscopy for adnexal masses in the second trimester of pregnancy. *J Am Assoc Gynecol Laparosc.* 2003;10(1):55-59.

106. ICON2: randomised trial of single-agent carboplatin against three-drug combination of CAP (cyclophosphamide, doxorubicin, and cisplatin) in women with ovarian cancer. ICON Collaborators. International Collaborative Ovarian Neoplasm Study. *Lancet.* 1998;352(9140):1571-1576.

107. Picone O, Lhomme C, Tournaire M, et al. Preservation of pregnancy in a patient with a stage IIIB ovarian epithelial carcinoma diagnosed at 22 weeks of gestation and treated with initial chemotherapy: case report and literature review. *Gynecol Oncol.* 2004;94(2):600-604.

108. Elit L, Bocking A, Kenyon C, Natale R. An endodermal sinus tumor diagnosed in pregnancy: case report and review of the literature. *Gynecol Oncol.* 1999;72(1):123-127.

109. Kwon YS, Mok JE, Lim KT, et al. Ovarian cancer during pregnancy: clinical and pregnancy outcome. *J Korean Med Sci.* 2010;25(2):230-234.

110. Beadle BM, Woodward WA, Middleton LP, et al. The impact of pregnancy on breast cancer outcomes in women < or = 35 years. *Cancer.* 2009;115(6):1174-1184.

111. Woo JC, Yu T, Hurd TC. Breast cancer in pregnancy: a literature review. *Arch Surg.* 2003;138(1):91-98; discussion 99.

112. Loibl S, von Minckwitz G, Gwyn K, et al. Breast carcinoma during pregnancy. International recommendations from an expert meeting. *Cancer.* 2006;106(2):237-246.

113. Albrektsen G, Heuch I, Kvale G. The short-term and long-term effect of a pregnancy on breast cancer risk: a prospective study of 802,457 parous Norwegian women. *Br J Cancer.* 1995;72(2):480-484.

114. Wohlfahrt J, Andersen PK, Mouridsen HT, Melbye M. Risk of late-stage breast cancer after a childbirth. *Am J Epidemiol.* 2001;153(11):1079-1084.

115. Nettleton J, Long J, Kuban D, Wu R, Shaefffer J, El-Mahdi A. Breast cancer during pregnancy: quantifying the risk of treatment delay. *Obstet Gynecol.* 1996;87(3):414-418.

116. Litton JK, Theriault RL, Gonzalez-Angulo AM. Breast cancer diagnosis during pregnancy. *Womens Health (Lond Engl).* 2009;5(3):243-249.

117. Yang WT, Dryden MJ, Gwyn K, Whitman GJ, Theriault R. Imaging of breast cancer diagnosed and treated with chemotherapy during pregnancy. *Radiology.* 2006;239(1):52-60.

118. Nicklas AH, Baker ME. Imaging strategies in the pregnant cancer patient. *Semin Oncol.* 2000;27(6):623-632.

119. Samuels TH, Liu FF, Yaffe M, Haider M. Gestational breast cancer. *Can Assoc Radiol J.* 1998;49(3):172-180.

120. Buchholz TA, Austin-Seymour MM, Moe RE, et al. Effect of delay in radiation in the combined modality treatment of breast cancer. *Int J Radiat Oncol Biol Phys.* 1993;26(1):23-35.

121. Lyman GH, Giuliano AE, Somerfield MR, et al. American Society of Clinical Oncology guideline recommendations for sentinel lymph node biopsy in early-stage breast cancer. *J Clin Oncol.* 2005;23(30):7703-7720.

122. Gentilini O, Cremonesi M, Toesca A, et al. Sentinel lymph node biopsy in pregnant patients with breast cancer. *Eur J Nucl Med Mol Imaging.* 2010;37(1):78-83.

123. Mondi MM, Cuenca RE, Ollila DW, Stewart JHt, Levine EA. Sentinel lymph node biopsy during pregnancy: initial clinical experience. *Ann Surg Oncol.* 2007;14(1):218-221.

124. Keleher A, Wendt R 3rd, Delpassand E, Stachowiak AM, Kuerer HM. The safety of lymphatic mapping in pregnant breast cancer patients using Tc-99m sulfur colloid. *Breast J.* 2004;10(6):492-495.

125. Amant F, Deckers S, Van Calsteren K, et al. Breast cancer in pregnancy: recommendations of an international consensus meeting. *Eur J Cancer.* 2010;46(18):3158-3168.

126. Hahn KM, Johnson PH, Gordon N, et al. Treatment of pregnant breast cancer patients and outcomes of children exposed to chemotherapy in utero. *Cancer.* 2006;107(6):1219-1226.

127. Giacalone PL, Laffargue F, Benos P. Chemotherapy for breast carcinoma during pregnancy: a French national survey. *Cancer.* 1999;86(11):2266-2272.

128. Azim HA Jr, Peccatori FA, Liptrott SJ, Catania C, Goldhirsch A. Breast cancer and pregnancy: how safe is trastuzumab? *Nat Rev Clin Oncol.* 2009;6(6):367-370.

129. Kelly H, Graham M, Humes E, et al. Delivery of a healthy baby after first-trimester maternal exposure to lapatinib. *Clin Breast Cancer.* 2006;7(4):339-341.

130. Ibrahim EM, Ezzat AA, Baloush A, Hussain ZH, Mohammed GH. Pregnancy-associated breast cancer: a case-control study in a young population with a high-fertility rate. *Med Oncol.* 2000;17(4):293-300.

131. Halaska MJ, Pentheroudakis G, Strnad P, et al. Presentation, management and outcome of 32 patients with pregnancy-associated breast cancer: a matched controlled study. *Breast J.* 2009;15(5):461-467.

132. Ives A, Saunders C, Bulsara M, Semmens J. Pregnancy after breast cancer: population based study. *BMJ.* 2007;334(7586):194.

133. Velentgas P, Daling JR, Malone KE, et al. Pregnancy after breast carcinoma: outcomes and influence on mortality. *Cancer.* 1999;85(11):2424-2432.

134. Mueller BA, Simon MS, Deapen D, Kamineni A, Malone KE, Daling JR. Childbearing and survival after breast carcinoma in young women. *Cancer.* 2003;98(6):1131-1140.

135. Gelber S, Coates AS, Goldhirsch A, et al. Effect of pregnancy on overall survival after the diagnosis of early-stage breast cancer. *J Clin Oncol.* 2001;19(6):1671-1675.

136. Azim HA Jr, Santoro L, Pavlidis N, et al. Safety of pregnancy following breast cancer diagnosis: a meta-analysis of 14 studies. *Eur J Cancer.* 2011;47(1):74-83.

137. Alexander A, Samlowski WE, Grossman D, et al. Metastatic melanoma in pregnancy: risk of transplacental metastases in the infant. *J Clin Oncol.* 2003;21(11):2179-2186.

138. Gupta A, Driscoll MS. Do hormones influence melanoma? Facts and controversies. *Clin Dermatol.* 2010;28(3):287-292.

139. Balch CM, Gershenwald JE, Soong SJ, et al. Final version of 2009 AJCC melanoma staging and classification. *J Clin Oncol.* 2009;27(36):6199-6206.

140. Lens MB, Nathan P, Bataille V. Excision margins for primary cutaneous melanoma: updated pooled analysis of randomized controlled trials. *Arch Surg.* 2007;142(9):885-891; discussion 891-883.

141. Rousseau DL Jr, Ross MI, Johnson MM, et al. Revised American Joint Committee on Cancer staging criteria accurately predict sentinel lymph node positivity in clinically node-negative melanoma patients. *Ann Surg Oncol.* 2003;10(5):569-574.

142. Chakera AH, Hesse B, Burak Z, et al. EANM-EORTC general recommendations for sentinel node diagnostics in melanoma. *Eur J Nucl Med Mol Imaging.* 2009;36(10):1713-1742.

143. Kirkwood JM, Strawderman MH, Ernstoff MS, Smith TJ, Borden EC, Blum RH. Interferon alfa-2b adjuvant therapy of high-risk resected cutaneous melanoma: the Eastern Cooperative Oncology Group Trial EST 1684. *J Clin Oncol.* 1996;14(1):7-17.

144. Kirkwood JM, Manola J, Ibrahim J, Sondak V, Ernstoff MS, Rao U. A pooled analysis of eastern cooperative oncology group and intergroup trials of adjuvant high-dose interferon for melanoma. *Clin Cancer Res.* 2004;10(5):1670-1677.

145. Eggermont AM, Suciu S, Santinami M, et al. Adjuvant therapy with pegylated interferon alfa-2b versus observation alone in resected stage III melanoma: final results of EORTC 18991, a randomised phase III trial. *Lancet.* 2008;372(9633):117-126.

146. Eggermont AM, Suciu S, MacKie R, et al. Post-surgery adjuvant therapy with intermediate doses of interferon alfa 2b versus observation in patients with stage IIb/III melanoma (EORTC 18952): randomised controlled trial. *Lancet.* 2005;366(9492):1189-1196.

147. Hauschild A, Weichenthal M, Rass K, et al. Efficacy of low-dose interferon {alpha}2a 18 versus 60 months of treatment in patients with primary melanoma of >= 1.5 mm tumor thickness: results of a randomized phase III DeCOG trial. *J Clin Oncol.* 2010;28(5):841-846.

148. Egberts F, Lischner S, Russo P, Kampen WU, Hauschild A. Diagnostic and therapeutic procedures for management of melanoma during pregnancy: risks for the fetus? *J Dtsch Dermatol Ges.* 2006;4(9):717-720.

149. Hiratsuka M, Minakami H, Koshizuka S, Sato I. Administration of interferon-alpha during pregnancy: effects on fetus. *J Perinat Med.* 2000;28(5):372-376.

150. Shuff JH, Siker ML, Daly MD, Schultz CJ. Role of radiation therapy in cutaneous melanoma. *Clin Plast Surg.* 2010;37(1):147-160.

151. Lee SM, Betticher DC, Thatcher N. Melanoma: chemotherapy. *Br Med Bull.* 1995;51(3):609-630.

152. Middleton MR, Grob JJ, Aaronson N, et al. Randomized phase III study of temozolomide versus dacarbazine in the treatment of patients with advanced metastatic malignant melanoma. *J Clin Oncol.* 2000;18(1):158-166.

153. O'Meara AT, Cress R, Xing G, Danielsen B, Smith LH. Malignant melanoma in pregnancy. A population-based evaluation. *Cancer.* 2005;103(6):1217-1226.

154. Lens MB, Rosdahl I, Ahlbom A, et al. Effect of pregnancy on survival in women with cutaneous malignant melanoma. *J Clin Oncol.* 2004;22(21):4369-4375.

155. Reintgen DS, McCarty KS Jr, Vollmer R, Cox E, Seigler HF. Malignant melanoma and pregnancy. *Cancer.* 1985;55(6):1340-1344.

156. Cooper DS, Doherty GM, Haugen BR, et al. Revised American Thyroid Association management guidelines for patients with thyroid nodules and differentiated thyroid cancer. *Thyroid.* 2009;19(11):1167-1214.

157. Mack WJ, Preston-Martin S, Bernstein L, Qian D, Xiang M. Reproductive and hormonal risk factors for thyroid cancer in Los Angeles County females. *Cancer Epidemiol Biomarkers Prev.* 1999;8(11):991-997.

158. Mazzaferri EL. Management of a solitary thyroid nodule. *N Engl J Med.* 1993;328(8):553-559.

159. Morris PC. Thyroid cancer complicating pregnancy. *Obstet Gynecol Clin North Am.* 1998;25(2):401-405.

160. Moosa M, Mazzaferri EL. Outcome of differentiated thyroid cancer diagnosed in pregnant women. *J Clin Endocrinol Metab.* 1997;82(9):2862-2866.

161. Wu M. A comparative study of 200 head and neck FNAs performed by a cytopathologist with versus without ultrasound guidance: evidence for improved diagnostic value with ultrasound guidance. *Diagn Cytopathol.* 2011;39(10):743-751.

162. Owen RP, Chou KJ, Silver CE, et al. Thyroid and parathyroid surgery in pregnancy. *Eur Arch Otorhinolaryngol.* 2010;267(12):1825-1835.

163. Mazzaferri EL, Jhiang SM. Long-term impact of initial surgical and medical therapy on papillary and follicular thyroid cancer. *Am J Med.* 1994;97(5):418-428.

164. McGriff NJ, Csako G, Gourgiotis L, Lori CG, Pucino F, Sarlis NJ. Effects of thyroid hormone suppression therapy on adverse clinical outcomes in thyroid cancer. *Ann Med.* 2002;34(7-8):554-564.

165. LeBeau SO, Mandel SJ. Thyroid disorders during pregnancy. *Endocrinol Metab Clin North Am.* 2006;35(1):117-136, vii.

166. Rosen IB, Korman M, Walfish PG. Thyroid nodular disease in pregnancy: current diagnosis and management. *Clin Obstet Gynecol.* 1997;40(1):81-89.

167. Doherty CM, Shindo ML, Rice DH, Montero M, Mestman JH. Management of thyroid nodules during pregnancy. *Laryngoscope.* 1995;105(3 Pt 1):251-255.

168. Herzon FS, Morris DM, Segal MN, Rauch G, Parnell T. Coexistent thyroid cancer and pregnancy. *Arch Otolaryngol Head Neck Surg.* 1994;120(11):1191-1193.

169. Yasmeen S, Cress R, Romano PS, et al. Thyroid cancer in pregnancy. *Int J Gynaecol Obstet.* 2005;91(1):15-20.

170. Vannucchi G, Perrino M, Rossi S, et al. Clinical and molecular features of differentiated thyroid cancer diagnosed during pregnancy. *Eur J Endocrinol.* 2010;162(1):145-151.

171. Hirsch D, Levy S, Tsvetov G, et al. Impact of pregnancy on outcome and prognosis of survivors of papillary thyroid cancer. *Thyroid.* 2010;20(10):1179-1185.

172. Leboeuf R, Emerick LE, Martorella AJ, Tuttle RM. Impact of pregnancy on serum thyroglobulin and detection of recurrent disease shortly after delivery in thyroid cancer survivors. *Thyroid.* 2007;17(6):543-547.

173. Hurley TJ, McKinnell JV, Irani MS. Hematologic malignancies in pregnancy. *Obstet Gynecol Clin North Am.* 2005;32(4):595-614.

174. Weisz B, Schiff E, Lishner M. Cancer in pregnancy: maternal and fetal implications. *Hum Reprod Update.* 2001;7(4):384-393.

175. Gelb AB, van de Rijn M, Warnke RA, Kamel OW. Pregnancy-associated lymphomas. A clinicopathologic study. *Cancer.* 1996;78(2):304-310.

176. Shapira T, Pereg D, Lishner M. How I treat acute and chronic leukemia in pregnancy. *Blood Rev.* 2008;22(5):247-259.

177. Vassilakopoulos TP, Angelopoulou MK, Siakantaris MP, et al. Combination chemotherapy plus low-dose involved-field radiotherapy for early clinical stage Hodgkin's lymphoma. *Int J Radiat Oncol Biol Phys.* 2004;59(3):765-781.

178. Rizack T, Mega A, Legare R, Castillo J. Management of hematological malignancies during pregnancy. *Am J Hematol.* 2009;84(12):830-841.

179. Connors JM. Challenging problems: coincident pregnancy, HIV infection, and older age. *Hematology Am Soc Hematol Educ Program.* 2008:334-339.

180. Pereg D, Koren G, Lishner M. The treatment of Hodgkin's and non-Hodgkin's lymphoma in pregnancy. *Haematologica.* 2007;92(9):1230-1237.

181. Aviles A, Diaz-Maqueo JC, Talavera A, Guzman R, Garcia EL. Growth and development of children of mothers treated with chemotherapy during pregnancy: current status of 43 children. *Am J Hematol.* 1991;36(4):243-248.

182. Greenlund LJ, Letendre L, Tefferi A. Acute leukemia during pregnancy: a single institutional experience with 17 cases. *Leuk Lymphoma.* 2001;41(5-6):571-577.

183. Wagner VM, Hill JS, Weaver D, Baehner RL. Congenital abnormalities in baby born to cytarabine treated mother. *Lancet.* 1980;2(8185):98-99.

184. Walker JW, Reinisch JF, Monforte HL. Maternal pulmonary adenocarcinoma metastatic to the fetus: first recorded case report and literature review. *Pediatr Pathol Mol Med.* 2002;21(1):57-69.

185. Lishner M, Zemlickis D, Degendorfer P, Panzarella T, Sutcliffe SB, Koren G. Maternal and foetal outcome following Hodgkin's disease in pregnancy. *Br J Cancer.* 1992;65(1):114-117.

186. Langagergaard V, Horvath-Puho E, Norgaard M, Norgard B, Sorensen HT. Hodgkin's disease and birth outcome: a Danish nationwide cohort study. *Br J Cancer.* 2008;98(1):183-188.

187. Bennett JM, Young ML, Andersen JW, et al. Long-term survival in acute myeloid leukemia: the Eastern Cooperative Oncology Group experience. *Cancer.* 1997;80(suppl 11):2205-2209.

188. Catanzarite VA, Ferguson JE 2nd. Acute leukemia and pregnancy: a review of management and outcome, 1972-1982. *Obstet Gynecol Surv.* 1984;39(11):663-678.

189. Boutselis JG. Intraepithelial carcinoma of the cervix associated with pregnancy. *Obstet Gynecol.* 1972;40(5):657-666.

190. Dudan RC, Yon JL, Ford JH, Averette HE. Carcinoma of the cervix and pregnancy. *Gynecol Oncol.* 1973;1:283.

191. Thompson JD, Caputo TA, Franklin EW, 3rd, Dale E. The surgical management of invasive cancer of the cervix in pregnancy. *Am J Obstet Gynecol.* 1975;121(6):853-B63.

192. Nisker JA, Shubat M. Stage IB cervical carcinoma and pregnancy: report of 49 cases. *Am J Obstet Gynecol.* 1983;145(2):203-206.

193. Greer BE, Easterling TR, McLennan DA, et al. Fetal and maternal considerations in the management of stage I-B cervical cancer during pregnancy. *Gynecol Oncol.* 1989;34(1):61-65.

194. Duggan B, Muderspach LI, Roman LD, Curtin JP, d'Ablaing G, 3rd, Morrow CP. Cervical cancer in pregnancy: reporting on planned delay in therapy. *Obstet Gynecol.* 1993;82(4 Pt 1):598-602.

195. Sorosky JI, Squatrito R, Ndubisi BU, et al. Stage I squamous cell cervical carcinoma in pregnancy: planned delay in therapy awaiting fetal maturity. *Gynecol Oncol.* 1995;59(2):207-210.

196. Sorosky J. Stage 1b cervical carcinoma in pregnancy: awaiting fetal maturity. *J Gynecol Tech.* 1996;2:155-158.

197. van Vliet W, van Loon AJ, ten Hoor KA, Boonstra H. Cervical carcinoma during pregnancy: outcome of planned delay in treatment. *Eur J Obstet Gynecol Reprod Biol.* 1998;79(2):153-157.

198. Traen K, Svane D, Kryger-Baggesen N, Bertelsen K, Mogensen O. Stage Ib cervical cancer during pregnancy: planned delay in treatment–case report. *Eur J Gynaecol Oncol.* 2006;27(6):615-617.

199. Germann N, Haie-Meder C, Morice P, et al. Management and clinical outcomes of pregnant patients with invasive cervical cancer. *Ann Oncol.* 2005;16(3):397-402.

200. Lee JM, Lee KB, Kim YT, et al. Cervical cancer associated with pregnancy: results of a multicenter retrospective Korean study (KGOG-1006). *Am J Obstet Gynecol.* 2008;198(1):92 e91-96.

201. Gonzalez Bosquet E, Castillo A, Medina M, Sunol M, Capdevila A, Lailla JM. Stage 1B cervical cancer in a pregnant woman at 25 weeks of gestation. *Eur J Gynaecol Oncol.* 2008;29(3):276-279.

202. Ishioka S, Ezaka Y, Endo T, et al. Outcomes of planned delivery delay in pregnant patients with invasive gynecologic cancer. *Int J Clin Oncol.* 2009;14(4):321-325.

203. Favero G, Chiantera V, Oleszczuk A, et al. Invasive cervical cancer during pregnancy:laparoscopic nodal evaluation before oncologic treatment delay. *Gynecol Oncol.* 2010;118(2):123-127.

204. Lai CH, Hsueh S, Chang TC, et al. Prognostic factors in patients with bulky stage IB or IIA cervical carcinoma undergoing neoadjuvant chemotherapy and radical hysterectomy. *Gynecol Oncol.* 1997;64(3):456-462.

205. Tewari K, Cappuccini F, Gambino A, Kohler MF, Pecorelli S, DiSaia PJ. Neoadjuvant chemotherapy in the treatment of locally advanced cervical carcinoma in pregnancy: a report of two cases and review of issues specific to the management of cervical carcinoma in pregnancy including planned delay of therapy. *Cancer.* 1998;82(8):1529-1534.

206. Marana HR, de Andrade JM, da Silva Mathes AC, Duarte G, da Cunha SP, Bighetti S. Chemotherapy in the treatment of locally advanced cervical cancer and pregnancy. *Gynecol Oncol.* 2001;80(2):272-274.

207. Caluwaerts S, K VANC, Mertens L, et al. Neoadjuvant chemotherapy followed by radical hysterectomy for invasive cervical cancer diagnosed during pregnancy: report of a case and review of the literature. *Int J Gynecol Cancer.* 2006;16(2):905-908.

208. Benhaim Y, Pautier P, Bensaid C, Lhomme C, Haie-Meder C, Morice P. Neoadjuvant chemotherapy for advanced stage cervical cancer in a pregnant patient: report of one case with rapid tumor progression. *Eur J Obstet Gynecol Reprod Biol.* 2008;136(2):267-268.

209. Bader AA, Petru E, Winter R. Long-term follow-up after neoadjuvant chemotherapy for high-risk cervical cancer during pregnancy. *Gynecol Oncol.* 2007;105(1):269-272.

210. Palaia I, Pernice M, Graziano M, Bellati F, Panici PB. Neoadjuvant chemotherapy plus radical surgery in locally advanced cervical cancer during pregnancy: a case report. *Am J Obstet Gynecol.* 2007;197(4):e5-6.

211. Seamon LG, Downey GO, Harrison CR, Doss B, Carlson JW. Neoadjuvant chemotherapy followed by post-partum chemoradiotherapy and chemoconsolidation for stage IIIB glassy cell cervical carcinoma during pregnancy. *Gynecol Oncol.* 2009;114(3):540-541.

212. Rabaiotti E, Sigismondi C, Montoli S, Mangili G, Candiani M, Vigano R. Management of locally advanced cervical cancer in pregnancy: a case report. *Tumori.* 2010;96(4):623-626.

17 Metastases to the Gynecologic Tract

S. Diane Yamada and Nita K. Lee

Metastases to the genital tract may occur as a result of recognizable widely disseminated disease from another site or as an isolated lesion. In the latter case, it may be difficult to distinguish between a primary tumor of the gynecologic tract or metastases to the gynecologic tract from a nongynecologic site. Because treatment planning and appropriateness of surgery may be dictated by the primary site of the tumor, it is important to make the distinction between primary and metastatic disease. This chapter focuses on common sites of metastases to the gynecologic tract, characteristic clinical presentations, and radiologic and pathologic considerations that may be clinically helpful in treatment planning.

EPIDEMIOLOGY

Key Points

1. Metastatic disease to the gynecologic organs most commonly arises from colorectal, breast, gastric, and appendiceal primary malignancies.
2. Within the reproductive tract, the ovaries and vagina are the organs most commonly affected by metastatic disease.
3. Malignant masses or lesions in the gynecologic organs should be considered as potential sites of metastases if an established primary malignancy is of advanced stage or demonstrates poor prognostic factors.

Metastatic disease to the genital tract from nongenital tract malignancies is relatively uncommon but is influenced by geographic differences in cancer incidence. For instance, in Asian countries where gastric cancer is more common, metastatic disease to the genital tract is more prevalent. In Japan, 18% to 29% of tumors found in the reproductive organs may be nongynecologic in origin; in Thailand, where cholangiocarcinoma is quite prevalent, 7% of all metastases to the genital tract may arise from the gallbladder or extrahepatic biliary tract.[1] A single-institution review from the United States of 445,000 accessioned cases identified 325 metastatic tumors to the genital tract over a 32-year time period; 149 (45.8%) were from extragenital sites including the colon and rectum, breast, stomach, and appendix. Additional primary sites included the bladder, ileum, and cutaneous melanoma. The remaining sites of metastases originated from other areas within the genital tract such as the endometrium.[2]

The ovaries and vagina are, by far, the structures most commonly involved with nongenital tract metastases. Although percentages may vary by geographic area, the most common primary sites of disease metastatic to the ovaries typically arise from the gastrointestinal (GI) tract (large intestine and stomach, pancreas, biliary tract, and appendix) and breast. These sites comprise 50% to 90% of the metastatic cancers to the ovaries (Table 17-1). Although the histology of a metastatic breast cancer may look uniquely like breast cancer, metastases from other sites, such as the pancreas and appendix, are mucinous and can be difficult to distinguish from a primary mucinous tumor of the ovary. Endometrioid-appearing histologies in the ovary can arise from metastatic colon cancer, and clear cell histology can be confused with signet ring

Table 17-1 Metastatic Tumor to the Ovaries

Primary Site of Cancer	Number (%)
Stomach	743 (76)
Colon and rectum	104 (11)
Gallbladder/biliary	28 (3)
Breast	44 (4)
Others[a]	59 (6)
Total	978 (100)

[a]Small intestine, appendix, pancreas, bladder, kidney.
Adapted from Kiyokawa et al.[16]

cells from a gastric cancer or a metastatic clear cell renal carcinoma. In the case of breast cancer, metastases to the ovary may remain completely occult and are detected only at autopsy or when they become symptomatic to the patient or identified on examination by her physician. With mucinous tumors, the metastases in the ovary can become quite large, leading to significant symptoms and typically dominating the clinical picture for the patient and the clinician.

Reproductive tract lesions are most likely to reflect metastatic disease when there is an established nongynecologic primary malignancy, especially if the primary tumor is advanced or has poor prognostic factors. This is true of metastatic breast, pancreatic, and colon cancer. In the case of some metastatic GI tract malignancies, however, the primary tumor may not be found for many years after the metastasis. The classic signet ring cell adenocarcinoma of the ovary is called a Krukenberg tumor, which represents fewer than 6% to 7% of all ovarian tumors in Western countries. The signet ring morphology was initially described in 1896 by a German pathologist and gynecologist, Friedrich Krukenberg. However, the extragenital origin of the Krukenberg tumor was not described until 6 years later. The stomach is the primary site of malignancy in 70% of cases of Krukenberg tumor. The route of spread to the ovaries is believed to be lymphatic due to the copious lymphatic plexus surrounding the gastric mucosa and submucosa. This lymphatic plexus, which communicates with the lymphatics along the ovarian vessels, provides a direct conduit for even small gastric cancers to spread to the hilum and cortex of the ovary.[3]

Primary appendiceal neoplasms, including low-grade mucinous neoplasms, signet ring adenocarcinomas, and mucinous carcinoid tumors, also may remain occult until they present with symptomatic ovarian masses or disseminated mucin consistent with pseudomyxoma peritonei. The rupture site of a primary low-grade appendiceal neoplasm may be small and contained with fibrotic mucus.[4] When this occurs, the resulting ovarian metastases are frequently bilateral and

occur as a result of implantation of tumor cells and mucin on the surface of the ovaries, which can then invade into the stroma. If there is unilateral involvement of the ovary, it is more frequently on the right side, adjacent to the appendix.[5]

Most patients with colorectal cancer, similar to those with breast cancer, will have their primary malignancy detected before the diagnosis of metastatic disease to the ovaries. In colorectal cancers, only 3% of patients initially present with an ovarian mass. In general, the majority of primary colon cancers occur distally in the sigmoid or rectum. In patients who develop ovarian metastases, most have a primary lesion in the colon that has full-thickness invasion of the bowel wall, direct invasion into adjacent structures, multiple positive lymph nodes, and/or involvement of other non-ovarian sites such as the omentum or liver.[6] Although ovarian involvement can occur by direct extension, other processes such as angiogenesis and stromal cell–cancer cell interaction have been proposed for the predilection of colorectal cancer to metastasize to the ovaries. In patients with pancreatic cancer, 4% to 6% will have ovarian metastases during the course of their disease.[4] In a small series of patients with metastatic pancreatic cancer, all patients had other sites of intraperitoneal disease, such as the omentum and bowel mesentery, when the ovarian involvement was detected.[7]

Carcinomas of the extrahepatic bile ducts and gallbladder are far more common in Asian countries. Ovarian metastases may present in a heterogenous manner, with nearly equal number of patients presenting at the time of primary tumor diagnosis and before or after detection of the primary tumor site. The vast majority of metastases are bilateral and mucinous, but the tumor may be infiltrative or primarily present on the surface of the ovaries and can be cystic, solid, or mixed in morphology.[8]

After the gastrointestinal tract, breast cancer is the most common site of origin of metastatic disease, especially to the ovaries. Because there are genetic mutations in *BRCA1*, *BRCA2*, and the DNA mismatch repair genes that predispose women to develop ovarian cancer, distinguishing a primary ovarian malignancy from a metastatic breast or colon cancer in women who harbor these genetic mutations may create a diagnostic dilemma. Nearly 10% of women who develop breast cancer before the age of 50 years will harbor a mutation in *BRCA1* or *BRCA2* that will place them at risk for ovarian cancer.[9] Distinguishing advanced primary ovarian cancer from metastatic breast cancer is critical in providing recommendations for the appropriateness of cytoreductive surgery, chemotherapy, or hormonal therapy.

In a review of 79 women with a history of breast cancer who presented with carcinomatosis and underwent surgery, the majority of patients (75%) were diagnosed with primary ovarian, tubal, or peritoneal cancers.[10]

Although not statistically significant, the authors suggested a trend favoring a new primary ovarian cancer in women with longer intervals since their breast cancer diagnosis and higher CA-125 values. In autopsy studies, 10% of patients with breast cancer have ovarian metastases.[11] The most significant risk factor for ovarian involvement is advanced-stage breast cancer. In a series of 31 patients with stage IV breast cancer who underwent laparoscopy for either an adnexal mass or therapeutic bilateral salpingo-oophorectomy, 21 patients (68%) were diagnosed with metastatic breast cancer.[12] Conversely, women diagnosed with early-stage breast cancer are more likely to have benign adnexal disease than metastatic disease in their ovaries. In a series of 129 women with breast cancer who underwent surgery for an adnexal mass, 88% were found to have benign ovarian cysts; of the remaining patients with malignant lesions, the majority were primary ovarian cancers rather than metastatic breast cancer.[10]

Metastatic melanoma and renal cell carcinoma frequently pose diagnostic problems. When metastatic to the ovaries or uterus, the majority of patients with melanoma have disseminated disease in other areas. The ovaries represent the majority (75%) of metastases. Usually, there is a history of removal of a cutaneous lesion or an ocular lesion. The time span to the development of metastatic disease that involves the ovaries and becomes clinically significant may be many years.

Metastases to the uterus, cervix, vagina, and vulva are exceedingly rare, with individual reports scattered throughout the literature. Primary sites that can metastasize to the uterine corpus or cervix include breast, stomach, colon, rectum, melanoma, lung, and kidney.[13] In patients with a history of breast cancer, distinguishing between a primary uterine malignancy and metastatic breast cancer can be challenging if the patient has received hormonal therapy for her breast cancer. Tamoxifen is associated with known uterine pathology, including hyperplasias, highly irregular polyps, and primary endometrial cancers, all of which may also present with vaginal bleeding. In general, women with metastatic breast cancer to the uterus have a poor prognosis, as the uterus is rarely the only site of disseminated disease.[14] Isolated metastases to the vagina have been described in breast, renal, pancreatic, biliary tract, and colon cancer. Reports of metastases to the vulva are even more unusual.

DIAGNOSIS

Key Points

1. Metastatic lesions to the reproductive organs typically present with similar symptoms of primary gynecologic cancers and include abnormal bleeding, pelvic pain, and bloating.

2. Ultrasound imaging may identify solid and bilateral ovarian masses that are suggestive of metastatic disease.

3. In women with pelvic masses or vaginal lesions, elevated serum markers, such as carcinoembryonic antigen (CEA) or CA–19-9, may suggest a nongynecologic primary malignancy.

Whenever a patient has a history of cancer and presents with a mass or lesion in the gynecologic tract, metastatic disease must be considered in the differential. Patients with metastatic disease to the ovaries are frequently younger than patients with primary ovarian cancer. On average, patients with Krukenberg tumors are in the 40- to 50-year age range.[15] Symptoms associated with ovarian involvement can include abdominal bloating, abdominal or pelvic pain, and weight loss. Gastric cancers, because of luteinization of the ovarian stroma, may produce virilization or, on occasion, irregular vaginal bleeding.[16] Occasionally, the patient may be asymptomatic and have a mass discovered on routine physical examination.[17] This can occur with metastatic breast cancer. In 30% of cases of metastatic disease to the ovaries, the mass may be the initial presenting feature before the diagnosis of the actual primary tumor site.[16] Any metastatic tumor that involves the uterus, cervix, vagina, or vulva may lead to symptoms of irregular or postmenopausal bleeding, discomfort due to the presence of a mass, or pain.

Symptoms or the finding of an unexplained mass in the reproductive tract should trigger a diagnostic work-up in the form of imaging and appropriate laboratory studies. Ultrasound or CT is usually the initial imaging study performed. Features of ovarian tumors on ultrasound that suggest a metastatic origin include bilateral involvement of the ovaries, a solid appearance, and a differential in the size of the ovaries. These features occur in 80% of patients of Krukenberg tumor. When there is a combined solid and cystic component, or cystic features only, distinction from a primary ovarian cancer becomes challenging (Figure 17-1). On CT scan or MRI, many of the same features found on ultrasound will be present, including a primarily solid component or solid and cystic components with septations (Figure 17-2). In the face of bilateral cystic ovarian masses and copious fluid on imaging studies, a low-grade appendiceal neoplasm resulting in pseudomyxoma peritonei should be suspected.

CT scan may identify the primary site of disease if a suspicious mass is found elsewhere in the GI tract. In addition, a radiographic abnormality on upper GI series may suggest an underlying gastric cancer. However, tumors in the gastric mucosa may be quite small when they metastasize and remain undetected for many years. Endoscopic examination may miss a small tumor that has extensively infiltrated into the submucosa.

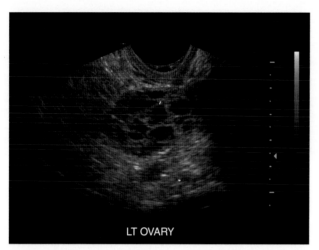

FIGURE 17-1. Transvaginal ultrasound of Krukenberg tumor involving the left ovary, metastatic cholangiocarcinoma.

Tumors arising from the pylorus may also be difficult to detect given their location.

Serum markers may help to distinguish the primary site of disease. CA-125 is elevated in 70% of advanced-stage ovarian cancers. Although CA-125 may be elevated in a patient with a Krukenberg tumor, it may not be elevated to the degree of epithelial ovarian cancers.[18] CEA is a marker for colon, appendiceal, and gastric cancers, whereas CA–19-9 can be a marker for pancreatic cancer. A CA-125 to CEA ratio of greater than 25 has also been used to help distinguish ovarian from metastatic colorectal cancer with an overall test accuracy of 94%.[19]

Metastatic lesions to the ovary from the breast frequently present as solid masses or generalized ovarian enlargement in postmenopausal women. This occurs more frequently in women who have stage IV breast cancer. When the masses are cystic and solid, however,

differentiating a primary ovarian cancer from a metastasis is more difficult. Positron emission tomography (PET)-CT, which is often used in breast cancer staging and restaging, can detect incidental lesions in the pelvis that require further investigation. The sensitivity and specificity of PET for metastatic lesions to the ovary is not well established. Although the standardized uptake value (SUV) is higher in breast cancer metastases to the ovaries compared with GI cancers, these results are based on very limited numbers of patients with overlapping SUV levels and should not be used to distinguish primary cancers from metastatic disease at this time.[20]

PATHOLOGY

Key Points

1. Mucinous adenocarcinomas of the ovary may represent metastases from a primary malignancy in the gastrointestinal tract or pancreas.
2. Krukenberg tumors are characteristically bilateral, solid, and exhibit a bosselated outer surface.
3. Immunohistochemical profiling, including CK7, CK20, CDX2, and S100, may distinguish a primary gynecologic malignancy from metastatic disease.

The majority of primary ovarian cancers are of papillary serous histology. In any instance where the ovarian cancer is a mucinous or endometrioid histology, it may be challenging to distinguish a primary malignancy of the ovary from a metastatic tumor. Metastatic colorectal cancers can mimic primary endometrioid ovarian carcinomas, whereas metastatic appendiceal and pancreatic cancers can be confused with primary mucinous or mucinous borderline tumors of the ovary. Frequently, however, primary mucinous or endometrioid cancers of the ovary are unilateral, not bilateral. When the tumor is bilateral, or small (< 10 cm) and unilateral, metastatic disease should be suspected. The classic Krukenberg tumor has pathologic criteria defined by the World Health Organization to include the presence of mucin-producing signet ring cells, stromal involvement, and ovarian stromal sarcomatoid proliferation.[21] The intracytoplasmic mucin of the signet ring cells typically stains with mucicarmine or a periodic acid-Schiff stain. Although Krukenberg tumors have typically been classified as metastatic gastric cancers, more recently the term has been applied to all metastatic GI cancers and can include colon or pancreatic cancers as well as metastatic tumors of any nongenital tract origin. When they result from metastatic gastric cancer, they are grossly solid with a smooth nodular or bosselated outer surface (Figure 17-3A). When cut,

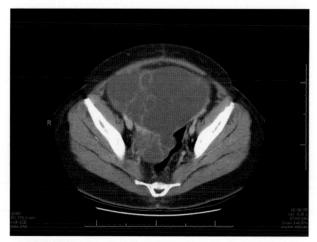

FIGURE 17-2. CT scan, Krukenberg tumor involving ovaries, metastatic colorectal carcinoma.

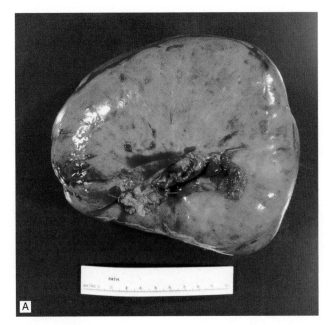
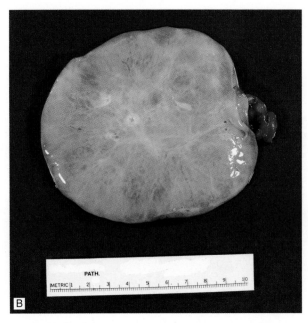

FIGURE 17-3. A. Krukenberg tumor, gastric cancer, gross section. **B.** Krukenberg tumor, gastric cancer, cut surface.

the surface is white or tan with areas of red or brown discoloration and a firm or gelatinous appearance (Figure 17-3B). Histologically, the tumors have an infiltrative, irregular growth pattern with single-cell invasion, signet ring cells, and surface mucin (Figure 17-4A, 4B).[22] Metastatic mucinous cancers tend to have a multinodular growth pattern that involves the ovarian surface. The presence of necrotic debris or "dirty necrosis," a higher degree of nuclear atypia in the well-formed glands, and desmoplasia are features of metastatic colon cancer and can be used to distinguish a metastatic lesion from a primary mucinous or endometrioid cancer (Figure 17-5A-C).[11] The size of the ovarian metastasis does not seem to be a distinguishing

factor in metastatic colorectal cancer, as the lesions can get quite large (> 10 cm) and be unilateral.[6]

Pancreatic ductal adenocarcinomas and cholangiocarcinomas (Figures 17-6A and 17-6B) are another source of mucinous tumors. Four to 6% of patients with pancreatic cancer will have metastases to the ovaries. They more commonly arise from the tail of the pancreas and may be confused with primary ovarian cancers, especially when there is diffuse peritoneal and omental involvement. The ovaries may become quite large (average size, 12.5 cm) and contain large mucinous cysts with smaller glands in the intervening stroma.[23]

The classification of appendiceal mucinous tumors has gone through some evolution. Tumors that are

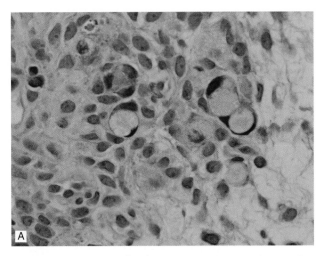
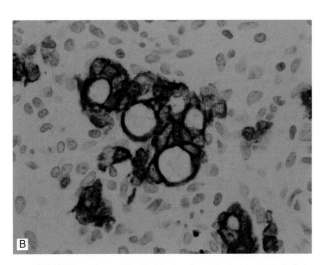

FIGURE 17-4. A. Krukenberg tumor, metastatic gastric cancer, AE1/AE3 stain, ×40. **B.** Krukenberg tumor, metastatic gastric cancer, AE1/AE3 stain ×400.

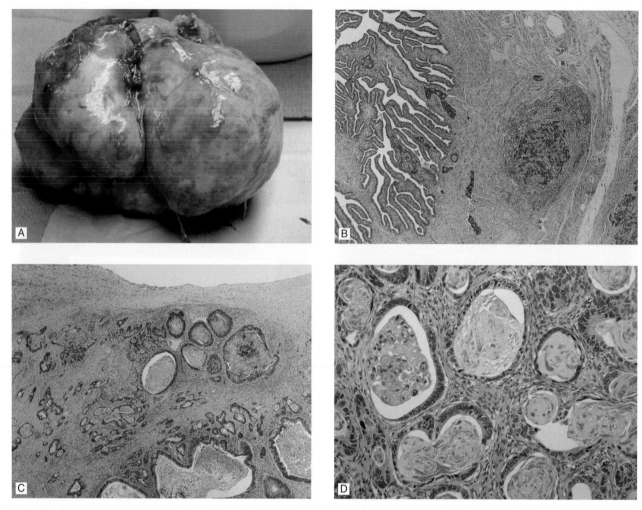

FIGURE 17-5. A. Krukenberg tumor, colon cancer, gross section. **B.** Metastatic colon cancer in the stroma of the fallopian tube demonstrating desmoplasia. **C.** Metastatic colon cancer involving the ovary, low power. **D.** Metastatic colon cancer involving the ovary, high power.

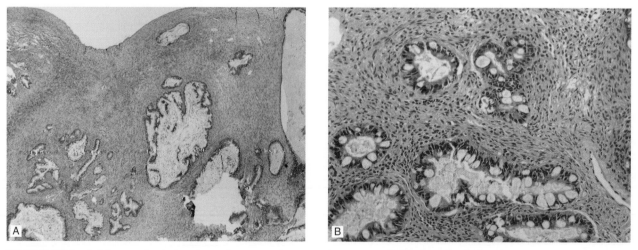

FIGURE 17-6. A. Metastatic cholangiocarcinoma to the ovary, low power. **B.** Metastatic cholangiocarcinoma to the ovary, high power.

confined to the appendix have been called adenomas or low-grade appendiceal mucinous neoplasms. If there is a breach in the muscularis mucosa, the tumor has been called a mucinous tumor of uncertain malignant potential. Tumors with high-grade cytology or with destructive invasion of the appendiceal wall are called appendiceal adenocarcinomas or invasive adenocarcinomas.[24] Primary appendiceal carcinomas are quite rare, representing fewer than 1% of all GI tract cancers. The primary tumor in the appendix may be small, or the appendix may rupture, leading to obliteration of the tumor altogether. In pseudomyxoma peritonei, there is diffuse gelatinous material present in the peritoneal cavity. Mucinous low-grade appendiceal neoplasms may produce secondary neoplasms in the ovary. Most commonly, there is bilateral involvement of the ovaries; if unilateral involvement is found, it is usually right sided. On cut section of the ovary, there is mucinous material in the stroma of the ovary (pseudomyxoma ovarii) and multiple cysts lined by low-grade, bland-appearing mucinous cells with minimal nuclear atypia. In a small number of cases, primary appendiceal carcinomas in the form of signet ring histology can metastasize to the ovaries as a Krukenberg tumor.

Application of an immunohistochemical profile using cytokeratin stains and other markers can distinguish the primary site of disease (Table 17-2). Primary ovarian carcinomas are typically cytokeratin (CK) 7 positive and CK 20 negative. In contrast, colon cancer is typically CK 7 negative and CK 20 positive. Other GI primaries such as appendiceal, gastric, and small intestinal cancers, like ovarian cancer, can be CK 7 positive. CA-125 is expressed in the majority of papillary serous ovarian cancers but is also positive in half of mucinous ovarian cancers, making it a less useful immunostain for mucinous tumors. Although CEA is positive in most mucinous tumors, this can occur regardless of whether the origin is ovarian or GI, also

making it a less useful distinguishing marker. CDX2 is a nuclear transcription marker that is frequently positive in lower GI tract cancers, which can be helpful in differentiating a metastatic GI primary from a primary mucinous ovarian cancer.[25] Other studies of mucinous markers such as MUC2 and MUC5AC have shown variable results. S100 is a marker for melanoma that is characteristically diffusely positive in metastatic lesions. Although immunostain profiles can be helpful, they are not mutually exclusive, and the patient's entire clinical picture must be taken into account when interpreting the results of stains.

In autopsy studies, metastatic breast cancer has been found in the ovaries in 10% of patients. Lobular carcinomas have a greater propensity to spread to the ovaries than infiltrating ductal carcinomas; however, given the higher overall frequency of ductal carcinomas, most metastases to the ovaries will be ductal in nature. The ovaries may be quite small when involved with metastatic disease. If the histology of the ovarian cancer is papillary serous, it is more likely to be a separate primary ovarian cancer. Lobular carcinomas can present with solid nests of tumor that may appear similar to adult type ovarian granulosa cell tumors. Ductal carcinomas can be challenging to differentiate from adenocarcinomas of the ovary or peritoneum and often require further work-up, including specific immunohistochemical stains. Breast carcinomas tend to have a similar cytokeratin profile to ovarian cancers and are often CK 7 positive and CK 20 negative. CA-125, WT1, and gross cystic disease fluid protein 15 (GCDFP-15) may be helpful in distinguishing primary ovarian cancer from metastatic breast cancer. In primary ovarian cancers, CA-125 is positive in 92% of cases, and WT1 is positive in 76% of cases, whereas GCDFP-15 tends to be negative in comparison with the breast cancer lesions.[26] More recently, PAX8, a transcription factor necessary for organogenesis in

Table 17-2 Immunostain Profile of Primary Versus Metastatic Carcinomas Involving the Ovaries

Primary Tumor	Histologic Resemblance	Immunophenotype				
		CK7	CK20	CA125	CEA	CDX2
Ovarian carcinoma						
Serous carcinoma		+	–	+	–	
Mucinous carcinoma		+	+	+/–	+	+/–
Endometrioid carcinoma		+	–	+	–	
Metastatic carcinoma						
Colon-rectum	Endometroid cancer	–	+	–	+	+
Stomach	Mucinous cancer	+	+/–	–	+	+/–
Appendix	Mucinous cancer	–/+	+	–	+	+
Pancreas	Mucinous cancer	+	+/–	+/–	+	+/–

Modified from Hart,[4] Vang et al,[25] and Prat.[34]

the thyroid, kidney, and Mullerian system, has been studied with WT1 to distinguish ovarian cancers from breast cancers. PAX8 staining performed better than WT1 and was diffusely positive in 87% of known ovarian cancers, whereas none of the breast cancers stained positive for Pax8.[27] Although it is a rare occurrence, when breast cancer metastasizes to the uterus, it often involves the myometrium and stroma while sparing the endometrial glands.

Renal cell carcinoma metastatic to the ovaries is quite rare, but when it occurs, it is invariably of the clear cell type. Therefore, making a distinction between a primary ovarian clear cell cancer from a metastatic renal cell carcinoma becomes a dilemma. In primary clear cell cancers of the ovary, there is a heterogeneity in the appearance of the cells, as there is an admixture of flattened cells, hobnail cells, and cuboidal cells. Primary clear cell cancers of the ovary may also be associated with endometriosis. In metastatic tumors, there is more homogeneity to the clear cells, and there may be a sinusoidal vascular pattern. Positive CK 7 immunostaining may help to distinguish a primary ovarian cancer from a metastatic renal cell cancer, which tends to be CK 7 negative.[28]

Cutaneous malignant melanoma can metastasize to nearly any organ in the body. Approximately 20% of such patients develop recurrent disease. However, metastases to the genital tract are exceedingly rare and represent only 2.5% of cases. Although the most frequent sites of recurrence are the primary site of disease followed by the regional lymph nodes, visceral spread can occur. In the genital tract, the ovaries are the most common metastatic site, but metastases to the endometrium and myometrium of the uterus have also been described.

Only 30% of ovarian metastases are pigmented. Immunostains such as S-100, HMB-45, and MART1 are positive in most melanomas and may be helpful in identifying the primary sites of disease.[11]

TREATMENT AND PROGNOSIS

Key Points

1. Surgical resection of metastatic lesions should be considered in symptomatic patients with good performance status and isolated masses.
2. Limited evidence suggests a potential survival benefit with resection of metastatic disease in colorectal, pancreatic, and breast cancers.

The treatment of patients with metastases to the genital tract depends on the performance status of the patient, whether the patient has a known primary site of disease, and whether the metastatic lesions are isolated or diffusely disseminated. Overall, the survival of patients with metastases to the ovaries is poor. Nearly 80% of patients succumb to their disease within 2 years. Despite this, metastatic tumor to the ovaries can create significant symptoms to warrant removal for palliation. In one recent retrospective series of patients, there was a significant difference in survival if patients had isolated metastases to the ovaries or disseminated disease. In patients with isolated ovarian metastases, median survival was 30.7 months as compared with those with extensive, disseminated disease, for whom the median survival was 10 months ($P = .02$). Patients with colon cancer had longer survivals compared with patients with gastric cancer (29.6 months vs. 13 months, respectively), and patients who underwent surgery and were left with microscopic disease also experienced longer survival as compared with those left with visible residual disease.[29] In another study of metastatic pancreatic cancer to the ovaries, the mean patient age was only 49 years. Those who underwent resection of their ovarian metastases had a median survival of 16.5 months, as compared with 8.5 months in those who received chemotherapy alone. In patients who received only chemotherapy, the ovarian metastases did not respond to treatment.[23] Patients with known ovarian metastases from colon cancer also showed a lack of response to chemotherapy, which may suggest that the ovaries are a sanctuary for metastatic disease.[30] In a Korean study of patients with a history of gastric cancer who developed Krukenberg tumors, the median age was also only 41 years. Patients who underwent either bilateral salpingo-oophorectomy or hysterectomy with bilateral salpingo-oophorectomy had median survivals of 10.9 months if there was no gross residual disease or 7.5 months if left with gross residual disease. There were 2 patients in this series of 34 patients who survived longer than 4 years after complete resection of their Krukenberg tumors. Additionally, there was a significant difference if the patient had disease confined to the ovaries (median survival, 13.1 months) as compared with disease in the pelvis (median survival, 7.5 months) or intra-abdominal disease (median survival, 3.6 months).[31] Therefore, a reasonable approach in a patient with good performance status and isolated metastatic disease would be to consider surgery to remove the ovaries.

Many of the same treatment strategies observed in metastatic GI cancer hold true for metastatic breast cancer. Several retrospective studies have identified a trend toward longer progression-free survival in women who can be optimally debulked even in the setting of metastatic breast cancer. This typically occurs in the setting of isolated metastatic disease and in patients without evidence of other metastatic disease. Garg et al[32] showed that in 19 patients who were found to have abdominal carcinomatosis due to breast cancer, those undergoing successful cytoreductive surgery (5 patients) had a longer median survival time than those with larger volume residual disease (14 patients; 34.4 vs. 3.9 months; $P = .0001$).[32] In another small study of 29 patients, 62% underwent nonoptimal surgery or biopsies and the remainder underwent complete resection of metastatic disease; median survival was 2 years in the former group and had not been reached at 2 years of follow-up in the latter group.[33] The subsequent development of metastatic disease in other sites such as the pelvis and liver occurred in the majority of patients after surgery. This should be considered in counseling patients about the risks and benefits of undergoing surgery and effect on palliation of symptoms. As chemotherapy regimens improve for nongynecologic cancers, however, the survival of these patients may be expected to improve.

Management of metastases to other areas of the genital tract will clearly depend on the patient's overall prognosis and symptoms. If a patient develops significant problems with vaginal bleeding from uterine or cervical metastases, it would be reasonable to perform a hysterectomy. A complete hysterectomy also allows for definitive diagnosis of the disease. Metastases to the vagina and vulva must be managed individually and with attention paid to minimizing complications in the face of a disease with poor prognosis. Primary resection and radiation have been described in the management of disease involving the vagina, but the numbers of patients treated are too small to provide any meaningful conclusions about the effectiveness of treatment.

FUTURE DIRECTIONS

In conclusion, patients who develop metastatic disease to the genital tract frequently have primary malignancies arising from the GI tract or breast, and the primary disease is usually advanced stage. Ovarian metastases are frequently bilateral; mucinous histologies, in particular, may be difficult to distinguish from primary mucinous ovarian cancers. Surgery to cytoreduce the metastatic lesions appear to be associated with longer survival if the metastatic disease is isolated and able to be completely cytoreduced. As molecular markers improve, it may become easier to distinguish primary gynecologic malignancies from nongynecologic malignancies. Although it would be preferable to have serum markers that could adequately determine the primary site of disease, often the decision to operate or treat with chemotherapy or hormonal therapy tailored to the primary site of disease becomes a function of patient performance status, symptoms, and the presence of other sites of disease.

REFERENCES

1. Khunamornpong S, Suprasert P, Chiangmai WNA, et al. Metastatic tumors to the ovaries: a study of 170 cases in northern Thailand. *Int J Gynecol Cancer.* 2006;16:132-138.
2. Mazur MT, Hsueh S, Gersell DJ. Metastases to the female genital tract. Analysis of 325 cases. *Cancer.* 1984;53:1978-1984.
3. Al-Agha OM, Nicastri AD. An in-depth look at Krukenberg tumor. *Arch Pathol Lab Med.* 2006;130:1725-1730.
4. Hart WR. Diagnostic challenge of secondary (metastatic) ovarian tumors simulating primary endometrioid and mucinous neoplasms. *Pathol Int.* 2005;55:231-243.
5. Young R, Gilks B, Scully R. Mucinous tumors of the appendix associated with mucinous tumors of the ovary and pseudomyxoma peritonei: a clinicopathologic analysis of 22 cases supporting an origin in the appendix. *Am J Surg Pathol.* 1991;15:415-429.
6. Lewis MR, Euscher ED, Deavers MT, Silva EG, Malpica A. Metastatic colorectal adenocarcinoma involving the ovary with elevated serum CA125: a potential diagnostic pitfall. *Gynecol Oncol.* 2007;105:395-398.
7. Young RH, Hart WR. Metastases from carcinomas of the pancreas simulating primary mucinous tumors of the ovary: a report of seven cases. *Am J Surg Pathol.* 1989;13:748-756.
8. Khunamornpong S, Lerwill MF, Siriaunkgul S, et al. Carcinoma of the extrahepatic bile ducts and gallbladder metastatic to the ovary: a report of 16 cases. *Int J Gynecol Pathol.* 2008;3:366-379.
9. Kwon JS, Gutierrez-Barrera AM, Young D, et al. Expanding the criteria for BRCA mutation testing in breast cancer survivors. *J Clin Oncol.* 2010;28(27):4214-4220.
10. Simpkins F, Zahurak M, Armstrong D, et al. Ovarian malignancy in breast cancer patients with an adnexal mass. *Obstet Gynecol.* 2005;105:507-513.
11. Young RH. From Krukenberg to today: the ever present problems posed by metastatic tumors in the ovary. Part II. *Adv Anat Pathol.* 2007;14:149-177.
12. Quan ML, Fey J, Eitan R, et al. Role of laparoscopy in the evaluation of the adnexa in patients with stage IV breast cancer. *Gynecol Oncol.* 2004;92(1):327-330.
13. Kumar NB, Hart WR. Metastases to the uterine corpus from extragenital cancers: a clinicopathologic study of 6 cases. *Cancer.* 1982;50:2163-2169.
14. Hara F, Kiyoto S, Takabatake D et al. Endometrial metastasis from breast cancer during adjuvant endocrine therapy. *Case Rep Oncol.* 2010;3:137-141.
15. Yook JH, Oh ST, Kim BS. Clinical prognostic factors for ovarian metastasis in women with gastric cancer. *Hepatogastroenterology.* 2007;54:955-959.
16. Kiyokawa T, Young RH, Scully RE. Krukenberg tumors of the ovary. A clinicopathologic analysis of 120 cases with emphasis on their variable pathologic manifestations. *Am J Surg Pathol.* 2006;30:277-299.
17. Moore RG, Chung M, Granai CO et al. Incidence of metastases to the ovaries from nongenital tract primary tumors. *Gynecol Oncol.* 2004;93:87-91.
18. Lewis MR, Deavers MT, Silva EG, Malpica A. Ovarian involvement by metastatic colorectal adenocarcinoma: still a diagnostic challenge. *Am J Surg Path.* 2006;30:177-184.
19. Yedema CA, Kenemans P, Wobbes T, et al. Use of serum tumor markers in the differential diagnosis between ovarian and colorectal adenocarcinomas. *Tumour Biol.* 1992;13:18-26.
20. Kitajima K, Suzuki K, Senda M, et al. FDG PET/CT features of ovarian metastasis. *Clin Radiol.* 2011;66:264-268.
21. Serov SF, Scully RE. Histologic typing of ovarian tumours, vol. 9. Geneva, Switzerland: World Health Organization; 1973: 17-18.

22. Lee KR, Young RH. The distinction between primary and metastatic mucinous carcinomas of the ovary: gross and histologic findings in 50 cases. *Am J Surg Pathol.* 2003;27:281-292.

23. Falchook GS, Wolff RA, Varadhachary GR. Clinicopathologic features and treatment strategies for patients with pancreatic adenocarcinoma and ovarian metastases. *Gynecol Oncol.* 2008; 108:515-519.

24. Misdraji J. Appendiceal mucinous neoplasms. Controversial issues. *Arch Pathol Lab Med.* 2010;134:864-870.

25. Vang R, Gown AM, Wu LSF. Immunohistochemical expression of CDX2 in primary ovarian mucinous tumors and metastatic mucinous carcinomas involving the ovary: comparison with CK20 and correlation with coordinate expression of CK7. *Modern Pathol.* 2006;19:1421-1428.

26. Tornos C, Soslow R, Chen S, et al. Expression of WT1, CA125 and GCDFP-15 as useful markers in the differential diagnosis of primary ovarian carcinomas versus metastatic breast cancer to the ovary. *Am J Surg Pathol.* 2005;29:1482-1289.

27. Nonaka D, Chiriboga L, Soslow RA. Expression of Pax8 as a useful marker in distinguishing ovarian carcinomas from mammary carcinomas. *Am J Surg Pathol.* 2008;32;10:1566-1571.

28. McCluggage WG, Wlkinson N. Metastatic neoplasms involving the ovary: a review with emphasis on morphological and immunohistochemical features. *Histopathology.* 2005;47:231-247.

29. Joang R, Tng J, Cheng X, Zang RY. Surgical treatment for patients with different origins of Krukenberg tumors: outcomes and prognostic factors. *Eur J Surg Oncol.* 2009;35:92-97.

30. Goere D, Daveau C, Elias D, et al. The differential response to chemotherapy of ovarian metastases from colorectal carcinoma. *Eur J Surg Oncol.* 2008;34:1335-1339.

31. Kim HK, Heo DS, Bang YJ, Kim NK. Prognostic factors of Krukenberg's tumor. *Gynecol Oncol.* 2001;82:105-109.

32. Garg R, Zahurak ML, Trimble ET, et al. Abdominal carcinomatosis in women with a history of breast cancer. *Gynecol Oncol.* 2005;99:65-70.

33. Bigorie V, Morice P, Duvillard P, et al. Ovarian metastases from breast cancer. *Cancer.* 2010;799-804.

34. Prat J. Ovarian carcinomas, including secondary tumors: diagnostically challenging areas. *Mod Pathol.* 2005;18:S99-S111.

Part III

Clinical Management Topics

Perioperative and Critical Care

18

Renata Urban and Lee-may Chen

PREOPERATIVE RISK EVALUATION

A thorough preoperative history and physical should be taken from all patients undergoing surgery. Preoperative testing may include a complete blood count and chemistries with additional testing being based on the findings of the preoperative history, physical examination, indication for surgery, and planned procedures. Special attention needs to be paid to the preoperative and intraoperative issues that arise in the care of obese patients, cardiac patients, respiratory-compromised patients, and any other patients with significant medical comorbidities including patients with venous thromboembolism or malnutrition. Counseling and postoperative management of patients and their families will be influenced by the unique surgeries and conditions encountered in gynecologic oncology.

In general, preoperative evaluation and testing are stratified based on a patient's comorbidities. All patients undergoing surgery for gynecologic cancer should undergo a thorough evaluation of other medical issues. Such evaluations will provide an individualized preoperative assessment. In addition, the identification of preoperative medical issues will allow these conditions to be medically optimized.

Preoperative Testing

Many patients with gynecologic malignancies will be of older age. As a result, they often have other medical comorbidities. In 2007, the leading causes of death in the United States were heart disease, cancer, stroke, chronic lower respiratory disease, and accidents. Given the prevalence of coronary artery disease, diabetes, peripheral vascular occlusive disease, and obesity in our population, many patients will require some preoperative testing to assess their cardiopulmonary function in anticipation of anesthesia and surgery.

In healthy patients, the likelihood of an unrecognized medical condition that will cause undue surgical risk is low. A review of studies investigating routine preoperative laboratory evaluations with subsequent likelihood of postoperative complications demonstrated that only hematocrit, creatinine, and electrolytes provided a modest benefit to predict for postoperative complications. Preoperative tests should be selected judiciously, because the addition of unnecessary tests has been found to add a significant cost burden.[1] Additionally, in patients who have had a recent laboratory evaluation, retesting will not likely lead to identification of new abnormalities. Our anesthesiologists recommend that preoperative laboratory tests be performed no more than 30 days before surgery to have an up-to-date baseline.

There is also little utility in screening electrocardiograms (ECGs) and chest radiographs (CXRs) in otherwise healthy patients. An abnormal preoperative ECG is not a useful predictor of postoperative cardiac complications, even in elderly patients. However, a preoperative ECG can be helpful as a baseline for comparison with postoperative ECG abnormalities. The 2007 American College of Cardiology/American Heart Association (ACC/AHA) guidelines on perioperative cardiac evaluation include a recommendation for a preoperative 12-lead resting ECG prior to intermediate-risk noncardiac or vascular surgery for patients with known cardiovascular disease, cerebrovascular disease, or peripheral artery disease.[2] Intermediate-risk procedures include intraperitoneal and intrathoracic procedures, which are commonly performed in the surgical staging and treatment of patients with gynecologic malignancies. The ACC/AHA guidelines also recommend preoperative ECG in patients with other cardiac risk factors, such as diabetes, renal insufficiency, compensated or prior heart failure, or ischemic heart disease.

Even in the healthiest of patients, the preoperative evaluation of patients undergoing surgery for gynecologic cancer will typically include a CXR for staging. Such an evaluation can be helpful in the detection of subclinical pulmonary disease, which may affect intra- and postoperative respiratory function. In addition, the presence of a preoperative pleural effusion is associated with a decreased likelihood of achieving optimal surgical cytoreduction.

When the preoperative suspicion of malignancy is low, there is little evidence supporting the benefit of preoperative CXR regardless of age, unless there is a history of prior or current cardiopulmonary disease. In a meta-analysis of 21 studies investigating the routine use of preoperative CXR, only 0.1% of all CXRs performed led to a change in management. The American College of Physicians recommends preoperative CXR in patients with known cardiopulmonary disease and those older than 50 years of age undergoing upper abdominal/thoracic surgery.[3] The AHA suggests a routine posteroanterior and lateral CXR prior to surgery in all patients with morbid obesity (body mass index [BMI] ≥ 40).[4]

Patients with suspected ovarian, fallopian tube, or peritoneal carcinomas are recommended to have an ultrasound and/or an abdominopelvic computed tomography (CT) scan. Preoperative imaging may also be of use in planning surgery, in order to appropriately counsel patients as to the extent of surgery and postoperative issues that may arise. In the management of ovarian cancer, certain features on CT scan have been associated with the feasibility of optimal cytoreduction. In 2 prospective studies, Bristow et al[5] and Ferrandina et al[6] both found that a predictive index incorporating features of peritoneal thickening, number of peritoneal implants, involvement of bowel mesentery, suprarenal para-aortic lymphadenopathy, omental extension to spleen and stomach, pelvic sidewall involvement, and/or hydroureter was accurate in the identification of patients unlikely to undergo optimal primary cytoreductive surgery. For patients with presumed ovarian or peritoneal cancer, a preoperative CT scan may allow for counseling of patients as to the likelihood that all

disease can be surgically removed and potential selection of patients for primary chemotherapy.

In uterine cancer, the role of lymphadenectomy remains controversial. Histology and depth of myometrial invasion have been associated with the likelihood of lymph node involvement. Unfortunately, imaging techniques have not been as reliable in the preoperative prediction of myometrial involvement or lymph node involvement. Positron emission tomography (PET)/CT, CT scan, and Doppler ultrasound have not been found to be sensitive means to assess depth of myometrial involvement.[7] However, magnetic resonance imaging (MRI) has been found to be sensitive in the assessment of cervical involvement[8]; preoperative knowledge of cervical involvement may indicate a need for radical hysterectomy, which in some series has been shown to improve outcome.[9] MRI may also play a role when trying to determine whether a tumor is originating from the cervix or endometrium. With the advent of more minimally invasive surgery, preoperative imaging may help anticipate the presence of suspicious or bulky retroperitoneal disease.

MRI and PET/CT are commonly used in the preoperative assessment of cervical cancer. In the American College of Radiology Imaging Network 6651/Gynecologic Oncology Group (GOG) 183 series of early cervical cancer patients, MRI was found to be superior to CT scan in the evaluation of uterine body involvement, tumor size, and parametrial involvement.[10] However, neither modality was accurate in the preoperative assessment of cervical stromal invasion. Although MRI has been demonstrated to have increased sensitivity compared with PET/CT in the preoperative assessment of patients with cervical cancer,[11] a retrospective study correlating pathology outcome of 38 patients with stage IB/II cervical carcinoma demonstrated a negative predictive value of 92% for PET/CT scan.[12] Another small prospective study found that PET/CT was superior to MRI in the preoperative detection of lymph node metastases in cervical cancer.[13]

Cardiovascular Issues

In general, the risk of a perioperative coronary event following major gynecologic oncology surgeries is approximately 1% to 5%. Clinical evaluation of patients undergoing noncardiac surgery includes a review of systems to evaluate whether patients are at significant risk for coronary artery disease. The Goldman Cardiac Risk Index, which is based on 9 risk factors, and the subsequent Revised Cardiac Risk Index, which is based on 6 independent predictors of cardiac complications, are both only estimates of risk (Table 18-1).[14] The 2007 ACC/AHA Guidelines recommend that "high-risk" cardiac patients, including those with unstable coronary

Table 18-1 Revised Cardiac Risk Index

Revised Cardiac Risk Index	Incidence of Major Cardiac Event (n = 1422)	OR of Major Cardiac Event (OR, 95% CI)
Ischemic heart disease	5%	3.8 (1.7-8.2)
Congestive heart failure	7%	4.3 (2.1-8.8)
Cerebrovascular disease	7%	3.0 (1.3-6.8)
Diabetes mellitus requiring insulin	5%	1.0 (0.3-3.8)
Renal insufficiency (serum creatinine >2 mg/dL)	5%	0.9 (0.2-3.3)
"High-risk" procedures (defined as intraperitoneal or intrathoracic procedures)	4%	2.6 (1.3-5.3)

Adapted from Lee TH, Marcantonio ER, Mangione CM, et al. Derivation and prospective validation of a simple index for prediction of cardiac risk of major noncardiac surgery. *Circulation.* 1999;100:1043-1049.

syndromes, decompensated heart failure, significant arrhythmias, and severe valvular disease, undergo further evaluation.[15] Patients deemed as being at "intermediate risk," including those with factors described in Table 18-1, should undergo a clinical evaluation to determine the need for preoperative noninvasive cardiac testing with methods such as transthoracic echocardiogram to evaluate left ventricular function or dobutamine stress echocardiography.

Preoperative heart failure can be an important determinant of postoperative cardiac complications. The ACC/AHA recommends that during the preoperative history and physical examination, an effort be made to assess for unrecognized heart failure.[16] Impaired exercise tolerance, which can be a sign of heart failure, can also be a predictor of adverse postoperative cardiac outcome. A prior study of 600 patients undergoing noncardiac surgery showed that simple self-reported measures (eg, ability to walk or climb stairs) were significantly predictive for postoperative cardiac events. However, adequate exercise tolerance may also obviate the need for additional perioperative cardiac testing.

The use of perioperative β-blockade for prevention of coronary events was initially studied in cardiovascular surgery, with subsequent application for patients undergoing noncardiac surgery. The initiation of perioperative β-adrenergic receptor blockade (atenolol or metoprolol) has previously been recommended to decrease perioperative myocardial infarction and mortality. In a randomized controlled trial of 8000 patients undergoing noncardiac surgery, metoprolol therapy did reduce the risk of myocardial infarction, but actually increased the risk of perioperative death and stroke.[17] The ACC/AHA has recommended that patients who are on β-blocker medications preoperatively be continued on the agent. For patients undergoing noncardiac surgery, only those who have existing coronary artery disease or 1 risk factor for coronary artery disease (as listed in Table 18-1) can

be considered for perioperative β-blockers.[18] Many patients do have indications for long-term β-blocker use including patients with known cardiac ischemia, and these patients may still be considered for initiation of β-blockade at the discretion of their primary care provided or cardiologist at least 2 weeks prior to surgery. Patients who are taking antihypertensive medications preoperatively should be continued on these drugs if possible, with careful follow-up of their blood pressure and heart rate because these are affected by perioperative pain and fluid management. Treatment with statins has also been associated with improved mortality after noncardiac surgery.

Pulmonary Issues

Any surgical procedure requiring intubation for general anesthesia increases the risk of pulmonary complications. The presence of an acute respiratory condition poses significant concerns in the perioperative patient. Acute infections should be treated before surgery in most nonemergent situations. Other patients with high-risk conditions, including asthma, bronchitis, emphysema, or smoking, should be optimized for their medical condition if possible. Preparing for surgery can also be a teachable moment to encourage a smoking patient to consider smoking cessation. However, prior case-control studies have suggested that a short period of smoking cessation may not abate and may actually increase the rate of pulmonary complications. Because a period of abstinence from smoking of 8 weeks or greater is not always possible prior to cancer surgery, awareness of an increased risk of pulmonary complications for smokers is necessary, even in the absence of chronic lung disease. Additionally, in the setting of a short period of smoking cessation, the evidence surrounding the increased risk is insufficient to dissuade patients from nicotine abstinence in the preoperative period.

Similar to the cardiac preoperative risk indices, pulmonary multifactorial risk indices have been developed and validated to identify patients at increased risk for postoperative pneumonia, so that appropriate respiratory interventions can be made. Age, poor functional status, upper abdominal surgery, general anesthesia, chronic obstructive pulmonary disease, transfusion, steroid use, and smoking all contribute to perioperative pulmonary risks. For patients with significant pleural effusions, consideration can be given to preoperative thoracentesis versus intraoperative chest tube placement to maximize pulmonary function during the time of surgery.

Endocrine Issues

The majority of gynecologic oncology patients with diabetes will have insulin-resistant, or type 2, diabetes mellitus. However, patients with type 1 diabetes will also be encountered. With autoimmune destruction of the pancreatic islets, such patients have a complete lack of endogenous insulin production. Type 1 diabetics are susceptible to frank ketoacidosis. All diabetic patients are also at risk of metabolic and wound complications following surgery. Furthermore, patients with type 2 diabetes have a higher incidence of concomitant coronary atherosclerosis and are at risk for "silent ischemia."[19] Type 2 diabetics can also be at risk for hyperosmolar nonketotic acidosis in the setting of extreme hyperglycemia.

Prior to surgery, baseline glucose levels should be assessed in diabetic patients. Consideration can be given for a glycosylated hemoglobin (HbA_{1c}) serum test. Elevated glucose values, as well as an abnormal HbA_{1c}, are associated with an increased risk of wound infections.[20] In addition, the medications and/or insulin used in management of diabetes should be recorded. For patients with evidence of poor glycemic control, aggressive management may include acute hospitalization and subcutaneous (or intravenous) insulin preoperatively. Patients taking oral hypoglycemic medications should be instructed to hold such medications(s) on the morning of surgery. For patients who require insulin and use long-acting insulin, one-third to one-half of their usual dose should be given the night prior to surgery. Scheduling diabetic patients for surgery earlier in the day may help minimize their risk of hypoglycemia while fasting.

Numerous medical conditions benefit from treatment with steroids, including patients with chronic obstructive pulmonary disease, asthma, and rheumatoid arthritis, and many organ transplantation survivors. As a result, some patients will be on chronic steroids prior to surgery. The ingestion of more than 20 mg of prednisone per day (or its equivalent) for ≥5 days leads to suppression of the hypothalamic-pituitary-adrenal (HPA) axis and subsequent inability of the adrenal gland to respond adequately to physiologic stress. Such adrenal suppression can result in hypotension and cardiovascular instability at the time of surgery. The use of 5 to 20 mg of prednisone a day is associated with variable suppression of the HPA axis. It is unclear whether high-dose steroids are necessary in the prevention of adrenal insufficiency. A summary of trials concluded that the use of a daily steroid dose (vs. a high dose of hydrocortisone) did not result in any difference in the incidence of perioperative hypotension or tachycardia.[21] Weighing against the concern for perioperative adrenal crisis, it is important to note that the chronic use of high-dose steroids can be associated with impaired glycemic control and wound healing.

Renal Issues

Chronic kidney disease is defined as a glomerular filtration rate of 60 mL/min, in the presence or absence of structural kidney disease. In 2010, there were estimated to be more than 600,000 patients with end-stage renal disease (ESRD) in the United States. In a large meta-analysis, patients with chronic kidney disease undergoing noncardiac surgery were found to have higher rates of cardiovascular events and perioperative death.[22] Patients with ESRD on dialysis have significant fluid management issues and have been found to have increased perioperative complications, including bleeding, infections, and electrolyte abnormalities, particularly hyperkalemia. Although dialysis performed immediately prior to and after surgery has been associated with improved outcomes in patients undergoing cardiac surgery, there has been no such investigation in patients undergoing abdominal surgery. Common goals in patients with chronic kidney disease include a focus on intraoperative euvolemia to maintain renal perfusion. Coordination with nephrologists may help to optimize the timing of perioperative dialysis.

Hepatic Issues

Given the improved care of patients with chronic liver disease and the advanced state of transplantation medicine, patients with chronic liver conditions may develop and require surgical intervention for staging of gynecologic malignancies. Patients with mild to moderate hepatitis, in the absence of cirrhosis, have no additional surgical risk. Cirrhotic patients are at significant risk of increased postoperative complications such as coagulopathy, hypoglycemia, hepatic decompensation with encephalopathy, and even death.[23] In patients with large esophageal varices, consideration should be given to delaying laparotomy until variceal banding or shunting can be performed. Although the overall risk of surgery to the varices is unclear, minimally invasive surgery has been performed safely in patients with varices and splenomegaly; in a recent series of 52 laparoscopic procedures in patients with cirrhosis, 4% required conversion to laparotomy.[24]

The Child-Pugh classification of hepatic cirrhosis has been found to be predictive of surgical outcome, and such clarification should be made in conjunction with the patient's hepatologist. Unfortunately, preoperative testing may not be helpful in assessing hepatic dysfunction, because transaminases may be normal even in the setting of cirrhosis.[23] Thrombocytopenia, prolonged prothrombin time, and hypoalbuminemia may portend increased perioperative risk as well. Although cirrhotic patients often share findings of ascites and splenomegaly with ovarian cancer patients, superficial vascular skin changes such as spider telangiectasias are unique to cirrhotic patients.

Nutritional Issues

Prior to surgery, many gynecologic oncology patients will have compromised nutrition. This can be due to prior chemotherapy and/or radiation, medical comorbidities, or the advanced nature of their disease. Perioperative nutritional assessment may help identify patients who are most likely to benefit from nutritional support. Preoperative weight loss should be quantitated, and the degree of malnutrition should be assessed. The presence of malnutrition has been demonstrated to be associated with prolonged hospitalization in gynecologic cancer patients,[25] as well as poor postoperative outcome in other surgical specialties. Albumin, a serum protein marker produced by the liver, is a widely used indicator of malnutrition and has been shown in numerous studies to be associated with increased complications during the postoperative period,[26] even when not associated with malnutrition cachexia. Extremely poor preoperative nutrition, as demonstrated by a prealbumin < 10 mg/dl, was shown to be significantly associated with intraoperative blood loss and perioperative morbidity in a series of more than 100 patients undergoing surgical cytoreduction.[27] Patients with poor nutrition, in conjunction with complicated medical comorbidities, should be considered to be at increased risk of intensive care (ICU) unit admission.

Special Considerations

Prior to surgery for gynecologic malignancies, patients should be made aware of possible complications in the postoperative period. Following surgery for ovarian cancer, 20% to 30% of patients will require admission to an ICU. The most common reasons for admission include respiratory support and fluid management. Consideration of such disposition in the preoperative period will also allow for appropriate resource allocation following surgery.

An important part of counseling prior to surgery for gynecologic cancer involves a discussion of postoperative sexual function and body image. Procedures that are unique to the surgical treatment of gynecologic malignancies are also associated with unique care issues in the intraoperative and postoperative period.

Patients may inquire as to the impact of cervical removal on sexual function; a prior randomized trial of supracervical versus total hysterectomy in benign gynecologic disease showed that there was no difference in postoperative sexual function.[28] However, the extent of pelvic dissection in radical hysterectomy may alter postoperative sexual function. Issues with sexual function, such as lubrication and arousal, have been noted after radical hysterectomy for cervical carcinoma.[29] In a series of 38 patients, the rate of postoperative sexual function was similar between those who underwent the procedure via laparotomy or laparoscopy.[30] "Nervesparing" radical hysterectomy has been suggested to minimize rates of postoperative sexual dysfunction. Radical vulvectomy and pelvic exenteration can both affect body image and sexuality, yet both surgeries are performed with a goal of cure and prolongation of life. Counseling with a focus on psychosexual issues may also help in the adjustment period.

The rates of urinary tract dysfunction following radical hysterectomy are estimated to be between 50% and 75%. Patients should be made aware of the possibility of prolonged catheterization. The mode of catheterization can be either by transurethral or suprapubic catheterization.

Depending on the type of surgery and the extent of cancer involvement, patients may require either a temporary or permanent fecal ostomy. Preoperative discussion of the likelihood and nature of such diversion is essential for both the short-term and long-term adaptation of patients and families to such devices. Furthermore, preoperative marking for stoma placement can allow for marking in lying, sitting, and standing positions to determine the optimal place for stoma placement.

Preparing both the patient and involved family for home care coordination in the postoperative period is also helpful, particularly if the need for a skilled nursing facility is anticipated.

SURGICAL PREPARATION

Infectious Disease Prophylaxis

Surgical Site Infection Prophylaxis

The majority of patients undergoing gynecologic oncology procedures will undergo a hysterectomy. Given the breach in the vaginal epithelium that occurs, such

Table 18-2 Prophylactic Antimicrobial Regimens

Procedure	Medication	Dose
Hysterectomy	Cefazolin (Acceptable alternatives: cefotetan, cefoxitin, cefuroxime, or ampicillin-sulbactam)	1 or 2[a] g intravenous (IV)
History of immediate sensitivity reaction to penicillin	Clindamycin plus	600 mg IV
	gentamicin or	1.5 mg/kg IV
	quinolone or	400 mg IV
	aztreonam	1 g IV
	Metronidazole plus	500 mg IV
	gentamicin or	1.5 mg/kg IV
	quinolone	400 mg IV
Intestinal operations	Ertapenem	1 g IV

[a] A 2-g dose is recommended in women with a body mass index greater than 35 or weight greater than 100 kg or 220 lb.
Adapted from Antibiotic Prophylaxis for Gynecologic Procedures. *Obstet Gynecol.* 2009; 113(5):1180-1189.

patients should receive preoperative antimicrobial prophylaxis. Table 18-2 lists possible antimicrobial regimens. Patients with a history of a hypersensitivity reaction to penicillins and/or cephalosporins are recommended to receive clindamycin or metronidazole, plus gentamicin or aztreonam or a quinolone.[31] Antimicrobial prophylaxis should be given within 60 minutes prior to the surgical incision to ensure that appropriate tissue levels are present. Many gynecologic debulking procedures will also include intestinal resection; coverage of gram-negative and anaerobic bacterium must be incorporated. According to the Surgical Care Improvement Project, cefazolin may still be considered for preoperative antibiotic prophylaxis[32]; cefoxitin or cefotetan can be considered given the improved coverage of bowel anaerobes. Recently, a randomized trial comparing ertapenem to cefotetan in elective colorectal surgery showed that ertapenem was associated with a significantly decreased rate of surgical site infectious; it was, however, associated with an increased risk of *Clostridium difficile*–associated diarrhea.[33]

Endocarditis Prophylaxis

The 2007 AHA guidelines incorporated major revisions to the groups of patients who will most benefit from endocarditis prophylaxis.[34] Antimicrobial prevention of endocarditis is now only recommended in patients with prosthetic valves, a prior history of infective endocarditis, unrepaired cyanotic congenital heart disease, repaired congenital heart disease with prosthetic material, and valvular disease in a transplanted heart. Such patients should receive endocarditis prophylaxis prior to invasive genitourinary procedures with ampicillin and gentamicin, substituting vancomycin for ampicillin in penicillin-allergic patients.

Thromboembolic Prophylaxis

Among cancer patients, those with gynecologic malignancies have the highest risk of thromboembolic disease. Prior to surgery, in addition to assessing the likelihood of malignant disease, patients should also be assessed for other risk factors for venous thromboembolism.[35] Patients with known cancer, or those in whom the preoperative suspicion is high, should be considered for preoperative thromboprophylaxis with unfractionated heparin (UFH) or low molecular weight heparin 2 hours prior to surgery, as recommended by the 2008 American College of Chest Physician guidelines.[36] Some gynecologic oncologists have expressed concern regarding preoperative administration of anticoagulants before major surgery, but continuous assessment for change in practice is indicated. Einstein et al[37] reported that a recent change in protocol that included administration of UFH 1 to 2 hours prior to surgery led to a significant decrease in the rate of thromboembolic events. In the event that patients should be interested in the use of regional anesthesia or neuroaxial blockade, discussion should be made with the anesthesia team before administration of preoperative heparin. Continuation of pharmacologic prophylaxis may also be indicated in high-risk patients.

Some patients may have a pre-existing diagnosis of thromboembolism or atrial fibrillation or have a mechanical heart valve in place and be on anticoagulation therapy, prior to surgery. Because there is a risk of hypercoagulability with discontinuation of warfarin, patients at significantly high risk for thrombosis should be transitioned to intravenous or low molecular weight heparin before and after surgery.[38] The international normalized ratio should decrease to less than 1.3 to 1.5 before elective surgery. Intravenous heparin should be stopped 6 hours prior to incision. Low molecular weight heparin should be stopped 12 hours prior to incision. Consultation with the patient's hematologist or cardiologist is also indicated.

Elective surgery is traditionally to be avoided in the first month after acute venous thromboembolism given the significantly increased risk of perioperative complications. A temporary inferior vena cava (IVC) filter should be considered in situations of acute venous thromboembolism to minimize the incidence of perioperative pulmonary emboli or if the risk of bleeding on intravenous heparin is high. If planned in advance with interventional radiology, an IVC filter can be removed within 2 weeks after surgery, even after a patient has resumed anticoagulation. A recent retrospective study from Adib et al[39] demonstrated not only that the use of perioperative IVC filters was feasible without a significant increase in the rate of recurrent venous thromboembolism or surgical complications, but also that surgery could be performed relatively soon after the placement of an IVC filter. After surgery, intravenous heparin should be restarted without bolus after at least 12 hours and potentially longer if there is continued concern for surgical bleeding. A temporary vena caval filter can be removed within 2 weeks after surgery, even after a patient has resumed anticoagulation.

Bowel Preparation

For decades, mechanical bowel preparation has been included in the surgical preparation process; the goal of such preparation is to evacuate stool, allowing for improved visualization and reduction of endogenous intestinal bacteria. Increasing evidence has suggested that such preparations not only lead to an increase in anastomotic leaks, but also are associated with an increase in surgical site infections. This was shown in a meta-analysis involving 13 randomized trials as well as a 2009 Cochrane review.[40,41] Magnesium citrate may also have risk in patients with renal impairment. Small volumes of polyethylene glycol may be considered if a bowel preparation is necessary.

In minimally invasive surgery, the use of mechanical bowel preparation may theoretically aid in surgical visualization through decompression of the bowels. However, in a series of patients undergoing gynecologic laparoscopy, the use of preoperative bowel preparation did not have a significant impact on the surgical field, operative difficulty, or operative time; however, preoperative discomfort was significantly elevated in the bowel preparation group.[42] In open tumor debulking cases, bowel preparation may help to eliminate solid boluses of stool that may potentially confound intra-abdominal exploration for tumor resection.

A recent Cochrane review found that the use of oral and intravenous antibiotics, in the setting of colorectal surgery, was superior to intravenous antibiotics alone.[43] This theoretical benefit is not seen in all series; furthermore, in a small series, the use of preoperative oral antibiotics was actually shown to be associated with an increased incidence of *C difficile*–associated diarrhea. The use of oral antibiotics may still be considered in gynecologic oncology patients who are likely to have intestinal surgery incorporated into surgery; however, given the gastrointestinal (GI) distress that may accompany oral antibiotics, parenteral antimicrobial prophylaxis may be preferred.

Surgery on the Obese Patient

The prevalence of obesity in the United States is increasing every year; 65% of the American population can now be classified as overweight (BMI ≥ 25) or obese (BMI ≥ 30). In addition to being at risk of multiple other malignances due to obesity, obese women are at particular risk of developing cancer of the endometrium. The practicing gynecologic oncologist is therefore extremely likely to operate upon patients with morbid obesity and should be familiar with the physiology and comorbidities that may be present.

The AHA recommends obtaining a preoperative 12-lead ECG and CXR in all morbidly obese patients prior to surgery.[4] The AHA proposes additional testing when signs of right ventricular hypertrophy or left bundle branch block are seen on preoperative ECG, because these may be indicative of existing pulmonary hypertension and occult coronary artery disease, respectively. Obese patients with no risk factors for coronary heart disease, such as hypertension, heart failure, vascular disease, or pulmonary hypertension, may not require any further testing. However, patients with 3 risk factors or those with current coronary heart disease will likely require additional invasive testing with exertional cardiac testing. Exercise stress testing is an appropriate assessment of functional capacity and can be predictive of postoperative cardiovascular complications.[44] If the patient's functional capacity is poor or cannot be assessed due to extreme obesity, a dobutamine stress echocardiogram can be considered.

In the presence of morbid obesity, the sheer weight of the chest wall can lead to a restrictive lung physiology, leading to a decreased functional residual capacity and expiratory reserve volume.[45] In addition, these patients may also have concomitant or unrecognized sleep apnea.[4] If patients are on ambulatory continuous positive airway pressure, this should be continued in the hospital.

The GOG LAP 2 trial demonstrated that minimally invasive surgery in obese patients was feasible; although a higher BMI was associated with an increased likelihood of conversion to laparotomy, this randomized trial demonstrates the feasibility of this technique.[46] In addition, a recent case-control study demonstrated that robotic-assisted laparoscopy in obese patients may also be feasible.[47] Minimally invasive surgery in the obese population is associated with unique risks. Prolonged steep Trendelenburg positioning, combined with carbon dioxide pneumoperitoneum, will lead to increased airway pressure and decreased airway compliance. In addition, careful positioning is necessary to prevent pressure necrosis given extremes of body weight.[48] Furthermore, prolonged surgical procedures may also increase the possibility of rhabdomyolysis. If this is a concern, a creatine kinase level may be obtained.

When minimally invasive approaches are not available or when the obese patient cannot tolerate the necessary positioning, the patient may be considered for a simultaneous panniculectomy, which may facilitate exposure during laparotomy. Such patients are at risk of wound breakdown, and wound infection rates following panniculectomy during gynecologic surgery have ranged from 3% to 33%. However, this procedure has been described in several series to be a beneficial addition to improve visualization in a morbidly obese patient; further, a long-term follow-up study of 42 such patients revealed that 91% of patients were pleased with their surgical outcome.[49]

CRITICAL CARE/POSTOPERATIVE EVALUATION

The ICU is an essential resource for the management of the most critically ill gynecologic cancer surgery patients. ICU utilization for gynecologic oncology patients ranges between 6% and 33%.[50] A multivariate analysis of ovarian cancer patients admitted to the ICU for short (<24 hours) versus longer stays found that the patients' preoperative medical condition was less important than perioperative factors in utilization of ICU resources. Patients requiring bowel resection, placement of a pulmonary artery catheter, and ventilator dependence were most likely to require ICU care. Preoperative factors such as hypoalbuminemia and significantly elevated CA-125 have also been associated with an increased likelihood of extensive disease and need for ICU admission.[26] Severity of illness by the Acute Physiology and Chronic Health Evaluation (APACHE) classification system has also been correlated with survival of critically ill gynecologic oncology patients.[50] Most patients admitted to the ICU after gynecologic oncology surgery have a short critical care course, although in single-institution reports, the 30-day postoperative mortality rate ranges between 11% and 27%. Identification of patients who may be at greatest risk for needing ICU care allows for appropriate anesthesia and perioperative planning to optimize care and outcomes for the patients.

The ICU must be a collaborative setting, involving interactions between the surgeon, critical care–trained physicians, subspecialty consultants (including palliative care), nurses, respiratory therapists, nutritionists, physical therapists, and other support staff, all working together for the common goals of the patient. Although the surgeon may know the acute issues of the patient and her family best, the internist may be able to add perspective to goals of care, particularly if there are conflicts in the level of care being provided to critically ill patients who may actually be facing the end of life. Regardless of an "open" model, where the surgical team continues to be the primary service, or a "closed" model, where the ICU team becomes the primary service while in the ICU, the involvement of an ICU physician can help coordinate patient care and improve patient outcome.

Cardiovascular Issues

The stresses and hemodynamic shifts related to gynecologic cancer surgery may have significant impact on the cardiovascular system. Cardiac events are estimated to account for more than 50% of perioperative deaths. Tachycardia is the most common hemodynamic abnormality associated with the postoperative period. This increase in heart rate both increases demand and decreases diastolic filling time; the subsequent imbalance between myocardial oxygen supply and demand results in ischemia. The incidence of myocardial infarction after noncardiac surgery in patients with ischemic heart disease is as high as 5% to 6%, with a peak incidence within 2 days of surgery.[51] Postoperative hypotension and tachycardia may be related to a relative hypovolemic state. Despite intraoperative fluid resuscitation and tumor cytoreduction, patients with advanced gynecologic tumors may reaccumulate ascites and "third-space" fluid for 2 to 3 days after surgery. Fluid replacement may either be with crystalloid or colloid solutions; however, a low serum albumin and oncotic pressure may lead to continued intravascular depletion. Fluid resuscitation with goal-directed therapy is recommended; a colloid in the form of hetastarch can be used.[52] After the second or third postoperative day, fluid mobilization begins; patients may require some assistance with diuretics if renal function is suboptimal or if clinically significant fluid overload is present.

Shock is a condition of inadequate tissue perfusion that may develop as a result of many conditions. Symptoms include hypotension, tachycardia, hypoxia, low urine output, and peripheral vasoconstriction. Depending on the underlying condition, there are various alternations seen on hemodynamic monitoring (Table 18-3). After surgery, the most common hemodynamic condition is hypovolemia. Treatment to improve oxygen

Table 18-3 Hemodynamic Parameters of Shock

	Pulmonary Artery Occlusion Pressure	Cardiac Output	Systemic Vascular Resistance
Hypovolemic	Low	Low	High
Cardiogenic	High	Low	Low
Sepsis (early)	Low	High	Low
Sepsis (late)	High	Low	High

delivery and decrease oxygen consumption should focus on volume replacement, keeping the patient warm, correcting coagulopathy, and controlling pain. Replacement of fluids can be done using either crystalloid or colloid solutions. Despite the hypoalbuminemia in many advanced ovarian cancer patients, albumin has not been consistently found to be superior to crystalloid in the resuscitation of hypovolemia.[53] Intermittent fluid boluses, rather than continuous infusion, are preferable to allow for evaluation of response. Vasopressor agents may act through increasing cardiac output (inotrope or chronotrope) or by increasing systemic vascular resistance. Dobutamine and intermediate-dose dopamine (5-15 µg/kg/min) are β-selective agonists ideally used in patients with a history of heart failure and may act to improve myocardial contractility and improve cardiac output.

Phenylephrine (Neo-Synephrine) and norepinephrine (Levophed) are vasoconstrictors that increase systemic vascular resistance and thus improve blood pressure. Both systemic and individual organ perfusion must be monitored in the pharmacologic management of shock. Hemorrhagic shock can be reversible with prompt replacement of circulating volume and oxygen delivery. Prolonged shock may trigger a cascade of local and systemic cytokines, resulting in a systemic inflammatory response syndrome, which may lead to multiple organ failure.

Sinus tachycardia is common in the postoperative ovarian cancer patient who may be volume depleted or experiencing pain. Treatment involves addressing the underlying physiologic condition. Supraventricular tachyarrhythmias are most commonly encountered and can include atrial fibrillation, atrial flutter, and other sinus node re-entrant tachycardias. Narrow complex tachycardias incorporate a wide variety of rhythm abnormalities, which may be difficult to distinguish on ECG. Initial management should focus on the hemodynamic impact of the rhythm disturbance by controlling the rapid ventricular rate, ruling out ischemia, and evaluating for underlying causes. Paroxysmal supraventricular tachycardia can be managed first with vagal maneuvers or adenosine for diagnosis.

Atrial fibrillation or atrial flutter should be managed first by controlling the ventricular response rate. In a hemodynamically stable patient, calcium channel blockers, β-blockers, digoxin, or amiodarone may be used for rate control. Cardioversion may also override and reset the abnormal pulse generator using low doses of electrical energy. Although it may occur in 4% to 12% of patients undergoing noncardiac surgery, atrial fibrillation most commonly occurs within 3 days following surgery.

Cardiac Monitoring

Regardless of the etiology, hypotensive patients may require central venous pressure monitoring, which may be helpful in assessing the patients' volume status. However, practitioners should be aware of the infectious, mechanical, and thrombotic complications associated with such catheters. Pulmonary artery (Swan-Ganz) catheters are rarely needed in the absence of significant cardiac disease or pulmonary hypertension. Increasingly, echocardiography is becoming a less invasive modality to evaluate left ventricular function and vascular pathology during both the intraoperative and postoperative period.

Ischemia

Myocardial ischemia may manifest itself as angina/pain or nausea, or it may be asymptomatic with ECG changes only. Tachycardia and elevated catecholamines are a common response to surgery; thus, control of pain and anxiety may help to decrease the incidence of postoperative cardiac events. The classic symptom of chest pain may actually be absent or may be seen in association with other symptoms in female patients; in a review of 515 female patients with a recent myocardial infarction, only 30% reported chest pain, whereas 58% reported shortness of breath and 55% reported weakness. Prompt recognition and treatment allow for the prevention of myocardial infarction and other complications including dysrhythmias, congestive heart failure, and death. Immediate treatment of suspected cardiac ischemia includes administration of supplemental oxygen, nitrates to decrease myocardial demand by venodilation, and β-blockers to decrease heart rate and contractility. Serial ECGs and measurements of serum troponin I can be reflective of the extent of myocardial ischemia. In surgical patients, use of anticoagulation such as heparin must be considered with respect to their recent surgical procedure. Aspirin and antiplatelet drugs are also to be considered at the discretion of the managing surgeon and cardiologist. Transthoracic echocardiography may also evaluate myocardial function to determine the need for additional cardiology interventions.

Pulmonary Issues

At the end of surgery, most patients are awakened from anesthesia and extubated. In cases of large fluid resuscitation or prolonged surgery, extubation may be delayed until the recovery room or ICU. Laryngeal edema can increase the likelihood of airway obstruction; such edema can be exacerbated by prolonged Trendelenburg positioning. In addition, bowel edema may increase the intra-abdominal pressure, which in turn limits respiratory excursion and functional residual capacity.

Pulmonary hygiene is emphasized in the postoperative period and is most easily accomplished by encouraging incentive spirometry and early ambulation. Atelectasis can result in retention of bronchial secretions and in fevers and increases the likelihood of pneumonia. Aspiration pneumonitis without infection is treated by support. Pneumonia in the postoperative period is a common cause of respiratory compromise, a leading cause of nosocomial infection, and ICU deaths. Clinical risk factors for pneumonia include thoracic or upper abdominal surgery, history of respiratory disease, and a bedridden status resulting in atelectasis. Patients requiring mechanical ventilation for greater than 24 hours have a higher risk of nosocomial pneumonia.

Chronic obstructive pulmonary disease is usually smoking related and may range from mild to severe. Bronchodilators remain the mainstay of therapy, with a role for inhaled steroids and antibiotics in acute exacerbations. The ventilator management of patients with chronic obstructive pulmonary disease should be modified for the risk of hyperinflation. Because of reduced elasticity, alveoli are prone to overdistention with early airway collapse causing air trapping and inadvertent positive end-expiratory pressure ("autoPEEP"). Such positive airway pressure can accumulate, resulting in hyperinflation of the lungs, barotrauma, and hemodynamic compromise. Extrinsic PEEP can be helpful to decrease intra-alveolar pressure, and the use of a low ventilator sensitivity setting can allow for triggering breaths.

Although acute respiratory distress syndrome (ARDS) is unusual after gynecologic cancer surgery, ovarian cancer patients may be particularly susceptible. Predisposing causes include direct lung injury from aspiration or pneumonia, as well as indirect phenomena of massive fluid shifts, coagulopathy, transfusion, and sepsis. ARDS is defined as a condition with acute onset, bilateral infiltrates on CXR, pulmonary artery wedge pressure <18 mm Hg in the absence of clinical evidence of left atrial hypertension, and a gradient of partial pressure of arterial oxygen (Pao_2) to fractional inspired oxygen (Fio_2) of <200. A Pao_2 to Fio_2 ratio of <300 is considered acute lung injury. Treatment consists of supportive care with ventilation and oxygenation, evaluation for underlying causes and nosocomial infection, and prevention of the development of multisystem organ failure. Because of the heterogenous process of ARDS, some areas of the lung may be normal while other areas may be poorly compliant. A positive pressure breath will go preferentially to normal lung; however, this may lead to overdistention of more compliant normal lung zones and subsequently greater stretch injury. Ventilator strategies include using lower tidal volumes and higher PEEP, thereby avoiding overdistension of normal alveoli. A phase III study by the Acute Respiratory Distress Syndrome Network demonstrated a 22% decrease in mortality using low tidal volumes when compared to the use of traditional volumes (6 mL/kg vs. 12 mL/kg).[54] Restricting fluids may decrease pulmonary edema, but studies have been negative. The use of glucocorticoids or surfactant has not shown any pharmacologic advantage.

Ventilator Support

Mechanical ventilation supports respiration by delivering positive pressure though either volume control or pressure control. Intermittent mandatory ventilation delivers a set rate and volume, with unassisted spontaneous breaths allowed in between. In pressure-controlled ventilation, the volume delivered is determined by a preset level of pressure; the patient's inspiratory effort triggers the ventilator to deliver the breath. Delivering PEEP or continuous positive airway pressure provides support to keep previously collapsed alveoli open and reduces the overall work of breathing. For patients intubated for airway management issues following surgery, the management of mechanical ventilation involves supportive care until a trial of weaning can be performed. The Fio_2 should be weaned to minimize injury from oxygen radicals, and the peak inspiratory pressure should be kept low to minimize barotraumas. As long as oxygen and carbon dioxide exchange is adequate, the patient may be extubated once the patient has demonstrated adequate oxygenation and intact neurologic status.

Reintubation

Reintubation is most frequently a result of an unplanned extubation, often due to patient self-extubation. Risk factors for unplanned extubation include inadequate sedation and subsequent agitation, as well as physical restraints. In the setting of planned extubation following a prolonged intubation, a positive fluid balance in the previous 24 hours can be a risk factor for reintubation[55]; this is particularly pertinent to ovarian cancer patients, who often have a positive fluid balance due to reaccumulation of ascites and/or pleural

Table 18-4 Commonly Used Parenteral Solutions

	pH	mOsm/L	kcal/L	Na (mEq/L)	K (mEq/L)	Ca (mEq/L)	Cl (mEq/L)	Lactate (mEq/L)
D$_5$ W	4.3	253	170	—	—	—	—	—
D$_5$ ½ NS	4.4	405	170	77	—	—	77	—
D$_5$ NS	4.4	560	170	154	—	—	154	—
NS	5.6	308	—	154	—	—	154	—
D$_5$ LR	5.0	530	170	130	4	3	109	28
LR	6.3	275	—	130	4	3	109	28

D$_5$, dextrose 5%; LR, lactated Ringer's; NS, normal saline; W, water.

effusions. Given that reintubation in the ICU setting is associated with worse posthospitalization outcome, patients requiring reintubation will benefit from a multidisciplinary care team involving anesthesiologists and critical care physicians. Of note, patients at risk for reintubation following planned extubation may be considered for noninvasive positive pressure ventilation (bilevel or continuous positive airway pressure), because this has been found to decrease rates of reintubation. Care for such patients should be done with communication with colleagues from anesthesia and critical care.

Fluid and Electrolyte Management

The daily fluid requirement for an average adult ranges between 2 and 3 L/d. Several formulas are available to estimate maintenance fluid requirements; a simple one includes 4 mL/kg/h for the first 10 kg of body weight, 2 mL/kg/h for the second 10 kg, and 1 mL/kg/h for each subsequent kilogram of weight. GI and urinary losses can be replaced with lactated Ringer's solution or normal saline crystalloid solution (Tables 18-4 and 18-5). Postoperative considerations of fluid management must include insensible losses related to the surgical procedure in addition to the usual insensible losses associated with skin, lung, and fecal material. Weighing the

patient daily is the best means of assessing total body fluid status. Supplemental intravenous fluids may be weaned off as the patient's oral intake increases.

The degree of fluid shifts into the extracellular "third space" reflects the severity of the surgical procedure. Postoperative sodium retention is a response to a decrease in extracellular volume. Fluid replacement during surgery should include 4 mL/kg/h of lactated Ringer's solution or normal saline for a minimally traumatic procedure, 6 mL/kg/h for a moderately traumatic procedure, and 8 mL/kg/h for an extremely traumatic procedure such as an extensive debulking procedure for a patient with significant ascites. In a procedure where blood loss is significant, replacement should emphasize colloid or blood products. If cardiac and renal functions are normal, the retained fluid should mobilize back into the intravascular space 2 to 3 days after surgery. However, if cardiac function and/or renal function are impaired, inadequate clearance of this fluid may result in pulmonary edema or congestive heart failure. A patient who is slow to spontaneously diurese may only need a single dose of furosemide to facilitate the process.

Clinical evaluation of hypovolemia includes looking for signs of oliguria, supine hypotension, and orthostatic hypotension. Urine output of 0.5 mg/kg/h suggests adequate renal perfusion. Laboratory parameters may include hemoconcentration, azotemia, or low urinary

Table 18-5 Gastrointestinal Fluid Content

	Na (mEq/L)	K (mEq/L)	Cl (mEq/L)	HCO$_3$ (mEq/L)	Daily Volume (mL)
Gastric	20	10	120	0	1000-2500
Pancreatic	140	5	75	80	500-1000
Bile	148	5	100	35	300-1000
Small bowel	110	5	105	30	1000-3000
Diarrheal stools	120	25	90	45	500-17,000

sodium. A ratio of blood urea nitrogen to serum creatinine that is greater than 20 may suggest dehydration. In prerenal oliguria, urine sodium is low, due to increased sodium and water resorption. A fractional excretion of sodium ($FE_{Na} = [(U_{Na} \times P_{Cr})/(P_{Na} \times U_{Cr})] \times 100$) of less than 1% is suggestive of a prerenal state that is best managed by volume expansion. This calculation may be less useful in patients who are elderly, have pre-existing renal disease, or have received diuretics. Even if the urine output is low while volume resuscitative efforts may be ongoing, continued urine production and a stable creatinine indicate adequate renal perfusion. Prevention of acute oliguria in the postoperative patient is best accomplished by recognition of prerenal events including blood loss, surgical trauma, and reaccumulation of ascites or effusions.

The goal of treating hypovolemia is to restore volume with fluid that is similar to the fluid that was lost. Patients with significant blood loss are managed by transfusion and administration of colloids intra- and postoperatively. Although blood products are required to treat anemia and coagulopathy, lactated Ringer's solution and normal saline without added dextrose are the crystalloid solutions of choice for continued hypotension or shock. However, large volumes of lactated Ringer's solution may result in hyperkalemia, whereas large volumes of normal saline may result in hyperchloremic acidosis. Intravenous albumin (250 mL of 5% concentration) may not be more effective than crystalloid solutions in the replacement of drained ascites and may eventually leak from the intravascular space into the peritoneal cavity.

Disorders of sodium concentration, hyponatremia and hypernatremia, reflect relative excesses or deficits of extracellular fluid. Pseudohyponatremia may occur with hyperproteinemia or hyperlipidemia, where protein or lipids displace water from plasma, producing a low plasma concentration of sodium. True hyponatremia (sodium < 136 mmol/L) may develop rapidly or chronically; acute hyponatremia can be associated with neurologic changes due to cerebral edema, whereas chronic hyponatremia may trigger compensatory mechanisms that then require slow correction. Serum sodium is frequently low in the postoperative patient with ovarian cancer. With the administration of crystalloid fluids during surgery, hyponatremia may be actually associated with increased total body sodium. In the immediate postoperative patient, there may still be a state of relative hypovolemia, which then results in secretion of antidiuretic hormone, which in turn preserves intravascular volume. Most patients with a serum sodium of greater than 125 mmol/L have few symptoms. A rapid decline of the sodium level to less than 130 mEq/L may result in mental status changes and even seizures; these patients will require rapid but controlled correction with hypertonic saline. An assessment of total body sodium may be made by measuring urine sodium and osmolarity. Although third spacing is ongoing during the immediate postoperative period, the urine sodium level is low (< 10-15 mEq/L), and urine osmolarity is high (> 400 mOsm/kg). Treatment of hyponatremia with high serum osmolarity is directed toward the restriction of both sodium and water. Hypovolemic hyponatremic patients are treated with 0.9% saline. Hypervolemic hyponatremic patients are managed with fluid restriction, occasionally increasing free water excretion with the administration of diuretics. Hypernatremia is usually associated with a total fluid deficit and may also result in neurologic changes. It can result from pure water loss (eg, diabetes insipidus) or hypotonic sodium loss (eg, nasogastric drainage) but may also be iatrogenic from hypertonic sodium loading. Correction of hypovolemia must be performed slowly with hypotonic solutions to avoid precipitating cerebral edema or seizures.

Disorders of potassium homeostasis may be affected by the balance of intake versus excretion. Specifically, potassium can enter the body through oral or parenteral means and leaves through renal excretion, which may be affected by acid-base status. Potassium is the major intracellular cation—plasma potassium may reflect total body potassium poorly. At the time of surgery, adrenergic stress may mobilize potassium from the intravascular to the intracellular space. Additional GI fluid losses will produce hypokalemia, unless the potassium deficit is adequately replaced. Hypokalemia interferes with muscle contractility; thus ileus and generalized weakness are common manifestations of hypokalemia (potassium < 3.0 mmol/L). Significant hypokalemia is associated with an increased risk of cardiac arrhythmias and can predispose to digitalis toxicity. Treatment of hypokalemia involves potassium replacement, and this must be performed cautiously (10-20 mEq/h) to avoid hyperkalemic complications. Hyperkalemia may occur through excess ingestion or intravenous administration, but more frequently occurs through renal impairment. The most lethal manifestations of hyperkalemia are cardiac conduction abnormalities, including prolongation of the PR interval, decrease in P-wave amplitude, and widening of the QRS complex resulting in ventricular fibrillation or asystole. Cardiac effects are negligible when the potassium level is less than 6 mEq/L. Indications for treatment include the presence of ECG changes or when the serum concentration of potassium is greater than 7 mEq/L. Treatment of hyperkalemia involves eliminating exogenous potassium, reversing myocardial membrane hyperexcitability, and removing potassium from the body. Acute therapy includes administration of calcium, insulin and glucose, sodium bicarbonate, diuretics, or cation exchange resins (via the GI tract). Dialysis should be reserved for patients with renal failure or life-threatening hyperkalemia resistant to conventional treatment.

Approximately 50% of serum calcium is free, whereas the remainder is complexed, primarily to albumin. Hypoalbuminemia, as seen in many ovarian cancer surgery patients, alters total serum calcium concentration; clinical decisions should thus be based on ionized calcium levels. If ionized calcium cannot be measured, the total serum calcium can be corrected by adding 0.8 mg/dL for each 1.0 g/dL that the serum albumin is below 4.0 g/dL. In the perioperative patient receiving multiple transfusions, hypocalcemia may be attributable to chelation by citrate. Hyperphosphatemia may precipitate calcium or decrease intestinal absorption of calcium. Hypomagnesemia may suppress the production of parathyroid hormone. Clinical manifestations of hypocalcemia (ionized calcium <0.7 mmol/L) include neuronal membrane irritability and tetany. Acute management includes replacement of calcium intravenously and correction of other electrolyte abnormalities. Hypercalcemia occurs most commonly with bone resorption, when calcium enters the extracellular volume more rapidly than can be excreted by the kidneys. Hypercalcemia (total serum calcium >13 mg/dL or ionized calcium >1.3 mmol/L) is less common in the perioperative gynecologic oncology patient; bone metastases, although uncommon in gynecologic oncology patients, should be considered in the differential of persistent hypercalcemia as well as a paraneoplastic syndrome.

Magnesium also plays an important role in neuronal conduction. Although hypomagnesemia is common in perioperative gynecologic oncology patients, symptoms are uncommon unless serum magnesium is less than 1.0 mg/dL, at which time patients may have symptoms of weakness, lethargy, muscle spasms, paresthesias, and depression. Causes of hypomagnesemia may include excessive losses through the GI tract or inability of the kidneys to conserve magnesium. The sodium–potassium pump is magnesium dependent; attempts to correct potassium deficits may not be successful unless the magnesium deficit is simultaneously corrected. Treatment is by replacing magnesium intravenously, with reduced doses given in patients with renal insufficiency. Most cases of hypomagnesemia are iatrogenic and will correct with urinary excretion.

Phosphate provides the primary energy bond in adenosine triphosphate, is an essential element of second messenger systems, and is a major component of cellular membranes and nucleic acids. Significant phosphate depletion also results in cellular energy depletion. Severe hypophosphatemia (<1 mg/dL) usually indicates total body phosphate depletion and may manifest with paresthesias, muscle weakness, malaise, encephalopathy, seizures, and coma. Moderate hypophosphatemia (1-2.5 mg/dL) is usually attributable to renal losses and a decrease in GI absorption. Hypophosphatemic patients are often hypokalemic and hypomagnesemic. Intravenous administration of phosphorus should also be given cautiously to patients with renal dysfunction or hypocalcemia. Hyperphosphatemia in the postoperative patient is usually due to decreased renal excretion.

Prompt recognition and treatment of acid-base disturbances and electrolyte imbalances are important to the homeostasis of postoperative patients. A pH of 7.4 refers to the normal hydrogen concentration, which is maintained in balance with arterial partial pressure of carbon dioxide ($Paco_2$) and bicarbonate (HCO_3^-). Acidemia can result from either an increased $Paco_2$ or a decreased HCO_3^- concentration. Alkalemia can result from either decreased $Paco_2$ or increased HCO_3^-. Most of the time, the clinical process is mixed.

Metabolic acidosis (pH <7.35) results from a decrease in HCO_3^- (<21 mEq/L) due to either loss of bicarbonate or accumulation of acid. Loss of HCO_3^- may be through diarrhea, biliary drainage, urinary diversion, or renal tubule losses—hyperchloremic metabolic acidosis is associated with a normal anion gap (calculated as: $Na^+ - [Cl^- + HCO_3^-]$). A high anion gap may be due to excess production of acids (lactic acidosis or ketoacidosis), increased retention of waste products (sulfate or phosphate), or ingestion of toxins (salicylic acid, ethylene glycol, or methanol). A compensatory response is seen through hyperventilation and a decrease in $Paco_2$. In the postoperative gynecologic cancer patient, metabolic acidosis may be most commonly due to GI fluid losses and renal failure. Treatment of metabolic acidosis should focus on correcting the underlying metabolic condition. In a mechanically ventilated patient, a compensatory hyperventilation should be included in ventilator settings. Administration of sodium bicarbonate or other alkalinizing agents should be reserved for severe acidemia.

Metabolic alkalosis (pH >7.45) results from either a loss of hydrogen (H^+) or a gain in HCO_3^- (>27 mEq/L). Loss of H^+ may be through nasogastric suction or diuretic administration. The reabsorption of HCO_3^- in the distal renal tubules results in hypokalemia and hypovolemia, resulting in a so-called "contraction alkalosis." Treatment of metabolic alkalosis therefore includes the replacement of volume and electrolytes. Fluid resuscitation with lactated Ringer's solution may be advantageous versus normal saline because HCO_3^- can be generated from lactate.

Respiratory acidosis (pH <7.35) is characterized by hypercarbia ($Paco_2 \geq 45$ mm Hg), which occurs when ventilation is insufficient to eliminate carbon dioxide. Over time, the kidneys compensate by excreting H^+ and retaining HCO_3^-. Postoperative patients are particularly at risk of respiratory depression with upper abdominal incisions or when receiving opiates for perioperative pain management. Supplemental oxygen minimizes the incidence of hypoxia, even when decreased ventilation increases the risk of hypercarbia. Severe respiratory acidosis is an indication for intubation and ventilatory support.

Respiratory alkalosis (pH >7.45) occurs with increased ventilation, causing hypocarbia ($Paco_2 \leq 35$ mm Hg). In a mechanically ventilated patient, overbreathing can also result in respiratory alkalosis. In the postoperative patient on the floor, pain, anxiety, central nervous system disease, and sepsis may all be causes of hyperventilation. An active approach may include interventions of sedation and reassurance if anxiety is the cause of hyperventilation.

Infectious Disease Issues

Postoperative fever is a common occurrence with potentially serious implications. Although infection must be considered, fever may also be a result of tissue inflammation. An accepted definition of fever in the postoperative period is a temperature elevation of greater than 38°C to 38.5°C in a 24-hour period. Reported incidences of postoperative fever range from 15% to 47%, with a source of infection identified in only 5% to 36% of patients and bacteremia identified in less than 3% of patients. A traditional "fever work-up" of complete blood count, urine culture, blood culture, and CXR may be an inefficient use of resources.

Following gynecologic surgery, the incidence of postoperative fever can be as high as 75%,[56] with increased occurrence in the gynecologic oncology population. However, the actual incidence of infection is low. Patients undergoing radical pelvic procedures, including radical hysterectomy and debulking, were found in a recent series to have a higher rate of postoperative fever, but no increased incidence of infection.[57] A separate series of 194 patients undergoing exploratory gynecologic surgery also found that surgery for malignancy, bowel resection, and higher postoperative fever or white blood cell count are associated with the presence of significant infection[56] and should be considered for a thorough evaluation, including complete blood count, urine culture, blood culture, and CXR. However, empiric evaluation of all patients may not be cost effective. Within the first 3 days after surgery, postoperative fevers are often attributable to atelectasis. Clinical history is important to help assess the patient's overall risk for postoperative infection. Length of surgery, blood loss, surgical contamination, pre-existing infection, nutritional status, immunocompromised state, and presence of malignancy all contribute to patient risk. Targeting cultures and laboratory tests to the population at highest risk helps to minimize excessive testing of low yield.

Foreign bodies can be a nidus for infection. Drains including Foley catheters, ureteral stents, and pelvic drains should be removed as soon as appropriate. Use of antibiotic-coated or antiseptic impregnated central venous catheters has been found to decrease the incidence of catheter colonization and catheter-related blood infections. Intra-abdominal and pelvic infections can be insidious in onset. Unfortunately, imaging studies may not always provide definitive evidence of infection, because the presence of free air on x-ray may persist for several days after abdominopelvic surgery. Furthermore an abscess may take time to consolidate before CT drainage can be undertaken.

Suspicion for intra-abdominal infection or systemic sepsis should prompt the initiation of broad-spectrum antibiotics. One-quarter of patients with clinical suspicion of sepsis will not be documented on microbiology; these patients have similar predisposing risk factors as those with positive cultures and also a similar risk for death. Antibiotics are essential for the management of septic shock but, unfortunately, are not sufficient for optimal treatment. Airway management, fluid management, and correction of hypoperfusion all contribute to maintaining organ function. Early recognition of systemic inflammatory response and organ dysfunction may identify patients who may benefit from recombinant activated protein C (drotrecogin alfa) but with a higher risk of significant bleeding. Serious bleeding occurred primarily in patients predisposed to bleeding, including patients with coagulopathy, severe thrombocytopenia (<30,000/μL), GI bleeding, or trauma. However, in a prospective, randomized, multicenter trial, use of drotrecogin alfa in septic patients with an APACHE score <25 or single-organ failure did not benefit from therapy; thus, the use in postsurgical patients must be considered carefully based on severity of illness.[58]

Selection of antimicrobial agents usually involves empiric and broad-spectrum agents. Wound infections are frequently due to staphylococcal or streptococcal organisms, which are frequently sensitive to penicillins or first-generation cephalosporins; clindamycin provides coverage of gram-positive organisms in patients with penicillin allergies. Intra-abdominal organisms such as *Escherichia coli* or *Bacteroides fragilis* may be treated with piperacillin with tazobactam, with the possible addition of an aminoglycoside. More virulent gram-negative rods may respond better to a third- or fourth-generation cephalosporins, a β-lactam/β-lactamase inhibitor, or a carbapenem. Fungal organisms may require treatment with fluconazole or caspofungin. If non-albicans *Candida* is suspected, caspofungin may preferred over fluconazole. Treatment should be continued for 14 days after bacteremia or fungemia is cleared.

Antimicrobial resistance is a serious concern, with increasing resistance to several classes of antibiotics. Methicillin-resistant *Staphylococcus aureus* is increasingly recognized as a cause of nosocomial bloodstream infection. Vancomycin-resistant *Enterococcus* is another common and difficult to treat hospital-acquired infection. Limiting the use of drugs such as fluoroquinolones and increasing the treatment dose to reduce the risk of mutant selection are strategies that may aid in maintaining the antibiotic armamentarium.

When pneumonia is suspected, the timeline of symptoms and risk factors for pneumonia must be considered, because the microbiology of hospital-acquired pneumonia is significantly different than that of community-acquired pneumonia. Severely ill patients have a higher risk of being colonized with gram-negative bacilli, and the bacteria are often polymicrobial. The usual presentation is that of fever, sputum production, evidence of pulmonary consolidation on physical examination, and a localized infiltrate on x-ray. However, the clinical picture may vary, especially in critically ill patients, because fevers or leukocytosis may be from one of several sources and infiltrates on CXR may be confounded by atelectasis or malignant pleural effusions. Gram stain is more valid as an index of pulmonary infection because most cultures will reveal airway flora. The antibiotic used for surgical prophylaxis should be considered as one to which the organism may be resistant. Second- or third-generation cephalosporins are effective regimens, as are β-lactamase inhibitors or fluoroquinolones.

Renal Issues

The perioperative setting in the hospital is associated with a high risk for acute renal failure. The overall incidence is highest in patients undergoing cardiac or vascular surgery, although patients with pre-existing renal disease, hypertension, cardiovascular disease, diabetes, and advanced age are all considered to be at higher risk. Elderly patients have a lower glomerular filtration rate and are more susceptible to volume depletion as well as other nephrotoxic insults. Mortality from acute renal failure remains high despite advancements in renal replacement therapy, perhaps because acute renal failure is often managed in the setting of multiorgan failure.

Traditionally, the evaluation of acute renal failure includes consideration of prerenal, intrarenal, and postrenal causes (Table 18-6). Prerenal injury to the kidney can be caused by ischemic or hypotensive insult, resulting in acute tubular necrosis. Full renal recovery can occur after several days, barring any further injury. Renal injury from nephrotoxic drugs is unusual in a healthy well-hydrated patient, but an older, volume-depleted woman with chronic renal insufficiency undergoing gynecologic cancer surgery is more vulnerable to renal injury. Attention should be paid to the use of nonsteroidal inflammatory drugs, aminoglycoside antibiotics, angiotensin-converting enzyme inhibitors, and angiotensin II receptor blockers, all of which may lead to renal injury. Radiographic contrast is also nephrotoxic, although this risk can be reduced with the administration of intravenous sodium bicarbonate or *N*-acetylcysteine before and after administering the contrast dye. Postrenal causes of renal failure include urinary retention and ureteral injury. Radical pelvic dissection in gynecologic cancer debulking can often result in bladder dysfunction. Although a thoracic-level epidural should not impede bladder function, a recent small series of female patients undergoing urologic surgery showed a high rate of postoperative urinary retention in the setting of thoracic epidural use.[59] In addition, high doses of opiates for pain control may delay spontaneous voiding. If ureteral obstruction is suspected, a transient rise may be seen in the serum creatinine level. A renal ultrasound may confirm hydroureteronephrosis, but a nondilated collecting system does not exclude the possibility of obstruction. For patients with a high index of clinical suspicion, a CT urogram may evaluate the entire urinary tract and also identify any associated postsurgical findings. Isolated renal failure may recover, but given that renal failure is often caused by a syndrome of multiple organ failure associated with hemodynamic compromise, dialysis or hemofiltration may be necessary.

Prerenal acute renal failure can be reversible if renal perfusion is maintained and additional renal insults are avoided. In administering the patient's medications, dosing of renally excreted drugs may require dose adjustment for creatinine clearance. Urinalysis, urine microscopy, and urine electrolytes may be helpful in the distinction between prerenal and intrarenal

Table 18-6 Common Causes of Acute Renal Failure in the Surgical Setting

Prerenal	Intrarenal	Postrenal
Hypotension Hypovolemia Arterial occlusion or stenosis Cardiac failure Sepsis	Drugs: nonsteroidal anti-inflammatory drugs, aminoglycosides, amphotericin B, radiographic contrast Toxins: endotoxins Pigment: myoglobin	Ureteral obstruction Bladder dysfunction Urethral obstruction

Adapted from Carmichael P, Carmichael AR. Acute renal failure in the surgical setting. *ANZ J Surg.* 2003;73(3):144-153.

processes. In renal failure due to prerenal causes, the specific gravity will be high (>1.020), urine sodium will be low (<20 mmol/L), and the fractional excretion of sodium will be less than 1%. In the setting of acute tubular necrosis, granular or epithelial cell casts may be seen on the urinalysis. The treatment of acute renal failure is mainly supportive, with treatment of the underlying cause of renal failure and correction of fluid and electrolyte imbalances. Low-dose dopamine (1-5 µg/kg/min) has not been shown to be effective in protecting or improving renal function. Loop diuretics are commonly used for converting oliguric to nonoliguric renal insufficiency, although response may be only a demonstration of less severe kidney damage. In severe renal failure, large doses of diuretics may be required, and recent studies have suggested that a furosemide infusion may be more effective than bolus therapy.

When planning renal replacement therapy, management of volume and solute toxicity are equal goals. Intermittent hemodialysis is the most common approach for renal replacement therapy. Indications for dialysis in the acute setting include severe fluid overload, hyperkalemia, metabolic acidosis, and uremia. In a stable patient with acute renal failure, hemodialysis allows for the rapid removal of fluids and toxic metabolites. In a critically ill patient after surgery, hypotension from sepsis or multiorgan failure often precludes the use of intermittent hemodialysis. Continuous hemofiltration or hemodiafiltration allows for a slower rate of fluid removal and theoretically results in fewer hemodynamic shifts in the unstable ICU patient.[60] In continuous venovenous hemofiltration, vascular access is achieved through a central vein, and anticoagulation with heparin is given to maintain the extracorporeal circuit. Despite these new technologies, however, renal replacement is only a means of support,

and ultimate mortality reduction still requires recovery of the kidneys and other affected organs.

Neurologic Issues

A cerebrovascular event is one of the most devastating neurologic complications of surgery; thankfully, the incidence of a stroke following noncardiac abdominal surgery is quite low and is estimated to be less than 1%.[61] Patients with a history of prior stroke and/or transient ischemic attack can be at increased risk of postoperative stroke. Additional risk factors for stroke that are pertinent to gynecologic cancer patients are listed in Table 18-7. Nearly 50% of strokes occur 24 hours after surgery, with the remainder occurring ≥2 days postoperatively. In the immediate setting of an embolic stroke, the use of thrombolytic therapy up to 4.5 hours after the event has been found to improve functional outcomes.[62] Although recent surgery is considered a contraindication to thrombolytic therapy, it has been performed safely in patients undergoing cardiac surgery. However, such an intervention should be emergently discussed with a neurologist.

Injury to peripheral nerves during surgery for gynecologic cancer may present with symptoms in the immediate or delayed postoperative period. The incidence of such injury is quite low; a recent prospective study of more than 600 patients undergoing gynecologic surgery found an overall rate of 1.8%, with the majority of injuries involving the femoral and lateral femoral cutaneous nerves.[63] In general, the majority of such neuropathies will resolve. In a series of 1210 patients, the only patients to not achieve full recovery were those with an unrepaired nerve transection or an injury to the lumbosacral nerve plexus.

Table 18-7 Risk Factors for Perioperative Stroke

Preoperative	Intraoperative	Postoperative
Advanced age (>70 years)	Type of anesthesia	Heart failure, myocardial infarction
Female sex	Duration of surgery	Arrhythmias (atrial fibrillation)
History of stroke or TIA	Arrhythmias	Dehydration and blood loss
Carotid stenosis	Hyperglycemia	Hyperglycemia
Ascending aortic atherosclerosis	Hypo/hypertension	
Abrupt discontinuation of antithrombotic therapy before surgery		
History of: hypertension, diabetes mellitus, renal insufficiency, smoking, COPD, PVD, cardiac disease and cardiac systolic dysfunction		

COPD, chronic obstructive pulmonary disease; PVD, peripheral vascular disease; TIA, transient ischemic attack.
Adapted from Selim M. Perioperative stroke. *N Engl J Med.* 2007;356(7):706-713.

Delirium is a common event in the postoperative setting; the overall incidence following noncardiac surgery is approximately 10%, although studies from the various surgical specialties have estimated the incidence to be 3% to 70%.[64] Given that many patients with gynecologic malignancies are elderly, they are particular susceptible to this issue. In contrast to dementia, which is often a chronic process, delirium is characterized by the acute onset of mental status change, accompanied by hallucinations, lack of orientation, and poor short-term memory. Risk factors for postoperative delirium include age, preoperative use of psychotropic medications, poor nutritional status, and preoperative impairment of cognitive and/or functional status. In addition, medications can precipitate delirium, as can metabolic disturbances, infection, dehydration, immobility, and malnutrition. In a recent prospective study of 103 patients on a gynecologic oncology service in which all patients underwent a pre- and postoperative Mini-Mental Status Examination, the overall incidence of postoperative delirium was 17.5%. Risk factors for delirium included age >70 years, use of more than 5 medications, and the need for additional narcotics for pain.[65] Interventions to minimize delirium are to orient the patient with cognitive stimulation, consider ambulation with minimal use of physical restraints, removing catheters and drains when medically appropriate, visual and hearing aids, and volume replacement for patients with dehydration. Undertreated pain can cause agitation, yet opiate use can precipitate delirium as well. Pain medications for modest surgical incisions can be started with acetaminophen, reserving opiates for breakthrough pain medications. Involving family members in postoperative care can help keep women recovering from ovarian cancer surgery oriented and active. In addition, the use of antipsychotic medications, as well as donepezil (Aricept), has been found to lessen the severity and time course of postoperative delirium.[66]

Blood Transfusion

Red blood cells are transfused for anemia and to increase the oxygen-carrying capacity of the patient (Table 18-8). Fresh frozen plasma is separated from whole blood and frozen within 6 hours of collection to minimize loss of coagulation factors V and VIII. Fresh frozen plasma is indicated for coagulopathy from transfusion and correction of warfarin effect. Platelets are usually pooled from 6 units of whole blood and transfused to treat thrombocytopenia or deficits of platelet function.[67] Typically, spontaneous bleeding is uncommon with platelet levels about 20,000/dL, although patients undergoing major operative procedures should generally have platelet counts of about 50,000/dL to 70,000/dL for effective hemostasis. Cryoprecipitated antihemophilic

Table 18-8 Contents of Blood Products

Component	Volume (mL)	Content	Response in Adult Patients
Red blood cells	250-350	50%-65% hematocrit	Increases hematocrit by 3%
		Small amount of plasma	
		Variable leukocyte content	
Whole blood	450	35%-45% hematocrit	Increases hematocrit by 3%
		Few platelets	
		Decreased factors V, VIII	
Platelets	40-60	$\geq 5.5 \times 10^{10}$ platelets	Increases platelets 5000-10,000/μL
		Small amount of plasma	
		Usually pooled as 4-10 packs	
Single-donor platelets	250	$3.5\text{-}4.0 \times 10^{11}$ platelets	Increases platelets 7.5×10^9/L
Fresh frozen plasma	200-275	Fibrinogen	Increases coagulation factors 2%
		Factors V, VII, IX, XI	
		Protein C and S	
		Antithrombin III	
Cryoprecipitate	5-10	Fibrinogen	
		Factor VIII	
		von Willebrand factor	Increases factor VIII activity 30%-50%

Adapted from American Red Cross. *Practice Guidelines for Blood Transfusion.* 2nd ed. Washington, DC: American Red Cross; 2007.

globulin is also pooled from whole blood and serves as a therapeutic source of fibrinogen. Although cryoprecipitate is rich in factor VIII, the treatment of choice for hemophiliacs currently is factor VIII concentrate. Current blood bank practice involves screening for disease transmission of syphilis, hepatitis B, hepatitis C, human immunodeficiency virus (HIV-1/2), human T-lymphotropic virus (HTLV-I/II), Chagas disease, and West Nile virus.

Adverse reactions to transfusion may include febrile reactions that may be caused by recipient antibodies to leukocyte antigens reacting to leukocyte fragments in the transfused blood.[67] These reactions are most commonly seen in patients with a history of multiple blood transfusions or pregnancies, which can stimulate the development of leukocyte antibodies. Allergic urticarial reactions are seen in approximately 1 in 100 transfusion recipients. This reaction is likely caused by foreign plasma proteins. Premedication with acetaminophen and diphenhydramine may help minimize febrile and allergic reactions. Fever is also the most frequent manifestation of acute hemolytic transfusion reactions. These reactions are most likely to occur when a group O patient is mistakenly transfused with group A, B, or AB blood. Symptoms may include fevers, chills, chest tightness, tachycardia, hypotension, and hemoglobinemia, with subsequent hemoglobinuria and hyperbilirubinemia. If a transfusion reaction is suspected, the transfusion must be stopped and supportive measures undertaken. Fluid and diuretic therapy may be indicated, and blood specimens from the patient and the transfused blood product should be collected to confirm hemolysis. Delayed hemolytic reactions may occur in patients who have developed antibodies from prior transfusion and may not manifest until 4 to 8 days after transfusion. Such delayed reactions may not be detected as the red cell destruction occurs slowly, and they are diagnosed only with a decreasing hematocrit and positive direct antiglobulin (Coombs) test. Transfusion-related acute lung injury (TRALI) is a rare (1 in 1333 to 1 in 5000) complication of transfusion manifested by abrupt noncardiogenic pulmonary edema. This reaction is likely associated with the presence of donor antibodies reactive to recipient leukocyte antigens or with inflammatory mediators in stored blood components; it is most commonly seen after transfusion with fresh frozen plasma or whole blood–derived platelet concentrates.[68] Severe cases may require ventilator support but usually resolve within 72 hours. Donors who have been implicated in a case of TRALI are usually deferred from future blood donation.

The popularity of autologous and designated donor blood programs has increased while the estimated rates of transfusion-related infections have decreased. Autologous and designated donor programs vary by institution but have been proposed for procedures where the mean transfusion requirement exceeds 1 unit, where more than 10% of patients undergoing the procedure require transfusion, and where the anticipated blood loss is greater than 20% of the patient's estimated blood volume. In most cases, however, it is probably not cost effective because surgical blood loss is difficult to predict.

The effects of anemia must be separated from those of hypovolemia. The likelihood of ongoing bleeding, the presence of underlying coagulopathy, and the pre-existing cardiovascular condition of the patient should be considered prior to transfusion. Multiple studies comparing conservative versus liberal transfusion strategies in critically ill patients have demonstrated that red blood cell transfusion is an independent predictor of death, associated with increased risk of infection, organ dysfunction, and ARDS.[69] In a nonbleeding patient with a hemoglobin concentration greater than 7.0 g/dL and without cardiac risk factors, the benefits of red blood cell transfusion are limited. An exception may be the patient who is going to receive chemotherapy soon after surgery.

Physical examination of the perioperative coagulopathic patient should include an assessment of bleeding from an anatomic site versus continued consumptive coagulopathy. In particular, there are large surfaces of tumor beds following debulking surgery in ovarian cancer where oozing may continue until the coagulation disorder is corrected. Inadequate surgical hemostasis may be considered if the patient's condition appropriately responds to transfusion but then deteriorates again. If the physical examination findings suggest a hematoma in a self-limited space, the bleeding should be self-limited, and transfusion should be continued to support the self-limited process. If the physical examination is consistent with a bleeding pedicle (increasing tense abdomen, gross blood in an abdominal drain), re-exploration may be necessary to control hemostasis.

Prophylaxis

Venous Thromboembolism

Deep venous thrombosis and pulmonary embolism continue to be the leading causes of postoperative morbidity and mortality in surgery. Gynecologic oncology patients are particularly at risk given the risk factors of malignancy, older age, longer surgical procedures, limited mobility after abdominal surgery, and frequent dissection around pelvic vessels, which are then prone to intimal injury. Clear cell ovarian cancers, in particular, are more commonly associated with venous thromboembolism when compared to other histologies.[70] In a prospective study of gynecologic cancer patients undergoing major radical surgery, the incidence of deep venous thrombosis detected by ^{125}I-fibrinogen scanning was 38%, the majority of which were evident within 24 hours of surgery. Only 10% of deep venous thromboses were

Table 18-9 American College of Chest Physicians Guidelines for Thromboprophylaxis in Gynecologic Oncology Patients

- Low molecular weight heparin daily or every 12 hours
- Low-dose unfractionated heparin 5000 units every 8 hours
- Intermittent pneumatic compression devices started before surgery and used continuously while the patient is not ambulating
- Alternative consideration: Combination of heparin and mechanical thromboprophylaxis, or fondaparinux

The duration of thromboprophylaxis should continue until discharge from the hospital and up to 28 days after discharge with low molecular weight heparin.

Adapted from Geerts WH, Bergqvist D, Pineo GF, et al. Prevention of venous thromboembolism: American College of Chest Physicians Evidence-Based Clinical Practice Guidelines (8th Edition). *Chest.* 2008;133(6 suppl):381S-453S.

clinically evident, and bilateral disease was present in 20% of cases. The clinical diagnosis of pulmonary embolism is equally inaccurate, with 70% of patients with fatal pulmonary embolism diagnosed at autopsy. A high index of suspicion is critical in the gynecologic oncology postoperative population, and prophylactic measures should be universally used.

Prophylactic interventions can decrease the incidence of deep venous thrombosis by 50% (16%-8%) and fatal pulmonary embolism by 75% (0.4%-0.1%).[71] Consensus panel guidelines from the American College of Chest Physicians recommend routine prophylaxis of gynecologic surgery patients with low molecular weight heparin once to twice daily.[35] Alternatively, low-dose UFH may be used, in combination with pneumatic compression devices (Table 18-9).

Compared to UFH, low molecular weight heparins have a better anticoagulation profile, based on better bioavailability, longer half-life, dose-independent clearance, and decreased binding to plasma proteins and endothelial cells. They have less antithrombin activity, more anti–factor Xa activity, and less effect on partial thromboplastin time. They also have less platelet inhibition and do not increase microvascular permeability; therefore, fewer bleeding complications are seen with their use. Patients with renal impairment may have increased serum levels after enoxaparin administration, and its dosage should be adjusted downward when creatinine clearance is less than 30 mL/min.

Venous thromboembolic events may be minimally symptomatic or attributed to other perioperative processes. Classic clinical findings of deep venous thrombosis include leg swelling, pain, increased warmth, and erythema. Doppler ultrasonography is the most commonly used diagnostic procedure to diagnose deep venous thrombosis (Figure 18-1).

Particularly after pelvic surgery, the Doppler ultrasound is limited to evaluation of veins below the inguinal ligament. In the situation of a negative or indeterminate study with high clinical suspicion, contrast venography still remains the standard. Negative quantitative enzyme-linked immunosorbent assay D-dimer assays combined with negative noninvasive imaging have been found to have high negative predictive value in outpatients, but these results are not yet confirmed to have validity in cancer patients. A negative test in a high-risk patient does not exclude pulmonary embolism, and a positive D-dimer in a postoperative coagulopathic patient may not be specific either.

Pulmonary embolism is the most serious potential consequence of deep venous thrombosis. Classic clinical findings include hypoxia, chest pain, hemoptysis, shortness of breath, and tachycardia. In a critically ill postoperative ovarian cancer patient, the differential diagnosis is broad and may include fluid overload, pneumonia, effusion, atelectasis, or a cardiac event. The most common findings on CXR include atelectasis, infiltrate, and small effusion, all of which are nonspecific in a perioperative setting. Findings in ECG may include ST-segment or T-wave changes, but few patients will have electrical changes suggestive of right

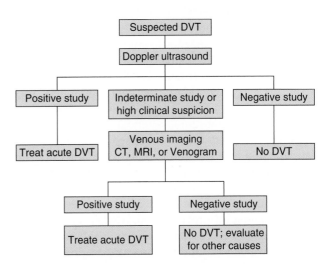

FIGURE 18-1. Diagnostic algorithm for evaluation of suspected postoperative deep venous thrombosis. CT, computed tomography; DVT, deep venous thrombosis; MRI, magnetic resonance imaging.

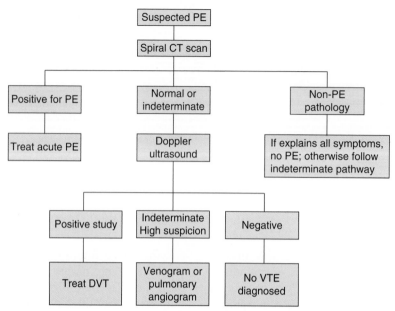

FIGURE 18-2. Diagnostic algorithm for evaluation of suspected postoperative pulmonary embolism. CT, computed tomography; DVT, deep venous thrombosis; PE, pulmonary embolism; VTE, venous thromboembolism.

heart strain. An arterial blood gas may help determine the degree of hypoxia and hypercapnea, although a quarter of patients with acute pulmonary embolism will have a normal Pao_2. A CT angiogram, or spiral CT, can reliably diagnose most clinically significant pulmonary emboli but is less sensitive in evaluating the subsegmental vessels (Figure 18-2). A ventilation/perfusion scan has the advantage of not using iodinated contrast but has the disadvantage of determining only indirect evidence of pulmonary embolism. In the Prospective Investigation of Pulmonary Embolism Diagnosis (PIOPED) study[72], only 14% of patients had a high probability scan, whereas 77% of patients had an indeterminate, nondiagnostic study. Pulmonary angiography remains the standard of diagnosis for pulmonary embolism but is considered rather invasive by requiring catheterization of the main pulmonary vessels and requiring a considerable contrast dye, which is particularly significant in a patient population whose renal function may be compromised from intravascular depletion or acute tubular necrosis. For a critically ill patient in the ICU, transesophageal echocardiography may also be performed at the bedside to evaluate for pulmonary embolism. Although transesophageal echocardiography provides poor visualization of the left pulmonary and lobar arteries, it is able to identify right ventricular volume and pressure overload associated with pulmonary embolism.

Clinically, the most practical examination may be spiral CT pulmonary angiography. Combining spiral CT of the chest with indirect CT venography may also exclude the need for lower extremity Doppler studies if either a pulmonary embolism or deep venous thrombosis is identified. Although a contrast dye load is still required, it is not as invasive and allows for evaluation of pelvic and lower extremity thrombi with greater than 90% sensitivity and specificity.

Heparin remains the primary therapy for postoperative patients with venous thromboembolic events. Failure to rapidly anticoagulate a patient with an acute event has been associated with late recurrence of thrombosis. However, the priority to anticoagulate a patient must be tempered with the knowledge of the patient's postoperative condition and the potential for ongoing bleeding or coagulopathy. If an epidural catheter is in place, it should be removed before the initiation of anticoagulation if the patient is stable enough to wait 1 hour before starting heparin. The short half-life of intravenous UFH allows for rapid reversal of anticoagulation in a patient at high risk of bleeding or requiring an invasive procedure (Figure 18-3). Once the patient is hemodynamically stable and therapeutically anticoagulated with heparin, low molecular weight heparin or warfarin can be started for a course of long-term anticoagulation. Patients with active bleeding may benefit from an IVC filter, which may prevent new or recurrent pulmonary emboli. Although the placement of a filter reduces the acute risk of pulmonary embolism, the filter may still become occluded, and once stable, patients typically require lifelong anticoagulation to minimize their later risk of recurrent deep venous thrombosis.

Labs prior to initiation of heparin: activated partial thromboplastin time (aPTT), prothrombin time (PT)/international normalized ratio (INR), platelets, urinalysis, stool guiac

Loading dose: 80 U/kg (minimum 5000 units, maximum 10,000 units)
Continuous infusion: 18 U/kg/h

Obtain first aPTT 4 hours after initiation of heparin therapy, If <55 seconds, follow table below. If ≥55 seconds, recheck aPTT in 4 hours. Adjust rate using table below. Recheck aPTT every 6 hours until 2 consecutive aPTT values within therapeutic range; then obtain daily complete blood count (CBC) with platelets and aPTT.

aPTT (seconds)	Re-bolus (units)	Hold drip (minutes)	Change drip (units per hour)	Repeat aPTT
<40	70 U/kg	0	+200	6 hours
40-47	0	0	+200	6 hours
48-54	0	0	+100	6 hours
Therapeutic range				
55-80	0	0	0	6 hours until stable, then every morning
81-90	0	0	−100	6 hours
91-100	0	30 minutes	−200	6 hours
>100	0	60 minutes	−300	6 hours

Therapeutic heparin level as measured by protamine titration assay: 0.2 to 0.4 units; or as measured by anti-Xa assay: 0.3 to 0.7 units.

Warfarin may be initiated on day 1 of heparin therapy. A minimum of 5 days is recommended. The therapeutic range for warfarin should be 2.0 to 3.0. A PT/INR should be ordered daily.

Day	INR	Warfarin dosage
1	<1.1	5 mg
2	<1.5	5 mg
	1.5-1.9	2.5 mg
	2-2.5	1-2.5 mg
	>2.5	0 mg
3	<1.5	5-10 mg
	1.5-1.9	1.5-5 mg
	2-3	0-2.5 mg
	>3	0 mg
4	<1.5	10 mg
	1.5-1.9	5-7.5 mg
	2-3	0-5 mg
	>3	0 mg
5	<1.5	10 mg
	1.5-1.9	7.5-10 mg
	2-3	0-5 mg
	>3	0 mg

Note that these guidelines are recommendations and are not intended to replace an individual clinician's judgment.

FIGURE 18-3. Anticoagulation of acute deep venous thrombosis or pulmonary embolism with high bleeding risk.

Several meta-analyses of clinical trials comparing low molecular weight heparin to UFH for the treatment of patients with deep venous thrombosis have shown that low molecular weight heparin provides greater reduction of thrombus size, as well as a decrease in recurrent venous thromboembolism.[73] Low molecular weight heparin also appears to be as safe and effective as UFH in the management of pulmonary embolism. The dose of low molecular weight heparin depends on the indications of prevention or treatment. A prophylactic dose of dalteparin is 5000 IU 10 to 12 hours before surgery and once daily after surgery. A prophylactic dose of enoxaparin is 40 mg 2 hours before surgery and once daily after surgery, whereas a therapeutic dose for anticoagulation is 1 mg/kg every 12 hours. Dalteparin was found to be comparable to tinzaparin in a randomized clinical study of treatment for deep vein thrombosis and pulmonary embolism. Monitoring is not required for prophylactic doses or in most patients for treatment, but measuring the anti–factor Xa level can be considered for patients with renal insufficiency or morbid obesity or patients who are refractory to therapy.

Arterial thrombotic events are rare occurrences in gynecologic cancer surgery patients; however, arterial emboli require prompt recognition as a vascular surgery emergency. Hypercoagulability, tissue trauma, and patient immobilization are risk factors that may exacerbate underlying vascular disease. Classic clinical signs include pain, pulselessness, paresthesia, pallor, and paralysis. Limb ischemia may lead to muscle necrosis and compartment syndrome within hours after onset. Prompt diagnosis and rapid revascularization allow the best opportunity for limb salvage and avoidance of amputation.

Gastrointestinal

In general, GI prophylaxis against stress ulcer formation is recommended to patients in the ICU with coagulopathy, patients with a history of recent upper GI bleed, or those who have been ventilated for ≥48 hours.[74] However, GI prophylaxis is often used inappropriately, as the frequency of GI bleeding outside of the ICU is quite low, and inappropriate use may result in increased rates of nosocomial pneumonia and *C difficile*–associated diarrheal illness. In the comparison of H_2 antagonists versus proton pump inhibitors, a recent meta-analysis showed these medications to be equivalent as prophylaxis against stress ulcers.[75]

Following surgery for advanced gynecologic malignancies, a nasogastric tube is sometimes left in place to decompress the stomach and avoid stress on gastric vascular pedicles. Such patients may be at risk of aspiration of gastric contents and should receive acid-reducing medications.

Pain Management

Following gynecologic oncology surgery, intravenous and/or epidural administration of analgesic medications may be used for pain control. An intravenous patient-controlled analgesia machine is an effective means of delivering opioids to treat postoperative pain. Early oral analgesia in gynecologic oncology patients is also safe and efficacious, but this depends on the use of early postoperative feeding. Epidural analgesia is also an effective therapy for the management of pain after major abdominal surgery and has been associated with decreased intraoperative blood loss, fewer thromboembolic events, and early ambulation.

More recently a prospective randomized study from Memorial Sloan-Kettering Cancer Center compared perioperative patient-controlled epidural analgesia (morphine and bupivacaine) to postoperative intravenous patient-controlled analgesia (morphine) in open gynecologic surgery.[76] Patients in the epidural arm had significantly less postoperative pain with no difference in time to discharge. In another nonrandomized prospective study, use of perioperative patient-controlled epidural analgesia (fentanyl and bupivacaine) did not improve pain management over postoperative patient-controlled analgesia (hydromorphone).[77] However, in this study, patients selected for epidurals were more likely to have a diagnosis of cancer and more complicated surgical procedure. With no difference in time to ambulation, tolerating diet, and readiness for discharge, the authors suggest that patient selection for epidural may influence the beneficial effects of neuraxial blockade.

Wound/Stoma Care

Patients should be cautioned on signs of wound infection, such as purulent drainage, erythema, or increased pain at the surgical site. Patients at increased risk of wound complications, such as the obese, diabetics, and the immunosuppressed, should take extra caution. In the setting of infection, hematoma, and/or seroma, large laparotomy incisions may open and require closure by secondary intention. Applying negative pressure to wounds, via the placement of a vacuum-assisted closure device, is a recent and novel means of debriding the wound while allowing for closure by secondary healing.[78] Following surgery for vulvar and vaginal cancer, meticulous care of the surgical site is a key factor in postoperative wound healing; issues such as sitz baths and perineal care should be addressed at multiple times during the perioperative period. Such supportive care includes strict instructions to keep the surgical site dry with heat, blow dryers, and the use of gauze fluffs. When inguinofemoral lymphadenectomy is performed, the use of drains in the lymphatic space has been found to decrease the risk of wound hematoma, seroma, or infection; however, patients should have necessary arrangements for home drain management when they leave the hospital.

The wide variety of procedures performed for patients with gynecologic malignancies can include leaving patients with urostomies and/or temporary or permanent fecal diversion stomas. In the postoperative period, patients can benefit from education on avoiding complications of stomas, such as the use of barrier systems for skin protection. In addition, patients with ileostomies or ascending colostomies should receive information on fluid intake and diet in order to avoid long-term complications with fluid and electrolyte balance. Patients with colostomies should be encouraged to learn techniques to avoid constipation.[79]

Lymphedema

Chronic lymphedema may occur following both pelvic and inguinal lymphadenectomy. In the setting of inguinal lymphadenectomy, early wound complications are not predictive of the incidence or severity of chronic lymphedema. Those with early and chronic lymphedema should be counseled on "complete decongestive therapy" (CDT), which includes manual lymphatic drainage, compression wraps and garments, skin care, and exercises to facilitate lymphatic drainage. Nurses and physicians may play critical roles in informing patients not only of the signs of lymphedema, but also early techniques of CDT.

Discharge Planning

The clinical team involved in the disposition of a patient following surgery for gynecologic cancer can include not only physicians, but also case managers, social workers, and physical and occupational therapists. Given the complexities that can arise due to the various procedures performed for women with gynecologic cancers, patients may benefit from a period of subacute nursing care. Attention should also be paid to the postoperative follow-up plan in which the pathology and treatment plan will be discussed in order to smooth the transition between the acute postoperative period and subsequent outpatient oncology care.

NUTRITIONAL SUPPORT

Following open surgery, patients have traditionally been restricted from oral intake until they have signs of improved bowel function. However, several studies have demonstrated that early feeding after laparotomy may actually improve GI function and overall perioperative outcome.

Placement of a nasogastric tube intraoperatively does not necessarily mean that the patient continues with nasogastric intubation in the postoperative period. Patients frequently complain of discomfort from the tube, and although traditional surgeons argue that nasogastric decompression decreases gastric and intestinal distention, these benefits have not been proven in clinical trials. In a prospective study of 110 gynecologic oncology patients undergoing intra-abdominal surgery randomized to postoperative nasogastric tube or intraoperative orogastric tube, there was no difference in bowel complications, time to tolerating a regular diet, or length of hospital stay. A meta-analysis of 26 clinical trials including 3964 patients evaluating nasogastric decompression also found that patients managed without nasogastric tubes had significantly less febrile morbidity, atelectasis, and pneumonia.[80] There was greater abdominal distension and vomiting, but this was not associated with any increase in complications (wound dehiscence, infection, or anastomotic leak) or length of stay.

Early oral feeding was first suggested to be safe in GI and colorectal surgery. Studying the safety and efficacy of early postoperative feeding in gynecologic oncology patients, 200 patients were randomized to clear liquids on postoperative day 1 versus nothing by mouth until passage of flatus. Time to development of bowel sounds (1.8 vs. 2.3 days, $P = .07$), tolerance of clear liquids (1.2 vs. 3.5 days, $P < .0001$), and regular diet (2.3 vs. 4.2 days, $P < .0001$) and length of hospital stay (4.6 vs. 5.8 days, $P = .001$) were significantly shorter in the early feeding group. These findings were confirmed by a separate prospective randomized study at Indiana University comparing clear liquids on postoperative day 1 with nothing by mouth until bowel sounds, flatus or bowel movement, or subjective hunger. The study group had a higher incidence of emesis but actually tolerated a regular diet 1 day earlier than the control group. In a recent retrospective review of 880 patients on a gynecologic oncology service at University of California, Irvine Medical Center, early feeding was well tolerated.[81] In this series, only 44 patients (5%) required readmission; 11 of these patients were readmitted with a diagnosis of ileus or small bowel obstruction. A recent prospective study of gynecologic oncology patients undergoing intestinal resection found that early feeding was not associated with any increase in postoperative complications.[82]

Beyond its digestive capacities, the GI tract is recognized as being an immunologic barrier against infection. Once tolerating a regular diet, patients may tolerate oral analgesics earlier.

Evaluation of Malnutrition

Malnutrition in gynecologic cancer patients may result from the physical compression of the bowel from tumor masses, omental caking, and ascites, resulting in decreased oral intake or partial bowel obstruction. In addition, cancer cachexia may cause metabolic changes, including increased resting energy expenditure, increased anaerobic glycolysis, and a high turnover of glycerol and free fatty acids. Patients who are nutritionally depleted are at greater risk of surgical morbidity, including increased risk of infection, prolonged hospital stay, and mortality. Patients with low serum albumin level on admission (< 3.4 g/dL) to an acute care hospital have been observed to have greater than a 3-fold increased risk for mortality when compared to patients with normal serum albumin. Whereas albumin levels represent the long-term nutritional status, prealbumin levels may represent short-term status.[83] Weight loss and diminished skinfold thickness are also indicators of malnutrition. Although many studies have demonstrated that nutritional support improved the nutritional parameters of patients, strong data are lacking to demonstrate improvement in clinically significant end points. Malnutrition is assessed more effectively in the preoperative setting, because nutritional parameters such as albumin may be altered from drainage of ascites and volume resuscitation and transferrin may be altered due to postoperative inflammation.

Nutritional Interventions

Total Parenteral Nutrition

Total parenteral nutrition may be considered in patients who are expected to remain without enteral feeding for a prolonged period of time, but the timing of nutrition support is also influenced by the hemodynamic stability of the patient in the postoperative period. The altered metabolic state of increased catecholamines, glucocorticoids, and glucagon favors the process of gluconeogenesis, glycogenolysis, and fatty acid oxidation. Nutritional support has become a standard of care for these patients, yet the length of tolerable starvation remains an unanswered question. Total parenteral nutrition is not recommended for patients with an intact and functional GI tract, but many gynecologic oncology patients requiring critical care may have also had bowel resection and can be expected to have a delayed return of bowel function. A meta-analysis of 26 prospective randomized trials including 2211 patients comparing total parenteral nutrition with (standard) oral diet and intravenous dextrose did not show any improvement in overall mortality of surgical or critically ill patients (risk ratio, 1.03; 95% confidence interval [CI], 0.81-1.31). The rate of major complications was lower among malnourished patients receiving total parenteral nutrition (risk ratio, 0.52; 95% CI, 0.31-0.91).[84]

Caloric requirements are assessed based on the patient's stored reserves and body catabolism. The Harris-Benedict equation is based on a basal energy expenditure calculated using the age, sex, height, and weight of the individual, and then multiplied by a ratio for stress and activity (Figure 18-4). A reasonable estimate of energy in a critically ill adult patient is 25 to 30 kcal/kg. Carbohydrates compose 60% to 70% of nonprotein calories, whereas fats constitute 25% to 30% of calories and include essential fatty acids. Protein needs range from 1.2 to 2.0 g/kg per day. Fluids, electrolytes, vitamins, and trace elements complete the daily formulation of total parenteral nutrition (Table 18-10). H_2-receptor antagonists and regular insulin are also compatible as additives in parenteral nutrition solutions. Central administration of parenteral nutrition is recommended due to hyperosmolarity and vein irritation. Concurrent administration of fat emulsion may reduce the amount of vein irritation.

Refeeding syndrome may occur in the feeding of severely malnourished patients. Intracellular incorporation of phosphate may result in severe hypophosphatemia and possibly respiratory failure. Potassium and magnesium shift intracellularly as well, resulting in hypokalemia and hypomagnesemia. Regular monitoring of laboratory profiles, including electrolytes, glucose, liver function, and lipid panels, can prevent metabolic complications of parenteral nutrition. Excess glucose can result in hyperglycemia and other hyperosmolar states. Excess lipids can result in hyperlipidemia, and excess protein can worsen azotemia or encephalopathy. Albumin, prealbumin, and C-reactive protein may be monitored weekly. Adjustments to rates of additional maintenance fluids given should also be made accordingly.

A 24-hour urine urea nitrogen excretion can be collected after stable protein intake for 3 to 5 days to calculate the patient's nitrogen balance. Nitrogen intake equals protein intake (in grams) divided by 6.25. Nitrogen output equals urine urea nitrogen plus insensible loses (constant of 3). A nitrogen balance of +4 to +5 g

---

For women, the Harris-Benedict equation:

Basal energy expenditure = 655 + 9.6 × weight (kg) + 1.7 × height (cm) − 4.7 × age (years)

Multiply by activity factor:

Confined to bed	1.2×
Out of bed	1.3×
Active	1.4×

Multiple by stress factor

Minor surgery	1.0-1.2×
Soft tissue trauma	1.1-1.4×
Peritonitis	1.2-1.5×
Major sepsis	1.4-1.8×
Sever burn patients	2.0×

FIGURE 18-4. Total estimated calorie requirement is based on the basal energy expenditure and stress and injury factors.

Table 18-10 Standard Parenteral Nutrition Formulations per Liter

	Central Formulation		Peripheral Formulation	
Dextrose	25%	250 g	10%	100 g
Amino acids	4.25%	42.5 g	2.5%	25 g
Sodium		45 mEq		41 mEq
Potassium		40 mEq		18 mEq
Calcium		4.5 mEq		4 mEq
Magnesium		5 mEq		5 mEq
Chloride		43 mEq		35 mEq
Phosphorus		15 mM		9 mM
Acetate		41 mEq		28 mEq
Trace elements				
Vitamin K (weekly)				
Osmolarity		1825 mOsm/L		880 mOsm/L
Calories		1020 kcal		440 kcal
Nitrogen content		6.7 g		4.0 g

is required for anabolism; nutrition specialists should be involved to help optimize parenteral nutrition orders. Calorie counts may help quantitate the patient's intake, and parenteral nutrition should be continued until the patient is taking at least 50% of calories through the enteric route.

Peripheral Parenteral Nutrition

Although small studies have suggested some benefit to peripheral parenteral nutrition when central venous access is not available, there is no evidence suggesting that peripheral parenteral nutrition is equivalent to total parenteral nutrition in providing nutritional support. To avoid thrombophlebitis, the concentrations of amino acids and dextrose are maintained at 3% and 10%, respectively.[85] Solutions that can be infused through a peripheral vein must often be diluted into a large volume to meet daily caloric needs, which may have adverse effects in postoperative patients. To meet optimal nutritional needs, parenteral nutrition solutions require either a volume or concentration that is too high for infusion into a peripheral vein. Lipids may be added to provide nonprotein calories; however, maintaining the stability of a mixture of lipids with the lower concentration of glucose in peripheral solutions is difficult.

Enteral Feeding

Compared to parenteral nutrition, enteral nutrition promotes decreased GI mucosal permeability and better wound healing. The enteral route is also associated with fewer metabolic disturbances and is less expensive than parenteral nutrition. Limitations in postoperative patients are its contraindication in patients with ileus and patients at risk for aspiration. Patients with short gut syndrome also may require parenteral supplementation until the remaining bowel adapts. Feeding into the small bowel may be preferable over gastric feeding; this avoids the risks of regurgitation and aspiration associated with delayed gastric emptying, particularly in an ovarian cancer surgery patient where gastric distention may compromise pedicles on the short gastric vessels from an infragastric omentectomy. However, bypassing the stomach does not necessarily increase the tolerance to feeds, and either approach to enteral feeding may be acceptable. Randomized trials of prokinetic agents have not shown them to be advantageous in improving postoperative ileus. In the immediate postoperative period, a critically ill, nutritionally depleted patient will more likely be considered for total parenteral nutrition, but enteral feeding should be considered after recovery of bowel function.

Appetite Stimulants

In the postoperative setting, appetite is often limited by the return of intestinal function. However, as neoadjuvant chemotherapy is increasingly incorporated into the treatment of gynecologic cancers, patients may have received cytotoxic treatment prior to surgery, which may also compromise their appetite. Megestrol acetate is commonly used and is effective in treating chemotherapy-induced anorexia. However, its use has also been associated with an increased risk for thromboembolic events; therefore, use in the postoperative period should be monitored closely. Corticosteroids such as dexamethasone have been found to have similar stimulatory effects on appetite, yet their use is also associated with mild agitation and insomnia, which can be difficult to tolerate in the postoperative period and may exacerbate delirium in elderly patients. Anabolic steroids have also been proposed.

REFERENCES

1. St Clair CM, Shah M, Diver EJ, et al. Adherence to evidence-based guidelines for preoperative testing in women undergoing gynecologic surgery. *Obstet Gynecol.* 2010;116(3):694-700.
2. Fleisher LA, Beckman JA, Brown KA, et al. ACC/AHA 2007 Guidelines on Perioperative Cardiovascular Evaluation and Care for Noncardiac Surgery: executive summary: a report of the American College of Cardiology/American Heart Association Task Force on Practice Guidelines developed in collaboration with the American Society of Echocardiography, American Society of Nuclear Cardiology, Heart Rhythm Society, Society of Cardiovascular Anesthesiologists, Society for Cardiovascular Angiography and Interventions, Society for Vascular Medicine and Biology, and Society for Vascular Surgery. *J Am Coll Cardiol.* 2007;50(17):1707-1732.
3. Smetana GW, Lawrence VA, Cornell JE. Preoperative pulmonary risk stratification for noncardiothoracic surgery: systematic review for the American College of Physicians. *Ann Intern Med.* 2006;144(8):581-595.
4. Poirier P, Alpert MA, Fleisher LA, et al. Cardiovascular evaluation and management of severely obese patients undergoing surgery: a science advisory from the American Heart Association. *Circulation.* 2009;120(1):86-95.
5. Bristow RE, Duska LR, Lambrou NC, et al: A Model for predicting surgical outcome in patients with advanced ovarian carcinoma using computed tomography. *Cancer.* 89:1532-1540; 2000.
6. Ferrandina G, Sallustio G, Fagotti A, et al. Role of CT scan-based and clinical evaluation in the preoperative prediction of optimal cytoreduction in advanced ovarian cancer: a prospective trial. *Br J Cancer.* 2009;101(7):1066-1073.
7. Ozdemir S, Celik C, Emlik D, et al. Assessment of myometrial invasion in endometrial cancer by transvaginal sonography, Doppler ultrasonography, magnetic resonance imaging and frozen section. *Int J Gynecol Cancer.* 2009;19(6):1085-1090.
8. Nagar H, Dobbs S, McClelland HR, et al. The diagnostic accuracy of magnetic resonance imaging in detecting cervical involvement in endometrial cancer. *Gynecol Oncol.* 2006;103(2):431-434.
9. Orezzoli JP, Sioletic S, Olawaiye A, et al. Stage II endometrioid adenocarcinoma of the endometrium: clinical implications of cervical stromal invasion. *Gynecol Oncol.* 2009;113(3):316-323.
10. Mitchell DG, Snyder B, Coakley F, et al. Early invasive cervical cancer: tumor delineation by magnetic resonance imaging, computed tomography, and clinical examination, verified by pathologic results, in the ACRIN 6651/GOG 183 Intergroup Study. *J Clin Oncol.* 2006;24(36):5687-5694.
11. Chung HH, Kang KW, Cho JY, et al. Role of magnetic resonance imaging and positron emission tomography/computed tomography in preoperative lymph node detection of uterine cervical cancer. *Am J Obstet Gynecol.* 2010;203(2):156:e1-5.
12. Boughanim M, Leboulleux S, Rey A, et al. Histologic results of para-aortic lymphadenectomy in patients treated for stage IB2/II cervical cancer with negative [18F]fluorodeoxyglucose positron emission tomography scans in the para-aortic area. *J Clin Oncol.* 2008;26(15):2558-2261.
13. Choi HJ, Roh JW, Seo SS, et al. Comparison of the accuracy of magnetic resonance imaging and positron emission tomography/computed tomography in the presurgical detection of lymph node metastases in patients with uterine cervical carcinoma: a prospective study. *Cancer.* 2006;106(4):914-922.
14. Ford MK, Beattie WS, Wijeysundera DN. Systematic review: prediction of perioperative cardiac complications and mortality by the revised cardiac risk index. *Ann Intern Med.* 2010;152(1):26-35.
15. Fleisher LA, Beckman JA, Brown KA, et al. 2009 ACCF/AHA focused update on perioperative beta blockade incorporated into the ACC/AHA 2007 guidelines on perioperative cardiovascular evaluation and care for noncardiac surgery: a report of the American College of Cardiology Foundation/American Heart Association Task Force on Practice Guidelines. *Circulation.* 2009;120(21):e169-e276.
16. Fleisher LA, Beckman JA, Brown KA, et al. ACC/AHA 2007 guidelines on perioperative cardiovascular evaluation and care for noncardiac surgery: executive summary: a report of the American College of Cardiology/American Heart Association Task Force on Practice Guidelines (Writing Committee to Revise the 2002 Guidelines on Perioperative Cardiovascular Evaluation for Noncardiac Surgery). *Anesth Analg.* 2008;106(3):685-712.
17. Devereaux PJ, Yang H, Yusuf S, et al. Effects of extended-release metoprolol succinate in patients undergoing non-cardiac surgery (POISE trial): a randomised controlled trial. *Lancet.* 2008;371(9627):1839-1847.
18. Fleischmann KE, Beckman JA, Buller CE, et al. 2009 ACCF/AHA focused update on perioperative beta blockade. *J Am Coll Cardiol.* 2009;54(22):2102-2128.
19. Scognamiglio R, Negut C, Ramondo A, et al. Detection of coronary artery disease in asymptomatic patients with type 2 diabetes mellitus. *J Am Coll Cardiol.* 2006;47(1):65-71.
20. Dronge AS, Perkal MF, Kancir S, et al. Long-term glycemic control and postoperative infectious complications. *Arch Surg.* 2006;141(4):375-380.
21. Marik PE, Varon J. Requirement of perioperative stress doses of corticosteroids: a systematic review of the literature. *Arch Surg.* 2008;143(12):1222-1226.
22. Mathew A, Devereaux PJ, O'Hare A, et al. Chronic kidney disease and postoperative mortality: a systematic review and meta-analysis. *Kidney Int.* 2008;73(9):1069-1081.
23. O'Leary JG, Yachimski PS, Friedman LS. Surgery in the patient with liver disease. *Clin Liver Dis.* 2009;13(2):211-231.
24. Cobb WS, Heniford BT, Burns JT, et al. Cirrhosis is not a contraindication to laparoscopic surgery. *Surg Endosc.* 2005;19(3):418-423.
25. Laky B, Janda M, Kondalsamy-Chennakesavan S, et al. Pretreatment malnutrition and quality of life: association with prolonged length of hospital stay among patients with gynecological cancer: a cohort study. *BMC Cancer.* 2010;10:232.
26. Diaz-Montes TP, Zahurak ML, Bristow RE. Predictors of extended intensive care unit resource utilization following surgery for ovarian cancer. *Gynecol Oncol.* 2007;107(3):464-468.
27. Geisler JP, Linnemeier GC, Thomas AJ, Manahan KJ. Nutritional assessment using prealbumin as an objective criterion to determine whom should not undergo primary radical cytoreductive surgery for ovarian cancer. *Gynecol Oncol.* 2007;106(1):128-131.
28. Kuppermann M, Summitt RL Jr, Varner RE, et al. Sexual functioning after total compared with supracervical hysterectomy: a randomized trial. *Obstet Gynecol.* 2005;105(6):1309-1318.
29. Cibula D, Velechovska P, Sláma J, et al. Late morbidity following nerve-sparing radical hysterectomy. *Gynecol Oncol.* 2010;116(3):506-511.

30. Serati M, Salvatore S, Uccella S, et al. Sexual function after radical hysterectomy for early-stage cervical cancer: is there a difference between laparoscopy and laparotomy? *J Sex Med.* 2009;6(9):2516-2522.

31. ACOG Committee on Practice Bulletins. ACOG Practice Bulletin No. 104: antibiotic prophylaxis for gynecologic procedures. *Obstet Gynecol.* 2009;113(5):1180-1189.

32. Bratzler DW, Hunt DR. The surgical infection prevention and surgical care improvement projects: national initiatives to improve outcomes for patients having surgery. *Clin Infect Dis.* 2006;43(3):322-330.

33. Itani KM, Wilson SE, Awad SS, et al. Ertapenem versus cefotetan prophylaxis in elective colorectal surgery. *N Engl J Med.* 2006;355(25):2640-2651.

34. Wilson W, Taubert KA, Gewitz M, et al. Prevention of infective endocarditis: guidelines from the American Heart Association: a guideline from the American Heart Association Rheumatic Fever, Endocarditis, and Kawasaki Disease Committee, Council on Cardiovascular Disease in the Young, and the Council on Clinical Cardiology, Council on Cardiovascular Surgery and Anesthesia, and the Quality of Care and Outcomes Research Interdisciplinary Working Group. *Circulation.* 2007;116(15):1736-1754.

35. ACOG Committee on Practice Bulletins. Practice Bulletin No. 84: prevention of deep vein thrombosis and pulmonary embolism. *Obstet Gynecol.* 2007;110(2 Pt 1):429-440.

36. Geerts WH, Bergqvist D, Pineo GF, et al. Prevention of venous thromboembolism: American College of Chest Physicians Evidence-Based Clinical Practice Guidelines (8th Edition). *Chest.* 2008;133(6 suppl):381S-453S.

37. Einstein MH, Kushner DM, Connor JP, et al. A protocol of dual prophylaxis for venous thromboembolism prevention in gynecologic cancer patients. *Obstet Gynecol.* 2008;112(5):1091-1097.

38. NCCN Clinical Practice Guidelines in Oncology (NCCN Guidelines TM) Venous Thromboembolic Disease. v.1.2010. Available at: http://www.nccn.org/professionals/physician_gls/f_guidelines.asp.

39. Adib T, Belli A, McCall J, et al. The use of inferior vena caval filters prior to major surgery in women with gynaecological cancer. *BJOG.* 2008;115(7):902-907.

40. Pineda CE, Shelton AA, Hernandez-Boussard T, et al. Mechanical bowel preparation in intestinal surgery: a meta-analysis and review of the literature. *J Gastrointest Surg.* 2008;12(11):2037-2044.

41. Guenaga KK, Matos D, Wille-Jorgensen P. Mechanical bowel preparation for elective colorectal surgery. *Cochrane Database Syst Rev.* 2009(1):CD001544.

42. Muzii L, Bellati F, Zullo MA, et al. Mechanical bowel preparation before gynecologic laparoscopy: a randomized, single-blind, controlled trial. *Fertil Steril.* 2006;85(3):689-693.

43. Nelson RL, Glenny AM, Song F. Antimicrobial prophylaxis for colorectal surgery. *Cochrane Database Syst Rev.* 2009(1):CD001181.

44. Wijeysundera DN, Beattie WS, Austin PC, et al. Non-invasive cardiac stress testing before elective major non-cardiac surgery: population based cohort study. *BMJ.* 2010;340:b5526.

45. Poirier P, Giles TD, Bray GA, et al. Obesity and cardiovascular disease: pathophysiology, evaluation, and effect of weight loss: an update of the 1997 American Heart Association Scientific Statement on Obesity and Heart Disease from the Obesity Committee of the Council on Nutrition, Physical Activity, and Metabolism. *Circulation.* 2006;113(6):898-918.

46. Walker JL, Piedmonte MR, Spirtos NM, et al. Laparoscopy compared with laparotomy for comprehensive surgical staging of uterine cancer: Gynecologic Oncology Group Study LAP2. *J Clin Oncol.* 2009;27(32):5331-5336.

47. Seamon LG, Bryant SA, Rheaume PS, et al. Comprehensive surgical staging for endometrial cancer in obese patients: comparing robotics and laparotomy. *Obstet Gynecol.* 2009;114(1):16-21.

48. Ebert TJ, Shankar H, Haake RM. Perioperative considerations for patients with morbid obesity. *Anesthesiol Clin.* 2006;24(3):621-636.

49. Wright JD, Rosenbush EJ, Powell MA, et al. Long-term outcome of women who undergo panniculectomy at the time of gynecologic surgery. *Gynecol Oncol.* 2006;102(1):86-91.

50. Leath CA 3rd, Kendrick JE 4th, Numnum TM, et al. Outcomes of gynecologic oncology patients admitted to the intensive care unit following surgery: a university teaching hospital experience. *Int J Gynecol Cancer.* 2006;16(5):1766-1769.

51. Auerbach A, Goldman L. Assessing and reducing the cardiac risk of noncardiac surgery. *Circulation.* 2006;113(10):1361-1376.

52. Vanacker B. Anaesthetic issues in women undergoing gynaecological cytoreductive surgery. *Curr Opin Anaesthesiol.* 2009;22(3):362-367.

53. Jacob M, Chappell D, Conzen P, et al. Small-volume resuscitation with hyperoncotic albumin: a systematic review of randomized clinical trials. *Crit Care.* 2008;12(2):R34.

54. The Acute Respiratory Distress Syndrome Network. Ventilation with lower tidal volumes as compared with traditional tidal volumes for acute lung injury and the acute respiratory distress syndrome. *N Engl J Med.* 2000;342(18):1301-1308.

55. Frutos-Vivar F, Ferguson ND, Esteban A, et al. Risk factors for extubation failure in patients following a successful spontaneous breathing trial. *Chest.* 2006;130(6):1664-1671.

56. de la Torre SH, Mandel L, Goff BA. Evaluation of postoperative fever: usefulness and cost-effectiveness of routine workup. *Am J Obstet Gynecol.* 2003;188(6):1642-1647.

57. Kendrick JE, Numnum TM, Estes JM, et al. Conservative management of postoperative fever in gynecologic patients undergoing major abdominal or vaginal operations. *J Am Coll Surg.* 2008;207(3):393-397.

58. Abraham E, Laterre PF, Garg R, et al. Drotrecogin alfa (activated) for adults with severe sepsis and a low risk of death. *N Engl J Med.* 2005;353(13):1332-1341.

59. Wuethrich PY, Burkhard FC, Panicker JN, Kessler TM. Effects of thoracic epidural analgesia on lower urinary tract function in women. *Neurourol Urodyn.* 2011;30(1):121-125.

60. Forni LG, Hilton PJ. Continuous hemofiltration in the treatment of acute renal failure. *N Engl J Med.* 1997;336(18):1303-1309.

61. Selim M. Perioperative stroke. *N Engl J Med.* 2007;356(7):706-713.

62. Lees KR, Bluhmki E, von Kummer R, et al. Time to treatment with intravenous alteplase and outcome in stroke: an updated pooled analysis of ECASS, ATLANTIS, NINDS, and EPITHET trials. *Lancet.* 2010;375(9727):1695-1703.

63. Bohrer JC, Walters MD, Park A, et al. Pelvic nerve injury following gynecologic surgery: a prospective cohort study. *Am J Obstet Gynecol.* 2009;201(5):531.e1-7.

64. Sieber FE. Postoperative delirium in the elderly surgical patient. *Anesthesiol Clin.* 2009;27(3):451-464.

65. McAlpine JN, Hodgson EJ, Abramowitz S, et al. The incidence and risk factors associated with postoperative delirium in geriatric patients undergoing surgery for suspected gynecologic malignancies. *Gynecol Oncol.* 2008;109(2):296-302.

66. Flinn DR, Diehl KM, Seyfried LS, et al. Prevention, diagnosis, and management of postoperative delirium in older adults. *J Am Coll Surg.* 2009;209(2):261-268.

67. American Red Cross. *Practice Guidelines for Blood Transfusion.* 2nd ed. Washington, DC: American Red Cross; 2007.

68. Silliman CC, Fung YL, Ball JB, Khan SY. Transfusion-related acute lung injury (TRALI): current concepts and misconceptions. *Blood Rev.* 2009;23(6):245-255.

69. Marik PE, Corwin HL. Efficacy of red blood cell transfusion in the critically ill: A systematic review of the literature. *Crit Care Med.* 2008;36(9):2667-2674.

70. Duska LR, Garret L, Henretta M, et al. When 'never-events' occur despite adherence to clinical guidelines: the case of venous thromboembolism in clear cell cancer of the ovary compared with other epithelial histologic subtypes. *Gynecol Oncol.* 2010;116(3):374-377.

71. Geerts WH, Heit JA, Clagett GP, et al. Prevention of venous thromboembolism. *Chest.* 2001;119(90010):132S-175S.

72. Stein PD, Fowler SE, Goodman LR, Gottschalk A, Halles CA, Hull RD, et al. PIOPED II Investigators: multidetector computed tomography for actue pulmonary embolism. N Engl J Med. 2006;354(22):2317-2327.

73. Siragusa S, Cosmi B, Piovella F, et al. Low-molecular-weight heparins and unfractionated heparin in the treatment of patients with acute venous thromboembolism: results of a meta-analysis. *Am J Med.* 1996;100(3):269-277.

74. Spirt MJ, Stanley S. Update on stress ulcer prophylaxis in critically ill patients. *Crit Care Nurse.* 2006;26(1):18-20, 22-28.

75. Lin PC, Chang CH, Hsu PI, et al. The efficacy and safety of proton pump inhibitors vs histamine-2 receptor antagonists for stress ulcer bleeding prophylaxis among critical care patients: a meta-analysis. *Crit Care Med.* 2010;38(4):1197-1205.

76. Ferguson SE, Malhotra T, Seshan VE, et al. A prospective randomized trial comparing patient-controlled epidural analgesia to patient-controlled intravenous analgesia on postoperative pain control and recovery after major open gynecologic cancer surgery. *Gynecol Oncol.* 2009;114(1):111-116.

77. Chen LM, Weinberg VK, Chen C, et al. Perioperative outcomes comparing patient controlled epidural versus intravenous analgesia in gynecologic oncology surgery. *Gynecol Oncol.* 2009; 115(3):357-361.

78. Schimp VL, Worley C, Brunello S, et al. Vacuum-assisted closure in the treatment of gynecologic oncology wound failures. *Gynecol Oncol.* 2004;92(2):586-591.

79. Doughty D. Principles of ostomy management in the oncology patient. *J Support Oncol.* 2005;3(1):59-69.

80. Cheatham ML, Chapman WC, Key SP, et al. A meta-analysis of selective versus routine nasogastric decompression after elective laparotomy. *Ann Surg.* 1995;221(5):469-476.

81. Chase DM, Lopez S, Nguyen C, et al. A clinical pathway for postoperative management and early patient discharge: does it work in gynecologic oncology? *Am J Obstet Gynecol.* 2008; 199(5):541:e1-7.

82. Minig L, Biffi R, Zanagnolo V, et al. Early oral versus "traditional" postoperative feeding in gynecologic oncology patients undergoing intestinal resection: randomized controlled trial. *Ann Surg Oncol.* 2009;16(6):1660-1668.

83. Devakonda A, George L, Raoof S, et al. Transthyretin as a marker to predict outcome in critically ill patients. *Clin Biochem.* 2008;41(14-15):1126-1130.

84. Keyland DK, MacDonald S, Keefe L, Drover JW. Total parenteral nutrition in the critically ill patient: a meta-analysis. *JAMA.* 1988;280(23):2013-2019.

85. Gura KM. Is there still a role for peripheral parenteral nutrition? *Nutr Clin Pract.* 2009;24(6):709-717.

Principles of Radiation Therapy

Wui-Jin Koh and Lindsay R. Sales

Radiotherapy plays an integral role in the care of many gynecologic cancers and can be used for definitive management, adjuvant therapy, or palliation. The principal basis of therapeutic radiation lies in its ability to cause ionization, or the creation of free electrons and free radicals, when absorbed by biologic matter. These highly reactive chemical species interact with critical molecules in a cell (in particular deoxyribonucleic acid [DNA]) and, if unrepaired, lead to loss of cellular reproductive capacity and eventual cell death. Ionizing radiation can be emitted from radioactive isotopes, both naturally occurring and man-made, or created using specialized high-voltage but nonradioactive equipment such as linear accelerators.

Optimal radiation for gynecologic malignancies often combines both teletherapy (external beam radiotherapy) and brachytherapy (internal radiation) with careful clinical judgment required to determine the proper weighting of each component. The challenge in radiation delivery is to deliver intended full dose(s) to selected target(s), while minimizing exposure to adjacent normal tissues. Sophisticated developments in imaging, computer-based treatment planning, and linear accelerator technology provide for ever-greater sophistication and accuracy in radiotherapy. However, such precision in dose delivery has to be accompanied by improvements in patient set-up immobilization, reproducibility, and regular tumor tracking to prevent marginal misses of the intended target volume. Advances in radiotherapy for gynecologic malignancies will be based on further integration with systemic agents (for both spatial cooperation and chemosensitization), as well as developments in targeting, tracking,

and adaptive processes, featuring radiation plans that may be modified during a course of therapy to conform to changes in patient and tumor geometry.

FUNDAMENTALS OF RADIATION PHYSICS

Structure of Matter

All matter is composed of individual units called elements. Each element is defined by the physical and chemical properties of its basic component—the atom. The atom consists of a central core, the nucleus, made up of positively charged particles, called protons, and neutrons, which have no charge. The nucleus is surrounded by a "cloud" of negatively charged particles, or electrons, which move in orbits around the nucleus. In the basic "resting" state of an atom, the number of protons in the nucleus is equal to the number of orbiting electrons, making the atom electrically neutral.

The formula $^A_Z X$ is used to identify each atom. X is the chemical symbol for the element, A is the mass number or number of nucleons (the number of neutrons *and* protons in the nucleus), and Z is the atomic number (the number of protons in the nucleus). The number of protons (Z) in an atom determines its chemical properties and its elemental name. Within the periodic table of elements, as Z increases, the number of accompanying neutrons increases proportionally more (ie, A:Z ratio > 2) to maintain nuclear stability. Atoms with the same Z, but with different numbers of neutrons, share the same element name and chemical properties but are called isotopes. When the A:Z ratio varies from the baseline (or lowest energy) form, these isotopes are often unstable and seek to achieve nuclear stability by giving off excess energy in the form of radiation, and are thus called radioisotopes (or radionuclides).

Hydrogen, carbon, oxygen, and nitrogen are the main elements that make up the human body. Each has a relatively small atomic number and mass number. The neutron-to-proton ratio for each of these elements is unity, and each exists at baseline in an electrically neutral and stable configuration.

The mass of subatomic particles is measured in terms of the atomic mass unit (AMU). An AMU is defined as one-twelfth of the mass of the carbon atom. In metric units of mass, 1 AMU = 1.66×10^{-27} kg. The mass of a proton is 1.00727 AMU, and that of a neutron is very similar at 1.00866 AMU. Electrons are significantly smaller, with a mass of 0.000548 AMU.

According to the atomic model proposed by Niels Bohr, the negatively charged electrons revolve around the positively charged nucleus, held in place by Coulombic force of attraction, in fixed orbits at specific distances from the nucleus. Electron orbits are referred to as shells, with the K shell being the inner most shell, followed radially by the L, M, N, and O shells. The maximum number of electrons in an orbit is defined as $2n^2$, where n is the integer specific to each shell and called the principle quantum number. In reality, the actual configuration and location of orbital electrons are rather complex and dynamic; however, this simplified model provides for an understanding of the basic concepts of atomic structure.

Electron orbits can also be considered as energy levels within an atom. When an electron moves to an orbit closer to the nucleus, energy is released. For an electron to move to an orbit farther from the nucleus, energy is required. The energy required to remove an electron *completely* from an atom (or ionization) is termed the binding energy of the electron. The binding energy of the electron depends on the magnitude of the Coulomb force of attraction between the nucleus and the electron. The binding energy for the higher Z atoms is greater because of the greater nuclear charge. Additionally, the binding energy is greater for electrons closer to the nucleus. However, on average, removal of an electron from an orbit requires 33 to 35 eV, where 1 eV, or electron volt, is defined as the kinetic energy acquired by an electron in passing through a potential difference of 1 V. This 33 to 35 eV range reflects the minimum amount of energy that an incident beam of radiation, or photon, must have to cause ionization.

Types of Radiation

The different forms of radiation are usually categorized into 2 groups: electromagnetic and particulate.

Electromagnetic radiation exists on a spectrum and is defined by its energy, or corresponding wavelength. In general order of increasing energy, the electromagnetic spectrum includes radio waves, microwaves, infrared, visible light, ultraviolet, and x-rays and γ-rays. All radiation within the electromagnetic spectrum has the same velocity (the speed of light, or 3×10^8 m/s). Although electromagnetic radiation has no mass or charge, it exists in a duality that can be considered either as a waveform (expressed as wavelength or frequency) or as packets of energy called photons (expressed as eV). These 2 properties of photons can be readily converted from one form to another using the following equation:

$$E = h\nu$$

where E is the photon energy (eV), ν is the frequency of the radiation (s^{-1}), and h is Planck's constant (4.1357×10^{-15} eV · s).

The frequency and wavelength of a photon are inversely related, with the correlation given by:

$$\nu = c/\lambda$$

where ν is the frequency of the radiation (s^{-1}), c is the speed of light (3×10^8 m/s), and λ is the wavelength (m).

As the wavelength of the photon becomes shorter, the frequency increases in inverse proportion. Hence, electromagnetic radiation of shorter wavelengths has higher energies. For the purposes of radiotherapy, it is only the photons that have sufficient energy to overcome the binding energy of electrons in biologic matter that are of specific interest; these are the ionizing x-rays and the γ-rays that exist in the higher energy portion of the electromagnetic spectrum. The lower energy forms of electromagnetic radiation do not cause ionizations but can result in heat and/or light, which are usually considered less injurious to biologic matter. Typically, electromagnetic radiation is considered to be ionizing when the photon energy exceeds 124 eV (or has a wavelength $<10^{-8}$ m).

There are no intrinsic differences in characteristics between x-rays and γ-rays—their names refer only to the specific photon source. Gamma rays (γ-rays) arise from within the nuclei of radioactive atoms, whereas x-rays come from extranuclear sources. In general, γ-rays are emitted from radioactive isotopes as they decay, whereas x-rays are produced "artificially" in high-voltage equipment, via bombardment of a target with high-speed electrons. Otherwise, they share the same physical properties and, if of similar energy, result in identical biologic effects.

Particulate radiation can be charged (electrons, protons, helium ions, carbon ions) or uncharged (neutrons). The charged particles have a defined and finite depth of penetration in matter, determined by their incident energy. This characteristic is exploited clinically to limit dose to the target range, sparing tissues beyond a specified depth. Of these particulate types, only electrons are commonly used in clinical radiotherapy for gynecologic cancers, although proton radiotherapy is an emerging technology that holds promise for ultra-precise delivery of radiation.

Radioactive Decay

Radioactive decay is a phenomenon in which radiation is given off by the nuclei of elements. As previously mentioned, certain combinations of protons and neutrons are less stable than others for a given element, with heavier elements requiring a specific neutron-to-proton ratio greater than 1 (or A:Z > 2) for maximal stability. When the A:Z ratio varies from the explicit baseline (or lowest energy) form, these isotopes (whether naturally occurring or artificially created by bombardment with neutrons in a reactor) are often unstable and seek to return to stability by nuclear disintegrations that result in the emission of ionizing radiation. This process is known as radioactive decay, in which a "parent" radioisotope achieves a more stable form by transforming to a lower energy "daughter" isotope of the same atom (same Z), or even to a completely different element (different Z). In general, the elements with high atomic numbers tend to be "naturally" radioactive, and all elements beyond lead (with a Z of 82) are radioactive, even if the decay rate is so slow as to be undetectable except with the most sophisticated equipment. However, any element, if bombarded with neutrons to perturb its baseline A:Z ratio, can be rendered radioactive, such as tritium (hydrogen 3) or carbon 14.

A common concept used in describing radioactive decay is the half-life ($T_{1/2}$), which is the time required for half the atoms of a specific parent radioisotope to have transformed into its daughter nuclide. The daughter nuclide, in turn, could be stable or remain unstable with further nuclear disintegrations, resulting in its own subsequent $T_{1/2}$ of decay. A related concept is the "activity," or the number of disintegrations per second of a given amount of a specific radioisotope. The greater the activity, the shorter the $T_{1/2}$, as the parent radionuclide is transformed more rapidly. The half-lives of radioisotopes vary tremendously and can range from femtoseconds (10^{-15} seconds) to billions of years.

There are 3 distinct types of radiation emitted by radioactive decay: α-particles, β-particles, and γ-rays. Each nuclear disintegration of a radioisotope can result in the emission of 1 or more of these types of radiation. Alpha decay occurs when the ratio of neutrons to protons is lower than the stable baseline, particularly in radionuclides with atomic numbers above 82. The emitted particle in α decay is a helium nucleus (2 protons and 2 neutrons) with a positive charge. These α-particles are relatively "heavy" and of low kinetic energy, such that their effective range is at most only a few centimeters of air or a few millimeters of tissue. In β decay, a β-particle is emitted; it typically has a negative charge and is also known as an electron. The distance range of electrons from nuclear decay is variable, depending on the kinetic energy with which they are ejected. Sometimes, the β-particle has a positive charge, and is then called a positron. Because positrons are readily attracted to surrounding negatively charged electrons in matter, they travel very short distances (typically < 1 mm) before reacting (or annihilating) with an electron, producing a pair of opposing 511-eV photons that can be detected by specialized scintillators. This forms the basis for positron emission tomography (PET), where fluorine 18, a positron emitter, is used to label glucose uptake in tissues. Finally, γ decay occurs when a nucleus undergoes a transition from a higher to lower energy state and a high-energy photon (or γ-ray) is emitted. The penetration capability of the γ-ray in tissue is dependent on the specific energy of the photon; these γ-rays can be used for diagnostic or therapeutic purposes.

The "hotness" of a radioisotope is a complex function of nuclear activity (disintegrations per second), the type(s) and energy of radiation emitted by that specific isotope, and the distance at which the radioactivity is measured.

Inverse Square Law

The inverse square law is represented as:

$$I \propto 1/d^2$$

where I is the intensity of radiation (or a force such as gravity) and d is the distance from the source of the radiation (or force).

When applied to ionizing radiation, the inverse square law strictly applies only to electromagnetic radiation (not to particulate radiation) and where the origin of radiation is a "relative" point source in relation to the distance at which the radiation is measured. When these conditions are met, it means that an increase in the distance from a radiation source results in a proportionately greater decrease in the radiation exposure. For example, doubling the distance from a radiation point source would result in only one-quarter of the dose at the original distance. When the radiation source is not at a "point" relative to the distance at which dose is measured (eg, when calculating vaginal mucosal and paravaginal doses with brachytherapy using a "line source" in the cylinder), the inverse square law does not hold, and the exposure may then be more proportional to $1/d$. Nonetheless, the impact of distance on dose remains, and this concept is critical in helping design shielding for rooms housing linear accelerators and/or brachytherapy radioisotope sources. It also explains why, when handling radioisotopes, that in addition to shielding, long-handled equipment is used where possible to maximize source distance and minimize dose exposure.

Interaction of Radiation With Matter

Electrons carry a negative charge and have mass. As a result, they rapidly interact with other electrons found in matter, resulting in rapid transfer of energy, ionization of atoms, and a relatively short, finite range (typically up to a few centimeters), depending on the energy of the incident electron.

When photon radiation enters matter, it is possible that it will pass through without interaction, or it may interact in 1 of several ways, including photoelectric effect, Compton effect, and pair production. In clinical radiotherapy, with the contemporary clinical use of high-energy, megavoltage photons, Compton effect is the dominant interaction of ionizing radiation with biologic matter.

In Compton interaction, the photon interacts with an orbital electron, where it provides enough energy to overcome the binding energy of the electron to the nucleus and further transfers additional kinetic energy to the "free" electron, which is then emitted from the atom. The photon is likewise deflected but continues with reduced energy and may react with additional electrons in a similar fashion along its new path, as long as it has sufficient residual energy to overcome the binding energies of other electrons. Figure 19-1 depicts the Compton effect, which thus results in ionization of biologic molecules and the production of fast electrons.

The electrons produced by the Compton effect can also go on to cause further ionization of additional atoms by interacting with other orbital electrons.

Ultimately, the primary basis of ionizing radiation is the production of these free electrons and ions, which are highly reactive and energetic. These ultimately react with important biologic molecules, especially DNA, and result in disruption of vital chemical bonds that may lead to cellular damage and death.

An important consequence of the Compton effect is that its interaction with matter is nearly independent of the atomic number (Z) of the absorbing matter. This is in contrast to the photoelectric effect, which prevails in lower energy photon–matter interactions, where absorption is proportional to Z^3. Diagnostic radiology uses lower energy photons (in the kilovoltage range), where photoelectric effect is significant, such that heavier elements (eg, calcium in bones) absorb much more radiation than soft tissue, giving rise to the characteristic tissue contrasts seen in radiographs. However, for therapeutic radiation, preferential absorption by bone (eg, the pelvic girdle in gynecologic cancers) would be detrimental. The relative independence of radiation absorption with respect to Z for the Compton effect (which predominates in megavoltage radiotherapy) means that although a radiograph taken with higher energy photons has reduced contrast, the absorbed dose is very similar in soft tissue, muscle, fat, and bone and, as such, allows better dose delivery to central pelvic structures.

Units Used in Radiation Oncology

Historically, the unit for radiation exposure has been the roentgen (R), defined as the amount of x-rays or γ-rays required to liberate positive and negative charges of 1 electrostatic unit of charge in 1 cubic centimeter of air. With the advent of Système International d'Unités (SI units), the roentgen is no longer used, and exposure is now expressed as coulomb per kilogram (C/kg), which is equivalent to approximately 3876 R. The SI-based definition for absorbed dose in tissue is measured in joule per kilogram (J/kg), which is also known as gray (Gy). As a unit of energy, 1 J is equal to 6.24×10^{18} eV. *Rad* had previously been used for absorbed dose and was equivalent to 0.01 J/kg. Hence 1 Gy equals 100 rad, and thus, the units centigray (cGy) and rad are often used interchangeably.

For radioisotopes, activity describes the number of disintegrations per unit of time interval. Curie (Ci) had been the historical unit of activity and was based on the number of nuclear events in 1 g of radium 226 (3.7×10^{10} disintegrations per second). Becquerel (Bq) is the SI unit now used for activity and is equal to 1 nuclear disintegration per second of any given radionuclide (1 Ci = 3.7×10^{10} Bq).

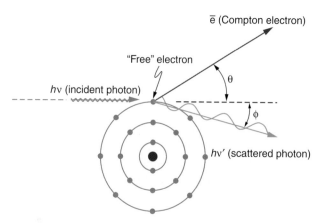

FIGURE 19-1. The Compton effect. (Reproduced, with permission, from Khan FM. *The Physics of Radiation Therapy.* 4th ed. Philadelphia, PA: Lippincott Williams & Wilkins; 2010:60, Figure 5.7.)

RADIATION BIOLOGY

Radiation Damage in Biologic Matter

Radiation biology is the study of the effects of ionizing radiation on biologic systems. The most important biologic effect of radiation appears to result from DNA damage, which can result in genetic mutations, chromosome aberrations, disturbed cell proliferation patterns, cell death, neoplastic transformation, or teratogenesis.

As previously mentioned, when radiation (in particular photons or electrons) enters a biologic system, it results in creation of kinetically energized free electrons (ionization). These electrons ultimately impact the cell by disrupting vital chemical bonds, either directly or indirectly via a cascade of free radical formation.

In direct action, the free electron (eg, produced via Compton effect) itself results in ionization of the nearby DNA strand, thus leading to DNA molecular damage. For x-rays or γ-rays, this accounts for only about one-third of the DNA damage produced. In indirect action, the electron interacts with water molecules (which comprise the vast majority of a cell volume), which become ionized as follows: $H_2O \rightarrow H_2O^+ + e^-$. The H_2O^+ ion radical has a relatively short lifetime, on the order of 10^{-10} seconds, but can react with surrounding water molecules to form additional free radicals ($H_2O^+ + H_2O \rightarrow H_3O^+ + OH\cdot$). These added free radicals, particularly the hydroxyl radical ($OH\cdot$), are highly reactive and have a longer lifetime of about 10^{-5} seconds, so they can diffuse some distance to the DNA and cause damage. Indirect action is estimated to account for two-thirds of the DNA damage produced by x-ray or γ-rays. Because of its "lengthier" course, indirect action is also the component of biologic effect that can be modified by chemical sensitizers and protectors. Figure 19-2 depicts both direct and indirect action of free electrons produced by ionizing radiation. This DNA damage occurs through physical and chemical processes that occur in fractions of seconds. If unrepaired, it then leads to a cascade of biologic events that may take hours, days, months, years, or even generations to be expressed.

Biologic Effects of Radiation: Repair and Cell Death

There is strong laboratory evidence that DNA is the principal target for the biologic effects of ionizing radiation. DNA is a very large and long molecule, which consists of 2 complementary strands of sequential bases held together by an alternating sugar and phosphate "spine," entwined in a double helical structure. Primarily, damage from radiation results in strand breaks in the DNA spine or backbone, although

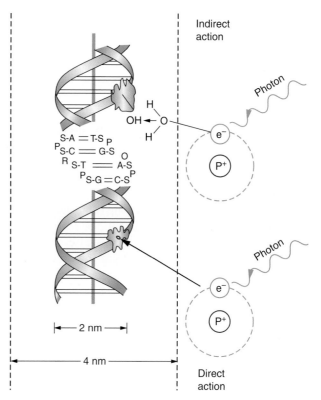

FIGURE 19-2. Direct and indirect action of free electrons created by ionizing radiation. (Reproduced, with permission, from Hall EJ, Giaccia AJ. *Radiobiology for the Radiologist.* 7th ed. Philadelphia, PA: Lippincott Williams & Wilkins; 2012:9, Figure 1.8.)

the induction of abnormal cross-links between DNA strands or between DNA and nuclear proteins can also play a role in the loss of normal replication and transcription. DNA strand breaks can be either single- or double-stranded. Single-stranded breaks are considered of little biologic consequence because they can be repaired readily using the opposite strand as a template, assuming no disruption of normal cellular repair mechanisms. Additionally, breaks in both strands that are well separated in the nucleotide base sequence are also readily repaired as independent breaks. However, DNA strand breaks that are directly opposite one another or separated by only a few base pairs lead to double-strand breaks, which are more difficult or impossible to repair and can result in the separation of the chromatin into 2 or more pieces.

It may be noted that cells are generally very efficient at repair of DNA damage, even with double-strand breaks, using a variety of repair pathways and enzymes. However, a great number of double-strand breaks can overwhelm a cell's repair processes. Individuals with defective DNA repair mechanisms, such as in ataxia telangiectasia, are more vulnerable to the effects of ionizing radiation. Cancer cells themselves often have mutations that can impact their DNA repair pathways; this increased susceptibility to unrepaired DNA double-strand breaks, as compared to normal cells, is one of the factors exploited with radiotherapy.

Unrepaired fragmented chromatin ends may reassort and rejoin other broken ends to give rise to grossly distorted structures or may fail to rejoin, ultimately giving rise to chromosomal aberrations. Several of these aberrations are lethal to cells. Others are not lethal but can lead to carcinogenesis and other mutations.

When exposed to a dose of ionizing radiation, a cell may survive or die. For nonsurviving cells, death while attempting to divide, known as mitotic or reproductive death, is the dominant process. In this case, the unrepaired DNA/chromosome damage in the parent cells does not allow creation of viable progeny cells. Other mechanisms of inactivation include apoptosis or programmed cell death (typically seen in lymphoid cells) and cellular senescence. Nevertheless, the most important end point for radiation-induced lethality is mitotic death, or the cell's loss of reproductive capability. The hallmark of a cancer cell is its immortalization, or the ability to continuously proliferate. Using this definition of cell kill, a tumor cell may remain physically and morphologically intact for some time, but if it ultimately dies at the time of attempted mitosis, it has lost its reproductive integrity and is no longer clonogenic.

Cell death, or conversely, survival, following exposure to ionizing radiation is often described by means of a cell survival curve. For a single cell type population, typically determined in vitro, the cell survival curve is represented on a semi-logarithmic scale, where the x-axis represents radiation dose and the y-axis denotes the log of the proportion of surviving cells (Figure 19-3). This is described as a linear-quadratic model of cell survival. As noted earlier, cell

death is linked to the frequency of unrepaired DNA double-strand breaks and chromosomal aberrations. At very low doses, both strand breaks may be caused by the same electron, in which case the probability of chromosomal disruption and cell death is linearly proportional to the dose. However, at higher doses, the 2 double-strand breaks are more likely to result from 2 separate electrons acting independently and stochastically, in which case the probability of an interaction is proportional to the square of the dose. The linear-quadratic cell survival curve is a simplified but useful model for evaluating radiation effects on proliferating cell systems and is described mathematically as:

$$-\ln S = \alpha D + \beta D^2$$

where S is the surviving fraction of cells, D is the dose of radiation delivered, α is the linear component of ionizing radiation cell kill, and β is the quadratic component of ionizing radiation cell kill.

The α and β values used in the linear-quadratic cell survival curve model vary by cell type and are measures of the DNA repair capacity of that cell. A high α means that for a given dose of radiation, there is less repair compared to cells with a high β. Because these 2 components of repair exist to a variable degree in most cells, this repair capability is often expressed as the ratio α/β. Cellular systems with high α/β ratios have a "steeper" cell survival curve, indicating less repair, and thus greater cell kill, for a given radiation dose than cells with lower α/β ratios. In general, tumors and acute-responding, rapidly cycling normal tissues (eg, hematopoietic cells, skin, hair follicles, and gastrointestinal mucosa) are considered to have high α/β ratios, approximating 10, whereas late-responding normal tissues (eg, visceral parenchyma and stroma) have lower α/β ratios of approximately 3. This difference in α/β ratios, representing the differential repair of tumor and various tissues to the effects of ionizing radiation, is critical and is exploited when using a course of fractionated radiotherapy of multiple lower-dose applications, rather than a single large dose of radiation (Figure 19-4). During fractionated radiotherapy, assuming sufficient time between doses to allow for repair, the initial slope of the cell survival curve is reprised with each subsequent dose of radiation. This allows the relatively small differences in the single-fraction cell survival curves to be magnified over a protracted course of radiation, allowing greater sparing of late-responding, dose-limiting tissues relative to tumor. Although fractionation may provide relatively little sparing of early-responding tissues, acute toxicity in clinical practice is often supported by compensatory proliferation and migration of neighboring cells from outside the radiation field. The linear-quadratic model and α/β ratios can also be used to "convert" one dose fractionation

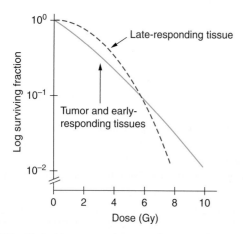

FIGURE 19-3. Linear-quadratic cell survival curves for tumor and early-responding tissues compared to late-responding tissues.

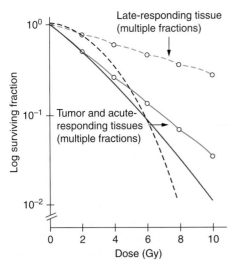

FIGURE 19-4. Effect of dose fractionation on radiation cell survival. As compared with single large doses, fractionation magnifies the difference in survival, or "sparing," of late-reacting normal tissues relative to tumor.

scheme to its biologic equivalent using a different fraction size.

A similar corollary to radiation dose size on cell survival, and the relative sparing impact of fractionation, can be seen for the effect of radiation dose rate (Figure 19-5). This is particularly germane in the use of brachytherapy sources.

Beyond ionization, DNA double-strand breaks, and cellular repair capacity, several other factors impact on the biologic effects of radiation. All proliferating cells, including tumors, travel through the cell cycle, with phases that have been defined as mitosis (M), gap1 (G1), DNA synthesis (S), and gap2 (G2). The nature

of the DNA molecule itself, the presence of cell cycle checkpoints to accommodate repair time, and the relative levels of repair, replicative, and transcriptive enzymes vary during the course of the cell cycle. In general, cells are considered most radiosensitive in M and late G2 phases, but are most resistant during the S phase. The presence of oxygen during radiation has profound impact on the subsequent biologic effects. It has been postulated that oxygen prolongs or perpetuates the free radical process initiated by ionization, leading to an approximately 3-fold increase in radiosensitivity in the presence of oxygen (known as the oxygen enhancement ratio) compared to hypoxic or anoxic conditions. Because many tumors have aberrant vasculature and regions of hypoxia, the study of oxygen effect on ionizing radiation, as well the potential to enhance tumor oxygenation during radiotherapy, has commanded a significant proportion of basic and clinical research efforts over the past few decades.

Much of the biologic effects of ionizing radiation described earlier relate to low linear energy transfer (LET) radiation, which include photons, electrons, and also protons. High-LET radiation, such as neutron and carbon ions, causes very dense ionization trails in biologic matter, which result in decreased DNA repair and reduction of both the cell cycle and oxygen effects. However, the expense, lack of broad clinical benefit, and often unacceptable normal tissue injury (because reduced repair affects both tumor and normal tissues) of high-LET radiation have led to very limited clinical use and applicability.

Genetic Effects of Radiation and Radiation's Impact on the Human Reproductive Process

In distinction to the reproductive or mitotic cell death in *any* tissue that can be induced by ionizing radiation, it also has direct impact on the human reproductive system. These effects can take the form of reduction or ablation of fertility or germline mutations that can be transmitted to future, yet unconceived offspring, or they can affect a developing embryo or fetus in a pregnant woman.

In women, the ovarian dose associated with permanent sterility is age-dependent, reflecting the maximum number of oocytes present at birth (with no further production) and accelerated decrease following the onset of menarche. In the prepubertal female, a radiation dose of 12 Gy or more is generally required to cause sterility, whereas a dose of only 2 Gy may cause the same consequence in a premenopausal woman. Unlike in men, ovarian gonadal function is tightly linked to hormonal production, such that the same doses that cause permanent sterility also result in menopause.

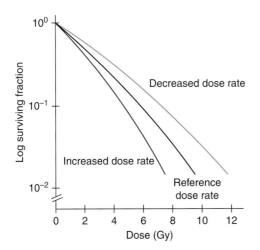

FIGURE 19-5. Effect of dose rate on radiation cell survival. For a given dose, a higher dose rate results in greater cell kill than lower dose rates.

If the female is not rendered infertile, radiation can cause nonlethal damage and mutations in oocyte DNA that may be inherited by subsequent generations, resulting in heritable, or genetic, diseases in offspring. It is important to remember that genetic mutations occur with some baseline frequency in the general population, independent of any radiation, and that not all mutations result in clinically apparent disease. Ionizing radiation does not result in unique or bizarre heritable diseases, but rather increases the frequencies of the same genetic mutations that already occur spontaneously. Hereditary diseases can be classified as single gene–based (eg, Huntington chorea and sickle cell anemia), chromosomal (eg, Down syndrome), or multifactorial (eg, neural tube defects, cleft lip). Information on the added hereditary effects of radiation exposure comes almost entirely from animal experiments; based on mouse data, the dose required to double the spontaneous germ cell mutation rate is approximately 1 Gy (100 cGy).[1]

The effect on ionizing radiation on an existing embryo or fetus depends on its gestational stage. In the first week to 10 days following fertilization and zygote formation (preimplantation phase), doses as low as 10 cGy can result in loss of the embryo. However, if the embryo survives, it may then develop normally, with few consequences (hence termed an "all-or-nothing" effect). Radiation exposure during the period of organogenesis, from approximately weeks 2 to 6, results in the highest likelihood of congenital malformations (teratogenesis), neonatal death, and growth retardation. After approximately week 6 (fetal stage of gestation), radiation can lead to permanent growth retardation and also mental retardation, as the central nervous system matures later in utero. Although the effect of radiation on the embryo and fetus is dose dependent, there is *no threshold dose* below which ionizing radiation can be stated to have no impact. Thus, the use of medical radiation in a pregnant patient should be avoided whenever possible or, if absolutely required, be given only after a full discussion of risk and informed consent. Although controversial, it has been suggested that 10-cGy in utero exposure, at least during the early first trimester, be used at the cutoff point beyond which a therapeutic termination of pregnancy should be considered.

Beyond 20 to 25 weeks (third trimester), low doses of radiation to the fetus may be "relatively" safe, although some have reported an increase in childhood malignancies. Obviously, pelvic or abdominal radiotherapy, as is used in gynecologic cancers, results in an unacceptably high dose to the fetus and would be associated with spontaneous abortion or require an evacuation. However, there are many case reports and small series of successful and healthy infant deliveries following radiotherapy to other sites during late pregnancy (eg, for breast cancer or supradiaphragmatic lymphomas). Careful blocking and patient set-up to limit scatter dose to the uterus, medical physics consult to optimize shielding and dose monitoring, and patient informed consent are clearly required.

Radiation-Induced Malignancies

Ionizing radiation has been shown to cause an increased risk of both solid tumors and hematologic malignancies. The induction of secondary cancer is considered to be a stochastic effect, that is, the probably of occurrence increases with dose, but there is no threshold dose, and the severity of the malignancy, once induced, is independent of the dose. The risk is also age dependent; younger patients may have developing tissues that are more susceptible to radiation carcinogenesis and may have a longer life span in which to manifest the secondary malignancy. There is often a long interval between exposure to radiation and the appearance of the induced malignancy. The shortest latencies are seen in leukemias, which may occur 5 to 7 years after radiation, whereas secondary solid cancers may take 10 to 40 years or more to develop. Radiation-induced malignancies also tend to appear at the same age as spontaneous malignancies of the same type.

Risk estimates of secondary malignancy after therapeutic radiation are somewhat controversial because patients undergoing radiation are often already at a higher risk of developing a second cancer based on lifestyle and/or genetic predisposition. However, studies do indicate that there is an increased risk of radiation-induced malignancies in cancer patients, regardless of underlying biases. Fortunately, the absolute risk of secondary malignancy induction by ionizing radiation is very low. In a recent large-population analysis of more than 485,000 irradiated patient survivors from the US Surveillance, Epidemiology, and End Results (SEER) database, it was estimated that therapeutic radiation resulted in a risk of 3 and 5 excess cancers per 1000 individuals at 10 and 15 years, respectively, after diagnosis and treatment. Germane to the field of gynecologic oncology, radiotherapy did result in a small risk of induced secondary malignancies in patients treated for cervical cancer (hazard ratio [HR], 1.34) and endometrial cancer (HR, 1.14), but this risk disappeared in patients radiated when they were 60 years of age or older.[2]

RADIATION INSTRUMENTATION

Cobalt Units

Up to about 1950, most external beam radiation was primarily carried out with x-rays generated from kilovoltage machines. These low-energy x-rays suffered from poor penetration for deeply seated tumors and resulted in excess dose deposit on the skin surface, as well as in bones (high photoelectric component of photon interaction). Indeed, skin toxicity was often the limiting factor in delivering adequate doses of kilovoltage therapeutic radiation.

The introduction of cobalt 60 (^{60}Co) therapy units in the 1950s represented a big step forward in radiation oncology. ^{60}Co, a radioactive isotope that is artificially created by neutron bombardment of the stable cobalt 59 in a reactor, undergoes nuclear decay with the emission of 2 clinically useful γ-rays of 1.17 MeV and 1.33 MeV and a half-life of 5.3 years. ^{60}Co radiotherapy units allowed the first routine use of megavoltage photons, with improved depth dose penetration, skin sparing, and abrogation of excessive bone absorption (via high-energy Compton effect). Other advantages of the ^{60}Co units were the relatively constant beam output, lack of day-to-day output fluctuations, well-defined half-life allowing for predictable decay, and introduction of an isocentric gantry system, in which the radiation source rotated about a stationary patient. However, the quest for even higher energy photons, the poor dose homogeneity for large fields, the need to replace the radioactive ^{60}Co isotope every 4 to 5 years, strict Nuclear Regulatory Commission requirements for shielding and securing of a source that cannot be "turned off," and costly licensing fees have led to its widespread replacement by linear accelerators (at least in developed countries) over the past 2 to 3 decades.

Linear Accelerators

The linear accelerator (linac) has now become the dominant radiotherapy treatment unit (Figure 19-6). It is a megavoltage machine and uses high-frequency electromagnetic waves to accelerate electrons to high energies through a linear tube, with the electron energy determined by the strength of the accelerating electromagnetic field. The units used to determine the energy of the produced radiation are MeV for electrons and MV for photons—both units refer to the millions of volts in electrical potential difference that is created for electron acceleration in a linac. The accelerated high-energy electron beam can be used by itself for treating superficial tumors, or it can be made to strike a metal target (typically tungsten), within the accelerator head, to produce x-rays for treating deeper tumors. This type of machine is often referred to as a multimodal linac because it can provide multiple electron beam energies (6-25 MeV), as well as 2 or 3 x-ray energies (6, 10, and 18 MV). The effective source of radiation in a linac is mounted on a gantry and can rotate 360° around a stationary patient. The point around which the gantry rotates is called the isocenter. It is typically sited in a patient within a tumor volume so that the target can be readily radiated from multiple different directions.

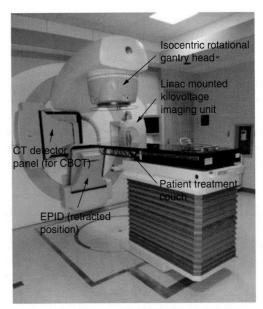

FIGURE 19-6. A contemporary linear accelerator (linac). Note that the gantry is mounted on a rotational mechanism that allows it to completely rotate about an isocentric point. Opposing the gantry is the electronic portal imaging device (EPID), which allows capture of digital radiographic portal images, predominantly emphasizing bony anatomical landmarks. Perpendicular to the gantry/EPID axis is a computed tomography (CT) imager and detector set, which allows for 3-dimensional cone beam CT (CBCT) of specified soft tissue targets for enhanced image-guided radiotherapy.

Within the accelerator tube, electrons are accelerated to extremely high speeds (and energies) via an electromagnetic microwave field. As the high-energy electrons emerge from the accelerator structure, they are monoenergetic and in the form of a pencil beam of about 3 mm in diameter. To produce x-rays, which are the most commonly used form of ionizing radiation, the electrons are directed toward a water-cooled metal target, typically consisting of tungsten. As the electrons "crash into" the tungsten target, they lose energy, resulting in the production of a spectrum of x-rays with a range of different energies, but with the maximum photon energy equal to the incident electron energy. These x-rays are typically referred to as Bremsstralung radiation, which results from the "braking," or rapid deceleration, of the high-energy electrons on encountering the metal target. The *average* photon energy of the beam thus created is approximately one-third of the monoenergetic incident electron energy. Photon energy is designated as MV because of its heterogeneous energy; the MV refers to the *maximum* photon energy. If electrons, rather than x-rays, are selected for clinical use, the tungsten target of the linac is withdrawn. Instead, as the thin electron beam exits the accelerator structure, it is made to strike a scattering foil to widen the beam to a clinically useful dimension and to get a uniform electron fluence across the treatment field. Electron beam energy is designated by MeV because it is monoenergetic.[3]

The treatment head of a linac also contains the collimation (or aperture) system for defining, or "shaping," the radiation beam. The primary collimator is created by pairs of heavy metal jaws (or blocks) that move in perpendicular directions, thus determining the length and width of the radiation field. Previously, secondary collimation to further shape the radiation beam into asymmetric shapes was achieved by poured blocks that were then mounted on the outside of the gantry head. New linacs have built-in secondary collimation that consists of multiple thin leaves, which can be designed to achieve the desired geometry of almost any radiation field shape. This system of multiple-leaf collimators (MLCs) now allows near-infinite computer-assigned positions that can remain static during a radiation exposure or can change shape in real time and, when coordinated with gantry and patient couch rotations, produce highly dynamic, conformal dose delivery such as with intensity-modulated radiation therapy techniques.

Simulators

A treatment simulator is an apparatus that uses diagnostic x-rays to display the treatment fields so that the target volume may be appropriately encompassed without delivering excessive radiation to the surrounding normal tissues. It duplicates the physical set-up characteristics of the linac itself, in terms of isocentricity and the ability to recreate patient and treatment machine alignments. Historically, simulators were based on fluoroscopic units, with plain radiographs obtained of the region to be treated. Areas to be avoided were then defined on the 2-dimensional films, which were then used as a template for cut blocks to shape the radiation beam. Today, computed tomography (CT) scans have almost completely replaced fluoroscopic simulators in developed countries. CT simulation allows the capture of more anatomic information and creation of 3-dimensional volumes that can be used to refine tumor coverage and normal tissue shielding.

Radiation Implants/Radioisotopes

Treatment of gynecologic cancer with radioactive material inserted against, or into, the tumor, has been used effectively for many decades. With rare exceptions, the radiation sources are not placed directly into the patient, but rather are contained indirectly within hollow, specialized applicators that are positioned within the target volume. Early applicators were preloaded with the radiation sources and were thus inserted "hot" into the patient, raising concerns for operator safety. Today, all gynecologic applicators are first inserted without radioactivity, allowing the clinician to take time to achieve optimal geometrical positioning. These hollow applicators are then "afterloaded" with the appropriate radioisotope, either manually (using long-handled equipment) or, increasingly, remotely by specialized machines.

The original radiation source used for gynecologic implants was radium 226 (^{226}Ra). ^{226}Ra itself does not produce any γ-rays appropriate for treatment. However, ^{226}Ra undergoes nuclear decay and transforms into radon gas (radon 222 [^{222}Rn]). The daughter products of the ^{222}Rn actually produce the higher energy γ-rays necessary for effective treatment. Due to these properties, the radium, along with the radon, had to be encapsulated and sealed to produce a suitable brachytherapy source. ^{226}Ra is a rare, naturally occurring isotope with an extremely long half-life. Several tons of ore material have to be refined to obtain enough ^{226}Ra for a single clinically useful source.

The typical activity for a ^{226}Ra source is 10 to 20 mCi. This corresponds to a mass of 10 to 20 mg of radium by definition (because 1 Ci is defined as the activity, or number of disintegrations per second, of 1 g of ^{226}Ra). Most treatments used between 2 and 5 sources, lasted about 48 hours, and were defined as low dose rate (LDR) brachytherapy. These ^{226}Ra sources had to be hand loaded into the applicators, and the patient was confined to bed during the entire treatment.

Much of our understanding regarding radiation implants, from applicator geometry, dose and dose rate, tumor control probably, and normal tissue tolerance, is based on the historical use of ^{226}Ra. However, the hazards of securing ^{226}Ra and ^{222}Rn and the disastrous consequences if the integrity of a source capsule is compromised became large-scale problems for institutions and regulators. Other radioisotopes were investigated as replacements, but with the intention of mimicking the geometry and dose distribution of ^{226}Ra. With the advent of nuclear reactors, a good clinical substitute was found in cesium 137 (^{137}Cs). This was a readily available reactor by-product refined from spent fuel rods. The sealed ^{137}Cs sources, without a gaseous daughter molecule, were much safer than the ^{226}Ra capsules. To recapitulate the size, shape, and activity of the ^{226}Ra sources, ^{137}Cs sources were calibrated in milligram-Ra-equivalent units (mgRaEq). For example, a 20-mgRaEq ^{137}Cs source did not specifically detail the amount of ^{137}Cs itself in the source; it was simply the amount of ^{137}Cs that gave the same amount of dose and activity, at a specified distance, as the previously used ^{226}Ra source. Because the size, shape, and activity of the ^{137}Cs sources reprised those of its corresponding ^{226}Ra capsule, the applicators generally were unchanged, and source loading and duration of treatment remained the same (ie, continued LDR brachytherapy).

The ^{137}Cs supply has now become increasingly restricted due to decreased reactor production. Additionally, techniques have been developed, using remote afterloading equipment, to effectively treat patients in a much shorter time, removing the necessity of a prolonged hospital stay. This required a very high activity source and a shielded procedure suite. This method of implant radiation delivery has become known as high dose rate (HDR) brachytherapy. The source developed for HDR brachytherapy was iridium 192 (^{192}Ir). ^{192}Ir is activated inside a nuclear reactor, without having to disturb the fuel core or spent fuel rods. To accommodate outpatient-based HDR brachytherapy, a source would have to be highly radioactive, as well as suitably small, such that it could fit in small-diameter tubes. This combination of source attributes is defined by an isotope's specific activity, which is the maximum achievable activity of an isotope per gram of material. The specific activity of ^{192}Ir is 100 and 10,000 times that of ^{226}Ra and ^{137}Cs, respectively, allowing it to have a very compact size while maintaining high activity. For HDR brachytherapy delivery, the ^{192}Ir source activity typically ranges between 4 and 10 Ci. For this activity range, ^{226}Ra or ^{137}Cs sources would have to be the size of grapes or larger, but ^{192}Ir, with its high specific activity, can be constructed into sources that measure 4 to 5 mm in length and < 1 mm in width, making it eminently suitable for HDR systems. A comparison of the physical properties of the 3 radioisotopes historically and currently used for gynecologic brachytherapy is provided in Table 19-1.

In addition to the sealed radiation material discussed earlier, "unsealed" radioisotopes may also be injected parenterally into a patient, with resulting large-volume or whole-body distribution. Of these, phosphorus 32 (typical dose of 15 mCi) was previously used intraperitoneally in the treatment of ovarian and endometrial cancer but has now lost favor secondary to high toxicity and questionable efficacy. Other current systemically administered unsealed radioisotopes include iodine 131 for thyroid cancer and strontium 89 for diffuse bone metastases.

CLINICAL RADIOTHERAPY CONSIDERATIONS: DOSE RESPONSE AND MODIFIERS OF DOSE EFFECT

Radiation Dose Response and the Therapeutic Ratio

The goal of therapeutic radiation is to maximize locoregional tumor control, while minimizing injury to surrounding normal structures. It has been previously discussed that increased doses of ionizing radiation cause increased DNA damage, and corresponding cell death, in both tumors and normal tissues. However, this relatively straightforward laboratory description of radiation effects on isolated cell populations does not take into account that in clinical radiotherapy, the ultimate impact on tumor and normal tissues is influenced by complex interactions among multiple cell types in both cancer and surrounding stroma, as well as volumetric and patient-specific considerations (see later section, Radiation Toxicity).

A useful clinical concept that guides the application of radiotherapy is the dose-response curve. This is an overall function that implicates the probabilistic impact of radiation dose on tumor control probability, as well as on normal tissue injury (Figure 19-7). In general, this function follows a sigmoid-shaped curve. There are 3 components to this curve: (1) a minimal dose below which radiation is "wasted," with no chance of tumor effect; (2) a steep portion of the curve where an increase in dose is associated with a significant increase in tumor response; and (3) a plateau region where further escalation in dose would result in little incremental tumor control probability. Note that the x-axis does not specify actual doses; it is the relative dose that matters

Table 19-1 Properties of Brachytherapy Isotopes Used in Gynecologic Cancer

Isotope	Half-Life	Average Energy (keV)	Half Value Layer (mm lead)	Typical Activity (mCi)	Density (g/mL)	Specific Activity (mCi/g)	Typical Clinical Size of Isotope Source
Radium 226	1622 years	830	8	20	5.50	9.75E + 02	22 mm × 3 mm cylinder
Cesium 137	30 years	662	5.5	50	1.87	8.70E + 04	22 mm × 3 mm cylinder
Iridium 192	74 days	380	4.5	10,000	22.40	9.19E + 06	5 mm × 0.6 mm cylinder

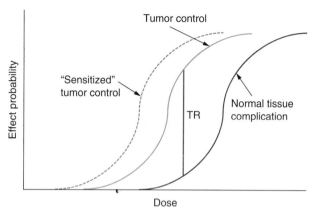

FIGURE 19-7. Dose-response curves for control of tumor and late-reacting normal tissues. The therapeutic ratio (TR) is defined as the probability of tumor control achieved, for a specified dose, for a given incidence of normal tissue damage. Sensitization of tumor to radiotherapy results in a "leftward" shift of the tumor control curve and increases the TR, as long as the normal tissue dose-response curve is not likewise shifted or is shifted to a lesser degree.

in this simplified concept. Actual doses will depend on the tumor type (intrinsic radiosensitivity), tumor volume, and the outcome being measure (long-term control and cure vs. palliative effect). Likewise, a similar sigmoid curve describes the risk of normal tissue injury. Empirically, the normal tissue injury dose-response curve often "sits to the right" of the tumor control curve, indicating that in many situations, a therapeutic benefit can be achieved at a correspondingly "lower risk" of complications. This difference, which forms the basis for clinical radiotherapy, is expressed as the therapeutic ratio (or index), defined as the probability of tumor control achieved for a specified dose, for a given incidence of normal tissue damage.

Much clinical effort has focused on improving the therapeutic ratio, in essence by separating the curves further apart. As noted previously, one approach is to optimize radiation fractionation to exploit the relatively small differences in radiation repair between cancer cells and late-responding normal tissues. Decades of clinical experience have established that, for most tumor systems, a fractionated dose of 1.8 to 2 Gy/d is feasible and effective for tumor control and normal tissue recovery, without the hazard of further prolonging treatment duration if smaller fraction sizes are used. However, other means of modifying the therapeutic ratio, both physically and biochemically, have been tried.

Physical Modifiers of Dose Response: The Impact of Surgery

Radiation is often combined with surgery in the treatment of gynecology cancers. Examples include radiotherapy following hysterectomy for cervical or endometrial cancers and wide local resection and inguinofemoral node dissection for vulvar cancer. By removing the bulk of tumor, the dose of radiation to achieve tumor control may be reduced in the adjuvant setting, in effect shifting the tumor dose-response curve to the left. Furthermore, susceptible normal tissues may be displaced (such as with transposition of the ovaries outside the radiation field). There are 2 caveats to this role of surgery. First, cell survival following radiation exposure is based on a logarithmic basis, and it has been estimated that a dose of approximate 6 to 7 Gy is required to achieve 1 log of clonogenic cell kill in a typical epithelial cancer. Hence, subtotal resection of a tumor (eg, of 50%-80%), or the presence of grossly positive margins, does not significantly impact on the dose of radiation required to maximize tumor control. Using this logic, it may be argued that surgery should remove at least 1.5 to 2 logs of existent tumor cells, or at least 95% to 99% of all disease, to meaningfully reduce the subsequent radiation dose prescribed. Second, surgery may itself cause injury to adjacent normal tissues or displace more normal tissue into the radiation volume (eg, adhesions and/or increased small bowel in the pelvis following hysterectomy), so that the normal tissue damage curve is also shifted leftward, indicating increased risk of late complications. Therefore, careful assessment of patient and tumor characteristics should be undertaken when integrating surgery and radiotherapy in clinical management.

Chemical Modifiers of Radiation Response and the Role of Chemotherapy

The historical definition of a radiosensitizer is that of a compound that in and of itself has little or no direct effect on tumor cells but, when combined with ionizing radiation, significantly enhances the lethality of the radiation. In the laboratory, oxygen is the archetypal radiosensitizer; it is a simple, widely available substance, and the presence of oxygen reduces the dose of radiation required to achieve a specified level of cell kill by approximately 3-fold compared to a hypoxic cell populations (sensitization ratio, or oxygen enhancement ratio, of 3). It was historically thought that the oxygen effect was mediated via promulgation of free radicals initiated by ionizing radiation, based on the affinity of oxygen to accept free electrons and thus contribute to the oxidative process. It was also shown that multiple experimental and human tumors had hypoxic elements, either due to aberrant vasculature or other factors, and this was felt to contribute to clinical radioresistance. In this scenario, molecular oxygen, or a chemical substitute, had to be present exactly at the time of radiation to interact with the free radicals formed. Multiple approaches at radiosensitization by trying to overcome hypoxia were developed in the laboratory and extended to clinical trials over the past 4 decades, including the use of hyperbaric oxygen, red cell enhancement by transfusion and erythropoietin administration, and the use of hypoxic cell radiosensitizers (chemicals that mimic the chemistry of oxygen by having high electron affinity), but unfortunately, these have overall not been found effective. More recent information indicates that the impact of hypoxia in tumor biology and radiation resistance is highly complex. In addition to its acute effect on free radical reactions during radiation, hypoxia induces other biochemical changes (eg, increased vascular endothelial growth factor production and induction of hypoxia-inducible factor) that create a cascade of downstream effects that lead to increased tumor aggressiveness and metastatic potential, regardless of whether the inciting hypoxic environment is subsequently corrected.

More recent attempts at radiosensitization have focused on the use of cytotoxic chemotherapy agents concurrent with radiotherapy. The initial rationale for combining radiation and chemotherapy was based on the concept of "spatial cooperation," where the drug and the ionizing radiation acted independently. This notion recognized that radiation could provide local control, but chemotherapy might address micrometastases not targeted by radiation. In this construct, the impact of chemotherapy and radiation on the local tumor was additive (ie, overall tumor kill was the sum of the effect of the individual modalities of chemotherapy and radiation).

More recent clinical efforts have focused on the potential synergistic interactions between chemotherapy and radiation. Although both modalities retain their independent influence, certain chemotherapeutic agents demonstrate a synergistic, or supra-additive, effect on local tumor control when combined with radiotherapy. This synergism results in tumor control rates that are higher than would be expected from the sum of the effect of each modality if used alone. The specific mechanisms for this interaction are complex and myriad, but they broadly relate to chemotherapy inhibition of repair following DNA damage induced by ionizing radiation. This has now led to the adoption of the term "chemosensitization" when discussing the integrated effects of concurrent chemotherapy and radiation.

For gynecologic cancers, the prototype drug used for chemosensitization is cisplatin. Cisplatin-based chemoradiation has become the standard of care in the management of advanced cervical cancer and has also been used in vulvar and endometrial cancers. Other chemotherapy agents that have shown benefit in combined-modality approaches include carboplatin, 5 fluorouracil, paclitaxel, and gemcitabine. Although the synergistic aspects of these drugs with radiation are clear, it is noteworthy to remember that spatial cooperation may remain an important component (especially in management of micrometastatic disease), because these are also generally the most active cytotoxic agents in gynecologic cancers.

Accelerated Repopulation and Its Detrimental Impact on Prolonged Duration of Radiation

Within a tumor, a variable proportion of the clonogenic cells exist in a rest, or G0, stage. Studies have indicated that during a course of radiation, many of these cells are recruited into the active cell cycle, causing accelerated repopulation of the cancer. This leads to an increased growth fraction of cycling clonogenic cells, which may occur even as the tumor is grossly shrinking. If the treatment ultimately fails to eradicate the clonogenic cells, then tumor persistence, or recurrence, occurs.

The phenomenon of accelerated repopulation implies that radiation, once started, should be completed as expeditiously as possible, with no elective treatment breaks. For example, in locally advanced cervical cancer, which arguably represents the most aggressive/complex use of radiotherapy for a gynecologic malignancy, the recommendation is for completion of all radiation in 8 weeks. The use of concurrent cisplatin-based chemotherapy is indicated during radiation, but care should be taken to monitor and mitigate acute combined-modality effects (including aggressive supportive care) such that treatment breaks for toxicities are avoided or minimized.

TECHNICAL ASPECTS OF RADIOTHERAPY

Teletherapy

Teletherapy (*tele* meaning from afar, Greek origin) is radiation delivered from a distance beyond the body (whether from a linac or a radioisotope such as ^{60}Co) and is now more commonly termed external beam radiotherapy (EBRT). The most common forms of EBRT used are photons, for deep structures within the body, and electrons, for superficial regions that do not extend more than a few centimeters below the skin surface (eg, superficial groin nodes).

For practical purposes, a linac radiation source may be considered a "point source," as the tungsten target used for producing x-rays is only a few millimeters in size, while the patient is treated, typically, at an isocentric distance of 100 cm. The most direct component of the radiation beam, which exits the source with 0° of deviation and usually reaches the patient at the shortest, perpendicular distance, is known as the central axis, or central ray. Within a radiation field, other portions of the beam diverge from this central axis, with the angle of divergence increasing as the field dimensions are increased.

Any given single beam of external radiation has an identifiable distribution pattern, known as the percent depth dose (PDD) characteristic, or beam profile. This is dependent on the type of radiation (clinically speaking, either photons or electrons), energy of the beam, size of the radiation field, and specific features of the linac that produces the beam. Therefore, these beam characteristics have to be individually measured for each energy, and varying field sizes, for each linac. The PDD of a beam describes the sequential decrease in measured doses at greater depths in tissue, as a result of both the inverse square law (increased distance from the radiation source) and, more importantly, absorption of some of the radiation itself by more superficial layers of tissue (known as attenuation). This PDD characteristic is determined along the central axis of the beam and is usually characterized by absorption in water, which accounts for the overwhelming proportion of human tissue composition. Examples of PDD curves for photons and electrons are shown in Figures 19-8 and 19-9. There are 3 notable features of the PDD curves: (1) the depth of penetration of a beam increases with energy; (2) electrons have a finite depth of dose deposition, whereas photons technically have infinite, but constantly decreasing, depth dose distribution; and (3) higher energy photons show increasing skin and superficial dose sparing. Rudimentary calculations of dose may be accomplished "by hand" from these depth dose distribution curves and measured patient parameters, as was done historically, but this was confined to dose along the central axis, with limited accounting for "off-axis" structures or correction

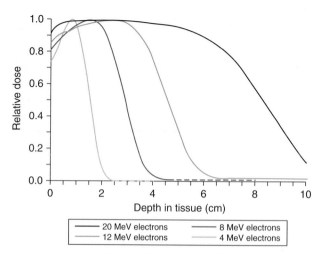

FIGURE 19-9. Percent depth dose curves for electrons of different energies. As opposed to photons, electrons have a relatively finite, and short, range in tissue.

for tissues of nonwater density. In treatment of gynecologic cancers, single photon beams are rarely used. Although high-energy photons have deep tissue penetration, multiple beams are required to appropriately concentrate dose to deep pelvic tumors without overdoing more superficial structures.

To more fully describe beam characteristics within a 3-dimensional (3D) volume, isodose curves are now used, which describe dose distribution at multiple points and depths within the total path of the beam (as opposed to just the central axis), and include the effect of beam divergence and corresponding scatter. The isodose characteristics for each beam are programmed into the dosimetry computer. Contemporary dosimetric planning allows the calculation of 3D dose distribution, integrating the contribution of multiple radiation beams (which may be of differing energies, fields sizes, and angles), when matched to anatomic structures and densities from the treatment planning CT, to create composite isodose distribution within a specified volume (see later section, Dosimetry).

EBRT allows for homogenous dose coverage of large target volumes. In practice, it is used when the volume of disease is diffuse and cannot be covered by brachytherapy alone. This would include nodal groups deemed at risk, as well as bulky primary tumors. For nodal coverage, EBRT can be extended beyond a standard pelvic volume (extended-field radiation) in patients with known extrapelvic retroperitoneal metastases or in patients with multiple pelvic nodes who are felt to be at high risk of harboring occult para-aortic disease. Although providing the widest coverage, a potential downside of EBRT is that all structures within the high-dose radiation volume, including normal tissues, receive essentially the same prescribed dose.

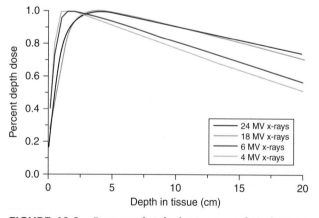

FIGURE 19-8. Percent depth dose curves for photons of different energies. Note the greater depth penetration and associated increased skin and superficial sparing with higher energy photons.

The challenge with EBRT is to precisely determine the volume at risk, so that as much normal tissue as possible can be excluded, or shielded. In the management of intact, locally advanced cervical cancer, a key role of EBRT is to shrink the primary lesion to such as size where it can be adequately encompassed by brachytherapy dosing. Other gynecologic sties may not be as amenable to brachytherapy, such as locally advanced vulvar primaries. In this situation, escalation of EBRT may be required to achieve optimal local control, but the volume of irradiated tissue needs to be carefully assessed. To avoid unacceptable normal tissue injury, the volume taken to increasingly high doses must be carefully minimized; this can be accomplished through a technique known as "sequential shrinking field boosts," whereby the external beam fields are decreased in size as the primary tumor regresses.

Brachytherapy

Brachytherapy (*brachy* meaning from a short distance, Greek root) is a term that has persisted in common clinical use and refers to radiation delivered from sealed radioactive sources placed on or within a patient's body. In the treatment of gynecologic cancers, this is synonymous with "internal radiation." Brachytherapy allows a high dose of radiation to be delivered locally (to the implanted or juxtaposed target volume), with rapid dose fall-off with small increases in distance. Unlike EBRT, brachytherapy dose distribution is inherently nonhomogenous within a given volume or target, but this rapid decrement in dose, or inhomogeneity, is exploited to escalate central dose while sparing nearby normal tissues.

As noted earlier, brachytherapy now involves the use of specialized applicators placed within a patient, which are then afterloaded, either manually or remotely, with the radiation source(s). The majority of brachytherapy procedures for gynecologic cancers are intracavitary, which means that the applicator is placed within an existing body space, such as the uterine cavity, endocervical canal, or vaginal tract (Figures 19-10 to 19-12). In rare instances where the tumor geometry is bulky, distorted, or asymmetrically oriented with respect to the central pelvis, especially in a posthysterectomy patient, an interstitial approach, where applicator needles are pierced into tumor stroma or connective tissue, may be required (Figure 19-13).

Historically, brachytherapy was performed using LDR exposure, with typical dose rates of 0.4 to 2.0 Gy/h to a selected point or volume. Treatment times for LDR brachytherapy range from 1 to 4 days and require the patient to be hospitalized and bed-bound for the entire duration. In the past 2 decades, HDR brachytherapy has gained widespread use in gynecologic and other cancers. With dose rates exceeding 12 Gy/h and

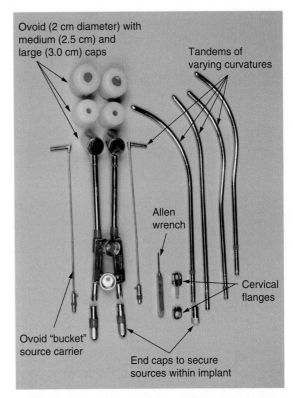

FIGURE 19-10. Components of a low dose rate, manually afterloaded Fletcher-Suit tandem and ovoids set, used for brachytherapy in intact cervical cancer. To accommodate variable tumor and patient geometry, tandems of variable angles and ovoid caps of different sizes are provided.

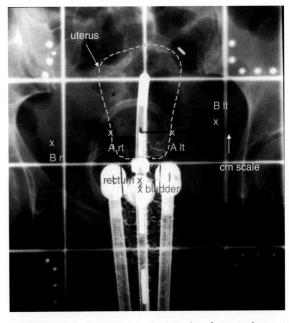

FIGURE 19-11. Anterior radiograph of a tandem and ovoids implant within a patient. The approximate position of the uterus is illustrated. Dose points corresponding to points A, points B, and bladder and rectum are defined.

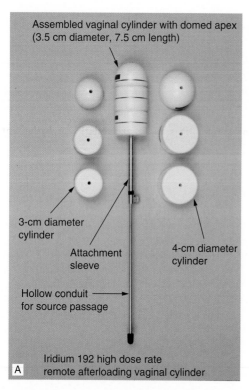
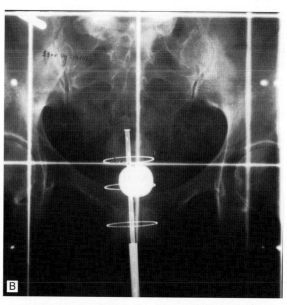

FIGURE 19-12. Vaginal cylinder applicator. A. Assembled high dose rate vaginal cylinder, with cylinder segments of varying diameters selected clinically. **B.** Radiograph of vaginal cylinder placement within a patient for adjuvant therapy of the vaginal cuff following hysterectomy for early-stage endometrial cancer.

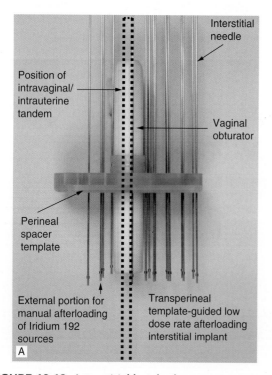
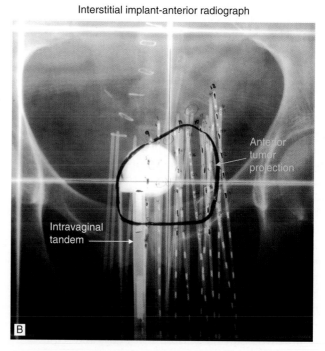

FIGURE 19-13. Interstitial brachytherapy apparatus. A. Perineal template-guided interstitial needles, combined with a central vaginal obturator/tandem. **B.** Radiograph of a manually afterloaded, low dose rate interstitial implant in a posthysterectomy patient with bulky vaginal canal tumor recurrence. The volume of intended tumor coverage is emphasized on the image.

radiation exposure times of only a few minutes, HDR brachytherapy can be performed in an outpatient setting and holds the promise of greater patient comfort, avoidance of prolonged bed rest, and possible better implant stability and reproducibility compared to protracted LDR exposures. Initial concerns were raised over the potential radiobiologic disadvantages of HDR brachytherapy (specifically in relation to normal tissue injury, because higher dose rates of radiation allow less cellular repair; see Figure 19-5). However, broad clinical experience and 4 randomized trials in intact cervical cancer have not substantiated this fear, and it is now generally accepted that HDR brachytherapy, when performed with care, proper fractionation, and technical attention to details, is a safe and effective alternative to traditional LDR approaches. An example of HDR intrauterine brachytherapy, using a tandem and ring applicator, with 3D dosimetry planning is illustrated in Figure 19-14.

Recognizing that historical understanding of tumor dose response and normal tissue injury risk are based on LDR experience, recommendations in textbooks and published guidelines continue to use LDR-based doses. Because HDR dose rates are intrinsically more biologically effective, it would be a mistake to apply these LDR-based dose guidelines to HDR brachytherapy without an appropriate dose modification. This conversion, from an HDR dose to an "LDR-equivalent" dose, or vice versa, can be achieved using a modification of the linear-quadratic equation previously discussed:

$$\text{BED} = \text{Total dose } [1 + \text{dose per fraction}/\alpha/\beta]$$

where BED is the biologically effective dose and α/β is the measure of cellular radiation repair (~10 for tumor and acute-responding normal tissue and ~3 for late-responding normal tissues).

Brachytherapy may be used by itself, independent of any EBRT, for management of gynecologic cancer. The most common example is when vaginal brachytherapy alone is given to reduce the risk of isolated cuff failures following hysterectomy for endometrial cancer. Additionally, tandem-based brachytherapy is sometimes used alone to treat nonoperable patients with small, very early stage cervical cancer.

Brachytherapy, combined with EBRT, is considered a critical component of radiation for locally advanced, intact cervical cancer. Historically, and persisting to today, brachytherapy dose is specified using the point A system. Point A identifies a paracervical location 2 cm superior and 2 cm lateral to the external cervical os, along the axis of the intrauterine tandem (Figure 19-15). In a highly simplified way, the dose at point A serves as a surrogate for minimal lateral dose to a cervix of no more than 4 cm in diameter. Point B identifies a lateral parametrial location, defined as 2 cm superior to the external os and 5 cm lateral to the midline of the patient. Specific designations for representative rectal and bladder dose points have also been developed by international consensus.

Although much has been made about the specific technique and system of brachytherapy for intact cervical cancer, it can be argued that *whether* intracavitary brachytherapy is used may be just as important, or even more so, than *how* it is placed. What is clear is that the introduction of radioactive sources into the endocervical and endometrial canal permits a central tumor dose intensification that is unachievable by any EBRT technique, regardless of the nuances of source placement (Figure 19-16). It is this very high radiation dose, placed in direct juxtaposition to tumor, within a radiation-tolerant organ, that allows for control of even large cervical cancers.

The dose distribution from a typical intracavitary implant for cervical cancer is centrally symmetrical and classically described as "pear-shaped." Recent efforts in image-guided brachytherapy, in particular using magnetic resonance imaging (MRI), have suggested that improved tumor control and decreased normal tissue injury may be achieved in some cases where the dose distribution is deviated from this traditional pattern and biased toward an asymmetrical region of residual tumor. However, these early experiences remain to be validated in routine clinical use, and concerns remain that such image-guided approaches would result in underestimation of the residual volume at risk or result in underdosage of tumor due to strict but indiscriminate adherence to normal tissue constraints.

Treatment Planning

In its most elemental form, radiation treatment planning is the technical calculation of dose (in Gy) to be delivered to a region in the body. However, this definition of treatment planning excludes the myriad variables that have to be considered in radiotherapy planning. The contemporary treatment planning process encompasses a series of steps, performed both sequentially and iteratively, to arrive at a comprehensive plan that will deliver specified doses(s) to carefully defined target(s), while minimizing exposure to adjacent normal tissues, often based on different correlative imaging tests and taking into account variable patient presentation, anatomy, and the impact of multimodality interventions.

The initial question posed in this expanded concept of treatment planning is whether the patient should be considered for radiotherapy based on clinical evaluation of tumor type, stage, location, other therapeutic interventions, and patient comorbidities. Localization

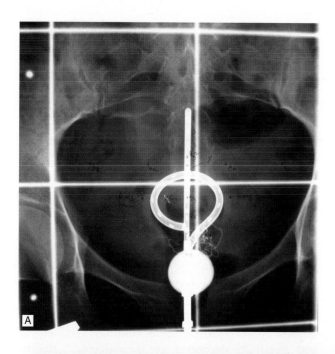
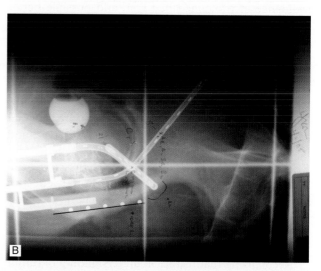
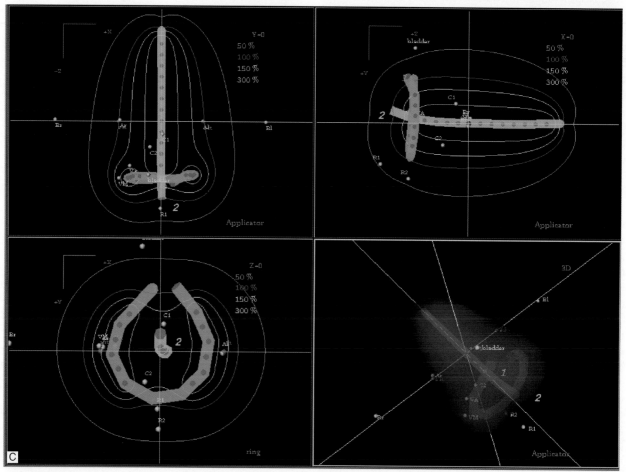

CHAPTER 19

FIGURE 19-14. Anterior (A) and lateral (B) radiographs of high dose rate (HDR) intracavitary brachytherapy in intact cervical cancer, using a tandem and ring applicator. **C.** Computerized dosimetry planning allows viewing of the dose distribution in multiple planes. Note that this HDR application reprises the "pear-shaped" dose distribution of traditional low dose rate brachytherapy by using only the lateral source dwell positions in the ring colpostat.

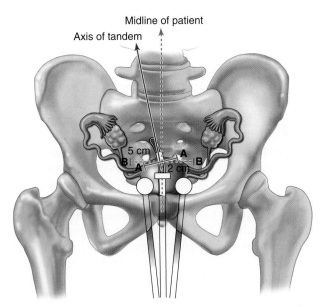

Midline of patient

Axis of tandem

5 cm

FIGURE 19-15. Schematic definitions of points A and B for intact cervix brachytherapy.

of the tumor and/or the region(s) at risk follows and includes integration of physical examination findings, assessment of surgical and pathologic reports, and often, tomographic imaging studies.

Simulation

A major recognizable part of treatment planning is simulation, where patient anatomy and geometry are

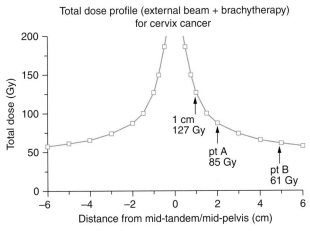

Total dose profile (external beam + brachytherapy) for cervix cancer

1 cm
127 Gy

pt A
85 Gy

pt B
61 Gy

Distance from mid-tandem/mid-pelvis (cm)

FIGURE 19-16. The central dose escalation achieved when combining intracavitary brachytherapy with external beam radiotherapy in intact cervical cancer. The "0" on the x-axis marks the position of the tandem, with dose fall-off as one moves laterally away from the tandem. This illustration assumes "standard" dose prescriptions of 45 Gy to the whole pelvis, 40-Gy low dose rate equivalent to point A using brachytherapy, and bilateral parametrial boosts of up to 9 Gy (with shielding of midline structures).

"captured" for further computerized evaluation and manipulation. Although fluoroscopic simulation is still used at times, CT simulators have become standard equipment in most radiation oncology centers. In addition to obtaining detailed 3D anatomic information, CT simulation also provides the tissue densities (in Hounsfield units) that determine radiation absorption characteristics used in subsequent dose calculations. Although a patient may perceive CT simulation as similar to a diagnostic scan, implicit in the simulation process is specific patient alignment and immobilization, such that the same position can be recapitulated each day during external beam therapy. The patient is usually simulated while supine; however, when clinically indicated, a prone or different position can be used, as long as that position is deemed reproducible on a daily basis. For pelvic malignancies, the lower extremities and/or torso are typically fitted to a custom-formed cradle to assist in daily positioning and set-up. Often, oral and/or intravenous contrast, as well as skin or internal markers, are used to help ascertain structures or volumes at risk (eg, a thin wire around a suspicious groin node or a cervical or vaginal clip to define the most inferior extent of a tumor). Simulation is usually set up to accommodate isocentric radiation treatment, centered on an axis or point around which the gantry, collimators, and couch of the linac will rotate. This isocenter is projected onto the patient surface by light lasers built into the CT simulator or within the imaging room. At this point, several skin marks are typically made on the patient, corresponding to the isocenter projections, and are used for daily treatment alignment. To prevent the marks from being erased, small permanent tattoos are usually etched to define the skin alignment points.

Dosimetry

The information and images collected from simulation are next transferred to a work station for computerized dosimetric planning. Within the dosimetry computer, all relevant information (ie, isodose distributions) for each radiation beam that may be used on a specific linac has been programmed (see earlier section, Teletherapy, for further details). As noted, ultimate radiotherapy dose distribution also depends on the CT images and the associated Hounsfield units that determine radiation absorption by tissues of different densities.

Volumes, or regions of interest (ROIs), are next defined within the dosimetry program, corresponding to tumor, pathway(s) or volume(s) of potential spread, and selected adjacent normal tissues. Several nomenclature terms have been coined that help in standardization and evaluation of dosimetric variables. The gross target volume (GTV) represents tumor that can be seen and/or palpated (eg, the grossly apparently tumor and bulky nodes in a locally advanced cervical cancer). It is important that physical examination findings, such as vaginal mucosal extension, which may not be well defined on imaging, be carefully integrated into GTV determination. At times, other imaging modalities, including PET or MRI, provide additional useful information, and these other imaging studies can be coregistered spatially and fused to the CT simulation scan to improve delineation of the GTV. A clinical target volume (CTV) is next defined and includes the GTV as well as possible pathways of spread that may harbor microscopic disease (eg, nodal echelons, parametria, vagina). The CTV is not simply a concentric expansion of the GTV, as routes of potential spread in gynecologic malignancies often follow asymmetrical paths away from the primary tumor. Even where there is no GTV (such as in a patient who has undergone radical hysterectomy for a node-positive cervical cancer), a CTV should be defined that encompasses vaginal, parametrial, and nodal tissues at risk. Finally, a planning target volume (PTV) is created, which includes the CTV plus a selected margin, to account for daily set-up variability as well as patient and internal organ mobility. Separate ROIs are also drawn on the computer that correspond with adjacent normal structures, such as rectum, bladder, small bowel, and femoral heads. These normal tissues are sometimes collectively referred to, in dosimetric parlance, as organs at risk (OARs).

Once the various volumes of interest are defined, radiation beams, with appropriate blocking to exclude as much normal tissue as possible while still maintaining tumor coverage, are created. These beams, or fields, are modeled within the dosimetry program and are later recreated on the actual patient on the linac. With the exception of very superficial structures that may be treated with single-field electrons (eg, skin metastases, groin nodes in a slender patient), 2 or more fields are typically used daily in the treatment of gynecologic cancers. When evaluating a plan, further adjustments in beam angle, energy, and blocking can be performed iteratively to refine the radiation dose distribution. In the past, blocking was accomplished on the linac by customized cut blocks; this has now been mostly replaced by MLCs built into the gantry head that can be programmed and shaped to the desired field geometry. Using computerized planning, the patient can be viewed at any selected beam angle, referred to as a beam's eye view, which may facilitate the clinician's ability to appreciate tumor and normal tissue juxtapositions distinct from a typical anterior or lateral projection.

With contemporary computer-based dosimetry, dose distribution can be evaluated by viewing isodose lines in multiple projections within a patient. An isodose line indicates a specific dose level within a volume of tissue, much like an isotherm line shows a particular temperature in a geographic region. A series of isodose lines thus show regions of varying doses, as well as their anatomic location and extent. This information can be further supplemented by dose-volume histograms (DVHs), which provide quantitative information regarding the doses received, as a function of fractional volume, by each of the defined targets and neighboring critical structures. The goal is to deliver uniformly high doses to the entire tumor target, while minimizing the dose and/or the volume radiated of the adjacent normal OARs. Figure 19-17 illustrates isodose distributions and a corresponding DVH in a patient treated for advanced pelvic cancer. Figure 19-18 shows isodose curves for a patient with metastatic cervical cancer to the anterior chest wall, demonstrating the use of a single superficial electron beam to avoid deeper underlying structures.

A historic technical approach for radiotherapy used opposing beams of radiation delivered anterior-to-posterior and posterior-to-anterior relative to the patient (often referred to as an APPA approach). To provide better dose distribution within the pelvis, current conventional radiation field arrangements often uses 4 incident photon beams, which typically include an anterior, a posterior, and 2 opposed lateral beams. This is often referred to as a 4-field box technique, although it should be emphasized that patient transaxial geometry is not routinely "box-shaped," and the beams do not have to be limited to specific right angles. An example of 4-field pelvic radiotherapy is illustrated later in Figure 19-20. The 4-field approach may allow for some increased sparing of normal tissues compared to an APPA approach, including the distal rectum or small bowel in the anterior portion of the pelvis. However, an APPA approach may still be found preferable in some circumstances, such as in a slender patient with limited bowel anterior to the uterus (see Figure 19-17) or in a very obese patient with severe lateral redundant tissues. The use of multiple radiation beams, when designed with specific blocking for individual fields, together with CT-based dosimetry calculations and evaluation of a DVH, is often referred to as 3D conformal treatment planning.

A critical component of treatment planning is the prescription of radiation dose. Obviously, the tumor targets, as defined by the GTV, CTV, and PTV, should be taken to "full" dose, where possible. It is important to note that several doses can actually be stipulated; for example, the GTV often is taken to a higher dose level, whereas the remainder of the CTV (the portion with presumably only microscopic disease) may be prescribed a more moderate dose. The impact of other interventions, including surgery and/or chemotherapy, and patient medical history (eg, inflammatory bowel disease, severe vascular compromise) influence decisions regarding dose.

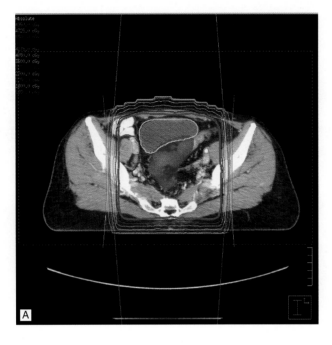

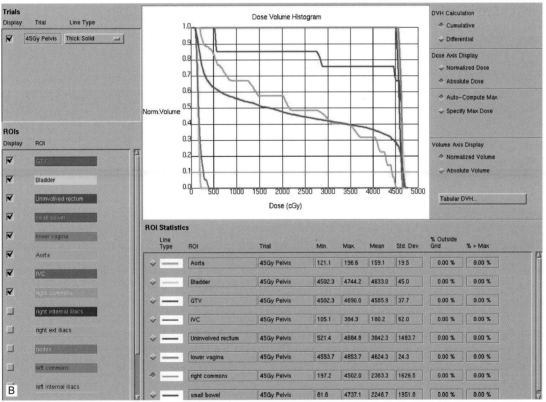

FIGURE 19-17. A. Transaxial isodose distribution in a patient treated with anterior-to-posterior and posterior-to-anterior (APPA) technique for a T4 rectal cancer with invasion into the vagina and bladder. The red-shaded region represents gross tumor volume (GTV) (primary tumor and right iliac nodes). Other delineated regions of interest include bladder (yellow), small bowel (pink), and internal and external iliac vessels as surrogates for nodal basins. Given the extent of the tumor in a thin patient, it was noted that a 4-field approach would not result in significant added sparing of normal tissue (and in fact would expose more pelvic marrow). **B.** The corresponding dose-volume histogram showing full prescribed dose to the GTV (red) and the vagina (green), with "sparing" of dose to the uninvolved rectum (brown) and small bowel (pink).

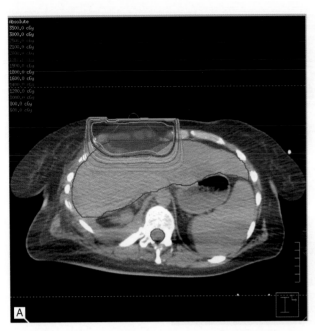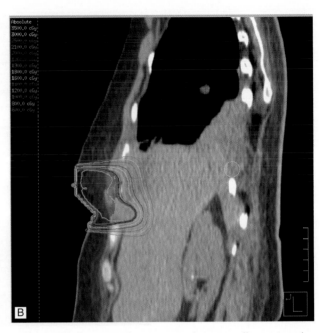

FIGURE 19-18. **Single anterior electron field used to treat a chest wall metastasis from cervical cancer,** illustrating the superficial dose distribution. Isodose curves are shown in the transverse **(A)** and sagittal **(B)** planes.

This recognizes that tumor and late normal tissue effects from radiation are not "all-or-nothing," but rather exhibit dose-response effects that may overlap to some degree (see Figure 19-7).

Linac Radiation Delivery and Treatment Set-Up Verification

When dosimetry planning is completed and approved, the patient is brought to the linac and positioned/immobilized as per the simulation, and the computer-designed radiation fields are then recreated on the patient, typically focused to the skin tattoos that define the treatment isocenter. Even when aligned to skin marks, further verification of accuracy in final targeting is obtained intermittently (at least weekly) by portal imaging, which compares internal landmarks (usually bony structures) on a megavoltage image taken by the linac, correlated with the x-ray or digitally reconstructed radiograph obtained during simulation. The use of radiographic film for port verification has now mostly been replaced by electronic portal imaging devices (EPID). EPID uses a silicon flat panel detector, built onto the linac itself, to capture portal images, provides software for digital enhancement and manipulation of image contrast, and allows the radiation oncologist to easily compare intended versus actual planned radiation fields simultaneously on a computer monitor (Figure 19-19). As radiation delivery has become ever more focused and anatomically constrained, with reduced margin for localization errors, some have proposed that patient field alignment

based on bony landmarks is insufficient and does not account for soft tissue mobility and structural deformation within the target volume. To accommodate this increased level of precision in radiation targeting and delivery, newer linacs have built-in kilovoltage x-ray units that can be used to obtain a tomographic image of the volume of interest, including relevant soft tissue, which can then be fully compared to the 3D information from the original CT simulation. This tomographic imaging obtained on the linac is created using cone beam CT (CBCT) technology. The location of the EPID and CBCT apparatus on a contemporary linac is shown in Figure 19-6. Although much of radiotherapy is clearly defined by imaging, even when using "plain" radiographs of bony anatomy, the use of tomographic imaging on a regular basis for reconciliation with the treatment planning CT is now known specifically as image-guided radiotherapy.

It is of interest that radiation dose is rarely measured in a patient herself. The beam characteristics used in dosimetry planning are calibrated regularly on the linac by medical physicists, using water or other anthropomorphic tissue-equivalent phantoms. However, for highly complicated set-ups, such as when patient anatomy is highly irregular and heterogeneous or in cases of reirradiation where extra precision is required, special dosimeters (eg, ion chambers, thermoluminescent detectors) can be placed on, or in, a patient while receiving treatment on the linac, and the actual delivered dose can be measured to confirm that it corresponds to the dosimetrically planned dose.

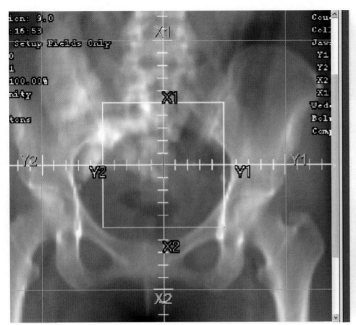
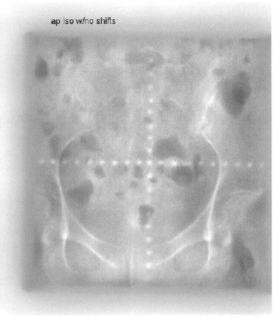

FIGURE 19-19. Standard patient alignment check using pelvic bony anatomic landmarks, comparing the computed tomography simulation–generated digitally reconstructed radiograph (DRR) (left) with the digitally captured megavoltage portal image from electronic portal imaging device (right). Note that secondary to the Compton effect of megavoltage photons, the portal image has less contrast compared to the kilovoltage-based DRR (photoelectric effect), but new technology allows digital enhancement of the portal image to improve viewing resolution.

Much of the preceding discussion has focused on the delivery of EBRT. However, given the importance of brachytherapy in the management of many gynecologic cancers, comprehensive treatment planning also needs to account for, and integrate, the internal radiation contribution. In particular, for patients with locally advanced cervical cancer, optimal treatment requires a balance between external beam and brachytherapy components, with the relative weight of each determined by consideration of multiple tumor and patient factors. The dose components delivered by EBRT and brachytherapy are sometimes added together to give a cumulative overall dose, but this can be done only for well-defined "surrogate" points or locations, such as at points A or the bladder and rectal points as designated by the International Commission on Radiologic Units (ICRU).

Adaptive (Dynamic) Treatment Planning

Currently, treatment planning mostly follows a sequential algorithm as described earlier, with the plan developed first, and then radiotherapy delivered in adherence to it throughout the entire course of treatment. However, there are nascent efforts in the development of adaptive treatment planning, in recognition of the fact that a plan created on a "static" set of images at a single time point prior to initiation of radiation may not accurately reflect subsequent alterations in patient anatomy, cancer regression leading to changes in volume and geometry, and variations in the relationships of tumor and normal tissues. In this situation, simulation and treatment planning may be repeated at various intervals, and radiation dose and volume may be adapted to the changes observed. Adaptive treatment planning is being investigated for both EBRT and brachytherapy.[4,5]

Intensity-Modulated Radiation Therapy

One of the most important recent technical advances in radiation delivery has been the development, and subsequent widespread adoption, of intensity-modulated radiation therapy (IMRT). Although most widely applied in prostate, head and neck, and central nervous system tumors, IMRT has found increasing use in gynecologic cancer radiotherapy.

An underlying premise for the use of IMRT is that gynecologic cancer targets are juxtaposed against, or surrounded by, multiple critical normal structures, including rectum, bladder, small bowel, femoral head and necks, and the pelvic bones. Given their anatomic relationships, a 4-field pelvic "box" technique often cannot maximally exclude these normal tissues, and everything within the "box" is radiated to the same dose as the tumor target. It would thus be attractive to have a technique that would permit "bending and shaping" of the radiation isodose lines to better conform to irregular contours. IMRT provides such a dosimetric capability.[6]

IMRT has been made possible through advancements in high-definition tomographic imaging (including fusion of different imaging modalities), dose algorithm computing, and linac technology (featuring computer-controlled MLCs that can continually change aperture shape in "real time" during an ongoing treatment). Precise definition of all target volumes and OARs is required at the outset of treatment planning. Multiple fields, typically 7 to 9, are used. Each beam is divided into multiple beamlets using the shifting MLCs, such that the fluence profile of each beam is not homogenous (unlike that in standard radiotherapy), and no 1 beam includes the entire target volume in its entirety. Traditional beam blocks are not defined by the clinician. The dose is not prescribed to a single point or even 1 fixed volume, but rather is calculated based on a "best fit" of multiple dose-volume objectives. Doses are specified for each target and may be at different levels for the GTV compared to the CTV. Doses to the OARs are designated with reference to the fractional volume of the normal structure that is permitted to receive that dose level. Once the dose-volume objectives and constraints are specified, the dosimetry program performs inverse planning, determining the linac output and field shapes that will result in a best-fit dose distribution to the defined parameters. In this setting, intuitive control of the radiation field geometry, as well as dose per field (or dose per beamlet within any field), is surrendered to the computer. Although each beam is heterogenous in dose distribution relative to the tumor target, the integrated doses from all beamlets and all beams allow for a highly conformal, shaped distribution that "bends" or "curves" around a nonuniform target contour.

There are challenges to IMRT, including the limitations of various imaging modalities in defining target volumes. Whereas tight isodose lines surrounding a target allow for exclusion of more adjacent normal tissues, they also permit less latitude in tumor coverage margins and run a higher risk of marginal misses. Patient positioning reproducibility and internal organ motion need to be accounted for. IMRT involves more physician and dosimetrist planning time and also requires stringent physics quality assurance of the plan and individualized phantom measures of the dose for each patient. Finally, although IMRT allows excellent shaping of the higher level isodoses, the lower dose levels are more diffusely spread out (given the multiple entry beams), resulting in larger volumes of tissues exposed to *lower* doses of radiation.

Despite the added technical demands imposed by IMRT, there is emerging consensus regarding its role in the posthysterectomy setting (where the target volume presents a highly concave geometry within the pelvis) for dose escalation to gross para-aortic nodes or bulky sidewall disease or for selected cases of reirradiation. Figure 19-20 illustrate 4-field versus IMRT

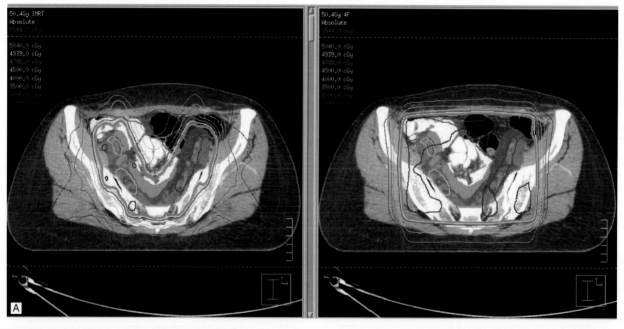

FIGURE 19-20. Transaxial isodose distributions for a patient undergoing adjuvant external beam radiotherapy following radical hysterectomy for stage I cervical adenocarcinoma, but with high-risk pathologic features. The intensity-modulated radiation therapy (IMRT) plan on the left is compared to its corresponding traditional 4-field plan on the right, for selected levels in the upper pelvis **(A)**, mid pelvis **(B)**, and low pelvis **(C)**. The clinical target volume is shaded in pink. Note that higher intensity isodose curves provide greater "shaping" or conformality surrounding the target volume, but the lower isodose lines are more spread out, secondary to the increased number of incident beams used with IMRT **(B)**.

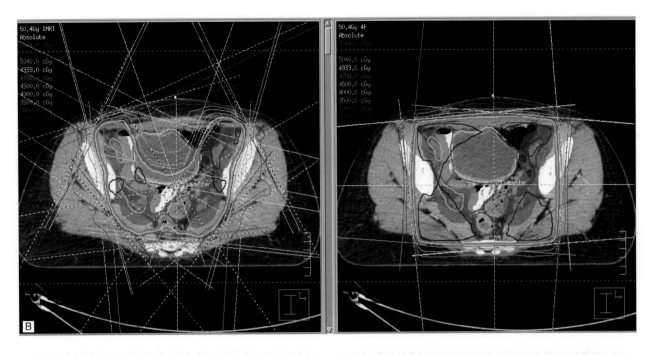

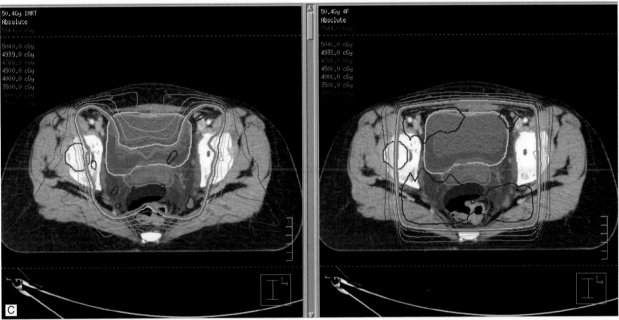

FIGURE 19-20. (Continued)

isodose distributions for a posthysterectomy patient, with the corresponding DVHs shown in Figure 19-21.

RADIATION TOXICITY

The effects of ionizing radiation on the embryo and fetus are covered earlier, in the section entitled Genetic Effects of Radiation and Radiation's Impact on the Human Reproductive Process.

Effects of Radiation on Normal Tissue

Radiation treatment side effects can be divided into acute (during treatment until 3 months afterward) and late or long-term toxicities (beyond 3 months). Radiation reactions are related to the specific normal structure radiated, as well as to the dose, dose per fraction, and volume of normal tissue exposed. Patient comorbid factors, such as hypertension, diabetes, and inflammatory bowel conditions, affect radiation toxicity. Concurrent chemotherapy and smoking also impact on radiation effects.

It has generally been felt that the acute and late complications of radiation are "decoupled." Early effects relate to acute-reacting normal tissues with rapidly dividing cell systems, such as skin, hair, gastrointestinal mucosa, and hematologic elements. These acute "irritative" symptoms are expected in most patients undergoing radiation and are exacerbated by the use of concurrent chemotherapy. However, when appropriately managed and supported, acute toxicity is expected to resolve within several weeks after completion of radiotherapy. It has also been discussed previously that although fractionation may provide relatively little sparing of early-responding normal tissues, acute toxicity in clinical practice is often "self-limited" by compensatory proliferation and migration of neighboring normal cells from outside the radiation field.

Late complications, on the other hand, are considered secondary to the depletion of normal tissue stem cells, as well as chronic microvasculature injury. These can occur months to year following radiation and are marked by decreased blood supply, stromal changes, and fibrosis. Late toxicity is generally felt to be independent of acute effects, except in cases where the acute complication is so severe that it does not sufficiently recover and then persists into a late effect (termed "consequential late effect"). The incidence of severe late complications in clinical radiotherapy is fortunately relatively infrequent. However, recent research has focused on lower-grade late changes that, although not catastrophic, may be much more frequent and impact on patients' long-term quality of life. Although concurrent chemotherapy does increase acute radiation toxicities, most studies have indicated that it does not increase late effects compared to radiotherapy alone.

Potential acute side effects that can occur during EBRT to the abdomen and/or pelvis include fatigue; decreased appetite; radiation dermatitis or hair loss in the treatment fields; cystitis causing polyuria, dysuria, or hematuria; bladder spasms potentially resulting in urinary incontinence; enteritis manifesting as diarrhea,

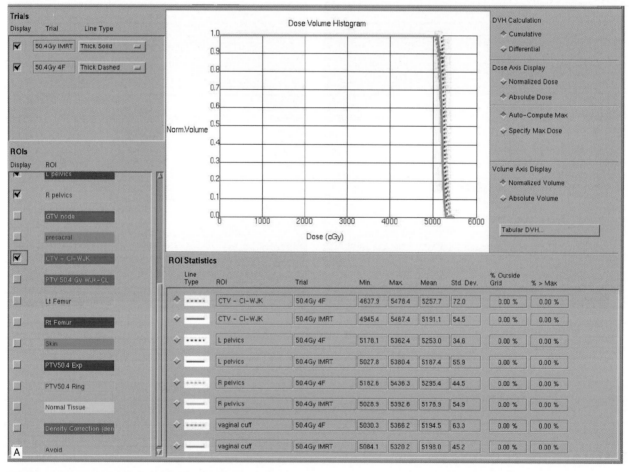

FIGURE 19-21. Comparative dose-volume histograms corresponding to the intensity-modulated radiation therapy (IMRT) (solid lines) and 4-field (dotted lines) plans for the patient illustrated in Figure 19-19. A. For the tumor targets, including the clinical target volume, pelvic nodes, and vagina, there is no discernible difference in radiation coverage. **B.** However, for the organs at risk, there is noticeable sparing (in dose and in volume) of rectum (brown), bladder (yellow), and small bowel (pink).

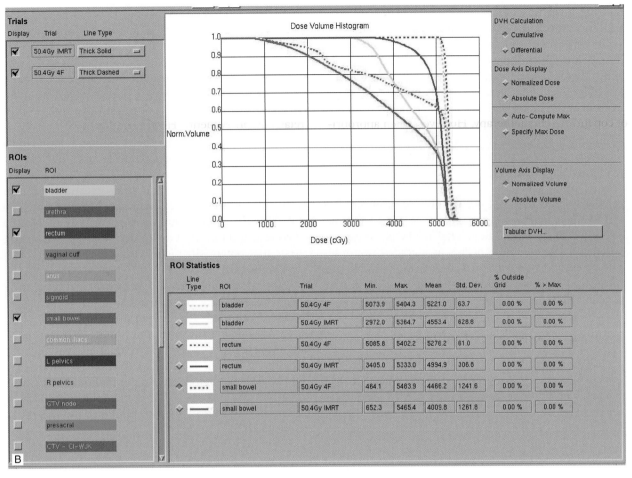

FIGURE 19-21. *(Continued)*

nausea, or vomiting; proctitis resulting in rectal pain, bleeding, or incontinence; vaginal mucositis causing pruritus, vaginal discharge, or discomfort; and hematologic or renal dysfunction. In many cases, these acute reactions respond well to supportive measures, including topicals, medications, and at times intravenous fluid and electrolyte replacement. As noted previously, all attempts should be made to complete the course of radiation or chemoradiation without prolonged treatment breaks, to avoid the hazard of accelerated tumor repopulation.

Potential long-term side effects of EBRT to the abdomen/pelvis include infertility, permanent skin changes or hair loss in the treatment fields, subcutaneous induration, vaginal and cervical stenosis, small bowel malabsorption or obstruction, stricture/fistula of bowel or bladder, femoral head necrosis, osteoporosis and pelvic insufficiency fracture, permanent kidney dysfunction, transverse myelitis, and the risk of a secondary malignancy. The generally low risk of high-grade late toxicity is increased in patients with pre-existing vascular disease (such as hypertension or diabetes) and in patients who have undergone previous surgery within the irradiated volume (presumably secondary to vascular compromise and/or the formation of adhesions). The risk of a permanent, severe complication varies according to the dose and volume of radiation delivered; for patients who receive moderate doses of adjuvant radiation, the incidence of a significant late injury is of the order of 5%, but this risk can increase to 10% to 15% following very high–dose radiotherapy, such as that required in definitive treatment of locally advanced cervical cancer.

The brachytherapy component of radiotherapy has its unique set of possible side effects, including the risks associated with sedation/anesthesia and the hazards of the procedure itself, including infection, bleeding, and uterine perforation.

Late radiation reaction is affected by the structural and functional organization of the tissue/organ in question. Conceptually, normal structures are organized into functional subunits (FSUs), which impact on perceived clinical complication by the patient, and influence the volume of an organ that can be "safely" irradiated without global harm. The FSUs of the spinal cord and peripheral nerves are arranged serially, such that the integrity of each link is critical to maintaining function throughout the chain. Radiation effect on such tissues shows a binary response, with a threshold dose below which there is normal function, but above which there is clearly appreciated and clinically relevant loss of function. The liver, lung, and kidney, on the other hand, have FSUs arranged in parallel. Inactivation of a proportion of parallel FSUs may not lead to whole-organ dysfunction, and thus, these organs have an increased tolerance to high-dose partial-volume radiation (similar to pulmonary lobectomy, partial hepatectomy, or partial nephrectomy). Clinically relevant functional damage to parallel systems does not occur until a critical number of FSUs are inactivated, implying a threshold volume below which no global functional injury is measured, but above which damage occurs as a graded response. The bowel and skin have no well-defined FSUs but are considered to share characteristics of both serial and parallel FSUs.

Tolerance of Organs to Radiation

Table 19-2 shows the widely accepted normal tissue tolerances of organs typically radiated in gynecologic malignancies. The data are based on the general consensus among expert radiation oncologists in the early 1990s.[7] Toxicity dose (TD) 5/5 is the dose that is estimated to result in a 5% risk of severe adverse outcome at 5 years. TD 50/5 refers to the dose that would cause an estimated 50% risk of high-grade injury at 5 years. The tolerance doses are presented as a function of the fractional volume of the normal organ irradiated, either 1/3, 2/3, or 3/3. The tolerance doses for skin are quantified in relation to the area of skin exposed, and for the spinal cord, to the length irradiated.

These normal tissue tolerance estimates have guided clinical radiotherapy for several decades but may be considered conservative, given the relative lack of shielding, dose conformality, and sophisticated dosimetry that was available at that time. More recently, the QUANTEC study (Quantitative Analysis of Normal Tissue Effects in the Clinic) was released, which suggests that potentially higher doses may be tolerable in several normal tissues.[8]

With particular relevance to brachytherapy, experience suggests that the upper one-third of the vaginal mucosa can tolerate radiation doses as high as 120 to 140 Gy, whereas the lower third of the vaginal mucosa should usually receive no more than 80 to 90 Gy. The combined dose of external beam and brachytherapy to the ICRU bladder reference point should not exceed 75 to 80 Gy, and the ICRU rectal point should ideally be limited to 70 to 75 Gy to minimize the risk of late complications.

Table 19-2 Tolerance Doses of Organs Typically Radiated in Gynecologic Malignancies

Organ	TD 5/5 (cGy) Volume			TD 50/5 (cGy) Volume			Clinical End Point
	1/3	2/3	3/3	1/3	2/3	3/3	
Colon	5500						Obstruction, perforation, ulceration, fistula
Rectum			6000			8000	Severe proctitis, necrosis, fistula, stenosis
Small intestine	5000		4000	6000		5500	Obstruction, perforation, fistula
Bladder		8000	6500		8500	8000	Symptomatic bladder contracture and volume loss
Kidney	5000	3000	2300		4000	2800	Clinical nephritis
Femoral head			5200			6500	Necrosis
	10 cm²	30 cm²	100 cm²	10 cm²	30 cm²	100 cm²	
Skin	7000	6000	5500			7000	Necrosis, ulceration
	5 cm	10 cm	20 cm	5 cm	10 cm	20 cm	
Spinal cord	5000	5000	4700	7000	7000		Transverse myelitis

Toxicity dose (TD) 5/5 is the dose that is estimated to result in a 5% risk of severe adverse outcome at 5 years. TD 50/5 refers to the dose that would cause an estimated 50% risk of high-grade injury at 5 years.
Data based on Emami B, Lyman J, Brown A, et al. Tolerance of normal tissue to therapeutic irradiation. *Int J Radiat Oncol Biol Phys.* 1991;21(1): 109-122.

CLINICAL USES OF RADIATION IN GYNECOLOGIC MALIGNANCIES

Cervical Cancer

The role of radiotherapy in cervical cancer is fairly well defined. Surgery is typically the standard of care for patients with early-stage disease (stage IA, IB1 tumors). However, for patients who have major illness precluding an operation or who decline surgery, radiation is an effective alternative. For patients with stage IA or small IB tumors (typically <2 cm), brachytherapy alone is an option, which might allow a medically compromised individual to be spared the potential toxicity of EBRT. When brachytherapy alone is used, doses of 70 to 80 Gy (LDR-equivalent specification) to point A are usually prescribed, depending on the volume of presenting disease.

For patients undergoing primary surgery, surgico-pathologic risk features may dictate the need for further adjuvant radiotherapy to reduce the likelihood of relapse. Conventionally, such patients are grouped into 2 risk categories. Those deemed at high risk (positive lymph nodes, parametrial invasion, or positive surgical margins), where collectively, the cancer may be considered to have extended beyond the anatomic limits of the cervix, have demonstrated survival benefit with adjuvant pelvic radiation (generally to a dose of 50 Gy) and concurrent cisplatin-based chemotherapy. For those at intermediate risk, where the pathologic findings remain "confined" to the cervix itself (large primary tumor size, deep cervical stromal invasion, or lymphovascular space invasion), adjuvant pelvic radiation alone to 50 Gy is appropriate and associated with decreased relapses and improved progression-free survival. Brachytherapy is typically not used in the posthysterectomy adjuvant radiation setting unless there are positive vaginal mucosal surgical margins, in which case a cylinder boost to the vaginal cuff, in addition to EBRT, may be considered.

For patients with more locally advanced disease (stage IB2 to IVA tumors), the standard of care is considered to be definitive chemoradiation. This entails the careful combination of EBRT and brachytherapy boost to deliver high doses to the cervix (point A dose of 80 to 85 Gy or higher), while limiting exposure (both in terms of dose and volume) to adjacent critical normal structures such as the bladder and rectum.

Endometrial Cancer

Hysterectomy remains the primary initial therapy for almost all patients with uterine cancer. Over the past 2 decades, the use of radiation in endometrial cancer has appropriately diminished. This decrease has been predicated on the impact of surgical staging, a better understanding of patterns of failure, and an appreciation of the contribution of systemic chemotherapy in advanced disease. Nonetheless, radiation continues to play a considerable role in the management of endometrial cancer.

For the infrequent medically inoperable patient, primary radiotherapy, using brachytherapy alone or in combination with EBRT, allows good relief of symptoms (such as bleeding or pain) and provides for a reasonable likelihood of local tumor control. The intra-uterine brachytherapy component of therapy may need modification from that used in cervical cancer (where dose is concentrated in the cervix and lower uterus by tandem and colpostat applicators), because endometrial cancer typically involves more of the superior fundus and is often associated with an enlarged uterine cavity. In this setting, the use of a double or split tandem set-up allows for broader dose distribution in the superior fundus.

In posthysterectomy patients with uterine-confined disease, the presence of certain pathologic features (high grade, deep myometrial invasion, cervical extension, and lymphovascular space infiltration) predicts for an increased risk of local failure, of which the majority are limited to the vaginal cuff. Although historically managed with EBRT, contemporary evidence suggests that most can be effectively and equally well treated with vaginal brachytherapy alone, with excellent prevention of cuff relapses and little associated acute and late toxicity. Brachytherapy, typically using a cylinder applicator (see Figure 19-12), delivers a high dose to the vaginal mucosa, but with rapid fall-off, exposure to bladder, rectum, and other pelvic tissues is minimized. Historically, LDR brachytherapy delivered a dose of approximately 60 to 70 Gy to the vaginal mucosa over 48 to 72 hours as an inpatient. Today, most vaginal brachytherapy is done with outpatient HDR; a common dose scheme prescribes 7 Gy for each of 3 cylinder insertions, with dose specified to a depth of 0.5 cm deep to the mucosal surface. A typical HDR vaginal brachytherapy application is often completed in an hour or less.

For patients with more advanced uterine cancers (stage III and IV), the use of chemotherapy has, to a great degree, supplanted the historical role of radiotherapy, especially when one considers the use of a single adjuvant treatment modality. Despite the benefit of chemotherapy, outcomes for these patients remain relatively poor. There remain unanswered questions regarding whether tumor control and survival for these patients (especially those with stage IIIC or nodal improvement) might be further improved by integrating appropriate tumor-directed EBRT, *in addition to* systemic chemotherapy. This question has formed the basis for a current phase III clinical trial (Gynecologic Oncology Group trial 258).

CHAPTER 19

Ovarian Cancer

In the preplatinum era, whole abdominal-pelvic radio-therapy (WAPRT) was often used in patients with ovarian cancer. Long-term survivals were seen in selected patients, in particular those with lower-grade disease and with minimal residual tumor burden after initial surgery. WAPRT requires significant technical expertise and great appreciation for the radiation tolerance of multiple normal tissues, especially in the upper abdomen (small bowel, liver, kidneys) and even the low thorax (lung base, heart). Ovarian cancers are generally radioresponsive, but this is balanced against the low doses achievable in the upper abdomen. The use of WAPRT has largely been abandoned, given its known increased risk of long-term bowel toxicity, the great difficulty of performing secondary surgery and instituting second-line therapy, and the very high response and progression-free survival rates now seen for primary platinum and, more recently, platinum- and taxane-based chemotherapy.

Radiotherapy may be considered in 2 scenarios in ovarian cancer, both using less extensive radiation coverage than that of WARPT. For patients with localized suboptimally debulked primary disease, the integration of locoregional radiation in addition to chemotherapy may increase the likelihood of tumor control. In this particular setting, radiation may be thought of as an "extension" to surgery, to complete an optimal tumor debulking that was surgically unachievable (eg, in a patient with residual but localized gross retroperitoneal adenopathy). Radiotherapy is also an effective, and perhaps underused, palliative treatment for patients with recurrent or metastatic disease. The response rate of locally treated tumors is high, and radiation can successfully provide durable palliation of symptoms such as bleeding, pain, and localized obstruction.

Vulvar Cancer

In the radiotherapeutic management of vulvar cancer, the approaches to the primary lesion and to the nodes are often "uncoupled," taking into account the different anatomic and clinical constraints. This paradigm also recognizes the general acceptance that localized vulvar relapses following surgery are readily salvageable, whereas metachronous groin failures following initial therapy carry a grave prognosis and are often ultimately fatal.

Primary therapy for early vulvar cancer is typically surgical resection, with associated inguinal-femoral node dissection. Patients found to have groin node metastases, especially if there is gross nodal disease or ≥2 positive nodes, clearly benefit from adjuvant radiation to the groin and pelvis. Various pathologic risk

factors also predict for primary site relapse following surgery (including deep invasion, close surgical margins, lymphovascular space involvement, and "spray pattern" histology), but the use of adjuvant radiotherapy to the vulvar resection bed has not been systematically evaluated.

To avoid the morbidity (especially lymphedema) of combined groin node dissection and postoperative radiotherapy, there have been attempts to evaluate "prophylactic" groin radiation (without surgery) in patients deemed to be at risk for occult nodal disease. Although criticized for technical shortcomings in EBRT delivery in previous clinical studies, there remains doubt about the effectiveness of prophylactic groin node radiotherapy. Ongoing attempts to improve on this approach include the use of contemporary high-resolution tomographic imaging as well as sentinel node evaluation.

Patients with advanced vulvar cancer were historically treated with ultraradical surgery, including exenteration. To reduce the morbidity of such debilitating surgery, investigators evaluated the role of neoadjuvant radiation and showed that radiotherapy could lead to significant tumor debulking and the successful incorporation of more limited, viscera-sparing resection. More recent studies have established the tolerability, benefit, and role of concurrent chemoradiation (using cisplatin with or without 5-fluorouracil), followed by biopsies or conservative excision, with avoidance of exenterative surgery in more than 90% of cases.

Vulvar cancer presents with highly diverse spatial geometry, where the volume at risk changes significantly in shape and distribution from the vulva to the groins to the pelvic nodes. This variability in geometry results in extra radiation dose to surrounding normal tissues when treated with conventional APPA or 4-field techniques and may lend itself well to the adaptable and conformal coverage provided by IMRT (Figure 19-22).

Vaginal Cancer

Given its rarity and varied clinical presentations, few prospective data and no phase III trials address therapeutic interventions in vaginal cancer. Due to the desire to spare closely adjacent bladder and/or rectum, with the exception of very small, localized tumors, radiotherapy (rather than surgery) is used for the primary treatment of most vaginal cancers. The treatment algorithm is extrapolated from that of cervical cancer and generally uses a combination of EBRT and brachytherapy. Vaginal cancers are frequently asymmetric in location, and the vagina does not have the geometric and biologic advantage of an intact uterus to accommodate extremely high intracavitary doses, while "displacing" adjacent normal structures. Hence, brachytherapy for vaginal cancers often emphasizes the role of interstitial implants to optimize radiation dose distribution, especially for tumors with residual thickness exceeding 0.5 to 1 cm. The role of chemoradiation has not been widely evaluated in vaginal cancer, but based on the cervical cancer data, it would be reasonable to consider this in patients fit enough to tolerate cisplatin-based chemotherapy.

NOVEL RADIATION MODALITIES

Hyperthermia

It has long been recognized that heat can denature proteins and lead to cellular disruption and depth. As a complement to radiotherapy, hyperthermia has been attractive because it is not impacted by the S-phase fraction or tumor hypoxia, which are 2 conditions

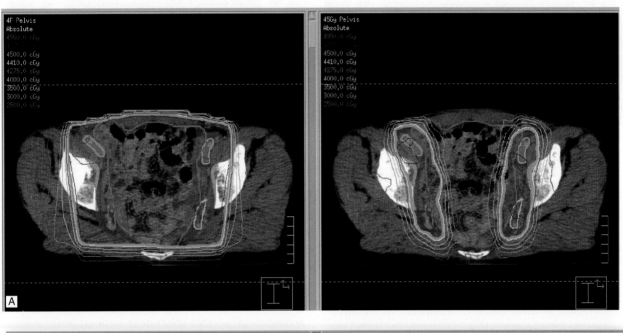

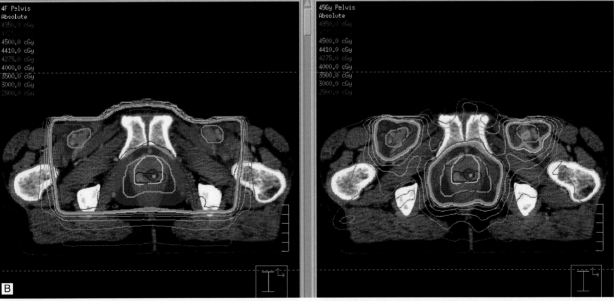

FIGURE 19-22. Comparison of "standard" 4-field dosimetry (left) with intensity-modulated radiation therapy (IMRT) plan (right) for a patient with locally advanced vulvar cancer and vaginal extension. The different spatial presentations of the volume at risk at varying transaxial levels within the patient lend to greater conformal sparing of normal tissues by IMRT, as seen in selected computed tomography slices: **(A)** mid pelvis, for coverage of pelvic nodes; **(B)** low pelvis, for coverage of the vagina and groin nodes; and **(C)** for coverage of the vulva.

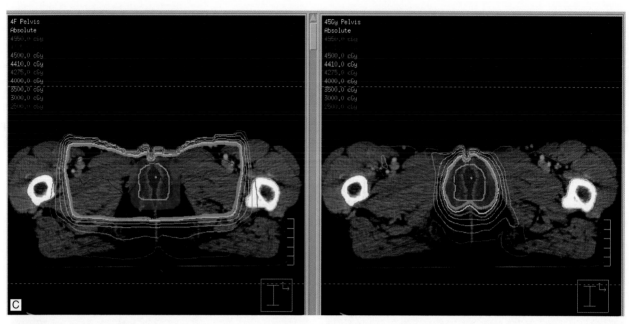

FIGURE 19-22. *(Continued)*

that render tumor cells relatively resistant to ionizing radiation. However, there is no consistent difference in inherent heat sensitivity between normal and malignant cells, unlike the disparities in cellular repair that can be exploited with ionizing radiation (see Figure 19-4). Furthermore, the localized and accurate delivery of heat, and monitoring/maintenance of a suitable stable temperature, in tissue has been hampered by technical limitations until recently, thus restricting the broad use of hyperthermia in oncologic applications.

Recent advances in heat delivery systems and in vivo thermometry, especially using noninvasive techniques, have created renewed interest in hyperthermia. Although heat to a temperature exceeding 50°C to 60°C will ablate tissues on its own, work has also focused on lower levels of hyperthermia (approximately 40°C-43°C) that may not be intrinsically cytotoxic but can enhance the effects of ionizing radiation and certain chemotherapeutic agents. Hyperthermia in combination with cytotoxic agents has been evaluated in isolated limb perfusions and intraperitoneal chemotherapy studies. In a prospective Dutch randomized trial of patients with advanced cervical cancer, the combination of hyperthermia and radiotherapy resulted in improved local control and overall survival compared to radiotherapy alone.[9] This approach has not been widely adopted, because chemoradiation has now been established as the standard of care for locally advanced cervical cancer. A new, ongoing international trial seeks to clarify the contribution of hyperthermia by randomizing patients with advanced cervical cancer to chemoradiation versus hyperthermia plus chemoradiation.

Stereotactic Radiosurgery and Stereotactic Body Radiotherapy

The use of stereotactic radiosurgery (SRS) is well established in the treatment of patients with intracranial tumors. This consists of a *single* ablative dose of radiation, delivered via a specialized gamma knife (which has approximately 200 individual ^{60}Co sources arranged in a semi-spheroidal helmet, with a focal point at an isocenter) or a modified linac. The spheroidal geometry of the skull lends itself well to these approaches, because it permits a centralized lesion to be targeted by multiple, surrounding, noncoplanar beams of radiation.

Stereotactic body radiotherapy (SBRT) is an adaptation of the principles and techniques developed in SRS, but focused on delivery of radiation to extracranial sites. The radiation is given in 1 to 5 fractions and is accomplished either with a specialized CyberKnife unit (which has the radiation source mounted on a free robotic arm that can move about the patient) or a modified linac. SBRT allows for more focal and precise delivery of radiation than conventional EBRT or even IMRT and is typically used for smaller, isolated lesions (<5 cm). It is important to remember that although SBRT delivers very high doses of radiation to an identified tumor, it, by definition, does not provide prophylactic or adjuvant coverage to adjacent tissues at risk of harboring microscopic disease. A primary challenge to SBRT planning is that because extracranial sites are not spheroidal in geometry, the degrees of freedom, or "angles" of radiation beam entrance, are limited compared to SRS for brain tumors. Furthermore, without the rigid head frame used in SRS, patient positioning reproducibility and internal organ motion (especially from respiration) have to be taken into account. Nonetheless, improvements in immobilization techniques, the use of 4-dimensional CT imaging (3D CT with integration of target volume over respiratory cycle time), sophisticated dosimetric and treatment planning tools, and near real-time image guidance such as CBCT on the linac have allowed for increasing application of SBRT in management of certain disease presentations. Germane to gynecologic malignancies, SBRT may be useful in treating oligometastatic lung or liver lesions or as a localized boost (in combination with more general EBRT) in addressing unresectable nodes or pelvic sidewall recurrences.

Protons

Protons are charged particles that can be very tightly focused to a target volume. The technique makes use of the Bragg peak effect, in which the proton beam has an extremely sharp, well-defined range in tissue, with little side scatter, to deliver radiation precisely to the intended target, with markedly reduced doses to the surrounding normal tissues. Proton beams have lower entry, and *no exit*, doses compared to standard megavoltage photons, giving rise to their dosimetric advantage. Furthermore, protons improve on the dose conformality of current technologies, by providing highly concentrated dose contours around tumor, without the "scatter" of lower doses to large volumes of surrounding tissues inherent with IMRT. The precision of protons requires extreme care in target definition and tracking of tumor volumes, similar to that for other highly conformal techniques such as IMRT. When absorbed by tissue, protons have the same ultimate biologic effect as that of photons for any given dose; the advantage of protons rests entirely on their superior physical dose distribution.

There is significant current interest and momentum in the installation of proton centers and the use of proton radiotherapy. Protons have shown clinical benefit in pediatric cancers, as well as in certain brain and spine tumors, but these represent relatively uncommon clinical presentations. It has been argued by some that protons represent the ultimate in physical radiation dose delivery and should be the radiotherapy technique of choice for many, if not most, cancers. However, there remain concerns regarding the widespread use of protons, mostly surrounding its high costs, indications, and the lack of randomized studies that confirm its clinical superiority.[10] Nonetheless, in an age of increasing combined-modality management of cancer, protons may allow for enhanced systemic therapy by reducing the locoregional toxicities of radiotherapy.

REFERENCES

1. Hall EJ, Giaccia AJ. *Radiobiology for the Radiologist.* 7th ed. Philadelphia, PA: Lippincott Williams & Wilkins; 2012.
2. de Gonzalez AB, Curtis RE, Fry SF, et al. Proportion of second cancers attributable to radiotherapy treatment in adults: a cohort study in the US SEER cancer registries. *Lancet Oncol.* 2011;12:353-360.
3. Khan FM. *The Physics of Radiation Therapy.* 4th ed. Philadelphia, PA: Lippincott Williams & Wilkins; 2010.
4. van de Bunt L, Van der Heide UA, Ketelaars M, de Kort GA, Jurgenliemk-Schulz IM. Conventional, conformal, and intensity modulated radiation therapy treatment planning of external beam radiotherapy for cervical cancer: the impact of tumor regression. *Int J Radiat Oncol Biol Phys.* 2006;64(1):189-196.
5. Potter R, Kirisits C, Fidarova EF, et al. Present status and future of high-precision image guided adaptive brachytherapy for cervix carcinoma. *Acta Oncologica.* 2008;47(7):1325-1336.
6. Loiselle C, Koh WJ. The emerging use of IMRT for treatment of cervical cancer. *J Natl Compr Canc Netw.* 2010;8(12):1425-1434.
7. Emami B, Lyman J, Brown A, et al. Tolerance of normal tissue to therapeutic irradiation. *Int J Radiat Oncol Biol Phys.* 1991;21(1):109-122.
8. Bentzen SM, Constine LS, Deasy JO, et al. Quantitative Analyses of Normal Tissue Effects in the Clinic (QUANTEC): an introduction to the scientific issues. *Int J Radiat Oncol Biol Phys.* 2010;76(3 suppl):S3-S9.
9. Franckena M, Stalpers LJ, Koper PC, et al. Long-term improvement in treatment outcome after radiotherapy and hyperthermia in locoregionally advanced cervix cancer: an update of the Dutch Deep Hyperthermia Trial. *Int J Radiat Oncol Biol Phys.* 2008;70(4):1176-1182.
10. Glatstein E, Glick J, Kaiser L, Hahn SM. Should randomized clinical trials be required for proton radiotherapy? An alternative view. *J Clin Oncol.* 2008;26(15):2438-2439.

Principles of Chemotherapy

Ursula A. Matulonis

GENERAL PRINCIPLES

Chemotherapy agents are grouped into different categories based on mechanism of action. These categories include alkylating agents, antimicrotubule agents, plant alkaloids, antimetabolites, anthracyclines, topoisomerase inhibitors, and others.

In addition to tumor site and diagnosis, individual patient factors such as age, organ function, comorbidities, and residual toxicities from the receipt of prior therapies will all influence the choice of chemotherapy regimens. Dose adjustments should be made when appropriate depending on goals of treatment and previous treatments the patient may have received. Physicians prescribing anticancer agents should understand the goals of care for the individual patient (curative vs. palliative) as well as the metabolism and toxicities of the agents prescribed. Patients and their families should be educated about the expected toxicities and goals of therapy.

Tumor Growth

Tumor growth is a complicated intricate process governed by genetic abnormalities within the cell and the tumor's interaction with its microenvironment. The understanding of cancer has accelerated significantly over the past decade, and Hanahan and Weinberg[1] have defined the distinguishing features of cancer detailing the following hallmarks in addition to genomic instability as an underlying premise of the make-up of cancer cells: promotion and sustaining proliferative signaling, evading growth suppressors, resisting cell death, allowing replicative immortality, induction of angiogenesis,

and activating invasion and metastasis. The proliferation and growth control of normal cells are not well understood, but the mitogenic signaling of cancer cells is increasingly better understood. Cancer cells acquire the ability to proliferate unchecked by several different mechanisms: self-production of growth factor ligands; control of the tumor microenvironment by signaling local stromal cells, which in turn produce factors leading to cancer growth; overexpression or enhanced signaling of transmembrane receptors; and growth factor independence via constitutive activation of tyrosine kinases within the receptor and/or downstream signaling molecules.[2] Enabling characteristics of cancer cells that allow the above changes to occur include overall genomic instability and the cancer cell's ability to avoid immune destruction.[3]

Cell Kinetics and Log Kill Hypothesis

Cell kinetics were originally described based on murine tumor models, but it is now accepted that most human solid tumors do not grow in an exponential manner. The log kill hypothesis was based on the L1210 murine leukemia model, which is a fast-growing leukemia where 100% of the cells are actively progressing through the cell cycle.[4] Logarithmic kill hypothesis states that a given anticancer drug should kill a constant proportion or fraction of cells in contrast to a constant number of cells, and cell kill is proportional regardless of the bulk of tumor. For example, if a drug can lead to a 3 log kill of cancer cells and can reduce the cancer burden from 10^9 to 10^6, the same drug and dose can also reduce the tumor burden from 10^6 to 10^3.

However, solid tumors tend to follow the Gompertzian model of tumor growth because most solid tumors do not grow and expand exponentially.[5] The Gompertzian model predicts that cell growth is faster at the start of the growth curve when a tumor is small compared to a larger tumor existing in the slower part of the growth curve, which thus has a lower growth fraction. The Gompertzian model also predicts that the sensitivity of a cancer to chemotherapy depends on where the tumor is in its growth phase and that growth decreases exponentially over time. Similarly, the log kill produced by chemotherapy is higher in small-volume tumors than large-volume tumors because of the differences in growth kinetics.

Drug Resistance

Resistance to chemotherapy ultimately occurs with all cancers except those that are curable. Multiple mechanisms exist, new mechanisms are being discovered, and overlapping mechanisms can occur simultaneously; tumor resistance to drug therapy results primarily from tumor growth and selection of existing resistant clones while sensitive cells are killed.[6,7] One of the original hypotheses explaining drug resistance is the Goldie and Coldman hypothesis reported initially in 1979, which served as the basis for drug regimens used in hematologic malignancies and more recently in gynecologic malignancies.[8] The tenets of the Goldie and Coldman hypothesis include the following: Treatment should begin as soon as possible in order to treat the smallest amount and bulk of tumor, multiple non–cross-resistant agents should be used in order to avoid selection of resistant clones, and drugs should be used as often as possible and in doses that are higher than minimally cytotoxic doses. In clinical trials that test features of the Goldie and Coldman hypothesis, adjuvant breast cancer therapy has shown improvements in outcome by using this tenet, but in upfront treatment of ovarian cancer, the use of sequencing non–cross-resistant agents did not result in improved progression-free survival or overall survival.[9] Examples of mechanisms of drug resistance include alteration of drug movement across the cell membrane with respect to both influx and efflux, increased repair of DNA to offset damage done by certain agents, defective apoptosis so cancer cells are not receptive to drug effects, alteration of drug targets such as topoisomerase II alteration by point mutation, deletions or overexpression, and other mechanisms. The mechanisms of resistance associated with specific agents are discussed within the individual drug descriptions.[6,10] Newly described drug resistance mechanisms include identification of secondary mutations that restore the wild-type *BRCA* reading frame, which is likely a mediator of acquired resistance to platinum-based chemotherapy.[11]

Dose Intensity

The therapeutic selectivity of chemotherapy is dependent on the outcome of dose response between normal tissue and cancer tissue. Dose intensity is the amount of drug delivered per unit of time, and the dose intensity of each regimen is based on the time period during which the treatment is actually administered. Calculations can be made regarding the intended dose intensity as well as the actual dose intensity that the patient receives in total. By reducing the dose intensity to decrease toxicity, clinicians may compromise the predicted outcome of a patient, and therefore, it is mandatory that clinicians state up front the intended outcome of administering chemotherapy (ie, curative vs. palliative). The importance of maintaining dose intensity has been demonstrated in early-stage breast cancer patients using adjuvant cyclophosphamide, methotrexate, and 5-fluorouracil, as well as cyclophosphamide and doxorubicin. In gynecologic cancers, the importance of dose intensity has been observed in older patients with ovarian cancer who may have worse outcomes compared to younger patients because of reduced dose intensity and less aggressive dosing of chemotherapy in older patients.[12]

Several mechanisms to deliver chemotherapy in a dose-intense fashion are available to clinicians. First, doses of drugs can simply be escalated. Second, the same doses of drugs can be given in a reduced interval of time (ie, "dose-dense administration"). For example, adjuvant cyclophosphamide and doxorubicin followed by paclitaxel in early breast cancer administered every 2 weeks rather than every 3 weeks demonstrated improvements in the dose-dense regimen.[13] The prophylactic use of myeloid growth factors has enabled chemotherapy to be delivered at higher doses safely without excess neutropenic events and has enabled chemotherapy to be delivered in a dose-dense manner.

Single Versus Combination Therapy

Decisions regarding choice of single versus combination therapy should be based on the objectives of therapy (curative vs. palliative treatment), published regimens for specific indications and dosing of agents, and predicted toxicities. Specific doses chosen should be based on published studies, but dose alterations can occur based on objectives of treatment; renal, hepatic, or bone marrow function; toxicities experienced by the patient during previous cycles; current performance status and comorbidities of the patient; direct measurement of drug levels in the individual patient when possible; and potential interactions with other concomitant medications. Although combination chemotherapy typically yields higher response rates overall compared to single agents, toxicities are usually higher; outcomes such as overall survival and progression-free survival may better with combinations.[14] Scheduling of drugs is such that the most myelosuppressive agents are given on day 1 and scheduled every 2 to 4 weeks depending on the timing of the myelosuppression nadir. This allows for recovery of bone marrow, gastrointestinal, dermatologic, and other organ toxicities without allowing significant tumor growth to occur. Mechanisms of action of the drugs and duration of infusion may also influence drug sequencing and toxicities.

PHARMACOLOGY

Chemotherapy agents are divided into classes based on their mechanism of actions.

Alkylating Agents

Alkylating agents work by interfering with the mechanisms of DNA and DNA repair, and their actions result in the covalent binding of an electrophilic alkyl group or a substituted alkyl group to different nucleophilic groups such as proteins, RNA, and DNA bases, leading to their cytotoxicity. Bifunctional alkylating agents that have 2 chloroethyl side chains undergo cyclization forming a covalent bond with an adjacent nucleophilic group, leading to DNA–DNA or DNA–protein cross-linking. The 7 nitrogen or 6 oxygen atoms of the base guanine appear to be susceptible to targeting with alkylating agents and may be targets that lead to the cytotoxicity and mutagenicity of treatment using these agents. Alkylating agents are typically highly reactive and overall have short half-lives. Alkylating agents are mostly metabolized via spontaneous hydrolysis, and several also are metabolized via enzymatic conversions. The toxicities of alkylating agents include bone marrow suppression and gastrointestinal toxicities. Contraindications to these agents include patients with significantly depressed bone marrow function as well as allergic reactions, although safe administration can be feasible in certain situations using desensitization protocols (see later section, Allergic or Infusion Reactions).

Hexamethylmelamine

Hexamethylmelamine (altretamine) is an alkylating agent that has an uncertain mechanism of action, and altretamine (Hexalen) capsules are indicated for use as a single agent for the palliative treatment of patients with persistent or recurrent ovarian cancer following first-line therapy with a cisplatin- and/or alkylating agent–based combination.

Following oral administration, hexamethylmelamine is well absorbed and undergoes rapid and extensive hepatic demethylation, resulting in variation of hexamethylmelamine levels. The main metabolites are pentamethylmelamine and tetramethylmelamine, and following administration of doses of 120 to 300 mg/m² in ovarian cancer patients, free fractions of hexamethylmelamine, pentamethylmelamine, and tetramethylmelamine were 6%, 25%, and 50%, respectively, all showing binding to plasma proteins. Peak plasma levels are reached between 0.5 and 3 hours and vary between 0.2 and 20.8 mg/L. There have been no formal studies of use of hexamethylmelamine in patients with hepatic and/or renal compromise. Hexamethylmelamine is administered in 4 divided doses, although there are no formal pharmacokinetic data for this schedule or information on the effect of food on absorption. Hexamethylmelamine has been used in ovarian cancer in varying schedules (either 14 or 21 days out of a 28-day cycle). Coadministration of hexamethylmelamine and monoamine oxidase inhibitors may result in orthostatic hypotension, especially in patients over the age of 60 years, and should be used with caution. Other toxicities of hexamethylmelamine include peripheral neuropathy, other central nervous system toxicities (ataxia, dizziness, and mood disorders), nausea, vomiting, fatigue, and importantly, myelosuppression. Blood count nadirs typically occur by 3 to 4 weeks when the schedule of 21 days out of 28 is used, and continuous dosing results in median nadirs of 6 to 8 weeks. However, because of variable oral absorption and difficulties assessing bone marrow tolerability of this drug, exact prediction of the extent and duration of the nadir is sometimes difficult. Thus, caution should be used in heavily pretreated patients, and counts should be monitored frequently, even weekly, in patients in whom it is uncertain when the exact nadir will occur. Toxicities necessitating changes in dose and perhaps schedule include gastrointestinal intolerance, other grade 3 or 4 toxicities, progressive neurotoxicity, and myelosuppression.

Melphalan

Melphalan is a bifunctional alkylating agent that is a phenylalanine derivative of nitrogen mustard and is also known as L-phenylalanine mustard, phenylalanine mustard, L-PAM, or L-sarcolysin. Melphalan's cytotoxicity results from cross-linking of DNA, likely by binding at the N⁷ position of guanine. Melphalan has been used in gynecologic malignancies, specifically ovarian cancer. Because of melphalan's toxicities and the institution of more effective and less toxic drugs, melphalan's use has diminished over time and is very limited. Toxicities include secondary malignancies, specifically acute nonlymphocytic leukemias and myelodysplastic syndrome. The cumulative dose impacts the risk of secondary hematologic malignancies. For cumulative doses above 730 mg and up to 9652 mg, the 10-year cumulative risk was 19.5%, and for doses below 600 mg, the cumulative risk of a secondary hematologic malignancy was less than 2%. Other toxicities include myelosuppression, fatigue, gastrointestinal toxicities, and mutagenesis. Because of melphalan's toxicities and the difficulty predicting them and the development of less toxic agents, melphalan is rarely used.

Platinum Drugs

Platinum drugs that have been tested in gynecologic cancers include cisplatin, carboplatin, and oxaliplatin. Cisplatin and carboplatin are 2 of the most important agents in treating gynecologic malignancies. All platinum drugs have a fixed, planar platinum core and are surrounded by both carrier ligands and leaving groups; all of the components exist in a 2-dimensional plane. Unlike alkylating agents, which use carbon as the main atom and have reactive arms that move around carbon, platinum compounds have fixed reactive groups relative to platinum, and thus the DNA that binds covalently to the platinum compound bends to conform to the platinum core and ends up being fixed. All of the platinum compounds result in similar DNA lesions: N7-d(GpG)-intrastrand adducts (representing approximately 60% of total DNA binding), N7-d(ApG)-intrastrand adducts (representing about 30% of total DNA binding), N7-d(GpXpG)-intrastrand adducts (representing about 10% of total DNA binding), and N7-d(X)-d(X)G-intrastrand cross-links (representing about <2% of total DNA binding). The different platinum drugs have different leaving groups and carrier ligands, and how these groups determine the individual behavior and toxicities of the platinum agents has not been determined. The leaving groups for cisplatin are the chloride atoms, which are positioned in the *cis* configuration of the molecule and dissociate from the molecule under physiologic pH conditions; the carrier ligands are ammonia atoms. The leaving group for carboplatin is the dicarboxylatocyclobutane entity, which does not dissociate as easily as the chloride atoms do in cisplatin and may require active cleavage by an esterase. The leaving group for oxaliplatin is the oxalate moiety, resulting in the parent platinum molecule with 2 reactive *cis* bonds (similar to cisplatin and carboplatin), and the carrier ligand of oxaliplatin is a diaminocyclohexane moiety and influences DNA repair in addition to inhibition of the platinum-DNA adduct's replication bypass. Platinum drugs are able to access the intracellular compartment by 2 mechanisms: passive diffusion through the lipid bilayer and carrier-mediated uptake. Described platinum influx transporters include copper transporter proteins, organic cation transporters that belong to the SLC22 family, and a *cis* configuration–specific platinum influx transporter; the exact roles that these transporters have in actual drug levels intracellularly in addition to platinum resistance and sensitivity mechanisms are unknown.

Mechanisms of resistance of cisplatin have been better studied than carboplatin, but available data suggest that the mechanisms of resistance are quite similar and can either be intrinsic resistance, as seen in cancers that have little initial platinum sensitivity such as prostate and colon cancer, or acquired resistance as is seen in ovarian cancer.[15,16] Examples of resistance mechanisms include increased efflux of drug, reduced influx of drug, decreased blood flow of drug to the tumor, intracellular detoxification by intracellular compounds such as glutathione and metallothioneins, changes in DNA repair such as loss of mismatch repair, enhanced nucleotide excision repair, intrastrand cross-link repair, and defective apoptosis.

Cisplatin

Cisplatin has shown anticancer activity against most gynecologic malignancies. Cisplatin is US Food and Drug Administration (FDA)–approved for metastatic ovarian cancers in established combination therapy with other approved chemotherapeutic agents in patients with advanced ovarian cancers who have already received appropriate surgical therapy and/or radiotherapy. Cisplatin, as a single agent, is indicated as secondary therapy in patients with metastatic ovarian tumors refractory to standard chemotherapy who have not previously received cisplatin therapy. Cisplatin is also indicated for metastatic testicular tumors in established combination therapy with other approved chemotherapeutic agents as well as in advanced bladder cancer as a single agent for patients with transitional cell bladder cancer that is no longer amenable to local treatments, such as surgery and/or radiotherapy.

Once injected intravenously (IV), 90% of the platinum parent drug is bound to plasma proteins including albumin, transferrin, and γ-globulin within 3 hours after a bolus infusion and 2 hours after the end of a 3-hour infusion. Drug concentrations of cisplatin are highest in the liver, kidney, and prostate, and platinum is present in tissues for as long as 180 days after the final administration of the drug. A drug concentration differential exists between the tumor and surrounding tissue; platinum levels are lower in the tumor than in surrounding tissues of the organ where the cancer is located.

Cisplatin can lead to cumulative nephrotoxicity; cisplatin is contraindicated in patients with preexisting renal impairment and should be used with caution in patients who are more prone to renal injury (ie, diabetes mellitus, long-standing hypertension, the elderly). All patients should be prehydrated with 1 to 2 L of normal saline immediately prior to receipt of cisplatin, either IV or intraperitoneal (IP). Failure to hydrate patients in accordance with guidelines and the

FDA package insert can and will lead to renal damage and perhaps renal failure. IV fluids should be given after infusion as well because cisplatin remains in tissues. Serum creatinine, blood urea nitrogen, creatinine clearance, magnesium, sodium, potassium, and chloride must be checked prior to each administration of cisplatin and in between cycles of administration if warranted, making certain that all laboratory tests are adequate to proceed to the next cycle. Other toxicities of cisplatin include peripheral neuropathy, loss of motor function, allergic reactions, ototoxicity, development of secondary leukemias, myelosuppression, electrolyte abnormalities, hyperuricemia, hepatotoxicity, other types of neurotoxicity (loss of taste, autonomic neuropathy, dorsal column neuropathy, and seizures), asthenia, cardiac abnormalities, hiccups, rash (may be secondary to an allergic reaction), and alopecia rarely. Neuropathy should be monitored for at each cycle administration, and patients should inform their treating team of the severity of any intracycle neuropathy because the neuropathy may have improved at the time of the start of the next cycle. Symptoms and signs of neuropathy and other central nervous system abnormalities most often occur during treatment, but symptoms of neuropathy can occur following the completion of cisplatin treatment; patients should be warned of this, although it is rare (see later section on neuropathic complications of anticancer agents). Significant and persistent peripheral neuropathy can occur for up to 1 year or more after the completion of IP treatment.[17] Cisplatin should be discontinued following the initiation of significant neuropathy. Peripheral neuropathy may be irreversible in some patients, and patients need to be counseled about this potentially long-term toxicity. Monitoring of auditory acuity may also be necessary, especially if patients have an already existing hearing deficit or if they develop ototoxicity during therapy.

Carboplatin

Carboplatin, much like cisplatin, produces cell cycle nonspecific intrastrand DNA cross-links rather than DNA-protein cross-links. The aquation of carboplatin leads to the active compound, and platinum from carboplatin is irreversibly bound to plasma proteins that are slowly eliminated with a half-life of approximately 5 days.

Carboplatin has an FDA indication for the initial treatment of advanced ovarian carcinoma in combination with other approved chemotherapeutic agents. Carboplatin is also indicated for the palliative treatment of patients with recurrent ovarian carcinoma after prior chemotherapy, including patients who have been previously treated with cisplatin.

The major route of elimination of carboplatin is via renal excretion. Glomerular filtration rate (GFR) determines creatinine clearance (CrCl). Thus, elimination varies based on CrCl; patients with a CrCl of ≥ 60 mL/min will excrete approximately 65% of a carboplatin dose in the urine within 12 hours and 71% of the dose within 24 hours. In patients with lower CrCl (<60 mL/min) and thus reduced renal clearance of carboplatin, the doses of carboplatin should be reduced. In the elderly population, because their renal function is often decreased, formula dosing of carboplatin based on estimates of GFR should be used to ensure predictable plasma carboplatin area under the curve (AUC) values and thereby minimize toxicity. Obese patients do not appear to have higher toxicities compared to nonobese patients, and in a Gynecologic Oncology Group study that examined carboplatin dosing using the Jelliffe equation to calculate GFR and using a carboplatin dose of AUC 7.5, obese patients appeared to have fewer toxicities compared to nonobese patients.[18] Obese patients with epithelial ovarian cancer appear to have a comparable prognosis to other patients, provided that they receive optimal doses of chemotherapy based on measured GFR and actual body weight.

The dosing of carboplatin has changed over the past 2 decades. Initial studies in ovarian cancer used milligram per meter squared dosing, but recognition that carboplatin elimination is based on GFR led to renal function and age-based dosing, leading to more accurate dosing. Calvert dosing uses AUC dosing in addition to GFR; the dosing is: total dose (mg) = (target AUC) × (GFR + 25). There are currently 2 ways to calculate GFR: the Jelliffe formula and the Cockcroft-Gault formula, and the decision to use one formula or the other should be based on published regimens. In October 2010, the FDA issued an alert on carboplatin dosing safety after discussions with the National Cancer Institute/Cancer Therapy Evaluation Program. By the end of 2010, all clinical laboratories in the United States would be using the new standardized isotope dilution mass spectrometry (IDMS) method for measurement of serum creatinine. The IDMS method appears to underestimate serum creatinine values compared to older methods when the serum creatinine values are relatively low (eg, ~0.7 mg/dL). Thus, measurement of serum creatinine by the IDMS method could result in an overestimation of the GFR in some patients with normal renal function. If a patient's GFR is estimated based on serum creatinine measurements by the IDMS method, the FDA recommends that physicians consider capping the dose of carboplatin for desired exposure (AUC) to avoid potential toxicity due to overdosing. The maximum carboplatin dose (mg) = target AUC (mg · min/mL) × (150 mL/min), which is based on a GFR estimate that is capped at 125 mL/min for patients with normal renal function. No higher estimated GFR values should be used.

Overall, carboplatin is better tolerated than cisplatin, and thus, carboplatin should be selected as the drug of choice when both carboplatin and cisplatin show equivalent results. Carboplatin has more minimal nephrotoxicity and a more tolerable nausea/vomiting profile compared to cisplatin. Toxicities of carboplatin include myelosuppression, nausea and vomiting, peripheral neuropathy, ototoxicity, electrolyte abnormalities (including hyponatremia, hypomagnesemia, hypokalemia, and hypocalcemia), allergic reaction, fatigue and malaise, and other more rare side effects such as secondary leukemia, vision loss, central neurotoxicity, alopecia, shortness of breath, cardiovascular toxicities, mucositis, and cancer-associated hemolytic uremic syndrome (FDA package insert). Bone marrow suppression is the dose-limiting toxicity of carboplatin and is more pronounced in patients with reduced CrCl and in those who have received prior chemotherapy or radiation therapy. Bone marrow suppression is cumulative, and blood counts should be monitored in between cycles if indicated; future cycles of carboplatin should only be administered when blood counts have recovered. Nadir toxicity when carboplatin is used as a single agent occurs at about day 21. Dose modifications are listed in the FDA package insert.

When carboplatin is combined with paclitaxel, myelosuppression, specifically neutropenia, is lessened if paclitaxel is administered first; this has been observed with cisplatin but should be followed with carboplatin as well. In addition, the less toxic sequence of paclitaxel followed by the platinum drug is also more cytotoxic to tumor cells in vitro, so paclitaxel should be administered first, and then the platinum drug thereafter.

Allergic reactions have been reported with carboplatin and tend to occur in patients who have had prior exposure to platinum. Allergic reactions may be mild, such as mild pruritus or flushing, or may include anaphylaxis. Allergic reactions most commonly occur during the infusion and less commonly occur after the infusion has been completed (hives or rash) (see specific toxicities later in this chapter).

Oxaliplatin

Oxaliplatin has not been found to be an active agent in gynecologic cancers. Oxaliplatin undergoes nonenzymatic conversion in physiologic solutions to active forms through displacement of the labile oxalate ligand, resulting in the formation of several transient reactive species including monoaquo- and diaquo-diaminocyclohexane platinum, which then covalently bind with DNA and other proteins. The terminal half-life of the drug is 38 to 47 hours. Current FDA-approved indications for oxaliplatin when used in combination with infusional 5-fluorouracil/leucovorin are: (1) adjuvant treatment of stage III colon cancer in patients who have undergone complete resection

of the primary tumor and (2) treatment of advanced colorectal cancer. Toxicities include myelosuppression, diarrhea and mucositis, peripheral neuropathy, hand-foot syndrome, and nausea and vomiting. Oxaliplatin, like the other platinum analogs, can cause anaphylaxis and other unusual toxicities including hemolytic uremic syndrome and anemia and others listed in the package insert. Oxaliplatin can also lead to injection site reactions, which can be severe; signs and symptoms of an injection site reaction include blistering, inflammatory changes, erythema, tenderness, and possibly ulceration and skin breakdown leading to possible skin grafting.

Cyclophosphamide

Cyclophosphamide is one of the most commonly used and successful chemotherapy drugs.[19] Cyclophosphamide was initially thought to selectively target cancer cells via activation of cancer cell phosphamidases, which was later found not to be its mechanism of action. After administration, the prodrug cyclophosphamide is hepatically activated to both active and inactive metabolites. Approximately 70% to 80% of cyclophosphamide are activated by hepatic microsomal P450 mixed function microsomal oxidases to form 4-hydroxycyclophosphamide and is in equilibrium with its tautomer aldophosphamide, and the name 4-hydroxycyclophosphamide applies to them both. Several cytochrome P (CYP) isoenzymes have been implicated in cyclophosphamide activation, including CYP2B6, CYP3A4, CYP3A5, CYP2C9, CYP2C18, and CYP2C19. CYP2B6 has the highest 4-hydroxylase activity. 4-Hydroxycyclophosphamide, which is very unstable, is able to diffuse into cells but is not cytotoxic itself. 4-Hydroxycyclophosphamide decomposes into phosphoramide mustard via β-elimination of acrolein, which are the 2 downstream metabolites of cyclophosphamide. Phosphoramide mustard is a bifunctional DNA alkylating agent that is likely responsible for most of the anticancer effect of cyclophosphamide by cross-linking with DNA in cancer cells. Extracellular phosphoramide mustard is not able to enter cells because it is ionized at physiologic pH. With oral dosing, cyclophosphamide is well absorbed, with a bioavailability greater than 75%, and the unchanged drug has an elimination half-life of 3 to 12 hours. Cyclophosphamide is eliminated primarily in the form of active metabolites, but from 5% to 25% of the dose is excreted in urine as unchanged drug. Following IV administration, metabolites reach a maximum concentration in plasma in 2 to 3 hours. Plasma protein binding of unchanged drug is low, but some metabolites are bound to an extent greater than 60%.

Several toxicities of cyclophosphamide exist, and toxicities are dependent on route of administration and dose. Higher doses of intravenously administered drug can result in myelosuppression, hemorrhagic cystitis, cardiac toxicity (ie, hemorrhagic carditis leading to cardiomyopathy and pericarditis), and anaphylactic reactions. Toxicities that are observed with more standard doses of the drug include myelosuppression; gastrointestinal toxicities such as nausea, vomiting, and mucositis; alopecia; hemorrhagic cystitis; interstitial pneumonia; and carcinogenic and teratogenic toxicities.

Cyclophosphamide's FDA indications are the following: ovarian cancer, malignant lymphomas, Hodgkin disease, lymphocytic lymphoma, mixed-cell type lymphoma, histiocytic lymphoma, Burkitt lymphoma, multiple myeloma, chronic lymphocytic leukemia, chronic granulocytic leukemia, acute myelogenous and monocytic leukemia, mycosis fungoides, neuroblastoma, retinoblastoma, and breast cancer.

Ifosfamide

Ifosfamide, much like cyclophosphamide, requires metabolic activation by microsomal liver enzymes that lead to biologically active metabolites. Hydroxylation at the ring carbon atom 4 leads to activation and forms 4-hydroxyifosfamide, an unstable metabolite that degrades to a more stable urinary metabolite, 4-ketoifosfamide. When the ring is opened, this forms another stable urinary metabolite, 4-carboxyifosfamide. Ifosfamide's half-life is 15 hours, and the urinary excretion of metabolites is 15% at 24 hours. Renal clearance of ifosfamide plays a minor role compared to hepatic clearance, but renal insufficiency may increase the risk of neurotoxicity because of more extensive deactivation of ifosfamide, and dose reduction in patients with renal insufficiency should be considered. Like cyclophosphamide, because of acrolein formation, ifosfamide can also lead to hemorrhagic cystitis, and the thiol compound mesna can be given IV or orally and is rapidly auto-oxidized in plasma at pH 7.4 to dimesna, which is inactive. In renal tubular epithelial cells, dimesna is converted back to mesna by glutathione reductase enzymes, and the free sulfhydryl groups of mesna bind to acrolein. The severity and incidence of hemorrhagic cystitis can be lowered with hydration and bladder irrigation if necessary. To protect against hemorrhagic cystitis, mesna should be given continuously before, during, and following ifosfamide administration to any patient receiving high-dose cyclophosphamide and any patient with pre-existing drug-induced cystitis. Other toxicities of ifosfamide include myelosuppression, encephalopathy (which is not observed with cyclophosphamide), nephrotoxicity, alopecia, nausea, vomiting, and rarely cardiotoxicity and interstitial pneumonitis. The encephalopathy observed with ifosfamide is likely due to chloroacetaldehyde, one of its metabolites, and chloroacetaldehyde closely resembles the structure of ethanol. If symptoms of encephalopathy do develop, such as confusion, the patient should be treated clinically via electrolyte correction, hydration, and potential hospitalization. Ifosfamide is indicated for relapsed germ cell tumors.

Antimicrotubule Agents

Microtubules are cellular organelles that play a vital role in cell shape, division, signaling, polarity, and the proper transport of other organelles and vesicles and are the conveyor belts of the cell. Structurally, microtubules are linear polymers of tubulin, and groups of these are called protofilaments. A protofilament is a linear row of tubulin dimers. Polymerization of tubules proceeds by a nucleation–elongation mechanism. The first stage of formation is called "nucleation," which requires tubulin, Mg^{++}, and guanosine triphosphate. This stage is relatively slow until the microtubule is initially formed. The second phase, called "elongation," proceeds much more rapidly. The ends of microtubules are distinct; the plus end is more active kinetically, whereas the opposite end is more inert and called the minus end. Microtubules participate in 2 important activities. The first is called treadmilling, resulting in net growth on one end and shortening at the opposite end. The second is called dynamic instability, during which the microtubule ends can switch spontaneously between slow growth and rapid shortening.

Because of their broad anticancer activity, the taxanes are one of the most important classes of anticancer drugs. Paclitaxel was originally identified from the extract of the bark from the Pacific yew tree, *Taxus brevifolia*, in 1963. Early development of this drug was slowed by limited supply, but eventually large-scale production became available, making widespread use of paclitaxel possible. Paclitaxel is an antimicrotubule drug that promotes assembly of microtubules from tubulin dimers and is obtained via a semi-synthetic process; its chemical name is 5β,20-epoxy-1,2α,4,7β,10β,13α-hexahydroxytax-11-en-9-one 4, 10-diacetate 2-benzoate 13-ester with (2R, 3S)-*N*-benzoyl-3-phenylisoserine. Paclitaxel stabilizes microtubules by preventing and blocking depolymerization, resulting in inhibition of normal reorganization of the microtubule network. This microtubule reorganization is necessary for interphase and cellular mitotic functions, and paclitaxel exposure also leads to abnormal arrays or bundles of microtubules in the cell cycle and during mitosis. The microtubules formed when paclitaxel is present are dysfunctional yet stable, and cell death arises from disruption of the normal microtubule interactions and dynamics required for cell division. Resistance mechanisms include presence of altered α- and β-tubulin in tumor cells that have an impaired ability to polymerize into microtubules and slowed microtubule assembly and presence of drug efflux pumps.[20,21] Other mechanisms of resistance to taxanes include mutations in tubulin isotype genes and gene amplification.

Docetaxel is synthesized by the addition of a side chain to 10-deacetylbaccatin III, which is an inactive taxane precursor found in the needles of other yew tree species. Commonalities exist in the structures of both paclitaxel and docetaxel. The taxane rings of paclitaxel and docetaxel are linked to an ester side chain, which is located on the C13 position of the taxane ring, and this is essential for the antimicrotubule and thus anticancer activity of both agents. These agents do have different substitutions at position C10 of the taxane ring and position C13 on the ester side chain. Paclitaxel binds to the interior surface of the lumen of the microtubule at binding sites that are distinct from those of the vinca alkaloids. Although docetaxel is more water soluble than paclitaxel, it has the same binding site on the microtubule as paclitaxel does. Both paclitaxel and docetaxel alter the tubulin dissociation rate constants at both microtubule ends, resulting in inhibition of both treadmilling and dynamic instability. Vinca alkaloids alter tubulin polymerization, whereas the taxanes do not.

Paclitaxel has been FDA approved for the following indications: (1) treatment of patients with suboptimally cytoreduced stage III or IV ovarian cancer when combined with a platinum compound as primary induction therapy; (2) recurrent ovarian cancer after failure of first-line or subsequent chemotherapy; (3) advanced breast cancer after failure of combination chemotherapy or at relapse within 6 months of adjuvant chemotherapy; (4) adjuvant combination chemotherapy of lymph node–positive breast cancer sequentially after standard doxorubicin-based chemotherapy; (5) second-line treatment of Kaposi sarcoma associated with acquired immunodeficiency syndrome; and (6) primary treatment of non–small-cell lung cancer in combination with cisplatin. Docetaxel has been approved for the following (1) metastatic breast cancer that has progressed or relapsed after anthracycline-based chemotherapy as well as a second-line indication; (2) adjuvant chemotherapy of lymph node–positive breast cancer in combination with doxorubicin-based chemotherapy; (3) first-line chemotherapy for locally advanced or metastatic breast cancer; (4) nonresectable, locally advanced or metastatic non–small-cell lung cancer after failure of cisplatin-based chemotherapy; (5) first-line treatment of nonresectable, locally advanced or metastatic non–small-cell lung cancer in combination with cisplatin; (6) androgen-independent, hormone refractory metastatic prostate cancer in combination with prednisone; (7) first-line treatment of gastric adenocarcinoma including gastroesophageal junction adenocarcinoma in combination with cisplatin and 5-fluorouracil; and (8) inoperable locally advanced squamous cell cancer of the head and neck in combination with cisplatin and 5-fluorouracil.

After administration of longer infusions of paclitaxel, plasma levels decline in a biphasic manner; the initial rapid decline is secondary to distribution in the peripheral compartment ($\approx$20-minute half-life), and the second phase represents slower efflux of paclitaxel from this peripheral compartment (6-hour half-life). When shorter infusions are given that are 3 hours or less, the pharmacokinetics of paclitaxel are nonlinear, resulting in small increases in drug dose and a disproportionate increase in drug levels and toxicities and dose reductions, leading to a disproportionate decrease in drug exposure and possible lack of anticancer activity. Most of paclitaxel is excreted via stool through enterohepatic circulation 5 days following administration, and renal clearance is minimal. Paclitaxel is metabolized to 6α-hydroxypaclitaxel and 3'p-hydroxypaclitaxel via the isoenzymes CYP2C8 and CYP3A4.

Docetaxel pharmacokinetics on a 1-hour administration schedule are triexponential and linear when given at doses $\leq$115 mg/m^2, and terminal half-lives between 11 and 18.5 hours have been demonstrated. CYP3A4 and CYP3A5 are important in biotransformation and metabolism of docetaxel.

The sequencing of paclitaxel and other anticancer agents has important implications on toxicity and anticancer activity as discussed in the alkylating section. Sequencing cisplatin prior to paclitaxel in vitro results in enhanced neutropenia in addition to diminished anticancer activity when paclitaxel is administered over a 24-hour infusion; therefore, in clinical practice, taxane administration should precede the platinum infusion when combination taxanes and platinum agents are used.

Neutropenia is a common side effect that in noncumulative, and the duration of plasma levels of paclitaxel that are above biologically active levels (0.05-0.10 μmol) is an important determinant in prolonged neutropenia. Other side effects include an approximately 3% risk of hypersensitivity reactions, which typically occur within the first 10 minutes of the first treatment, although infusion reactions can occur at any time regardless of how many prior paclitaxel treatments the patient has received; the patient should be reminded of the signs and symptoms of paclitaxel reactions periodically. These reactions are thought to be secondary to Cremophor, which allows solubilization of paclitaxel. A standard premedication regimen for paclitaxel includes oral dexamethasone 20 mg 12 and 6 hours before infusion, an H$_1$-receptor antagonist such as diphenhydramine (Benadryl) 50 mg IV 30 minutes prior to infusion, and an H$_2$-receptor antagonist (ie, famotidine 20 mg, ranitidine 150 mg, or cimetidine 300 mg, all IV) given 30 minutes before infusion; this regimen was implemented originally when severe reactions were being observed during early clinical testing of this drug, some of which were fatal. Another single dose of a corticosteroid may be administered 30 minutes prior to paclitaxel infusion as well. Despite use of this premedication regimen, hypersensitivity reactions still can occur, and patients and treating staff must be aware of these reactions, which can be life threatening.

Paclitaxel also causes neuropathy that manifests in a stocking and glove distribution. Cardiac arrhythmias can also occur; the most common is asymptomatic bradycardia, but other abnormal rhythms can occur such as sinus tachycardia, atrial fibrillation, and other more malignant atrial and ventricular rhythms. Other toxicities include mild nausea, vomiting and diarrhea, hepatotoxicity, pulmonary toxicity with pneumonitis present on lung imaging, alopecia, nail changes, and rarely optic nerve disturbances. Docetaxel toxicities include neutropenia; hypersensitivity reactions; edema and fluid retention; palmar-plantar erythrodysesthesia; fatigue; mild gastrointestinal toxicities such as nausea, vomiting, and diarrhea; peripheral neurotoxicity; nail changes; and rarely stomatitis. Fluid retention is from increased capillary permeability and leaking and is cumulative with docetaxel, leading to peripheral edema and third-space fluid accumulation such as ascites or pleural effusions that are not malignant but related to docetaxel. Early treatment with diuretics and prophylactic use of corticosteroids are recommended, and the signs and symptoms of the fluid retention syndrome resolve after discontinuation of docetaxel.

Albumin-bound paclitaxel (ABI-007) is a formulation of paclitaxel that is solvent free, is a colloidal suspension with nanoparticle albumin, and has limited study in gynecologic cancers. Advantages of its use are that hypersensitivity reactions are markedly reduced because it is solvent free and no premedication with steroids is required, which is an advantage when treating patients with diabetes mellitus. Toxicities appear to be similar to equivalent doses of paclitaxel, but this drug has not been adequately studied in gynecologic cancers, and safety of its use has not been studied in patients with prior hypersensitivity reactions to either paclitaxel or docetaxel.

Vinca Plant Alkaloids

This class of agents includes vincristine, vinorelbine, and vinblastine. Vinca alkaloids were originally isolated from the leaves of the periwinkle plant, *Catharanthus roseus G. Don*, and were discovered in the late 1950s. The mechanism of action of the vinca alkaloids at clinically relevant concentrations is to block mitosis by binding to the β subunit of tubulin dimers at the vinca-binding domain. Vinca alkaloid binding of tubulin leads to a conformational change and altering treadmilling or growth/shortening of the microtubules which ultimately blocks mitosis. Vinca alkaloids enter cancer cells by simple diffusion, which is temperature independent and nonsaturable. Lipophilicity also plays a role in how the drug is able to enter cells. Vinca alkaloids are administered intravenously, and the drugs within this class have in common large volumes of distribution and long terminal half-lives. Metabolism and elimination of these drugs are predominantly via the hepatobiliary system and predominantly via the hepatic cytochrome CYP3A. Because of the importance of CYP3A metabolism, concomitant administration of vinca alkaloids with inhibitors and inducers of CYP3A may alter vinca alkaloid metabolism, and the treating clinician should know about these potential interactions. In addition, vinca alkaloids are potent vesicants, and extravasation could lead to significant tissue damage. If extravasation occurs, the drug infusion should be stopped immediately, and aspiration of any remaining drug in the soft tissues should be performed.

The vinca alkaloids differ with respect to toxicities. Neurotoxicity is more common with vincristine than the other vinca alkaloids, although neurotoxicity can occur with any of the agents. Neurotoxicity is most common with vincristine, can occur quickly, and is cumulative, and any patients with pre-existing neuropathic disorders or altered hepatic metabolism will predispose that patient to enhanced neurotoxicity. Vinorelbine and vinblastine also can cause neuropathy, and mild to moderate neuropathy can occur in up to 30% of patients. Gastrointestinal autonomic dysfunction can be observed with any of the vinca alkaloids, and these symptoms are manifested by constipation, bloating, abdominal pain, and an ileus. Patient education at the start of therapy is important, and patients should be encouraged to avoid narcotics that slow peristalsis, if possible, and take laxatives, if necessary. Neutropenia is the main toxicity of vinorelbine and vincristine, and myelosuppression is not cumulative. Other rare side effects include alopecia, hand-foot syndrome, acute cardiac ischemia, hepatic and pulmonary toxicity, and syndrome of inappropriate antidiuretic hormone (SIADH).

Antimetabolites

Methotrexate

Methotrexate (MTX) is the most widely used antifolate in cancer treatment; it binds and inhibits dihydrofolate reductase (DHFR), which is a critical enzyme in folate metabolism. DHFR maintains the intracellular folate pool in the reduced form as tetrahydrofolates, which serve as precursors for de novo production of thymidylate and purine nucleotides. The purported mechanism of MTX is the irreversible binding of DHFR, resulting in stoppage of thymidylate and purine nucleotide synthesis as well as other amino acid synthesis through the lack of reduced folates. Through polyglutamation, the cytotoxic effects of MTX are prolonged because MTX polyglutamated forms have a longer half-life with a higher propensity to have effects in malignant rather than normal cells. MTX polyglutamates themselves are direct inhibitors of several folate-dependent enzymes such as DHFR and thymidylate synthase (TS).

MTX is metabolized and cleared renally, and the majority of the dose is excreted unchanged (80%-90%) in the urine. Therefore, patients with reduced renal clearance (CrCl < 60 mL/min) should not receive high-dose MTX; MTX is not significantly hepatically metabolized, so hepatic impairment will not alter MTX dosing. Renal excretion of MTX is inhibited by several drugs, including aspirin, penicillins, cephalosporins, probenecid, and nonsteroidal anti-inflammatory medications. MTX is third-spaced, and the presence of large-volume ascites or pleural effusions can alter the pharmacokinetics of MTX by slowing elimination. Clinicians should consider draining large third-space volumes prior to MTX administration.

MTX metabolism, when administered IV, results in a 3-phase elimination pattern, and absorption is optimal when given IV, with oral doses above 25 mg/m² more inconsistent. The initial phase of IV infusion lasts a few minutes; the second phase lasts 12 to 24 hours, during which the drug has a half-life of 2 to 3 hours; and during the third phase, MTX clearance is prolonged with a half-life of 8 to 10 hours. The second and third phases of clearance are affected and lengthened in patients with renal impairment. High-dose MTX is considered to be any dose of MTX that is 500 mg/m² or higher and is given over 6 to 42 hours. These doses are considered lethal and should not be administered to patients with impaired renal function. When administering high-dose MTX, care must be given to adequate IV hydration of the patient, alkalinization of urine, careful monitoring of MTX levels, and adequate administration of leucovorin. Following high-dose MTX administration, MTX levels should be monitored every 24 hours. Leucovorin should be given until the MTX level is 50 nM or less; excessive leucovorin can negatively affect the levels of MTX. Leucovorin can be administered orally or IV; higher doses are more effectively administered IV because oral absorption is impaired at doses of ≥40 mg.

Toxicities of MTX are predominantly myelosuppression and gastrointestinal, and these toxicities are dose and schedule dependent; even small doses of MTX can result in significant renal toxicity in patients with impaired renal function. Mucositis precedes myelosuppression, and these toxicities resolve usually within 14 days unless MTX clearance is impeded. High-dose MTX administration can lead to elevated hepatic enzymes, and bilirubin can be observed, which typically resolves within 10 days. Other side effects include pneumonitis, which is manifested by fevers, pulmonary infiltrates, and a cough. In addition, high-dose MTX can give rise to cerebral dysfunction with behavioral changes, paresis, seizures, and aphasia. Chronic MTX administration can lead to chronic neurotoxicity after 2 to 3 months of therapy, and symptoms include encephalopathy, motor paresis, and dementia; the etiology of MTX-induced neurotoxicity is unknown.

Pemetrexed

Pemetrexed is a multitargeted antifolate drug that inhibits several enzymes important for folate production such as DHFR, TS, ribonucleotide formyltransferase, and aminoimidazole carboxamide formyltransferase.[22] Pemetrexed enters cells mainly via the reduced folate carrier system and via the folate receptor transporter as a more minor component of entry. Intracellularly, pemetrexed undergoes polyglutamation, making its potency 60-fold higher than the nonpolyglutamated parent compound. Pemetrexed is cleared renally, has a half-life of 3.1 hours, and must be used with caution with impaired renal function. Dose reduction in patients with renal dysfunction should be considered. Toxicities include myelosuppression, skin rash, and mucositis, with the latter 2 toxicities being significant in patients who are not pretreated with folic acid and vitamin B_{12}. Other toxicities include fatigue, anorexia, and reversible transaminitis. Patients pretreated with folic acid (350 μg/d) and vitamin B_{12} (1000 μg intramuscularly given at least 1 week prior to starting drug) exhibit decreased rates of toxicities, specifically rash and mucositis.

5-Fluorouracil

5-Fluorouracil (5-FU) was originally synthesized in 1957 and remains one of the most widely used anticancer drugs. 5-FU enters the intracellular compartment via facilitated uracil transport and is metabolized. 5-FU is mainly metabolized by dihydropyrimidine dehydrogenase (DPD). 5-FU is cytotoxic through several mechanisms, including inhibition of TS and incorporation into both RNA and DNA, leading to changes in mRNA translation, RNA processing, and inhibition of DNA function and synthesis. 5-FU may also exert cytotoxicity through Fas signaling pathways. The main mechanisms of resistance are through alterations in the target enzyme TS and its level of expression and degree of enzymatic activity, which can be altered by mutations. The toxicities of 5-FU are schedule and dose dependent, with the main toxicities being gastrointestinal toxicity and myelosuppression. When 5-FU is given daily for 5 days every 4 weeks, the main toxicities are diarrhea and mucositis. When given weekly, toxicities include myelosuppression and diarrhea, and when given as a continuous infusion, the toxicities are diarrhea and hand-foot syndrome. Other toxicities include rash, mild nausea and vomiting, and a rare acute neurologic syndrome, which includes ataxia, somnolence, and upper motor neuron signs. 5-FU can also rarely lead to chest pain, electrocardiogram changes, and elevations in cardiac enzymes. DPD is the main and rate-limiting enzyme in the catabolism of 5-FU, and deficiencies of this enzyme can lead to significant and, at times, life-threatening toxicities such as diarrhea and neurotoxicity. If a patient is known to have a DPD deficiency or if the toxicities with 5-FU are more significant than expected and DPD levels are found to be decreased, appropriate dose reductions should be done or the drug should not be given.

Capecitabine

Capecitabine is an oral fluoropyrimidine carbamate that was originally approved for metastatic breast cancer by the FDA in 1998 that is resistant to both taxanes and anthracyclines. Capecitabine has 80% oral bioavailability, is inactive in its parent compound, and must undergo 3 enzymatic steps before activation. First, it is hydrolyzed intrahepatically by carboxylesterase to the intermediate 5′-deoxy-5-fluorocytidine, which is then converted by cytidine deaminase to 5′-deoxy-5-fluorourodine. The third activation is performed by the enzyme thymidine phosphorylase (TP), which is located at higher concentrations in the cervix, breast, colon, head and neck, and stomach; TP converts 5′-deoxy-5-fluorourodine to 5-FU. Capecitabine and its metabolites are predominantly renally cleared, so clinicians should use caution when dosing this drug in patients with renal impairment, and it is contraindicated in patients with a CrCl < 30 mL/min.

Toxicities of capecitabine include hand-foot syndrome and diarrhea. Other toxicities associated with 5-FU such as myelosuppression, alopecia, nausea, and vomiting are much lower in incidence with capecitabine. Alternate dosing with capecitabine has been explored given the high toxicities associated with the FDA-approved dosing of this drug,[23] and clinicians should carefully choose a starting dose of this drug and educate patients about the specific toxicities of this drug. Patients should be instructed to call their physician if diarrhea starts and be told to hold the drug if diarrhea becomes severe. Interestingly, patients in the United State are less able to tolerate starting doses of capecitabine compared to European patients, and this may be related to vitamin supplementation in US diets.

Gemcitabine

Gemcitabine (2′,2′-difluorodeoxycytidine [dFdC]) has shown activity in many gynecologic tumors and is a radiation sensitizer. Gemcitabine is administered IV and undergoes deamination to a catabolic metabolite, difluorodeoxyuridine. Gemcitabine in its parent form is inactive and requires intracellular metabolism and activation intracellularly to become cytotoxic. Cytarabine and gemcitabine have similar enzymatic activation patterns; the enzyme deoxycytidine kinase converts dFdC into gemcitabine monophosphate, and this molecule is phosphorylated by nucleoside monophosphate and diphosphate kinases to di- (dFdCDP) and triphosphate (dFdCTP) metabolites. Ultimately, dFdCTP is incorporated into DNA, resulting in the inhibition of DNA synthesis and normal functioning as well as interference with DNA repair and chain elongation. Resistance to gemcitabine includes the presence of nucleoside transport-deficient cells or cells that have decreased quantities of these transporters, deficiency of enzymes that are involved in the intracellular metabolism of gemcitabine, and increased amount or activity of certain catabolic enzymes.

Greater than 90% of the drug following IV administration is found in the urine. Gemcitabine clearance is lowered in the elderly, and increased hepatic toxicity is observed when gemcitabine is given when total bilirubin levels are > 1.6 mg/dL; gemcitabine doses should be lowered in this setting. Toxicities of gemcitabine are dose dependent, and longer infusions lead to more myelosuppression. Toxicity includes myelosuppression, and both neutropenia and thrombocytopenia are observed. Other side effects include fevers, transient elevation of transaminases, myalgias, and asthenia. Rarer complications that require discontinuation of gemcitabine include dyspnea and hemolytic uremic syndrome. Both of these toxicities should be recognized early and treated, and gemcitabine should be stopped.

Topoisomerase Inhibitors

Topoisomerases are enzymes that alter the topology of DNA. During replication, transcription, and recombination, the double helix DNA is separated, resulting in torsional stress, and DNA topoisomerases reduce and resolve torsional stress. Type I and type II topoisomerases exist, and they differ based on the number of DNA strand breaks they can make. Type I topoisomerases cleave a single DNA strand and alter DNA linking number by 1 per activity cycle. Type II topoisomerases cleave both DNA strands and change DNA linking number by 2. Mammalian cells contain 1 type IB topoisomerase, topoisomerase I (Top1); 2 type IA topoisomerases, topoisomerase IIIα (Top3α) and topoisomerase IIIβ (Top3β); and 2 type II topoisomerases, topoisomerase IIβ (Top2β) and topoisomerase IIα (Top2α). These different topoisomerases perform different functions; Top1, Top2α, and Top2β are essential for cell viability. Top1 is also important in replication fork movement during DNA replication as well as relaxing supercoiled DNA that is formed during transcription. Top2α also allows DNA relaxation during transcription as well as unlinking daughter duplexes during DNA replication and helps remodel chromatin structure.

Camptothecin

Camptothecin was identified in the 1960s and is a naturally occurring alkaloid derived from the *Camptotheca acuminata* tree. Initial studies of camptothecin were complicated by severe toxicities of myelosuppression and hemorrhagic cystitis and showed only minimal anticancer activity. Active lactone forms that are water-soluble derivatives of camptothecin, irinotecan and topotecan, are currently FDA approved for cancer treatment. Camptothecins work by stabilizing the typically transient reaction in which the enzyme is covalently linked to DNA. Resistance to camptothecins is likely multifactorial and result from inadequate intracellular drug levels, impaired metabolism of the prodrug such as occurs with irinotecan, changes in the cell's response to the drug–Top1 interaction, and alterations in the normal topoisomerases themselves.

Irinotecan

Irinotecan is a prodrug that possesses a large dipiperidino side chain at C10 that must be cleaved intrahepatically as well as in other tissues by a carboxylesterase-converting enzyme in order to form the active metabolite, SN-38. Renal excretion accounts for 25% of irinotecan, and excretion is through hepatic metabolism and biliary excretion. Thus, dose reductions should be performed for patients with hepatic impairment. In addition, SN-38 is metabolized via glucuronidation intrahepatically by the enzyme UGT1A1, and patients who are homozygous for the UGT1A1 allele should undergo dose reductions of irinotecan. An FDA-approved test for the detection of UGT1A1 allele exists. The most common toxicities of irinotecan are diarrhea and myelosuppression. Irinotecan-induced diarrhea is predominantly caused by 2 mechanisms, which are also temporally different. Acute cholinergic effects caused by the prodrug's inhibition of acetylcholinesterase can lead to diarrhea and abdominal cramping within 24 hours, which can be treated with atropine. Direct mucosal cytotoxicity can also lead to diarrhea, which is usually observed greater than 24 hours after drug administration and is treated with loperamide.

Patients with deficiencies of UGT1A1 may experience more side effects of diarrhea and myelosuppression.

Topotecan

Topotecan is a semisynthetic analog of camptothecin that binds Top1. Topotecan undergoes reversible, pH-dependent hydrolysis of the active lactone moiety, forming an open-ring hydroxyacid, which is inactive. The terminal half-life of topotecan in patients with normal renal function is 2 to 3 hours, and this is increased to 5 hours in patients with renal dysfunction; topotecan clearance is decreased by approximately 25% in patients with moderate renal function impairment (CrCl, 20-39 mL/min). Toxicities are dependent on dose and schedule, and toxicities include myelosuppression, including neutropenia, anemia, and thrombocytopenia; mild nausea; fatigue; alopecia when given on the 5 days in a row schedule; and less commonly transient hepatic transaminitis, rash, and low-grade fevers. Receipt of heavy pretreatment with other cytotoxic drugs and prior radiation therapy can worsen myelosuppression, so clinicians may consider dose reduction in those patients. Because renal clearance is the predominant clearance of topotecan, clinicians should dose reduce topotecan in patients with renal impairment or choose an alternative therapy. Entry of topotecan into the cerebrospinal fluid (CSF) is higher than other camptothecins, but that does not appear to contribute to its toxicities; CSF levels of topotecan are approximately 30% of plasma levels. Topotecan has been approved for the treatment of recurrent ovarian cancer, lung cancer, and stage IVB recurrent or persistent carcinoma of the cervix cancer that is not amenable to curative treatment with surgery and/or radiation therapy.

Anthracyclines and Anthracenediones

Anthracyclines are derived from *Streptomyces peucetius* var. *caesius*. These drugs target Top2 through DNA intercalation leading to RNA and DNA synthesis inhibition and DNA–Top2 complex stabilization resulting in DNA double-stranded breaks. In addition, anthracyclines also enhance the catalysis of oxidation–reduction reactions through their quinone structure and promote the generation of oxygen free radicals, thereby leading to additional anticancer effect via DNA and cell membrane damage. Anthracyclines enter cells through passive diffusion and are hydrophobic. They are substrates for P-glycoprotein and Mrp-1. Major mechanisms of resistance include drug efflux, mutations in Top2 enzymes or reduced expression, overexpression of Bcl-2, *p53* mutations, and increase in neutralizing molecules such as glutathione or glutathione transferase. The different anthracyclines are doxorubicin, pegylated liposomal doxorubicin, daunorubicin, epirubicin, and idarubicin; anthracyclines are metabolized hepatically and excreted in the bile. Dose reductions are mandatory in patients with decreased hepatic function and elevated total bilirubin levels. Urinary excretion of anthracyclines is minimal and represents about 10% or less of the dose administered.

Doxorubicin

Doxorubicin is available in a standard salt form or as a liposomal formulation. The major toxicity of anthracyclines is cardiac toxicity, and both acute and chronic toxicities can be observed with this class of anticancer agents. Acute doxorubicin toxicity, which is typically reversible and occurs within a few days of the infusion, is clinically manifested by hypotension, dropped left ventricular ejection fraction, tachycardia, and electrocardiogram changes. Chronic toxicity is more common than acute toxicity and is cumulative and usually irreversible. Direct myocardial damage occurs via reactive oxygen species generated during election transfer from the semiquinone to quinone moieties and production of hydrogen peroxide and the peroxidation of myocardial lipids. Chronic cardiac damage is manifested by congestive heart failure from congestive cardiomyopathy, and cardiac biopsies in patients with chronic cardiac damage and congestive heart failure show interstitial fibrosis and occasional vacuolated myocardial cells. Myocytes hypertrophy and degenerate, along with loss of cross-striations. Risk factors for chronic cardiomyopathy include the dose, schedule of drug administration, cumulative dosing, and other risk factors such as previous heart disease history, radiation to the mediastinum, age younger than 4 years old, prior use of other cardiac toxins, concomitant administration of other chemotherapy such as paclitaxel or trastuzumab, and a history of hypertension. When doxorubicin is given as an IV bolus infusion every 3 to 4 weeks, the risk of congestive heart failure is 3% to 5% once the cumulative dose of doxorubicin reaches 400 mg/m^2, 5% to 8% when the dose reaches 450 mg/m^2, and 6% to 20% when the dose reaches 500 mg/m^2. Cardiac function should be monitored during treatment with anthracyclines by echocardiography or radionuclide scans. If arrhythmias are suspected, electrocardiograms should be monitored. Left ventricular ejection fraction (LVEF) should be checked prior to starting an anthracycline. Anthracyclines become contraindicated when either the baseline LVEF in patients is <50% or the LVEF drops by more than 10% during therapy. Dexrazoxane is a metal chelator that can lessen myocardial toxicity of doxorubicin by chelating iron and copper and thus interferes with redox reactions that can generate free radicals and damage myocardial lipids. Other toxicities of doxorubicin include myelosuppression, alopecia, nausea, vomiting, mucositis, and fatigue, and all of these toxicities are dose and schedule dependent.

Doxorubicin is a vesicant, and care should be taken to avoid extravasations; central venous catheters should be placed if peripheral venous access is poor. Extravasations of doxorubicin can lead to skin and local tissue necrosis that may be treated with ice and dimethylsulfoxide to minimize the extravasation and possible surgical debridement and/or skin grafts if the extravasation is extensive enough. Flare reaction consisting of erythema around the injection site is a benign reaction. Other toxicities of doxorubicin include radiation recall, which consists of an inflammatory, erythematous reaction that occurs at sites of previous radiation leading to skin rash, pericarditis, and pleural effusions. Careful attention to ruling out other causes of skin rash besides a recall reaction such as inflammatory breast cancer, skin metastases, or other drug reactions or systemic disorders should occur. Secondary leukemias or myelodysplastic syndrome have been reported in patients treated with doxorubicin, and this risk is increased in patients who are treated concomitantly with other DNA-damaging anticancer agents or radiotherapy or with escalated doses of anthracyclines and when patients have been heavily pretreated with cytotoxic drugs. The risk of acute myeloid leukemia or myelodysplastic syndrome is more sharply elevated with intensified doses of cyclophosphamide in combination with standard doses of doxorubicin.

Pegylated Liposomal Doxorubicin

Pegylated liposomal doxorubicin (PLD) (doxorubicin HCl liposome injection; Doxil or Caelyx) is doxorubicin that has been encapsulated in extended-circulating liposomes. Liposomes are microscopic vesicles, composed of a phospholipid bilayer, that encapsulate active drugs, and PLD consists of a liquid suspension of vesicles with a mean size of 80 to 90 nm. Doxorubicin is encapsulated in the internal compartment of the liposome, and a single lipid bilayer membrane separates the internal compartment from the external one. There are approximately 10,000 to 15,000 doxorubicin molecules per liposome, and polyethylene glycol is located on the liposome surface for liposome stability. Most of the doxorubicin is present as a crystalline-like precipitate without osmotic effects, and this gives stability to the entrapment of doxorubicin. During circulation, at least 90% of PLD remains encapsulated, and the drug has a half-life of approximately 30 to 55 hours depending on the study reported, patient population, and patient age. PLD is eliminated via 2 phases, the distribution phase, where a minor fraction of drug is cleared from the circulation with a half-life of approximately an hour, and the elimination phase, which is significantly longer. Approximately 95% of PLD in the plasma remains encapsulated within liposomes and is not bioavailable. The volume of distribution is approximately the total blood volume, and the AUC is increased approximately 60-fold higher compared to free doxorubicin.

PLD is considered an irritant, and precautions should be taken to avoid extravasation. The most common adverse events associated with PLD are hand-foot syndrome (also known as palmar-plantar erythrodysesthesia) and stomatitis, and these adverse events are schedule and dose dependent. Patients should be carefully monitored for toxicity. Adverse reactions, such as hand-foot syndrome, hematologic toxicities, and stomatitis, may be managed by dose delays and adjustments. Following the first appearance of a grade 2 or higher adverse reaction, the dosing should be adjusted or delayed. Once the dose has been reduced, it should not be increased at a later time. Following administration of PLD, small amounts of the drug can leak from capillaries in the palms of the hands and soles of the feet. The result of this leakage is redness, tenderness, and peeling of the skin that can be uncomfortable and even painful. Other side effects include some nausea and fatigue; the cardiac effects of PLD are less than doxorubicin. For patients with hepatic impairment, it is recommended that the PLD dosage be reduced if the bilirubin is elevated as follows: serum bilirubin 1.2 to 3.0 mg/dL, give 50% of normal dose; serum bilirubin >3 mg/dL, give 25% of normal dose (package insert). Dose reductions for skin toxicity are listed in the package insert.

Mitoxantrone

Mitoxantrone was originally synthesized in the 1970s. It is a DNA intercalator and stabilizes the Top2–DNA complex, which leads to breaks in double-stranded DNA. Unlike anthracyclines, mitoxantrone undergoes oxidative–reduction reactions and formation of free radicals less frequently, so cardiac toxicity is less. Currently, mitoxantrone is FDA approved for hormone-refractory prostate cancer and acute myeloid leukemia. Toxicities include myelosuppression and, less commonly, nausea, vomiting, alopecia, and mucositis. Cardiac toxicity can be observed at cumulative doses greater than 160 mg/m². Dose reductions should be undertaken for patients with hepatic dysfunction.

Actinomycin

Actinomycin was originally isolated from the culture broth of *Streptomyces* in the 1940s. Dactinomycin is FDA approved for Ewing sarcoma, gestational trophoblastic disease (GTD), metastatic testicular cancer, rhabdomyosarcoma, and nephroblastoma. Dactinomycin is indicated as a single agent or in combination with other chemotherapeutic agents for treatment of GTD. Dactinomycin consists of a planar phenoxazone ring that is attached to 2 peptide side chains, and its mechanism of action is DNA intercalation between adjacent guanine–cytosine bases. This intercalation results in inhibiting Top2 and leads to double-stranded DNA breaks. Dactinomycin is transported by P-glycoprotein and represents a resistance mechanism. Its half-life is 36 hours. Toxicities include myelosuppression, nausea, vomiting, alopecia, mucositis, hepatotoxicity including veno-occlusive disease, fatigue, and acne. Elimination of dactinomycin is predominantly biliary and in feces and, to a lesser extent, renal; dactinomycin is typically excreted via these routes unchanged.

Epipodophyllotoxins

This class of drugs is comprised of etoposide and teniposide, both of which poison Top2 as their mechanism of anticancer activity. These drugs are glycoside derivatives of podophyllotoxin, which is an antimicrotubule agent originally extracted from the mandrake plant. Etoposide's chemical formula is 4′-demethylepipodophyllotoxin 9-[4,6-0-(R)-ethylidene-β-D-glucopyranoside]. Etoposide can be administered either orally or IV, and it has FDA approval for use in small-cell lung cancer and refractory testicular cancer. In gynecologic cancers, etoposide has activity in recurrent ovarian cancer, germ cell tumors, GTD, and small-cell tumors of the gynecologic tract.

Teniposide is FDA approved in refractory pediatric acute lymphoid leukemia but is not used in gynecologic cancers. In adults, clearance of etoposide is correlated with CrCl, serum albumin concentration, and nonrenal clearance. Thus, patients with impaired renal function receiving etoposide have exhibited reduced total body clearance, increased AUC, and a lower volume of distribution at steady state. The IV route is typically administered daily for 3 to 5 days every 3 to 4 weeks, and the main toxicities include myelosuppression, nausea, vomiting, diarrhea, fatigue, and alopecia. Other side effects include transient hypotension following rapid IV administration, which has been reported in 1% to 2% of patients; this has not been associated with cardiac toxicity or electrocardiographic changes. To prevent this rare toxicity, it is recommended that etoposide be administered by slow IV infusion over a 30- to 60-minute period. Another rare side effect is the development of anaphylactic-like reactions characterized by chills, fever, tachycardia, bronchospasm, dyspnea, and/or hypotension, which have been reported in 0.7% to 2% of patients receiving IV etoposide and in less than 1% of patients treated with oral capsules. These reactions typically respond to cessation of the infusion and administration of pressor agents, corticosteroids, antihistamines, or volume expanders, as appropriate; however, the reactions can be fatal.

Epipodophyllotoxins are associated with the development of secondary acute myeloid leukemias (French-American-British [FAB] class M4 and M5) due to balanced translocations affecting the breakpoint cluster region of the *MLL* gene at chromosome 11q23. The cumulative risk of secondary acute myeloid leukemias with this drug is approximately 4% over 6 years. The bioavailability of oral etoposide is very variable, with an average bioavailability of 50%. Etoposide is primarily cleared unchanged in the kidneys, and dose reductions are recommended; as per the package insert, a 25% dose reduction should be done for patients with a CrCl between 15 and 50 mL/min, and a 50% dose reduction should be done for patients with a CrCl <15 mL/min.

Miscellaneous Chemotherapy Agents

Bleomycin

Bleomycin sulfate is comprised of a mixture of glycopeptide antineoplastic antibiotics, bleomycin A_2 and bleomycin B_2, which are isolated from the fungus *Streptomyces verticillus*. Bleomycin's anticancer mechanism is derived from oxygen-free radical formation that then lead to single-stranded and double-stranded DNA breaks. The presence of a redox-active Fe^{2+} metal ion is necessary to generate the active free moieties. Bleomycin's effects are cell cycle specific and are specific for G2 and M phases of the cell cycle. Bleomycin is used as part of germ cell tumor regimens and is used intracavitary to treat malignant pleural effusions. Mechanisms of resistance to bleomycin include decreased drug accumulation intracellularly because of altered cell uptake, increased drug inactivation through increased expression of bleomycin hydrolase, and enhanced repair of DNA through the increased expression of DNA repair enzymes. Interestingly, bleomycin hydrolase is widely distributed in normal tissues with the exception of the skin and lungs, both targets of bleomycin toxicity. Bleomycin is given IV or intramuscularly and has an initial half-life of 10 to 20 minutes with a terminal half-life of 3 hours. Excretion is predominantly renal, and most of the drug is eliminated unchanged in the urine. The major toxicities of bleomycin are pulmonary. Pulmonary toxicity can occur in up to 10% of patients, and this toxicity is related to the cumulative dose received. The incidence of this toxicity is higher in patients above the age of 70 and in those who have received a total cumulative dose of 400 units. Additional risk factors include smoking, any underlying previous lung disease, prior chest irradiation, exposure to high concentrations of oxygen, and use of granulocyte colony-stimulating factor (G-CSF). The use of G-CSF and risk of pulmonary toxicity may be related to neutrophil presence and infiltration within areas of lung injury. The use of pulmonary function testing to monitor for pulmonary toxicity is controversial. It is recommended that the diffusing capacity of the lung for carbon monoxide (D_{LCO}) be monitored monthly if it is to be used to detect pulmonary toxicities, and the drug should be discontinued when the D_{LCO} falls below 30% to 35% of the pretreatment value. Frequent serial chest imaging via chest x-ray or computed tomography should also be performed. Signs and symptoms include dyspnea and cough, evidence of inspiratory crackles on physical examination, and pulmonary infiltrates or interstitial changes on chest imaging. A hypersensitivity reaction with fevers, chills, and urticaria is observed in up to 25% of patients; in 1% of lymphoma patients, a severe idiosyncratic reaction (similar to anaphylaxis) consisting of hypotension, mental confusion, fever, chills, and wheezing has been reported.

Because of bleomycin's sensitization of lung tissue, patients who have received bleomycin and who will receive oxygen administered at surgery are at greater risk of developing pulmonary toxicity. Even following bleomycin administration, lung damage can occur at lower concentrations of oxygen that are usually considered safe. Suggested preventive measures include maintaining fractional inspired oxygen (Fio_2) at concentrations approximating that of room air (25%) during surgery and the postoperative period and careful monitoring of fluid replacement. Skin toxicities can occur in up to 50% of treated patients, and this side effect consists of erythema, rash, hyperpigmentation, and tenderness of the skin. Hyperkeratosis, nail changes, alopecia, pruritus, and stomatitis have also been reported. Skin toxicities rarely result in discontinuation of bleomycin (2% of cases). Skin toxicity is a late manifestation and usually develops in the second and third week of treatment after 150 to 200 units of bleomycin have been administered; it appears to be related to the cumulative dose. Fevers can occur with the infusion or following completion of the infusion and can be quite elevated. Other rare toxicities include vascular toxicities such as myocardial infarction, cerebrovascular accidents, thrombotic microangiopathy (hemolytic uremic syndrome), or cerebral arteritis.

Renal insufficiency markedly alters bleomycin elimination. The terminal elimination half-life increases exponentially as the CrCl decreases. Dosing reductions have been proposed by the package insert for patients with CrCl values of <50 mL/min, with incremental dose reductions for each 10 mL/min drop below 50 mL/min.

PRINCIPLES OF CHEMOTHERAPY MANAGEMENT AND SIDE EFFECTS

All patients with gynecologic malignancies should be encouraged to participate in clinical trials when appropriate and available. Prior to administration of chemotherapy, requirements for adequate organ function and patient performance status should be met depending on drug pharmacology; the goals of therapy should be reviewed with the patient and documented in the medical record. Informed consent from the treating physician must be obtained prior to drug administration. During chemotherapy treatment, patients need to be observed closely for any treatment-related complications, and appropriate dose reductions should be made depending on the prior cycle's toxicities, goals of therapy, and organ function at that time. Patients need to understand both short-term and long-term toxicities of treatment and should be followed long term for treatment-related toxicities that may develop after the end of therapy such as peripheral neuropathy and secondary bone marrow abnormalities like myelodysplasia and secondary leukemias.

Neutropenia and Myelosuppression

Each chemotherapeutic agent has its own nadir point of bone marrow suppression based on metabolism and half-life. Based on published regimens and their toxicities, clinicians should monitor blood counts as appropriate for the regimen. In addition, certain populations are more prone to complications from prolonged neutropenia; these include patients with age greater than 65 years, poor performance status, poor nutritional status, past history of fever and neutropenia, extensive prior therapy with chemotherapy and/or radiation therapy, previous administration of combined chemoradiotherapy, bone marrow involvement with tumor, presence of open wounds or active infections, advanced cancer, and other serious comorbidities. In such clinical situations, the American Society of Clinical Oncology (ASCO) guidelines recommend primary prophylaxis with colony-stimulating factors (CSFs) even when administering a regimen that has febrile neutropenia (FN) rates <20%.[24] ASCO guidelines state that CSF use is appropriate when the FN risk of a regimen is 20% or higher. Secondary prophylaxis with CSF is recommended for patients who develop FN during a prior cycle of chemotherapy, and a dose reduction may compromise the treatment outcome. Dose reduction may also be a recommended next step in the setting of a previous episode of FN if medically appropriate. Three forms of CSFs exist for the prevention of FN: (1) G-CSF (filgrastim) is started 24 to 72 hours following the administration of chemotherapy, the dose is 5 μg/kg/d, and the drug is continued until the absolute neutrophil count (ANC) is at least 2 to 3×10^9/L; (2) pegylated G-CSF (pegfilgrastim) is administered as a single 6-mg subcutaneous injection 24 hours after the completion of chemotherapy; and (3) granulocyte-macrophage colony-stimulating factor is administered not less than 24 hours from the last chemotherapy and given at a dose of 250 μg/m^2/d until the ANC is $>1.5 \times 10^9$/L for 3 consecutive days.

Treatment of Anemia

For anemia treatment and prevention, erythropoiesis-stimulating agents (ESAs) have been tested to both prevent and treat anemia, but the routine use of ESAs has lessened in clinical practice because of observed toxicities and increased rates of death with use; guidelines exist for use of ESAs in cancer.[25] A recent meta-analysis by Bohlius et al[26] examined studies where ESAs were concomitantly administered with chemotherapy, and the meta-analysis demonstrated that ESAs increase mortality in patients who have cancer. A black box warning added to ESAs in 2008 states that ESAs shorten survival and increase risk for cancer progression in patients with breast, non–small-cell lung, head and neck, lymphoma, and cervical cancers. The package insert also warns that ESAs should be used only to treat cancer patients receiving chemotherapy, stopped when the chemotherapy is completed, and given at the lowest dose that corrects the anemia. This addition to the package insert also stated that ESAs should not be used when chemotherapy is used with curative intent, regardless of the type of cancer. Reasons for increased mortality in patients receiving ESAs are not completely understood but may include the stimulation by ESAs of erythropoietin receptors that are expressed on cancer cells and/or development of thromboembolic events associated with higher hemoglobin levels.

Nausea and Vomiting

Chemotherapy drugs are typically divided into categories based on risk for nausea and vomiting. ASCO divides risk into 4 categories: high emetic risk (>90%), moderate risk (30%-90%), low risk (10%-30%), and minimal risk (<10%).[27] Recommendations for antiemetic use are based on these drug risk categories. Antiemetics that have the greatest activity include 5-HT$_3$ serotonin receptor antagonists, dexamethasone, and aprepitant. Several different 5-HT$_3$ serotonin receptor antagonists exist, and these drugs appear to have equivalent safety and efficacy. They can also be used interchangeably. Oral formulations of the 5-HT$_3$ serotonin receptor antagonists are equally effective and safe compared to IV administration of these agents.

Peripheral Neuropathy and Other Nervous System Toxicities of Chemotherapy

One of the most problematic and long-lasting complications of chemotherapy is chemotherapy-induced peripheral neuropathy.[28] The affected areas are typically a stocking-and-glove distribution, and the neuropathy tends to worsen with repetitive chemotherapy cycles and will usually subside when the offending drug is discontinued. Chemotherapy drugs used to treat gynecologic malignancies that can cause peripheral neuropathy include the taxanes, platinum agents, and vinca alkaloids.

The taxanes can lead to a peripheral neuropathy that is manifested by sensory symptoms such as paresthesias, numbness, and pain in a stocking-and-glove distribution. Both large fibers (proprioception and vibration) and small fibers (pinprick and temperature) can be affected in a symmetric pattern and are thought secondary to axonal loss. Rarely, patients can experience involvement of the arms and legs and even the face suggestive of a neuronopathy. Motor and autonomic dysfunction can also occur with orthostasis and ataxia; the extent and severity of neuropathy are worse in patients who are predisposed to neuropathy such as those with diabetes mellitus and alcoholism.

Vinca alkaloids can lead to peripheral neuropathy and autonomic neuropathy, especially vincristine, and toxicities include peripheral sensorimotor loss and autonomic dysfunction with paralytic ileus, orthostasis, and sphincter abnormalities. Central nervous system side effects can also lead to ataxia, cranial nerve palsies, cortical blindness, and seizures.

Of the platinum analogs, carboplatin, cisplatin, and oxaliplatin can all lead to peripheral neuropathy. In approximately 80% of patients, oxaliplatin will additionally lead to distal paresthesias and mild muscle contractions. Other less common neurologic toxicities of oxaliplatin include voice and visual changes, perioral paresthesias, and pseudolaryngospasm.

Treatment of peripheral neurotoxicity or other nervous system toxicities includes either cessation or decreasing the dosage of the offending drug. Multiple pharmacologic interventions have been attempted to treat peripheral neurotoxicity, but thus far, the data for these various drugs are insufficient to recommend any agents.[29]

Teratogenesis and Gonadal Toxicity

Many chemotherapy agents will have unintended toxicities on reproductive organs in women, and effects on gonadal function will depend on the age of the patient, specific anticancer agents used, and doses of these drugs.[30] With respect to pregnancy, all women of reproductive age and capability should be questioned about their likelihood of pregnancy before beginning any chemotherapy regimen, and pregnancy should be ruled out even if the chance is small. If a cancer is diagnosed during pregnancy, in general, all chemotherapy agents are completely contraindicated during the first trimester of pregnancy, and some drugs may be given during the second and third trimesters depending on the agent.[31] The patient must be counseled about all toxicities to her and the developing fetus, the possibility of terminating the pregnancy if the patient's life is immediately endangered or the possibility of forgoing therapy until the pregnancy is complete, and all other treatment options.

Alkylating agents can have significant toxic effects on reproductive organs. Pathology of ovaries that have been exposed to alkylating agents demonstrated absence of primordial follicles and postmenopausal hormonal levels with decreased estrogen and progesterone levels and elevated follicle-stimulating hormone and luteinizing hormone levels. First-trimester exposure of the fetus to alkylating agents can result in a malformed fetus; chemotherapy exposure during the first trimester resulted in a 17% risk of malformations with single-agent chemotherapy and a 25% risk with combination chemotherapy. Exposure during the second and third trimesters with most alkylating agents does not appear to increase fetal malformation risk above that observed for a patient's age. Taxanes are used widely to treat gynecologic malignancies, but very little is known about their safety during pregnancy even during the second and third trimesters.

If a patient does opt to receive chemotherapy during her second or third trimester, besides the potential teratogenic toxicities and the known toxicities of the chemotherapy drug, the patient must be counseled about other possible side effects such as increased risk of intrauterine growth retardation, low birth weight, increased risk of fetal or neonatal death, and premature delivery.[31]

Allergic or Infusion Reactions

Nearly any drug used in oncology has the potential to result in either an infusion reaction or an allergic reaction. Infusion reactions are characterized by milder symptoms such as flushing, back pain, fever, and chest tightness, whereas hypersensitivity (allergic) reactions are characterized by more severe symptoms such as shortness of breath, edema, hives, pruritus, and hemodynamic changes. Drug reactions can occur either during chemotherapy administration or after the drug infusion has been completed. Anaphylaxis is a rare type of severe allergic reaction that can occur with the taxanes and platinum agents (other drugs much less commonly) and can lead to cardiovascular collapse and even death. Adverse infusion reactions associated with taxane agents (ie, paclitaxel, docetaxel) tend to occur at first exposure or during the first few cycles of therapy; occasionally, patients can develop a reaction with more prolonged or future use. However, re-exposure to carboplatin and/or cisplatin increases a patient's risk of a hypersensitivity reaction or an allergic reaction that could be life threatening.[32] Risk factors for developing a hypersensitivity reaction include having allergies to other drugs, reintroduction of the drug after a period of no exposure, receipt of multiple previous cycles, and intravenous exposure to the drug rather than oral or IP exposure. Patients should be counseled that either an infusion reaction or allergic reaction could occur, and this should be part of the consenting process. Patients should also be educated about the signs and symptoms of hypersensitivity reactions and should be treated by medical personnel familiar with these toxicities in a medical setting that has appropriate medical equipment and staff that can handle these potential life-threatening emergencies.[33] Standing orders should be written in advance in case an allergic or infusion reaction occurs. Mild infusion reactions (eg, flushing, back pain) could be rechallenged with the taxane if the patient, physician, and nursing staff agree with the plan to rechallenge; the patient has been counseled as to the risks and benefits; and the clinic area has emergency-trained personnel and emergency equipment. Usually, the taxane is infused at a slower rate, and many institutions have already existing nursing policies that stipulate how the drug will be infused. For more severe reactions, such as shortness of breath, hemodynamic changes, urticaria, or hypoxia, or for repetitively occurring infusion reactions, an allergist should be consulted. If it is deemed necessary for the patient to continue to receive the drug and there are no alternatives, the allergist can decide upon drug desensitization for future infusions.

Desensitization refers to a drug delivery process that renders the patient less likely to respond to an allergen and can be considered for patients who have had a prior reaction and in consultation with an allergist.[32] However, if the patient has developed a severe life-threatening reaction to a drug, it is recommended that the patient not be rechallenged with the implicated drug. If desensitization is recommend by the allergy team, the patient must receive the implicated drug through a desensitization with each infusion.

Chemotherapy Sensitivity and Resistance Assays

The routine use of chemotherapy sensitivity and resistance assays is not supported because of insufficient level of evidence, and these assays should not supplant standard of care chemotherapy.[33,34] In addition, most of the clinical studies testing in vitro chemotherapy

sensitivity and resistance were retrospective, and to date, 1 small study testing the adenosine triphosphate–tumor chemosensitivity assay compared to empiric selection demonstrated no significant survival benefit for the use of the assays. Although an accurate chemosensitivity or resistance assay would have great clinical utility in helping to select optimal therapy, no such assay is widely available at this time.

REFERENCES

1. Hanahan D, Weinberg RA. Hallmarks of cancer: the next generation. *Cell*. 2011;144:646-674.
2. Lemmon MA, Schlessinger J. Cell signaling by receptor tyrosine kinases. *Cell*. 2010;141:1117-1134.
3. Negrini S, Gorgoulis VG, Halazonetis TD. Genomic instability: an evolving hallmark of cancer. *Nat Rev Mol Cell Biol*. 2010;11:220-228.
4. Skipper HE. Kinetics of mammary tumor cell growth and implications for therapy. *Cancer*. 1971;28:1479-1499.
5. Norton LA. A Gompertzian model of human breast cancer growth. *Cancer Res*. 1988;48:7067-7071.
6. Raguz S, Yague E. Resistance to chemotherapy: new treatments and novel insights into an old problem. *Br J Cancer*. 2008;99:387-391.
7. Gerlinger M, Swanton C. How Darwinian models inform therapeutic failure initiated by clonal heterogeneity in cancer medicine. *Br J Cancer*. 2010;103:1139-1143.
8. Goldie JH, Coldman AJ. A mathematical model for relating the drug sensitivity of tumors to their spontaneous mutation rate. *Cancer Treat Rep*. 1979;63:1727-1733.
9. Bookman MA, Brady MF, McGuire WP, et al. Evaluation of new platinum-based treatment regimens in advanced-stage ovarian cancer: a phase III trial of the Gynecologic Cancer InterGroup. *J Clin Oncol*. 2009;27:1419-1425.
10. Tan DS-W, Gerlinger M, The B-T, et al. Anti-cancer drug resistance: understanding the mechanisms through the use of integrative genomics and functional RNA interference. *Eur J Cancer*. 2010;46:2166-2177.
11. Sakai S, Swisher EM, Karlan BY, et al. Secondary mutations as a mechanism of cisplatin resistance in BRCA2-mutated cancers. *Nature*. 2008;451:1116-1121.
12. Cress RD, O'Malley CD, Leiserowitz GS, et al. Patterns of chemotherapy use for women with ovarian cancer: a population based study. *J Clin Oncol*. 2003;21:1530-1535.
13. Citron ML, Berry DA, Cirrincione C, et al. Randomized trial of dose-dense versus conventionally scheduled and sequential versus concurrent combination chemotherapy as postoperative adjuvant treatment of node-positive primary breast cancer: first report of Intergroup Trial C9741/Cancer and Leukemia Group B Trial 9741. *J Clin Oncol*. 2003;21:1431-1439.
14. Pfisterer J, Plante M, Vergote I, et al. Gemcitabine plus carboplatin compared with carboplatin in patients with platinum-sensitive recurrent ovarian cancer: an intergroup trial of the AGO-OVAR, the NCIC CTG, and the EORTC GCG. *J Clin Oncol*. 2006;24:2699-2707.
15. Burger H, Loos WJ, Eechoute K, et al. Drug transporters of platinum-based anticancer agents and their clinical significance. *Drug Resist Updat*. 2011;14:22-34.
16. Stewart DJ. Mechanisms of resistance to cisplatin and carboplatin. *Crit Rev Oncol Hematol*. 2007;63:12-31.
17. Armstrong DK, Bundy B, Wenzel L, et al. Intraperitoneal cisplatin and paclitaxel in ovarian cancer. *N Engl J Med*. 2006;354:34-43.

18. Wright JD, Tian C, Mutch DG, et al. Carboplatin dosing in obese women with ovarian cancer: a Gynecologic Oncology Group study. *Gynecol Oncol.* 2008;109:353-358.

19. Emadi A, Jones RJ, Brodsky RA. Cyclophosphamide and cancer: golden anniversary. *Nat Rev Clin Oncol.* 2009;11:638-647.

20. Kavallaris M. Microtubules and resistance to tubulin-binding agents. *Nat Rev Cancer.* 2010;10:194-204.

21. Galletti E, Magnani M, Renzulli ML, et al. Paclitaxel and docetaxel resistance: molecular mechanisms and development of new generation taxanes. *Chem Med Chem.* 2007;2:920-942.

22. Villela LR, Stanford BL, Shah SR. Pemetrexed, a novel antifolate therapeutic alternative for cancer chemotherapy. *Pharmacotherapy.* 2006;26:641-654.

23. Traina TA, Theodoulou M, Feigin K, et al. Phase I study of a novel capecitabine schedule based on the Norton-Simon mathematical model in patients with metastatic breast cancer. *J Clin Oncol.* 2008;26:1797-1802.

24. ASCO practice guidelines for the use of white blood cell growth factors. *J Clin Oncol.* 2006;24:3187-3205.

25. Rizzo JD, Somerfield MR, Hagerty KL, et al. Use of epoetin and darbepoetin in patients with cancer: 2007 American Society of Clinical Oncology/American Society of Hematology clinical practice guideline update. *J Clin Oncol.* 2008;26:132-149.

26. Bohlius J, Schmidlin K, Brillant C. Erythropoietin or darbepoetin for patients with cancer: meta-analysis based on individual patient data. *Cochrane Database Syst Rev.* 2009;8(3):CD007303.

27. American Society of Clinical Oncology guideline recommendations for antiemetics in oncology. *J Clin Oncol.* 2006;24:2932-2947.

28. Kannarkat G, Lasher EE, Schiff D. Neurologic complications of chemotherapy agents. *Curr Opin Neurol.* 2007;20:719-725.

29. Wolf S, Barton D, Kottschade L, et al. Chemotherapy-induced peripheral neuropathy: prevention and treatment strategies. *Eur J Cancer.* 2007;44:1507-1515.

30. Oktay K, Sönmezer M. Chemotherapy and amenorrhea: risks and treatment options. *Curr Opin Obstet Gynecol.* 2008;20(4):408-415.

31. Pereg D, Koren G, Lishner M. Cancer in pregnancy: gaps, challenges, and solutions. *Cancer Treat Rev.* 2008;34:302-312.

32. Castells MC, Tennant NM, Sloane DE, et al. Hypersensitivity reactions to chemotherapy: outcomes and safety of rapid desensitization in 413 cases. *J Allergy Clin Immunol.* 2008;122:574-580.

33. Morgan RJ Jr, Alvarez RD, Armstrong DK, et al. Epithelial ovarian cancer. *J Natl Compr Canc Netw.* 2011;9:82-113.

34. Karam AK, Chiang JW, Fung E, Nossov V, Karlan BY. Extreme drug resistance assay results do not influence survival in women with epithelial ovarian cancer. *Gynecol Oncol.* 2009;114(2):246-252.

21 | Targeted Therapy and Immunotherapy

Robert L. Coleman and Paul J. Sabbatini

COMPONENTS OF THE IMMUNE SYSTEM

While simplistic in its view, the effectors of the immune system are generally divided into those components that support innate immunity and those that support acquired immunity. The classification suggests a dichotomous relationship, but there is necessary and frequent cross-talk between the 2 arms. Innate immunity is active from birth, is the first line of defense against most pathogens, and does not require modification for activity. Acquired immunity largely requires activation of B lymphocytes and T lymphocytes and uses a complex process of activation, modification, expansion, and suppression in response to changing stimuli.

Innate immunity includes physical barriers (skin, mucous membranes), chemical components (hydrolytic enzymes and complement), and several cellular components. For example, polymorphonuclear lymphocytes are phagocytic cells with lysosomes containing enzymes and generally fight infection. Recent data suggest that neutrophil survival is modulated by T-cell responses, thus illustrating 1 area of cross-communication between the innate and acquired immunity systems. Monocytes are heavily granulated cells that migrate from blood to various tissues and differentiate depending on site. They become Kupffer cells in the liver, microglial cells in the central nervous system, and macrophages in the lung, spleen, and peritoneal surface. Collectively, these differentiated cells (histiocytes and macrophages) become part of the reticuloendothelial system with a major function

of phagocytosis of invading entities. The role of the macrophage is much more complex, however, because it produces proinflammatory proteins (cytokines and chemokines) that stimulate the growth of specific immune and inflammatory cells and positions them where needed. They mediate inflammatory responses during wound healing and, after consuming pathogens, can present them to the corresponding T-helper cell. This is another example of communication between traditionally defined innate and acquired immunity effectors. This presentation is done in conjunction with attaching to a major histocompatibility complex (MHC) class II molecule to identify the macrophage as self despite the foreign antigens on its surface. Macrophages can also play a counterproductive role in tumor elimination through the production of molecules that promote tumor growth and angiogenesis (eg, vascular endothelial growth factor [VEGF] and basic fibroblast growth factor [FGF]). Because they promote inflammation, they also release compounds such as tumor necrosis factor (TNF), resulting in nuclear factor-κB activation, which inhibits apoptosis.

Natural killer (NK) cells are granular lymphocytes (10%-15% of total blood lymphocytes) that recognize and destroy tissues that have been altered or stressed, typically by viruses or by malignant transformation. They differ from T lymphocytes in that they do not have antigen-specific receptors. Instead, they have inhibiting receptors that can recognize the MHC class I molecules on normal cells preventing activation. MHC-I expression is absent or aberrant on many virus- and tumor-infected cells. In another example of cooperation between innate and acquired immunity, NK cells

427

participate in the process of antibody-dependent cell-mediated cytotoxicity (ADCC). Immunoglobulin (Ig) G antibodies can bind to infected cells. Fc receptors found on NK cells (also are present on macrophages, neutrophils, and eosinophils) bring the NK cell into contact with the antibody-coated target cell. Upon contact, NK cells release modified cytoplasmic granules containing perforin and granzymes, which promote apoptosis.

The primary effector components of the acquired immune systems are T and B lymphocytes and involve their interaction with antigens. Antigens are any agents that can bind to a component of the immune system, such as binding with an antibody. This is distinct from an immunogen, which also produces an immune response. In general, for an antigen to be immunogenic, it has to be recognized as foreign (ie, tolerance must be broken), has to be large and complex enough (this can sometimes be rectified by using carriers), and for T-cell activation, has to interact with MHC on the antigen-presenting cells. Factors such as dose, schedule, adjuvant therapy, and route of administration have also been shown to have an impact on immunogenicity. A variety of entities may serve as antigens with varying immunogenicity, with common ones including carbohydrates (these can also induce antibody responses without T-cell help), lipids and nucleic acids (both require protein carriers), and proteins.

Biologic Response Modifiers

Cytokines are secreted substances that facilitate a variety of immune response functions. Many are well characterized, and as examples, a few will be discussed here. Classifications are arbitrary because most are pleiotropic in function. Chemokines are chemoattractant cytokines, which are low molecular weight proteins, that direct the movement of a variety of effector cells to needed locations. Interleukin (IL)-8, for example, which is secreted by macrophages, mobilizes and activates neutrophils and promotes angiogenesis.[1] Colony-stimulating factors cause the differentiation of progenitor cells in the bone marrow, with many produced for clinical use (granulocyte colony-stimulating factor, granulocyte-macrophage colony-stimulating factor, erythropoietin, and thrombopoietin).[2] Interferons are produced by lymphocytes, macrophages, and dendritic cells and have a wide variety of functions. The interferon-γ produced by T_H1 cells activates NK cells and macrophages and induces the expression of MHC class II on many cell types. Many cytokines also promote inflammation such as IL-1, IL-6, IL-23, and TNF-α.[3] Despite diverse functionality, cytokines generally bind and induce polymerization of a cell surface receptor, which activates a signal transduction pathway. It is not well understood how 2 cytokines with diverse functions retain specificity when using the same signal transduction pathway.

PRINCIPLES OF IMMUNOTHERAPY

Humoral Immunity

B lymphocytes (B cells) produce secreted *antibodies* that can recognize soluble and cell surface molecules in response to an antigen. Each B cell expresses immunoglobulin against a single antigenic determinant, with the immunoglobulin expressed at the cell surface of the B cell. The diversity of specificities in different B cells is generated by rearrangements of the immunoglobulin genes, and new antibody specificities continue to be generated in response to new antigens.[4] The antigen binds to the B-lymphocyte surface receptor and activates the B cell. B lymphocytes are mobile and migrate to the T-cell rich areas where T-cell help can be provided to promote increased antibody diversity and increased affinity through immunoglobulin gene rearrangements and class switching. Many antigens require costimulation from CD4+ helper T cells (T-cell–dependent antigen), but other antigens do not, including nonprotein antigens such as glycolipids (T-cell–independent antigen). Clonal expansion ensues to make multiple copies of the antigen-specific B cell. Differentiation then occurs to form either plasma cells of short duration (antibody-producing cells), memory cells (which are responsible for the amnestic response), or a small population of B cells expressing germline immunoglobulins that have not undergone rearrangement (which are found in the CD5+ B-cell population). Antibodies are produced by the plasma cells of 1 of 5 isotypes (IgG, IgA, IgM, IgE, or IgD). The immunoglobulin variable region (called the Fv region) determines antibody specificity and is located in the Fab domain of immunoglobulins. A conformational change in the Fc portion occurs after binding of antibody to antigen, leading to the activation of several effector mechanisms including complement activation. The early antibody response is IgM, but if T-cell help is available, antibody responses mature through immunoglobulin gene rearrangements into the higher affinity IgG classes. These IgG molecules are capable of improved binding to antigen as well as receptors on the bone marrow–derived cells through their Fc domain, thereby expanding effector functions. The response to most nonprotein antigens are IgM class and generally do not mature to IgG responses. IgM is pentameric and has increased avidity to bind multimeric antigens.

It then activates complement as its main effector function.[5] The complement system consists of a variety of blood components with different enzymatic properties, which cause opsonization (coating of pathogens by complement components); recognition by complement receptors on macrophages, monocytes, neutrophils, and dendritic cells; and subsequent activation of these cells, leading to phagocytosis and/or killing. In addition, complement can cause local and direct killing by forming a membrane attack complex that creates holes in membranes of target pathogens and cancer cells, producing complement-dependent cytotoxicity.

IgG antibodies are synthesized following immunoglobulin gene rearrangements, with switches in Fc domains, as the B cell matures in response to T-cell help. IgG antibodies usually have higher affinity than IgM antibodies and can be found in the extracellular space and in the blood. Subclasses of IgG antibodies in humans are especially effective at activating complement and also sensitizing pathogens for killing by NK cells, macrophages, and other cells with complement receptors and immunoglobulin Fc receptors.

The cross-linking of Fc receptors can also lead to activation of the cells and can produce ADCC of tumor cells through the production of cytotoxic molecules such as perforin and granzymes by NK cells. Monoclonal antibodies are commonly used for cancer therapy. Antitumor effects can be in part mediated by antibody binding to critical molecules on the surface of tumor cells, for example by inhibiting tumor cell attachment or growth receptors. However, generally more than 1 mechanism is at work, and Fc receptor–mediated effector mechanisms such as ADCC are also activated.

Cellular Immunity

T lymphocytes arise in the bone marrow and migrate to the thymus, where they differentiate and develop T-cell receptors and CD4 and CD8 coreceptors. The coreceptors bind to the MHC complex (CD4 cells bind to MHC class II molecules, and CD8 cells bind to MHC class I complexes), as shown in Figure 21-1. The MHC binding is required as a first step to ensure the immune attack is directed at the appropriate target and self can be recognized. Antigens must be processed by antigen-presenting cells for recognition (dendritic cells are 1 major example). The combined antigen/MHC molecules are then trafficked to the cell surface for recognition by T-cell receptors, which are encoded by genes of the immunoglobulin family. Just as with antibodies, the diversity of T-cell receptors is generated by rearrangements of these immunoglobulin family genes. Each monoclonal T-cell receptor binds to its

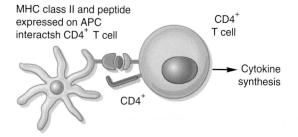

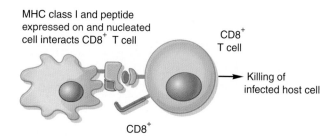

FIGURE 21-1. Cells expressing major histocompatibility complex (MHC) class II cells interact with CD4+ T cells, which produce cytokines. Cells expressing MHC class I cells interact with CD8+ T cells, which destroy infected host cells.

appropriate antigen/MHC complex presented on the surface of the antigen-presenting cell. Two signals are required for T-cell activation. The first is the binding of the antigen/MHC complex. The second is a costimulatory signal that comes from the T-cell surface molecule CD28. CD28 engages B7 molecules found on the antigen-presenting cells. Therefore, successful activation of a T cell requires engagement of the T-cell receptor by an appropriately presented antigen/MHC complex in conjunction with CD28 engagement, with B7 as a "safety lock" to be certain activation occurs only in the correct setting.[6]

Ox40 and 4-1BB are examples of 2 other costimulatory molecules that are upregulated on the surface of activated T cells, which promote survival of T cells and generate T-cell memory responses.[7] Multiple effector functions are available to T cells once appropriately activated by professional antigen-presenting cells (primarily dendritic cells), including the production of cytokines and cytotoxic molecules, which lead to death of target cells.

The immune response must be suppressed when the threat has resolved. Natural CD4+/CD25+ T regulatory cells constitute approximately 10% of CD4+ cells and participate in this function. Cytotoxic T-lymphocyte antigen 4 (CTLA-4) is expressed on these cells. CTLA-4 also binds B7 molecules, but with much higher affinity, thus displacing the required CD28 activation signal. CTLA-4 signaling leads to downregulation of the T-cell

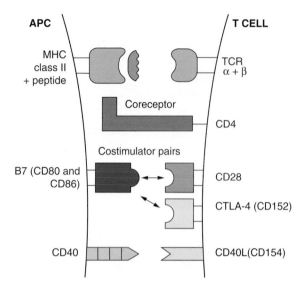

FIGURE 21-2. Selected paired interactions required at the surface of an antigen-presenting cell (APC) and a CD4+ T cell that lead to activation and proliferation with cytokine production. MHC, major histocompatibility complex; TCR, T-cell receptor. (Reproduced, with permission, from Dubinett SM, Lee JM, Sharma S, Mule JJ. Chemokines: can effector cells be redirected to the site of the tumor? *Cancer J.* 2010;16(4):325-335.)

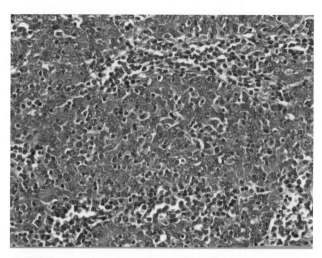

FIGURE 21-3. Tumor-infiltrating lymphocytes found in epithelial ovarian cancer specimens. (Images contributed by R. Soslow [Memorial Sloan-Kettering Cancer Center, Pathology]).

response. The manipulation of CTLA-4 expression is being investigated as a novel therapeutic maneuver, with recent data supporting its usefulness in treating patients with melanoma.[8] Depletion of T regulatory cells may be particularly useful in enhancing the response to tumor vaccines. The multiple opportunities for paired interactions during the T-cell activation process are illustrated in Figure 21-2.

Immunosurveillance

The notion that the immune system may identify and destroy tumors is long-standing. William B. Coley first observed regression in some patients with sarcoma contracting "accidental erysipelas" as early as 1891. Because the rate of spontaneous regression for tumors is rare and patients with functioning immune systems still develop cancer, the confidence in the ability of the immune system to control cancerous growths has varied over the decades. More sophisticated animal models showing the development of carcinoma in animals deficient in various immunologic components, however, allowed the concept of immunosurveillance to grow. Observations noting CD4+ and CD8+ tumor-infiltrating lymphocytes (TILs) in patients with epithelial ovarian cancer further support its role, as illustrated in Figure 21-3. For example, the 5-year overall survival in epithelial ovarian cancer has been related to the presence or absence of TILs (38% vs. 4.5%,

$P < .001$).[9] A second study also showed improved survival in patients with increased frequencies of intraepithelial CD8+ TILs (55 months vs. 26 months; hazard ratio, 0.33; 95% confidence interval [CI], 0.18-0.60; $P = .0003$). In contrast, patients with increased numbers of immune-suppressive CD4+CD25HI regulatory T cells have reduced survival.[10] The process is made more complex when we recognize that not only can the immune system protect the host against tumor development, but also some select cancer cells of lower immunogenicity can escape early immunity due to changes in gene expression. This actually leads to an outgrowth of tumors with the capacity to escape recognition, and this process has been termed immunoediting. The immunoediting or "immune sculpting" process, therefore, is responsible for shaping the immunogenicity of the tumors that will eventually form. Considering the effectors of the immune system in the context of both of these processes is important to develop immune-directed therapies with the greatest chance of success.

Escape From Surveillance

An alteration in the function of almost every process discussed herein to facilitate immune activation has been postulated to participate in the ways tumors can evade immune detection. In some cases, antigen presentation is downregulated, or gene deletions or rearrangements may cause reduced expression of the MHC-I complex, thus preventing T-lymphocyte activation. Tumors can also secrete proteins that inhibit T-cell effector action or that promote the development of regulatory T cells that suppress immune function.

A recent novel observation showed that certain melanomas can actually remodel their stromal microenvironment so it resembles lymphoid tissue, which recruits regulatory cells to promote tolerance and allow tumor progression.[11] Other mechanisms include the downregulation of intracellular adhesion molecules, changes in molecules responsible for apoptosis signaling, and the development of peripheral tolerance. Based on the increasing number of interacting mechanisms with putative activity that allow immune escape, approaches directed against multiple mechanisms will likely be needed to eradicate immune-tolerant tumor cells.[12]

Immunoprophylaxis

The development of most immunotherapeutic strategies for investigation requires deciding which of the tumor-associated antigens one will target (often multiple). The next step is to select the strategy that will be used (such as dendritic cell vaccination or autologous cell lysates) to generate the proposed effector cells. Some assessment that the effector cells are indeed directed at the target is then prudent. Finally, the clinical merit of the approach must be assessed.

Ongoing advances using newer technologies including serologic analysis of recombinant cDNA expression libraries (SEREX), robust applications of bioinformatics, and seromic profiling techniques have allowed the further characterization of tumor-associated antigens in multiple tumor types.[13,14] There are more than 2000 candidate tumor-associated antigens, and they are generally classified as follows: (1) differentiation antigens, (2) mutational antigens (that are altered forms of proteins), (3) amplification antigens, (4) splice variant antigens, (5) glycolipid antigens, (6) viral antigens, and (7) cancer-testis antigens. Representative examples of each group are provided in Table 21-1.

Table 21-1 Tumor-Associated Antigen Categories With Representative Examples

Antigen Category	Representative Examples
Differentiation antigens	Tyrosinase, Melan/MART-1, gp-100
Mutational antigens	CD4, β-catenin, caspase
Amplification antigens	Her-2/neu, p53
Slice variant antigens	NY-CO-37/PDZ 45, ING1
Glycolipid antigens	MUC1
Viral antigens	HPV
Cancer-testis antigens	MAGE, NY-ESO-1, LAGE-1

Table 21-2 Cancer Vaccine Strategies

I. Antigens alone with or without adjuvants
  Peptides
  Protein
  Gangliosides
  Immunoglobulin idiotypes

II. Dendritic cells
  Peptides, immunoglobulin idiotype
  Tumor lysates
  DNA or RNA
  Protein

III. Tumor cells unmodified or modified
  Autologous
  Allogeneic
  Mixed autologous-allogeneic

IV. Tumor-APCs hybrid

V. Whole tumor cell vaccines (modified)

VI. DNA alone (naked DNA), recombinant viruses (adenovirus, vaccinia, others)

APCs, antigen-presenting cells.

In addition to selecting the appropriate targets, the next step is to determine the strategy to be used for vaccination. Multiple approaches have been considered, including: a variety of antigens can be given alone or with adjuvant treatment; modified or unmodified tumor cell lysates can be administered (autologous or allogeneic); dendritic cells can be primed with a variety of agents; tumor hybrids with antigen-presenting cells can be made; or DNA alone or in a recombinant fashion can be administered. A variety of cancer vaccine strategies are listed in Table 21-2.

It is important to evaluate the effector cells for the ability to interact with the target. This may be simple and straightforward, or a variety of surrogate approaches may be used to identify whether the biologic end point is being achieved. This may be the most challenging area in immunotherapy because a traditional dose-limiting toxicity finding model does not apply. Radioimmunoassays (enzyme-linked immunosorbent assays [ELISA]) are used to measure antigens, antibodies, or antigen–antibody complexes if appropriate. Antibodies are generally tested for specificity against certain cell surface antigens using fluorescence-activated cell sorting techniques (FACS), or following stimulation with specific antigens in vitro, they can be cultured in the enzyme-linked immunosorbent spot (ELISPOT) assay. Assays for T-cell proliferation and activation are more complex. A cytotoxicity assay (cytotoxic T lymphocytes) measures the ability of cytotoxic T or NK cells to kill radiolabeled target cells (often chromium-51) expressing the appropriate antigen that was initially targeted. The percentage of chromium release can be measured.

Possible effector responses (depending on the strategy selected) are varied and include enhancing phagocytosis, antibody and complement activation, loss of adhesive properties of tumor cells promoted by antibody administration, cytotoxic and helper T lymphocytes, ADCC, activated macrophages, neutrophils, NK/T cells, lymphokine-activated killer cells, and NK cells. More than 1 mechanism is generally at work through direct stimulation or via cross-talk between systems.

CLINICAL PRACTICE IN GYNECOLOGIC ONCOLOGY

Suitability for Immunotherapy

Opportunities to improve the outcome for patients exist by making primary therapy more effective or by exploring the application of "consolidation" or "maintenance" approaches to patients in a complete primary or subsequent remission. One important issue in evaluating immunotherapeutic approaches in ovarian cancer is deciding where in the disease course the novel agent should be evaluated. In general, the minimal disease state is sought, and the remission populations are best suited. The value of treatment in clinical complete remission was first established in acute leukemia, and additional "consolidation" or "maintenance" chemotherapy dramatically improved the outcome for some of these patients. These concepts have not found a place in solid tumor therapy, and the nomenclature remains confusing. Strictly speaking, "consolidation" is best applied to those strategies that are of limited duration, such as a fixed immunization course, and "maintenance" is best used to describe interventions that continue for years (or until progression) such as with trastuzumab. In ovarian cancer, no randomized consolidation study has provided a statistically significant improvement in overall survival, although many attempts have been made. Negative randomized consolidation approaches include both subcutaneous and intraperitoneal interferon-α, high-dose chemotherapy, continued intravenous carboplatin versus whole abdominal radiotherapy (WART), chemotherapy versus observation versus WART, intraperitoneal radioactive phosphorus (phosphorus 32), "non–cross-resistant" chemotherapy in the form of cisplatin and 5-fluorouracil for 3 cycles or topotecan for 4 cycles, the monoclonal antibody oregovomab, which targets CA-125, and the SMART study.[15-17] Consolidation strategies have generally been used in the first remission population; investigational strategies in the second and third remission groups have been rare and all likewise negative to date.[18] Patients with ovarian cancer in remission are ideal candidates for an immunotherapeutic strategy. Recent data highlight the homogeneity of the second and third remission groups who have a progression-free survival (PFS) interval of less than 12 months so that hints of efficacy from a given immunotherapeutic approach could be recognized with a shorter follow-up interval than that required in first remission.

The number of therapeutic strategies under investigation for immunotherapy in patients with ovarian cancer is large. Most trials are pilot studies or phase 1 trials with the goal of assessing safety and immunogenicity. Some have correlated improved outcome with a surrogate such as antibody or T-cell response, and most current trials aim to produce cellular responses. The number of adequately powered randomized trials is few, however, and none has shown definitive efficacy to date. We will consider several examples of immunotherapeutic approaches that are being evaluated in the clinics, but the list is not exhaustive, and many other approaches have merit.

Antibodies Used as Immunogens

Although some antibodies are administered in the treatment of patients with cancer to convey passive immunity, they may also be used as immunogens and can elicit a complex immune response. Oregovomab (MAb B43.13), which is an IgG1k subclass murine monoclonal antibody that binds with high affinity (1.16×10^{10}/M) to circulating CA-125, has been evaluated. Both cellular and humoral immune responses have been seen with the production of anti-oregovomab antibodies (Ab2), T-helper cells, and cytotoxic T cells in addition to the human anti-mouse antibody (HAMA) response. Nonrandomized clinical studies to date have consistently associated a longer overall survival with immune response. A randomized placebo-controlled trial in patients with stage III or IV epithelial ovarian cancer in first clinical remission receiving oregovomab or placebo showed no benefit using the intent-to-treat population. However, a favorable subgroup of patients (≤2 cm residual at debulking, CA-125 ≤65 U/mL before third cycle, and CA-125 ≤35 U/mL at entry) showed a time to progression advantage favoring vaccination of 24 months versus 10.8 months (hazard ratio, 0.543; 95% CI, 0.287-1.025). This subgroup was appropriately considered to be hypothesis generating, and a follow-up study enrolled 354 patients using the characteristics of this group as eligibility criteria. The median time to progression was 10.3 months (95% CI, 9.7-13.0 months) for the oregovomab group and 12.9 months (95% CI, 10.1-17.4 months) for the placebo group ($P = .29$), showing no benefit to oregovomab immunotherapy.[17]

Another antibody strategy is immunization with an anti-idiotype vaccine. The hypothesis is that the antigenicity of the immunogen (in this case, the antibody) can be increased by presenting the desired epitope to the now tolerant host in a different molecular environment. The "immune network hypothesis," which provided the foundation for this approach, was first proposed in the early 1970s and describes an interconnected group of idiotypes expressed by antibodies. The proposed mechanism assumes that immunization with a given antigen will generate the production of antibodies against this antigen (termed Ab1). Ab1 can generate anti-idiotype antibodies against Ab1, classified as Ab2. Some of the anti-idiotypic antibodies (Ab2β) express the internal image of the antigen recognized by the Ab1 antibody and can be used as surrogate antigens. Immunization with Ab2β (the anti-idiotype antibody) can cause the production of anti-anti-idiotype antibodies (classified as Ab3) that recognize the corresponding original antigen identified by Ab1. Ab3 antibodies are also denoted Ab1' to show that they may differ in their other epitopes compared with Ab1. The relationships of these antibodies to each other are illustrated in Figure 21-4. A previous phase 1/2 study of abagovomab, the anti-idiotype monoclonal antibody whose epitope mirrors CA-125, suggested that Ab3 production was associated with overall survival. Other studies have shown an increase in interferon-γ expression of CA-125–specific CD8+ T cells following immunization, but there has been no specific correlation between the induction of Ab3 and frequencies of CA-125–specific cytotoxic T lymphocytes and T-helper cells. The efficacy of abagovomab in patients in first remission is currently being evaluated in an international phase 3, randomized, double-blind, placebo-controlled study ongoing in approximately 120 study locations (MIMOSA Trial). Outcomes are recurrence-free survival, overall survival, and safety. Preliminary blinded immunogenicity results were reported with 888 patients enrolled onto the study

and showed that 68% and 69% of all patients were positive for Ab3 (median values, 62,000 ng/mL and 337,000 ng/mL, respectively), whereas 53% and 63% of patients were positive for HAMA (median values, 510 ng/mL and 644 ng/mL, respectively). Efficacy results will be available in early 2011.[19]

Cancer-Testis Antigen Vaccines

The *cancer-testis antigens* are a distinct class of differentiation antigens. The family has grown from the original melanoma-associated antigen 1 (MAGE-1) identified in a melanoma cell line to 100 cancer-testis genes or gene families identified in a recent database established by the Ludwig Institute for Cancer Research.[20] These antigens share several characteristics, including preferential expression in normal tissues on the testis and expression in tumors of varying histology (including ovarian cancer), and many are members of multigene families that are mostly encoded on chromosome X. Cancer-testis antigen expression has been correlated with clinical and pathologic parameters in a variety of tumors. MAGE-A4 expression shows an inverse correlation between expression and patient survival, for example, in ovarian cancer ($P = .016$).

The NY-ESO-1 antigen, initially defined by SEREX in esophageal cancer, is expressed in several tumors, including 40% of epithelial ovarian cancers. NY-ESO-1 MHC class I and II restricted epitopes (recognized by CD8+ cytotoxic and CD4+ helper T cells) have been characterized, including those recognized in conjunction with human leukocyte antigen (HLA)-A2 as well as with other haplotypes. Both NY-ESO-1 peptides and full recombinant protein have been administered to patients on protocols with immunogenicity as the primary end point with various adjuvants. Vaccination has been shown to induce both humoral and T-cell responses.[21] In a phase 1 trial in patients with epithelial

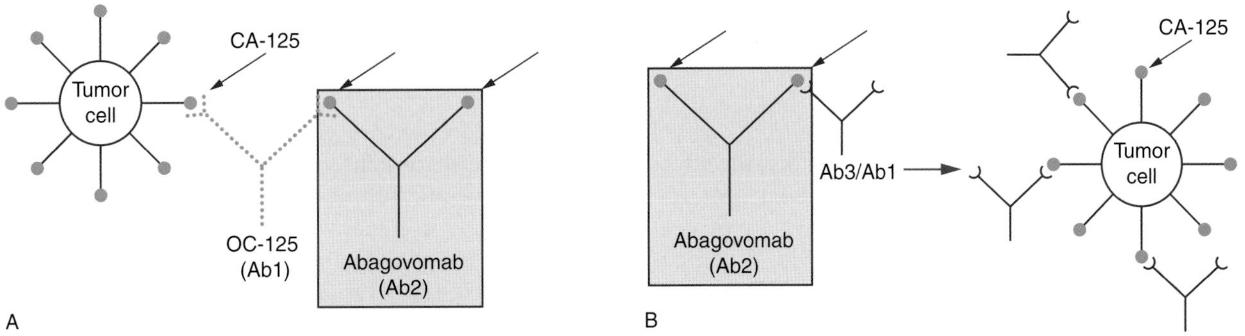

FIGURE 21-4. The relationship of antibodies in an anti-idiotypic vaccine strategy. A. The injection of a tumor-associated antigen (TAA) binding antibody (Ab1) leads to an immune response containing antibodies (Ab2) mimicking the structure of the original antigen. **B.** Vaccination with a TAA-mimicking antibody (Ab2) leads to an immune response directed to the original antigen.

ovarian cancer in first remission immunized with HLA-A*0201–restricted NY-ESO-1b peptide with montanide ISA-51 as the adjuvant,[22] treatment was well tolerated. Seven (77%) of 9 patients showed T-cell immunity by tetramer and ELISPOT analyses. Multiple approaches have been used to try and enhance the inherently limited immunogenicity of these peptide vaccinations. Some have included amino acid substitution at the anchor positions of Melan-A/MART-1$_{26-35}$2L; terminal modification of MART-1$_{27-35}$; substitution of cysteine residues for NY-ESO-1; modification of T-cell receptor interacting amino acid residues for carcinoembryonic antigen; and loading of peptides onto autologous dendritic cells. In addition, cytokines and costimulatory molecules have been administered.

Dendritic Cell–Based Vaccines

Dendritic cells are professional antigen-presenting cells. They endocytose, process, and then present tumor antigens to T cells. Many strategies are currently under way to manipulate the dendritic cell for use in immunotherapy. Dendritic cells have been pulsed with tumor-associated peptides or proteins and mRNA-encoded receptors such as folate receptor-α.[23] Other vaccines have been developed by the viral transduction of dendritic cells with tumor-specific genes or through transfection with liposomal DNA or RNA. Another strategy that has been tried to avoid the need to specifically define the effective tumor-associated antigens is to pulse them with tumor lysates or tumor protein extracts. In many cases, preclinical models have suggested protective immunity to subsequent tumor challenge, which supports further interest in investigating the approach.

A specific example includes a study by Czerniecki et al,[24] in which advanced breast and ovarian cancer patients were treated with dendritic cells pulsed with HER-2/*neu* or MUC-1–derived peptides. In 50% of patients, peptide-specific cytotoxic T-cell lymphocytes were generated. Side effects were minimal. Gong and colleagues[25] fused human ovarian cells to human dendritic cells and likewise showed the proliferation of autologous T cells, including cytotoxic T-cell activity with lysis of autologous tumor cells by an MHC class I restricted mechanism (ie, demonstrating that the effector cells had the desired activity). Heat shock proteins, which are molecular chaperones that facilitate protein folding, have also been isolated, along with accompanying peptides, and used as immunogens. Heat shock peptide complexes have been shown to interact with dendritic cells via the CD91 receptor. The heat shock proteins are taken up by endocytosis, are cross-presented by MHC-I molecules on the dendritic cells, and result in activation of naïve CD8[+] cells along with

upregulation of costimulatory molecules and the production of cytokines.

Many reported studies have similar immunologic end points, but the clinical interpretation is often difficult from phase 1/2 trials without comparators. Further issues under study include the choice of dendritic cell subtype and maturational status at immunization, antigen loading method, preparation of the cells loaded on the dendritic cells, and route and frequency of administration.

Vaccines Designed to Generate Antibody Responses

Most current vaccines seek to generate cellular responses (often with an accompanying humoral response), but a vaccine is currently in a phase 2 randomized trial in ovarian cancer (Gynecology Oncology Group [GOG] Study 255) that evaluates a vaccine approach primarily designed to augment antibodies. Techniques for the chemical and enzymatic synthesis of carbohydrate and glycopeptide antigens have permitted the development of a variety of synthetic vaccines that depend on antibody production and ADCC as the primary effectors. A variety of options such as different adjuvant therapies, schedules, and methods of conjugation have been tried to enhance immunogenicity. A proposed optimal construct has consisted of an antigen (single or multiple) with the carrier protein keyhole limpet hemocyanin (KLH) and the saponin adjuvant QS-21 (or OPT-821).[26] GOG 255 is a randomized trial in patients with second or third complete clinical remission receiving either the adjuvant therapy alone (OPT-821) or a multivalent antigen construct plus OPT-821. The end point is the proportion of patients disease free at 12 months, and accrual is ongoing.

Adoptive Cellular Therapy

Using the adoptive cellular therapy approach, one selects and activates large numbers of lymphocytes and introduces them into a manipulated host environment with a selected target. One way T cells may be modified to recognize tumor-associated antigens is to introduce ex vivo a gene encoding artificial T-cell receptors termed chimeric antigen receptors (CARs) against a specific tumor-associated antigen. The first phase 1 study in patients with epithelial ovarian cancer using gene-modified autologous T cells with reactivity against the ovarian cancer–associated antigen α-folate receptor (FR) has been reported.[27] Cohort 1 received T cells with IL-2, and cohort 2 received dual specific T cells followed by allogeneic peripheral blood mononuclear cells. No reduction in tumor burden was seen in any patient. Polymerase chain reaction analysis showed that gene-modified T cells were present in the circulation 2 days after transfer but then declined. An inhibitory factor developed in the serum of 3 of 6 patients tested over the period of treatment that significantly reduced the ability of gene-modified T cells to respond against FR-positive tumor cells. Future studies need to use strategies to increase T-cell persistence. The chimeric receptor approach continues to evolve in specificity against targets expressed in ovarian cancer such as the LeY carbohydrate antigen (expressed on 70% of ovarian cancer cells) or HER-2/*neu*. Most recently, receptors have been engineered to target the extracellular domain (termed MUC-CD) of MUC16 (CA-125), which is expressed in most ovarian carcinoma.[28] In vitro, these CAR-modified, MUC-CD–targeted T cells showed MUC-CD–specific cytolytic activity against ovarian cell lines, and infusion into severe combined immunodeficiency (SCID)-beige mice bearing orthotopic human MUC-CD–positive ovarian carcinoma tumors showed delayed disease progression or eradication. Clinical trials are planned. One necessary challenge to overcome is how to circumvent the multiple mechanisms in the tumor microenvironment that inhibit tumor-targeted T cells. Options under investigation include administering T cells after lymphodepleting chemotherapy, antibody-based blockade of inhibitory ligands, and infusion of proinflammatory cytokines such as IL-12.

Whole Tumor Antigen Vaccines

This strategy seeks to overcome some of the potential problems associated with trying to generate specific immune responses. In the latter case, the response may simply miss the target, it can be limited to only the epitopes provided on the stimulating antigen and actually drive variants of tumor cells that can evade the immune response (immunoediting), or it may be restricted to small numbers of patients of a certain HLA type, as in the case of using HLA-restricted peptides.[22] The reason for using whole tumor antigen vaccines is that it allows one to immunize without needing to define the tumor-associated antigens. They can be derived from autologous tumor cells or using an allogeneic strategy. One obvious challenge in using whole tumor antigen vaccines is that the tumor is currently residing in a host where tolerance to the tumor is already present. This tolerance is likely produced in multiple ways, including the production of IL-10 and transforming growth factor (TGF)-β to inhibit T-cell and dendritic cell functions, VEGF to inhibit dendritic cell maturation and differentiation, and soluble Fas ligand, which induces lymphocyte apoptosis. The whole tumor immunogen, therefore, is processed or modified in some way in an attempt to overcome this. Strategies have included using apoptotic whole tumor cells (developed with a lethal dose of irradiation), using necrotic tumor cell lysates (created with repetitive freezing and thawing and often administered as pulsed dendritic cells), and constructing dendritic cell/tumor fusion vaccines.[29] The issue of how to increase the immunogenicity of whole tumor vaccines remains a priority. One effective approach has been the use of a replication-deficient herpes simplex virus to infect tumor cells, which are subsequently engulfed and show enhanced ability to both activate NK cells and provide a costimulatory signal for T cells.

TARGETED THERAPIES

The principal tenets of optimal disease management in women with gynecologic malignancies have been the strategic utilization of surgery, cytotoxic chemotherapy, hormonal therapy, and radiotherapy. Although substantial progress has been realized from these practices, disease-specific mortality from gynecologic malignancies still accounts for about 9% of all cancer-related deaths and underscores the need for the development of new therapeutic modalities. Investigation into the mechanisms governing cancer initiation, proliferation, metastases, autophagy, and apoptosis have uncovered a wealth of new opportunities, many of which harbor the potential of reversing the malignant phenotype, selectively inducing cancer cell death, overcoming primary and induced drug resistance, and optimistically improving overall outcomes for patients. Ability to pharmacologically and pharmacodynamically interact with these new "targets" has fostered rapid drug development, some of which is beginning to show merit in the treatment of women with gynecologic malignancy. Because the biology of cancer growth often shares homology across different tumor types, targeted therapies are being investigated where the pathway of aberration is suspected to play an important or dominant role in disease pathogenesis. Although an "Achilles' heel," or a solitary activated pathway, is not present in most solid tumors, the opportunity to selectively target key regulatory and survival mechanisms in the tumor microenvironment holds great promise in expanding our therapeutic armamentarium for these women. We review some of these pathways and agents in this section.

Mechanisms of Action

One of the most common events defining the cancer process is dysregulation of protein kinases that govern normal cellular function. In light of this observation, proteins are frequently the targets of anticancer agents. Although there are many ways to affect protein kinase function, including small molecules, monoclonal antibodies, antagomirs, antisense, RNA interference, immuno- and receptor drug conjugates, decoy receptors, allosteric inhibitors, and nanotubes, the intent is to target these aberrancies either restoring normal host function or inducing cell death. The principle challenge is to affect tumor cells without impacting the function of normal host cells. Three relevant mechanisms are important to review.

Interruption of Signal Transduction Pathways

Signal transduction is the process where a ligand, usually lipophobic (eg, a growth factor), meets a receptor or channel on the cell surface and initiates a cascade of events such as kinase activity or dissociation of G-coupled proteins resulting in some cellular response. In contrast, lipophilic ligands (eg, steroids) can penetrate the cell membrane and may affect cellular functions by direct binding to cytoplasmic or nuclear targets. Many of the "small molecules" being developed for cancer therapy involve blocking the tyrosine kinase activity of membrane-bound receptors that are usually influenced by a number of promoting

ligands. The prototypical example of a relevant ligand-receptor signal transduction pathway in carcinogenesis is the epidermal growth factor receptor (EGFR) (Figure 21-5). This receptor family is overexpressed and activated in many tumor types, including gynecologic malignancies, and appears to play a key role in disease pathogenesis.[30] Binding of the epidermal growth factor (EGF) ligand to the receptor induces tyrosine kinase activity, which leads to receptor dimerization and activation of the pathway driving multiple cellular functions such as cellular proliferation, enhanced cellular motility, resistance to apoptosis, and angiogenesis. Because of the broad spectra of activity, there has been intense interest in developing therapeutics against this pathway. Typically, these targeted agents are classified in 2 broad categories: competitive adenosine triphosphate (ATP)–pocket small-molecule inhibitors and monoclonal antibodies to the receptor's extracellular domain. The clinical experience of these molecules in gynecologic cancer will be discussed later; however, the crafted directive of these targeted agents is to disrupt ligand/receptor activation in the hopes of blocking the signal transduction pathways leading to cancer cell survival.

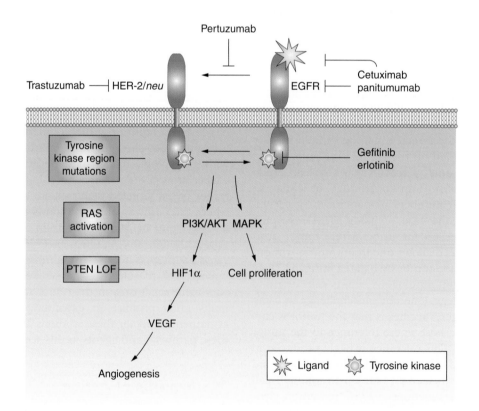

FIGURE 21-5. The epidermal growth factor receptor (EGFR) pathway. Ligand binds with the extracellular domain of the EGFR and causes the receptor to dimerize. Upon this, activation of the pathway drives several downstream events including angiogenesis, proliferation, cellular motility, and resistance to apoptosis. Various agents to block this pathway are depicted. See text. LOF, loss of function; VEGF, vascular endothelial growth factor.

Induction of Apoptosis

Normal development and functional physiology are dependent on tight regulation of cellular growth and death. The representation of cancer as "uncontrolled cellular proliferation" attests to the importance dysregulated cellular programmed cell death, or apoptosis, plays in human disease. Phenotypical transformation of normal cell to cancer cell is likely highly influenced by loss of apoptotic function. In addition, resistance to chemotherapy-induced cytotoxicity is frequently the result of cellular escape from apoptotic inducement. Two dominant pathways govern cellular apoptosis: extrinsic, induced via a receptor-ligand interaction (death receptor), and intrinsic, induced via mitochondria-apoptosome signaling (Figure 21-6). The converging points for both pathways are the effector caspases, which are closely regulated by upstream signaling proteins either inducing apoptosis or preventing it. A caspase-independent pathway also exists and appears to be mediated through apoptosis-inducing factor (AIF), which is released from mitochondrial pores under control of Bcl-2 and induces nuclear chromatin clumping. The ultimate declaration of apoptosis is largely the balance of proapoptotic proteins (BAX, BID, BAK, and BAD) and antiapoptotic proteins (Bcl-XI and Bcl-2). Numerous ligands have been identified as substrates for the death receptor including TNF, TNF-related apoptosis-inducing ligand (TRAIL), and Fas. Recently, novel targeted agents harboring agonist activation of this pathway at both the ligand and receptor levels have entered clinical trials.[31]

The intrinsic pathway may be initiated by a number of cellular stressors such as radiation therapy, chemotherapy, hypoxia, infection, and starvation. Mitochondria contribute to the apoptotic process either by increasing permeability, leading to the release of important regulators such as second mitochondrial-derived activator of caspases (SMACs) and nitric oxide, or by developing membrane pores causing the organelle to swell, which can lead to release of cytochrome C. This latter process has been shown to contribute to the formation of the apoptosome, which converts pro-caspase-9 to its active form, which in turn promotes caspase 3 activation, an effector caspase. Proteins belonging to the BCL-2 family primarily govern the mitochondrial pathway. This is an extensive family that may be divided functionally (pro- or antiapoptotic) or structurally (those that share BCL-2 homology and those expressing only the BH3 domain).[32] This latter domain, BH3, is the natural ligand for the BCL-2 family's protein–protein interaction and has become of great interest in drug therapeutic development.

Finally, *p53*, the most commonly mutated gene in human malignancy, functions as a transcription factor regulating downstream genes involved in DNA repair, cell cycle arrest, and both the intrinsic and extrinsic apoptotic pathways. *p53*, when activated, promotes the proapoptotic genes of the BCL-2 family, which inhibit Bcl-2 at the mitochondrial membrane, as well

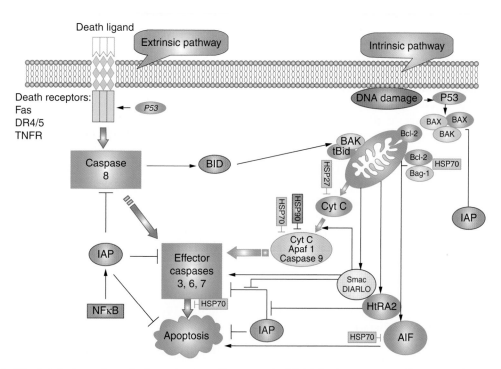

FIGURE 21-6. The intrinsic and extrinsic pathways of apoptosis. Multiple downstream effectors and cross-talk relationships are depicted and are current targets of drug therapy development.

as activate expression of the death receptors, such as DR$_5$.[31] In this manner, cross-talk between the intrinsic and extrinsic pathways is extensive. When *p53* is dysfunctional, one or both of these pathways may drive carcinogenesis; thus, this serves as rationale to consider combinatorial treatment approaches, such as targeted therapy of the death receptor ligand in combination with cytotoxic chemotherapy.

Stimulation of the Immune Response

As was previously presented, the immune system is a highly complex and interactive network of specialized cells and organs working in conjunction to maintain health. It is of no surprise that attempts at leveraging innate response or inducing a heightened response to cancer cells has been the subject of cancer therapeutic investigation for decades. The slow, albeit measured, clinical progress in this regard is a reflection of the complexity of the system, the evasiveness of cancer cells, and the imperfect models to preclinically study the system. However, the efficiency, selectivity, and sensitivity of the immune response make it one of the most promising avenues of targeted therapy and worthy of the effort.

Key effectors of the immune response include cytokines, such as interferons and interleukins, and antibodies. Contemporary understanding of the interplay between cancer and the immune system suggests that although cancer cells are immunogenic, they do not always elicit a response. This "immunotolerance" is not well understood but may be mediated in part by local anti-inflammatory tumor cytokine production, which may prevent dendritic cells from properly processing tumor cell antigens for a robust immune, anticancer response. Nevertheless, several avenues of investigation have been pursued; the agents used in this regard are called biologic response modifiers (BRMs).

The first BRMs to be created and used in cancer therapy were the interferons. As discussed earlier, this class of compounds has both direct and indirect activity on cancer cells. For example, the interferons can slow cancer cell growth or induce phenotypic transformation into normal cell behavior. Interferons also stimulate NK cells, T cells, and macrophages, which may increase the efficiency of the immune response to effect better anticancer treatment. Several interferon compounds (α, β, and γ) have been US Food and Drug Administration (FDA) approved for cancer therapy, and many have entered mature clinical investigation, including for gynecologic cancers, albeit with mixed results. For instance, an Austrian phase 3 study randomized 148 women with International Federation of Gynecology and Obstetrics stage IC-IIIC disease to cisplatin/cyclophosphamide with or without subcutaneously administered interferon-γ. PFS at 3 years was significantly improved (17 vs. 48 months; $P = .031$; Relative

Risk (RR), 0.48; 95% CI, 0.28-0.82), and toxicity was considered comparable between the arms. However, a much larger phase 3 study (N = 847) conducted by the GRACES clinical trial consortium investigating combination paclitaxel/carboplatin with or without interferon-γ-1b in women with advanced-stage ovarian cancer was terminated early due to an interim futility analysis suggesting detrimental effects in the experimental cohort.[33] Clearly, more work in this area is needed.

A second class of cytokines being investigated as cancer therapeutics is the interleukins (IL). These naturally occurring families of compounds have a vast cache of activities in multiple host systems, including lymphoproliferative organs and angiogenesis and immune system effectors, such as lymphocytes and platelets. Currently, IL-2 (aldesleukin), an IL that stimulates growth and differentiation of the T-cell response, is FDA approved for the treatment of metastatic renal cell carcinoma and melanoma. However, in light of the numerous functions ILs drive in the immune and host response to cancer cells, investigators continue to search for key treatment opportunities. For example, it has been known that IL-6, a proinflammatory cytokine that impacts hematopoietic stem cells, is a poor prognostic factor (associated with advanced disease, chemotherapy resistance, early recurrence, and short survival) of several solid tumors, including the gynecologic cancers, and is closely linked to angiogenesis, particularly in ovarian cancer, where high levels are also identified in ascites.[34] It also may be an important mediator of the paraneoplastic thrombocytosis phenotype, which is commonly identified in patients with advanced-stage ovarian cancer (Anil Sood, MD, personal communication in 2010). In light of these observations, IL-6–targeted therapies are being developed, including highly selective silencing through short interfering RNA.

MONOCLONAL ANTIBODIES

Antibodies with a specific target created from clones of a unique parent cell are called monoclonal antibodies (MoAbs). Their specificity for a unique target has made them highly desired for cancer therapeutics for which several, such as trastuzumab, bevacizumab, and cetuximab, are already FDA approved. These compounds have been often referred to as the "magic bullets" of disease therapy, a modern realization of the initial hypothesis of selective cytotoxicity forwarded by Paul Ehrlich in 1908.

Development

MoAbs were first developed in murine systems by injecting human cells of interest (eg, cancer cells)

Table 21-3 Biologically Targeted Monoclonal Antibody Class and Nomenclature

Suffix	Antibody Class	HAMA Potential	Example
"-omab"	Murine	+++	
"-ximab"	Chimeric	+/++	Cetuximab
"-zumab"	Humanized	+	Bevacizumab
"-mumab"	Fully human	−	Panitumumab

HAMA, human anti-mouse antibody.

and collecting murine plasma containing antihuman murine antibodies. Expansion of these antibodies was initially accomplished in hybridomas created from myeloma cells lacking the ability to secrete antibodies fused with healthy B cells, which were immunized by an antigen of interest. These murine antibodies were largely ineffective as treatment due to poor induction of immune cytotoxicity and the development of HAMAs, which rapidly degraded these agents and, in some cases, led to catastrophic circulatory collapse with repeated exposure. Murine MoAbs are usually represented by the suffix "-omab" (Table 21-3).

Humanization

To reduce the immunogenicity associated with murine MoAbs and to enhance their effectiveness, specific modifications were subsequently developed. Three types of MoAbs fall into this "humanization" process: chimeric antibodies, humanized antibodies, and fully human antibodies. All 3 types are used in clinical practice today, including oncology therapeutics. The class of MoAbs can be generally recognized by its nomenclature suffix: chimeric, by "-ximab" (eg, EGFR MoAb, cetuximab); humanized, by "-zumab" (eg, VEGF receptor [VEGFR] MoAb, bevacizumab); and fully human, by "-mumab" (EGFR MoAb, panitumumab). Chimerics are derived by fusing murine variable regions with human constant regions. Humanized MoAbs are created by grafting a small portion (~5%) of the immunized murine antibody to a human antibody backbone. The resulting molecule retains specificity for the human target, but due to the latter, largely evades the HAMA response. Although affinity for the primary target may be reduced in the process, several contemporary technologies have been developed to enhance antigen recognition. Fully human MoAbs are produced via transgenic mice, which are genetically engineered to produce human MoAbs following vaccination or by phage display technology. As will be presented later, this class of therapeutic has been central to some of the most important recent cancer treatment advances in gynecologic malignancies.

CLINICAL TARGETS IN GYNECOLOGIC ONCOLOGY

Estrogen Receptor

In light of the central role hormonal steroids play in developmental and adult physiology, it is not surprising that investigation into the role these elements play in proliferative disorders was the basis for some of the earliest forms of cancer therapeutics, particularly in gynecologic malignancies. It is generally well accepted that the bioactivity of estrogen is mediated through either or both estrogen receptors (α and β), which are predominately located in the nucleus. The principal ligand for the estrogen receptor is estrogen, but it may be activated by several growth factors including the epidermal growth factor, insulin, insulin-like growth factor-1, and TGF-α.[35] Upon binding of ligand, the estrogen receptor forms either homodimers or heterodimers (in the presence of estrogen receptor-β), which activate transcription of specific genes containing estrogen response elements. In many tissues, this transcription drives proliferation, which if unfettered, can induce aberrations leading to carcinogenesis. This is one of the hypotheses for the development of type I endometrial cancer and may well describe early events in the initiation of ovarian/tubal carcinogenesis and, more recently, metastases. Cells not expressing the estrogen receptor may also respond to estrogen ligand through nongenomic signaling via G-coupled proteins and an associated second messenger. In addition, membrane-bound estrogen receptor-α can activate Akt signaling via interaction with PI3K, particularly in endothelial cells. Conversely, estrogen-independent activation of the estrogen receptor can be induced through the Ras/Raf/ERK pathway in cells that overexpress ErbB2. It is interactions such as these that are suspected to contribute to an endocrine-resistant phenotype in breast and ovarian cancers (Figure 21-7). Estrogen receptor-α is predominately expressed in endometrial tissues and stroma, whereas estrogen receptor-β is observed more prevalently in ovarian tissues, although both receptors are expressed there. The function role of these 2 receptors in response to

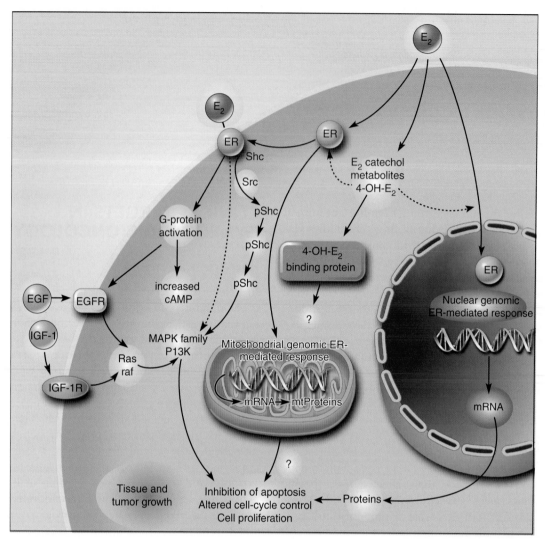

FIGURE 21-7. Estrogen receptor (ER) signaling may occur through nuclear or cytoplasmic interactions. Inhibition of apoptosis and aberrant cellular growth can occur via estrogen ligand-independent activation of the ER via Ras/Raf/ERK activation.

ligand can be complementary or opposing depending on the tissue site. In light of these observations, therapy antagonizing the estrogen receptor/ligand axis has been of interest in many tumors.

The clinical activity of hormonal therapy in endometrial and ovarian cancer is discussed in detail in other chapters; however, it is of interest to comment on the interaction between the estrogen hormone receptor and microRNAs (miRNA). miRNAs are short double-stranded RNA fragments that have near perfect complementarity to a number of genes and are predominately associated with translational repression or degradation.[36] Recently, a number of miRNAs have been discovered to reduce estrogen receptor protein translation from estrogen receptor-α, which in turn regulates the expression of controlling miRNAs. The feedback loop is important in tumors where regulatory

miRNAs are under suppressive control by estrogen receptor-α overexpression. The relevance of these discoveries will likely be elucidated as therapeutic RNA interference strategies are developed for systemic administration.

Epidermal Growth Factor Receptor

EGFR, like VEGFR, is a tyrosine kinase receptor in the cell membrane. Its ligand, EGF, binds EGFR, which then dimerizes and initiates signal transduction pathways that affect cellular proliferation, motility and invasion, apoptosis, and angiogenesis. EGFR is overexpressed in 60% to 80% of endometrial cancers, 73% of cervical carcinomas, and 68% of vulvar malignancies and is associated with advanced stage and poor prognosis.[37] Initial in vivo studies of EGFR inhibitors showed increased chemo- and radiosensitivity of tumors.

Cetuximab is an MoAb against EGFR that has improved survival in patients with head and neck and colorectal carcinoma. This antibody has been tested in combination with carboplatin in patients with EGFR-positive recurrent epithelial ovarian cancer with a response rate of 35% (12% with complete response).[38] A trial of cetuximab in combination with carboplatin and paclitaxel in patients with advanced ovarian or peritoneal cancer achieved a complete response of 70%, but 18-month PFS was 38.8% and was not considered a meaningful improvement in outcome over expected activity of carboplatin and paclitaxel alone. Several clinical trials in nearly all gynecologic primaries have now been completed, with both MoAbs and small-molecule tyrosine kinase inhibitors (eg, erlotinib and gefitinib) of this pathway showing modest or limited clinical efficacy. Although overexpression of EGFR would appear to define some aspects of tumor biology, multiple collateral activation pathways below the receptor level are likely contributing to the disconnect between receptor silencing and continued pathway signaling.

Human epidermal growth factor receptor 2 (HER-2) is also a membrane-bound tyrosine kinase receptor in the same family as EGFR. Like EGFR, HER-2 dimerizes upon activation to mediate cell survival, proliferation, and angiogenesis. Approximately 5% to 23% of epithelial ovarian cancers and up to 44% of endometrial cancers overexpress HER-2.[39] *HER-2* gene amplification has been found to directly correlate with poor clinical outcomes in many malignancies including breast and ovarian cancer. Trastuzumab is a humanized MoAb against HER-2 that has been effective for the treatment of many patients with HER-2–positive breast cancer. In patients with recurrent or progressive epithelial ovarian cancer positive for HER-2 overexpression, 7.3% achieved a clinical response with single-agent trastuzumab, but only 95 of 837 patients screened positive for HER-2, and only 41 patients were eligible for the study. The combination of trastuzumab with paclitaxel and carboplatin for patients with progressive advanced ovarian cancer resulted in a complete response rate of 43%; however, only 7 patients were included in the trial, and only 22 of 321 patients screened showed positive *HER-2* gene amplification.[40] No clinical response has been observed with single-agent trastuzumab in patients with advanced or recurrent endometrial cancer and *HER-2* gene amplification.

Pertuzumab is a humanized MoAb that inhibits ErbB2 dimerization with the other ErbB receptors, independent of ErbB2 expression. In a recently completed phase 2 trial of pertuzumab in patients with refractory ovarian cancer, the overall response rate was 4.3%, with 6.8% of patients reporting stable disease at 6 months.[41] A randomized, placebo-controlled, double-blind phase 2 trial investigating pertuzumab in combination with gemcitabine revealed similar rates of PFS between patients treated with or without pertuzumab (3.0 vs. 2.6 months). Interestingly, relative expression of ErbB2 to ErbB3 appeared to indicate clinical benefit by response and PFS criteria. Because ErbB2:ErbB3 heterodimerization is a preferred and potent mitogenic signaling initiator, ErbB3 mRNA appears to reflect efficacy of "on target" pertuzumab binding and may explain the clinical observation. Unfortunately, at this point, it is unclear whether there will be a development plan for the agent in gynecologic cancers.

VEGF-targeted agents appear to have greater activity against cervical cancer than EGF-, EGFR-, and HER-2–blocking agents. A phase 2 trial compared the 2 approaches head to head using pazopanib, a tyrosine kinase inhibitor that blocks VEGFR and platelet-derived growth factor receptor (PDGFR), versus lapatinib, a tyrosine kinase inhibitor that targets EGFR and HER-2 activity. Pazopanib was superior to lapatinib, with improved PFS and overall survival and minimal toxicity. In a multicenter phase 2 trial of bevacizumab in combination with erlotinib in patients with recurrent ovarian cancer, a response rate of 15% was noted, consistent with the response rate observed with bevacizumab alone.[42] A randomized phase 2 clinical trial of vandetanib (dual VEGFR/EGFR inhibitor) followed by docetaxel versus vandetanib plus docetaxel is being launched by the Southwest Oncology Group (Trial S0904, ClinicalTrials.gov identifier: NCT00872989).

Despite the apparent lack of activity of EGFR inhibitors in gynecologic cancer, there is rationale for further evaluation of these drugs. Given the high expression of EGFR in gynecologic malignancies and the increased sensitivity of tumors to other cytotoxic therapies when given in combination with EGFR inhibitors, further studies may prove highly beneficial. As illustrated by the discovery that *KRAS* mutations in colorectal tumors made the tumors resistant to EGFR inhibition, continued strides toward effective oncologic treatment require a better molecular understanding of carcinogenesis.

Vascular Endothelial Growth Factor

VEGF, also known as vascular permeability factor (VPF), is one of the most well-characterized angiogenesis mediators. VEGF comprises a family of proteins, of which VEGFA (often implied by the term "VEGF") is the dominant factor in tumor angiogenesis[43] (Figure 21-8). There are 3 tyrosine kinase receptors for VEGF, of which VEGFR-2 appears to have the most significant effects on angiogenesis. VEGF is ubiquitous in most

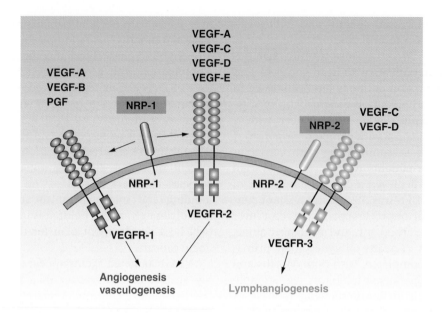

FIGURE 21-8. The vascular endothelial growth factor (VEGF)/VEGF receptor (VEGFR) pathway. Ligands for the 3 VEGF receptors are depicted above their respective receptor. The neuropilins (NRPs) may act as coreceptors or activators of the pathway and are found on mesenchymal vascular supporting cells called pericytes. PGF, placental growth factor.

human tissue and is upregulated in response to injury or stress. Interaction of VEGFR-2 with its ligand causes homo- or heterodimerization of the receptors, resulting in activation of a cascade of downstream signaling pathways. VEGF activation also results in increased production of nitric oxide and prostaglandin I_2, both vasodilators.[44] Increased production of VEGF and other growth factors is frequently observed in regions of hypoxia or inflammation and in the presence of activated oncogenes or downregulated tumor suppressor genes. Human papillomavirus (HPV), for example, is the root cause of virtually all cervical cancers. HPV's E6 protein increases VEGF production by downregulating the tumor suppressor gene *p53* and enhancing induction of hypoxia-inducible factor (HIF) 1-α.[45] Overexpression of VEGF results in increased endothelial cell proliferation, decreased apoptosis, and increased fenestration of endothelial cells. High VEGF expression has been shown to be associated with poor prognosis in most gynecologic malignancies including cervical, endometrial, ovarian, and vulvar cancers.

Bevacizumab

Bevacizumab is a humanized MoAb against VEGFA that is approved by the FDA for the treatment of metastatic colorectal, non–small-cell lung, renal cell, and breast cancers. Several phase 2 trials of this VEGFA antibody have been performed to assess its activity in gynecologic cancers. Bevacizumab has been most extensively studied in recurrent ovarian cancer patients, where response rates have ranged from 16% to 24%

and median overall survival is 10.7 to 17 months when administered either as a single agent or in combination with metronomic cyclophosphamide.[46-48] It has also been shown to have activity in patient with recurrent or persistent endometrial cancer and in patients with progressive or recurrent cervical cancer (Figure 21-9).[49,50]

Most studies of bevacizumab in gynecologic cancer have been conducted in patients with recurrent or progressive disease. Following encouraging data in phase 2 studies compared with historical controls, 2 randomized phase 3 studies in untreated advanced ovarian cancer patients have been conducted: GOG 218 (NCT00262847) and ICON-7 (NCT00483782). Each of these trials included an experimental arm with a maintenance treatment phase, which was placebo controlled in GOG 218 and open label in ICON-7. Both trials demonstrated superior clinical activity (hazard for progression) over control and, in the case of GOG 218, over combination paclitaxel, carboplatin, and bevacizumab followed by placebo maintenance. Of interest, the PFS of these "winning" arms is substantively less than that reported by earlier phase 2 data despite a similar proportion of suboptimal stage IIIC patients.

Toxicities associated with bevacizumab in phase 2 trials include hypertension, proteinuria, hemorrhage, neutropenia, venous thromboembolism, pulmonary embolus, congestive heart failure, myocardial infarction, and cerebrovascular ischemia (Table 21-4). Hypertension is the best characterized and most common side effect of the drug. It is thought to be caused

On presentation   **Following 3 courses of therapy**

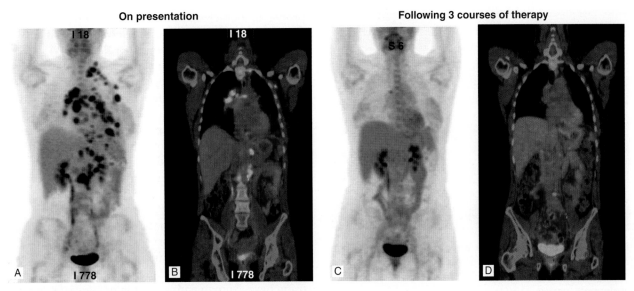

FIGURE 21-9. A-D. Dramatic response to combination paclitaxel and carboplatin with bevacizumab in a patient with widely metastatic recurrent squamous cell carcinoma of the cervix. She had previously been treated with cisplatin-based chemoradiation.

by blocking nitric oxide production via inhibiting activation of VEGFR-2 and by endothelial dysfunction in normal tissue. The severity of hypertension is directly correlated with the dose of bevacizumab and the baseline blood pressure of the patient before initiating therapy. The degree of hypertension may also be a biomarker for response to therapy.[51]

One of the most alarming potential adverse events associated with bevacizumab is gastrointestinal (GI)

perforation and fistula (Figure 21-10). Two phase 2 trials of bevacizumab in treatment of ovarian cancer were stopped early due to a high rate of GI perforation (11% and 15%).[42,47] A retrospective review at Memorial Sloan-Kettering Cancer Center of patients with ovarian carcinoma receiving bevacizumab either in combination or as monotherapy revealed a GI perforation rate of 4% (6 of 160 patients). This is comparable to a compilation of published ovarian cancer

Table 21-4 High-Grade (Grade 3-5) Toxicities of Biologic Therapies Reported as Related to Investigational Agent Listed According to Agent and Frequency

Agent	GI Perf	HTN	TE	Heme	Bleed[a]	Pain	Wound[b]	HFS
Bevacizumab monotherapy	0%-11%	8%-15%	2%-11%	2%-17%	0%-2%	5%-13%	0%-5%	0%
Bevacizumab combination therapy	3%-15%	8%-16%	1%-3%	3%-11%	0%-1%	0%-19%	0%-1%	0%-3%
Sorafenib monotherapy	0%	3%-13%	0%-4%	0%-7%	0%-5%	0%	0%-2%	0%-13%
Sorafenib combination therapy	0%	21%	0%	32%	0%	0%	0%	0%
Sunitinib	0%	11%-31%	0%	42%	0%	0%	0%	0%
Cediranib	0%	33%-46%	0%	0%	7%	7%	0%	0%
Pazopanib	0%	3%	0%	0%	0%	3%	0%	0%
Aflibercept	1%-18%	9%	1%-8%	0%	0%	0%	0%	0%

GI Perf, gastrointestinal perforation; heme, hematologic toxicities; HFS, hand-foot syndrome; HTN, hypertension; TE, thromboembolism.
[a]Includes any hemorrhage.
[b]Wound complications including fistulas.

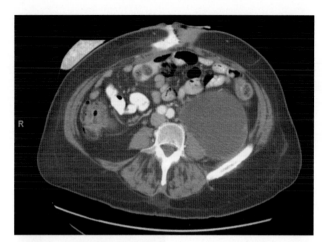

FIGURE 21-10. Patient who developed a fistula while on bevacizumab for therapy of recurrent ovarian cancer. The orally administered contrast dye is seen in the anterior abdominal wound.

trials of bevacizumab that estimates a GI perforation risk of 5.4% (16 of 298 patients). Many of the enrolled patients were heavily pretreated. Some studies have suggested that bowel involvement with ovarian carcinoma, bowel wall thickening, or bowel obstruction on computed tomography imaging; prior radiation therapy; and recent surgery may predispose patients to GI perforation, but strong evidence of association with these factors is still lacking. There are also reports of GI perforations associated with diverticulitis, ulcers, recent anastomosis, or bowel stricture or ischemia.[52] The etiology of these events is not fully understood but may be related to vascular compromise following VEGF blockade. Although it has yet to be validated in whom bevacizumab administration is without safety concerns, it is prudent to consider these known toxicities relative to benefit and in the context of pre-existing medical infirmity prior to treatment.

Other Therapeutics Against VEGF and VEGFR

Sorafenib and sunitinib are 2 tyrosine kinase inhibitors that block the activity of VEGFR, and both are approved by the FDA for targeted cancer therapy in renal cell carcinoma. Sorafenib inhibits several proteins including VEGFR-1, VEGFR-2, VEGFR-3, and PDGFR-α. Clinical investigation of sorafenib in gynecologic malignancies has revealed modest objective tumor responses and significant stable disease. Another multikinase inhibitor that blocks VEGFR and PDGFR, sunitinib, has been found to promote stable disease in women with recurrent ovarian cancer and recurrent or metastatic endometrial or cervix cancer.[53] Sorafenib clind sunitinib have a similar side effect

profile to bevacizumab, with the addition of hand-foot syndrome, which occurs as grade 3 or higher in approximately 13% of recipients (Table 21-4).

In light of the cross-talk pathways that contribute to cancer cell survival, interest has flourished in evaluating combinations of anti-angiogenic agents. An analysis of sorafenib with bevacizumab in patients with ovarian cancer yielded an impressive 43% response rate; however dose reductions of sorafenib were required in 74% of patients due to toxicities.[54] Eighty-four percent of the ovarian cancer patients in this study experienced grade 1 to 3 hypertension, and grade 1 to 2 hand-foot syndrome occurred in 95%. The toxicities experienced with the drugs in combination were greater than the additive effects of each drug alone. Similar trends of increased response with increased toxicity requiring dose reduction or discontinuation have been observed using bevacizumab with sunitinib or sorafenib in renal cell carcinoma.

Other small-molecule tyrosine kinase inhibitors that target VEGFR include AZD2171, pazopanib, and BIBF-1120. AZD2171 (cediranib) is an oral tyrosine kinase inhibitor of VEGFR-1, VEGFR-2, VEGFR-3, PDGFR-α, and c-kit that has been evaluated in phase 2 trials for patients with recurrent epithelial ovarian cancer, fallopian tube carcinoma, or peritoneal cancer. The partial response rate in this population was 10% to 17%, and stable disease was achieved in 13% to 34%.[55] ICON-6 (NCT00544973) is currently evaluating AZD2171 in a randomized, placebo-controlled, phase 3 trial in patients with recurrent ovarian cancer. Pazopanib is an inhibitor of VEGFR-1, VEGFR-2, VEGFR-3, PDGFR-α, PDGFR-β, and c-kit and has been tested in patients with advanced epithelial ovarian, fallopian tube, or primary peritoneal carcinoma. Response rate, as measured by CA-125 decline, was 47%, and 27% of patients had stable disease.[56] Pazopanib is currently being evaluated as a maintenance therapy in a double-blind, placebo-controlled, phase 3 clinical study in women who have achieved a partial or complete response to primary platinum-based adjuvant chemotherapy (NCT00866697). BIBF-1120, an inhibitor of VEGFR-1, VEGFR-2, VEGFR-3, PDGFR-α, PDGFR-β, and FGF, has been investigated as a single agent in the maintenance setting. Eighty-four patients with best outcome to 1 or 2 previous lines of chemotherapy of either partial or complete response were randomized to either placebo or BIBF-1120. The primary end point was PFS. Overall, patients on placebo had a PFS of 2.8 months compared to 4.8 months in patients treated with BIBF-1120.[57] These data have prompted a larger phase III trial (NCT01015118) and exploration of chemotherapy combinations as primary therapy for women with ovarian cancer. These agents have similar side effects, the most frequent being hypertension, fatigue, and GI complaints (Table 21-4).

Table 21-5 Comparison of Bevacizumab to Aflibercept

Characteristic	Bevacizumab	Aflibercept
Molecule	Humanized chimeric murine monoclonal antibody	Fusion protein
Target	VEGF	VEGF, placental growth factor
$T_{1/2}$	21 days	25 days
FDA approval?	Yes, but not for gynecologic malignancies	No

Note. Both agents bind VEGF ligand with high affinity but have slightly different characteristics.
$T_{1/2}$, half-life; VEGF, vascular endothelial growth factor.

Aflibercept

VEGF Trap, or aflibercept, is a protein containing the VEGF binding regions of VEGFR-1 and VEGFR-2 fused to the Fc region of a human IgG1. This inhibitor resulted in a partial response rate of 11% in women with recurrent platinum-resistant epithelial ovarian carcinoma. Aflibercept was also studied as a single agent in women with refractory ascites. In this trial, the agent was significantly associated with reduced need for paracentesis.[58] In patients with uterine sarcoma, a phase 2 trial of aflibercept showed that 16% of patients with leiomyosarcoma experienced stable disease for over 6 months, but no response and no stable disease were observed in those with carcinosarcoma.[59] Similar to bevacizumab, aflibercept is also associated with fatigue, hypertension, and GI complaints; a comparison of the 2 is shown in Table 21-5.

PI3K/mTOR/Akt Pathway

The tumor suppressor gene *PTEN* (phosphate and tensin homolog detected on chromosome 10) is important for normal cellular function. Mutations in *PTEN* result in decreased apoptosis and are found in up to 83% of endometrioid carcinomas of the uterus. Decreased transcription due to mutation leads to decreased phosphatidylinositol 3-kinase (PI3K) inhibition, increased activity of Akt, and uncontrolled function of mammalian target of rapamycin (mTOR). Elevated activity of mTOR is seen in a vast majority of endometrial cancers as well as approximately 50% of cervical adenocarcinomas and 55% of ovarian carcinomas.[60] mTOR is a kinase that regulates cell growth and apoptosis.[37] Temsirolimus, ridaforolimus, and everolimus are mTOR inhibitors that have been tested as single agents in phase 2 studies and found to promote stable disease in 44% of patients with metastatic or recurrent cancer of the endometrium.[61] Side effects of these drugs consist mostly of myelosuppression, hyperlipidemia, hypercholesterolemia, and fatigue. Because aberrations in the PI3K/Akt/mTOR pathway are prolific in

gynecologic cancers, drug discovery is keeping pace with several new agents entering the clinical domain (Figure 21-11). These drugs are being studied as single agents and in combination with chemotherapy and hormonal therapy.[37]

Poly(ADP-Ribose) Pathway

There are a total of 17 members of the poly(ADP-ribose) polymerase (PARP) family, of which PARP-1 and PARP-2 orchestrate repair of single-stranded breaks in DNA.[62] These enzymes bind to DNA at the site of damage and then initiate repair by ribosylation of nearby proteins, leading to base-excision repair at the site of damage and downstream effects on transcription and differentiation (Figure 21-12). Inhibition of PARPs via competitive blockade of the catalytic domain results in accumulation of DNA damage and cell death. *BRCA1* and *BRCA2* are tumor suppressor genes also important in DNA repair at sites of double-stranded breaks. Homologous recombination at DNA-damaged sites is a high-fidelity method of DNA repair mediated by Rad51 that is dependent on normal *BRCA* function. Mutations of *BRCA* genes force the cellular machinery to rely on lower fidelity methods of DNA repair and thus promote genomic instability. The initial studies of PARP inhibitors in *BRCA*-deficient tumors noted that, although mutations in *BRCA* increased tumor sensitivity to certain cytotoxic therapies, PARP inhibition causes cell death in this population approximately 3-fold over traditional treatment. By leaving single-stranded breaks unchecked by PARP inhibition, double-stranded DNA breaks are promoted in cells already lacking DNA repair capability, a process known as synthetic lethality. Normal cells with intact *BRCA* function will be able to repair their double-stranded DNA breaks, making tumor cells more susceptible to this treatment than normal tissue (Figure 21-12). Additionally, PARP inhibition, itself, has been found to suppress expression of *BRCA1* and Rad51. Since the discovery of synthetic lethality in

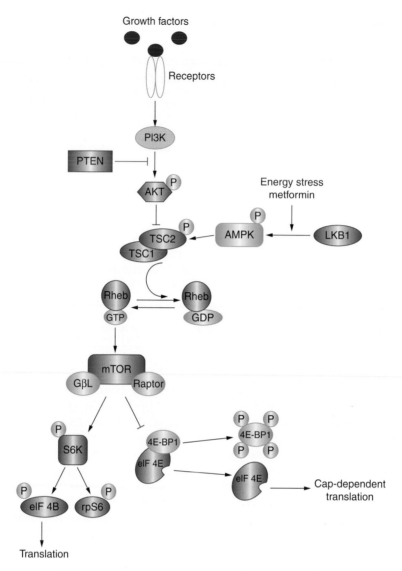

FIGURE 21-11. The PI3K/Akt/mTOR pathway is frequently altered in human malignancy. The multiple effectors of this pathway provide important targets for therapeutic intervention.

2005, inhibitors of PARP have been studied in *BRCA*-positive breast cancer and have been found not only to enhance the cytotoxic effects of chemotherapy and radiation, but also to improve outcomes when used as single agents.[63]

PARP inhibitors are now being tested in patients with *BRCA*-positive ovarian cancer. AZD2281 (olaparib) is an oral small-molecule PARP-1 and PARP-2 inhibitor that was tested in 2 phase 1 trials. Among patients with *BRCA* mutations and ovarian carcinoma treated with olaparib, a response rate of 41% to 53% was noted.[64] A phase 2 study of AZD2281 in patients with *BRCA*-positive recurrent ovarian cancer yielded a response rate of 33% at a dose of 400 mg twice a day and 12.5% at a dose of 100 mg twice a day. Side effects of olaparib include GI complaints, fatigue, and myelosuppression. Continued trials of AZD2281 and other PARP inhibitors alone and in combination with

chemotherapy are ongoing in patients with *BRCA*-positive and -negative ovarian and primary peritoneal cancer. Newly developed PARP inhibitors, such as ABT-888, MK4827, and BSI-201, are also currently being tested in gynecologic and nongynecologic tumors.

The activity of PARP inhibitors may not be limited to patients with germline *BRCA* mutations. Approximately 50% of undifferentiated and high-grade serous ovarian cancers have loss of *BRCA1* function.[65] Many tumors have *BRCA*-like functional losses such as inactivation of *BRCA* genes or defects in other genes needed for *BRCA*-associated DNA repair that yield a clinical outcome similar to cancers with *BRCA* mutations. There is also increasing evidence that PARP inhibitors enhance the cytotoxic effects of chemotherapy and radiation without regard to *BRCA* function. These alternative mechanisms of propagating cytotoxic DNA damage may expand the utility of PARP

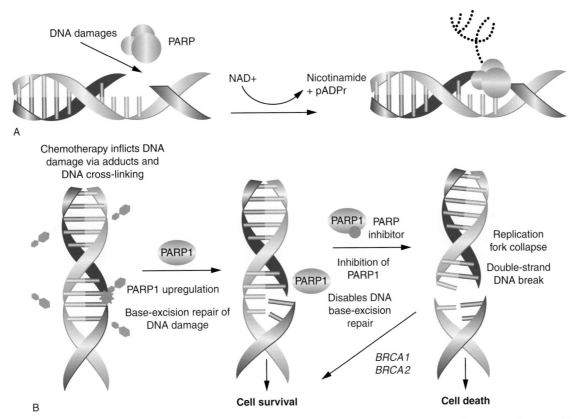

FIGURE 21-12. Poly(ADP-ribose) pathway (PARP). A. The enzyme is important for repair of DNA single-strand breaks. **B.** In the absence of high-fidelity homologous recombination, such as exists in women whose tumors carry *BRCA* mutations, tumors engage PARP for continued cell growth and proliferation. This makes them vulnerable to catastrophic damage under the influence of PARP inhibition unless *BRCA* function returns via reversion mutation.

inhibitors to a substantial number of malignancies. PARP inhibitors are currently being tested alone and in combination with chemotherapeutic agents, which may induce a vulnerable tumor homologous recombination phenotype, to evaluate the potential risks and benefits of these drugs among patients with impaired and normal *BRCA* function.

FUTURE DIRECTIONS

Over the last 5 to 10 years, there has been rapid development and evaluation of molecularly targeted therapies in oncology. The goal of these endeavors is to identify agents against aberrant pathways common among specific tumors that can improve current treatments. Initial phase 2 trials show some promising results, and large phase 3 trials are under way to confirm activity of these agents. There is concern that molecular targeting in treatment of cancer may provide evolutionary pressure to select for tumor cells that are highly resistant to therapy. Targeting multiple pathways of oncogenesis and using molecular inhibitors in combination with other cytotoxic treatments

may overcome these selective processes to achieve higher cure rates for patients.

The evolution of investigation of immunotherapy for the treatment of patients with ovarian cancer is following a similar path. Finding targets specific for tumor cells has proven difficult. The range of immune strategies under investigation is wide. They include efforts to increase the effector cell response in specificity, number, and duration, as well as manipulating factors responsible for tolerance and terminating the immune attack. A favorable toxicity profile remains the hallmark of many approaches, and investigating these strategies in an attempt to prolong remission is ongoing. Evolving knowledge regarding the mechanisms of evasion of novel targeted treatments, including those targeting the immune response and other signaling pathways, should lead to better combinations that will hopefully surpass current standard therapy.

REFERENCES

1. Dubinett SM, Lee JM, Sharma S, Mule JJ. Chemokines: can effector cells be redirected to the site of the tumor? *Cancer J.* 2010;16(4):325-335.

2. Metcalf D. The colony-stimulating factors and cancer. *Nat Rev Cancer.* 2010;10(6):425-434.

3. Kopf M, Bachmann MF, Marsland BJ. Averting inflammation by targeting the cytokine environment. *Nat Rev Drug Discov.* 2010;9(9):703-718.

4. Boyd SD, Gaeta BA, Jackson KJ, et al. Individual variation in the germline Ig gene repertoire inferred from variable region gene rearrangements. *J Immunol.* 2010;184(12):6986-6992.

5. Kojouharova M, Reid K, Gadjeva M. New insights into the molecular mechanisms of classical complement activation. *Mol Immunol.* 2010;47(13):2154-2160.

6. Smith-Garvin JE, Koretzky GA, Jordan MS. T cell activation. *Annu Rev Immunol.* 2009;27:591-619.

7. Sharma RK, Schabowsky RH, Srivastava AK, et al. 4-1BB ligand as an effective multifunctional immunomodulator and antigen delivery vehicle for the development of therapeutic cancer vaccines. *Cancer Res.* 2010;70(10):3945-3954.

8. Hodi FS, O'Day SJ, McDermott DF, et al. Improved survival with ipilimumab in patients with metastatic melanoma. *N Engl J Med.* 2010;363(8):711-723.

9. Zhang L, Conejo-Garcia JR, Katsaros D, et al. Intratumoral T cells, recurrence, and survival in epithelial ovarian cancer. *N Engl J Med.* 2003;348(3):203-213.

10. Dietl J, Engel JB, Wischhusen J. The role of regulatory T cells in ovarian cancer. *Int J Gynecol Cancer.* 2007;17(4):764-770.

11. Shields JD, Kourtis IC, Tomei AA, Roberts JM, Swartz MA. Induction of lymphoidlike stroma and immune escape by tumors that express the chemokine CCL21. *Science.* 2010;328(5979):749-752.

12. Yigit R, Massuger LF, Figdor CG, Torensma R. Ovarian cancer creates a suppressive microenvironment to escape immune elimination. *Gynecol Oncol.* 2010;117(2):366-372.

13. Chatterjee M, Wojciechowski J, Tainsky MA. Discovery of antibody biomarkers using protein microarrays of tumor antigens cloned in high throughput. *Methods Mol Biol.* 2009;520:21-38.

14. Piura B, Piura E. Autoantibodies to tumor-associated antigens in epithelial ovarian carcinoma. *J Oncol.* 2009;2009:581939.

15. Alberts DS, Hannigan EV, Liu PY, et al. Randomized trial of adjuvant intraperitoneal alpha-interferon in stage III ovarian cancer patients who have no evidence of disease after primary surgery and chemotherapy: an intergroup study. *Gynecol Oncol.* 2006;100(1):133-138.

16. Verheijen RH, Massuger LF, Benigno BB, et al. Phase III trial of intraperitoneal therapy with yttrium-90-labeled HMFG1 murine monoclonal antibody in patients with epithelial ovarian cancer after a surgically defined complete remission. *J Clin Oncol.* 2006;24(4):571-578.

17. Berek J, Taylor P, McGuire W, Smith LM, Schultes B, Nicodemus CF. Oregovomab maintenance monoimmunotherapy does not improve outcomes in advanced ovarian cancer. *J Clin Oncol.* 2009;27(3):418-425.

18. Sabbatini P. Consolidation therapy in ovarian cancer: a clinical update. *Int J Gynecol Cancer.* 2009;19(suppl 2):S35-S39.

19. Sabbatini P, Berek J, Casado A, et al. Abagovomab maintenance therapy in patients with epithelial ovarian cancer after complete response post first line chemotherapy: preliminary results of the randomized double blind, placebo controlled multi-center MIMOSA trial. *J Clin Oncol.* 2010;28(suppl 15). Abstract 5036.

20. Old LJ. Ludwig Institute for Cancer Research. 2007. Available at: http://www.licr.org/. Accessed March 3, 2012.

21. Odunsi K, Qian F, Matsuzaki J, et al. Vaccination with an NY-ESO-1 peptide of HLA class I/II specificities induces integrated humoral and T cell responses in ovarian cancer. *Proc Natl Acad Sci U S A.* 2007;104(31):12837-12842.

22. Diefenbach CS, Gnjatic S, Sabbatini P, et al. Safety and immunogenicity study of NY-ESO-1b peptide and montanide ISA-51 vaccination of patients with epithelial ovarian cancer in high-risk first remission. *Clin Cancer Res.* 2008;14(9):2740-2748.

23. Hernando JJ, Park TW, Fischer HP, et al. Vaccination with dendritic cells transfected with mRNA-encoded folate-receptor-alpha for relapsed metastatic ovarian cancer. *Lancet Oncol.* 2007;8(5):451-454.

24. Czerniecki BJ, Koski GK, Koldovsky U, et al. Targeting HER-2/neu in early breast cancer development using dendritic cells with staged interleukin-12 burst secretion. *Cancer Res.* 2007;67(4):1842-1852.

25. Gong J, Apostolopoulos V, Chen D, et al. *J Immunol.* 2000;101(3):316-324.

26. Sabbatini PJ, Ragupathi G, Hood C, et al. Pilot study of a heptavalent vaccine-keyhole limpet hemocyanin conjugate plus QS21 in patients with epithelial ovarian, fallopian tube, or peritoneal cancer. *Clin Cancer Res.* 2007;13(14):4170-4177.

27. Kershaw MH, Westwood JA, Parker LL, et al. A phase I study on adoptive immunotherapy using gene-modified T cells for ovarian cancer. *Clin Cancer Res.* 2006;12(20 Pt 1):6106-6115.

28. Chekmasova AA, Brentjens RJ. Adoptive T cell immunotherapy strategies for the treatment of patients with ovarian cancer. *Discov Med.* 2010;9(44):62-70.

29. Hatfield P, Merrick AE, West E, et al. Optimization of dendritic cell loading with tumor cell lysates for cancer immunotherapy. *J Immunother.* 2008;31(7):620-632.

30. Rocha-Lima CM, Soares HP, Raez LE, Singal R. EGFR targeting of solid tumors. *Cancer Control.* 2007;14(3):295-304.

31. Wiezorek J, Holland P, Graves J. Death receptor agonists as a targeted therapy for cancer. *Clin Cancer Res.* 2010;16(6):1701-1708.

32. Lessene G, Czabotar PE, Colman PM. BCL-2 family antagonists for cancer therapy. *Nat Rev Drug Discov.* 2008;7(12):989-1000.

33. Alberts DS, Marth C, Alvarez RD, et al. Randomized phase 3 trial of interferon gamma-1b plus standard carboplatin/paclitaxel versus carboplatin/paclitaxel alone for first-line treatment of advanced ovarian and primary peritoneal carcinomas: results from a prospectively designed analysis of progression-free survival. *Gynecol Oncol.* 2008;109(2):174-181.

34. Giuntoli RL 2nd, Webb TJ, Zoso A, et al. Ovarian cancer-associated ascites demonstrates altered immune environment: implications for antitumor immunity. *Anticancer Res.* 2009;29(8):2875-2884.

35. Keely NO, Meegan MJ. Targeting tumors using estrogen receptor ligand conjugates. *Curr Cancer Drug Targets.* 2009;9(3):370-380.

36. Tessel MA, Krett NL, Rosen ST. Steroid receptor and microRNA regulation in cancer. *Curr Opin Oncol.* 2010;22(6):592-597.

37. Bansal N, Yendluri V, Wenham RM. The molecular biology of endometrial cancers and the implications for pathogenesis, classification, and targeted therapies. *Cancer Control.* 2009;16(1):8-13.

38. Secord AA, Blessing JA, Armstrong DK, et al. Phase II trial of cetuximab and carboplatin in relapsed platinum-sensitive ovarian cancer and evaluation of epidermal growth factor receptor expression: a Gynecologic Oncology Group study. *Gynecol Oncol.* 2008;108(3):493-499.

39. Grushko TA, Filiaci VL, Mundt AJ, Ridderstrale K, Olopade OI, Fleming GF. An exploratory analysis of HER-2 amplification and overexpression in advanced endometrial carcinoma: a Gynecologic Oncology Group study. *Gynecol Oncol.* 2008;108(1):3-9.

40. Tuefferd M, Couturier J, Penault-Llorca F, et al. HER2 status in ovarian carcinomas: a multicenter GINECO study of 320 patients. *PLoS One.* 2007;2(11):e1138.

41. Gordon MS, Matei D, Aghajanian C, et al. Clinical activity of pertuzumab (rhuMAb 2C4), a HER dimerization inhibitor, in advanced ovarian cancer: potential predictive relationship with tumor HER2 activation status. *J Clin Oncol.* 2006;24(26):4324-4332.

42. Nimeiri HS, Oza AM, Morgan RJ, et al. Efficacy and safety of bevacizumab plus erlotinib for patients with recurrent ovarian, primary peritoneal, and fallopian tube cancer: a trial of the Chicago, PMH, and California Phase II Consortia. *Gynecol Oncol.* 2008;110(1):49-55.

43. Ellis LM, Hicklin DJ. VEGF-targeted therapy: mechanisms of anti-tumour activity. *Nat Rev Cancer.* 2008;8(8):579-591.

44. Curwen JO, Musgrove HL, Kendrew J, Richmond GH, Ogilvie DJ, Wedge SR. Inhibition of vascular endothelial growth factor-a signaling induces hypertension: examining the effect of cediranib (recentin; AZD2171) treatment on blood pressure in rat and the use of concomitant antihypertensive therapy. *Clin Cancer Res.* 2008;14(10):3124-3131.

45. Monk BJ, Willmott LJ, Sumner DA. Anti-angiogenesis agents in metastatic or recurrent cervical cancer. *Gynecol Oncol.* 2010; 116(2):181-186.

46. Burger RA, Sill MW, Monk BJ, Greer BE, Sorosky JI. Phase II trial of bevacizumab in persistent or recurrent epithelial ovarian cancer or primary peritoneal cancer: a Gynecologic Oncology Group study. *J Clin Oncol.* 2007;25:5165-5171.

47. Cannistra SA, Matulonis UA, Penson RT, et al. Phase II study of bevacizumab in patients with platinum-resistant ovarian cancer or peritoneal serous cancer. *J Clin Oncol.* 2007;25(33):5180-5186.

48. Garcia AA, Hirte H, Fleming G, et al. Phase II clinical trial of bevacizumab and low-dose metronomic oral cyclophosphamide in recurrent ovarian cancer: a trial of the California, Chicago, and Princess Margaret Hospital phase II consortia. *J Clin Oncol.* 2008;26(1):76-82.

49. Aghajanian C, Sill MW, Darcy KM, et al. A phase II evaluation of bevacizumab in the treatment of recurrent or persistent endometrial cancer: a Gynecologic Oncology Group (GOG) study. *J Clin Oncol.* 2009;27(suppl 15S). Abstract 5531.

50. Monk BJ, Sill MW, Burger RA, Gray HJ, Buekers TE, Roman LD. Phase II trial of bevacizumab in the treatment of persistent or recurrent squamous cell carcinoma of the cervix: a Gynecologic Oncology Group study. *J Clin Oncol.* 2009;27(7):1069-1074.

51. Scartozzi M, Galizia E, Chiorrini S, et al. Arterial hypertension correlates with clinical outcome in colorectal cancer patients treated with first-line bevacizumab. *Ann Oncol.* 2009;20(2): 227-230.

52. Chen HX, Cleck JN. Adverse effects of anticancer agents that target the VEGF pathway. *Nat Rev Clin Oncol.* 2009;6(8):465-477.

53. Biagi J, Oza A, Grimshaw R, et al. A phase II study of sunitinib (SU11248) in patients (pts) with recurrent epithelial ovarian,

fallopian tube or primary peritoneal carcinoma: NCIC CTG IND 185. *J Clin Oncol.* 2008;26(suppl 20S). Abstract 5522.

54. Azad NS, Posadas EM, Kwitkowski VE, et al. Combination targeted therapy with sorafenib and bevacizumab results in enhanced toxicity and antitumor activity. *J Clin Oncol.* 2008;26(22): 3709-3714.

55. Matulonis UA, Berlin S, Ivy P, et al. Cediranib, an oral inhibitor of vascular endothelial growth factor receptor kinases, is an active drug in recurrent epithelial ovarian, fallopian tube, and peritoneal cancer. *J Clin Oncol.* 2009;27(33):5601-5606.

56. Friedlander M, Hancock KC, Rischin D, et al. A phase II, open-label study evaluating pazopanib in patients with recurrent ovarian cancer. *Gynecol Oncol.* 2010;119(1):32-37.

57. Ledermann J, Rustin G, Hackshaw A, et al. A randomized phase II placebo-controlled trial using maintenance therapy to evaluate the vascular targeting agent BIBF 1120 following treatment of relapsed ovarian cancer (OC). *J Clin Oncol.* 2009;27(suppl 20S). Abstract 5501.

58. Moroney JW, Sood AK, Coleman RL. Aflibercept in epithelial ovarian carcinoma. *Future Oncol.* 2009;5(5):591-600.

59. Townsley CA, Hirte H, Hoskins P, et al. A phase II study of aflibercept (VEGF trap) in recurrent or metastatic gynecologic soft-tissue sarcomas: a study of the Princess Margaret Hospital Phase II Consortium. *J Clin Oncol.* 2009;27(suppl 15S). Abstract 5591.

60. Faried LS, Faried A, Kanuma T, et al. Expression of an activated mammalian target of rapamycin in adenocarcinoma of the cervix: a potential biomarker and molecular target therapy. *Mol Carcinog.* 2008;47(6):446-457.

61. Slomovitz BM, Lu KH, Johnston T, et al. A phase 2 study of the oral mammalian target of rapamycin inhibitor, everolimus, in patients with recurrent endometrial carcinoma. *Cancer.* 2010; 116(23):5415-5419.

62. Miwa M, Masutani M. PolyADP-ribosylation and cancer. *Cancer Sci.* 2007;98(10):1528-1535.

63. Drew Y, Plummer R. PARP inhibitors in cancer therapy: two modes of attack on the cancer cell widening the clinical applications. *Drug Resist Updat.* 2009;12(6):153-156.

64. Fong PC, Boss DS, Yap TA, et al. Inhibition of poly(ADP-ribose) polymerase in tumors from BRCA mutation carriers. *N Engl J Med.* 2009;361(2):123-134.

65. Press JZ, De Luca A, Boyd N, et al. Ovarian carcinomas with genetic and epigenetic BRCA1 loss have distinct molecular abnormalities. *BMC Cancer.* 2008;8:17.

Integrative Oncology, Quality of Life, and Supportive Care

Diljeet K. Singh and Vivian E. von Gruenigen

The World Health Organization (WHO) defines health broadly as "a state of complete physical, mental and social well-being and not merely the absence of disease or infirmity."[1] This far-reaching definition reminds us of the powerful influence we can have as practitioners not only on the number of days our patients live but also on the quality and depth of their lives. For many patients, a cancer diagnosis provides an opportunity to examine their mortality and their lives. For some, this may enable them to make considerable health-supporting changes in their lifestyle including discontinuing tobacco use, improving their diet, and adding physical activity and stress management techniques to their health regimens. Others may find themselves exploring their spiritual beliefs and examining other aspects of their life. As health care providers, we can support our patients in their efforts to achieve their optimal health throughout the life cycle.

An understanding of integrative oncology, quality of life (QOL), supportive and palliative care, symptom management, and end-of-life (EOL) care can inform our ability to address our patients' global health needs (Figure 22-1).

INTEGRATIVE ONCOLOGY

Definitions

The National Center for Complementary and Alternative Medicine (NCCAM) at the National Institutes of Health defines complementary, alternative, and integrative medicine (CAM) as follows: Complementary medicine refers to use of CAM together with conventional medicine. Alternative medicine refers to use of CAM in place of conventional medicine. Integrative medicine refers to a practice that combines both conventional and CAM treatments for which there is evidence of safety and effectiveness. Practitioners describe integrative oncology as both a science and a philosophy that focuses on the complexity of the well-being of cancer patients and proposes a multitude of approaches to accompany conventional therapies to facilitate health.[2] In addition, integrative oncologists strive to support the innate healing abilities of the individual, using techniques for self-empowerment, individual responsibility, and lifestyle changes that could potentially reduce both cancer recurrence and second primary tumors. Integrative medicine includes biologically based practices (eg, diet, dietary supplements, herbs), mind-body medicine (eg, guided imagery, hypnosis, meditation, stress management), manipulative or body-based practices (eg, massage therapy, chiropractic, reflexology), energy medicine (eg, acupuncture, qigong, Reiki, yoga), and whole system approaches (eg, Ayurveda, traditional Chinese medicine [TCM], homeopathy) (Table 22-1).

For a number of reasons, ongoing tension exists between some aspects of integrative medicine and conventional medicine. Although the impact of diet, exercise, and stress management techniques on health is relatively well accepted, limited research and differing philosophical underpinnings have fostered distrust and knowledge gaps among conventional providers, which contribute to reluctance on the part of patients to discuss their usage with their providers. Data from well-conducted trials on the risks and benefits of complementary modalities

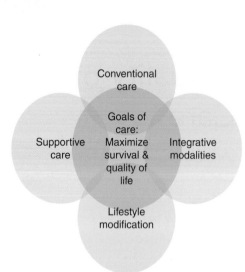

FIGURE 22-1. Holistic care for the gynecologic oncology patient.

are limited for several reasons. First, the NCCAM was only relatively recently established in 1999 as a consistent source of guidance and funding for research and training. Researchers have also identified lack of quality and substantial variability of dietary supplements as significant challenges to conducting research. The US Food and Drug Administration regulates dietary supplements as foods, not drugs, and thus does not analyze the content of dietary supplements. Whereas synthetic, single-entity drugs are relatively easy to characterize, the complexities of herbal preparations and our incomplete knowledge regarding the active components hinder research efforts. Traditional evidence-based medical research focuses on 1 variable and its impact on 1 outcome. By definition, integrative approaches imply a whole system with multiple component parts that work together toward the maximum

Table 22-1 Integrative Modalities

Biologically based practices
Diet, dietary supplements, herbs
Mind-body medicine
Guided imagery, hypnosis, meditation, stress management, biofeedback, social support
Manipulative or body-based practices
Massage therapy, chiropractic, reflexology
Energy medicine
Acupuncture, qigong, Reiki, yoga, healing touch
Whole system approaches
Ayurveda, traditional Chinese medicine, homeopathy

benefit of the patient. Thus, the best-suited research programs would evaluate a whole systems approach to patients. Studies and their analysis might include psychological interventions, physical exercises, nutritional variations, and combinations of botanicals. For example, in a series of work with prostate cancer patients, Ornish et al[3] used a mixed-interventions approach described as comprehensive lifestyle changes including nutritional changes, physical activity, and meditation and found decreases in prostate-specific antigen and cell and serum level changes thought to inhibit cancer progression.

Usage

The widespread use of CAM represents a challenge and an opportunity to our field; we must balance safety with our commitment to allow our patients to avail themselves of all potentially beneficial modalities. In 2008, the National Center for Health Statistics indicated that 38% of all Americans use some form of CAM.[4] A 2005 Institute of Medicine report detailed this trend and reported that Americans were spending at least $27 billion out of pocket for CAM products and services.[5] Use of CAM is particularly common among people with cancer. Studies indicate that up to 80% of all cancer patients use some form of CAM most commonly including acupuncture, massage, yoga, energy healing, TCM, Ayurveda, mind-body interventions, and a wide variety of vitamins, mineral supplements, antioxidants, and herbs.[6] Studies reveal that 40% to 70% of patients do not report CAM use to their physicians for a wide variety of reasons and that most patients are willing to discuss CAM use with their physicians, but they are concerned that their physician will not understand, approve of, or have interest in these modalities. Furthermore, although increasing numbers of physicians express open attitudes toward CAM therapies, they may be hesitant to discuss this with patients because of their lack of knowledge and a desire not to appear uninformed. A survey of ovarian cancer patients revealed significant use of herbs and a perceived need among patients for guidance from their physicians.[7]

Several concerns regarding the use of herbs and antioxidants are relevant to providers of women with a gynecologic malignancy. Quality of herbal preparations has not been well governed, and contamination of preparations has been reported. However, reported cases of complications with herb use are quite rare, and with trained guidance, safe, effective products can be identified. Antiplatelet effects and prolongation of coagulation parameters can theoretically occur with ginkgo biloba, garlic, ginseng, fish oils, vitamin E, dong quai, and feverfew. Holding these herbs before surgery is reasonable; it is unclear whether their potential bleeding effects warrant prohibiting their use during chemotherapy. Neuroprotective effects of vitamin E may outweigh the theoretical risks (see Symptom Management section). Cardiovascular effects of ephedra include tachycardia, hypertension, and palpitations, and pharmacologic doses of garlic may cause hypotension. Hypoglycemia has been reported with ginseng. Pharmacodynamic herb–drug interactions include potentiating the sedative effect of anesthetics by kava and valerian, and these may be held perioperatively as well. St. John's wort induces cytochrome P450, leading to increased metabolism of many drugs including warfarin, irinotecan, cyclosporine, oral contraceptives, digitalis, midazolam, lidocaine, and calcium channel blockers. Echinacea, goldenseal, and licroice may inhibit cytochrome P450, thus increasing circulating concenetrations of these same medications. Herbs that induce or inhibit drug metabolism should be used with caution during chemotherapy, as should other drugs known to alter metabolism.

Substantial controversy exists regarding the safety of supplemental antioxidant administration during chemotherapy and radiation.[8] Some practitioners have raised the concern that antioxidants may decrease the efficacy of chemotherapy by interfering with its mechanism of action. Others site data that antioxidant supplements are useful in conjunction with chemotherapy because they enhance the efficacy of the chemotherapy and alleviate toxic side effects, allowing patients to tolerate chemotherapy for the full course of treatment and possibly at higher doses. From the 19 randomized controlled trials of antioxidant use during chemotherapy reviewed by Block et al, no evidence was found that supported concerns that antioxidant supplementation given with chemotherapy diminished the efficacy of the chemotherapy in study populations comprising mostly advanced or relapsed patients.[9] In contrast, 17 of the 19 trials included in this review showed a statistically significant advantage or nonsignificantly higher survival and/or treatment response in patients given antioxidants. General and neurologic toxicities were also improved by antioxidant supplementation.

IMPACT OF LIFESTYLE ON GYNECOLOGIC CANCER

Multiple aspects of lifestyle impact on cancer risk and prognosis, including stress, social support, physical activity, and nutrition. Researchers postulate that stress-induced immunosuppression or dysregulation may contribute to the development and progression of malignancy. For example, in ovarian cancer patients, depressed and anxious mood is associated with a greater impairment of the cellular immune response and an increase in tumor progression.[10] Stress can be a cofactor for the initiation and progression of cancer.

The catecholamine stress hormone norepinephrine may influence tumor progression by modulating the expression of factors implicated in angiogenesis and metastasis.[11] Strategies to address stress in cancer patients include relaxation training, meditation, graded exercise, yoga, tai chi, and other mind-body interventions that induce the relaxation response. Social isolation is associated with an increased risk of death from cancer; thus, support groups and social connection can benefit cancer patients.

Weight, diet, and exercise are interrelated and modifiable risk factors for many diseases including cancer. Risk factors for endometrial cancer include obesity and sedentary lifestyle. Half of all endometrial cancers in postmenopausal women are attributable to being overweight (body mass index [BMI] >25 kg/m^2) or obese (BMI >30 kg/m^2). In a study of 1.2 million women enrolled in the Million Women Study in the United Kingdom, risk of endometrial cancer in obese women was almost triple that of normal-weight women.[12] Data from more than 32,000 women participating in the Women's Health Study confirmed the relationship between BMI and risk of endometrial cancer.[13] Women reporting any vigorous activity had lower risk than those reporting none. A large, prospective cohort study of more than 250,000 women from 9 European countries found little association between physical activity and endometrial cancer risk, although a potential risk reduction in premenopausal women was identified.[14] Data from the National Institutes of Health–American Association of Retired Persons Diet and Health Study of more than 100,000 women found a dose-response relationship between vigorous activity and endometrial cancer risk but no association with light/moderate, daily, routine or occupational physical activities. The relationship between physical activity and endometrial cancer risk was also examined in the American Cancer Society Cancer Prevention Study II Nutrition Cohort of more than 40,000 postmenopausal women.[15] They found that light and moderate physical activity were associated with lower endometrial cancer risk, although BMI attenuated the association. Physical activity was strongly associated with reduced risk in overweight and obese women in this study. The extent to which differences in level of physical activity contribute to endometrial cancer risk is not clear. In contrast, the relationship with BMI is unambiguous. Regardless of the direct effect of physical activity on endometrial cancer risk, women should be encouraged to maintain appropriate levels of physical activity to help maintain body weight.

BMI may influence patient outcomes and survival. In an analysis of nearly 400 early-stage endometrial cancer patients from a randomized trial of surgery with or without adjuvant radiation therapy, mortality was increased in obese patients and in morbidly obese patients, compared with lighter-weight women.[16]

In an analysis of patients with advanced or recurrent endometrial cancer from 5 Gynecology Oncology Group (GOG) trials who had been treated with adjuvant chemotherapy, no overall significant associations between progression-free survival (PFS) and BMI were detected. However, increased BMI was significantly associated with an increased risk of death in women with stage III/IV endometrial cancer, but not in patients with recurrent disease. Although some endometrial cancer patients gain weight after diagnosis, the effect of this weight gain on recurrence or mortality is unknown.

A recent review and meta-analysis examined the relationship between consumption of a high glycemic index or glycemic load (GL) diet and endometrial and ovarian cancer.[17] The estimates for endometrial cancer showed an increased risk for high GL consumers, which was further elevated in obese women. Only 2 studies examined ovarian cancer, and results also indicate positive associations for GL.

Data evaluating obesity as a risk factor for epithelial ovarian cancer have been mixed. In a recent meta-analysis of 28 eligible studies, 24 studies reported a positive association between obesity and ovarian cancer, and in 10 studies, this reached statistical significance.[18] In the European Prospective Investigation Into Cancer and Nutrition cohort of more than 200,000 women, the associations of measured anthropometric factors, including general and central adiposity and height, with ovarian cancer risk were evaluated with attention to menopausal status and specific histologic subtypes. There were approximately 600 incident cases of primary, malignant, epithelial ovarian cancer diagnosed during a mean follow-up of 9 years. Compared to normal-weight women, obesity was associated with an excess ovarian cancer risk for all women combined and for postmenopausal women, although the association was weaker for premenopausal women.[19] Other studies have analyzed the relationship between obesity and ovarian cancer in regard to the duration of obesity. A study of Danish women diagnosed with ovarian cancer found that women who had been overweight during the previous 5 years had an increased risk of death compared with normal-weight women. A prospective study in China of women diagnosed with ovarian cancer also found that increased BMI 5 years prior to diagnosis was associated with reduced survival. A retrospective US study of advanced-stage ovarian cancer patients noted that obesity (BMI >25 kg/m²) was independently associated with shorter disease-free survival and overall survival (OS).[20] These studies suggest that overweight/obesity is associated with reduced survival from ovarian cancer; however, the role of physical activity and benefits of modifying weight after diagnosis are not addressed in these studies.

If weight is a poor prognostic indicator, it may be postulated that these patients perhaps are receiving subtherapeutic treatment. Inconsistencies in dosing chemotherapy for obese patients have included use of body surface area, dosing at ideal body weight, dose capping, and differing measurements of renal function, all of which can underestimate dose and consequently negatively influence survival. However, in the Scottish Randomized Trial in Ovarian Cancer I study, in which more than 1000 patients received front-line chemotherapy, BMI was not associated with PFS, OS, or completeness of debulking surgery.[21] In a separate study of nearly 800 advanced ovarian cancer patients, no association between prechemotherapy BMI and survival was observed. Weight gain was associated with improved survival; however, 50% of the patients had a BMI of <25 kg/m², which would include women who were underweight and likely to benefit from weight gain.

Diet and Cancer Prevention

Studies of diet, nutrition, and cancer risk are restricted by retrospective collection of data, difficulty in correlating specific nutrients in food diaries, and the limitations of epidemiologic studies. In addition, advocates of integrative health approaches have objected to the reductionism of studying specific nutrients (vitamin A and β-carotene) instead of whole foods (yellow and orange fruits and vegetables), where the interactions of food components may be important. A holistic option is to study regional diets such as the Mediterranean diet.

Mediterranean Diet

The concept of the Mediterranean diet as a healthy diet was developed in the 1950s and referred to dietary patterns found in olive-growing areas of the Mediterranean region (Table 22-2). Although countries around the Mediterranean basin have different diets, religions, and cultures, common dietary characteristics have been identified and studied. The following scale was developed to determine adherence: (1) high monounsaturated-to-saturated lipid ratio, (2) high consumption of fruits, (3) high consumption of vegetables,

Table 22-2 Components of Mediterranean Diet

Omega-3–containing fats (olive oil, fish, nuts)
Protein predominantly from plant and fish sources
High consumption of fruits and vegetables
Low consumption of meat
Low to moderate consumption of dairy
Moderate consumption of red wine with meals

(4) high consumption of legumes, (5) high consumption of cereals, (6) moderate to high consumption of fish, (7) low consumption of meat and meat products, (8) low to moderate consumption of milk and dairy products, and (9) moderate consumption of ethanol, mostly in the form of wine at meals. Many epidemiologic studies have demonstrated reduced risks of overall mortality, cardiovascular diseases, and several common neoplasms in adherents of the Mediterranean diet. A recent meta-analysis showed that increased adherence to the Mediterranean diet was associated with a significant reduction of overall mortality, cardiovascular incidence or mortality, cancer incidence or mortality, and neurodegenerative diseases.[22] Mechanistically, researchers have proposed that the health benefits of this diet are based on bioactive compounds and their interactions, specifically monounsaturated-to-saturated fatty acid ratio, dietary fiber, antioxidant capacity of the whole diet, and phytosterol intake.

La Vecchia examined the relationship between the gynecologic cancers and specific components of the Mediterranean diet.[23] He found a significant decreased risk for endometrial and ovarian cancer when comparing lowest vegetable intake to highest. The risk for ovarian cancer was statistically decreased for women with an increase of 1 g/wk of omega-3 fatty acids (found in fish and olive oil). Highest consumption level of whole grain foods was associated with decreased risk of endometrial and ovarian cancer. Previous work by this group also showed an increase in risk of both endometrial and ovarian cancer associated with ≥7 servings of red meat compared with consumption of ≤3 servings per week.

Individual Dietary Components

Additional work has evaluated the relationship between specific dietary components and gynecologic malignancies. A review of the literature on variation in meat and fish intake found that low consumption of processed meat and higher consumption of poultry and fish may reduce the risk of ovarian cancer.[24] In contrast, high fish intake was associated with a reduced risk of ovarian cancer, and a frequent intake of poultry was associated with borderline significant reductions in risk of ovarian cancer. A systematic review of the role of diet on the risk of human papillomavirus (HPV) persistence and cervical neoplasia was conducted and included 23 observational studies and 10 randomized clinical trials.[25] The studies on HPV persistence showed a possible protective effect of fruits, vegetables, vitamins C and E, β- and α-carotene, lycopene, lutein/zeaxanthin, and cryptoxanthin.

An association between decreased vitamin D levels and increased rates of cancer has been described. Researchers have postulated that the known north-south gradient in age-adjusted mortality rates of ovarian cancer in the United States are attributable to lower solar irradiance and thus lower serum vitamin D levels. In support of this, laboratory findings have suggested that low levels of vitamin D metabolites could play a role in the etiology of ovarian cancer. The association of solar ultraviolet B irradiance, stratospheric column ozone, and fertility rates at age 15 to 19 years with incidence rates of ovarian cancer in 175 countries was examined. Age-adjusted ovarian cancer incidence rates were highest in countries located at higher latitudes. A review of the literature found that approximately half of the ecologic and case-control studies reported reductions in incidence or mortality of ovarian cancer with increasing geographic latitude, solar radiation levels, or dietary/supplement consumption of vitamin D, whereas the other half reported null associations with ovarian cancer risk.[26] In addition, no overall risk reduction was seen with increasing dietary/supplement consumption of vitamin D or with plasma levels of vitamin D prior to diagnosis; however, vitamin D intakes were relatively low in all studies. A serum study was performed to clarify the mixed data from ecologic studies. A case-control study of more than 7000 subjects from the National Health and Nutrition Examination Surveys demonstrated that ovarian cancer patients were 3 times more likely to have low serum vitamin D. These authors concluded that deficiency in vitamin D provides an etiologic link between the long-known ecologic findings regarding latitude.[27]

Botanicals

Several botanicals are being investigated as agents to inhibit cancer development; they include green tea, curcumin, *Astragalus*, and resveratrol. A systematic review of publications on green tea research concludes that green tea may have beneficial effects on cancer prevention and that further studies, such as large and long-term cohort studies and clinical trials, are warranted. Curcumin, a component of turmeric or curry powder, has been shown to downregulate several pathways of cancer initiation and promotion. Oral curcumin is well tolerated and has biological activity in some patients with pancreatic cancer. The dried root of *Astragalus membranaceus* (huang qi), a traditional Chinese herbal medicine, demonstrated improvements in survival, tumor response, and performance status in a meta-analysis of randomized trials of almost 3000 lung cancer patients on platinum-based chemotherapy.[28] Resveratrol is a polyphenol found in numerous plant species, including grapes, that has been shown to possess chemopreventive properties against several cancers through inducing apoptosis. Additional studies of these agents in gynecologic cancer are warranted.

Researchers analyzed the association between intake of 5 common dietary flavonoids and the incidence of epithelial ovarian cancer in more than 60,000 women in the Nurses' Health Study.[29] Although no clear association was found between total intake of the 5 flavonoids and ovarian cancer, there was a significant 40% decrease in ovarian cancer incidence for the highest versus lowest quintile of kaempferol intake and a significant 34% decrease in incidence for the highest versus lowest quintile of luteolin intake. An inverse association with consumption of nonherbal tea and broccoli, the primary contributors to kaempferol intake in our population, further supported this association. A study of epithelial ovarian cancer patients in China showed that habitual green tea intake was protective, and the benefit was dose- and duration-dependent. A recent prospective cohort study in more than 60,000 Swedish women followed for more than 15 years provided evidence that green tea intake reduced the risk for the development of epithelial ovarian cancer in a dose-dependent manner. A case-control study of diet and ovarian cancer in western New York involving ovarian cancer cases and controls found that compared with women in the lowest quintile of intake, reduced risks were observed for women in the highest quintile of intake of dietary fiber (57% decrease), carotenoids (67% decrease), stigmasterol (58% decrease), total lignans (57% decrease), vegetables (53% decrease), and poultry (55% decrease).

Epidemiology studies have reported associations between increased soy intake and decreased risk of endocrine-related gynecologic cancers. Myung et al[30] performed a meta-analysis examining the relationship between soy food intake and the risk of endometrial cancer and ovarian cancer. Compared with the lowest soy intake, the highest soy intake group had a 39% decrease in risk of all endocrine-related cancers, a 30% decrease in the risk of endometrial cancer, and a 48% decrease in risk of ovarian cancer. A case-control study of 500 women with endometrial cancer evaluated the associations between dietary intake of 7 specific compounds representing 3 classes of phytoestrogens (isoflavones, coumestans, and lignans) and risk. When comparing highest to lowest intake groups, isoflavone intake was associated with a 41% decrease in risk. In postmenopausal women, protection from isoflavones was even stronger, and a 43% reduction in endometrial cancer risk was also seen for lignan intake. Obese postmenopausal women consuming relatively low amounts of phytoestrogens had a 7-fold increase in the risk of endometrial cancer.

Diet and Cancer Prognosis

There is a paucity of research regarding nutrition and prognosis in ovarian cancer patients. In a longitudinal study of more than 300 women with ovarian cancer, longer survival was associated with total fruits and vegetables and vegetables separately. Subgroup analyses showed only yellow and cruciferous vegetables to significantly favor survival. In a population-based cohort of more than 600 women with epithelial ovarian cancer followed for up to 5 years, death was reduced in women who reported higher intake of vegetables and cruciferous vegetables. Inverse associations were seen between protein, red meat, and white meat and survival. There are no published studies of diet and endometrial cancer survival.

Regarding the relationship between individual dietary components and cancer prognosis, research has been done on vitamin D, green tea, and selenium. Studies in Norway and England found that individuals diagnosed with any cancer in summer or fall, when serum 25-hydroxyvitamin D levels are highest, had a milder clinical course and longer survival than those diagnosed in winter or spring. However, there are no vitamin D studies focused on gynecologic cancer survival after diagnosis. A small cohort study following more than 200 women with epithelial ovarian cancer demonstrated that habitual green tea consumption caused a significant dose-dependent increase in survival rate. Researchers evaluated the impact of randomized selenium supplementation in more than 30 patients with ovarian cancer undergoing chemotherapy. At 3 months, patients had significant increases in their white blood cells. After 2 to 3 months of selenium, significant decreases in hair loss, abdominal pain, weakness, and loss of appetite were noted among selenium-supplemented patients. Thus, promising data demonstrate the need for additional research to evaluate the potential for dietary modification and supplementation to improve survival and side effects in women with gynecologic malignancies.

Lifestyle and Quality of Life

Lifestyle decisions regarding nutrition, physical activity, tobacco use, and stress management not only affect cancer prevention and prognosis, but may also enhance QOL and improve patient outcomes. Physical activity may improve QOL, morbidity, and mortality in ovarian cancer patients.[31] A study examining ovarian cancer survivors who were on and off active treatment found that those meeting public health guidelines for physical activity had lower self-reported levels of fatigue and better scores for peripheral neuropathy, depression, anxiety, and sleep quality than women not meeting guidelines. An additional study of women undergoing gynecologic surgery found that baseline characteristics such as physical and mental health, age, and body weight affect QOL scores. Therefore, regular physical activity may enhance survival by increasing

QOL and improving ability to tolerate surgery and chemotherapy.

A recent study enrolled newly diagnosed ovarian cancer patients receiving adjuvant intraperitoneal (IP) or intravenous (IV) chemotherapy to a QOL lifestyle intervention trial.[32] Patients were counseled in physical activity and nutrition quality. Assessments were obtained at entry to the study, during therapy (cycle 3), and after chemotherapy. Walking is the preferred mode of exercise for ovarian cancer patients. The median number of steps during the week of chemotherapy administration was less than 5000; 1 week after chemotherapy, steps increased to nearly 6000; and 2 weeks after chemotherapy, steps increased by nearly 5300. Steps were lowest after the first cycle of chemotherapy. QOL and emotional and functional well-being scores increased linearly during each cycle of chemotherapy. Therefore, it is feasible for ovarian cancer patients on adjuvant chemotherapy to increase physical activity that may improve QOL.

Lack of exercise and obesity are associated with lower QOL in endometrial cancer survivors. A survey of nearly 400 endometrial cancer survivors found that lack of exercise and excess body weight were associated with lower QOL. Approximately 70% of the women surveyed were obese and were not meeting public health exercise guidelines. Analyses showed that both exercise and BMI were independently associated with QOL. Another survey of 120 endometrial cancer survivors demonstrated that pain and fatigue decreased while physical functioning increased with physical activity. von Gruenigen et al[33] conducted a prospective observational trial in newly diagnosed endometrial patients preoperatively and 6 months postoperatively. Again, there was a correlation between weight and QOL. Weight, exercise, and fruit and vegetable intake did not change over time; however, CAM use increased significantly at 6 months. Although small, this study highlighted an important observation that may apply to endometrial cancer patients: Without intervention, survivors of endometrial cancer who are sedentary and/or obese are unlikely to spontaneously modify their exercise and nutrition behaviors after diagnosis and treatment.

It is important to implement lifestyle interventions to improve survivorship of endometrial cancer patients who are at increased risk for poor QOL and premature death secondary to obesity-driven comorbidities. A randomized controlled study of an interventional lifestyle program in 45 endometrial cancer survivors demonstrated that patients can lose weight and improve their exercise after the intervention.[31] At 12 months, the intervention group lost 3.5 kg, compared to a 1.4-kg gain in the control group, and significantly increased physical activity. Therefore, a lifestyle intervention program in obese endometrial cancer patients is feasible and can result in sustained behavior change and weight loss over a 1-year period. This same research group is presently enrolling more than 100 endometrial cancer survivors to an intervention trial that includes both aerobic exercise and strength training.

QUALITY OF LIFE

QOL is a multidimensional concept that continues to be defined over time. QOL has been defined as an individual's physical, functional, emotional, and social well-being and how it is impacted by a medical condition and its treatment. QOL measures are reported directly by patients and hence are termed "patient-reported outcomes." They are not subject to interpretation by either health care providers or research professionals. QOL measurements can provide information about the impact of the disease and its treatment in cancer patients to aid physicians in selecting both antineoplastic and supportive care therapy. A recent meta-analysis of 30 randomized controlled trials from the European Organization for Research and Treatment of Cancer that included survival data for more than 10,000 patients with 11 different cancer sites found that QOL could help to predict survival in patients with cancer.[34]

There is a paucity of data regarding QOL in early-stage ovarian cancer patients because it is not as common as advanced-stage disease. Traditionally, treatment of ovarian cancer involves removal of both ovaries and the uterus, which puts younger women into menopause and ends their chance of bearing a child. Although women with early-stage ovarian cancer often have an excellent prognosis (5-year survival >90%), the loss of reproductive potential and lingering psychological survivorship sequelae may result in serious disruptions in QOL. A recent study by Wright et al[35] demonstrated that 5-year survival rates for stage I ovarian cancer patients were the same for women who had both ovaries removed and women who had just the cancerous ovary removed, suggesting that ovarian conservation may be considered in select patients.[33] This more conservative approach may result in improvements in QOL for women with early-stage disease. Matulonis et al[36] studied the QOL of early-stage ovarian cancer patients and observed that even though patients reported good physical QOL scores, one-third of the patients received treatment for family or personal problems, and nearly 60% reported anxiety associated with testing of CA-125.[34] Therefore, women with early ovarian cancer clearly benefit from support and interventions for their QOL needs.

Treatment advances for ovarian cancer patients have led to improvements in survival, allowing a broadening of care goals to include maximizing QOL. A single-institution study, in which the majority of ovarian cancer patients had advanced-stage disease, revealed that surgery significantly impacts QOL. QOL markedly decreased after surgery, with a slow improvement during adjuvant chemotherapy, specifically in the physical, functional, and fatigue domains.

Over the past 10 years, several international and GOG randomized trials have included QOL end points for evaluation. The National Cancer Institute of Canada OV10 randomized trial of nearly 700 patients identified that baseline performance status and global QOL were independent predictors of PFS and OS.[37] Two large-scale GOG studies (152 and 172) included QOL assessments at several time points in ovarian cancer patients with advanced disease. Wenzel et al compared QOL in patients enrolled in a randomized trial of interval secondary cytoreduction in advanced ovarian carcinoma (GOG 152). The baseline QOL score was positively associated with OS. GOG 172 randomized optimal stage III epithelial ovarian cancer patients to IV paclitaxel plus IP cisplatin and paclitaxel versus IV cisplatin and paclitaxel and found an improved OS in the IP arm.[38] Physical and functional well-being and ovarian cancer symptoms were significantly worse in the IP arm during and after treatment. In addition, during treatment, patients on the IP arm experienced more QOL disruption, abdominal discomfort, and neurotoxicity. However, 12 months after treatment, only neurotoxicity remained significantly greater for IP patients. In an ancillary analysis of GOG 152 and GOG 172, patients with lower QOL scores had declines in physical, functional, and emotional well-being. In the physical domain, significant differences were observed in physical symptoms (nausea, pain, feeling ill, and being bothered by the side effects of treatment), as well as more general effects (lack of energy, meeting needs of family, and forced to spend time in bed). These patients were least likely to sleep well. Regarding emotional well-being, there were significant differences in feeling nervous and worrying about dying.

Limited studies have been performed specifically assessing QOL in women with endometrial cancer. Limitations of prior research have included heterogeneous gynecologic populations and different adjuvant therapies, and the studies have not been well controlled. A recent, large study compared QOL among 5- to 10-year survivors of stage I to II endometrial cancer treated with surgery alone or surgery with external beam adjuvant therapy.[39] Comorbidity appeared to be the only variable that was negatively associated with all QOL subscales. On multivariate analyses, adjuvant radiation was negatively associated with vitality and physical and social well-being scale scores. Unfortunately, BMI was not a controlled variable. In addition,

the current adjuvant treatment for endometrial cancer patients at intermediate risk for recurrence is vaginal radiation not pelvic radiation. In addition, no studies have assessed obesity as the key variable of QOL in endometrial cancer.

QOL is compromised in endometrial cancer survivors, but not for the same reasons as in ovarian cancer patients. A recent ancillary analysis of 2 prospective endometrial cancer QOL trials revealed that scores were similar to normative data in age-matched women without cancer. BMI was inversely correlated with functional, physical, and social well-being and with several decreases in line items within the functional domain, including ability at work and being content. BMI also had an inverse relationship with the "lack of energy" item in the physical domain. Fatigue was present in nearly 30% of survivors, which increased as weight increased.

SUPPORTIVE CARE

Supportive care recognizes that life-threatening illness, whether it can be cured or controlled, carries with it significant burdens of suffering for patients and their families and that this suffering can be effectively addressed by modern palliative care (Table 22-3). Palliative care focuses on management of symptoms, psychosocial support, and assistance with decision making and has the potential to improve quality of care and reduce the use of futile medical services. However, palliative care has traditionally been delivered late in the course of disease. In a recent study of more than 100 patients with metastatic non–small-cell lung cancer, early palliative care led to significant improvements in survival, QOL, and mood.[40] As compared with patients receiving standard care, patients receiving early palliative care had less aggressive care at the EOL but longer survival. Researchers conducting a survey at a cancer center found that providers perceived the term "palliative care" as distressing and reducing hope to patients and families. These health

Table 22-3 Goals of Supportive Care Model

Improve quantity of life
Improve quality of life
Minimize disease-specific and treatment-related symptoms
Facilitate open, ongoing conversation with the patient and family regarding shifting treatment focus as appropriate
Utilize consultation and other expertise as needed to meet the above goals

care professionals significantly preferred the term "supportive care" over "palliative care" and were more likely to refer patients on active primary and advanced cancer treatments. This renaming has been embraced by other practitioners who also hope it reinforces the concept of an integrated-care model in which receipt of cancer therapies and symptom management are addressed concurrently.

Palliative Care

The term "palliative care" refers to those aspects of medical care concerned with the physical and psychosocial issues faced by a patient with cancer and his or her family. The WHO defines palliative care as an approach that supports and improves the QOL of patients and their families facing the problems associated with a life-threatening illness, such as cancer, through the prevention and treatment of distressing symptoms and attention to psychological and spiritual aspects of patient care. Although all patients with gynecologic cancer may benefit from attention to the physical and psychosocial consequences of a cancer diagnosis, for those with advanced or recurrent disease, this care is imperative. This type of care may be provided while patients are on medical therapy and/or when patients transition off treatment. Palliative care embraces the medical ethics of patient choice and the value of well-being.

Ethical Obligations

Physicians and health care providers have ethical obligations to all patients, and those on palliative care for cancer are no different. However, the provider may be more reflective of their obligations during this stage of a patient's disease. The ethical principles of autonomy, beneficence, and nonmaleficence have long been accepted as providing a framework for study of moral problems in medicine. Autonomy directs us to respect the choices, values, and life plans of patients and generates the requirements for informed consent. Beneficence forms the fundamental duty to promote patients' well-being. Nonmaleficence, the duty to refrain from harm, reflected in the Hippocratic Oath, is thought to be the most inflexible of medical ethical principles. Each of these will have different implications for palliative care depending on the sense of the term. Most hospitals have ethical committees that can help the physician or health care provider if there is an ethical dilemma in a patient's care.

Assessment

There are many options in the clinical delivery of palliative care. The most traditional and frequently used is the medical model of the physician assessing the patient in his/her office and addressing the patient's needs or directing the patient to other health care providers who can prescribe specific care. Multidisciplinary care has been criticized in the past because of poor communication, cost, and fragmentation of care. However, with the development of electronic medical records, the communication flaw may be rectified. Another medical model is interdisciplinary care, which involves a team of health care professionals including, as needed, the primary physician, a palliative care physician, nurse(s), social worker, physical and occupational therapist, dietician, speech pathologist, pastoral care, pharmacy professionals, bereavement providers, and volunteers. Depending on the hospital, institution, or health system, this model will vary along with collaborators, but among all, the goal is to embrace collaboration and open communications. In addition, as the trajectory of a patient's disease changes, the patient's needs and collaborative providers may change. Specific components of a patient's evaluation will include history of illness, treatment responses, obtaining an understanding of the patient's decision-making capacity (especially in the elderly), and physical, psychological, social, and spiritual assessments. This type of robust assessment takes time and may require multiple providers.

Discussion of Prognosis

Communication and understanding between the physician, patient, and family are pivotal to supportive cancer care. Physicians inform their patients well regarding cancer treatment; however, they differ in their ability to discuss prognosis and alternatives to anticancer treatments. The majority of cancer patients report a preference for detailed information about their disease, although some prefer to negotiate the extent and timing of the information they receive from oncologists.

Few physicians have received training in the communication skills necessary to discuss palliative care and EOL. It is imperative that physicians start by choosing the appropriate setting to hold these conversations. Physicians do not need to hold these conversations alone; often it is supportive to both patient and physician to have the patient's family, primary chemotherapy nurse, or social worker in the room. Others can be helpful in reframing or restating terminology for the patient and her family. Physicians need to be aware of the time commitment of such discussions and schedule sufficient time in the office or on hospital rounds. Options for beginning the conversation include starting with a warning phrase, such as "I'm afraid I have bad news." More than 1 session may be needed, and it can be an ongoing conversation from clinic visit to clinic visit. Physicians should discuss options of care with patients in an honest, sensitive, and straightforward way. They should also be willing to talk about dying and to use the words "death" and "dying." During the conversation, providers should confirm that patients understand the information being conveyed. As disease progresses, the frame of reference of hope will change. For example, the hope of prolongation of life will change to the hope of a good QOL at the EOL, minimization of symptoms, and opportunity to accomplish whatever activities or goals are important to the patient. If these discussions are not held, patients may seek others who offer false hope with ineffective and potentially harmful therapies.

Decision Making: Role of the Patient, Family, and Physician

Studies of decisions about treatment during palliative care and at the EOL have suggested that there are numerous personal characteristics of physicians, patients, and their families that influence decisions independently of actual prognosis. These include age, sex, education, religion, and personality characteristics. At times, patients and their families report a willingness to continue to seek aggressive therapies even in the face of progressive disease. Although this persistence may reflect the positive effects of maintaining hope, there is also some evidence that treatments thought to be life extending are more likely to be chosen over comfort-oriented treatment plans when patients and even physicians overestimate survival time.

Evaluation of Outcomes

The literature is sparse when assessing outcomes in women receiving palliative care for gynecologic cancer. It is unclear at what point in the course of disease a patient accesses palliative care; however, from the literature, we can deduce that it is quite variable. In addition, most of the research in ovarian cancer patients is directed toward the EOL. A retrospective multi-institutional study of more than 100 patients revealed that ovarian cancer patients have increased hospitalizations and palliative clinical events as they approach the EOL.[41] Significant clinical events in the study were defined as ascites, bowel obstruction, and pleural effusion. Many of these patients were treated for palliative intent with paracentesis, thoracentesis, and medical/surgical management of bowel obstructions. In this study, patients who received aggressive care did not have improvement in survival. The authors concluded that short chemotherapeutic remissions and increasing hospitalizations with significant clinical events are indicators to reduce cure-oriented therapies and increase palliative and supportive topics.

Symptom Management

Throughout the disease course, aggressive symptom management can improve patients' QOL and their ability to tolerate and continue to receive treatment.

Pain Management

Pain is a common symptom in cancer patients that can affect both QOL and other symptoms, but it is not always well addressed. The WHO advocates following a "3-step management ladder." In the setting of pain, there should be prompt oral administration of drugs in the following order: (1) nonopioids (aspirin and acetaminophen); then (2), as necessary, mild opioids (codeine); then (3) strong opioids such as morphine, until the patient is free of pain. To maintain freedom from pain, drugs should be given on a schedule such as every 2 to 6 hours rather than when requested or "on demand." Adjuvant analgesics are also commonly used and are defined as medications with a primary indication other than pain that have analgesic properties in some painful conditions. The group includes numerous drugs in diverse classes. Some adjuvant analgesics are useful in several painful conditions and are described as multipurpose adjuvant analgesics (eg, antidepressants, corticosteroids, α_2-adrenergic agonists, neuroleptics), whereas others are specific for neuropathic pain (eg, anticonvulsants, local anesthetics, N-methyl-D-aspartate receptor antagonists), bone pain (eg, calcitonin, bisphosphonates, radiopharmaceuticals), musculoskeletal pain (eg, muscle relaxants), or pain from bowel obstruction (eg, octreotide, anticholinergics). In a multisite, randomized clinical trial, nearly 400 patients with advanced cancer who were experiencing moderate to severe pain received 6 30-minute massage or simple-touch sessions over 2 weeks.[42] Although both groups demonstrated immediate improvement in pain and mood, massage led to larger improvements in both.

Nausea and Vomiting

Nausea and vomiting in the gynecologic oncology patient may be disease- or treatment-related. Nausea arising from stimuli in the gastrointestinal tract associated with slowing of the gut should respond to gastrokinetic antiemetics, such as metoclopramide, that promote gastric emptying and increase gut motility. However, bowel obstruction must be considered in patients with intra-abdominal disease; in these patients, stimulating agents may worsen symptoms.

Chemotherapy-induced nausea and vomiting (CINV) occurs based on the intrinsic emetogenicity of a given chemotherapeutic agent and the age and sex of the patient and may occur in 70% to 80% of patients

Table 22-4 Chemotherapy-Induced Nausea and Vomiting (CINV)

Types of CINV
Acute, delayed, anticipatory, breakthrough
First-line therapy
5-Hydroxytryptophan, serotonin receptor antagonists, corticosteroids, aprepitant, a neurokinin-1 receptor antagonist
Second-line or adjuvant options
Prokinetic agents (metoclopramide and ginger), phenothiazines, butyrophenones, cannabinoids, benzodiazepines, acupuncture, vitamin B_6

receiving chemotherapy (Table 22-4).[43] A number of chemotherapy regimens for gynecologic oncology patients include medications with high (cisplatin) and moderate (carboplatin, cyclophosphamide, doxorubicin, ifosfamide) risk of emesis. CINV can be divided into 4 subcategories: acute, delayed, anticipatory, and breakthrough CINV. The National Comprehensive Cancer Network (NCCN) defines acute nausea as that occurring shortly after chemotherapy administration but resolving within 24 hours. Delayed nausea occurs after 24 hours, peaks between 48 and 72 hours, and resolves by the day 6 or 7. Anticipatory nausea is described as a learned or conditioned response prior to chemotherapy. Finally, breakthrough CINV can occur when a patient experiences symptoms despite appropriate treatment.

First-line therapy of CINV consists of agents with high therapeutic index that are chosen based on a regimen's emetogenic potential and incidence of delayed emesis and includes 3 main classes of drugs: 5-hydroxytryptophan ($5-HT_3$) serotonin receptor antagonists, corticosteroids, and aprepitant, a neurokinin-1 receptor antagonist. For breakthrough CINV, agents with a lower therapeutic index (eg, metoclopramide, phenothiazines, butyrophenones, cannabinoids) may be considered when first-line therapeutics fail. Ideally, anticipatory CINV is prevented by avoiding or minimizing acute and delayed emesis. When anticipatory CINV does occur, benzodiazepines and behavioral therapy are suggested. A recent Cochrane review of the literature supports the efficacy of acupuncture point stimulation for acute CINV as well as for postoperative nausea.[44] In a randomized study of ovarian cancer patients, all of whom were receiving a standard antiemetic regimen, the combination of vitamin B_6 and acupuncture led to significantly fewer emesis episodes and a greater proportion of emesis-free days when compared with acupuncture or vitamin B_6 alone. In a randomized, double-blinded crossover study

in nearly 50 gynecologic cancer patients receiving cisplatin-based chemotherapy, ginger in capsule form was found to be equivalent to metoclopramide for delayed nausea.

Gastrointestinal Symptoms

Gastrointestinal (GI) symptoms that physicians will encounter include nausea and vomiting (discussed in the previous section), constipation, GI hypomotility progressing to bowel obstruction, oral and intestinal mucositis, and ascites. GI symptoms are common in patients with ovarian cancer even in early stages prior to diagnosis.

GI Hypomotility

Constipation in the gynecologic oncology patient may be disease related or may be an adverse effect of medications including narcotics or selective $5-HT_3$ antagonists. Perioperative and medication-related constipation can be avoided though anticipation, hydration, and the use of laxatives. Stool softeners, peristaltic agents, and osmotic laxatives may be used. Bulking agents may not be appropriate in patients who are not able to hydrate, have radiation-related dysfunction, or have extensive intra-abdominal disease. Women with extensive intra-abdominal disease with involvement of the mesenteric plexus may present with GI hypomotility, and treatment is aimed at increasing bowel peristalsis with medications such as metoclopramide and avoidance of constipation and impaction with hydration and appropriate laxatives.

Bowel Obstruction

Bowel obstruction in gynecologic malignancy is a complex issue in the setting of recurrent disease, and given the heterogeneity of patients and their clinical courses, literature to date offers limited guidance.[45] Many ovarian cancer patients will experience a bowel obstruction and, with their physicians, will have to make decisions regarding therapeutic options (surgical, medical, or supportive). Management decisions should be based on the patient's prognosis, performance status, and current goals of care. For patients focusing on managing discomfort, a combination of methods can be used, including pain management, antiemetics, corticosteroids, percutaneous gastrostomy placed endoscopically or by interventional radiology, and medications for decreasing intestinal secretions. Octreotide for this purpose has been shown to control emesis and to improve QOL and decrease hospitalization.

In 2010, Cochrane reviewers examined the literature and found only low-quality evidence comparing palliative surgery and medical management for bowel obstruction in ovarian cancer identifying only

1 study that met their inclusion criteria. They were unable to reach definite conclusions about the relative benefits and harms of the 2 forms of treatment or to identify subgroups of women who are likely to benefit from one treatment or the other.[45] In the only study that met the Cochrane reviewer's inclusion criteria, Mangili et al[46] analyzed retrospective data for 47 women who received either palliative surgery or medical management with octreotide and reported OS and perioperative mortality and morbidity. Although 6 surgical patients (22%) had serious complications of the operation and 3 patients (11%) died of complications, multivariable analysis found that women who received surgery had significantly better survival than women who received octreotide. However, the patients were not randomized, and women in the surgery group had significantly better performance status. Researchers recently reported on a small highly selected group of patients with ovarian cancer undergoing palliative endoscopic or operative procedures whose symptoms they followed prospectively. They noted symptomatic improvement or resolution within 30 days in 23 (88%) of 26 patients, with 1 (4%) postprocedure mortality. At 60 days, 10 (71%) of 14 patients who underwent operative procedures and 6 (50%) of 12 patients who had endoscopic procedures had symptom control. Median survival from the time of the palliative procedure was 191 days for those undergoing an operative procedure and 78 days for those undergoing an endoscopic procedure.

For large bowel obstruction, less invasive strategies like colonic stenting can help patients with recurrent malignant disease, although limited data on their use are available for gynecologic oncology patients. A recent study by Caceres et al[47] demonstrates the feasibility of this strategy in acutely ill gynecologic cancer patients who had successful stent placement.

Oral and Intestinal Mucositis

Oral and intestinal mucositis in the gynecologic oncology patient can be related to chemotherapy, radiation, or disease and can present with oral and esophageal ulceration, diarrhea, and tenesmus. Pathophysiology remains unclear, although recent work suggests that disturbances in bacterial microflora may contribute. Cochrane reviewers evaluated a wide range of preventive interventions for oral mucositis and found that compared with a placebo or no treatment, the following treatments showed benefit: amifostine, TCM, hydrolytic enzymes, and ice chips.[48] Other interventions showing some benefit with only 1 study were benzydamine, calcium phosphate, etoposide bolus, honey, iseganan, oral care, and zinc sulphate. In addition, L-glutamine has shown promise as a preventive and therapeutic agent for treatment-related mucositis. Palifermin, a human keratinocyte growth factor, reduced the duration and severity of oral mucositis after intensive chemotherapy

and radiotherapy for hematologic cancers. In a review of 32 treatment trials for oral mucositis involving 1500 patients, no benefits were seen with benzydamine HCl versus placebo or sucralfate versus placebo. Only low-level laser showed a reduction in severe mucositis when compared with a sham procedure. Opioid pain management has also been shown to be effective for mucositis-related pain.[49] A gynecologic cancer–specific study evaluated the impact of circadian rhythms on radiation-related mucositis manifesting as diarrhea in cervical cancer patients. More than 200 patients with cervical carcinoma were randomized to morning and evening arms. Although radiation response rates were similar, overall (grades 1-4) and higher-grade (grades 3 and 4) diarrhea was found to be significantly increased in the morning arm compared with the evening arm.

Gynecologic cancer patients with diarrhea and tenesmus also need to be evaluated for disease progression. Loperamide may be beneficial in the setting of radiation- or chemotherapy-induced diarrhea when disease progression and *Clostridium difficile* infection have been excluded. Tenesmus usually responds to anticholinergic agents, corticosteroids, and opioids, often in combination. In severe cases of radiation enteritis and proctitis, surgical intervention may be required.

Ascites

Ascites is a frequent issue in ovarian cancer patients, and the approach to symptom management will depend on the patient's current goals of care. Diuretics, intermittent IP paracentesis, permanent indwelling catheter, and sparing diuretics may be used. Malignant ascites often has a profound impact on the QOL of patients with refractory and heavily treated ovarian cancer. In retrospective studies, indwelling IP catheters appear to be a safe and effective palliative strategy to manage refractory malignant ascites, without overwhelming infection rates.[50] Some practitioners use IP cisplatin with success in highly selected patients to palliate symptomatic ascites. New biologic therapeutics may be a future option of treatment. Laboratory research demonstrates that a high content of vascular endothelial growth factor in ascites might be responsible for increased peritoneal permeability, resulting in the production of ascites. Case reports have studied the successful use of bevacizumab in palliative treatment of ascites in ovarian cancer patients. Toxicity was manageable, and no therapeutic paracenteses were required after initiation of therapy. Further prospective trials should consider evaluation of these agents as a tool for palliation treatment of ascites during the EOL.

Respiratory Symptoms

Respiratory symptoms in gynecologic oncology patients may be related to pulmonary tumor burden from lung metastasis or from pleural effusion. In addition, cancer-related cachexia, malnutrition, fatigue, anemia, and metabolic acidosis may contribute to dyspnea. In the setting of pleural effusion, decisions regarding interventions should be made based on patient prognosis and goals of care. Interventions such as thoracentesis, placement of indwelling catheter, and chemical pleurodesis may be considered. The American Thoracic Society consensus statement defines dyspnea as "a subjective experience of breathing discomfort that consists of qualitatively distinct sensations that vary in intensity," not necessarily related to hypercapnia or hypoxia.[51] A systematic review of the evidence for the efficiency of pharmacologic and nonpharmacologic treatments in alleviating dyspnea in terminal cancer patients revealed a paucity of randomized controlled trials on interventions for alleviation of dyspnea. Their review supported the use of opioids for dyspnea relief in cancer patients, but the use of supplemental oxygen to alleviate dyspnea was recommended only in patients with hypoxemia. A review of pharmacologic approaches to dyspnea confirmed benefits of systemic opioids, administered orally or parenterally. In addition, authors found that oral promethazine may also be used as a second-line treatment. Nursing-led nonpharmacologic interventions such as counseling, relaxation, and teaching coping strategies seemed to provide benefit although studies were limited.

Urinary Tract Symptoms

Urinary tract symptoms in the gynecologic oncology patient may be disease- or treatment-related. Women with both early- and late-stage ovarian cancer may present with symptoms of urinary urgency and frequency. Cervical cancer patients may have ureteral obstruction and bladder involvement by tumor; in addition, treatment-related symptoms include bladder dysfunction after radical hysterectomy, radiation cystitis, and ureterovaginal or vesicovaginal fistulas. Ureteral obstruction, with subsequent infection, pain, and acute renal failure (in the setting of bilateral obstruction), may justify mechanical measures such as nephrostomy or ureteric stent insertion in selected cases. When prognosis is otherwise limited, these invasive procedures may introduce unnecessary morbidity. Bladder dysfunction may be associated with radical hysterectomy, and some authors have advocated nerve-sparing approaches to decrease incidence. Radiation for cervical and endometrial cancer can cause urinary tract symptoms including immediate effects (bladder irritation or cystitis) and late effects (hematuria, fibrosis and contraction, or fistulas). In cervical cancer, the 10-year bladder complication rate in a series from the MD Anderson Cancer Center was 3%. On multivariate analysis, a central pelvic dose of external beam radiation >50 Gy, black race, smoking, and obesity were significantly associated with increased risk of bladder complications. Bladder symptoms may be treated with nonsteroidal anti-inflammatory medications for detrusor irritability or drugs with an anticholinergic action to reduce bladder contractility. Infection should also be assessed. Fistulas are ideally treated with surgical diversion; however, in settings of limited prognosis, urinary catheterization may ameliorate symptoms.

Edema

Thromboembolic disease, lymphedema, and severe nutritional deficiency can contribute to acute and chronic edema in the gynecologic oncology patient. In addition, recurrent or progressive tumor may contribute to edema. Cancer diagnosis, advanced age, abdominopelvic surgery, obstructing lesions, and treatment with thrombogenic chemotherapy regimens all put gynecologic oncology patients at high risk for venous thromboembolism (VTE). The reported rate of VTE in gynecologic cancer patients ranges from 11% to 18%, with the rate of pulmonary embolism (PE) between 1% and 2.6%. Among postoperative ovarian cancer patients, the rate of PE is as high as 7%. Perioperative prevention is essential, and the authors support a regimen similar to those advocated in the literature of dual prophylaxis with sequential compression devices plus heparin every 8 hours or daily low molecular weight heparin with extended prophylaxis for 2 to 4 weeks after surgery for high-risk patients. For the patient who has been diagnosed with a VTE, prolonged use of a low molecular weight heparin over oral anticoagulants to decrease VTE recurrence is supported by a current Cochrane review.[52]

A population-based study in Australia found that 10% of gynecologic cancer survivors who responded to a survey reported being diagnosed with lymphedema, and a further 15% reported undiagnosed "symptomatic" lower limb swelling.[51] The highest prevalence (36%) of diagnosed lymphedema was found in vulvar cancer survivors. For cervical cancer survivors, radiation and lymphadenectomy conferred increased risk of developing swelling. For uterine and ovarian cancer survivors, those who had lymph nodes removed or who were overweight or obese had the greatest chance of developing swelling. Treatment for lymphedema in the gynecologic oncology patient has been poorly studied, and most experience has been gained from breast cancer patients. Complete decongestive therapy for lymphedema consists of an acute treatment phase and a lifelong maintenance phase and combines manual lymph drainage, compression bandaging, and therapeutic exercise. Skin and nail care with inspection for cuts, scratches, irritation, or infection is also essential given risk of cellulitis. In the gynecologic patient with a limited life span, nutritional deficiency, hypo-albuminemia, immobility, and progressive obstructive tumor may all contribute to edema.

Fatigue

Cancer-related fatigue (CRF) is a prevalent and disabling symptom experienced by both cancer patients and cancer survivors. CRF is a multifaceted condition characterized by diminished energy and an increased need to rest, disproportionate to any recent change in activity level. It is accompanied by other clinical characteristics, including generalized weakness, diminished mental concentration, insomnia or hypersomnia, and emotional reactivity. Decrements in physical, social, cognitive, and vocational functioning; adverse mood changes; sleep disturbances; treatment noncompliance; and emotional and spiritual distress for both patients and their family members are among the consequences of CRF. The etiology and risk factors for CRF are multifactorial, and in an excellent recent review, Mitchell describes potentially contributing factors, including direct treatment-related effects, cancer-related conditions, and the adverse effects of medications.[53] Specific etiologies that are implicated include anemia; myeloid suppression; mood disorder; concurrent symptoms such as pain or sleep disturbances; electrolyte disturbances; cardiopulmonary, hepatic, or renal dysfunction; hypothyroidism; hypogonadism; adrenal insufficiency; infection; malnutrition; deconditioning; and skeletal muscle atrophy/weakness. Evidence-based guidelines from the NCCN recommend a symptom-oriented and individualized approach to each patient. A combination of exercise, psychoeducational interventions, efforts to manage concurrent symptoms, interventions to improve sleep quality, judicious use of medications such as modafinil and methylphenidate, and complementary therapies such as relaxation, massage, healing touch, and acupuncture is thought to offer the greatest likelihood of success.[49]

There are limited studies specific to fatigue in the gynecologic oncology population. Thirty-two women treated for recurrent gynecologic cancer and fatigue were prescribed methylphenidate at morning and noon over an 8-week period. Patients reported significant declines in fatigue and improvement in both mood and QOL at the end of the study when compared with baseline scores.[54] Forty-three women with gynecologic cancer receiving platinum chemotherapy were followed longitudinally in a trial of warm water footbath for CRF. Participants in the experimental group reported a significant reduction in fatigue and improvement in sleep quality from the second session of chemotherapy and continued to improve during the 6-month study period. Fifty-one women with ovarian

cancer (n = 37) or breast cancer (n = 14) participated in 10 weekly 75-minute restorative yoga classes that combined physical postures, breathing, and deep relaxation. Significant improvements were seen for depression, negative effect, state anxiety, mental health, and overall QOL. QOL improved and fatigue decreased between baseline and follow-up.[55]

Peripheral Neuropathy

Like other cancer-related symptoms, neuropathy can be due to both cancer and cancer treatment. In gynecologic malignancies, involvement of the sacral plexus by tumor can produce significant neuropathic pain. In addition, radiation treatment for endometrial and cervical cancer can lead to neuropathy when the sacral plexus is in the treatment field. Many agents cause chemotherapy-induced peripheral neuropathy (CIPN); the most common causes in the gynecologic oncology population are cisplatin, carboplatin, paclitaxel, and docetaxel. The functional effects of CIPN can significantly reduce a patient's QOL by introducing limitations such as not being able to hold a baby safely, button a shirt, or type on a keyboard. Pain, paresthesia (numbness), and reduced proprioception can all occur; symptoms may be constant or intermittent and vary in severity. The pain may be characterized as tingling, cold, burning, or dull.

In patients receiving treatments that put them at risk for CIPN, prevention, treatment, and maintaining functionality and safety should all be considered. Preventive agents still in the preclinical phase of study include acetyl-L-carnitine, α-lipoic acid, and ethosuximide, a selective antagonist of calcium channels. Clinical trials of preventive agents have been limited by small sample sizes, inconsistent methods for assessment, lack of randomization, and/or inclusion of multiple chemotherapeutic agents with potential neurotoxic effects. Several trials of glutathione in ovarian cancer patients receiving cisplatin have shown neuroprotective effects. Randomized clinical trials have shown protective effects of vitamin E supplementation in patients receiving cisplatin or cisplatin-paclitaxel combinations.[56] Oral glutamine, an amino acid that induces the transcription of nerve growth factor mRNA, was evaluated in a randomized controlled trial and found to significantly reduced incidence and severity of oxaliplatin-related peripheral neuropathy without a reduction in the efficacy of chemotherapy. Treatment of CIPN includes the use of opioids and adjuvant analgesics. Opioids have demonstrated efficacy for relieving various types of neuropathic pain in randomized controlled studies. Adjuvant analgesics used for CIPN include corticosteroids, anticonvulsant agents, tricyclic antidepressants, local anesthetics, and anticancer therapies. Corticosteroids have efficacy in reducing neuropathic pain; however, their side effect profile limits their use in patients with prolonged survival. Although anticonvulsant agents have been used with significant benefit for CIPN, anecdotally and in case reports, randomized controlled trials do not support their use. Tricyclic antidepressants may have efficacy for neuropathic pain, but their anticholinergic and histaminergic side effects may limit use. Of note, a randomized, double-blind, phase 2 trial of nortriptyline failed to show a significant benefit. Local anesthetics have demonstrated efficacy for several neuropathic pain syndromes, including diabetic neuropathy. Finally, acupuncture has shown improvement in nerve conduction studies in peripheral neuropathy and showed promising results in a case series of CIPN.[57]

Safety precautions are important for women suffering from neuropathy. Patients should be aware that water temperature might be hotter than they sense when they are bathing or washing dishes. Clearing hallways and stairwells and making sure they are well lit may also be important when proprioception is affected. In addition use of nonskid mats in bathtubs and wide-based soles may be beneficial.

Hypercalcemia

Hypercalcemia of malignancy occurs in 10% to 30% of patients with cancer, and etiologies include humoral hypercalcemia of malignancy (HHM), which may or may not be mediated by the paraneoplastic secretion of parathyroid hormone–related peptide (PTHrP), and local osteolytic hypercalcemia in the setting of bone metastasis. In gynecologic cancer, hypercalcemia has been reported with ovarian small-cell carcinoma, papillary serous carcinoma, clear cell carcinoma, and dysgerminoma, as well as with uterine leiomyosarcoma and endometrial, cervical, and vulvar carcinoma. A review of more than 5000 gynecologic cancer patients identified 256 patients with hypercalcemia (5%).[58] Most patients (82%) had mild hypercalcemia. Severity of hypercalcemia was associated with disease stage, use of hypercalcemia treatment, and survival duration. A review of the published cases in the gynecologic oncology literature identified 34 patients with HHM that was PTHrP mediated, of whom 22 had ovarian cancer, 6 had uterine cancer, 3 had vulvar cancer, and 3 had cervical cancer. Clear cell carcinoma was the predominant histology.

Although mild hypercalcemia may be asymptomatic, moderate to severe hypercalcemia can be associated with life-threatening neurologic, cardiac, GI, and renal signs. The treatment of hypercalcemia depends on the level, chronicity, and origin of the condition. General measures used in the treatment of moderate to severe hypercalcemia in patients with cancer include aggressive volume replacement with saline diuresis and inhibitors of bone resorption such as the bisphosphonates. Additional treatments include glucocorticoids and oral phosphate. Response to hypocalcemic treatment is gauged by resolution of symptoms and decrease in serum calcium concentrations.

End-of-Life Care

QOL During Palliative Care

QOL during palliative care is particularly challenging as physicians confront the crucial decision of whether to prescribe therapies that may be futile in prolonging life. However, palliative therapy can be justified when the goal is to improve QOL and specific symptoms. Cancer patients frequently receive chemotherapy near the EOL, and the literature suggests no association between aggressiveness of care and OS. The role of chemotherapy at the EOL was questioned in a pilot study of advanced recurrent ovarian cancer patients in which patients believed that psychosocial issues play a greater role in determining their QOL than their physical QOL. A retrospective study of more than 100 deceased ovarian cancer patients showed that patients with a shorter survival time had a trend toward increased chemotherapy during their last 3 months of life and had increased overall aggressiveness of care. Short disease remissions and clinical events such as frequent hospitalizations and procedures for pleural effusions and ascites were indicators for reducing cure-oriented therapies and increasing palliative interventions.[41] A prospective observational trial, GOG-QLM0301 is being developed by the GOG to study QOL and care needs in patients with platinum-resistant ovarian, fallopian tube, or peritoneal cancer.

Goals of Care at EOL

As with palliative care, the purpose of assistance at the EOL is to relieve any type of suffering. The obligation of the physician to serve is particularly focused when death is eminent. Spirituality is an important aspect of palliative care at the EOL. If the physician is not comfortable addressing these issues, then the appropriate services, such as pastoral care, must be involved. Bereavement care should also be accessed during palliative care but before the immediate EOL. Hospice services, whether inpatient or at home, can help the physician facilitate this transition. The goal of hospice is to provide compassionate, holistic care for patients and their families and to maximize patients' QOL at the EOL.

Site of Care

The majority of gynecologic cancer patients prefer EOL care at home. Brown et al[59] performed a survey and asked the patients to envision being informed by their physicians that efforts to cure or control the spread of their disease were failing. Fifty-seven percent of the gynecologic cancer patients, regardless of disease status, preferred to be treated at home. However, patients' preferences do not always translate into reality. In a multi-institutional retrospective analysis, von Gruenigen et al[39] revealed that 46% of ovarian cancer patients died at home, 21% died in hospice, and 17% died in a hospital. A study of gynecologic oncology patients in Toronto found that 51% of ovarian cancer patients, 49% of uterine cancer patients, and 53% of cervical cancer patients died in an acute care bed.[60] Therefore, it is imperative that the physician and the health care team have transparent communication with patients about their preferences and needs.

As health care providers for women with gynecologic malignancies, we can simultaneously maximize survival and QOL for our patients. We have a wide range of continuously evolving tools at our disposal, including conventional therapies, lifestyle modification, integrative modalities, and supportive care. Appropriate use of these therapies throughout the life cycle can enable us to support the innate healing abilities of our patients and help them achieve their life goals.

REFERENCES

1. Callahan D. The WHO definition of "health". *Stud Hastings Cent.* 1973;1(3):77-88.
2. Sagar SM, Lawenda BD. The role of integrative oncology in a tertiary prevention survivorship program. *Prev Med.* 2009;49(2-3):93-98.
3. Ornish D, Magbanua MJ, Weidner G, et al. Changes in prostate gene expression in men undergoing an intensive nutrition and lifestyle intervention. *Proc Natl Acad Sci USA.* 2008;105(24):8369-8374.
4. Barnes PM, Bloom B, Nahin R. *Complementary and Alternative Medicine Use Among Adults and Children: United States.* Bethesda, MD: National Center for Health Statistics; 2008. National Health Statistics Reports No. 12.
5. Institute of Medicine. *Complementary and Alternative Medicine in the United States.* Washington, DC: The National Academies Press; 2005.
6. Geffen JR. Integrative oncology for the whole person: a multidimensional approach to cancer care. *Integr Cancer Ther.* 2010;9(1):105-121.
7. Powell CB, Dibble SL, Dall'Era JE, Cohen I, Powell CB. Use of herbs in women diagnosed with ovarian cancer. *International Journal of Gynecological Cancer.* 2002;12(2):214-217.
8. Lawenda BD, Kelly KM, Ladas EJ, Sagar SM, Vickers A, Blumberg JB. Should supplemental antioxidant administration be avoided during chemotherapy and radiation therapy? *J Natl Cancer Inst.* 2008;100(11):773-783.
9. Block KI, Koch AC, Mead MN, Tothy PK, Newman RA, Gyllenhaal C. Impact of antioxidant supplementation on chemotherapeutic toxicity: a systematic review of the evidence from randomized controlled trials. *Int J Cancer.* 2008;123(6):1227-1239.
10. Lutgendorf SK, Lamkin DM, DeGeest K, et al. Depressed and anxious mood and T-cell cytokine expressing populations in ovarian cancer patients. *Brain Behav Immun.* 2008;22(6):890-900.
11. Yang EV, Kim SJ, Donovan EL, et al. Norepinephrine upregulates VEGF, IL-8, and IL-6 expression in human melanoma tumor cell lines: implications for stress-related enhancement of tumor progression. *Brain Behav Immun.* 2009;23(2):267-275.
12. Reeves GK, Pirie K, Beral V, Green J, Spencer E, Bull D. Cancer incidence and mortality in relation to body mass index in the Million Women Study: cohort study. *BMJ.* 2007;335(7630):1134.
13. Conroy MB, Sattelmair JR, Cook NR, Manson JE, Buring JE, Lee IM. Physical activity, adiposity, and risk of endometrial cancer. *Cancer Causes Control.* 2009;20(7):1107-1115.
14. Friedenreich C, Cust A, Lahmann PH, et al. Physical activity and risk of endometrial cancer: the European prospective investigation into cancer and nutrition. *Int J Cancer.* 2007;121(2):347-355.
15. Patel AV, Feigelson HS, Talbot JT, et al. The role of body weight in the relationship between physical activity and endometrial cancer: results from a large cohort of US women. *Int J Cancer.* 2008;123(8):1877-1882.
16. von Gruenigen VE, Tian C, Frasure H, Waggoner S, Keys H, Barakat RR. Treatment effects, disease recurrence, and survival in obese women with early endometrial carcinoma: a Gynecologic Oncology Group study. *Cancer.* 2006;107(12):2786-2791.
17. Mulholland HG, Murray LJ, Cardwell CR, Cantwell MM. Dietary glycaemic index, glycaemic load and endometrial and ovarian cancer risk: a systematic review and meta-analysis. *Br J Cancer.* 2008;99(3):434-441.
18. Olsen CM, Green AC, Whiteman DC, Sadeghi S, Kolahdooz F, Webb PM. Obesity and the risk of epithelial ovarian cancer: a systematic review and meta-analysis. *Eur J Cancer.* 2007;43(4):690-709.
19. Lahmann PH, Cust AE, Friedenreich CM, et al. Anthropometric measures and epithelial ovarian cancer risk in the European Prospective Investigation into Cancer and Nutrition. *Int J Cancer.* 2010;126(10):2404-2415.
20. Pavelka JC, Brown RS, Karlan BY, et al. Effect of obesity on survival in epithelial ovarian cancer. *Cancer.* 2006;107:1520-1524.
21. Barrett SV, Paul J, Hay A, Vasey PA, Kaye SB, Glasspool RM. Does body mass index affect progression-free or overall survival in patients with ovarian cancer? Results from SCOTROC I trial. *Ann Oncol.* 2008;19(5):898-902.
22. Sofi F, Abbate R, Gensini GF, Casini A. Accruing evidence about benefits of adherence to the Mediterranean diet on health: an updated systematic review and meta-analysis. *Am J Clin Nutr.* 2010;92(5):1189-1196.
23. La Vecchia C: Assocation between Mediterranean dietary patterns and cancer risk. *Nutr Rev.* 2009;67(1):1126-1129.
24. Kolahdooz F, van der Pols JC, Bain CJ, et al. Meat, fish, and ovarian cancer risk: results from 2 Australian case-control studies, a systematic review, and meta-analysis. *Am J Clin Nutr.* 2010;91(6):1752-1763.
25. Garcia-Closas R, Castellsague X, Bosch X, Gonzalez CA. The role of diet and nutrition in cervical carcinogenesis: a review of recent evidence. *Int J Cancer.* 2005;117(4):629-637.
26. Cook LS, Neilson HK, Lorenzetti DL, Lee RC. A systematic literature review of vitamin D and ovarian cancer. *Am J Obstet Gynecol.* 2010;203(1):70 e71-e78.
27. Bakhru A, Mallinger JB, Buckanovich RJ, Griggs JJ. Casting light on 25-hydroxyvitamin D deficiency in ovarian cancer: a study from the NHANES. *Gynecol Oncol.* 2010;119(2):314-318.
28. McCulloch M, See C, Shu XJ, et al. Astragalus-based Chinese herbs and platinum-based chemotherapy for advanced non-small-cell lung cancer: meta-analysis of randomized trials. *J Clin Oncol.* 2006;24(3):419-430.

29. Gates MA, Tworoger SS, Hecht JL, De Vivo I, Rosner B, Hankinson SE. A prospective study of dietary flavonoid intake and incidence of epithelial ovarian cancer. *Int J Cancer.* 2007; 121(10):2225-2232.

30. Myung SK, Ju W, Choi HJ, Kim SC. Soy intake and risk of endocrine-related gynaecological cancer: a meta-analysis. *BJOG.* 2009;116(13):1697-1705.

31. Arriba LN, Fader AN, Frasure HE, von Gruenigen VE. A review of issues surrounding quality of life among women with ovarian cancer. *Gynecol Oncol.* 2010;119(2):390-396.

32. von Gruenigen V, Kavanagh M, Nieves-Arriba L, et al. Physical activity may improve quality of life in women with ovarian cancer on adjuvant chemotherapy. *Gynecol. Oncol.* 2010;116(3):S140.

33. von Gruenigen VE, Courneya KS, Gibbons HE, Kavanagh MB, Waggoner SE, Lerner E. Feasibility and effectiveness of a life-style intervention program in obese endometrial cancer patients: a randomized trial. *Gynecol Oncol.* 2008;109(1):19-26.

34. Quinten C, Coens C, Mauer M, et al. Baseline quality of life as a prognostic indicator of survival: a meta-analysis of individual patient data from EORTC clinical trials. *Lancet Oncol.* 2009;10(9):865-871.

35. Wright JD, Shah M, Mathew L, et al. Fertility preservation in young women with epithelial ovarian cancer. *Cancer.* 2009;115(18):4118-4126.

36. Matulonis UA, Kornblith A, Lee H, et al. Long-term adjustment of early-stage ovarian cancer survivors. *Int J Gynecol Cancer.* 2008;18(6):1183-1193.

37. Carey MS, Bacon M, Tu D, Butler L, Bezjak A, Stuart GC. The prognostic effects of performance status and quality of life scores on progression-free survival and overall survival in advanced ovarian cancer. *Gynecol Oncol.* 2008;108(1):100-105.

38. Wenzel LB, Huang HQ, Armstrong DK, Walker JL, Cella D. Health-related quality of life during and after intraperitoneal versus intravenous chemotherapy for optimally debulked ovarian cancer: a Gynecologic Oncology Group study. *J Clin Oncol.* 2007;25(4):437-443.

39. van de Poll-Franse LV, Mols F, Essink-Bot ML, et al. Impact of external beam adjuvant radiotherapy on health-related quality of life for long-term survivors of endometrial adenocarcinoma: a population-based study. *Int J Radiat Oncol Biol Phys.* 2007;69(1):125-132.

40. Temel JS, Greer JA, Muzikansky A, et al. Early palliative care for patients with metastatic non-small-cell lung cancer. *N Engl J Med.* 2010;363(8):733-742.

41. von Gruenigen V, Daly B, Gibbons H, Hutchins J, Green A. Indicators of survival duration in ovarian cancer and implications for aggressiveness of care. *Cancer.* 2008;112(10):2221-2227.

42. Kutner JS, Smith MC, Corbin L, et al. Massage therapy versus simple touch to improve pain and mood in patients with advanced cancer: a randomized trial. *Ann Intern Med.* 2008;149(6): 369-379.

43. Hesketh PJ. Chemotherapy-induced nausea and vomiting. *N Engl J Med.* 2008;358(23):2482-2494.

44. Lee A, Fan LT. Stimulation of the wrist acupuncture point P6 for preventing postoperative nausea and vomiting. *Cochrane Database Syst Rev.* 2009;2:CD003281.

45. Kucukmetin A, Naik R, Galaal K, Bryant A, Dickinson HO. Palliative surgery versus medical management for bowel obstruction in ovarian cancer. *Cochrane Database Syst Rev.* 2010;7:CD007792.

46. Mangili G, Franchi M, Mariani A, et al. Octreotide in the management of bowel obstruction in terminal ovarian cancer. *Gynecol Oncol.* 1996;61(3):345-348.

47. Caceres A, Zhou Q, Iasonos A, Gerdes H, Chi DS, Barakat RR. Colorectal stents for palliation of large-bowel obstructions in recurrent gynecologic cancer: an updated series. *Gynecol Oncol.* 2008;108(3):482-485.

48. Worthington HV, Clarkson JE, Eden OB. Interventions for preventing oral mucositis for patients with cancer receiving treatment. *Cochrane Database Syst Rev.* 2007;4:CD000978.

49. Clarkson JE, Worthington HV, Furness S, McCabe M, Khalid T, Meyer S. Interventions for treating oral mucositis for patients with cancer receiving treatment. *Cochrane Database Syst Rev.* 2010;8:CD001973.

50. Fleming ND, Alvarez-Secord A, Von Gruenigen V, Miller MJ, Abernethy AP. Indwelling catheters for the management of refractory malignant ascites: A systematic literature overview and retrospective chart review. *J Pain Symptom Manage.* 2009;38(3):341-349.

51. Ryan M, Stainton MC, Slaytor EK, Jaconelli C, Watts S, Mackenzie P. Aetiology and prevalence of lower limb lymphoedema following treatment for gynaecological cancer. *Aust N Z J Obstet Gynaevcol.* 2003;43(2):148-151.

52. Akl EA, Barba M, Rohilla S, et al. Anticoagulation for the long term treatment of venous thromboembolism in patients with cancer. *Cochrane Database Syst Rev.* 2008;2:CD006650.

53. Mitchell SA. Cancer-related fatigue: state of the science. *PM R.* 2010;2(5):364-383.

54. Johnson RL, Block I, Gold MA, Markwell S, Zupancic M. Effect of methylphenidate on fatigue in women with recurrent gynecologic cancer. *Psychooncology.* 2010;19(9):955-958.

55. Danhauer SC, Tooze JA, Farmer DF, et al. Restorative yoga for women with ovarian or breast cancer: findings from a pilot study. *J Soc Integr Oncol.* 2008;6(2):47-58.

56. Pace A, Giannarelli D, Galie E, et al. Vitamin E neuroprotection for cisplatin neuropathy: a randomized, placebo-controlled trial. *Neurology.* 2010;74(9):762-766.

57. Schroder S, Liepert J, Remppis A, Greten JH. Acupuncture treatment improves nerve conduction in peripheral neuropathy. *Eur J Neurol.* 2007;14(3):276-281.

58. Jaishuen A, Jimenez C, Sirisabya N, et al. Poor survival outcome with moderate and severe hypercalcemia in gynecologic malignancy patients. *Int J Gynecol Cancer.* 2009;19(2):178-185.

59. Brown D, Roberts JA, Elkins TE, Larson D, Hopkins M. Hard choices: the gynecologic cancer patient's end-of-life preferences. *Gynecol Oncol.* 1994;55(3[1]):355-362.

60. Barbera L, Elit L, Krzyzanowska M, Saskin R, Bierman AS. End of life care for women with gynecologic cancers. *Gynecol Oncol.* 2010;118(2):196-201.

23 Surgical Instrumentation and Sutures

John C. Elkas and Addie Alkhas

It is imperative that surgeons understand the choice and limitations of their instruments and sutures with regard to a planned surgery. This knowledge will often make the difference between struggling or proceeding with purpose. Keeping current on the rapid and ongoing development of instrument technology can be difficult for the busy clinician. Yet taking advantage of these innovations can contribute significantly toward efficiently completing a challenging case. Surgical proficiency requires a well-planned approach with an appreciation and knowledge of the instruments and sutures to be used.

SURGICAL INSTRUMENTATION

Every surgeon has a preference for selecting particular instruments as a result of training and experience. Later, these choices are often modified by acquired habits and limits imposed by cost. Surgical instruments are an extension of a surgeon's hands and are designed to facilitate the operative procedure. The list of instruments provided in this chapter is neither comprehensive nor complete. What follows is a functional description of the basic tools for the gynecologic surgeon.

Scalpels

The Bard-Parker handle is usually fitted with a disposable blade that is attached using a needle holder. Commonly, the #10 or #20 blade is used for the skin incision and can then be used to extend the incision through the fascia. The #15 blade has a small area useful for confined spaces or small skin incisions. The #11 blade

has a straight edge useful for its pointed design in placing drains or opening abscesses. There are also long and curved handles to facilitate dissection in the deep pelvis.

Scissors

Scissors, with their long handles and strong blades, serve multiple functions in the operative field from cutting sutures, excising scar tissue, and transecting pedicles to fine dissection of adhesions involving intra-abdominal viscera. Surgical scissors usually come in various sizes and lengths, with straight and curved blades having chamfered or rounded ends. Examples of these are the Mayo and Metzenbaum scissors. The Jorgenson scissors are heavy scissors with sharply curved blades that facilitate the amputation of the cervix off the vaginal cuff.

Forceps

Thumb forceps, as the term suggests, act as an extension of the surgeons thumb and index finger for grasping tissue, steadying needles, or exploration. Spring tension keeps the tips apart until pressure is applied to close them. Forceps have a variety of widths and lengths, making them versatile and universally applicable in the operative field. The blade's design and surface configuration will determine its intended use. Adson forceps are used for manipulating the skin, whereas Bonney or Martin forceps have teeth for handling fascia. DeBakey or smooth forceps with a cross-serrated grasping surface make them ideal for handling peritoneum or vascular pedicles. Singley forceps with their fenestration

469

are ideal in atraumatic handling of tissue bundles during lymphatic dissection. Hemostatic forceps (clamps) are light instruments with spring handles, ratcheting closing mechanisms, and fine tips, making them ideal for isolating bleeding points, grasping small vascular pedicles, and careful dissection in the pelvis. They come in an assortment of sizes and lengths, making them very useful instruments. The Halsted mosquito forceps, Kelly clamps, Tonsils, Rochester-Ochsner, and Mixter forceps are a few other often-used forceps.

Hysterectomy Clamps

Because of the rich, extensive, and collateralized blood supply to the uterus, these clamps are designed to secure and maintain large vascular pedicles within their jaws while minimizing the trauma to the surrounding tissue. A ratchet locking device in the handle, serrations in the jaw, and teeth at the tips allow for a pedicle to be transected and ligated safely. Tissue slippage can result in extensive bleeding that is difficult to control, risking injury to the ureters as well as larger vessels. These clamps are generally at least 20 cm long and have curved or straight jaws or angled handles. The longitudinal serrations tend to be preferred because they prevent slippage of tissue from the clamp. Examples include the Heaney-Ballentine clamps, which have teeth at their tips to ensure secure bite at the cost of crushing the tissue; the Masterson clamp, which was designed to generate less crushing force by lacking the toothed tip; and the Zeppelin clamps, which may best satisfy the requirements for the use in complex pelvic procedures—greater holding force and minimal tissue trauma and slippage. In addition to the full range of abdominal Zeppelin clamp configurations, different sizes and curves are also available for vaginal surgery (Figure 23-1).

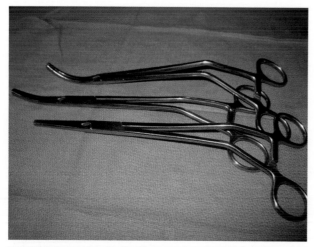

FIGURE 23-1. Zeppelin clamps.

Clip Applicators

Clip applicators are effective in obtaining hemostasis of small vessels deep in the pelvis or when performing a lymph node dissection to prevent lymphatic drainage. The applicator comes as a reusable single clip applicator with straight or angled head or as a disposable instrument with multiple loads. The applicators usually come in 3 sizes: small, medium, and large. After clip application, caution should be used with the use of the electrosurgical unit or suction device because of potentially unrecognized injury by thermal spread or dislodged clips causing rents in serosal surfaces or vascular structures.

Retractors

Surgery for ovarian cancer is normally performed through a midline laparotomy because evaluation of both pelvic and abdominal structures is required. A self-retaining retractor is essential to optimizing exposure, maximizing patient safety, and reducing surgeon fatigue. Of the available models of self-retaining retractors, those with a fixed arm attaching the retractor ring to the operating table are best suited for ovarian cancer surgery. The Bookwalter retractor is the standard self-retaining fixed-ring retractor and is versatile enough to be adapted to a variety of operative requirements. The retractor clips that attach the blades to the ring allow for 2-dimensional adjustments of the blade position in relation to the surgical field. The oval ring of the Bookwalter is most commonly used for ovarian cancer surgery, but circular and hinged rings are also available depending on the exposure needed. For example, the hinged ring can be used to surgical advantage when operating in the upper abdomen (eg, diaphragm, liver, spleen) by increasing the angulation of the retractor blade to provide more pronounced ventral displacement of the costal margin, improving exposure.

The Omni retractor has 2 adjustable "boomerang-shaped" arms that are attached to a fixed post. Each arm can be moved in 3 dimensions, and finer modifications in exposure can be achieved with the adjustable retractor blades as opposed to the fixed ring. The Omni retractor is especially helpful when operating on obese patients, because the extent of lateral retraction is not limited by the width of a retractor ring (eg, Bookwalter). Nonfixed, self-retaining retractors, such as the Balfour and O'Connor-O'Sullivan retractors, can also be used, but they are more limited in their field of exposure and are less steady than the fixed models because they are stabilized only by creating pressure on the opposing sides of the abdominal wall incision. In addition to limited exposure, self-retaining retractors have been associated with iatrogenic nerve injury due to compression of the femoral nerve in as many as 7.5%

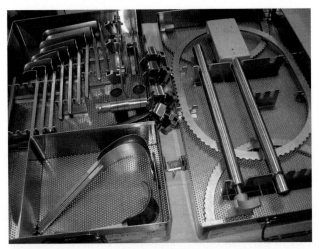

FIGURE 23-2. Bookwalter self-retaining retractor.

of cases.[1] Although retractors such as the Omni and Bookwalter may be associated with nerve injury as well, the elevation of the abdominal wall provided by these retractors may help to minimize this risk. With any self-retaining or fixed retractor, the surgeon must exercise particular attention when placing the blades along the lateral abdominal wall so as not to compress the psoas muscle and traumatize the underlying femoral nerve. The risk of femoral nerve injury may also be increased by extended Pfannenstiel incisions, thin habitus (body mass index < 20 kg/m²), narrow pelvis, and prolonged surgical time greater than 4 hours (Figure 23-2).

Needle Holders

The needle holder serves to guide and place a needle through tissue and then retrieve it. They are designed with various lengths and straight or curved jaws to facilitate their placement. A fine locking mechanism and serrated jaws assist with control of the needle to prevent unnecessary bleeding and tissue damage. Considerations for correct needle choice and caution with grasping the needle can prevent the needle from bending or breaking. Curved tips are preferred in vaginal surgery to aide with visualization and placement of the needle. However, the straight tip allows for better control of the needle with more precise placement. The Mayo-Hegar and DeBakey's are 2 commonly used needle holders.

The Electrosurgical Unit and Vessel Sealant Devices

The electrosurgical unit (ESU) (Force 2; ValleyLab, Boulder, CO) consists of a generator and electrodes and is probably the most commonly used instrument in ovarian cancer surgery. The ESU uses radiofrequency electrosurgery to oscillate intracellular ions, which converts electromagnetic energy to mechanical energy and then to thermal energy. The ESU can be configured with either monopolar or bipolar electrodes. The monopolar electrode is versatile and can be used for cutting, desiccation, and fulguration. With cutting current, a continuous high-frequency flow leads to a rapid buildup of heat and vaporization of intracellular water, resulting in local tissue disintegration without a significant coagulative effect but with minimal lateral heat transfer. In contrast, coagulation mode uses an interrupted current of lower energy, which leads to a slower heating of intracellular water, increasing the resistance to flow and producing a more pronounced coagulative effect on small blood vessels. Often a combination (or blended) current produces the most satisfactory tissue effect. Generally the lowest effective generator settings should be used to avoid excessive thermal damage to surrounding tissues. Customary settings for blended currents range from 30 to 50 W. With monopolar electrodes, a grounding or dispersive pad needs to be applied to non–hair bearing, well-perfused, and dry skin close to the surgical site. The bipolar electrode uses a dual paddle design that conducts current to produce a tissue-coagulating effect. Bipolar devices conduct current only between the 2 paddles of the instrument, limiting the risk of electrical injury, especially when used during laparoscopy.

Automated Stapling Devices

Advanced-stage ovarian cancer commonly involves the intestinal tract by contiguous extension or distant peritoneal metastasis. Consequently, the surgeon must be familiar with a variety of techniques of bowel resection and anastomosis. Traditionally, these procedures were performed using hand-sewn suture techniques. The introduction of automated surgical stapling devices permits the same procedures to be performed with comparable efficacy, greater simplicity, and increased speed. There are multiple brands of commercially available automated stapling devices; however, all use the same basic principle of compressing an inverted "U-shaped" staple into a "sideways B" in the closed position. The closed staple position secures the tissue contained within but does not constrict the vascular supply to the resulting staple line with the exception of the vascular load staplers.

There are 3 basic categories of automated stapling devices used for bowel surgery as well as other purposes. All contemporary stapling devices are single-use and disposable. The first category is the thoracoabdominal (TA) stapler, which lays down a double row of titanium staples staggered in an overlapping fashion. The TA stapler does not have a cutting component and therefore is used to close a segment of intestinal tract distal to the point of division or to close an enterotomy or colostomy created during one of various anastomotic techniques. The TA stapler is available in 3 different sizes (40, 60, and 90 mm) depending on the width of tissue to be secured. There are 2 standard staple sizes for the TA stapler, with the choice being dependent on the compression thickness of the stapled tissue. The 3.5-mm staple (open position) compresses to a thickness of approximately 1.5 mm in the closed position, whereas the 4.8-mm staple (open position) should be used for tissue that will compress to approximately 2.0 mm in the closed position. The Roticulator stapling device is a variation of the standard TA stapler that incorporates a rotating shaft and hinged cartridge head to allow greater flexibility of application. It is particularly useful when dividing a segment of colon or rectum deep in the pelvis. The Roticulator lays down a double row of 4.8-mm titanium staples 55 mm in length.

The second category of automated stapling devices is the gastrointestinal anastomosis (GIA) stapler, which lays down 2 double rows of staggered titanium staples and has a self-contained cutting blade that divides the tissue between the 2 staple lines. The GIA stapler is used to simultaneously secure and divide a segment of bowel or other tissue such as mesentery and is available in 2 lengths (60 and 80 mm) depending on the width of tissue. The basic staple sizes adapted for use in the GIA stapler are 3.8 mm, which compresses to 1.3 mm in the closed position, and 4.8 mm, which compresses to 2.0 mm in the closed position. Vascular load staple cartridges are also now in use with the GIA-type staplers that have a staple size of 2.5 mm, which compresses to 1.0 mm in the closed position. The staple line thus created is hemostatic for most small-caliber vascular pedicles.

The third category of automated stapling devices is the circular end-to-end anastomosis (CEEA) stapler. The CEEA stapler lays down a double row of circular staples and has a self-contained circular cutting blade that simultaneously excises the inverted internal tissue. The 4.8-mm staples compress to a tissue thickness of approximately 2 mm. The CEEA stapler is most commonly used to create end-to-end anastomosis of the colon but is also applicable to small bowel–small bowel and small bowel–colon anastomosis. Both straight and curved shafts are available variations of the CEEA stapler, although when performing a low colorectal anastomosis, navigation of the pelvic curvature is usually easier with the curved model. A low-profile detachable anvil is also available for the CEEA stapler, which is easier to place within the bowel lumen in some circumstances (eg, stapled end-to-side anastomosis). The standard CEEA stapler comes in 5 sizes that reflect the outer diameter of the circular stapler cartridge: 21, 25, 28, 31, and 33 mm. In general, the functional luminal diameter is approximately 10 mm smaller than the size of the stapler used to create the anastomosis.

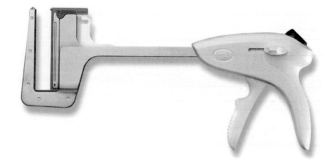

FIGURE 23-3. Thoracoabdominal stapling device.

Successful outcomes using automated surgical stapler to perform bowel anastomosis including colorectal anastomosis below the levator muscles have been reported in the gynecologic literature since the late 1970s. The rate of enteric anastomotic-related complications following trauma-related intestinal surgery has been confirmed to be similar regardless of whether an automated stapler or hand-sewn technique is used. In one of the largest case series documenting the use of end-to-end anastomosis stapling devices in the setting of radical gynecologic surgery, the 2 anastomotic breakdowns reported were noted in patients who had previously undergone radiation therapy.[2] Some authors argue that the favorable outcomes associated with the use of automated stapling devices in patients with gynecologic malignancies are due, at least in part, to the improved blood flow to the anastomosis, a contention that has been confirmed in an animal model. It must be stressed that, in all instances, the method of anastomosis elected should reflect the technique with which the surgeon is the most comfortable. The specifications of the 3 types of automated stapling devices are depicted in Figures 23-3, 23-4, and 23-5.

Recent innovations have been made to the GIA stapler to address issues related to bleeding at the staple line and enteric leakage. Many of these studies have been done in thoracic and bariatric surgery with

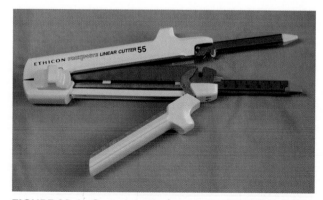

FIGURE 23-4. Gastrointestinal anastomosis stapling device.

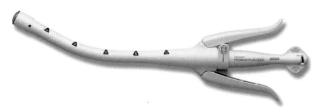

FIGURE 23-5. Circular end-to-end anastomosis stapling device.

endoscopic stapling devices but have applicability to open and hand-held devices as mentioned earlier. The new Ethicon Endo-Surgery Linear Cutter is the only linear cutter with 6-row, 3-dimensional surgical staple technology. It is a sterile, single-patient-use instrument that simultaneously staples and divides tissue. It may be used for transection, resection, and the creation of anastomoses. The 6-row stapling line is thought to provide superior hemostasis through added tissue compression. However, a recent German study of 362 patients comparing 4-row stapling in 148 patients to 6-row stapling in 214 patients noted a nonsignificant difference in anastomotic leak rate of 2.7% versus 3.7%, respectively. There was also a nonsignificant improvement in hemostasis.

A second innovation has been the use of reinforcement material in the staple line that is thought to redistribute tension evenly throughout, sealing off the staple holes and narrowing the spaces between the staples. Presently, several types of available reinforcement materials exist, such as Gore Seamguard, which contains a nonabsorbable and absorbable sleeve placed over each arm of the stapler prior to firing; Peri-Strips Dry with Veritas collagen matrix, which is an absorbable staple line made from bovine pericardium that is attached to the stapler with a gel; and the Duet TRS Reload with Tissue Reinforcement, which uses an absorbable polymer called Biosyn. The Duet TRS system has a preloaded Biosyn film attached to disposable staples, which makes use of this system rather straightforward. It also has the thinnest film thickness at 0.7 mm, potentially reducing misfiring on thick or edematous tissue. Several studies in animals and humans have demonstrated an increased burst pressure and decreased blood loss and leakage with reinforced staple lines. In a study by Jones et al[1] published in 2008, bioabsorbable staple line reinforcement for circular staples in a gastrojejunal anastomosis using Gore Seamguard showed a significant reduction in the incidence of anastomotic strictures from 9.3% to 0.7%, which may improve the morbidity from low anterior resections during ovarian cancer tumor debulking. Large prospective trials comparing these staple systems to conventional systems are ongoing, so firm conclusions as to their cost effectiveness cannot yet be made.

Argon Beam Coagulator

Compared with the standard ESU, which conducts current through air, the argon beam coagulator (ABC) (Conmed Corp., Utica, NY) conducts radiofrequency current to the target tissue through a coaxial stream of inert argon gas that is regulated automatically. ABC power settings range from 70 to 150 W and are selected according to the type of tissue being treated (eg, 70-80 W for cauterizing small-caliber vessels, 110-120 W for treating the surface of the liver or spleen). The ABC does not come into direct contact with tissue; rather, as the current contacts the tissue with the stream of argon gas, individual arc tunnels are formed within the target tissue. It is the formation of these arc tunnels that is thought to account for a more uniform distribution of current within the tissue and therefore a more uniform coagulative effect with less thermal injury. The ABC can effectively cauterize vessels of up to 3 mm in diameter. The jet of argon gas serves to improve visualization of the operative field by displacing blood and debris. In addition to its utility in achieving hemostasis, the underlying coagulative necrosis generated by application of the ABC is an efficient means of destroying small-volume implants of metastatic ovarian cancer and may facilitate optimal cytoreduction of disease in sites inaccessible to conventional resection. Tumor destruction has been documented in areas such as bowel mesentery, the diaphragm, ureters, vagina, presacral space, and iliac vessels. When used for ovarian cancer tumor implant ablation, the depth of tissue destruction is dependent on both the power setting and tissue interaction time.

Ultrasonic Instruments

Recently, a group of surgical instruments referred to as "vessel sealers" have demonstrated clinical utility by simultaneously cauterizing a tissue pedicle and cutting it with a self-contained surgical knife (eg, Ligasure; ValleyLab) or with ultrasound energy (Harmonic ACE; Ethicon, Cincinnati, OH). The energy generated from these instruments reforms the collagen in the vessel walls and connective tissue, producing a permanent seal that can effectively cauterize vessels.

Specifically with the Harmonic ACE device, also available as a hand-held device, when tissue with high water content is exposed to low-frequency ultrasonic energy, intracellular vibrations cause the tissue shear stress threshold to be exceeded and tissue proteins to denature and cells to destruct. The Harmonic scalpels achieve tissue temperatures in the range of 60 to 80°C, resulting in coagulum formation without the desiccation and charring caused by temperatures of ≥80°C that are produced using electrosurgical methods. Because these effects are a product of mechanical vibration propagating in the direction of the applied force, collateral tissue damage is minimal. The device consists of a generator, reusable handpiece, and ultrasonic blade that vibrates at a specific frequency and at a programmable excursion. The generator has an acoustic transducer that converts the electrical energy into high-frequency vibrations. This energy is then transmitted through the aluminum handpiece to the tip of the blade. An advantage of the Harmonic ACE is that because of minimal collateral spread, it is ideal for use close to bowel and ureter, but caution must be used during prolonged use at high frequency because of the thermal damage that may be caused to adjacent tissue. Because of the mechanism for tissue coagulation, it produces minimal smoke and provides for better visualization of the operative field. It does require longer coagulation time for sealing of vessels as opposed to cauterizing instruments such as the LigaSure, but it may allow more versatility for dissection in lymphatic beds adjacent to major vasculature due to decreased thermal spread.

The LigaSure device uses bipolar electrothermal energy to seal vessels. It is an alternative to clips, staplers, suture ligatures, and ultrasonic devices. The collagen and elastin within the vessel wall are denatured through the application of a high-current and low-voltage (monopolar sources use a low-current, high-voltage energy source) electrical system, resulting in a wide seal. The pressure applied within the jaws reforms the denatured proteins within the apposed vessel into a translucent seal that is transected by a deploying knife. The electrosurgical circuit for the LigaSure device is a tissue response generator that senses the density of the tissue bundle held within the forceps housing the active and return electrodes. The generator's circuitry automatically adjusts for an appropriate amount of energy to be delivered to the tissue, thereby effectively sealing it. The hemostatic plug is made from partially denatured and reformed collagen and elastin within the tissue bundle and blood vessels. Microscopically, the vessel wall fuses, obliterating the lumen. The recent development of the LigaSure Impact system using the TissueFect sensing technology with a ForceTriad energy platform has made it a formidable hand-held open surgical instrument. Its curved jaw and 180-degree rotating shaft allow for access into the deep pelvis. The electrode length is 36 mm, and its cutting length is 34 mm, allowing for substantial pedicles. When fired, it creates a seal width of 3.3 mm at its tip and 4.7 mm at the angle of the forceps. It is hand activated with a fusion cycle of 2 to 4 seconds and improved energy distribution, thus minimizing thermal spread. It uses an audible activation tone that changes from a continuous tone to a single short tone when the seal cycle is complete.

Vessel sealers can be adapted for both laparoscopic and open applications and are particularly useful for

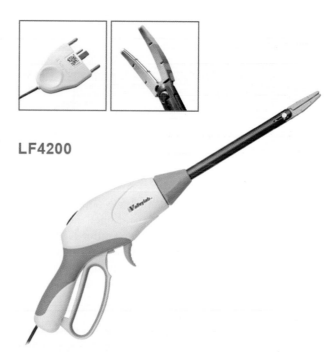

LF4200

FIGURE 23-6. The LigaSure (Impact) vessel sealer.

controlling vascular pedicles in areas that are difficult to reach. When using these instruments, 2 clinical issues must be considered. First, the maximal size of vessel capable of being effectively sealed and burst pressure must be known. The LigaSure device has been compared to the Harmonic ACE in the laboratory setting and found to be able to seal larger vessels (up to 7 mm in size vs. 5 mm) with a higher burst pressure. Second, peripheral energy spread must be known to minimize the risk of adjacent tissue injury. Although LigaSure has been shown to seal larger vessels at higher burst pressures, the Harmonic ACE has less than 1 mm of lateral thermal spread compared to the LigaSure, with as much as 6 mm lateral spread in some studies. Kyo et al,[3] in a recent study citing their experience with the use of the LigaSure device during radical hysterectomies and exenterations, demonstrated decreased mean operative time and a significant decrease in blood loss and transfusion rates. In the general surgical literature, the LigaSure device has been instrumental in successfully completing laparoscopic splenectomies with a significant reduction in operative time and an average blood loss of less than 100 mL (Figure 23-6).

Carbon Dioxide Laser

Laser is an acronym for "light amplification and stimulated emission of radiation." The laser beam possesses a single wavelength with all the elements in phase and parallel to each other, which allows for precise and focused ablation of targeted tissue that has minimal lateral tissue damage. The power density is measured in watts per centimeter squared and is inversely proportional to the spot size. The system is composed of a power source, lasing medium such as carbon dioxide (CO_2) or neodymium, an optical cavity consisting of reflective mirrors, and a delivery device that also uses aligned mirrors or fiber optic cables. For CO_2 lasers, the mirrors allow for adjustment of spot size to facilitate desired tissue effect. The water within the tissue absorbs the photons from the laser beam and is vaporized, ablating the tissue. Special precautions should be taken when using the laser. The heat generated from the laser can potentially cause drapes and towels to catch fire. The CO_2 laser beams can cause corneal damage, and protective eyewear should be worn. Masks with filtering capacity for particulate matter 2 to 5 μm in size should be worn to prevent the potential risk of transmission of human immunodeficiency virus or human papillomavirus in the plume. Constant smoke evacuation is necessary.

Clinically, in gynecologic applications, the CO_2 laser has been used extensively for ablation of endometriosis lesions and lower genital tract lesions. In the setting of ovarian cancer, cytoreductive efforts toward no gross residual disease in the primary and recurrent setting have demonstrated in retrospective studies and meta-analyses to offer the best survival for patients. Some retrospective and small prospective studies suggest a benefit to using the laser in aiding the removal of all gross disease without significant increase in complication rates. This benefit included removal of miliary disease (<1.5 cm) on peritoneal and diaphragmatic surfaces as well as bowel serosa and mesentery, potentially facilitating optimization for intraperitoneal chemotherapy. Operative time for the laser ablation was reported in terms of minutes of application with minimal blood loss, and the laser is extremely useful in anatomically challenging areas such as the porta hepatis and hepatic veins.

Cavitron Ultrasonic Surgical Aspirator

The Cavitron Ultrasonic Surgical Aspirator (CUSA) (ValleyLab) is another surgical adjunct that can be used during cytoreduction of advanced-stage ovarian cancers. The CUSA handpiece encloses a hollow titanium tube that vibrates at high frequency in a longitudinal axis; the variable amplitude of longitudinal vibration determines the depth of tissue disruption when the handpiece is placed in contact with tissue. The handpiece also contains an irrigation and aspiration system to remove tissue fragments and reduce heat buildup. The extent of tissue disruption is also dependent on the water content of the target tissue, with the CUSA causing relatively greater damage to tissue with a high water content (eg, visceral parenchyma, nodal

tissue, tumor implants) compared to tissue composed of predominately connective tissue (eg, muscle, ureter, vessel wall adventitia). The CUSA can be used to resect ovarian cancer metastases on the diaphragm, bowel serosa, liver and splenic capsules, and peritoneum. Several reports have cited the efficacy and safety of the CUSA as an adjunctive procedure in achieving optimal cytoreduction in areas inaccessible by more standard surgical techniques. In a prospective trial, the CUSA was associated with lower perioperative blood loss, shorter hospital stay, and less overall morbidity versus when the CUSA was not used during the cytoreductive effort. Although the safety of CUSA has been established in multiple studies, extensive and prolonged use of the CUSA for ovarian cancer cytoreduction should be approached with caution due to the potential for contributing to the development of disseminated intravascular coagulopathy in some patients.

Radiofrequency Ablation

Radiofrequency ablation (RFA) is a minimally invasive technique used to ablate or destroy tumor tissue and is occasionally used in ovarian cancer to cytoreduce intraparenchymal liver implants when liver resection is not feasible or the patient is not a candidate for such an effort. Reports in the literature suggest low rates of optimal cytoreductive efforts with hepatic intraparenchymal involvement, with concomitant decreased survival and need for multidisciplinary surgical approach to the liver resections.[4] RFA involves placing a needle probe into the tumor and passing high-frequency alternating current through the probe to increase the temperature of the tumor, resulting in tissue destruction. The procedure has low morbidity (<5%) and mortality (<1%) while allowing for rapid recovery and expediting treatment with systemic chemotherapy. Complications include thermal injury to adjacent structures like stomach and colon, portal vein thrombosis, biliary tract fistula or strictures, and hemorrhage requiring surgical intervention.

SUTURES

Surgical Needles

Choosing the right surgical needle depends on the type of tissue that is being sutured, accessibility to the tissue, size of suture material, and cosmetic factors. The purpose of surgical needles is to guide suture through tissue while causing minimal injury. Three essential properties of a needle guide its performance: its strength, its malleability, and its sharpness. The needles are manufactured from stainless steel, resist corrosion, and are easily made sterile. Surgical needles are divided into 3 areas, called the point, body (portion grasped by the needle clamp), and shank, which contains the eye. Most commonly, for ease of handling and maintaining, the shank lacks an eye, and instead, the suture is swaged to the shank as a continuous unit. There are also controlled-release sutures, also known as pop-offs, that allow the separation of suture from the needle; these are often used during hysterectomy while securing vascular pedicles. Needles with an open eye for threading are seldom used primarily because of the added inconvenience in handling and need to match the needle to the suture size. They are still sometimes used in vaginal surgery during a Burch suspension or uterosacral ligament fixation.

There are generally 2 needle shapes: curved and straight. The curved needles are called by their curvature: 1/4 (used in microsurgery), 3/8 (vascular pedicles, skin), or 1/2 (fascia or deep body cavities) circle. Their size is reflected by the depth of the wound and the suture size needed, with larger needles corresponding to larger sutures. The needle point is designed for the type of tissue handling required. The points are categorized as conventional cutting, reverse cutting, and round or tapered, depending on their cross-sectional shape. The reverse cutting needle has its cutting edge on the outside, allowing the needle edge to pass away from the wound and resulting in less tendency for the suture to tear through tissue. The round needles are ideal for fascial closure because they tend to leave small holes that resist tearing. The blunt tips were designed to supplement the tapered suture while minimizing needle stick injuries but require more precise tissue placement. The straight Keith needle uses a cutting point and is useful for rapid skin closure of abdominal wounds.

Suture Materials

For the surgeon, the choice of suture material depends on its purpose (ie, fascial closure, securing vascular pedicles, or skin reapproximation). In addition, wound closure and healing depend significantly on patient characteristics such as age, tissue, location of the wound, and medical conditions such as diabetes or steroid use that contribute to postsurgical complications such as infection, seroma, dehiscence, and hernia formations. Incisional hernias occur more often in women than men and are difficult to treat. This incidence can vary from 9% to 20%. Risk factors for incisional hernias include obesity; older age; medical comorbidities such as diabetes, corticosteroid use, or chronic pulmonary disease; malnutrition; and ascites, all which increase intra-abdominal pressure. Excessive tension on the closure and postoperative infection can lead to poor or inadequate healing; delayed complications such as pain, bowel obstruction, incarceration (6%-15%), and strangulation (2%) necessitating repeat surgical measures; and increased risk of recurrence. Incisional hernias can also enlarge

over time, leading to loss of abdominal domain with its potential respiratory dysfunction. Prevention of this complication should be considered the primary goal. Incidentally, small prospective studies in the repair of incisional hernia suggest that laparoscopic approaches yield decreased recurrence and complication rates (specifically infections) versus an open approach.

Historically, there were few surgical options for wound closure. From catgut, silk, and cotton, there is now an ever-increasing array of sutures, including antibiotic-coated and knotless sutures. There are often multiple choices available, and surgeon preference and experience with the material will guide this choice. An ideal suture material and method would prevent dehiscence, pain, infection, and suture sinus and incisional hernias. It is imperative that the surgeon understand the physical properties and tissue handling of the suture material (strength, durability, ease of handling, and resistance to infection)[5] as well as appreciate the dynamics of wound healing. The surgeon must use evidence-based data that were available to select fascial closure technique and suture material to minimize potential complications. Although extremely complex, traditionally wound healing has been described in 3 phases: hemostasis and inflammation (injury to days 4-6), proliferation (day 4-2 weeks), and maturation and remodeling (1 week-1 year.) It is in the last phase when ordered collagen deposition increases, translating to increasing tensile strength in the wound. According to Douglas, abdominal wounds will achieve 50% of normal strength at 2 months, 65% at 4 months, and between 60% and 90% at 1 year.[6] Wounds will never regain their full strength (Figures 23-7 and 23-8 and Table 23-1).

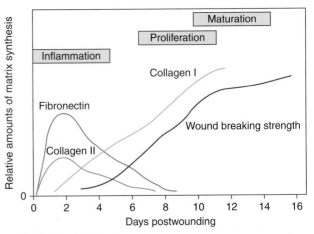

FIGURE 23-7. Wound matrix deposition over time. Fibronectin and type III collagen constitute the early matrix. Type I collagen accumulates later and corresponds to the increase in wound-breaking strength. (Reproduced, with permission, from Witte MB, Barbul A. General principles of wound healing. *Surg Clin North Am.* 1997;77:509-528.)

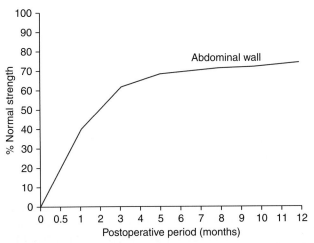

FIGURE 23-8. Healing of laparotomies. (Reproduced, with permission, from Rath AM, Chevrel JP. The healing of laparotomies: Review of the literature. Part 1. Physiologic and pathologic aspects. *Hernia.* 1998;2:145-149.)

The preferred suture material for laparotomy closure should maintain at least half of its strength during the 4 or 5 months following operation. The choice of suture material and closure technique play a large part in the complications and concomitant comorbidities encountered such as fascial dehiscence, fistulas, infection, hernia formation, incisional/chronic pain, and scarring. This has to be balanced with closure methods that are facile, efficient, and secure. Several meta-analyses have demonstrated that the simple mass closure technique of fascial closure such as a looped 1-0 polydioxanone (PDS) suture as opposed to a layered closure has shown reduction in dehiscence

(3.8%-0.8%) and suture sinus formation while being technically easier and taking less operative time. In our experience, the looped PDS has been a reliable suture for the mass closure of vertical incisions, offering all the advantages described in the following sections. Also, in the recent INLINE systematic review and meta-analysis, there was an increased rate of incisional hernias (12.6% vs. 8.4%), with odds ratio of 0.59 (95% confidence interval, 0.43-0.82; $P < .001$), with continuous versus interrupted suture closures. However, rates of wound dehiscence (1.6% vs. 2.6%), suture sinus (0% vs. 1.7%), wound infection (8.0% vs. 4.1%), and wound pain (1.2% vs. 1.7%) were not statistically significant when comparing continuous versus interrupted techniques.[7]

General Characteristics of Suture Materials

As mentioned, an ideal suture would have the following characteristics: ease of handling, high tensile strength, minimal tissue reaction and injury, favorable absorption properties, resistance to infection, and ability to hold a knot securely. However, given the heterogeneity of tissue composition and differences in requirements for wound closure, different suture characteristics are necessary. The following are general characteristics that pertain to categories useful to consider in surgical cases.

Suture Size

There are 2 standards currently in use to describe suture size: the US Pharmacopoeia (USP) classification system, established in 1937 for standardization and comparison of suture materials, and the European

Table 23-1 Absorption Rates of Absorbable Sutures

Suture	Time to 50% Loss of Tensile Strength (days)	Time to Complete Loss of Tensile Strength (days)	Time to Complete Mass Absorption (days)
Plain surgical gut[a]	3-5	14-21	70
Fast-absorbing coated polyglactin 910 (Vicryl Rapide)	5	14	42
Poliglecaprone 25 (Monocryl)	7	21	91-119
Chromic surgical gut[a]	7-10	14-21	90-120
Coated polyglycolide (Dexon II)	14-21	28	60-90
Coated polyglactin 910 (Vicryl)	21	28	56-70
Polyglyconate (Maxon)	28-35	56	180
Polydioxanone (PDS II)	28-42	90	183-238

[a]Extreme variability based on tissue type, infection, and other biologic conditions. Dexon II and Maxon, Covidien AG, Mansfield, MA; Monocryl, PDS II, Vicryl, and Vicryl Rapide, Ethicon, Inc., Somerville, NJ.
Modified, with permission, from Greenberg JA, Clark RM. Advances in suture material for obstetric and gynecologic surgery. *Rev Obstet Gynecol.* 2009;2(3):146-158.

Pharmacopoeia (EP). The USP system is more commonly used or listed. There are 3 classes of sutures generally used: collagen, synthetic absorbable, and nonabsorbable. Size refers to the diameter of the suture strand and is denoted by zeroes. The more zeroes characterizing a suture size, the smaller the resultant strand diameter (eg, 2-0, or 00, is larger than 4-0, or 0000).

Tensile Strength

Tensile strength is the measured force required force to break the suture usually and is measured in pounds or kilograms of force. There is a direct relationship between the suture size and tensile strength. The larger the suture size is, the greater the tensile strength of the strand. Suture material should have, and maintain, adequate tensile strength for its specified purpose, which is to prevent disruptive forces during wound healing.[8] Smaller sutures with smaller diameters have a higher tendency to tear through tissue, whereas larger strands with more material can lead to increased tissue reactivity. Tensile strength measurements are noted as straight pull or knot-pull, also known as "effective tensile strength," and measured as the force required to break a strand that has a knot in it. The knot-pull tensile strength is considered to represent true tissue-holding capacity and is always approximately one-third lower than the straight-pull strength.[8]

Absorption

Sutures are categorized as absorbable or nonabsorbable, depending on their ability to undergo degradation and absorption via proteolysis or hydrolysis. Most foreign material will to some degree undergo degradation. It as an important characteristic for the suture material to maintain tensile strength to allow for wound healing to take place while undergoing absorption to prevent late complications associated with nonabsorbable materials. Nonabsorbable sutures tend to resist absorption and maintain their tensile strength, whereas absorbable sutures tend to lose most of their tensile strength within 60 days. They are then subclassified into rapidly or slowly absorbed sutures. It should be noted that absorption is a suture characteristic distinct from the rate of tensile strength loss. A suture may display rapid loss of tensile strength yet be absorbed slowly.[8] The recent INLINE meta-analysis indicated that slowly absorbable sutures, versus nonabsorbable sutures, had significantly decreased rates of incisional hernias (6.1% vs. 26.3%) and suture sinus (0% vs. 9.0%). With regard to slowly versus rapidly absorbable sutures, a decreased rate of incisional hernias was seen with slowly absorbable sutures (8.1% vs. 10.8%). There were no statistically significant differences in wound dehiscence, infections, or pain.[7]

Multifilament Versus Monofilament

Multifilament sutures are constructed from more than 1 fiber by braiding (eg, polyglycolic acid [Dexon] and polyglactin 910 [vicryl]) or twisting (eg, plain or surgical gut) the strands together. Monofilament sutures, such as nylon and PDS, are made from a single strand of material. Multifilament sutures do not offer significant advantage from a wound healing aspect. Their enhanced capillarity and fluid absorption make them more prone to the transport and spread of infection. Because of their construction, they tend to have a rougher surface, leading to an increased drag coefficient, causing microtrauma as they are pulled through tissue and inciting an inflammatory response. All vicryl and Dexon sutures are now manufactured with a coating of lubricant to enhance their handling and performance. Generally, multifilament sutures tend to exhibit a better "stiffness" and "flexibility" profile compared with monofilaments, which also provides better knot security. It is counterintuitive that monofilaments exhibit characteristics opposed to those possessed by multifilament sutures. Their main disadvantage is their stiffness and elasticity, which requires multiple knots to be placed for securing the suture in tissue. Nylon's high memory has a tendency to loosen the knot, whereas polypropylene's (Prolene) plasticity, the capacity to be permanently molded or altered, could potentially loosen the suture in tissue undergoing expansion with edema. Their significant inertness, however, makes them desirable.

Historically, the number of suture materials that were available was quite limited. Collagen, from sheep or cow intestine, and silk sutures were dominant prior to World War II. With advances in polymer chemistry, new synthetic fibers were discovered, leading to nylon, polyester, and polypropylene sutures. However, these were nonabsorbable sutures. It was not until the 1970s that synthetic absorbable sutures were introduced that possessed improved and reliable tensile strength while eliciting less intense tissue reactions. A decade later, in the 1980s, newer polymers were manufactured (PDS and polyglycolide-trimethylene carbonate [Maxon]) that had adequate handling characteristics while being absorbable and monofilaments.[7] More than a decade ago, new absorbable monofilament sutures were developed constructed with segmented block copolymers consisting of soft and hard segments, such as poliglecaprone 25 (Monocryl); these sutures have better handling, maintaining their tensile strength while reducing absorption rates (see Table 23-1). Recent addition of the barbed suture to the list of available suture materials, such as the barbed PDS (PD0), offers the potential for a knotless suture with improved strength profile across the incision, decreased tissue reaction, and improved operative times. It is an expensive suture to use, and more experience needs to be gleaned for its applicability.

Suture Knots

Basic knot tying skill is essential. Techniques include 2-handed or single-handed methods as well as an instrument tie. As we have mentioned, the knot decreases the tensile strength of the tie being placed. Use of synthetic monofilament sutures also decreases knot security and increases possible slippage, requiring extra throws to ensure a secure knot. Regarding knot strength, sliding knots with extra throws are as secure as square knots, and surgeon's knots are no more secure than square knots for smaller diameter sutures.

CONCLUSIONS

Fluency in surgical techniques implies an understanding of the advantages and limitations within the arsenal of surgical instruments at the surgeon's disposal. Nothing is more essential than a preplanned case with instruments immediately available to the surgeon. Recent developments in instrument technology have been important in reducing operative time and surgical morbidity, but these should not be substitutes for a comprehensive knowledge of basic surgical skills.

REFERENCES

1. Jones WB, Myers KM, Traxler LB, Bour ES. Clinical results using bioabsorbable staple line reinforcement for circular staplers. *Am Surg.* 2008;74(6):462-467; discussion 467-468.
2. Harris WJ, Wheeless CR Jr. Use of the end-to-end anastomosis stapling device in low colorectal anastomosis associated with radical gynecologic surgery. *Gynecol Oncol.* 1986;23(3):350-357.
3. Kyo S, Mizumoto Y, Takakura M, et al. Experience and efficacy of a bipolar vessel sealing system for radical abdominal hysterectomy. *Int J Gynecol Cancer.* 2009;19(9):1658-1661.
4. Bosquet JG, Merideth MA, Podratz KC, Nagorney DM. Hepatic resection for metachronous metastases from ovarian carcinoma. *HPB (Oxford).* 2006;8(2):93-96.
5. Ceydeli A, Rucinski J, Wise L. Finding the best abdominal closure: an evidence-based review of the literature. *Curr Surg.* 2005;62(2):220-225.
6. Douglas DM. Wound healing. *Proc R Soc Med.* 1969;62(5):513.
7. Diener MK, Voss S, Jensen K, Buchler MW, Seiler CM. Elective midline laparotomy closure: the INLINE systematic review and meta-analysis. *Ann Surg.* 2010;251(5):843-856.
8. Greenberg JA, Clark RM. Advances in suture material for obstetric and gynecologic surgery. *Rev Obstet Gynecol.* 2009;2(3):146-158.

24 Ovarian and Fallopian Tube Procedures

Eric L. Eisenhauer and Jeffrey M. Fowler

SALPINGO-OOPHORECTOMY

Procedure Overview

Unilateral salpingo-oophorectomy (USO) and bilateral salpingo-oophorectomy (BSO) are performed for a wide variety of indications. In gynecologic oncology, there is a fundamental distinction between USO/BSO performed for an identified lesion (eg, pelvic mass, ovarian cyst) and risk-reducing salpingo-oophorectomy (RRSO) performed to decrease the risk of subsequent ovarian and breast cancer in women at increased genetic risk. Indications for USO/BSO for symptoms or suspected ovarian malignancy are detailed more completely in Chapter 11. Recommendations for RRSO should be based on the individual woman's risk for ovarian cancer. In the recent report of the Society of Gynecologic Oncologists Clinical Practice Committee, Berek et al[1] detail these risk groups. Women with *BRCA1* and *BRCA2* mutations may reduce their risk of an associated gynecologic cancer by 96% and their risk of an associated breast cancer by 50% to 80% by undergoing RRSO after completion of desired childbearing. Women without a germline mutation who are at higher than average risk because of a strong family history of breast or ovarian cancer may also benefit from RRSO, but the absolute risk reduction is less clear. In premenopausal women at average risk for ovarian cancer undergoing hysterectomy for benign disease, the decision for oophorectomy should be individualized based on the patient's personal risk factors.

Clinical outcomes after salpingo-oophorectomy as an isolated procedure are determined by both the surgical approach and menopausal status of the patient. Minimally invasive USO/BSO is generally an outpatient procedure with a short recovery period and low complication rate, whereas recovery after USO/BSO requiring laparotomy is longer as determined by the larger incision. Oophorectomy in premenopausal women results in menopausal symptoms in the majority of patients. Subsequent therapy for surgical menopause is determined by the severity of symptoms, specific risks related to hormone therapy, and patient choice. There are several studies suggesting an overall negative health impact when BSO is performed before the age of menopause. Among other findings, an observational study from the Nurse's Health Study found that women younger than 50 years who had BSO and never used estrogen had increased rates of all-cause mortality, coronary heart disease, and stroke.[2]

Preoperative Preparation

Preoperative evaluation for most patients consists of physical examination and radiologic and/or serologic studies. Pertinent examination findings include the size and mobility of a palpable mass, associated or referred pain symptoms, or the presence of adjacent cul-de-sac nodularity. Ultrasound, computed tomography (CT), and magnetic resonance imaging (MRI) can each play a role in preoperative characterization of adnexal findings and associated abnormalities within and outside of the pelvis. Serologic studies can include both standard preoperative testing (eg, complete blood count, chemistry, type and screen, and pregnancy test, as appropriate) and testing directed toward the risk of malignancy (eg, tumor markers, as detailed in Chapter 11). Preanesthesia risk assessment should be individualized by cardiopulmonary risk factors and other relevant medical issues.

Considerations for informed consent include those specific to the surgical approach, as well as those determined by menopausal status and hereditary risk factors. Blood loss is generally minimal, but may be higher for large masses or those associated with endometriosis. Wound infection risk is low for both minimally invasive and open approaches, but may be increased by obesity, diabetes, and other risk factors. Because several studies have suggested an overall negative health impact when BSO is performed before menopause, clear discussion of expected benefits and risks should be held before surgery. Finally, women with *BRCA1* and *BRCA2* mutations should be informed that despite the substantial ovarian and breast cancer risk reduction, the risk of peritoneal carcinoma after RRSO remains approximately 1%. A small tubal remnant remains in the uterine cornua after the fallopian tube is divided medially. However, fallopian tube cancers generally originate in the fimbriated portion, and the risk for subsequent cancer developing in this retained segment is uncertain but probably low.[3]

Patients should have nothing by mouth for 6 to 8 hours before surgery. Bowel preparation is not required but may be preferred by some surgeons to improve exposure for minimally invasive approaches. Intravenous antibiotics prior to skin incision should be administered to decrease wound infection risk. The myriad tools available to perform USO/BSO result in similar outcomes and are determined by availability and preference, but should be requested when the case is scheduled to limit delays on the day of surgery.

Operative Procedure

Box 24-2	Caution Points

- The position of the ipsilateral ureter varies, but generally passes under the infundibulopelvic (IP) vessels to descend over the pelvic brim medial to the IP.
- Ovarian tissue may extend into the IP ligament up to 1.5 cm from the visible margin.
- A small tubal remnant remains in the uterine cornua after the fallopian tube is divided medially.

The patient may be positioned in modified dorsal lithotomy in Allen stirrups if vaginal access is required for dilation and curettage or if use of uterine manipulator is preferred. Alternatively, supine positioning is appropriate if these procedures are not required. A Foley catheter should be placed, and an oral-gastric tube is preferred before minimally invasive port placement to decrease the risk of gastric injury. Open approaches generally involve a midline incision extended as necessary for the pelvic mass, and a fixed retractor may be helpful. For minimally invasive approaches, port placement will depend on the mode favored (laparoscopic or robotic) but should be arranged superior to the known ovarian mass. At a minimum, these approaches require a camera port and at least 2 instrument ports, and ports should be spaced to allow instruments to be moved independently. The diameter of the ports is determined by preference and availability; cameras, instruments, and cautery devices can range from 3 to 10 mm. Incorporating at least one 10-mm port facilitates removal of the surgical specimen. The camera port is placed first, and either open placement of a Hasson cannula or closed insufflation with a Veress needle may be used. The remaining ports are placed under direct visualization. Recently, successful outcomes have been reported after laparoendoscopic single-site RRSO.[4] This approach involves multiple ports closely placed within a single 2-cm umbilical incision and is a viable approach worthy of further study.

Regardless of approach, the remaining steps involve safely dividing the ovaries and tubes from their supportive and vascular attachments. Peritoneal washings are taken and sent for cytology. Adnexal and other adhesions are dissected free to maximize exposure and biopsied if suspicious for malignancy. The lateral pelvic peritoneum is divided from the round ligament to the level of the infundibulopelvic (IP) ligament (Figure 24-1). At

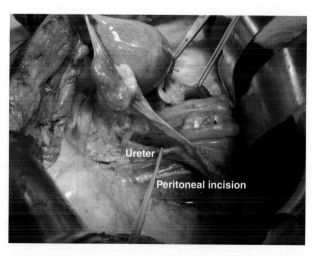

FIGURE 24-1. Peritoneal incision with identification of ureter and infundibulopelvic ligament.

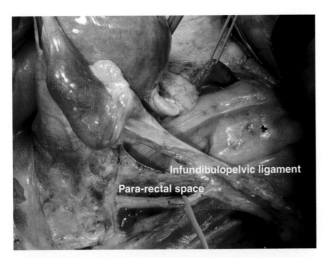

FIGURE 24-2. Salpingo-oophorectomy. Development of para-rectal space and relationship of ureter and infundibulopelvic ligament.

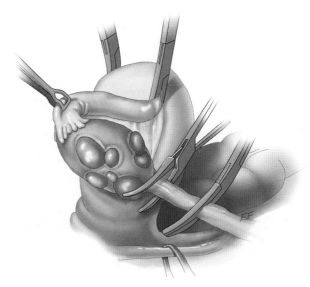

FIGURE 24-3. Salpingo-oophorectomy. Clamping of infundibulopelvic ligament (ovarian vessels).

laparotomy, the broad ligament is opened using sharp scissor dissection or the electrosurgical unit. At laparoscopy, laparoscopic scissors, harmonic scalpel, or argon beam coagulator can be used. The medial leaf of the broad ligament is retracted toward the midline, the para-rectal space is developed toward the pelvic floor, and the ureter is identified at the pelvic brim and traced distally along the broad ligament or vice versa (Figure 24-2). It is important to determine the proximity of the ureter at the pelvic brim to the IP ligament and the proximal ovarian border. Because ovarian tissue can be extended within the IP up to 1.5 cm from the visible ovarian border, the IP should be divided approximately 2 cm from the ovary.[5] Identifying the ureteral position at the pelvic brim ensures that this can be done safely. The IP ligament is then mobilized from the pelvic sidewall vessels and isolated by creating a window in the medial leaf of the broad ligament between it and the ureter. The ovary can be elevated and the IP safely divided between clamps (Figure 24-3). A single or double suture ligature of 0 or 2-0 delayed absorbable suture is used to secure the infundibulopelvic ligament pedicle (Figure 24-4). Laparoscopic options for dividing and sealing the IP include bipolar cautery, LigaSure (Covidien, Mansfield, MA), harmonic scalpel, stapling devices, and laparoscopic or open ties (Figures 24-5 and 24-6).

The broad ligament is then divided medially along the superior border of the round ligament to the uterine cornua. The fallopian tube and utero-ovarian ligament are divided individually when using a minimally invasive surgical approach or divided as a combined unit if approached via laparotomy and secured with a Heaney transfixion stitch of 0 or 2-0 delayed absorbable suture (Figures 24-7 and 24-8). Any of the

previously mentioned laparoscopic instruments can be used for this purpose. Consideration should given to cauterizing the tubal remnant in the uterine cornua for all women at increased genetic risk; this is most easily performed with the bipolar cautery or LigaSure. For minimally invasive procedures, the specimen is placed in an endoscopic bag and delivered through the 10-mm port site. Larger cystic ovarian masses can be decompressed once the open end of the bag is brought out through the incision. Solid masses may require extending the skin and fascial incisions for removal. Instrument ports should be removed under

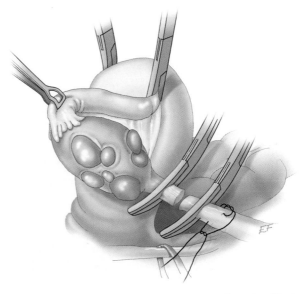

FIGURE 24-4. Salpingo-oophorectomy. The infundibulopelvic ligament is secured with a suture ligature.

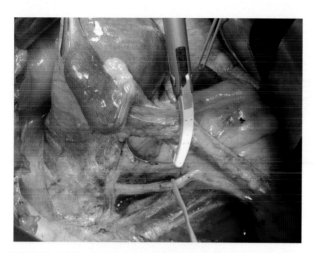

FIGURE 24-5. Salpingo-oophorectomy. The infundibulopelvic ligament is divided using a vessel-sealing device (LigaSure).

laparoscopic visualization to prevent bowel or omentum being drawn up into the defect. The fascia at all port sites larger than 8 mm should be closed laparoscopically or directly to decrease the risk of port site hernia, and the skin should be closed with subcuticular suture, skin adhesive, or both.

Postoperative Care

Box 24-3	Complications and Morbidity

- Ureteral injury at the pelvic brim
- Occult bowel injury from trocar placement or instrument
- Port site or incisional hernia
- Bleeding from inadequately secured infundibulopelvic ligament

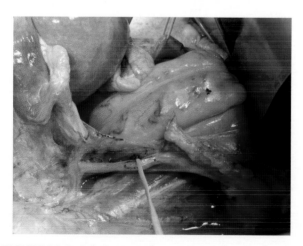

FIGURE 24-6. Salpingo-oophorectomy. Infundibulopelvic ligament is divided by a vessel-sealing device.

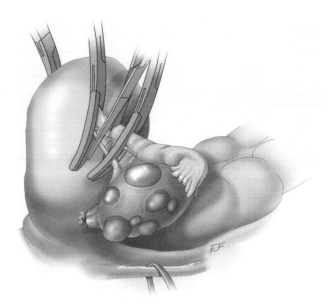

FIGURE 24-7. Salpingo-oophorectomy. Division of utero-ovarian ligament and fallopian tube.

For minimally invasive USO/BSO, patients are generally discharged home with instructions and oral pain medication, whereas after open procedures, patients may be admitted for 1 to 2 days. Complications after USO/BSO are rare but generally appear after this period. Bleeding from an unsecured IP ligament may initially cause low urine output and weakness from associated anemia. If left undetected, patients will acutely worsen as they develop hemorrhagic shock. Ureteral injuries can occur through ligation, transection, or

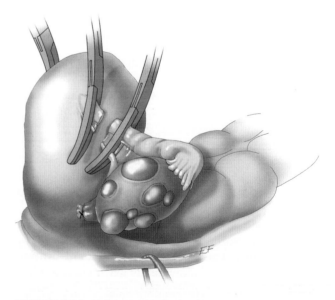

FIGURE 24-8. Salpingo-oophorectomy. Utero-ovarian ligament and fallopian tube pedicle secured with a transfixion stitch.

devascularization. Ligation injuries may manifest after several days with ipsilateral flank pain due to hydroureter, hydronephrosis, or pyelonephritis. Transection or devascularization injuries may manifest later with fever or drainage through the vaginal cuff if a hysterectomy was also performed. Unless both ureters are ligated, any increase in serum creatinine is likely to be transient and may be missed after the first postoperative day. Occult bowel injury will usually present with signs of infection as peritonitis develops and may be detected by contrast-enhanced CT scan. Port site hernias can develop early or late and may be found when the patient has either incisional or gastrointestinal discomfort. If incarcerated, these patients may become acutely worse and require bowel resection. Fortunately, by investigating the patient symptoms, hernias can often be detected and reduced before bowel resection is required.

OVARIAN TRANSPOSITION

Procedure Overview

Box 24-4	Master Surgeon's Corner

- Radiation exposure should decrease the further the ovary is mobilized from the radiation field.
- Ovarian transposition itself can cause ovarian failure if the gonadal vessels are compromised through excessive angulation or tension.
- The ovary should therefore be secured as high above the pelvic brim as mobilization of the gonadal vessels allows.

Ovarian transposition, or oophoropexy, is a procedure performed in premenopausal women who will or potentially will undergo pelvic radiation therapy. In gynecologic oncology, this is most commonly indicated for cervical cancer, although it is also performed for a wide variety of hematologic and solid malignancies in girls and young women. Preservation of ovarian function depends on a number of factors, including the reproductive age of the patient and corresponding ovarian reserve, total dose of radiation therapy, the fractionation schedule, and which chemotherapy agents are used.[6] Depending on the patient's age, ovarian irradiation doses from 12 to 20 Gy will generally cause permanent ovarian ablation, and if the ovaries remain within the radiation field, the received dose will typically exceed this. The goal of transposition is to limit the ovarian radiation exposure by surgically moving them as far as possible from the target field. Historical rates of ovarian failure after transposition have run as high as 50% and are likely a function of both radiation scatter and

vascular compromise to the gonadal vessels from the transposition procedure itself. Better patient selection and minimally invasive techniques may improve these rates in the future.

Preoperative Preparation

Because ovarian reserve declines with age, younger patients are more likely to have successful preservation of ovarian function after radiation therapy. In patients with other risk factors for ovarian failure, it may be appropriate to evaluate gonadal function prior to ovarian transposition. Risk tables based on age and expected radiation dose are available and can be useful for providing preoperative informed consent (Table 24-1).[7] The patient should also be informed that in addition to standard surgical complications, the procedure itself carries a risk of causing ovarian failure and/or chronic pain.

Patients should have nothing by mouth for 6 to 8 hours before surgery. Bowel preparation is not required but may be helpful to improve exposure for minimally invasive approaches. Intravenous antibiotics prior to skin incision should be administered to decrease wound infection risk. Instruments required vary by surgeon preference, but for minimally invasive approaches should include a laparoscopic clip applier so that the lower ovarian poles can be tagged for radiographic identification.

Operative Procedure

Box 24-5	Caution Points

- Limit direct cautery exposure to the ovary during mobilization.
- Remove attached fallopian tube unless doing so will compromise ovarian blood supply.
- How high the ovary can be fixed and the degree of angulation to the infundibulopelvic vessels can be competing concerns.

The positioning of the patient and setup for operative access are the same as described for a USO/BSO procedure. Ovarian transposition is frequently performed as part of a larger primary procedure and, if performed by laparotomy, will generally involve a midline incision extended as necessary for the primary procedure. For minimally invasive approaches, port placement will depend on the mode favored (laparoscopic or robotic) but should allow both for mobilization of the ovary in the pelvis and placement and fixation in the paracolic gutter.

Table 24-1 Predicted Age at Ovarian Failure With 95% Confidence Limits for Ages at Treatment From 0 to 30 Years and for Doses of 3, 6, 9, and 12 Gy

Age	3 Gy			6 Gy			9 Gy			12 Gy		
	Low	Mean	High	Low	Mean	High	Low	Mean	High	Low	Mean	High
0	31.2	35.1	39.0	18.7	22.6	26.5	9.8	13.7	17.6	4.0	7.9	11.8
1	31.3	35.2	39.1	19.0	22.9	26.8	10.4	14.3	18.2	4.8	8.7	12.6
2	31.5	35.4	39.3	19.3	23.2	27.1	10.9	14.8	18.7	5.5	9.4	13.3
3	31.6	35.5	39.4	19.7	23.6	27.5	11.5	15.4	19.3	6.2	10.1	14.0
4	31.7	35.6	39.5	20.1	24.0	27.9	12.1	16.0	19.9	6.9	10.8	14.7
5	31.9	35.8	39.7	20.5	24.4	28.3	12.7	16.6	20.5	7.7	11.6	15.5
6	32.1	36.0	39.9	20.9	24.8	28.7	13.3	17.2	21.1	8.4	12.3	16.2
7	32.2	36.1	40.0	21.3	25.2	29.1	13.9	17.8	21.7	9.1	13.0	16.9
8	32.4	36.3	40.2	21.7	25.6	29.5	14.6	18.5	22.4	9.9	13.8	17.7
9	32.6	36.5	40.4	22.1	26.0	29.9	15.2	19.1	23.0	10.6	14.5	18.4
10	32.8	36.7	40.6	22.6	26.5	30.4	15.8	19.7	23.6	11.4	15.3	19.2
11	33.0	36.9	40.8	23.0	26.9	30.8	16.5	20.4	24.3	12.1	16.0	19.9
12	33.2	37.1	41.0	23.5	27.4	31.3	17.1	21.0	24.9	12.9	16.8	20.7
13	33.4	37.3	41.2	23.9	27.8	31.7	17.8	21.7	25.6	13.6	17.5	21.4
14	33.6	37.5	41.4	24.4	28.3	32.2	18.5	22.4	26.3	14.4	18.3	22.2
15	33.9	37.8	41.7	24.9	28.8	32.7	19.1	23.0	26.9	15.1	19.0	22.9
16	34.1	38.0	41.9	25.4	29.3	33.2	19.8	23.7	27.6	15.9	19.8	23.7
17	34.3	38.2	42.1	25.9	29.8	33.7	20.5	24.4	28.3	17.0	20.5	24.4
18	34.6	38.5	42.4	26.4	30.3	34.2	21.2	25.1	29.0	18.0	21.3	25.2
19	34.9	38.8	42.7	27.0	30.9	34.8	21.8	25.7	29.6	19.0	22.0	25.9
20	35.1	39.0	42.9	27.5	31.4	35.3	22.5	26.4	30.3	20.0	22.8	26.7
21	35.4	39.3	43.2	28.0	31.9	35.8	23.2	27.1	31.0	21.0	23.5	27.4
22	35.7	39.6	43.5	28.6	32.5	36.4	23.9	27.8	31.7	22.0	24.3	28.2
23	36.0	39.9	43.8	29.1	33.0	36.9	24.6	28.5	32.4	23.0	25.0	28.9
24	36.3	40.2	44.1	29.7	33.6	37.5	25.3	29.2	33.1	24.0	25.7	29.6
25	36.7	40.6	44.5	30.3	34.2	38.1	25.9	29.8	33.7	25.0	26.5	30.4
26	37.0	40.9	44.8	30.8	34.7	38.6	26.6	30.5	34.4	26.0	27.2	31.1
27	37.3	41.2	45.1	31.4	35.3	39.2	27.3	31.2	35.1	27.0	27.9	31.8
28	37.7	41.6	45.5	32.0	35.9	39.8	28.0	31.9	35.8	28.0	28.7	32.6
29	38.0	41.9	45.8	32.5	36.4	40.3	29.0	32.6	36.5	29.0	29.4	33.3
30	38.3	42.2	46.1	33.1	37.0	40.9	30.0	33.2	37.1	30.0	30.1	34.0

Reproduced, with permission, from Wallace WH, Thomson AB, Saran F, Kelsey TW. Predicting age of ovarian failure after radiation to a field that includes the ovaries. *Int J Radiat Oncol Biol Phys.* 2005;62(3):738-744.

Regardless of approach, the remaining steps involve safely dividing the ovary or ovaries from uterine and tubal attachments and mobilizing the gonadal vessels to prevent vessel angulation. Adnexal and other adhesions are dissected free to maximize exposure and biopsied if suspicious for malignancy. The lateral pelvic peritoneum is divided from the round ligament to the level of the IP ligament. This can be safely performed with laparoscopic scissors, harmonic scalpel, or argon beam coagulator. The medial leaf of the broad ligament is retracted medially, and the ureter is identified and separated from the IP ligament. The broad

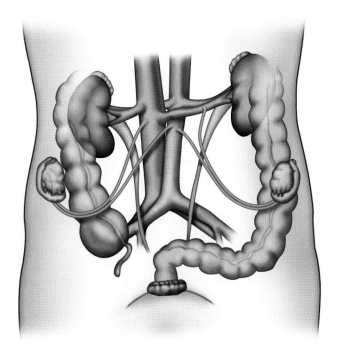

FIGURE 24-9. Diagram illustrating the location of the transposed adnexa to a nonpelvic site where they can be spared from pelvic irradiation.

ligament is then divided medially along the superior border of the round ligament to the uterine cornua. The fallopian tube is divided at the cornua, followed by the utero-ovarian ligament.

Freed of its uterine attachments, the fallopian tube is elevated, and if an adequate plane exists within the mesosalpinx, the fallopian tube can be separated from the ovary. If a plane is not present or removing it might risk devascularization of the ovary, the tubal segment is not removed. The ovary is then elevated gently, and the gonadal vessels are separated from the underlying ureter to a level above the pelvic brim. Once this plane is developed, the gonadal pedicle can be mobilized superiorly from its peritoneal attachments, while keeping the underlying ureter in the visual field. The position of the ovary in the lateral paracolic gutter is tested to ensure that the gonadal vessels will not be placed under excessive angulation. The para-ovarian tissue is then sutured to the peritoneum in the paracolic gutter, and the inferior pole is tagged with a metal clip for future radiologic identification (Figure 24-9).[8] If performed as part of an open procedure, the sutures can be placed directly. As a minimally invasive procedure, the sutures can either be placed and tied intracorporeally or placed, grasped with an EndoClose (Covidien) needle placed through a small lateral skin incision, and tied extracorporeally. Instrument removal and port closure procedures are the same as described for the USO/BSO procedure.

Postoperative Care

Box 24-6	Complications and Morbidity

- Resultant ovarian failure
- Pain from subsequent benign ovarian cyst
- Occult bowel or ureteral injury
- Port site hernia

For minimally invasive ovarian transposition prior to definitive chemoradiation, patients are generally discharged home the same day. If performed as part of a larger open procedure, patients may be admitted for a period of time commensurate with their primary procedure. Complications related to the ovarian transposition generally develop after this period. The risk of subsequent benign ovarian cysts, often necessitating additional surgery, may be as high as 25%, and the risk of resultant ovarian failure has been reported as high as 50%.[9] For patients with cervical adenocarcinoma, there is a small but significant risk of occult ovarian metastases that are now mobilized out of the radiation field. The risks of occult bowel and ureteral injury and of port site herniation are as detailed in the previous Salpingo-Oophorectomy section.

OVARIAN REMNANT SURGERY

Procedure Overview

Box 24-7	Master Surgeon's Corner

- Resection of an ovarian remnant often involves a difficult complete sidewall dissection.
- Identification and mobilization of the pelvic ureter are essential. Temporary ureteral stents may be helpful.
- Placing an EEA sizer in the vagina may assist in the surgical dissection by providing counter-tension and assists in identifying critical anatomy.
- The ovarian remnant must be removed completely with a margin of normal tissue.

Ovarian remnant syndrome (ORS) develops in women after BSO who have ovarian tissue left behind, distinguishing these patients from women who have a residual ovary left intentionally behind after prior USO. Patients frequently present with pelvic pain,

pain associated with a pelvic mass, or an asymptomatic pelvic mass. Risk factors relate to conditions that cause pelvic adhesive disease, such as endometriosis, pelvic inflammatory disease, and prior gynecologic surgery. Because of these predisposing factors, surgery for ORS is frequently a difficult procedure, requiring at least a modest pelvic sidewall dissection with a higher risk for ureteral, bowel, and vascular injury.

Preoperative Preparation

Preoperative evaluation includes history, examination, and imaging findings consistent with ORS. Premenopausal levels of follicle-stimulating hormone and estradiol may be present in 60% to 70% of patients but are not uniformly diagnostic.[10] Because ORS often develops in the setting of prior adhesive disease, MRI may be useful to delineate the relative positions of the ovarian remnant, ureter, and bowel. Assessment of integrity of the urinary collecting system with CT urography may be helpful. Preoperative bowel preparation is helpful both for ease of exposure and reducing the risk of bowel injury.

Informed consent should convey a modest risk of injury to the bladder, ureter, and bowel.[10,11] Although reported incidence for each is generally less than 5%, it is significantly higher than for standard oophorectomy. Blood loss is higher, with approximately 10% of patients requiring transfusion. With pathologic demonstration of removal, the recurrence risk should be low.

Operative Procedure

Box 24-8	Caution Points

- First restore normal anatomy by freeing adhesions in the pelvic sidewall and posterior cul-de-sac.
- Assume that the ovarian remnant was retained because it was initially in a difficult position. Identify the borders of the ureter, bowel, and iliac vessels early because the remnant is likely to be adherent.
- In the setting of a densely adherent sidewall mass, ureteral stents may help delineate normal anatomy.

The procedure is preferably performed in the modified dorsal lithotomy position, so that manual access to the vagina and rectum is available if required. Temporary ureteral stents are placed cystoscopically if desired and inserted through the side of the Foley catheter to drain into the same bag. An oral-gastric tube is placed prior to minimally invasive procedures.

Open approaches generally involve a midline incision extended as necessary for the pelvic mass, and a fixed retractor is usually helpful. For minimally invasive approaches, port placement will depend on the mode favored (laparoscopic or robotic), but should be arranged superior to the field of dissection. Choice of instruments is determined by surgeon preference and by surgical approach. For laparoscopic procedures, endoshears with monopolar cautery, argon beam coagulator, LigaSure, and harmonic scalpel can all be used with good effect. Cold dissection without cautery is preferred for dissection in close proximity to ureter and bowel. Additional ports to improve exposure and suction may be required.

The first step is to restore as much of the normal anatomy as possible and may require extensive lysis of adhesions to free the sidewall and cul-de-sac. The ureter should be identified at or above the pelvic brim and dissected down below the ovarian mass, if seen, and down to the distal pelvis if the remnant ovary cannot yet be delineated. A retroperitoneal approach is preferred by dividing the lateral peritoneum along the iliac vessels and proceeding medially so that the position of the iliac vessels is lateral to the direction of dissection. Mobilizing the rectum medially from the mass should aid greatly with exposure; this may require sharp dissection along the rectal border, and superficial defects created in the rectal wall may require suture reinforcement. Once the ovarian remnant and normal tissue margin is dissected free from the ureter, rectum, and iliac vessels, the blood supply at the superior border can be divided and the ovarian remnant removed in an endoscopic bag or directly for open procedures. Assessment of ureteral integrity with indigo carmine and confirmation of rectal integrity with a bubble test may be helpful. Closure is determined by initial approach as detailed earlier.

Postoperative Care

Box 24-9	Complications and Morbidity

- Ureteral injury at or below pelvic brim
- Enterotomy during dissection or mobilization
- Intraoperative or postoperative bleeding
- Port site hernia

For minimally invasive procedures, patients are generally discharged home when stable with instructions and oral pain medication. If performed as an open procedure, patients may be admitted for a period of time appropriate to their incision and postoperative symptoms. Injuries recognized intraoperatively will be repaired; unrecognized injuries generally present after hospital discharge. Bleeding complications may be recognized sooner and may require transfusion or reoperation. Occult ureteral and bowel injuries generally present later as described earlier for salpingo-oophorectomy. Ureteral injuries will be more frequently due to devascularization if ureteral integrity was confirmed intraoperatively. Port site hernias can present after minimally invasive procedures and can be recognized early with an appropriate index of suspicion.

REFERENCES

1. Berek JS, Chalas E, Edelson M, et al. Prophylactic and risk-reducing bilateral salpingo-oophorectomy: recommendations based on risk of ovarian cancer. *Obstet Gynecol.* 2010;116(3):733-743.
2. Parker WH, Broder MS, Chang E, et al. Ovarian conservation at the time of hysterectomy and long-term health outcomes in the Nurses' Health Study. *Obstet Gynecol.* 2009;113(5):1027-1037.
3. Cass I, Walts A, Karlan BY. Does risk-reducing bilateral salpingo-oophorectomy leave behind residual tube? *Gynecol Oncol.* 2010;117(1):27-31.
4. Escobar PF, Starks DC, Fader AN, et al. Single-port risk-reducing salpingo-oophorectomy with and without hysterectomy: surgical outcomes and learning curve analysis. *Gynecol Oncol.* 2010;119(1):43-47.
5. Fennimore IA, Simon NL, Bills G, et al. Extension of ovarian tissue into the infundibulopelvic ligament beyond visual margins. *Gynecol Oncol.* 2009;114(1):61-63.
6. Stroud JS, Mutch D, Rader J, et al. Effects of cancer treatment on ovarian function. *Fertil Steril.* 2009;92(2):417-427.
7. Wallace WH, Thomson AB, Saran F, Kelsey TW. Predicting age of ovarian failure after radiation to a field that includes the ovaries. *Int J Radiat Oncol Biol Phys.* 2005;62(3):738-744.
8. DiSaia PJ. Surgical aspects of cervical carcinoma. *Cancer.* 1981;48(suppl 2):548-559.
9. Gershenson DM. Fertility-sparing surgery for malignancies in women. *J Natl Cancer Inst Monogr.* 2005(34):43-47.
10. Magtibay PM, Nyholm JL, Hernandez JL, Podratz KC. Ovarian remnant syndrome. *Am J Obstet Gynecol.* 2005;193(6):2062-2066.
11. Nezhat C, Kearney S, Malik S, Nezhat C, Nezhat F. Laparoscopic management of ovarian remnant. *Fertil Steril.* 2005;83(4):973-978.

25 Uterine Procedures

John O. Schorge and David M. Boruta II

ABDOMINAL HYSTERECTOMY

Procedure Overview

Approximately 600,000 hysterectomies are performed annually—second only to cesarean delivery as the most frequently performed major surgical procedure for women of reproductive age in the United States. An estimated 20 million US women have had a hysterectomy, more than one-third of them by age 60. Approximately half will undergo concomitant bilateral oophorectomy.[1]

The 5 classes (or types) of hysterectomy were originally defined by Piver et al[2] to more accurately describe the technical features involved when tailoring surgical treatment of women with cervical cancer. Type I hysterectomy, also known as *extrafascial* or *simple hysterectomy*, removes the uterus and cervix, but does not require excision of the parametrium or paracolpium. Within gynecologic oncology, a simple hysterectomy is usually performed for benign conditions, preinvasive cervical disease, stage IA1 cervical cancer, and most instances of endometrial or ovarian cancer. Occasionally, a planned simple hysterectomy must be adapted to a type II or III procedure based on intraoperative findings.

Abdominal hysterectomy was the foundation of gynecologic surgery for the latter half of the 20th century. However, several recent developments have resulted in fewer of these procedures being performed each year, a trend that is expected to continue into the future. Nonoperative techniques, such as office endometrial ablation, insertion of levonorgestrel-releasing intrauterine devices, and outpatient uterine artery embolization, have enabled many women to avoid hysterectomy. Additionally, the rapid introduction of minimally invasive surgery over the past decade has decreased the number of abdominal hysterectomies being performed. In many training programs, abdominal cases are now often mainly performed in extreme circumstances, such as a frozen pelvis or massively enlarged uteri. As a result, residents currently graduating may have more experience using a laparoscopic approach. Since trainees in obstetrics and gynecology are increasingly confronted with a wider range of techniques that must be mastered, and fewer hysterectomies are being performed each year, the need for improved surgical education to achieve competency is increasingly recognized.[3]

Despite the recent paradigm shift to minimally invasive surgery, approximately two-thirds of uteri in the United States are still removed through an abdominal incision. As high-volume surgeons, the majority of gynecologic oncologists have increasingly incorporated laparoscopic and robotic techniques into their practice.[4] However, one-quarter of hysterectomies are performed by gynecologic surgeons who perform fewer than 10 per year. Such lower volume surgeons continue to perform the vast majority of their hysterectomies abdominally.[5]

Abdominal hysterectomy allows the greatest ability to manipulate pelvic organs and thus is often preferred to a minimally invasive approach if large pelvic organs or extensive adhesions are anticipated. Moreover, abdominal hysterectomy typically requires less operating time than laparoscopic or robotic hysterectomy, and no advanced instrumentation or expertise is needed. However, the duration of inpatient hospital stay is longer, and postoperative complications are more prevalent.

Preoperative Preparation

A spectrum of tests may be required to reach the preoperative diagnosis. These tests vary depending on the clinical setting and are discussed within the respective chapters covering those etiologies. Review of all pertinent information and office pelvic examination are crucial to form the best possible surgical plan.

After deciding to perform a hysterectomy, the next decision is to confirm that laparotomy is the best option based on patient circumstances. Abdominal surgery can result in major short- and long-term morbidity, generally exceeding a minimally invasive or vaginal approach. The other major decision in surgical planning is whether a vertical or transverse incision is best. When there is a pre-existing abdominal incision, it may or may not be appropriate for the planned operation. Morbidly obese patients should be examined supine in the office to map out and show where the intended incision will be located. Thereafter, the surgeon can effectively counsel the patient about abdominal hysterectomy via the intended incision. The consent should reflect the thought process behind the approach, as well as all related factors specific to the diagnosis. Concurrent illnesses, prior abdominal surgery, and a poor performance status are potential mitigating circumstances that should be taken into consideration during the consenting process.

Frequently, intra-abdominal findings of gynecologic oncology patients cannot be reliably predicted based on examination or imaging tests. In general, intraoperative bladder injuries are more likely with a history of cesarean section or a large uterus, whereas bowel injuries are more commonly associated with adhesiolysis.[6] Patients should be fully informed that such gastrointestinal or genitourinary injuries are possible, as are unexpected bleeding and the need for transfusion.

Postoperative wound dehiscence, infection, or other unanticipated sequelae are important to discuss.

When performing a hysterectomy abdominally, or by any other route, a blood sample should be typed and crossed for potential transfusion. Pneumatic compression devices, subcutaneous heparin, or both are particularly important due to the anticipated length of the operation and longer duration of postoperative recovery. Bowel preparation with a polyethylene glycol–electrolyte solution (GoLYTELY) is no longer commonly used. Inadvertent bowel injury should be rare unless extenuating circumstances are identified such as previous bowel surgery, known adhesions, or prior pelvic infections. Similarly, the addition of ureteral stenting varies widely, based on surgeon experience and patient circumstances.

A single dose of perioperative antibiotic prophylaxis with a third-generation cephalosporin such as cefoxitin is ordered to be given prior to incision. This is sufficient to prevent most postoperative surgical site infections, but the dose may need to be repeated if the operation continues beyond 4 hours or excessive bleeding is encountered.

Fortunately, abdominal hysterectomy is largely not dependent on specific instrumentation. In general, a self-retaining retractor, such as the Balfour or Bookwalter, is required. However, the surgeon may have particular requests, such as the Bookwalter extender with deep blades for an obese patient, certain coagulation sealing devices, or other relevant items required for an individual case.

Operative Procedure

Box 25-2	Caution Points

- Ensure self-retaining retractor blade tips do not rest on psoas muscles and underlying femoral nerves, especially in thin patients.
- Identify the ureter and understand its location during all phases of the procedure.
- Dense adhesions between the bladder and cervix require sharp, not blunt dissection.
- Stay inside the uterine artery pedicle when clamping the cardinal ligaments to avoid ureteral injury.

Anesthesia and Patient Positioning

Lower extremity compression devices are placed on the patient for venous thrombosis prophylaxis. General endotracheal or regional anesthesia is administered. Many gynecologic oncologists routinely position all abdominal surgery patients in dorsal lithotomy rather than supine position, mainly in the event that access to the perineum for intravaginal manipulation or transrectal placement of stapling devices is required. Frequently, the extent of pelvic disease cannot be anticipated with certainty based on examination findings and preoperative imaging. When positioning in dorsal lithotomy, the patient's legs are placed in Allen stirrups, the buttocks brought down to the table break, and arms secured laterally. Bimanual rectovaginal examination should always be performed to familiarize oneself with the anatomy and to make a final decision on the type of incision.

The abdomen and vagina are surgically prepared, and a Foley catheter is placed. When there is any perceived possibility of bladder injury, a 3-way Foley provides additional access to easily backfill with methylene blue–colored saline, and the integrity of the bladder should be confirmed before abdominal closure.

Abdominal Entry

Abdominal hysterectomy may be safely performed through a midline vertical, Pfannenstiel, Maylard, or Cherney incision. Many factors go into determining which is most appropriate for the particular patient, but adequate exposure is absolutely critical to prepare for unanticipated findings, excessive adhesive disease, or the unexpected need for cancer staging.

Once the fascia has been incised and the abdominal cavity entered, the undersurface of the abdominal wall is palpated to search for omental or intestinal adhesions. To maximize exposure, the peritoneal incision is sharply dissected as cephalad and caudad as possible within the limits of the skin incision. Peritoneal washings, if appropriate, are collected, and a comprehensive abdominal exploration is performed. Occasionally, the incision will be perceived as inadequate and may need to be further extended before proceeding. Bowel adhesions may need to be dissected away from the pelvic organs.

Next, the surgeon's preferred self-retaining retractor is assembled. Meticulous care of blade placement and bowel packing is critical to provide excellent visualization, decrease the likelihood of femoral nerve palsy, and allow for surgical efficiency in performing the subsequent surgical steps.

Retroperitoneal Dissection

Curved Kelly clamps are placed bilaterally at the uterine cornua, incorporating the round ligament. An Allis clamp is used to grasp the round ligament, and a single 0-vicryl is tied and held on a clamp laterally. Tagging the round ligament is particularly helpful whenever pelvic lymphadenectomy is to be later performed. The uterus is held medially to put the round ligament on stretch so that it can be divided with cautery. A right angle clamp is used to guide further cautery dissection of the anterior and posterior leaves of the broad ligament. Occasionally, the round ligament cannot be clearly identified due to pelvic disease or anatomical distortion. In this circumstance, the Allis clamp is used to grasp a section of peritoneum laterally on the pelvic sidewall, cautery is used to incise a small opening, the posterior broad ligament is opened, and the round ligament can be identified later in the dissection.

Loose areolar retroperitoneal connective tissue is bluntly dissected until the external iliac artery is palpated just medial to the psoas muscle. The index and middle fingers then are placed on either side of the artery, and the areolar connective tissue is dissected bluntly by a "walking" motion toward the patient's head (Figure 25-1). The medial peritoneal leaf of the broad ligament is elevated and placed on traction to permit direct identification of the common iliac bifurcation and origins of the external and internal iliac arteries. Blunt dissection with a finger or suction tip is used in a sweeping motion from top to bottom along the medial peritoneal leaf to identify and sufficiently mobilize the ureter crossing at the bifurcation. As a general rule, it is inadequate to just palpate the ureter or assume its location without directly visualizing unequivocal peristalsis. When the peritoneum is held on traction, and the tubular structure presumed to be the ureter is not seen to undergo peristalsis, the surgeon may need to further mobilize it by blunt dissection along its course and relax the peritoneum until its identity is confirmed.

Consistently performing a comprehensive retroperitoneal dissection has a number of potential advantages, including immediate ability to perform hypogastric artery ligation in case of hemorrhage and defining the anatomy when the pelvis is distorted by endometriosis, malignancy, or adhesions. Small vessel bleeding during this dissection can be quickly controlled with directed cautery, or a small sponge can be firmly placed into the space to tamponade general oozing, while switching to work on the contralateral side of the pelvis.

In the presence of diffuse fibrosis or other extenuating circumstances, it may be advisable to tag the ureter for visualization throughout the abdominal hysterectomy procedure. When the ureter is sufficiently mobilized off the medial peritoneal leaf, a right-angle clamp is used to "pop" through the underlying avascular space. Typically, the clamp is placed in a lateral to medial direction to avoid inadvertent injury to the sidewall vasculature. If the ureteral location does not easily allow this, a Babcock clamp can be used to grasp the ureter gently without crush injury and facilitate clamp placement underneath. Next, a ¼-in-wide Penrose drain is guided by a forceps to the right angle tip and slid back underneath the ureter, and the 2 ends are held on a clamp laterally. It is critical to directly

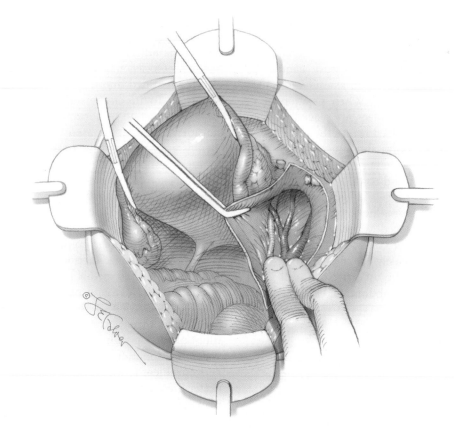

FIGURE 25-1. Finding the ureter. (Redrawn, with permission, from Schorge JO, Schaffer JI, Halvorson LM, et al, eds. *Williams Gynecology*. New York, NY: McGraw-Hill; 2008.)

observe unequivocal peristalsis before moving on to the subsequent surgical steps.

Utero-Ovarian Ligament Transection

The next part of the operation depends on whether the adnexa are to be concurrently removed or not. Once the ureter has been identified, the infundibulopelvic (IP) ligament may be divided and peritoneal attachments dissected, as described in Chapter 24. When the adnexa are to be temporarily or permanently left in situ, division of the utero-ovarian ligament is performed.

Development of the retroperitoneal spaces and transection of the round ligament should enable the surgeon to wrap a finger around the utero-ovarian ligament and identify an avascular space underneath. Cautery is used to open the space sufficiently to place a curved Heaney clamp laterally. The clamp should be placed with tips pointed toward the uterus in order to best secure the lateral vascular pedicle. Usually, the Kelly clamp originally placed on the uterine cornua can simply be repositioned into the opened space to prevent back-bleeding (Figure 25-2). The intervening tissue is divided, followed by a 0-vicryl free tie to crush the vessels while the Heaney clamp is "flashed" (opened and

closed), and then a second 0-vicryl transfixion stitch is placed on the lateral pedicle. A segment of adjacent peritoneum may also be sharply dissected so that the adnexa can be packed away from the operative field. The identical procedures are repeated on the contralateral side.

Bladder Flap

The uterus is pulled upward and cephalad in the midline position to best visualize the vesicouterine fold. The peritoneum that connects the superior edge of the bladder to the uterine isthmus should have been cut when the anterior leaf of the broad ligament was opened. Only loose areolar connective tissue joins the posterior surface of the bladder and anterior surface of the uterine isthmus and cervix. Many gynecologists will bluntly dissect the bladder distally, using either a thumb or sponge stick. However, the complicated circumstances wherein a gynecologic oncologist is performing an abdominal hysterectomy frequently dictate the necessity of careful sharp dissection instead. Tumor infiltration, tissue induration, and postsurgical fibrosis all increase the likelihood of bladder injury or deserosalization with blunt dissection.

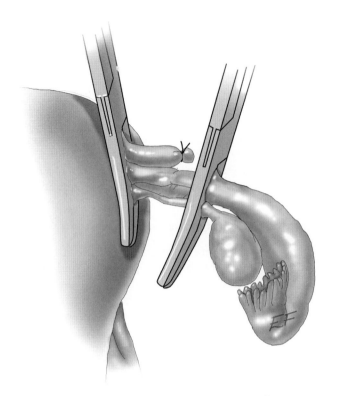

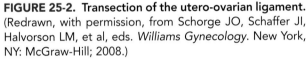

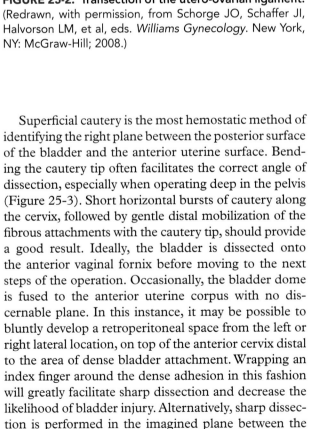

FIGURE 25-2. Transection of the utero-ovarian ligament. (Redrawn, with permission, from Schorge JO, Schaffer JI, Halvorson LM, et al, eds. *Williams Gynecology*. New York, NY: McGraw-Hill; 2008.)

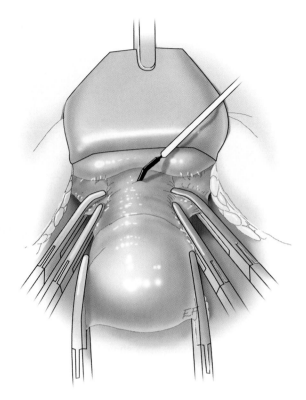

FIGURE 25-3. Dissecting the bladder flap. (Redrawn, with permission, from Schorge JO, Schaffer JI, Halvorson LM, et al, eds. *Williams Gynecology*. New York, NY: McGraw-Hill; 2008.)

Superficial cautery is the most hemostatic method of identifying the right plane between the posterior surface of the bladder and the anterior uterine surface. Bending the cautery tip often facilitates the correct angle of dissection, especially when operating deep in the pelvis (Figure 25-3). Short horizontal bursts of cautery along the cervix, followed by gentle distal mobilization of the fibrous attachments with the cautery tip, should provide a good result. Ideally, the bladder is dissected onto the anterior vaginal fornix before moving to the next steps of the operation. Occasionally, the bladder dome is fused to the anterior uterine corpus with no discernable plane. In this instance, it may be possible to bluntly develop a retroperitoneal space from the left or right lateral location, on top of the anterior cervix distal to the area of dense bladder attachment. Wrapping an index finger around the dense adhesion in this fashion will greatly facilitate sharp dissection and decrease the likelihood of bladder injury. Alternatively, sharp dissection is performed in the imagined plane between the bladder and uterus, with frequent attempts to identify a plane distally. Almost invariably, once the uppermost fibrotic attachments are dissected, the correct plane is encountered at some point thereafter, greatly facilitating distal mobilization of the bladder.

Uterine Artery Ligation

The uterus is again held on medial traction to skeletonize the uterine vessels in order to further drop the ureter laterally and allow an isolated vascular pedicle to be secured. Peritoneal attachments and excess connective tissue are gently retracted laterally with fine, smooth forceps and cauterized in a direction perpendicular toward the vessels. The uterine artery and vein are then visualized along the lateral aspect of the uterus at the level of the isthmus. In extenuating circumstances, a uterine vessel may be lacerated in the course of skeletonizing and lead to brisk bleeding. However, because the bladder flap has been taken down in advance, the vessel can be quickly secured by prompt clamp placement.

A curved Heaney clamp is opened, placed across the uterine vessels inferiorly to the planned site of transection, and purposefully slides off the lateral cervix as it is closed. The clamp tip must be placed as close to the cervix as possible to secure the entire lumen of both artery and vein. Additionally, the clamp should be placed as perpendicular as possible across the vertical axis of the uterine vessels (Figure 25-4). A Kocher or other straight clamp is placed to control back-bleeding above the planned uterine vessel transection

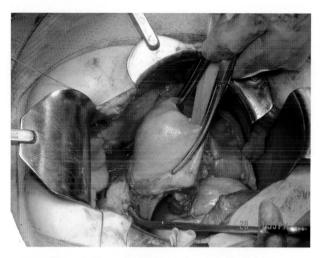

FIGURE 25-4. Clamping the uterine vessels.

so that its tip abuts the tip of the Heaney clamp and crosses the vessels at an approximate 45-degree angle. The uterine vessels are then sharply transected with curved Mayo scissors with blades pointed up, sliding along the Heaney clamp until reaching the distal tip, when the scissors are turned around to gently divide the last remaining tissue and fully isolate the uterine pedicle. The scalpel may be used in place of scissors but may be an inferior choice in some instances. When visualization is limited by obesity, a bulky uterus, or other mitigating circumstances, the uterine vessels may still be divided safely by the surgeon's "feel" of the Mayo scissors along the Heaney clamp to reach its tip, whereas the scalpel is a less-controlled approach.

A simple stitch of 0-gauge delayed-absorbable suture is placed below the tip of the Heaney clamp, with the needle directed posteriorly away from the bladder. The suture ends are wrapped to the heel of the clamp and tied directly against the back of the Heaney clamp with release upon cinching the knot. Next, the uterus is again pulled upward, and a straight Heaney or Zeppelin clamp is placed medially, inside the uterine pedicle, vertically and directly adjacent to the cervix. Upon closing the clamp onto the paracervical tissue, the handle is gently directed laterally to further press the tip against the cervix and laterally displace the uterine pedicle. The pedicle is similarly cut and ligated, before repeating these steps on the contralateral side.

Supracervical Hysterectomy

The surgeon may choose to amputate the uterus from the midcervix at this point in the operation due to benign disease and patient preference, limited visibility from a bulky uterus, or dense adhesions making cervix removal too risky to proceed. Regardless of the indication, the cautery tip is bent at an angle, its

energy source turned up, and suction brought into the field to remove the smoke plume. Often it is advisable to place a hand-held retractor posteriorly to prevent inadvertent cautery injury to the rectum. The uterine fundus is detached and handed off the field.

If the cervix is to remain in situ, the upper endocervix may be further resected or cauterized to prevent cyclic bleeding, which may otherwise be observed postoperatively in premenopausal women. Interrupted 0-gauge delayed-absorbable suture may be placed to achieve hemostasis, but otherwise is not required.

Removal of the Cervix

If the uterus has not been amputated from the cervix, then lateral straight clamp placement and pedicle ligation continue as before. Otherwise, single-toothed Kocher clamps are placed on the anterior and posterior walls of the remaining cervix for upward traction. The bladder flap is further advanced, if needed, by sharp dissection. The cardinal ligaments are successively clamped, cut, and ligated to reach the lateral aspect of the upper vaginal vault. The cervical distance to the vaginal fornix should be checked intermittently by placing a gloved hand into the pelvis, directly grasping the cervix in the palm, and palpating the cervical portio between the thumb and index finger. Otherwise, it is possible to inadvertently perform an upper vaginectomy or prematurely cut into the cervix before reaching the vagina. Further sharp dissection is performed anteriorly to be confident the bladder is sufficiently mobilized distally.

Once the lateral vaginal vault has been reached, upward and lateral traction is again exerted by the Kelly clamps holding the uterine cornua. A curved Heaney clamp is placed in front of the lateral tip of the cervix and swung posteriorly to incorporate the uterosacral ligament. A second Heaney clamp is similarly placed on the contralateral vaginal angle. The lateral vaginal fornices and intervening anterior and posterior vaginal attachments can be divided under direct visualization using a knife (Figure 25-5) or sharply curved scissors. The clamped pedicles are each secured with a transfixing 0-gauge delayed-absorbable stitch. The remainder of the upper vagina can then be closed by either interrupted or continuous running, 0-gauge delayed-absorbable suture.

On occasion, a bulky cervix, lateral tissue induration, or a cervix flush with the vaginal apex will dictate the need for a different approach. With the bladder flap dissected distally onto the anterior vaginal fornix, a Kocher clamp is placed anteriorly in the midline beyond the cervical portio. A second, more proximal Kocher clamp is similarly placed and cautery used in between to enter the vaginal vault (Figure 25-6). A right-angle clamp is inserted into the opening

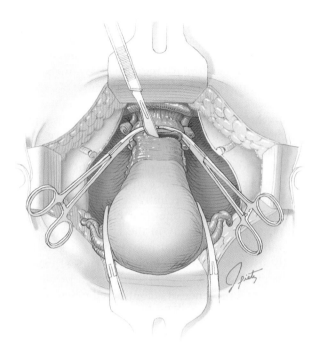

FIGURE 25-5. Detaching the uterus and cervix from the upper vagina. (Redrawn, with permission, from Schorge JO, Schaffer JI, Halvorson LM, et al, eds. *Williams Gynecology*. New York, NY: McGraw-Hill; 2008.)

(colpotomy) and used to facilitate bilateral cautery dissection. The proximal Kocher is repositioned to grasp the anterior lip of the cervix, reflecting it upward, where cautery or scissors can be used to detach it laterally and posteriorly. The vaginal cuff is grasped with Kocher or Allis clamps and closed, as described earlier.

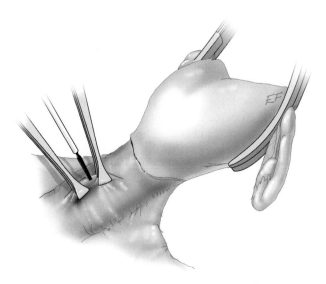

FIGURE 25-6. Entering the anterior vaginal fornix.

Final Steps

Once the abdominal hysterectomy has been performed, strict hemostasis should be achieved. The course of both ureters and all pedicle sites are re-inspected. Further abdominal exploration may be performed, as needed. Intraoperative drain placement is at the discretion of the surgeon, depending on concurrent ancillary procedures, the amount of blood loss, and other specific concerns. Copious irrigation of warmed saline is advisable, followed by careful attention to closure of the abdominal incision.

Postoperative Care

Box 25-3	Complications and Morbidity

- Intraoperative
  - Hemorrhage
  - Cystotomy
  - Ureteral transection, ligation, or "kinking"
  - Bowel deserosalization or enterotomy
- Postoperative
  - Ileus (more pronounced with vertical incision)
  - Vaginal or intraperitoneal bleeding
  - Neurologic deficit (ie, retractor injury)
  - Wound infection, separation, or fascial dehiscence
  - Thromboembolic event
  - Genitourinary fistula (rare)
  - Incisional hernia (more likely in obese patients)

Abdominal hysterectomy is generally associated with longer patient recovery and hospital stays, increased incisional pain, and a greater risk of postoperative febrile morbidity and wound infection compared to other approaches.[7] However, sometimes it is the best, or possibly the only, option for effective surgical management of the patient. Only extenuating circumstances, such as intraoperative hemorrhage, multiple concurrent procedures, or severe medical comorbidities, should prompt the surgeon to request specialized services within the intensive care unit for the immediate postoperative recovery.

All patients should be examined by a member of the health care team within several hours, with visualization of the dressing. Most dressings can be safely removed on postoperative day 1. In patients with vertical incisions above the umbilicus, it is often advisable to wait an additional day to remove the dressing as long as it remains dry. Thereafter, the incision site is checked frequently looking for signs of infection.

Typically, Foley catheter drainage may be discontinued on the first postoperative day. However, many gynecologic oncology patients may need to have catheter removal postponed due to difficulty with ambulation, fluid shifts resulting in borderline urine output, or related issues. When an intraoperative bladder injury has been repaired, the catheter should remain in place to keep the bladder decompressed from several days to 2 weeks, depending on the size of the injury. Although meticulous ureteral dissection should reduce the risk, the majority of ureteral injuries will be recognized postoperatively. Thus, symptoms of urinary incontinence or vaginal fluid leakage should alert the surgeon to this possibility.

Abdominal hysterectomy will result in a delay of return to normal bowel function for an unknown duration. In the absence of extensive concurrent surgery, a nasogastric tube is not necessary. The timing of when to advance diet past nothing by mouth (NPO) depends on numerous factors, including the individual surgeon's experience and specific preferences. Patients with a high vertical incision will be at higher risk of ileus and should be advanced more slowly. In uncomplicated circumstances, sips of clear liquids may be initiated on postoperative day 1 if the patient's examination is appropriate. Beyond that, advancing the diet is a day-to-day decision until flatus is passed, when a full diet may be allowed. Any signs of abdominal distention, nausea, or emesis should be taken into consideration throughout the hospital stay, with the patient potentially made NPO again if necessary.

Early ambulation is among the most critical interventions to facilitate rapid recovery. Discharge planning should be discussed early, especially when postdischarge rehabilitation is anticipated.

VAGINAL HYSTERECTOMY

Procedure Overview

Box 25-4	Master Surgeon's Corner

- Vaginal hysterectomy avoids the significant morbidity associated with abdominal incisions.
- Median episiotomy may facilitate exposure when limited by a small vaginal introitus.
- If salpingo-oophorectomy is indicated but difficult due to high location of the adnexa, laparoscopic instruments such as a ligature loop with slip knot may be useful.

Vaginal hysterectomy offers a number of potential advantages over abdominal or laparoscopic surgery, especially when pelvic organs are small, some degree of uterine descensus is present, and access to the upper abdomen is not required.[8] Operating time is reduced, regional anesthesia may be an option, inpatient hospitalization is brief, major morbidity is less, and a shorter postoperative recovery may be anticipated, especially when the procedure is performed by high-volume vaginal surgeons.[9,10] Moreover, because no abdominal incisions are required, vaginal hysterectomy could rightly be considered more of a minimally invasive operation than laparoscopy or robotic surgery.

In a previous era when the rate of cesarean delivery was very low and the number of births per woman was higher, the prevalence of pelvic organ prolapse made vaginal hysterectomy a popular technique. Currently, less than one-quarter of hysterectomies are performed vaginally in the United States. There are numerous additional reasons why it is not currently used more often, including lack of expertise of the gynecologic surgeon, anticipated pelvic adhesive disease, presence of a contracted pelvis, or other problematic factors. Within gynecologic oncology, even fewer patients are treated by this approach, mainly because the indications for hysterectomy often require intra-abdominal evaluation with or without staging. For the gynecologic oncologist, pre-invasive cervical disease is one of the more common indications, as well as the occasional elderly or excessively obese woman with complex atypical hyperplasia or grade 1 endometrial cancer.[11] Conceptually, the operational steps are in reverse order compared to abdominal hysterectomy.

Preoperative Preparation

The preoperative evaluation for vaginal hysterectomy largely mirrors that of the abdominal approach. Preoperative pelvic examination is especially important. With careful assessment, the potential for needing laparoscopic assistance or likelihood of converting to a laparotomy should be low. However, intraoperative findings often cannot be reliably predicted based on examination or imaging tests. As when performing other types of hysterectomy, patients should be fully informed that gastrointestinal or genitourinary injuries are possible, as is unexpected bleeding.

Vaginal hysterectomy is not dependent on specific instrumentation. However, sidewall retractors, such as the Breisky, are often helpful. Curved-tip needle drivers may also facilitate suture ligation of pedicles. The individual surgeon may have specific requests, such as certain coagulation sealing devices, to maximize efficiency. Frequently, a dilute saline solution containing vasopressin (20 units diluted in 20 mL of saline) is used to reduce blood loss.[12] Alternatively, some surgeons prefer using just saline due to concerns that intracervical vasoconstrictor usage may increase the risk of postoperative infection.

Operative Procedure

Box 25-5	Caution Points

- Excess bleeding during dissection between the bladder and cervix generally implies that dissection is proceeding in the wrong plane
- Place clamps close to the cervix, inside the uterosacral pedicles, when dividing the cardinal ligament in order to avoid the ureter laterally.
- Avoid transfixion sutures on vascular pedicles.

Anesthesia and Patient Positioning

One of the important advantages of vaginal hysterectomy is that it can be comfortably performed under regional anesthesia in patients who have a heightened surgical risk. Once regional or general anesthesia has been administered, positioning is particularly important. Access to the perineum is limited, and visualization is critically important. The patient is placed in dorsal lithotomy position with her feet comfortably positioned in stirrups. Candy-cane stirrups are preferred in order to provide maximal exposure to the operative field and allow room for 1 or 2 assistants. Extra care, including alternative stirrups (such as Allen), is sometimes necessary but may result in imperfect exposure. Next, the patient's hips are brought over the edge of the operating room table, and leg positioning is reassessed to confirm appropriate padding. Improper positioning can lead to sciatic, peroneal, and/or femoral nerve palsies.

Bimanual rectovaginal examination is performed before prepping to familiarize oneself with the anatomy. The vagina is surgically prepared, and a Foley catheter is placed. When there is any perceived possibility of bladder injury, a 3-way Foley may be indicated. It is often good practice to prep the abdomen as well, in case circumstances dictate the need to look laparoscopically or convert to an abdominal approach.

Vaginal Wall Incision

The operating table is raised to the appropriate height for the surgical team. A weighted vaginal speculum is placed posteriorly, and a right-angle or other suitable retractor is placed along the anterior vaginal wall to be held by the surgical assistant. A Lahey thyroid clamp is used to grasp both the anterior and posterior cervical lips, and the cervix is placed on downward and outward traction. The margin of the bladder can be identified as a crease in the overlying vaginal epithelium and accentuated by in-and-out movement of the cervix. Between 10 and 15 mL of diluted vasopressin solution is injected circumferentially beneath the mucosa at a level above the cervicovaginal junction, but below the inferior margin of the bladder to aid in defining tissue planes.

The location of the vaginal wall incision is crucial to facilitate the subsequent steps of the operation. If the incision is made too close to the cervical os, it results in unnecessary difficulty in entering the peritoneal cavity. Alternatively, an incision too far away from the os can lead to inadvertent bladder or rectal injury. Bending the cautery tip 45 degrees and using it on "cut" mode will facilitate dissection into the appropriate tissue planes. With the cervix pulled forward, the incision is started at the point of the posterior fornix attachment to the cervix. The anterior retractor is rotated to provide exposure so that the circular (or diamond-shaped) incision can be performed circumferentially.

Entering Posteriorly

Frequently, the peritoneal cavity is first entered posteriorly because it is easiest. Although it is tempting to bluntly dissect posteriorly after the vaginal incision has been made, that maneuver pushes the peritoneum farther away, making it much harder to enter the cul-de-sac. Instead, the cervix is pulled anteriorly to expose the posterior vaginal vault, and an Allis clamp is placed on the incised edge of the posterior vaginal wall. The Allis clamp is pulled downward to create tension across the exposed posterior peritoneum, and the posterior vaginal vault is boldly cut with curved Mayo scissors, with tips pointed up (Figure 25-7). If the peritoneal cavity is not entered with a single stroke, then the Allis clamp can be used to regrasp the posterior vaginal wall and the process repeated. If there is any concern for proximity to the rectum, a rectal examination can be performed to help guide the dissection. Inordinate difficulty in entering the peritoneal cavity posteriorly is unusual and may indicate an unanticipated obliteration of the cul-de-sac.

Upon entering the peritoneal cavity, the opening is expanded laterally by placing the Mayo scissors within the defect and opening widely. An index finger should be inserted to confirm position within the peritoneal cavity and gently palpate for adhesive disease or other pathology. The midportion of the posterior peritoneum is sutured to the posterior vaginal wall incision with a single 0-gauge delayed-absorbable suture and held on a straight snap. The weighted speculum is removed and ideally replaced by one with a longer blade (such as the "duckbill"), which is inserted through the opening into the cul-de-sac. The tie is maneuvered underneath the speculum to be used later during closure of the peritoneum at the procedure's end.

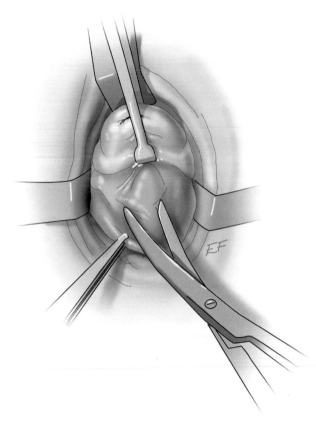

FIGURE 25-7. Entering the posterior cul-de-sac.

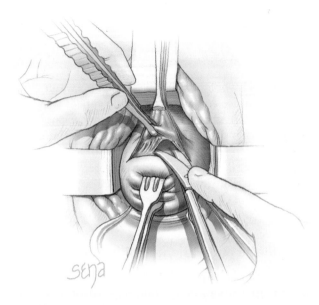

FIGURE 25-8. Sharp dissection between bladder and cervix. (Redrawn, with permission, from Schorge JO, Schaffer JI, Halvorson LM, et al, eds. *Williams Gynecology.* New York, NY: McGraw-Hill; 2008.)

Entering Anteriorly

The cervix is again held downward, and the bladder is mobilized anteriorly with the right-angle retractor. Brief horizontally directed strokes of cautery with intermittent upward mobilization using the tip should allow the tissue to fall away and facilitates identification of the correct plane of dissection. When the cautery dissection is too vigorous, the cervical stroma may be entered. To re-establish the correct plane, meticulous fine dissection is required above and distal to the inadvertent stromal entry. The anterior vaginal wall is next grasped and elevated with an Allis clamp. This traction will reveal fibrous bands still connecting the bladder and cervix. Typically, the cautery is exchanged for Metzenbaum scissors at this point to allow more precise dissection of these fibers (Figure 25-8). Blunt dissection with a finger or surgical gauze should be limited, if performed at all, to avoid pushing the anterior peritoneum farther away and making it harder to reach. Additionally, when the fibrous bands are thick and the fascial plane is hard to visualize, it is possible to create a cystotomy with blunt dissection that is more difficult to repair than when a small entry is made with sharp scissor dissection.

If a cystotomy is made, it will often allow the correct tissue plane to be more easily identified inferiorly.

Once the hysterectomy is completed, cystoscopy can be performed to assess the injury's proximity to the trigone, and then typically it can be easily repaired vaginally. Injuries near the trigone may require ureteral stent placement.

The bladder dissection is continued until the vesicouterine fold is reached. Usually, it can be identified as a transverse white line across the anterior cervix. Palpation reveals 2 thin smooth layers of peritoneum slipping against one another. The vesicouterine fold is grasped and elevated to place this peritoneal layer on tension. If there is any concern for the tissue fold representing bladder mucosa, the bladder can be backfilled and the presumed vesicouterine fold re-examined. The peritoneum then is incised (Figure 25-9).

The surgeon's index finger next explores the opening to confirm peritoneal entry and to palpate for any unanticipated pathology. The anterior retractor is then repositioned with its distal blade entering the peritoneal cavity, thereby elevating the bladder.

Dividing the Lateral Ligaments and Vessels

Once the peritoneum has been safely entered anteriorly and posteriorly, the hardest part of the operation is over. Firm lateral traction on the Lahey thyroid clamp both pulls the supporting uterine ligaments into view and prevents ureteral injury. Especially in obese patients, the Breisky sidewall retractor is often helpful at this point in the operation to facilitate visualization of

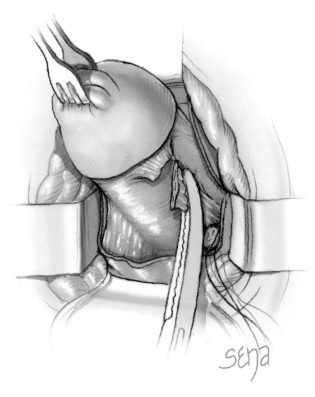

FIGURE 25-10. Cardinal ligament transaction. (Redrawn, with permission, from Schorge JO, Schaffer JI, Halvorson LM, et al, eds. *Williams Gynecology*. New York, NY: McGraw-Hill; 2008.)

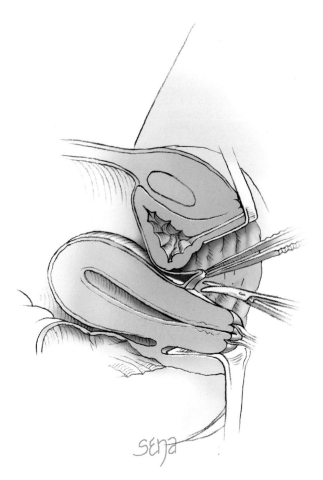

FIGURE 25-9. Vesicouterine fold incision. (Redrawn, with permission, from Schorge JO, Schaffer JI, Halvorson LM, et al, eds. *Williams Gynecology*. New York, NY: McGraw-Hill; 2008.)

the lateral pedicles. The uterosacral ligament is identified, clamped using a curved Heaney with tips pressed against the cervix, transected, and suture ligated with a transfixing stitch. The suture is tagged with a curved Kelly clamp, and the procedure is repeated on the contralateral side. Tissue sealing and cutting devices may be used instead of clamping and suturing to perform the steps more quickly, but the ligaments cannot be tied together later to provide vault support.

Next, the cardinal ligaments are similarly clamped, cut, and suture ligated (Figure 25-10). When feasible, the anterior jaw of the Heaney clamp should be positioned around the cardinal ligaments, incorporating the anterior peritoneal edge into the pedicle. The cardinal ligaments are held with curved hemostats to distinguish them later from the uterosacral pedicles. Frequently, the supportive ligaments are not easy to distinguish individually, and more than 2 clamp placements are required bilaterally to divide all of the connective tissue.

The uterine vessel pedicle, which contains the uterine artery and vein and the broad ligament peritoneum anterior and posterior to these vessels, is clamped with a single curved Heaney clamp, cut, and ligated with a single ligature. A transfixion suture should not be used on this vascular pedicle because of the possibility of injuring a vessel and causing a broad ligament hematoma. When the uterus is larger, it may be beneficial after securing the uterine vessels to deliver the uterine corpus posteriorly in order to expose the round and utero-ovarian ligaments (Figure 25-11). To accomplish this, tenaculum clamps can be used in tandem to pull the fundus into the vagina.

If the uterus is small and descensus adequate, 2 curved Heaney clamps are placed in tandem across the utero-ovarian and round ligaments, as close to the uterine fundus as possible. Often the surgeon's index finger can be looped around the pedicle to help guide the final clamps safely in place, avoiding omentum or loops of bowel. When visibility is limited, clamps may be placed bilaterally with removal of the uterus and cervix before securing the pedicles. A free tie is used first to ligate the lateral pedicle and occlude all vessels. Next, a transfixion suture ligature is placed with removal of the medial clamp (the one closest to the

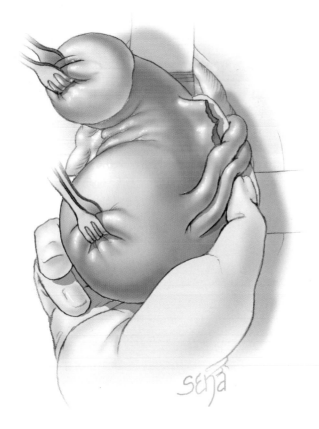

FIGURE 25-11. Delivery of the uterine corpus posteriorly. (Redrawn, with permission, from Schorge JO, Schaffer JI, Halvorson LM, et al, eds. *Williams Gynecology*. New York, NY: McGraw-Hill; 2008.)

uterus). The ties are again held laterally with matching clamps to help identify them later.

Oophorectomy

If removal of the ovaries is desired, the adnexa is grasped with a Babcock clamp and gently pulled toward the incision. An index finger is wrapped around the IP ligament to isolate it from surrounding structures. The IP ligament is clamped and ligated similarly to the utero-ovarian pedicle (Figure 25-12). The ends of the transfixing suture may be held by matching hemostats.

Vaginal Cuff Closure

The surgical pedicles should be inspected for bleeding and resecured if necessary with additional free ties or suture ligature. If hemostasis is adequate, then the utero-ovarian (or IP) ligament ties are cut. The peritoneum may be closed in a purse-string manner using 2-0 delayed-absorbable suture in order to extraperitonealize the pedicles. However, this is not a required

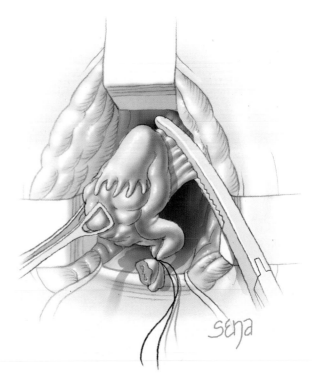

FIGURE 25-12. Salpingo-oophorectomy. (Redrawn, with permission, from Schorge JO, Schaffer JI, Halvorson LM, et al, eds. *Williams Gynecology*. New York, NY: McGraw-Hill; 2008.)

step, and it can certainly be skipped when visualization is limited.

The easiest and quickest way to provide apical support is to tie both cardinal ligaments together in the midline, and then to do the same for the uterosacral ligaments. Finally, the cardinal ligament suture is tied to the uterosacral suture. Alternatively, a suspensory suture may be included in which the cardinal or uterosacral or both ligaments are sutured to the lateral vaginal cuff on each side. More complex variations of preventing future vault prolapse are at the discretion of the surgeon. Strict hemostasis should be observed prior to cuff closure. The vaginal mucosa is closed from anterior to posterior with running suture, ultimately securing it to the posterior peritoneal stitch placed at the beginning of the operation.

Final Steps

Vaginal packs are not required at the completion of vaginal hysterectomy, but some surgeons will use them on occasion to tamponade surface oozing in the immediate postoperative period. When the abdominal entry is particularly challenging anteriorly or there is any other concern for injury to the genitourinary tract, diagnostic cystoscopy should be performed prior to extubation.

Postoperative Care

Box 25-6   Complications and Morbidity

- Intraoperative
  - Rectal injury during posterior dissection
  - Cystotomy during anterior dissection
  - Enterotomy due to unanticipated obliteration of the cul-de-sac or incorrect clamp placement
  - Ureteral transection, ligation, or "kinking"
  - Hemorrhage
- Postoperative
  - Vaginal or intraperitoneal bleeding
  - Neurologic deficit from hyperflexion of the hips
  - Vaginal cuff complications (ie, cellulitis, abscess, or dehiscence)
  - Genitourinary fistula
  - Vaginal vault prolapse

Vaginal hysterectomy patients typically have faster return of normal bowel function, easier ambulation, decreased analgesia requirements, shorter duration of hospital stay, and speedier return to normal activities compared to abdominal hysterectomy patients.[10] Rarely, signs of excessive vaginal bleeding and/or hemodynamic instability may necessitate a return to the operating room to achieve hemostasis. The Foley catheter is removed on the first postoperative day, the diet quickly advanced, and the patient discharged.

LAPAROSCOPIC HYSTERECTOMY

Procedure Overview

Box 25-7   Master Surgeon's Corner

- Abdominal hysterectomy principles of retroperitoneal dissection should be maintained (eg, identification of the ureters).
- A carefully placed, well-functioning uterine manipulator facilitates appropriate angles of approach for laparoscopic instruments.
- Use of a colpotomy cup to define the cervicovaginal junction pushes the ureters laterally and provides a consistent landmark.
- Skeletonization of vascular pedicles allows the tissue to be sealed/cauterized more effectively and protects nearby structures such as the ureter.

Several laparoscopic techniques have been developed for hysterectomy and vary depending on the degree of laparoscopic dissection versus vaginal surgery required to remove the uterus and the instrumentation used, including the robotic platform. Laparoscopically assisted vaginal hysterectomy (LAVH) was the most popular method for several years, until being recently largely supplanted by total laparoscopic hysterectomy (TLH). Numerous surgeons routinely perform these operations with robotic assistance rather than using "straight-stick" instrumentation. Relatively few gynecologic oncologists have mastered the technology involved to offer single-incision laparoscopic surgery (SILS) to their patients, but that method may be more common in the future.[13]

Appropriate patient selection is critical to successfully perform any variation of laparoscopic hysterectomy and concurrent surgery, including lymphadenectomy or other cancer staging. Limiting factors include morbid obesity, previous pelvic infection, and extensive or bulky disease. In addition, laparoscopy creates unique physiologic cardiopulmonary changes that stem mainly from hypercarbia and pulmonary compliance changes. Patients with significant cardiac or pulmonary disease may not tolerate a laparoscopic approach, especially for long durations. Extensive prior abdominal surgeries with subsequent dense adhesions limiting exposure may significantly lengthen operative times and ultimately require conversion to laparotomy. Uterine size can also affect the surgical approach. Specifically, a large bulky uterus may be difficult to manipulate, may block visualization, and may be too large for vaginal removal. Importantly, morcellation should be avoided when dealing with uterine or adnexal malignancy. Just as important, determining the extent of disease and potential spread of cancer to other organs is essential before proceeding with laparoscopic hysterectomy.

In gynecologic oncology, the use of and perceived indications for minimally invasive surgery, particularly with robotic assistance, continue to increase. The most common indication for laparoscopic hysterectomy among gynecologic oncologists is for the treatment and staging of endometrial cancer.[4] Despite longer operative time when compared to laparotomy, laparoscopic hysterectomy offers less postoperative pain, a shorter hospital stay, shorter recovery time, fewer complications, and vastly lower surgical site infection rates.[14,15] Laparoscopic hysterectomy is otherwise appropriate for a wide range of other gynecologic diagnoses.

Preoperative Preparation

The basic preoperative evaluation for laparoscopic hysterectomy is similar to that of either the abdominal or vaginal approach. Preoperative pelvic examination is important to determine uterine size and mobility. Although there are no specific upper limits, a wide bulky uterus (width >8 cm) with minimal mobility may be difficult to remove vaginally. Fortunately, findings such as a narrow introitus, a cervix flush with the vaginal apex, or a contracted pelvis are less problematic than when considering vaginal hysterectomy. Once a patient has been deemed eligible for a laparoscopic approach, the same preoperative evaluation as for an open procedure applies.

Laparoscopic hysterectomy is *very* dependent on specific instrumentation. The setups for LAVH, TLH, robotic-assisted hysterectomy, or SILS hysterectomy are quite different. Basic laparoscopic instruments include trocars, a video laparoscope, and laparoscopic devices for suturing, suction/irrigation, and coagulation, cutting, and sealing of tissue. Bariatric trocars may be needed for excessively obese patients. A number of suitable electrosurgical and ultrasonic energy-based devices are available and used according to surgeon preference and local availability. The da Vinci Surgical System (Intuitive Surgical, Inc., Sunnyvale, CA) is the only currently available robotic-assisted laparoscopy platform. It provides 3-dimensional imaging for the surgeon as well as a wide selection of "wristed" instruments that provide additional degrees of freedom of movement compared to traditional "straight-stick" instruments. To perform SILS, a port system allowing passage of 3 to 4 instruments, a deflecting tip laparoscope, articulating instruments, and other individualized equipment must be available. Regardless of the laparoscopic technique, access to a suitable uterine manipulator, such as the RUMI (CooperSurgical, Inc., Trumbull, CT) or V-Care (ConMed Corp., Utica, NY), as well as a colpotomy cup, such as the KOH Colpotomizer ring (CooperSurgical), is also important.

Operative Procedure

Box 25-8	**Caution Points**

- Consider alternate trocar entry points (ie, left upper quadrant) in patients with scars at the umbilicus.
- Directly observe all subsequent trocar placements with the laparoscope.
- Frequently ensure that the colpotomy cup is being pressed firmly into the vagina by the assistant.
- Insist upon good visualization and tissue retraction by regular communication with your assistant throughout the procedure.

Anesthesia and Patient Positioning

The introductory steps for laparoscopy are described in Chapter 31. Lower extremity compression devices are placed, and general endotracheal anesthesia is administered. To avoid stomach puncture by a trocar during primary abdominal entry, an orogastric tube should be placed to decompress the stomach. The patient is placed in dorsal lithotomy position using Allen stirrups, and the buttocks are brought to the edge of table. If very steep Trendelenburg position is anticipated, placement of the patient on beanbags or foam pads specially designed to prevent patient movement should be considered. The use of shoulder blocks or tape across the chest may be considered as well, but should be done with caution given the risk of brachial plexus injury and limitation on ventilation, respectively.

After sufficient vascular access is confirmed, the patient's arms are gently tucked and padded alongside her body. The use of toboggans designed to support the patient's arms may be necessary in morbidly obese women. Special attention is given to securing the patient's hands because they often are in the vicinity of where the Allen stirrup is positioned. Bimanual rectovaginal examination is performed before prepping to familiarize oneself with the anatomy. The abdomen and vagina are surgically prepped and draped.

Placement of the Uterine Manipulator

An open-sided speculum is inserted into the vagina to visualize the cervix. The anterior lip is firmly grasped with a single-toothed tenaculum. With outward traction provided by the tenaculum, the cervical canal is progressively and generously dilated, followed by uterine sounding. The measured distance from the external os to the fundus will determine the length of the uterine manipulator. When a RUMI is used for manipulation, the appropriate-size tip is selected (usually 8 or 10 cm in length) and attached to the manipulator. If there is a question between 2 sizes, it is preferable to request the larger size when also using a colpotomy cup. Next, the vaginal occluder balloon is placed over the uterine manipulator tip. An appropriately sized colpotomy cup (usually the medium) is placed over the end of the manipulator tip and occluder balloon (Figure 25-13). Metal colpotomy cups are appropriate when colpotomy is to be performed using ultrasonic energy, whereas blue plastic cups should be used when electrocautery is planned. The speculum is removed with the tenaculum remaining on the anterior lip of the cervix. The manipulator is grasped in the right hand with the index finger at the tip, and by providing downward traction of the tenaculum using the left hand, the manipulator tip is guided into the dilated

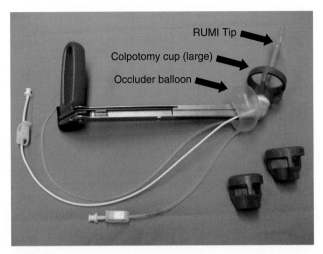

FIGURE 25-13. Uterine manipulator with attached colpotomy cup.

cervix. The uterine manipulator tip is advanced toward the pelvis as the colpotomy cup is slid into the vagina. While maintaining pressure toward the pelvis on the manipulator, the tenaculum is removed, allowing the colpotomy cup to advance flush to the cervicovaginal junction. The manipulator tip balloon and vaginal occluder balloon are filled. The manipulator handle is adjusted to test placement and moved upward to provide extreme anteversion of the uterus, thereby helping to prevent the manipulator from inadvertently being displaced or falling out.

Mitigating patient factors can make an otherwise straightforward manipulator placement very challenging. An introitus too narrow to allow insertion of a colpotomy cup may be expanded by performing an episiotomy. Cervical stenosis prohibiting dilation may prompt the surgeon to postpone further attempts until the camera has been placed and intraperitoneal visualization is possible. If the vagina is too contracted to permit placement of any colpotomy cup, the uterine manipulator can be placed without it. Occasionally no manipulator placement is possible, in which case a rectal probe can be placed vaginally to assist with upward uterine movement and demarcation of the cervicovaginal junction.

The Foley catheter is inserted after placement of the uterine manipulator so that it does not get in the way during placement. When there is any perceived possibility of bladder injury, a 3-way Foley may be indicated.

Port Placement

The primary surgeon stands on his or her preferred side of the patient, and the first assistant stands across the operative table. A second assistant, if available, sits or stands between the patient's legs. Ideally, the surgeon and first assistant should have a video screen directly in front of them, usually adjacent to the leg contralateral to their position.

The scope of the anticipated operation is very important when selecting where to begin the primary trocar entry and subsequently other port sites. The primary trocar can be placed using one of several methods, including the open technique, direct trocar insertion, or transumbilical insertion of a Veress needle. An umbilical or supraumbilical site is usually preferred for primary entry, unless planning for a robotic-assisted para-aortic node dissection, when the port is typically placed a few centimeters cephalad to the umbilicus. In the presence of known or anticipated adhesive disease near the umbilicus, initial access may be most appropriate by left upper quadrant Veress needle insertion in the midclavicular line.

In the open technique, a 1- to 2-cm skin incision is made just below (or within) the umbilicus. A combination of Mayo scissor dissection and retraction using S-shaped retractors is used to reach the fascia. A Kocher clamp is placed, and the fascia is further dissected free of subcutaneous tissue until a second clamp is placed. The fascia is elevated and entered sharply between the 2 clamps. Once the fascia is entered, the peritoneum is grasped with hemostats and incised sharply. The fascial edges are tagged with 0-gauge delayed-absorbable sutures. An index finger should be inserted to confirm intraperitoneal location and sweep along the anterior wall for adhesions or omental attachments. The tip of the S-shaped retractor is inserted into the peritoneal opening and used to guide a 10- or 12-mm Hasson trocar into the abdominal cavity. The trocar is twisted in place and secured laterally with the fascial-anchoring sutures, and the obturator is removed. When performing SILS, a similar technique is performed, although a slightly larger periumbilical incision is required for insertion of the specialized multiport device. Insufflation of the abdomen can begin through this umbilical port by connecting the carbon dioxide (CO_2) tubing to the side port of the trocar. High flow is appropriate for insufflation, and the intra-abdominal pressure should be maintained at 15 mm Hg. The laparoscope is then placed through the trocar. The abdomen and pelvis are thoroughly inspected to assess the extent of disease and adhesions. At this point, discovery of unanticipated metastatic disease or pelvic tumor extension may prompt the surgeon to convert to laparotomy. Trendelenburg position is used to facilitate pelvic exposure by movement of bowel into the upper abdomen. Additional ports are placed under direct laparoscopic visualization.

Four port sites are preferred for complex laparoscopic gynecologic procedures performed with traditional instruments (ie, not robotic-assisted or SILS). The umbilical port most often holds the laparoscope. Often, the remaining ports consist only of 5-mm trocars, thus decreasing the risk of postoperative port-site hernia. If specimens need to be removed or a needle inserted, a 5-mm laparoscope can be inserted through a lateral port. Usually the primary surgeon will use 2 ports to allow for work with both hands simultaneously. This is best facilitated with 2 laterally placed ports, but may also be accomplished with use of a suprapubic port and 1 lateral port. However, the ports must be spaced far enough apart to prevent instrument collision outside the patient. The assistant will typically hold the camera and have an additional lateral port. The second assistant provides uterine manipulation and should ensure that the uterus is pushed up into the pelvis during the entire procedure. The current setup for robotic-assisted procedures involves placement of 2 or 3 8.5-mm robotic ports, in addition to a 10- to 12-mm right upper quadrant "first assistant" trocar.

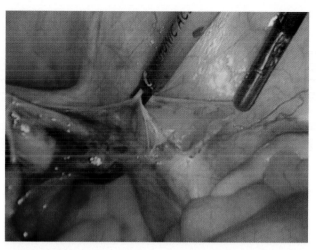

FIGURE 25-14. Opening the posterior broad ligament. (Reproduced, with permission, from Schorge JO, Schaffer JI, Halvorson LM, et al, eds. *Williams Gynecology*. New York, NY: McGraw-Hill; 2008.)

Retroperitoneal Access and Lateral Dissection

Either the da Vinci Surgical System is docked with the surgeon operating via the console, or the procedure continues laparoscopically. The following operative steps will describe traditional, "straight-stick" technique, but are generally applicable to robotic surgery. The uterus is mobilized to 1 side by movement of the uterine manipulator and/or by an intraperitoneal blunt grasper holding 1 cornu. In doing so, the contralateral round ligament should be stretched. The first assistant holds the contralateral fallopian tube medially to provide further exposure and stretch of the broad ligament. The surgeon tents up either the round ligament or the pelvic peritoneum above the psoas muscle. The tissue is sealed and cut with the surgeon's instrument of choice in order to obtain initial access to the retroperitoneum. The peritoneal incision is extended cephalad in parallel to the IP ligament (Figure 25-14). The ureter is conclusively identified retroperitoneally along the medial leaf of the broad ligament, usually most easily at the pelvic brim.

An avascular space within the medial leaf of the broad ligament is identified above the ureter and below the adnexal structures. An opening within this space is made using either blunt, sharp, or energy-based dissection. The surgeon expands the opening by placing 2 instruments within it and gently stretching the peritoneum by moving the instruments in opposite directions parallel to the IP ligament. Development of this opening ensures separation between the ureter and the adnexa. The IP or utero-ovarian ligament is then transected depending on whether the adnexa are to be removed or retained. While cauterizing or sealing the vascular pedicle, tension on the pedicle should be minimized to ensure a hemostatic transection. The uterus is then deflected in the opposite direction, and a similar dissection is performed on the other side.

Anterior Dissection and Bladder Mobilization

The uterine manipulator is adjusted to provide retroflexion, as pressure is maintained by firmly pushing the uterus cephalad from below. A peritoneal incision is made bilaterally within the anterior leaf of the broad ligament and extended across the anterior cul-de-sac at the vesicouterine fold. The surgeon elevates the peritoneum over the bladder centrally, placing the underlying fibrous attachments on stretch. A combination of blunt and sharp or energy-based dissection is used to develop the plane between the cervix and bladder (Figure 25-15). Although the bladder flap is most often initially developed centrally, the presence of scar, usually as a result of prior cesarean section, may necessitate approaching the plane of dissection laterally. It is crucial to adequately mobilize the bladder beyond the colpotomy cup to facilitate safe colpotomy and cuff closure.

Posterior Dissection

The uterine manipulator is adjusted to provide mild anteflexion and is slightly directed to 1 side, exposing the uterosacral ligament and uterine isthmus and cervix laterally. The peritoneum of the medial leaf of the broad ligament is incised toward the uterosacral ligament with care to remain above the ureter. The

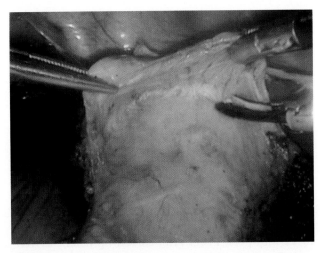

FIGURE 25-15. Mobilization of the bladder distally.

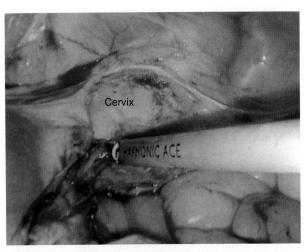

FIGURE 25-16. Sealing and dividing the uterine vessels.

incision should be directed toward the underlying colpotomy cup, which should be identified posteriorly. Gentle traction by the surgeon on the peritoneum medially and posteriorly will allow for its separation from the uterine isthmus. The uterine vasculature may be visible lateral to the uterine isthmus above the level of the colpotomy cup. After adjustment of the uterine position, the identical procedure is repeated on the contralateral side. Although a peritoneal incision extending across the posterior cul-de-sac is not necessary, it may facilitate development of the rectovaginal space in cases where the rectum is adherent to the cervix posteriorly. When performing an LAVH, the operation can be converted to the vaginal portion at this point or after dividing the uterine vessels.

Division of the Uterine Vessels

After ensuring adequate development of the bladder flap and following posterior dissection, the location of the uterine vessels will be in between, along the lateral uterine isthmus. When used, the colpotomy cup serves as a landmark at which the uterine vasculature should be transected. The uterus and cup should be directed firmly cephalad into the pelvis during the upcoming steps in order to ensure proper position and to minimize risk of injury to the ureters or bladder.

Peritoneal and fibrous attachments are dissected away to skeletonize the uterine vasculature. The isolated vessels are then coagulated or sealed (Figure 25-16). Performing this step bilaterally prior to transection of the vessels minimizes back-bleeding. The vessels are divided perpendicular to their course at the level of the underlying colpotomy cup. The uterine vessels are

dissected so that they fall laterally away from the cervix and underlying colpotomy cup.

Laparoscopic Supracervical Hysterectomy

If desired, the corpus can be amputated from the cervix following division of the uterine vasculature. The corpus is incised at a point just below the internal os and superior to the uterosacral ligaments once the uterine vessels have been divided. A conical incision is extended down into the cervix to limit the possibility of residual endometrium (Figure 25-17). Adjunctive coring or ablation of the endocervical canal also may be performed to decrease the risk of long-term postoperative bleeding. Although a uterine manipulator is used during performance of a laparoscopic supracervical hysterectomy, a colpotomy cup is not usually necessary. The uterine manipulator tip will be identified during the amputation of the corpus and is removed vaginally. The uterine corpus is removed either through an enlarged skin incision or via laparoscopic morcellation. The procedure is performed in limited fashion within gynecologic oncology given concerns regarding morcellation in the setting of known or suspected malignancy.

Detachment of the Cervix From the Vagina

The uterine manipulator is adjusted to provide maximum anteflexion and is directed centrally, pushing the colpotomy cup up firmly against the cervicovaginal junction below. The vaginal occluder balloon should be inflated to prevent loss of pneumoperitoneum during colpotomy incision. The upper vagina is incised anteriorly immediately over the underlying colpotomy cup.

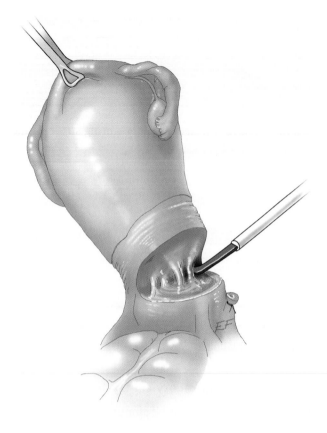

FIGURE 25-17. Uterine amputation. (Redrawn, with permission, from Schorge JO, Schaffer JI, Halvorson LM, et al, eds. *Williams Gynecology.* New York, NY: McGraw-Hill; 2008.)

The incision is extended circumferentially by adjustment of the uterine manipulator and intra-abdominal retraction of the uterus. The uterus and cervix, with or without adnexa, are completely detached and removed vaginally.

Occasionally, the manipulator will come out without removal of the uterus due to a small vaginal incision, a bulky uterus, or other circumstances. In this instance, the specimen can usually be grasped with a tenaculum and removed through the vagina. The tenaculum should be placed while visualizing the cervix either vaginally or laparoscopically to avoid injury to the rectum or bladder. If the indication for hysterectomy is benign, a large uterus can be laparoscopically bivalved or divided into pieces to facilitate removal vaginally. Very rarely, an abdominal incision will be required for removal of the uterus.

Closure of the Vaginal Cuff

Closure of the vaginal cuff following laparoscopic hysterectomy may be performed either vaginally or laparoscopically. If a laparoscopic approach is planned, pneumoperitoneum must be reinstituted by occlusion of the vagina using the uterus, the vaginal occluder balloon, a bulb syringe, or a glove stuffed with sponges. Irrigation and suction should be performed to clear the vaginal cuff of blood or small clots.

Laparoscopic closure of the vaginal cuff can be performed by multiple methods. For the method described below, the surgeon stands on the patient's right side. Two lateral ports are used, allowing the surgeon to work naturally with both hands. A 0- or 2-0–gauge delayed-absorbable suture is trimmed to about the length of a laparoscopic instrument. The suture on a CT-1 needle is introduced through the umbilical 10- to 12-mm port. Pistol grip, curved-tip needle drivers, with the curves directed inward at each other, facilitate efficient suturing and intracorporeal knot tying in the deep pelvis. The lateral vaginal angle on the right side is grasped, and the suture is passed through the full-thickness vagina anteriorly and then posteriorly. The stitch is pulled through until a 3- to 4-cm tail is present. The suture is tied using intracorporeal technique, and the tail is left for later use. The surgeon holds the trailing strand of suture to assist in positioning the vaginal cuff and creating resistance for passage of suture. The needle is passed through the full-thickness vagina from anterior to posterior in a running fashion progressing from right to left. Upon closure of the left vaginal cuff angle, a second running layer is accomplished from left to right. The assistant holds the trailing strand to follow the surgeon while the surgeon holds the initial suture tail, both working to elevate the cuff. Upon reaching the right-side angle, the suture is tied to the initial tail using intracorporeal knot tying. To confirm integrity of the cuff closure, a gloved hand is placed vaginally and the apex probed for defects.

Final Steps

Once the laparoscopic hysterectomy and any other operative procedures have been completed, a final inspection for hemostasis is performed. When robotic assistance has been used, it is undocked and backed away from the operating field. Ports are then removed under direct visualization, and the patient is taken out of Trendelenburg position. All fascial defects 10 mm or greater should be closed with delayed-absorbable suture to avoid a port-site hernia. Various methods of skin closure are available and include subcuticular suturing, skin adhesive (Dermabond; Ethicon, Cornelia, GA), or surgical tape strips (Steri-Strips; 3M, St. Paul, MN) plus tincture of benzoin. If difficulty in delivering the uterus was encountered, the vagina should be inspected prior to reversal of anesthesia and any vaginal lacerations repaired. Diagnostic cystoscopy is at the discretion of the surgeon.

Postoperative Care

Box 25-9	Complications and Morbidity

- Intraoperative
  - Trocar injury to bowel or blood vessels
  - Hemorrhage
  - Ureteral transection
  - Vaginal or periurethral laceration from initial colpotomy cup placement or later attempts at removing uterus
- Postoperative
  - Vaginal or intraperitoneal bleeding
  - Vaginal cuff complications (ie, cellulitis, abscess, or dehiscence)
  - Port-site bowel herniation or infection
  - Delayed thermal injury to bowel or genitourinary tract
  - Genitourinary fistula

Laparoscopic hysterectomy patients typically have the same fast return of normal bowel function, easier ambulation, and decreased analgesia requirements as those undergoing vaginal hysterectomy.[7] Postoperatively, the care is also very comparable. Intravenous narcotics are often unnecessary, and oral narcotic medication may be required for only 1 or 2 days.

Within a few hours after surgery, the abdominal bandages should be checked for excessive bleeding or serous fluid. Longer cases may result in facial swelling, periorbital edema, subcutaneous edema, and shoulder pain from extended Trendelenburg positioning, all of which usually resolve without complication over the first 24 hours postoperatively.

Although select patients may be discharged on the same day as surgery, typically patients leave the hospital within 24 hours. The Foley catheter is removed early in the morning on the first postoperative day, the diet quickly advanced, and ambulation encouraged.

Patients should be counseled to report heavy vaginal bleeding, fever, increased abdominal pain, or nausea and vomiting. A low threshold of suspicion for the presence of a bowel injury should exist in women who underwent extensive adhesiolysis should they present with fever and increasing abdominal pain. Rarely, women will present semi-emergently with vomiting and abdominal pain and be diagnosed with a trocar-site hernia.

Upon discharge, strict precautions should be reinforced not to resume sexual activity or place anything within the vagina until complete healing has taken place, approximately 6 to 8 weeks later. Laparoscopic hysterectomy is associated with a higher risk of vaginal cuff dehiscence compared to the abdominal or vaginal approach. This may be due to cautery effect near the suture line or technical limitations during surgery that prevent including sufficient tissue within the closure. Regardless of etiology, surgical repair can be performed either vaginally or laparoscopically.[16]

MODIFIED RADICAL ABDOMINAL HYSTERECTOMY (TYPE II)

Procedure Overview

Box 25-10	Master Surgeon's Corner

- Type II hysterectomy principles may be necessary in some benign conditions, such as a large cervical fibroid or a distended lower uterine segment.
- Development of the pararectal and paravesical spaces allows for assessment of the parametria and pelvic lymph nodes.
- With limited resection of the cardinal and uterosacral ligaments compared to type III procedures, less bladder and bowel dysfunction is anticipated.

Modified radical hysterectomy represents the second of 5 types of extended hysterectomy originally defined by Piver et al.[2] The anatomic landmarks distinguishing a type II hysterectomy are somewhat vague and thus allow a surgeon to tailor the procedure to a patient's specific situation.[17] Type II modified radical hysterectomy is increasingly being performed using a minimally invasive approach.

The purpose of the type II hysterectomy is to remove more paracervical tissue, while still preserving the blood supply to the distal ureters and bladder. Four main procedural differences distinguish a type II hysterectomy. First, the uterine artery is transected just medial to the ureter to ensure preservation of the distal ureteral blood supply. Second, the medial half of the cardinal ligament is resected. Third, the uterosacral ligament is divided halfway between the uterus and sacrum. Lastly, the upper one-third of the vagina is removed. When performed abdominally, these modifications serve to reduce surgical time and associated morbidity compared to a type III hysterectomy, while still enabling complete resection of smaller cervical tumors.

Absolute indications for performing a modified radical hysterectomy are relatively few and often controversial. Frequently, stage IA2 cervical cancer is the presenting diagnosis. Type II hysterectomy is also performed on occasion for (1) preinvasive or microinvasive cervical disease when a more invasive lesion cannot be excluded, (2) selected stage IB1 cervical cancers with lesions smaller than 2 cm, and (3) small central postirradiation recurrences.[18] Occasionally, extensive uterine cancer will also require a variation of this procedure. In addition, adaptation of the type II hysterectomy may be required if more extensive dissection is required to remove benign disease in the presence of tissue induration or other complicated circumstances.

Preoperative Preparation

Preoperative preparation is similar to that for abdominal hysterectomy. If the patient has had a diagnostic loop or cold knife conization, then it is prudent to wait 6 weeks for tissue healing before attempting radical surgery.

After deciding to perform a modified radical abdominal hysterectomy, the next decision in surgical planning is whether a vertical or transverse incision is best. When there is a pre-existing abdominal incision, it may or may not be appropriate for the planned operation. Whereas a Pfannenstiel incision may be appropriate in some situations, a bulky uterus or morbidly obese patient may suggest the necessity of a Maylard, Cherney, or vertical incision to obtain adequate exposure.

Significant morbidity and potentially unforeseen short- and long-term complications are more likely compared to a simple type I hysterectomy. These complications are more likely in women with obesity, prior pelvic infections, previous radiation therapy, and prior abdominal surgery. Of potential intraoperative complications, the most common is acute hemorrhage. Due to a more limited dissection, subacute postoperative complications, including ureterovaginal or vesicovaginal fistula and significant postoperative bladder or bowel dysfunction, are less likely than with the more radical type III hysterectomy.[18] Additionally, potential long-term effects on sexual function, loss of fertility, and other body functions should be candidly reviewed.

Modified radical abdominal hysterectomy is not dependent on specific instrumentation. In general, a self-retaining retractor, such as the Balfour or Bookwalter, is needed. However, the surgeon may have specific requests, such as cervical tunneling clamps, certain coagulation sealing devices, or other relevant items required for an individual case.

Operative Procedure

Anesthesia and Patient Positioning

General endotracheal anesthesia is administered, and the patient is positioned similarly, whether the planned operation is a type I, II, or III abdominal hysterectomy. Bimanual rectovaginal examination should always be performed in the operating room before scrubbing to familiarize oneself with the anatomy and to make a final decision on the type of incision. The abdomen and vagina are surgically prepared, and a Foley catheter is placed.

Abdominal Entry

Modified radical hysterectomy may be safely performed through a midline vertical or transverse incision. Following entry to the peritoneal cavity and abdominal exploration, the self-retaining retractor is assembled.

Retroperitoneal Dissection

The initial steps of modified radical abdominal type II hysterectomy mirror those of the type I or III procedure. However, the round ligament is sutured and divided more laterally than in a type I hysterectomy. The anterior and posterior leaves of the broad ligament are incised, exposing the retroperitoneum. The ureter is identified, mobilized, and tagged with a ¼-in Penrose drain. The pararectal space is developed by placing an index finger between the internal iliac artery and ureter. Pressure is directed medially and along the sacral curve toward the coccyx using a gentle swirling motion (Figure 25-18). As a result, the ureter, medial leaf of the broad ligament, and ultimately pararectal tissues are separated from the lateral pelvis.

Next, the paravesical space is developed by elevating the lateral tie on the round ligament and dissecting bluntly following the external iliac artery to the pelvic

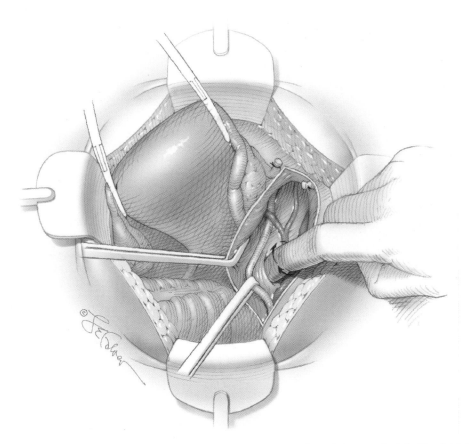

FIGURE 25-18. Making the pararectal space. (Redrawn, with permission, from Schorge JO, Schaffer JI, Halvorson LM, et al, eds. *Williams Gynecology*. New York, NY: McGraw-Hill; 2008.)

bone. The index, middle, and ring fingers of the right hand then are swept horizontally toward the midline, but remaining lateral to the umbilical vessels. By placing the index finger in the paravesical space and the surgeon's middle finger in the pararectal space, the parametria can be assessed for tumor extension before proceeding with this less radical operation. Otherwise, a type III hysterectomy might be more appropriate.

Utero-Ovarian Ligament Transection

The next operative step depends on whether the adnexa are to be concurrently removed or not. Once the ureter has been identified, the IP or utero-ovarian ligament may be divided and peritoneal attachments dissected, as described in the Abdominal Hysterectomy section.

Uterine Artery Ligation

Ligation of the uterine artery in a type II hysterectomy is performed medial to the ureter, necessitating less radical dissection of sidewall tissues than in a radical type III procedure. The superior vesical artery does not have to be identified, nor does the entire extent

of the internal iliac artery need to be dissected free of adventitial tissue. The ureter should be followed along the broad ligament, and the ureteral tunnel opening through the cardinal ligament should be palpated. The uterine vessels are divided at that location using clamps and delayed-absorbable ties (Figure 25-19) or a coagulation sealing device. Ligation of the uterine artery as it crosses the ureter allows preservation of distal ureteral blood supply.

Cardinal Ligament Resection

The bladder is mobilized distally off the cervix and onto the upper vagina as described for a type I abdominal hysterectomy. The ureteral tunnel through the cardinal ligament is unroofed with division of the medial half of the cardinal ligaments and anterior leaf of the vesicouterine ligament. The tissues are clamped, cut, and suture ligated with care to avoid the ureter (Figure 25-20). In contrast to the type III hysterectomy, the ureter is not dissected out of the tunnel bed, but is rolled laterally to expose the medial cardinal ligament. Maintenance of the posterior attachments between the ureter and the cardinal ligament further preserves its blood supply.

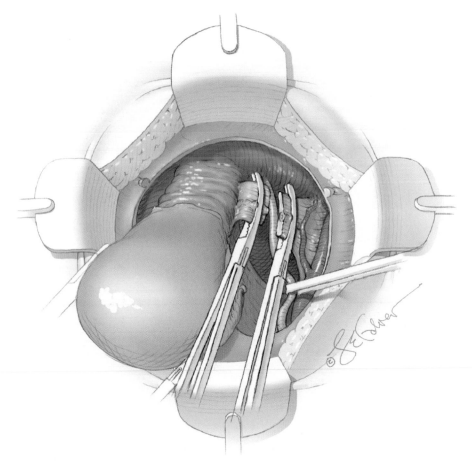

FIGURE 25-19. Uterine artery ligation. (Redrawn, with permission, from Schorge JO, Schaffer JI, Halvorson LM, et al, eds. *Williams Gynecology.* New York, NY: McGraw-Hill; 2008.)

Uterosacral Resection

Posterior radical dissection often is best performed near the end of the procedure because exposed retroperitoneal tissues typically bleed until the vaginal cuff is closed. The cervical external os is palpated, and cautery is used to superficially incise the peritoneum between the uterosacral ligaments.

A plane is developed by gently pressing a finger toward the vaginal wall without poking through into the vault. This rectovaginal plane should be developed by gentle pressure toward the sacrum and enlarged laterally until 3 fingers can be inserted comfortably. This maneuver frees the rectosigmoid away from the uterosacral ligaments and prevents inadvertent bowel injury. Remaining peritoneal attachments are dissected sharply to fully expose the rectovaginal space. The uterosacral ligaments are clamped halfway to the pelvic sidewall (instead of at the pelvic sidewall for a type III hysterectomy), transected, and ligated with 0-gauge delayed-absorbable suture, or sealed and divided with a coagulating sealing device. The uterus and adjacent parametrium can then be lifted well out of the pelvis,

and any additional tissues can also be clamped, cut, and ligated.

Vaginal Resection

At this point in surgery, the modified radical hysterectomy specimen should be held in place only by the paracolpium and vagina. The bladder and ureters are further bluntly and sharply dissected free until at least 2 cm of upper vagina are included in the specimen (instead of 3 to 4 cm as is the case for a type III hysterectomy). Curved clamps are placed on the lateral paracolpium, which is then cut and suture ligated (Figure 25-21). The upper vagina can then be closed with a continuous running method using 0-gauge delayed-absorbable suture. The specimen should be carefully examined to ensure an adequate upper vaginal segment and grossly negative margins.

Final Steps

Once the modified radical abdominal hysterectomy has been performed, a final review of the operative field should be performed, as for any type of abdominal

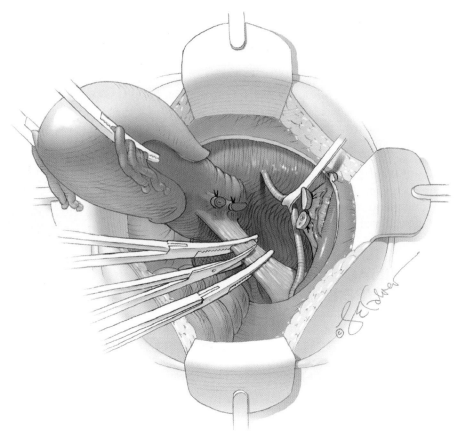

FIGURE 25-20. Cardinal ligament resection. (Redrawn, with permission, from Schorge JO, Schaffer JI, Halvorson LM, et al, eds. *Williams Gynecology*. New York, NY: McGraw- Hill; 2008.)

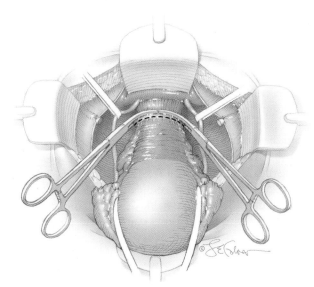

FIGURE 25-21. Upper vaginal resection. (Redrawn, with permission, from Schorge JO, Schaffer JI, Halvorson LM, et al, eds. *Williams Gynecology*. New York, NY: McGraw-Hill; 2008.)

surgery. Intraoperative drain placement is not required, unless the blood loss has been excessive or other extenuating circumstances warrant it.

Postoperative Care

Box 25-12	Complications and Morbidity

- Intraoperative
  - Hemorrhage
  - Bladder or rectal injury
  - Ureteral transection, ligation, or "kinking"
- Postoperative
  - Ileus (more pronounced with vertical incision)
  - Vaginal or intraperitoneal bleeding
  - Neurologic deficit (ie, retractor injury)
  - Wound infection, separation, or fascial dehiscence
  - Thromboembolic event
  - Genitourinary fistula (infrequent)
  - Incisional hernia (more likely in obese patients)
  - Long-term bladder or rectal dysfunction (limited)
  - Sexual dysfunction (limited)

Modified radical abdominal hysterectomy is associated with longer patient recovery and hospital stays, increased incisional pain, and a greater risk of postoperative febrile morbidity compared to laparoscopic or robotic approaches. In general, postoperative care should not be much different than that for simple type I abdominal hysterectomy. Overall, the incidence of complications is lower than compared to the more extensive type III radical operation.[18] Partial sympathetic and parasympathetic denervation should be much less extensive. Thus, bladder dysfunction is much less likely, and successful voiding occurs much earlier. Foley catheter drainage may be discontinued on the second postoperative day and is followed by a voiding trial.

RADICAL ABDOMINAL HYSTERECTOMY (TYPE III)

Procedure Overview

Box 25-13	Master Surgeon's Corner

- Type III hysterectomy principles may be necessary in a variety of surgical situations not involving malignancy.
- If suspicion of metastatic disease is present in the parametria or lymph nodes, intraoperative pathologic assessment should be considered if confirmation will change the operative plan.
- Obesity and extreme depth to the pelvis hinder the exposure essential to safe performance of a type III procedure; ensure availability of adequate retractors and longer instrumentation.

Radical hysterectomy refers to the third of 5 types of extended hysterectomy originally defined by Piver et al.[2] Type I and II hysterectomies were reviewed in the Abdominal Hysterectomy and Modified Radical Abdominal Hysterectomy (Type II) sections, respectively. Type IV hysterectomy involves excision of the superior vesicle artery and three-fourths of the upper vagina. Type V hysterectomy includes portions of the distal ureter or bladder. The aim of the type III operation involves wide radical excision of the parametrial and paravaginal tissues in addition to removal of intervening pelvic lymphatics. Type III radical hysterectomy is increasingly being performed by a minimally invasive approach (see Laparoscopic Radical Hysterectomy section).

Four main procedural differences distinguish a "true" radical hysterectomy. First, the uterine artery is ligated as it originates from the internal iliac artery (rather than where it crosses the ureter, as in a type II procedure). Second, dissection of the ureter from the

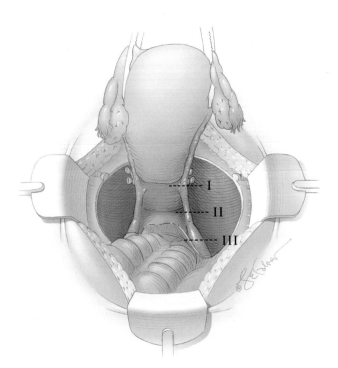

FIGURE 25-22. Extent of uterosacral ligament resection by hysterectomy type. (Redrawn, with permission, from Schorge JO, Schaffer JI, Halvorson LM, et al, eds. *Williams Gynecology.* New York, NY: McGraw-Hill; 2008.)

pubovesicle ligament (ie, the "tunnel") is completed until its entry into the bladder, except for a small lateral portion between the lower end of the ureter and the superior vesicle artery, thereby maintaining some distal ureteral blood supply. Third, the uterosacral ligaments are resected at their sacral attachments (instead of directly adjacent to the uterus as in a type I procedure, or halfway between the uterus and sacrum as in the type II procedure; Figure 25-22). Lastly, the upper one-third, about 3 to 4 cm, of the vagina is removed. This operation is chiefly indicated for stage IB1 to IIA cervical cancer, small central recurrences following radiation therapy, or clinical stage II endometrial cancer when tumor has extended to the cervix.

Radical hysterectomy is a dynamic operation that always requires significant intraoperative decision making. Every step requires a focused, consistent surgical approach. In many ways, radical abdominal hysterectomy initially defined the field of gynecologic oncology. Familiarity with its concepts continues to be critically important in developing expertise in complex pelvic surgery.

Preoperative Preparation

A spectrum of tests may be required to reach an accurate preoperative diagnosis, but typically, radical abdominal hysterectomy is performed for early-stage cervical cancer. Pelvic examination under anesthesia with cystoscopy and proctoscopy is not mandatory for smaller lesions, but accurate clinical staging of cervical cancer with appropriate imaging is critical prior to surgery. Other tests vary depending on the clinical setting and are discussed in Chapter 5. Unfortunately, there are limitations in what can be reliably detected preoperatively, and occasionally, unanticipated metastases will be discovered intraoperatively. If the patient has had a diagnostic loop or cold knife conization, it is often prudent to wait 6 weeks for tissue healing.

Radical abdominal hysterectomy can result in major short- and long-term morbidity, generally exceeding the minimally invasive approach.[19,20] Thus, the reasoning for laparotomy should be clearly communicated to the patient. The other major decision in surgical planning is whether a vertical or transverse incision is best. When there is a pre-existing abdominal incision, it may or may not be appropriate for the planned operation. Whereas a Pfannenstiel incision may be appropriate for type I or II hysterectomy, most gynecologic oncologists find it provides inadequate exposure to the lateral pelvis when performing a type III procedure.

Significant morbidity and potentially unforeseen short- and long-term complications are certainly more likely compared to a type I or II hysterectomy. These complications may develop more frequently in obese women and those with prior pelvic infections or prior abdominal surgery. Of potential intraoperative complications, the most common is acute hemorrhage. Blood loss averages 500 to 1000 mL, and transfusion rates are variable but relatively high.[21] Subacute postoperative complications may include ureterovaginal or vesicovaginal fistula (1%-2%) and significant postoperative bladder or bowel dysfunction (20%).[22] Additionally, long-term effects on sexual function, loss of fertility, and other body functions should be candidly reviewed.[23] The tone of the consenting process should reflect the extent of the operation required to hopefully cure or at least begin treatment of the malignancy. In addition, the patient must be advised that the procedure may be aborted if unexpected metastatic disease or pelvic tumor extension is found.

Other preoperative preparations follow as described for any type of abdominal hysterectomy. However, due to the potential for intraoperative hemorrhage, it may be prudent to have 2 units of packed cells typed and crossed in case they are urgently needed. Fortunately, radical abdominal hysterectomy is not dependent on specific instrumentation. In general, the equipment is similar to that used for a type II hysterectomy. Two doses of perioperative antibiotic prophylaxis with a third-generation cephalosporin such as cefoxitin may need to be given at spaced intervals if excessive bleeding occurs, due to the rapid clearance of antibiotics from the operative site.

Operative Procedure

Box 25-14	Caution Points

- Type III hysterectomies can be associated with large intraoperative blood loss, much of which occurs at a few select steps in the procedure:
  - Ligation and transaction of uterine vasculature, especially venous structures deep to the artery
  - Ligation and transection of the vesicouterine ligaments while unroofing the ureter
  - Ligation and transection of the uterosacral ligaments posteriorly
- Identify and tag the ureter early, especially while transecting the cardinal and uterosacral ligaments.

Anesthesia and Patient Positioning

General endotracheal anesthesia is administered, and the patient is positioned similarly, whether the planned operation is a type I, II, or III hysterectomy. Bimanual rectovaginal examination should always be performed in the operating room before scrubbing to familiarize oneself with the anatomy and to make a final decision on the type of incision. The abdomen and vagina are surgically prepared, and a transurethral Foley catheter is placed.

Abdominal Entry

A midline vertical abdominal incision provides excellent exposure but typically prolongs hospital stays and increases postoperative pain. Alternatively, Cherney or Maylard incisions offer postoperative advantages found with transverse incisions and allow increased access to the lateral pelvis. However, upper para-aortic nodes are not readily accessible through these transverse incisions. Following entry into the peritoneal cavity, the surgeon thoroughly explores the abdomen for obvious metastatic disease. Suspicious lymph nodes and any other lesions should either be removed or biopsied. Confirmation of metastatic disease or pelvic tumor extension should prompt an early decision about whether to proceed or abort an operation based on the overall intraoperative findings and clinical situation.

Entering the Retroperitoneal Space

The initial steps of a type III hysterectomy mirror those of the type I or II procedure except that, in this case, the round ligament is sutured with 0-gauge delayed-absorbable suture as far laterally as possible to facilitate the excision of parametrial tissue out to the pelvic sidewall. The anterior and posterior leaves of the broad ligament are sharply dissected, the ureter is placed on a ¼-in Penrose drain, and the paravesical and pararectal spaces are opened, as described earlier for type II hysterectomy.

Utero-Ovarian Ligament Transection

The next operative step depends on whether the adnexa are to be concurrently removed or not. Cervical cancer spread to the adnexa is much less common than via the lymphatics. Thus, removal of the adnexa should depend on a woman's age and potential for metastases. In candidates for ovarian preservation, transposition of ovaries out of the pelvis may be considered in premenopausal women if postoperative radiation is anticipated. However, symptomatic periadnexal cysts are common in transposed ovaries, and sustained ovarian function may not result. Regardless, once the ureter has been identified, the uteroovarian or IP ligament may be divided and peritoneal attachments dissected, as described in the Abdominal Hysterectomy section.

Uterine Artery Ligation

The superior vesical artery serves as the medial boundary for the paravesical space, which has been thoroughly developed. A narrow curved Deaver retractor is placed into the space and used to elevate and retract the artery medially. The vessel is both bluntly and sharply dissected on its lateral aspect down to its bifurcation off of the internal iliac artery. Placement of the surgeon's hand into the pelvis with the middle finger in the paravesical space and the index finger in the pararectal space allows for assessment of the parametria. Medial traction of the parametrial tissue and uterus places the uterine vasculature on stretch and exposes the medial surface of the internal iliac artery. From its bifurcation with the external iliac artery, parametrial attachments and areolar tissue are dissected along the internal iliac artery and reflected medially. During this dissection, the uterine artery will become apparent at its origin.

The uterine artery is one of several branches from the anterior division of the internal iliac artery; in the course of a radical hysterectomy, the posterior division should not be visible. The tissues immediately proximal and distal to the uterine artery are bluntly dissected, and a right-angle clamp is placed beneath this artery to retrieve a 2-0 silk suture (Figure 25-23). The uterine artery tie is placed as close as possible to its origin from the internal iliac artery. The process is repeated to place a separate silk suture far enough medial to enable vessel transection. Silk ties help identify the proximal and distal portions of the uterine

artery throughout the remainder of the operation. A small vascular clip can also be placed lateral to the silk tie on the proximal uterine artery for additional security of hemostasis. The uterine artery is then cut. The underlying uterine vein may also then be isolated, clipped or tied, and cut.

Uniting Paravesical and Pararectal Spaces

Once the uterine artery has been divided, it must be mobilized medially over the ureter along with surrounding parametrial tissue. Placement of a finger in both the paravesical and pararectal spaces results in the parametrial tissues being pressed together. Medial mobilization of the parametrial tissue unites these spaces and can be performed by several methods: (1) clamping, cutting, and suturing (Figure 25-24); (2) stapling with the gastrointestinal anastomosis stapler; (3) electrosurgical blade dissection to the pelvic sidewall using a right-angle clamp to elevate and isolate parametrial tissue; or (4) use of an electrothermal bipolar coagulator. Dissection is continued until the parametrial tissue is able to be fully mobilized medially over the ureter.

Ureter Mobilization

To detach the ureter from the medial leaf of the peritoneum, the tips of a right-angle clamp are positioned perpendicular to and just above the ureter. By opening the tips parallel to the ureter, a plane is created that permits it to be further bluntly dissected away from the peritoneum. The ureter is placed on gentle traction using the previously placed Penrose drain. An index finger placed medial to the ureter carefully sweeps it downward and laterally until the opening of the "tunnel" into the paracervical tissue is palpated ventromedially (Figure 25-25). Additional parametrial dissection is often required to ensure that the uterine artery and surrounding soft tissue have been entirely lifted medially over the ureter.

Unroofing the Ureteral Tunnel

The bladder is mobilized distally off of the anterior cervix as described for a type I or II hysterectomy, but will need to be additionally dissected several centimeters onto the upper vagina to allow for the more radical margin associated with a type III procedure. The uterus is placed on medial traction, and the proximal ureter is held laterally on traction by gently pulling on the Penrose drain. The tunnel opening should be palpated. Concurrently, a right-angle clamp is inserted above the ureter on its medial side with tips directed upward. Direct visualization of the underlying ureter is confirmed. The tips are directed medially toward the cervix, parallel to the course of the tunnel, and "popped" through the paracervical tissue ventrally. A

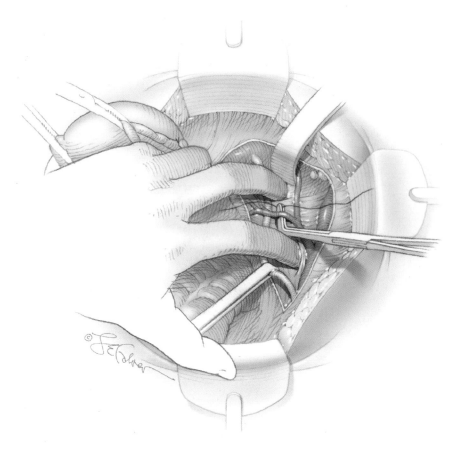

FIGURE 25-23. Ligating the uterine artery. (Redrawn, with permission, from Schorge JO, Schaffer JI, Halvorson LM, et al, eds. *Williams Gynecology.* New York, NY: McGraw-Hill; 2008.)

second clamp is placed through the opening. The ureter can be bluntly dissected and pushed posteriorly toward the tunnel floor. It should be visible below before cutting the overlying paracervical tissue (Figure 25-26). Delayed-absorbable 3-0 suture ties are placed to secure the paracervical tissue pedicles. Significant bleeding is commonly encountered during these steps. The same procedure may need to be repeated several times to completely unroof the tunnel and fully expose the course of the ureter. The dissection should proceed in a proximal to distal fashion with direct visualization of the ureter at all times, because this is the part of the operation where the ureter is most at risk for transection or other types of injury. Increasingly, the use of new technologies, such as an ultrasonic shear, can be used to secure and divide the pedicles, thereby decreasing operating time and blood loss. After unroofing the ureter, it is retracted upward and laterally. Filmy attachments between the ureter and tunnel bed are sharply divided.

Uterosacral Resection

Posterior radical dissection is generally performed as described for a type II hysterectomy, but the uterosacral

ligaments are clamped at the pelvic sidewall (Figure 25-27). The tissue is transected and ligated with 0-gauge delayed-absorbable suture or sealed and divided with a coagulating sealing device. This procedure may need to be repeated to complete transection of the entire uterosacral ligament and adjacent supportive tissues. The uterus and adjacent parametrium can then be lifted well out of the pelvis and any additional tissue attachments divided.

Vaginal Resection

At this point in the operation, the radical hysterectomy specimen should be attached only by the paracolpium and vagina. The bladder and ureters are further bluntly and sharply dissected free until at least 3 to 4 cm of upper vagina can be included with the resected specimen. Curved clamps are placed on the lateral paracolpium. The ureter should be lateral and directly visible. Tissue is then cut and suture ligated with 0-gauge delayed-absorbable suture. The upper vagina can then be incised circumferentially at the point of desired margin and closed with either continuous or interrupted 0-gauge delayed-absorbable suture. The specimen should be carefully examined to ensure an

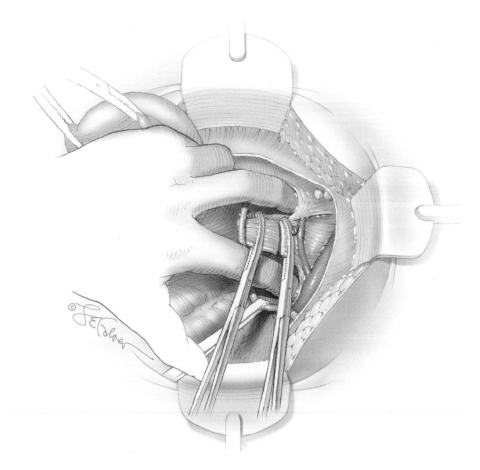

FIGURE 25-24. Uniting the spaces, division of parametrial tissue. (Redrawn, with permission, from Schorge JO, Schaffer JI, Halvorson LM, et al, eds. *Williams Gynecology.* New York, NY: McGraw-Hill; 2008.)

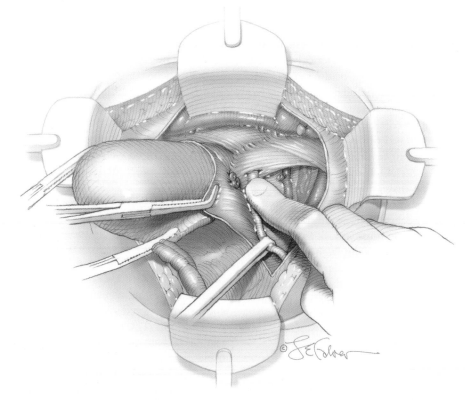

FIGURE 25-25. Mobilizing the ureter. (Redrawn, with permission, from Schorge JO, Schaffer JI, Halvorson LM, et al, eds. *Williams Gynecology.* New York, NY: McGraw-Hill; 2008.)

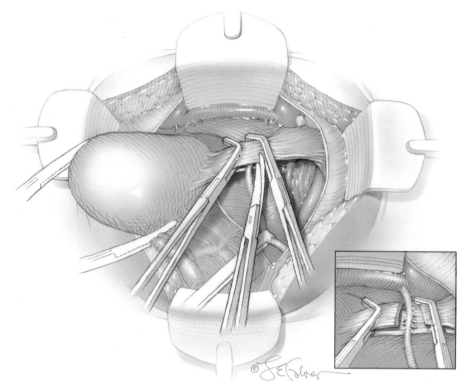

FIGURE 25-26. Unroofing the ureteral tunnel. (Redrawn, with permission, from Schorge JO, Schaffer JI, Halvorson LM, et al, eds. *Williams Gynecology.* New York, NY: McGraw-Hill; 2008.)

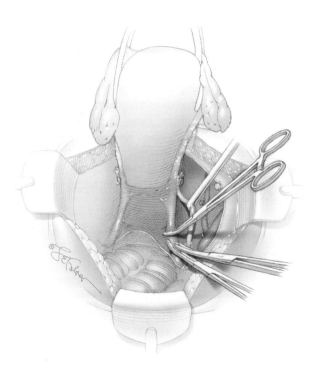

FIGURE 25-27. Uterosacral resection. (Redrawn, with permission, from Schorge JO, Schaffer JI, Halvorson LM, et al, eds. *Williams Gynecology.* New York, NY: McGraw-Hill; 2008.)

adequate upper vaginal segment and grossly negative margins.

Suprapubic Catheter Placement

The radical resection of the parametrial tissues in a type III procedure commonly results in early postoperative difficulty with voiding, necessitating bladder drainage for an extended period. In general, the transurethral Foley catheter will be satisfactory for postoperative management. However, placement of a suprapubic catheter may aid postoperative voiding trials in carefully selected, motivated patients. The tip of a second Foley catheter is brought through a stab incision in the lateral abdominal wall. The Foley catheter already within the bladder is held firmly and anteriorly in a distal extraperitoneal location. A 5-mm transverse incision is made through the bladder wall using an electrosurgical blade set to cutting mode. The Foley bulb should be directly visible to confirm entry through the mucosa. After being incised, the bladder mucosal edges are held with 2 Allis clamps. The second Foley catheter tip is inserted, and the balloon is inflated. A snug, but not overly tight, purse-string 3-0 chromic suture is used to close the bladder defect around the catheter. If the knot is placed too tightly, it may result in difficulty when removing the catheter postoperatively.

Delayed-absorbable suture in a running fashion is used to "bury" the visible intra-abdominal portion of the Foley catheter tubing in a tunnel of overlying peritoneum until its exit at the lateral anterior abdominal wall. The Foley catheter should be secured at the skin with a permanent suture that does not occlude the tubing. The urethral Foley catheter can be discontinued postoperatively when urine is seen to be draining from the suprapubic catheter.

Final Steps

Active bleeding should be controlled by cautery or ligature when the radical hysterectomy specimen has been removed. With bleeding controlled, ovarian transposition (Chapter 24) and/or lymphadenectomy (Chapter 28) may be performed next.

Once all planned surgical procedures have been completed, the surgeon should assess the vascular support to the ureter and other sidewall structures. If any structures appear particularly devascularized, an omental J-flap may be mobilized to provide additional blood supply. If ovarian transposition has been performed, the ovaries should be carefully inspected before abdominal closure to exclude vascular compromise. Routine pelvic suction drainage and closure of the peritoneum are not necessary in the absence of extenuating circumstances.[24]

Postoperative Care

Box 25-15 Complications and Morbidity

- Intraoperative
  - Hemorrhage
  - Bladder or rectal injury
  - Ureteral transection, ligation, or "kinking"
- Postoperative
  - Ileus (especially with vertical incision or excess blood loss)
  - Vaginal or intraperitoneal bleeding
  - Neurologic deficit (ie, retractor injury)
  - Wound infection, separation, or fascial dehiscence
  - Thromboembolic event
  - Genitourinary fistula (significantly more likely than for type II hysterectomy, especially when postoperative radiation is used)
  - Incisional hernia (more likely in obese patients)
  - Long-term bladder or rectal dysfunction (common)
  - Sexual dysfunction (common, particularly following postoperative radiation)

Radical abdominal hysterectomy is associated with longer patient recovery and hospital stays, increased incisional pain, and a greater risk of postoperative febrile morbidity compared to laparoscopic or robotic approaches.[19-21] Admission to the intensive care unit is uncommon but may be indicated for intraoperative hemorrhage, hemodynamic instability, or other medical comorbidities that might prompt the need for increased surveillance. In general, postoperative care is not dramatically different than for type I or II hysterectomy, or any type of abdominal surgery with a few exceptions.

Bladder tone typically returns slowly and is thought to be related to the degree of sympathetic and parasympathetic denervation during radical dissection. Foley catheter drainage is commonly continued until the patient is at least passing flatus, because improving bowel function typically accompanies resolving bladder hypotonia. Removal of the catheter or clamping of the suprapubic tube should be followed by a voiding trial, either prior to hospital discharge or at the first postoperative visit. A successful trial involves voiding more than 100 mL with a postvoid residual volume measuring less than 100 mL. When the trial is unsuccessful, it can be reattempted in several days. To remove the suprapubic tube, the skin stitch is cut, and the catheter should gently slide out. The small bladder opening will heal spontaneously.

Patients should be counseled that successful voiding may take several weeks to achieve. Unfortunately, in some cases, postoperative bladder dysfunction is permanent. Frequently, these patients had pre-existing abnormal urodynamic findings that were simply exacerbated by radical hysterectomy. For the less than 5% of women who develop long-term bladder hypotonia or atony, the preferred management is intermittent self-catheterization rather than indwelling urinary catheterization. Although most instances of long-term bladder dysfunction are unavoidable and simply represent a known risk of radical hysterectomy, some surgeons advocate a nerve-sparing technique as a way to reduce the likelihood.[25]

Tenesmus, constipation, and episodes of fecal incontinence are common immediate symptoms that should improve significantly months or years later. More than half of surgical patients report a worse sex life, at least in the short-term. Fortunately, patients treated by surgery alone can eventually expect a quality of life and overall sexual function similar to peers without a history of cancer.[26]

Although development of a fistula should be rare, the incidence increases 2- or 3-fold when patients require postoperative pelvic radiation. In addition, cervical cancer survivors treated with radiotherapy have much worse sexual functioning. Severe orgasmic problems, uncomfortable intercourse due to a reduced vaginal capacity, and severe dyspareunia may develop, sometimes resolving to some degree within 6 to 12 months. However, a persistent lack of sexual interest and lubrication often persist long-term.

LAPAROSCOPIC RADICAL HYSTERECTOMY (TYPES II AND III)

Procedure Overview

> **Box 25-16**   **Master Surgeon's Corner**
>
> - The position of the laparoscope within the pelvis provides excellent views of deep pelvic anatomy often not achievable by laparotomy.
> - The wristed instrumentation available with the robotic platform permits an ease of angulation to approach challenging anatomy. More effort is required to achieve similar results with traditional laparoscopic instruments.
> - The current robotic platform lacks haptic feedback, which many gynecologic oncologists find useful during open abdominal and traditional laparoscopic procedures.

Laparoscopic type II or III radical hysterectomy encompasses the identical anatomic boundaries as described for the corresponding abdominal procedures [see Modified Radical Abdominal Hysterectomy (Type II) and Radical Abdominal Hysterectomy (Type III) sections]. A minimally invasive laparoscopic approach, whether performed with traditional "straight-stick" instrumentation or with robotic assistance, is advantageous due to shorter recovery time, less postoperative pain, and decreased length of hospital stay.[19,20] Although initial series suggest similar oncologic outcomes compared to procedures performed abdominally, more long-term survival data are needed.[27] Laparoscopic radical hysterectomy, especially the type III procedure, is associated with initial long operative times and a flat learning curve. Utilization of a robotic platform in performance of the procedure is associated with accelerated skill acquisition. The currently available platform offers 3-dimensional imaging and wristed instrumentation, both of which are greatly beneficial given the meticulous dissection required. As a result, the majority of gynecologic oncologists use robotic assistance when performing laparoscopic radical hysterectomies.[21]

Selecting appropriate candidates is critical to successful minimally invasive surgery. In general, potentially problematic factors and other limitations are similar to those described earlier for laparoscopic type I hysterectomy. However, prior pelvic infections or other causes of retroperitoneal fibrosis may be particularly challenging to overcome when performing laparoscopic type II or III procedures due to the need for extensive dissection and development of tissue planes. Large cervical tumor size may limit the ability to place and use a uterine manipulator. A bulky uterus may be difficult to manipulate, block visualization within the pelvis, and be too large for vaginal removal. Patients with these findings may require an open, abdominal approach.

Preoperative Preparation

The basic preoperative evaluation for laparoscopic type II and III radical hysterectomy is similar to that of the abdominal approach. Preoperative pelvic examination is important to determine cervical appearance, uterine size, and mobility. Once a patient has been deemed appropriate for minimally invasive surgery, the same preoperative evaluation as for an open procedure applies. The consent should reflect the potential for needing to convert to laparotomy if exposure and organ manipulation are limited, the risks of gastrointestinal or genitourinary injuries, and other possible complications. Complications specific to laparoscopy include entry injury to the major vessels, bladder, ureters, and bowel.

Even more so than with performing a simple laparoscopic type I hysterectomy, the type II and III procedures are *very* dependent on specific instrumentation. Currently, the only commercially available robotic system is the da Vinci Surgical System (Intuitive Surgical). The specifics of this system and fundamentals of robotically assisted surgery are described in detail in Chapter 31. Important robotic instruments for radical hysterectomy include the EndoWrist monopolar scissors and the EndoWrist bipolar Maryland grasper. A PK Dissecting forceps is available as an alternative bipolar cautery source. The Harmonic Scalpel is also available but lacks the benefit of wristed movements. Various additional graspers and retractors can be used in the fourth robotic arm as desired for the procedure. The surgical assistant uses traditional laparoscopic instruments through a 12-mm assistant port. Some gynecologic oncologists prefer not to use a uterine manipulator in the setting of a cervical tumor, relying instead on the fourth arm of the robot to hold the uterus with a grasper. Others find use of a suitable uterine manipulator, as well as a modified colpotomy cup, to be indispensible.

Operative Procedure

Box 25-17 | **Caution Points**

- The ureter must be consciously, consistently held laterally during critical laparoscopic steps because it cannot be tagged as it is during abdominal surgery.
- Dissect the ureter out of the cardinal ligament tunnel with surgical effort directed just over and medial to the ureter. Dissecting under a ureter that is off tension can lead to accidental laceration just ahead of the leading edge of dissection.
- Although essential in maintaining a hemostatic operative field during laparoscopy, energy should be used in careful moderation in close proximity to the ureter and other fragile tissues.

Anesthesia and Patient Positioning

Administration of anesthesia and positioning are as previously described. After positioning the patient in dorsal lithotomy and before she is prepped and draped, a test of steep Trendelenburg should be performed to confirm secure positioning on the table. Bimanual rectovaginal examination is performed before prepping to familiarize oneself with the anatomy. Finally, the abdomen and vagina are surgically prepped and draped.

Placement of the Uterine Manipulator

When a bulky cervical cancer prevents insertion of a uterine manipulator, a blunt rectal probe may be inserted vaginally to facilitate the operation. Otherwise, whenever feasible, placement of an effective uterine manipulator is helpful. The technique is further described in the Laparoscopic Hysterectomy section. A modification of colpotomy cup placement has been described that facilitates incision of the vagina with a margin sufficient for radical hysterectomy.[28] Briefly, the smallest of 3 commonly available colpotomy cups is placed within the largest, and both are then placed on the uterine manipulator. The smaller cup exerts force directly on the cervix, while the ring of the larger demarcates the vagina at about 2 cm distal to the cervicovaginal junction. Because manipulator placement can often be difficult, the Foley catheter is inserted afterward so that it does not get in the way during placement. When there is any perceived possibility of bladder injury, a 3-way Foley provides additional access to easily backfill with methylene blue–colored

saline, and the integrity of the bladder should be confirmed at the end of the procedure.

Port Placement

The surgeon and assistant(s) are positioned around the patient, and abdominal entry is performed as described earlier in the Laparoscopic Hysterectomy section. The abdomen and pelvis are thoroughly inspected to assess the extent of disease and adhesions. At this point, discovery of unanticipated metastatic disease or pelvic tumor extension may prompt the surgeon to convert to laparotomy. Otherwise, additional ports are placed under direct intra-abdominal visualization. The patient is placed in steep Trendelenburg. Either the da Vinci Surgical System is docked with the surgeon operating via the console, or the procedure continues laparoscopically. The following technique is applicable regardless of whether or not robotic assistance is used. Instrumentation will differ according to approach and availability, but the general principles and steps should replicate an open, abdominal procedure.

Opening the Paravesical and Pararectal Spaces

Entering the retroperitoneum to identify the underlying structures is the initial step. As described for laparoscopic type I hysterectomy, the uterus is mobilized to 1 side by movement of the uterine manipulator and/or by an intraperitoneal blunt grasper holding 1 cornu. In doing so, the contralateral round ligament should be stretched. The surgeon tents up the round ligament, which is sealed and cut far laterally with the surgeon's instrument of choice, and initial access to the retroperitoneum is achieved. When performing robotic surgery, the Maryland bipolar forceps and monopolar scissors are used, whereas with traditional laparoscopy, ultrasonic shears are favored. The peritoneal incision is extended cephalad in parallel to the IP ligament.

While the first assistant holds and retracts the medial peritoneal edge medially, the surgeon uses 2 instruments in tandem to bluntly develop the retroperitoneum. Areolar tissue is separated easily, while small fibrous and vascular strands are sealed and cut. The lateral portion of the round ligament is elevated, and areolar tissue underneath is bluntly dissected. The external iliac vasculature is identified and exposed with extension of the peritoneal incision along the pelvic sidewall to above the bifurcation of the common iliac artery. The ureter is identified at the pelvic brim and exposed with retraction of the medial leaf of the broad ligament under the IP medially (Figure 25-28). The internal iliac artery is thus exposed down to the origin of the superior vesical

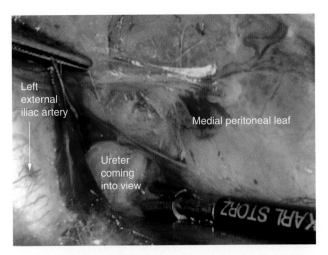

FIGURE 25-28. Identifying the retroperitoneal structures.

artery. Development of the pararectal space between the ureter and internal iliac vasculature is performed by the surgeon with 2 instruments working in tandem, bluntly retracting tissue in opposite directions. The dissection proceeds cautiously and is directed medially along the sacral curve. The uterine artery is usually identified in doing so.

Development of the paravesical space is facilitated by retraction of the medial umbilical ligament in the anterior pelvis medially by the first assistant. This places traction on the superior vesical artery to enable the surgeon to identify the correct plane of dissection. Blunt dissection beginning under the lateral portion of the cut round ligament directed medially toward the retracted medial umbilical ligament will initiate opening of the space. Tissue is then bluntly mobilized laterally away from the superior vesical artery all the way to its origin. Lastly, the obturator nerve is identified within the obturator fossa. Once the paravesical and pararectal spaces are opened, the parametria are now isolated between these 2 spaces. The uterus is then deflected in the opposite direction, and similar dissection is performed on the other side.

Adnexectomy or Ovarian Preservation

The utero-ovarian or IP ligament will be transected as previously described following identification of the ureter and development of an avascular space within the medial leaf of the broad ligament, depending on whether the adnexa are to be removed or retained. The procedure is repeated on the contralateral side.

Ureteral Isolation

The first assistant holds and retracts the medial edge of the cut medial leaf of the broad ligament medially,

exposing the ureter. The surgeon bluntly develops the plane between the ureter and peritoneum. The act of opening a closed fine grasper placed immediately medial to the ureter is a useful technique to safely begin development of this plane, which is then extended all the way until the uterine vasculature is to be encountered. Occasional cautious use of energy (ie, short bursts of monopolar cautery or use of ultrasonic shears) will be necessary to separate the ureter from more dense fibrovascular attachments. Later, the ureter will be further dissected in stages from surrounding attachments, depending on whether a type II or III hysterectomy is performed.

Bladder Mobilization

The bladder is mobilized laparoscopically as previously described, but to a greater degree compared to in a type I procedure. Fibrous attachments are divided with an energy source from proximal to distal between the posterior bladder and the uterus/anterior vagina. As the bladder is pushed inferiorly, the colpotomy cup, if present, will be palpable. Alternatively, a rectal probe can be used within the vagina both to provide vaginal landmarks and a firm surface on which to dissect. It is crucial to adequately mobilize the bladder onto the upper vagina to provide a satisfactory distal margin of the resection. Although the technique for performing laparoscopic type II and III hysterectomy has been identical to this point, the operative steps begin to diverge.

Uterine Artery Ligation and Ureteral Dissection

Type II Modified Radical Hysterectomy

The ureter has been dissected to a level near the uterine artery. Although the intent of a type II procedure is to transect the uterine artery where it crosses the ureter, it is often easiest to first identify the artery at its origin. Blunt dissection along the internal iliac and superior vesical arteries along with medial tension on the uterus will assist in its identification. In the case of a type II procedure, the uterine artery path is traced back to its intersection with the ureter. The ureter is then dissected so that it falls a short distance from the vessel, which can then be safely cauterized or sealed, and cut (Figure 25-29). The medial cut end of the uterine vessels along with the associated parametrial tissue are then elevated and held medially by the first assistant. The ureter is held on gentle lateral traction while the surgeon works to separate it from any medial attachments to the parametria. The tunnel of the ureter is encountered, comprised of cardinal

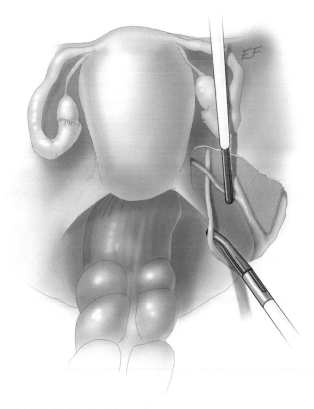

FIGURE 25-29. Dividing the uterine artery as it crosses the ureter (type II procedure).

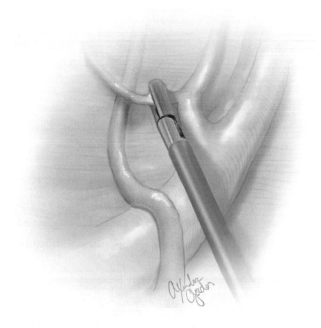

FIGURE 25-30. Dividing the uterine artery at its origin (type III procedure). Instrument used should be harmonic scalpel. (Redrawn, with permission, from Schorge JO, Schaffer JI, Halvorson LM, et al, eds. *Williams Gynecology*. New York, NY: McGraw-Hill; 2008.)

and vesicouterine ligaments. The medial half of these ligaments is incised by successive sealing and dividing the paracervical tissue medially, until reaching the upper vaginal margin. It is essential that the ureter be held laterally on slight tension while the tunnel is dissected to avoid cutting into a curve of ureteral tissue off tension. This is the most demanding step in a laparoscopic radical hysterectomy and where the wristed instrumentation of the robotic platform is most helpful. The ureter is unroofed and rolled medially, but not completely removed of its lateral attachments.

Type III Radical Hysterectomy

The ureter has been dissected to a level near the uterine artery. At this point, the artery is identified at its origin. Blunt dissection along the internal iliac and superior vesical arteries along with medial tension on the uterus will assist in its identification. With blunt dissection, the uterine artery is isolated, slightly skeletonized, and then ligated as close to its origin from the internal iliac artery as possible using clips, cautery, or ultrasonic shears, followed by transection (Figure 25-30). Once the uterine artery has been ligated, it is mobilized medially over the ureter along with its associated parametrial tissue. The medial cut end of the uterine vessels along with the associated parametrial

tissue are then elevated and held medially by the first assistant. The ureter is held on gentle lateral traction while the surgeon works to separate it from any medial parametrial attachments. The tunnel of the ureter is encountered, comprised of the cardinal and vesicouterine ligaments. The medial half of these ligaments is incised by creating a space ventrally (Figure 25-31), then successive sealing and dividing of the paracervical tissue medially, until reaching the upper vaginal margin. It is essential that the ureter be held laterally on slight tension while the tunnel is dissected to avoid cutting into a curve of ureteral tissue off tension. This is the most demanding step in a laparoscopic radical hysterectomy and where the wristed instrumentation of the robotic platform is most helpful. The ureter is unroofed and completely detached of all lateral and dorsal attachments to the cardinal ligament. It is then mobilized along with the bladder well off the vagina in preparation for later vaginotomy.

Uterosacral Transection

The pararectal space has been previously well developed, and the ureter has been dissected off of the broad ligament and pararectal tissues. The uterosacral ligaments can now be isolated and transected. First,

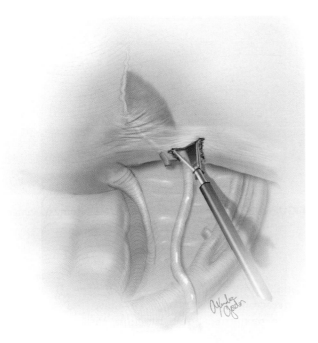

FIGURE 25-31. Unroofing the ureter (type III procedure). (Redrawn, with permission, from Schorge JO, Schaffer JI, Halvorson LM, et al, eds. *Williams Gynecology.* New York, NY: McGraw-Hill; 2008.)

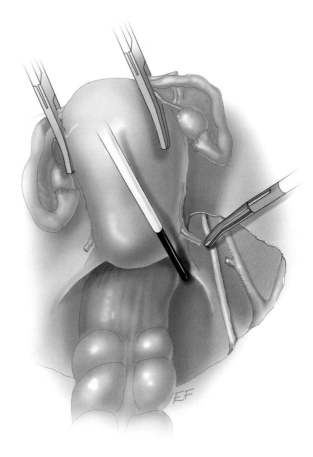

FIGURE 25-32. Dividing the uterosacral ligament. (Redrawn, with permission, from Schorge JO, Schaffer JI, Halvorson LM, et al, eds. *Williams Gynecology.* New York, NY: McGraw-Hill; 2008.)

the uterus is severely anteverted and the peritoneum within the posterior cul-de-sac incised from side to side. The rectovaginal space is developed with a combination of blunt dissection and focused use of cautery or the ultrasonic shears. The appropriate plane is best achieved beginning on the left side, further away from the rectal mesentery. In developing this space, the uterosacral ligaments will become evident bilaterally. The uterosacral ligaments, now isolated, can then be ligated halfway (type II procedure) or close to the sacrum (type III) using ultrasonic shears (Figure 25-32) or bipolar coagulation and scissors. The ureters should be retracted laterally before transecting the uterosacral ligament.

Vaginal Resection

With complete mobilization of the bladder and rectum, the anterior and posterior vagina should be easily identified. The radical hysterectomy specimen is now held in place only by the paracolpium and vagina, and manipulation of the specimen should be facile. If a modified colpotomy cup is present, it serves as a 2-cm marker within the vagina. Alternatively, a rectal probe can be used to direct the incision. The upper vagina is incised distally on the vaginal wall to allow resection of a portion of proximal vagina (1-2 cm for a type II; 3-4 cm for a type III; Figure 25-33). This

incision is extended circumferentially, and the specimen is removed vaginally. The specimen should be inspected for adequate margins (Figure 25-34), and an additional vaginal margin should be removed if necessary.

Final Steps

Laparoscopic closure of the vaginal cuff can be performed by multiple methods as previously described. Other procedures, such as lymphadenectomy or ovarian transposition, may be performed, depending on patient circumstances. Once procedures have been completed, an inspection for hemostasis is performed. If used, the robotic platform is undocked. Ports are next removed under direct visualization. All fascial defects 10 mm or greater should be closed with delayed-absorbable suture to avoid hernia development at the site. Skin incisions are closed by the surgeon's preferred method. Diagnostic cystoscopy is at the discretion of the surgeon.

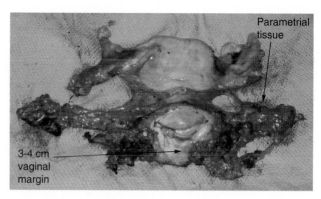

FIGURE 25-34. Laparoscopic radical hysterectomy specimen.

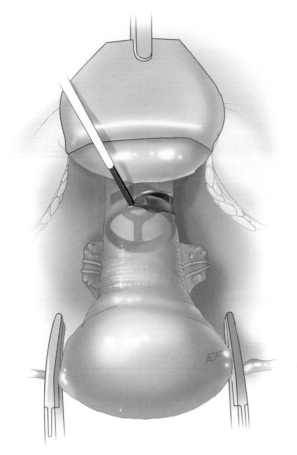

FIGURE 25-33. Upper vaginal resection. (Redrawn, with permission, from Schorge JO, Schaffer JI, Halvorson LM, et al, eds. *Williams Gynecology.* New York, NY: McGraw-Hill; 2008.)

Postoperative Care

Box 25-18   Complications and Morbidity

- Intraoperative
  - Trocar injury to the bowel or vessels
  - Hemorrhage
  - Bladder or rectal perforation
  - Ureteral transection, ligation, or "kinking"
- Postoperative
  - Vaginal or intraperitoneal bleeding
  - Neurologic deficit (eg, brachial plexus or peroneal nerve injury)
  - Port-site bowel herniation or infection
  - Delayed thermal injury to bowel or genitourinary tract
  - Genitourinary fistula (comparable to abdominal types II and III)
  - Long-term bladder or rectal dysfunction (comparable to abdominal types II and III)
  - Sexual dysfunction (comparable to abdominal types II and III)

Laparoscopic and robotic-assisted type II and III hysterectomy patients typically have the same fast return of normal bowel function, easier ambulation, and decreased analgesia requirements as those undergoing a type I procedure. Often pain is adequately controlled with oral medications, and intravenous narcotics are not needed.

Postoperatively, the care is also very comparable. The diet may be advanced quickly, and early ambulation is encouraged. The same principles for retaining a Foley catheter apply as described for the comparable abdominal procedures [see Modified Radical Abdominal Hysterectomy (Type II) and Radical Abdominal Hysterectomy (Type III) sections]. Patients undergoing type II hysterectomy may have the Foley catheter removed on day 2 with a voiding trial. Type III patients are typically sent home with the Foley catheter and return to clinic for a voiding trial in about 1 week. Overall, laparoscopic and robotic-assisted radical hysterectomy techniques appear to be equally adequate and feasible.[29]

REFERENCES

1. Whiteman MK, Hillis SD, Jamieson DJ, et al. Inpatient hysterectomy surveillance in the United States, 2000-2004. *Am J Obstet Gynecol.* 2008;34.e1-34.e7.
2. Piver MS, Rutledge F, Smith JP. Five classes of extended hysterectomy for women with cervical cancer. *Obstet Gynecol.* 1974;44:265-272.
3. Pulliam SJ, Berkowitz LR. Smaller pieces of the hysterectomy pie: current challenges in resident surgical education. *Obstet Gynecol.* 2009;113:395-298.
4. Mabrouk M, Frumovitz M, Greer M, et al. Trends in laparoscopic and robotic surgery among gynecologic oncologists: a survey update. *Gynecol Oncol.* 2009;112;501-505.
5. Boyd LR, Novetsky AP, Curtin JP. Effect of surgical volume on route of hysterectomy and short-term morbidity. *Obstet Gynecol.* 2010;116:909-915.
6. Brummer TH, Jalkanen J, Fraser J, et al. FINHYST, a prospective study of 5279 hysterectomies: complications and their risk factors. *Hum Reprod.* 2011;26:1741-1751.

7. Matthews CA, Reid N, Ramakrishnan V, et al. Evaluation of the introduction of robotic technology on route of hysterectomy and complications in the first year of use. *Am J Obstet Gynecol.* 2010;203:499.e1-5.

8. ACOG Committee opinion No. 444: choosing the route of hysterectomy for benign disease. *Obstet Gynecol.* 2009;114: 1156-1158.

9. Rogo-Gupta LJ, Lewin SN, Kim JH, et al. The effect of surgeon volume on outcomes and resource use for vaginal hysterectomy. *Obstet Gynecol.* 2010;116:1341-1347.

10. Nieboer TE, Johnson N, Lethaby A, et al. Surgical approach to hysterectomy for benign gynaecological disease. *Cochrane Database Syst Rev.* 2009;3:CD003677.

11. Smith SM, Hoffman MS. The role of vaginal hysterectomy in the treatment of endometrial cancer. *Am J Obstet Gynecol.* 2007;197:202.e1-6.

12. Ascher-Walsh CJ, Capes T, Smith J, et al. Cervical vasopressin compared to no premedication and blood loss during vaginal hysterectomy: a randomized controlled trial. *Obstet Gynecol.* 2009;113:313-318.

13. Boruta DM 2nd, Growdon WG, Schorge JO. Single-incision laparoscopic staging for endometrial cancer. *J Am Coll Surg.* 2011;212:e1-e5.

14. Tenney M, Walker JL. Role of laparoscopic surgery in the management of endometrial cancer. *J Natl Compr Canc Netw.* 2009;7:559-567.

15. Walker JL, Piedmonte MR, Spirtos NM, et al. Laparoscopy compared with laparotomy for comprehensive surgical staging of uterine cancer: Gynecologic Oncology Group Study LAP2. *J Clin Oncol.* 2009;27:5331-5336.

16. Ceccaroni M, Berretta R, Malzoni M, et al. Vaginal cuff dehiscence after hysterectomy: a multicenter retrospective study. *Eur J Obstet Gynecol Reprod Biol.* 2011;158:308-313.

17. Fedele L, Bianchi S, Zanconato G, et al. Tailoring radicality in demolitive surgery for deeply infiltrating endometriosis. *Am J Obstet Gynecol.* 2005;193:114-117.

18. Cai HB, Chen HZ, Zhou YF, et al. Class II radical hysterectomy in low-risk squamous cell carcinoma of cervix: a safe and effective option. *Int J Gynecol Cancer.* 2009;19:46-49.

19. Frumovitz M, dos Reis R, Sun CC, et al. Comparison of total laparoscopic and abdominal radical hysterectomy for patients with early-stage cervical cancer. *Obstet Gynecol.* 2007;110: 96-102.

20. Ko EM, Muto MG, Berkowitz RS, et al. Robotic versus open radical hysterectomy: a comparative study at a single institution. *Gynecol Oncol.* 2008;111:425-430.

21. Estape R, Lambrou N, Diaz R, et al. A case matched analysis of robotic radical hysterectomy with lymphadenectomy compared with laparoscopy and laparotomy. *Gynecol Oncol.* 2009;113: 357-361.

22. Hazewinkel MH, Sprangers MA, van der Velden J, et al. Long-term cervical cancer survivors suffer from pelvic floor symptoms: a cross-sectional matched cohort study. *Gynecol Oncol.* 2010;117:281-286.

23. Serati M, Salvatore S, Uccella S, et al. Sexual function after radical hysterectomy for early-stage cervical cancer: is there a difference between laparoscopy and laparotomy? *J Sex Med.* 2009;6:2516-2522.

24. Franchi M, Trimbos JB, Zanaboni F, et al. Randomised trial of drains versus no drains following radical hysterectomy and pelvic lymph node dissection: a European Organisation for Research and Treatment of Cancer-Gynaecological Cancer Group (EORTC-GCG) study in 234 patients. *Eur J Cancer.* 2007;43:1265-1268.

25. Ditto A, Martinelli F, Mattana F, et al. Class III nerve-sparing radical hysterectomy versus standard class III radical hysterectomy: an observational study. *Ann Surg Oncol.* 2011;18: 3469-3478.

26. Frumovitz M, Sun CC, Schover LR, et al. Quality of life and sexual functioning in cervical cancer survivors. *J Clin Oncol.* 2005;23:7428-7436.

27. Cantrell LA, Mendivil A, Gehrig PA, et al. Survival outcomes for women undergoing type III robotic radical hysterectomy for cervical cancer: a 3-year experience. *Gynecol Oncol.* 2010;117:260-265.

28. Ramirez PT, Frumovitz M, Dos Reis R, et al. Modified uterine manipulator and vaginal rings for total laparoscopic radical hysterectomy. *Int J Gynecol Cancer.* 2008;18:571-575.

29. Kruijdenberg CB, van den Einden LC, Hendriks JC, et al. Robot-assisted versus total laparoscopic radical hysterectom in early cervical cancer, a review. *Gynecol Oncol.* 2011;120:334-339.

26 Cervical Procedures

Danielle Vicus and Allan Covens

CERVICAL CONIZATION

Procedure Overview

Box 26-1	Master Surgeon's Corner

- The size and histologic cell type of the lesion, together with the desire for future fertility, help guide the technique and extent of the procedure.

A cervical conization refers to the surgical excision of the squamous-columnar junction. The indications are both therapeutic and diagnostic. It is a therapeutic procedure in cases of cervical intraepithelial neoplasia grade 2 or 3 and microinvasive carcinoma of the cervix (negative margins). Diagnostic indications include unsatisfactory colposcopy, positive endocervical curettage, persistent positive cytology for dysplasia in the presence of a normal colposcopy, and a cervical biopsy positive for microinvasion. The full management paradigm has been discussed in previous chapters and will not be reviewed here (see Chapters 4 and 5). A knife cone biopsy is the gold standard and has the advantage of proper evaluation of the margins because no thermal energy is used; however, for the most part, a loop electrosurgical excision procedure (LEEP) is sufficient. The exception is in cases in which a precise margin is essential. LEEP is usually performed as an outpatient procedure under local anesthesia, whereas in cases of knife cone biopsy, general or regional anesthesia is used.

Knife Cone Biopsy

Preoperative Preparation

Preoperatively a colposcopic evaluation of the cervix is performed to evaluate the extent of disease. Biopsies from appropriate areas are sent, and if a conization is indicated, formal informed consent is obtained with emphasis on possible complications including cervical incompetence, bleeding, and infection. The patient is admitted to the hospital on the day of surgery.

Operative Procedure

Box 26-2	Caution Points

- Optimal visualization is important in order to properly evaluate the extent of the lesion and thus minimize the need for repeat procedures.
- The size of the excision should be sufficient to remove the entire lesion; however, it should be kept in mind that the deeper the conization, the greater is the likelihood of future cervical incompetence.
- The use of relatively large loop electrodes can lead inadvertently to removal of large amounts of the cervix.

The procedure is performed under general or regional anesthesia. The patient is put in the semilithotomy position, and a bimanual examination is performed. The patient is then prepped and draped and the bladder emptied via a catheter. A speculum is inserted into the vagina for maximum visualization. Lugol's stain may be used to help delineate the dysplasia. A single-tooth tenaculum is used to grasp the anterior aspect of the cervix. Bleeding from the cervix can be minimized by injecting a dilute solution of vasopressin in lidocaine into the 4 quadrants of the cervical stroma. Figure-of-eight "stay" stitches of 1-0 delayed-absorbable suture can be placed at the 3 o'clock and 9 o'clock positions on the cervix just below the cervicovaginal junction. These stitches will aid in hemostasis and can be used to manipulate the cervix during conization. A #11 or a #15 blade is used to make a circumferential incision incorporating the demarcated area and the entire transformation zone. A cone-shaped incision should be made to the depth of approximately 2 to 2.5 cm, depending on the depth of the cervix (Figure 26-1). The cone should preferably be excised in a single piece and a suture placed at 12 o'clock to facilitate orientation of the specimen by the pathologist. Once the cone has been removed, an endocervical curettage is performed.

Hemostasis of the cone bed can be obtained using one of many techniques. Electrocautery, either with a ball electrode or a regular cautery tip, is commonly used. Monsel's solution applied generously to the cone bed can also control the bleeding. An additional option is suturing the bed of the cone with either a running lock absorbable suture or interrupted figure-of-eights that also approximate the proximal and distal edges. A combination of techniques, together with direct pressure or hemostatic agents (eg, Surgicel), may be used in case of heavy bleeding.

Loop Electrosurgical Excision Procedure

Loop diathermy has been shown to be an effective and reliable alternative to cold knife conization with the advantages of it being performed in an outpatient setting without the need for general anesthesia. It has been found to be technically easier and less time consuming than cold knife conization.[1,2]

The LEEP probe consists of a wire loop (stainless steel or tungsten), which comes in multiple sizes, attached to an insulated T-bar. It is performed with a blend of coagulation and cutting. The size of the loop is chosen with respect to the volume of the lesion. Most commonly, loop sizes of 10 to 20 mm are used. Although there is an advantage in obtaining the entire specimen in 1 pass because it helps the pathologist identify the surgical margins, the depth required usually entails a minimum of 2 passes of the loop (Figure 26-2). The procedure is performed under colposcopic guidance, and therefore, the margins can be re-examined before completion of the procedure. Bleeding from the cone bed can be controlled with the same techniques mentioned earlier for knife cone biopsy.

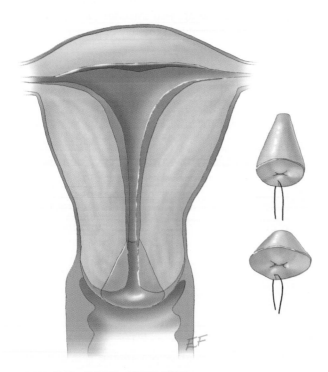

FIGURE 26-1. Knife cone biopsy.

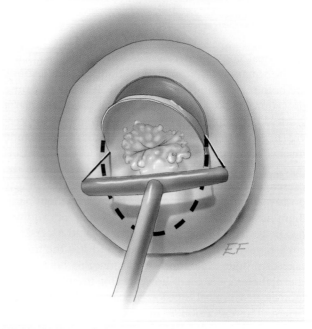

FIGURE 26-2. Loop electrosurgical excision procedure (LEEP).

Postoperative Care

CHAPTER 26

Box 26-3 — Complications and Morbidity

- Significant bleeding may occur 10 to 21 days after the procedure (5%-10% of cases) and is more common when using a larger loop and when a vasoconstrictive agent is not injected prior to the procedure.
- Cervicitis and ascending endometritis are rare but can occur.
- Cervical incompetence and, as a result, premature delivery have been reported to be doubled (approximately 6%) after a cervical excisional procedure.[3] However, no increase in neonatal morbidity or mortality has been shown.
- Cervical stenosis is an uncommon result (3%) of a cervical excisional procedure.

Patients usually tolerate cervical excisional procedures well and are discharged home on a regular diet the same day.

RADICAL TRACHELECTOMY

Procedure Overview

Box 26-4 — Master Surgeon's Corner

- The oncologic outcomes of the radical trachelectomy are comparable to those of radical hysterectomy; therefore, patients wishing to preserve fertility who meet the eligibility criteria should be offered this procedure.

The radical trachelectomy is a fertility-sparing procedure that consists of removing the majority, if not all, of the cervix jointly with the parametrium and the upper portion of the vagina. It can be performed by an abdominal or vaginal approach. The latter was initially described by Dargent and, when performed together with a laparoscopic pelvic lymph node dissection, has been shown to have low morbidity, comparable oncologic outcomes to the radical hysterectomy, and good obstetric outcomes.[3-5] The indications are desire to preserve fertility, tumor size less than 2 cm, International Federation of Gynecology and Obstetrics (FIGO) stage IA1 disease with lymph vascular space involvement, stage IA2 or IB1 tumors, squamous cell or adenocarcinoma, no involvement of the upper endocervical canal, and no metastasis to regional lymph nodes on computed tomography or magnetic resonance imaging.[6]

Radical Abdominal Trachelectomy

Preoperative Preparation

Once a patient is diagnosed with cervical cancer and expresses a desire to retain fertility, thorough evaluation is warranted to help decide whether a radical trachelectomy is appropriate. Because the FIGO staging of cervical cancer is clinical (as previously discussed in Chapter 5), the first step is a complete history, physical, and pelvic examination. When the pelvic examination is challenging, an examination under anesthesia should be performed. In patients with early-stage disease, a chest x-ray, complete blood count (CBC), and kidney function (creatinine) are frequently performed preoperatively. Additional imaging and blood work are left to the discretion of the treating oncologist while taking into consideration the patient's symptoms, comorbidities, and results of the clinical examination.

Once a decision is made to proceed with a radical trachelectomy and pelvic lymph node evaluation, informed consent is obtained. It is important to discuss the possibility of bladder dysfunction, urinary tract injury, and lymphedema and the option of a radical hysterectomy, in addition to bleeding, infection, and injury to other adjacent organs.

The patient is admitted to the hospital on the morning of the operation. Prophylactic antibiotic is administered prior to surgery.

Operative Procedure

Box 26-5 — Caution Points

- The height of the cervical amputation should be as far away from the internal os as possible, as long as a surgical margin of 5 mm is obtained.
- In a radical abdominal trachelectomy, the uterine artery is identified; however, attempts to preserve it should be made, and only the descending branches of the uterine artery should be ligated.

The patient is put in semilithotomy position, and general anesthesia is induced. Care is taken to place the legs appropriately to avoid pressure on the peroneal nerves. A bimanual examination is performed to assess the extent of disease to further guide the procedure. The abdomen and perineum are prepped and draped, and an indwelling Foley catheter is inserted into the bladder.

The incision can be either transverse (Pfannenstiel, Maylard, or Cherney) or a low midline incision from the umbilicus to the pubic bone. This is decided both by the extent of disease and the patient's habitus.

Once the peritoneal cavity is entered, a full abdominal and pelvic exploration is performed to look for metastatic disease. Special attention to the retroperitoneal nodes and to penetration of the tumor through the cervix toward the parametrium and pelvic sidewalls is noted. The patient is then put in Trendelenburg position, a self-retaining retractor is inserted, and the bowel is packed off to facilitate maximum exposure of the pelvis. Care must be taken to avoid undue pressure on the psoas muscles by the blades of the retractor to avert a femoral nerve injury secondary to compression. Thin patients are particularly vulnerable.

A bilateral pelvic lymph node dissection is usually performed prior to the trachelectomy. The retroperitoneum is entered either by dividing the round ligament or by opening up the peritoneum overlying the psoas muscle. Clamps may be placed on the round ligament stumps to facilitate uterine manipulation; however, clamps should not be placed across the fallopian tube/utero-ovarian ligament complex. This window to the retroperitoneum is then extended caudally toward the bladder reflection and cephalic toward the infundibulopelvic ligament. The retroperitoneal structures, including the psoas muscle and the external iliac vessels, are exposed while the uterus is retracted to the opposite side. The ureter is then identified as it crosses over the iliac bifurcation. The anterior peritoneum overlying the bladder is then dissected off the anterior wall of the vagina.

The paravesical and pararectal spaces are then developed (Figure 26-3). Care must be taken not to damage the adnexa, the uterus, or the ovarian vessels when manipulating the uterus. The pararectal space is found by carefully developing the space between the ureter and the internal iliac artery posterior to the cardinal ligament (ie, the uterine artery). The dissection is parallel to the sacrum and slants medial. The borders of the pararectal space are composed of the rectum medially, the internal iliac artery laterally, the cardinal ligament anteriorly, and the sacrum posteriorly. Care must be taken when developing the space in order to avoid bleeding from the lateral sacral or hemorrhoidal vessels and internal iliac vein. The paravesical space is then developed by gently dissecting between the obliterated hypogastric artery medially and the external iliac vein laterally. The dissection is carried to the level of the pelvic floor. Although this is potentially an avascular space, an aberrant obturator vein (24% of patients) may occupy this space and cause bleeding; therefore, care must be taken. The paravesical space is bordered by the obliterated umbilical artery medially, the obturator internus muscle laterally, the cardinal ligament posteriorly, and the pubic symphysis anteriorly.

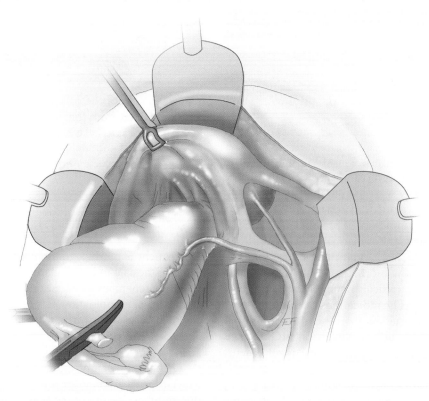

FIGURE 26-3. Radical abdominal dissection. The paravesical and pararectal spaces have been developed, and the ureter, parametrium, and retroperitoneal structures are under direct visualization.

Once the paravesical and pararectal spaces have been properly developed, the cardinal ligament and the uterine vessels are easily identified. The uterine artery is then identified; ideally, it should be preserved, and only the descending branches of the uterine artery should be ligated. This can be performed in a number of fashions (eg, using 2 hemoclips and cutting in between or alternatively passing 2 ties under the artery and dividing in the middle). It is useful to be able to identify the medial side of the uterine artery later while dissecting out the parametrium.

The ureter is then unroofed from the vesicouterine ligament. This is facilitated by gently dissecting superior and medial to the ureter, with either Metzenbaum scissors or a right angle clamp. This forms a tunnel under the cardinal ligament. It is important to take caution to stay superior to the ureter and confirm that the tip of the dissecting instrument protrudes cephalic to the bladder. The tunnel is then enlarged laterally by opening and closing the right angle clamp. A tie or hemoclip is inserted into the tunnel and is tied or clipped as laterally as possible. Medial to the tie (clip), the tunnel is divided.

Attention is then brought to the posterior aspect of the uterus by sharply drawing the uterus anteriorly exposing the cul-de-sac and putting the uterosacral ligaments on stretch. The uterosacral ligaments are identified, and a small window in the peritoneum is made approximately 1 cm beneath the inferior margin of the cervix in the midline. This opens the rectovaginal space that can further be deepened by either blunt or sharp dissection. The ureter is then separated from the medial peritoneum. Once the rectum is pushed down and the ureter is freed from the medial peritoneum, the uterosacral ligaments are clamped, divided, and sutured.

The paravaginal fascia is then dissected to further obtain the tissue between the cervix and the upper vagina. The vagina is then examined both anteriorly and posteriorly to verify that adequate vaginal margins will be obtained when the specimen is transected from the vagina. If the anterior margin is insufficient, further sharp dissection of the base of the bladder is to be freed from the anterior vagina.

When the specimen is ready, 2 clamps are placed across the vagina approximately 2 cm inferior to the level of the cervix. The cervix is then divided from the vagina above the clamps.

An estimation of the level of the lower uterine segment is made, and clamps are placed on the uterus at the level of the internal os. A knife is then used to transect the cervix approximately 5 mm below the level of the internal os (Figure 26-4). The specimen is then released and sent for frozen section to verify a negative endocervical margin. For patients with a positive margin or a margin less than 5 mm,

an additional resection is performed. A #5 French catheter is inserted and sutured into the os to maintain patency. This is removed at the patient's postoperative clinic visit. A permanent cerclage (Shirodkar) suture (Mersilene) is subsequently placed around the inferior edge of the uterus at the level of the internal os and the knot tied posteriorly. The uterus is then reapproximated to the vaginal cuff with 6 to 8 1-0 delayed-absorbable interrupted sutures (Figure 26-5). Hemostasis is obtained, and the abdomen is closed in the normal fashion.

Radical Vaginal Trachelectomy

The patient is put in semilithotomy position, and general anesthesia is induced. Care is taken to place the legs appropriately to avoid pressure on the peroneal nerves. A bimanual examination is performed to assess the extent of disease to further guide the procedure. The abdomen and perineum are prepped and draped, and an indwelling Foley catheter is inserted into the bladder. The operating room is prepared for laparoscopy and vaginal surgery.

The procedure is initiated with a laparoscopic bilateral lymph node evaluation by either a lymph node dissection or a sentinel lymph node biopsy. If a sentinel lymph node biopsy is performed, the vaginal procedure is performed while waiting for the result of the frozen section; however, the laparoscopic equipment remains sterile.

The patient is then put in high lithotomy position, and the cervix is visualized. The vaginal mucosa around the cervix is injected with a dilute solution of vasopressin in lidocaine. A scalpel is used to circumferentially incise the vaginal mucosa taking care to leave an adequate margin of 1 to 2 cm from the cervical portio. The posterior cul-de-sac is entered, while the vesicovaginal space anteriorly is developed, but the bladder peritoneum is not incised. The paravesical spaces are created by dissecting at the small indentation created by retracting the anterior vaginal cuff at the 12 o'clock position and the lateral vaginal cuff at the 3 (or 9) o'clock position. Using a long curved Kelly clamp or Metzenbaum scissors, the paravesical space is developed by gently spreading in a superior-anterior-lateral direction (Figure 26-6). Cooper's ligament is then palpable anteriorly. Krobach clamps are then placed horizontally on the vagina, which is closed over the cervix, facilitating traction of the cervix. The distal portion of the uterosacral ligaments can be safely clamped in their mid portion without identifying the ureter at this point. A Breisky retractor is placed in the paravesical space, and with a finger in the vesicouterine space, the ureter can be palpated against the retractor. The tissue between the paravesical and vesicouterine space is the

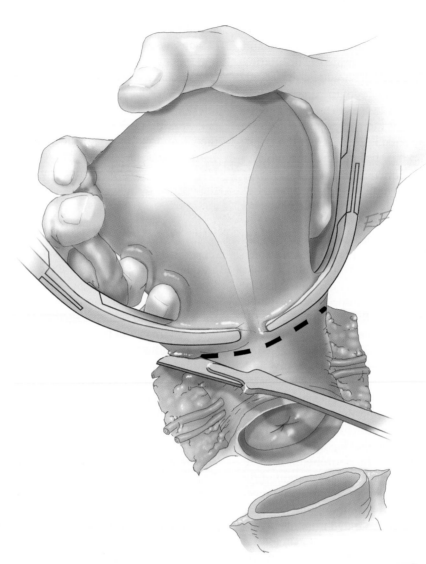

FIGURE 26-4. Radical abdominal trachelectomy. The cervix with parametria and upper vagina have been separated from the vagina and are detached from the uterine fundus.

vesicouterine ligament. The distal aspect of the vesico-uterine ligament can be transected up to the level of the ureter. This is preferably done with 1 hand palpating the ureter while the other hand dissects the vesicouter-ine ligament. Once the dissection reaches the ureter superiorly, the ureter can be mobilized anteriorly, and the knee of the ureter is identified (Figure 26-7).

The parametrium is identified, clamped, divided, and ligated to obtain an adequate margin. The cer-vicovaginal branch of the uterine artery is clamped, divided, and ligated. Once the parametrium and the cervicovaginal branch of the uterine artery have been divided, the cervix can be transected. By palpating pos-teriorly, the cervicouterine junction can be identified, and an appropriate portion of the cervix is transected from the uterus.

The cervical specimen is sent for frozen section to confirm a tumor-free margin of at least 5 mm. For

patients with a positive margin or a margin less than 5 mm, an additional resection is performed. A #5 French catheter is inserted and sutured into the os to maintain patency. This is removed at the patient's postoperative clinic visit. To prevent cervical incompetence, a Mersilene (Shirodkar cerclage) suture is placed around the lower uterine segment and tied posteriorly. The vaginal cuff is then sutured to the most lateral portions of the "neo-cervix" while burying the Mersilene suture.

Laparoscopic Radical Trachelectomy

The laparoscopic radical trachelectomy may be per-formed using a variety of laparoscopic instruments. This specific procedure will be described using the argon beam coagulator and the LigaSure.

The patient is put in semilithotomy position, and general anesthesia is induced. The patient is prepped

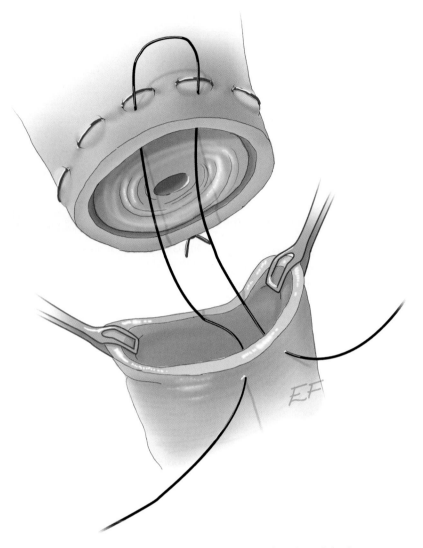

FIGURE 26-5. Radical abdominal trachelectomy. Cerclage has been placed, and the lower uterine segment is approximated to the upper vagina.

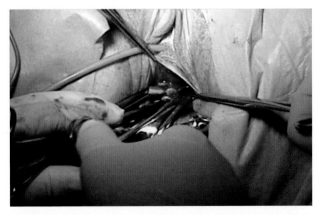

FIGURE 26-6. Radical vaginal trachelectomy. The left paravesical space is created by dissecting at the small indentation created by retracting the anterior vaginal cuff at the 12 o'clock position and the lateral vaginal cuff at the 9 o'clock position. Using a long curved Kelly or Metzenbaum scissors, the paravesical space is then developed by gently spreading in a superior-anterior-lateral direction.

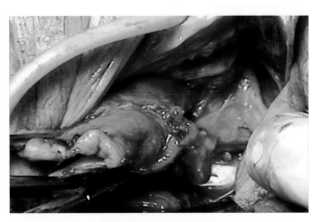

FIGURE 26-7. Radical vaginal trachelectomy. The distal aspect of the vesicouterine ligament is transected up to the level of the ureter. Once the dissection reaches the ureter superiorly, the ureter can be mobilized anteriorly, and the knee of the ureter is identified.

and draped in the usual fashion with the patient's arms tucked by her sides. Entry into the abdomen can be obtained by inserting a Veress needle either 1 cm above or below the umbilicus or through the Hasson open technique, as per the surgeon's preference. A pneumoperitoneum is obtained, and the camera is inserted through a 5-mm (high-definition laparoscope) or 10-mm trocar at the umbilicus. Patients with a previous midline incision can be managed using either an alternate entry site or a needle laparoscope at the umbilicus. The patient is then put in steep Trendelenburg position. A 10-mm trocar is placed suprapubically in the midline, and two 5-mm trocars are placed laterally approximately 2 cm medial to the anterior superior ischial spine and at the level of the umbilicus.

The pelvis and abdomen are then fully explored to rule out any macroscopic disease. The argon beam coagulator is inserted, along with a grasper and the LigaSure. A decision is made to start with the pelvic lymph node dissection or with the radical trachelectomy. Lymph node dissection is described in Chapter 28.

The peritoneum overlying the psoas muscle is grasped and put on tension. A continuous suction or venting of gases is advisable. This can be as simple as wall suction attached to the gas valve of one of the trocars. The peritoneum is then cauterized with the argon beam coagulator and then further opened parallel to the infundibulopelvic ligament exposing the iliac vessels and the psoas muscle. The argon beam is then used to further open the anterior peritoneum caudally up to the level of the bladder reflection. The infundibulopelvic ligament is retracted medially to facilitate exposure of the ureter, adjacent to the medial peritoneum, as it crosses over the iliac bifurcation.

The bladder peritoneum is then dissected off the anterior vagina and incised with the LigaSure or with the argon beam coagulator. The bladder is reflected inferiorly with sharp and blunt dissection until the bladder is adequately reflected off the anterior vaginal wall.

The paravesical and pararectal spaces are now developed bilaterally as described for radical abdominal trachelectomy. Care is taken to cauterize any small vessels encountered because bleeding highly impairs visualization.

Once the paravesical and pararectal spaces have been properly developed, the uterine vessels are easily identified (Figure 26-8). Ideally, an attempt should be made to preserve the uterine artery and ligate only the descending branches using the LigaSure. However, the significance of ligating the uterine artery at its origin, during a trachelectomy, is unclear.

The ureter is then unroofed from the vesicouterine ligament. This is facilitated by gently dissecting superior and medial to the ureter, with the tip of the LigaSure or a Maryland grasper. This forms a tunnel under the cardinal ligament. It is important to take caution to

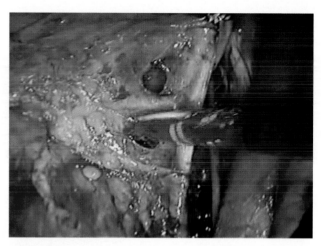

FIGURE 26-8. Laparoscopic radical trachelectomy. Visualization of the right uterine artery.

stay superior to the ureter and confirm that the tip of the dissecting instrument is directed cephalic to the bladder. Each step consists of gentle dissection, cauterization (or hemoclip), and then division. Inserting the Colpotomizer at this stage helps to identify the level of the cervix and to verify that the bladder is adequately dissected inferiorly off the vaginal wall.

Once the tunnel is complete and the ureter is unroofed up to the bladder, attention is brought to the posterior aspect of the uterus. The uterus is anteverted, and the cul-de-sac and uterosacral ligaments are exposed. A grasper is used to hold up the posterior peritoneum inferior to the cervix in the cul-de-sac. A window is made with the argon beam coagulator, and the rectovaginal space is entered. The space is then developed with blunt dissection, thus pushing the rectum posteriorly. The ureter is then separated from the medial peritoneum, and the uterosacral ligaments are cauterized and divided (Figure 26-9). The specimen is then examined to confirm that there are ample margins both anteriorly and posteriorly and the position of the ureters. Once this has been confirmed, the vagina is incised with the argon beam coagulator on the Colpotimizer. The cervix is then transected from the vagina. The next step is identifying the cervicouterine junction to define an appropriate level of the cervix to be transected from the uterus. This step can be performed with monopolar cautery or, alternatively, can be facilitated using a vaginal approach.

The cervical specimen is removed through the vagina and sent for frozen section to confirm a tumor-free margin of at least 5 mm. For patients with a positive margin or a margin less than 5 mm, an additional resection is performed.

The patient is then put in high lithotomy position. A #5 French catheter is inserted and sutured into the

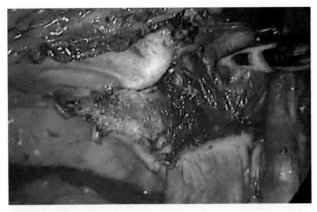

FIGURE 26-9. Laparoscopic radical trachelectomy. The ureter is seen separated from the medial peritoneum, and the uterosacral ligaments are ready to be cauterized and divided.

os to maintain patency. This is removed at the patient's postoperative clinic visit. To prevent cervical incompetence, a Mersilene (Shirodkar cerclage) suture is placed around the lower uterine segment and tied posteriorly. The vaginal cuff is then sutured to the most lateral portions of the "neocervix" while burying the Mersilene suture.

Hemostasis is obtained, the gas is let out of the abdomen, and the port sites are sutured closed.

Robotic-Assisted Radical Trachelectomy

The robotic-assisted radical trachelectomy is performed in a similar fashion to the laparoscopic radical trachelectomy; however, the port placement and the instruments may differ. The instruments commonly used in the robotic procedure are the monopolar scissors, bipolar cautery, and a grasper. Once the patient is under general anesthesia, prepped, and draped and a Foley catheter is inserted into the bladder, maximum Trendelenburg position is obtained. The procedure is then initiated by insufflation of the abdomen and placement of the trocars. A subumbilical stab can facilitate insertion of the Veress needle, and a pneumoperitoneum is obtained. A supraumbilical trocar, approximately 25 cm superior to the symphysis pubis, is then placed to accommodate the robotic camera. Two right lateral 8-mm ports are then placed; it is important to verify that there is a minimum of 10 cm between each port in order for the robotic arms to be able to maneuver optimally during the procedure. An additional 2 left lateral ports are inserted: one 8 mm and one 12 mm. The 12-mm port will act as the accessory port and be used by the assistant. The robot is then docked, and the procedure is begun. The steps of the procedure are identical to those previously noted for the laparoscopic radical trachelectomy.

Postoperative Care

> **Box 26-6 Complications and Morbidity**
>
> - Neurogenic bladder dysfunction: Radical trachelectomy can cause denervation of the bladder and a portion of the urethra; the degree is in direct correlation to the extent of the dissection.
> - Vesicovaginal fistula is a rare complication but can heal spontaneously (if small).
> - Ureteric or bladder injury can occur intraoperatively.
> - Patients who undergo a full lymph node dissection are at risk of developing leg lymphedema.

Patients commonly do well postoperatively, and the mode of surgical entry correlates with the postoperative management. Patients who undergo radical vaginal trachelectomy or minimally invasive surgery can be discharged the same evening or the following day on a regular diet, and mobilization is initiated once they recover from the anesthesia. After all radical procedures, there is some degree of denervation of the bladder and urethra; therefore, an indwelling Foley catheter is left in and then discontinued on postoperative day 3 to 6 after a postvoid residual (PVR) of less than 100 mL is demonstrated confirming normal bladder function. Patients who undergo a laparotomy usually tolerate a full diet and normal activity in approximately 3 days and can therefore be discharged home at that time. The Foley catheter can be left draining the bladder until the discharge day in which it is removed and a PVR is performed. Alternatively, a trial with a PVR can be performed on postoperative day 1 and the catheter reinserted if the PVR is greater than 100 mL. This can also be determined on an individual basis as per the extent of dissection.

The rubber catheter that was placed in the cervical os is removed after 3 weeks.

SIMPLE TRACHELECTOMY

Procedure Overview

> **Box 26-7 Master Surgeon's Corner**
>
> - The size of the cervical stump together with the habitus, parity, and previous surgeries of the patient assist in deciding on the preferred surgical approach.

A simple trachelectomy is surgical removal of the cervix. It can be performed vaginally or abdominally in cases of early cervical cancer, rare cases of persistent endocervical dysplasia after multiple excisions, or in patients who underwent a subtotal hysterectomy and subsequently require surgical excision of the cervix. In the majority of cases, the initial indication for the hysterectomy was benign; however, the final pathology identified a malignancy (eg, endometrial cancer or uterine sarcoma). Because radical trachelectomy has been discussed previously in this chapter, we will focus here on removal of the cervix in patients who had a prior subtotal hysterectomy.

Preoperative Preparation

Patients with an indication for a simple trachelectomy undergo a physical and pelvic examination, a chest x-ray, CBC, and kidney function (creatinine) preoperatively. Additional imaging and blood work are left to the discretion of the surgeon while taking into consideration the patient's symptoms, comorbidities, and results of the clinical examination.

Once a decision is made to proceed with a simple trachelectomy, informed consent is obtained. It is important to discuss the possibility of complications including bleeding, infection, and injury to adjacent organs.

The patient is admitted to the hospital on the morning of the operation. Prophylactic antibiotic is administered prior to surgery.

Operative Procedure

Simple Abdominal Trachelectomy

Box 26-8	Caution Points

- The proximity of the ureters to the cervix should be kept in mind when performing a vaginal or abdominal trachelectomy.

The patient is put in semilithotomy position, and general anesthesia is induced. Care is taken to place the legs appropriately to avoid pressure on the peroneal nerves. A bimanual examination is performed to assess the cervix and to further guide the procedure. The abdomen and perineum are prepped and draped, and an indwelling Foley catheter is inserted into the bladder.

The incision can be either transverse (Pfannenstiel, Maylard, or Cherney) or a low midline incision from the umbilicus to the pubic bone.

Once the peritoneal cavity is entered, a full abdominal and pelvic exploration is performed. The patient is then put in Trendelenburg position, a self-retaining

retractor is inserted, and the bowel is packed off to facilitate maximum exposure of the pelvis.

The cervical stump is then identified; however, commonly the bladder and/or bowel are adherent superiorly to the cervical stump, and these must be taken down carefully before the cervix can be visualized. Once the cervix is exposed, it can be grasped with a single-tooth tenaculum to allow manipulation. The retroperitoneum is opened by incising the peritoneum overlying the psoas muscle. The retroperitoneal structures, including the psoas muscle and the external iliac vessels, are exposed, and the ureter is identified. A right angle clamp can be used to gently dissect the ureter off the peritoneum, and a vessel loop is placed under the ureter to assist in orientation of its position throughout the procedure. The cervix is then elevated and the bladder dissected off anteriorly. A heavy clamp (eg, Kelly or curved Rogers) is used to clamp the cardinal ligament on either side. The ligament is then cut and tied. The uterosacral ligaments are then clamped, divided, and sutured. The paravaginal fascia is then dissected to further obtain the tissue between the cervix and the upper vagina. When the specimen is ready, 2 heavy clamps (eg, curved Rogers, Heaney) are placed across the vagina. The uterus and cervix are then divided from the vagina above the clamps. The specimen is sent to pathology.

A delayed-absorbable suture is then placed under each clamp to assure hemostasis of the vaginal angles. The opening of the vaginal cuff is then closed with either a running locking suture or, alternatively, with multiple interrupted figure-of-eights with special attention to include the vaginal mucosa of both the anterior and posterior wall. If the mucosa is not obvious at the time of closure, a long straight Kocher can be placed on each wall to verify that they are both incorporated in the suture.

Simple Vaginal Trachelectomy

In general, the vaginal approach is easier and less morbid than the abdominal approach. The patient is put in lithotomy position, and general anesthesia is induced. Care is taken to place the legs properly as to avoid pressure on the peroneal nerves. A bimanual examination is performed to assess the remaining cervix as to further guide the procedure. The perineum is prepped and draped, and an indwelling Foley catheter is inserted into the bladder.

The vaginal mucosa around the cervix is injected with a dilute solution of vasopressin in lidocaine. A scalpel is used to circumferentially incise the vaginal mucosa. The posterior cul-de-sac is entered, and the vesicovaginal space is developed. The bladder peritoneum is not incised. The cervix is grasped with a single-tooth tenaculum, facilitating traction of the cervix. The uterosacral ligaments are then clamped, cut, and sutured bilaterally. The cardinal ligaments are then clamped, divided, and ligated bilaterally. The cervix is now free of its attachments, and gentle traction on the cervical stump facilitates removal of the cervix. If additional tissue is adherent to the superior aspect of the cervix, care is taken while dissecting off the adhesions because the bladder and bowel are commonly adjacent.

The cervical specimen is sent for pathology. The vaginal cuff is then sutured closed with a running delayed-absorbable suture.

Laparoscopic Simple Trachelectomy

The laparoscopic simple trachelectomy may be performed using a variety of laparoscopic instruments. This specific procedure will be described using the argon beam coagulator and the LigaSure.

The patient is put in semilithotomy position, and general anesthesia is induced. The patient is prepped and draped in the usual fashion with the patient's arms tucked by her sides. Entry into the abdomen and trocar placement are the same as described for laparoscopic radical trachelectomy.

The argon beam coagulator is inserted, along with a grasper and the LigaSure. The peritoneum lying over the psoas muscle is grasped and put on tension. A continuous suction or venting of gases is advisable. This can be as simple as wall suction attached to the gas valve of one of the trocars. The peritoneum is then cauterized with the argon beam coagulator and then further opened parallel to the infundibulopelvic ligament exposing the retroperitoneal structures (ie, the iliac vessels and the psoas muscle). The argon beam is then used to further open the anterior peritoneum caudally up to the level of the bladder reflection. The infundibulopelvic ligament is retracted medially to facilitate exposure of the ureter, adjacent to the medial peritoneum, as it crosses over the iliac bifurcation.

The bladder peritoneum is then dissected off the anterior vagina and incised with the LigaSure or with the argon beam coagulator. The bladder is reflected inferiorly with sharp and blunt dissection until the bladder is adequately reflected off the anterior vaginal wall.

The cervical stump is then grasped and pulled cephalic using a single-tooth tenaculum and a Colpotimizer in the vagina to further delineate the correct planes. The LigaSure is used to cauterize and cut the cardinal ligaments bilaterally. The uterosacral ligaments are then cauterized and divided.

The vagina is incised with the argon beam coagulator on the Colpotimizer. The cervix is then transected from the vagina, and the specimen is removed through the vagina and sent to pathology. The vaginal cuff is sutured laparoscopically, taking care to incorporate both sides of the vaginal cuff mucosa.

Hemostasis is obtained, the gas is let out of the abdomen, and the port sites are sutured closed.

Postoperative Care

Box 26-9	Complications and Morbidity

- The retroperitoneum should be opened and the ureters identified in order to prevent an inadvertent ureteric injury.
- The bladder and/or bowel are frequently adhesed to the superior aspect of the cervical stump; these should be dissected off carefully before clamping the cervix.

Patients commonly do well postoperatively, and the mode of surgical entry correlates with the postoperative management. Patients who undergo simple vaginal trachelectomy can be discharged the same evening or the following day as the catheter is removed on completion of the surgery; a regular diet and mobilization are initiated once they recover from the anesthesia. Patients who undergo a laparotomy usually tolerate a full diet and normal activity in approximately 3 days and can therefore be discharged home at that time.

REFERENCES

1. Mathevet P, Chemali E, Roy M, Dargent D. Long-term outcome of a randomized study comparing three techniques of conization: cold knife, laser, and LEEP. *Eur J Obstet Gynecol Reprod Biol.* 2003;106(2):214-218.
2. Mathevet P, Dargent D, Roy M, Beau G. A randomized prospective study comparing three techniques of conization: cold knife, laser, and LEEP. *Gynecol Oncol.* 1994;54(2):175-179.
3. Beiner ME, Covens A. Surgery insight: radical vaginal trachelectomy as a method of fertility preservation for cervical cancer. *Nat Clin Pract Oncol.* 2007;4(6):353-361.
4. Marchiole P, Benchaib M, Buenerd A, Lazlo E, Dargent D, Mathevet P. Oncological safety of laparoscopic-assisted vaginal radical trachelectomy (LARVT or Dargent's operation): a comparative study with laparoscopic-assisted vaginal radical hysterectomy (LARVH). *Gynecol Oncol.* 2007;106(1):132-141.
5. Dargent D, Martin X, Sacchetoni A, Mathevet P. Laparoscopic vaginal radical trachelectomy: a treatment to preserve the fertility of cervical carcinoma patients. *Cancer.* 2000;88(8):1877-1882.
6. Piver MS, Rutledge F, Smith JP. Five classes of extended hysterectomy for women with cervical cancer. *Obstet Gynecol.* 1974;44(2):265-272.

Vulvar and Vaginal Excisional Procedures

Mark A. Morgan, Sarah H. Kim, and Sameer A. Patel

SIMPLE AND SKINNING VULVECTOMY

Procedure Overview

Simple vulvectomy involves the excision of vulvar skin with subcutaneous tissue, without dissection to the deep fascia of the vulva and perineum.[1] This procedure is indicated for extensive in situ or microinvasion carcinoma of the vulva (<1 mm of invasion), vulvar dystrophy, and Paget disease, where the lesions are not amenable to local excision or other forms of conservative therapy. For noninvasive lesions (except Paget disease), it may be acceptable to just remove the skin (a skinning vulvectomy) without removal of any underlying subcutaneous fat.[2] A total vulvectomy includes excision of the entire vulva, clitoris, and perineal tissue. For preinvasive lesions of the vulva, total vulvectomy (simple or skinning) is rarely used now, with wide local excision or even more conservative treatments such as laser ablation being much more common.[1]

Box 27-1   Master Surgeon's Corner

- For multifocal disease, several local excisions with primary closure may be preferable to extensive vulvectomy.
- Z-plasty and rhomboid flaps are often useful for closing larger defects. This is especially true near the perineum where primary closure may cause introital strictures and dyspareunia.

Preoperative Preparation

Bowel preparation is usually not required but may be used when perineal and perianal excision is required.

Operative Procedure

Initial Steps

General or regional anesthesia using epidural or spinal anesthesia is used for extensive resections. For limited excisions, local anesthesia and deep sedation or laryngeal mask anesthesia may be adequate. The patient is placed in dorsal lithotomy position using "candy cane" or Allen stirrups. Bladder catheterization is recommended for complete vulvectomy. Prophylactic antibiotics are given. After the skin is prepared and sterile draping is applied, excision margins are marked on the vulva with a pen.

Incision and Dissection

It is helpful to inject the proposed incision line lesion with a dilute lidocaine and epinephrine solution (eg, 1% lidocaine with 1:100,000 epinephrine), and then the superficial skin incision is made. The incision starts from above the labial folds on the mons pubis and is extended down the lateral fold of the labia majora and across the posterior fourchette (Figure 27-1). The clitoris is spared when possible. A dry pack is used to occlude the small bleeding vessels in the skin until this incision is completed, and cautery may be used for simple vulvectomy. If a skinning vulvectomy is performed, the dissection should be with the scalpel

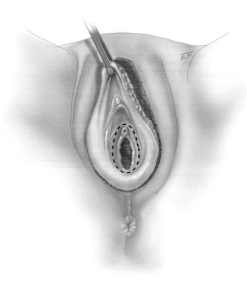

FIGURE 27-1. Simple vulvectomy removes the skin plus underlying dermis but does not reach the deep fascia.

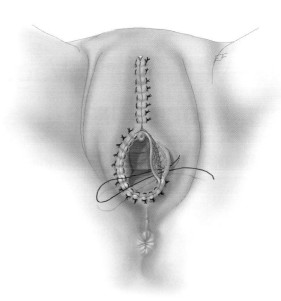

FIGURE 27-2. Primary closure after simple vulvectomy.

or sharp curved scissors to avoid cautery artifact. If the clitoris is excised, the suspensory ligament and the crura of the clitoris are divided and ligated. Depending on the depth of the incision, as the 4 and 8 o'clock positions on the vulva are approached, the pudendal artery and vein may be identified and clamped. The periurethral and vaginal incisions are made if necessary to complete the excision. Depending on the location of the lesion, the clitoris and labia minora may be spared. If the dissection involves the perineum, care must be taken to avoid the anal sphincter. The specimen should be oriented with marking stitch for pathologic evaluation.

Closure

Primary closure of the simple vulvectomy is made by using interrupted 2-0 or 3-0 synthetic absorbable sutures (Figure 27-2). Skinning vulvectomies usually require split-thickness skin grafts for closure. During closure of a simple vulvectomy, it is important to eliminate tension on the suture line, and this is often best done with vertical mattress sutures. Vulvar skin and subcutaneous tissues can be undermined and mobilized using sharp scissors or electrocautery. The posterior wall of the vagina is undermined and brought out to the posterior fourchette so that contracture of the vaginal introitus is avoided. The closure of the wound is continued superiorly to the mons pubis, and the periurethral mucosa is everted and sutured to the skin. If the defect is large, local advancement or transposition flaps can be used (see Chapter 32C). Transposition flaps such as the Z-plasty or the rhomboid flap are useful to prevent introital stenosis if there is a large perineal defect. Dressings are not necessary and difficult to

keep in place. An antibiotic ointment may be useful, however, in keeping the incision line moist.

Box 27-2 | Caution Points

- Bleeding is most likely around the urethra and posterolaterally from pudendal vessels.
- Closing the mons over the urethral meatus will result in distortion of the urinary stream.
- Introital stricture is most likely to occur when closing the perineum under tension and may be prevented by using transposition flaps.

Postoperative Care

The bladder catheter may be removed on postoperative day 1 unless there is concern regarding the periurethral closure. The patient can usually ambulate the day after surgery. Perineal hygiene with saline rinse, especially after urination and bowel movements, is useful. Sitz baths should be avoided for 3 to 4 weeks to prevent the synthetic absorbable sutures from dissolving prematurely. Stool softeners are helpful, but attempts at constipating are usually unsuccessful and can lead to fecal impaction.

Box 27-3 | Complications and Morbidity

- Wound separation/breakdown
- Cellulitis
- Stricture of vaginal introitus
- Distortion of urethral meatus

RADICAL VULVECTOMY

Procedure Overview

Historically, vulvar cancer has been treated by en bloc radical vulvectomy with bilateral dissection of the inguinal nodes.[3] Because of the high complication rate and psychosexual implications of such radical surgery, this approach has been replaced by radical local excision and ipsilateral groin dissection for unilateral, small tumors.[4] For posterior lesions, this may allow preservation of the clitoris. For centrally located tumors, bilateral groin dissection is recommended and can be performed through separate incisions (3-incision technique). An attempt should be made to obtain 2-cm margins, although a recent study suggested that 8-mm margins may be adequate.[5] Conservative surgery tailored to the lesion location and size has the advantage of preserving vulvar tissue and allowing primary closure of the wound defect. This results in less psychosexual disturbance, fewer wound complications, and a shorter hospital stay without compromising survival.[6]

Box 27-4	**Master Surgeon's Corner**

- The incisions may be individualized according to the location and size of the tumor, but the dissection should extend to the deep fascia, and at least 1-cm margins should be obtained.
- Vertical mattress sutures close the deep layer and skin. This method reduces tension on the skin, provides flexibility in closing irregular wounds, is fast, and results in good cosmesis.
- Although inguinal lymphadenectomy is usually performed prior to the vulvar procedure, in medically frail patients, it may be prudent to do the vulvar excision first in case the operation needs to be abandoned prematurely.
- If possible, leave at least 1 cm or more of mucosa surrounding the urethra to facilitate the closure and avoid distortion of the urethral meatus.

Preoperative Preparation

Women undergoing radical vulvectomy should be counseled about the altered appearance and effect on sexual sensation and function. Preoperative urinary or fecal continence should be evaluated, and the potential for an altered urinary stream and incontinence should be explained. The risk and consequences of wound breakdown and infection should be explained. A mechanical bowel preparation is recommended to avoid fecal soilage during or immediately after the surgery.

Operative Procedure

Initial Steps

General or regional anesthesia is required. The patient is placed in modified dorsal lithotomy position using Allen stirrups, giving adequate exposure to the lower abdomen, perineum, and inner thighs. Prophylactic antibiotics and heparin are given prior to the incision. A urethral catheter is placed in the bladder after the skin is prepared and sterile draping is applied.

A radical vulvectomy performed through an incision separate from the inguinal lymphadenectomy is most common, but the dissection can be tailored to the size and location of the lesion as long as adequate margins are obtained and a deep dissection to the fascia or symphysis pubis is performed (Figure 27-3).

Incision and Dissection

The skin incision may start superiorly or inferiorly (Figure 27-4). Starting superiorly has the advantage of using the symphysis pubis as a guide to the deep fascia of the vulva. The incision continues laterally in the labiocrural folds to the deep fascia, and then the dissection proceeds medially to the mons pubis and vagina at the level of the inferior fascia of the urogenital diaphragm (Figure 27-5). Electrocautery can be used for much of the dissection. At the 4 and 8 o'clock positions on the posterolateral vulva, the internal pudendal vessels are identified and ligated. If the clitoris needs to be excised, the suspensory ligament is clamped, transected, and ligated. It may also be necessary to suture the rich vascular network surrounding the clitoris. The labia minora are retracted laterally, and an inner elliptical

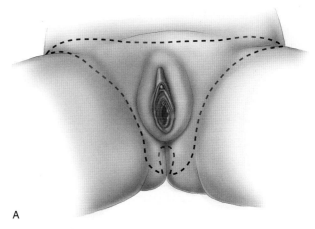

A

FIGURE 27-3. Types of radical vulvectomy incisions. A. Classic "single-incision" radical vulvectomy with bilateral groin node dissection (en bloc). **B.** Left partial radical vulvectomy with unilateral groin node dissection. **C.** "Triple-incision" radical vulvectomy with bilateral groin node dissection. **D.** Anterior partial radical vulvectomy with bilateral groin node dissection. **E.** Posterior partial radical vulvectomy with bilateral groin node dissection.

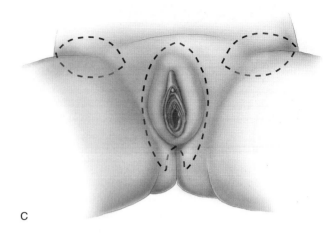

B

C

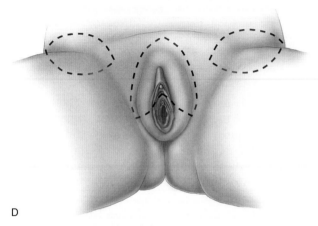

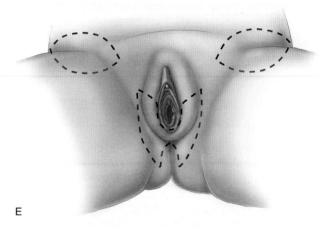

D

E

FIGURE 27-3. (*Continued*)

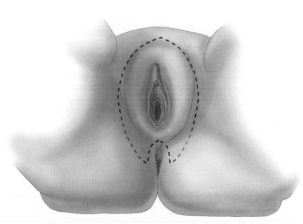

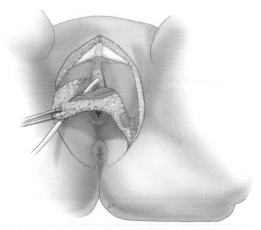

FIGURE 27-4. Radical vulvectomy without en bloc inguinal node dissection.

FIGURE 27-5. Radical vulvectomy. The incision is carried down to the inferior fascia of the urogenital diaphragm.

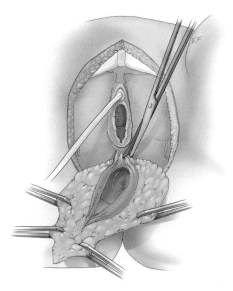

FIGURE 27-6. Radical vulvectomy, posterior dissection.

incision then circumscribes the vaginal introitus and vulvar vestibule. Medially, the vascular vestibular tissue along the vagina is clamped, divided, and ligated. During the posterior dissection, it is important to avoid damaging the anal sphincter (Figure 27-6). A finger in the rectum may help guide the dissection and clarify the location of the rectum and anal sphincter. If necessary, the anterior third of the anal sphincter or distal third of the urethra can be removed and continence maintained.

Closure

In most cases, the wound can be closed primarily (Figure 27-7). Vertical mattress sutures are useful to

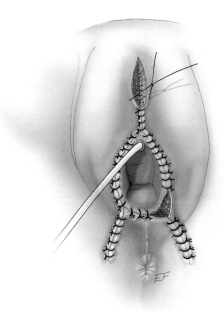

FIGURE 27-7. Radical vulvectomy, primary closure.

reduce tension on the suture line. The periurethral mucosa can be everted and secured to the skin closure to reduce urinary stream obstruction. If the dissection extended to the anus, a perineum should be reconstructed by plicating the superficial transverse perineal muscles in the midline and closing the skin with vertical mattress sutures. The vaginal mucosa should then be everted and sutured to the perineum. Primarily, 2-0 and 3-0 synthetic absorbable sutures are used, but in areas of increased tension, carefully placed permanent suture can be used to help prevent delayed wound separation as the absorbable sutures dissolve. Closed suction drains are usually not necessary, but can be placed in the ischiorectal fossa or under the closure of the vagina and brought out through the perineum.

Box 27-5	Caution Points

- Bleeding is most likely to occur around the urethra and posterolaterally from the internal pudendal vessels.
- The anal sphincter is at risk for injury when dissecting posteriorly.
- Avoid excessive undermining of the vulvar skin to prevent devascularization.

Postoperative Care

The patient is kept on bed rest for the first 2 to 3 days of the initial postoperative period. The Foley catheter is left in place at least until the patient becomes ambulatory. If a complete radical vulvectomy has been performed or the dissection is close to the urethra, the patient may be discharged to home with a catheter for 1 to 2 weeks. Deep vein thrombosis prophylaxis is recommended until discharge but may be continued for 1 month. Perineal hygiene with saline rinses may be used, but Sitz baths should be avoided for 3 to 4 weeks to prevent the absorbable sutures from dissolving prematurely.

Box 27-6	Complications and Morbidity

- Wound separation/breakdown
- Wound cellulitis
- Stricture of vaginal introitus
- Sexual dysfunction
- Hematoma/seroma
- Venous thromboembolism
- Rectovaginal or rectoperineal fistula
- Urinary or fecal incontinence

Vulvar Reconstruction

Local excision of vulvar cancers will result in defects involving skin and subcutaneous tissue with minimal mucosal resection. The defects can often be closed primarily in layers or with vertical mattress sutures. Several alternative options for reconstruction exist, and selection of the appropriate method of reconstruction is dependent on the size of the defect, location of the defect, and the amount of laxity and excess tissue in the surrounding area. Options for vulvar reconstruction using advancement flaps and transposition flaps are described in Chapter 32C.

INGUINOFEMORAL LYMPHADENECTOMY

Procedure Overview

Vulvar cancer spreads through local extension and in predictable pattern along lymphatic channels that course through the labia majora, medial to the labiocrural folds. The lymphatics then travel laterally to the superficial lymph nodes in the groin and then to the deep femoral lymph nodes below the cribriform fascia of the upper, inner thigh (Figure 27-8). From there, cancer can spread via the femoral canal to the lymphatics surrounding the external iliac vessels and cephalad to the para-aortic lymph node chain. It is believed that most early lymphatic spread is by embolization rather than direct permeation along lymph channels, so currently inguinofemoral lymphadenectomy is most often performed through separate incisions at the time of a radical local resection of vulvar cancer.[7] Historically, this lymphadenectomy was performed en bloc as part of a radical vulvectomy. Crossover lymphatic drainage to the contralateral groin is rare, except for midline lesions, so a unilateral dissection may be sufficient for lateralized lesions. Spread is almost always to superficial nodes initially, so sentinel lymph node techniques may be applicable (see Sentinel Lymph Node Dissection section). Aberrant channels have been found that go directly to deep femoral nodes, so a slightly increased recurrence rate may be seen when omitting a deep dissection.[8] A higher recurrence rate has been noted if only superficial nodes are dissected.[9]

Patients with resectable vulvar squamous carcinoma and a depth of invasion greater than 1 mm or with lymphovascular invasion should be considered for surgical evaluation of the inguinal lymph nodes either by inguinofemoral lymph node dissection or by sentinel node techniques. Unilateral groin dissection is sufficient for lateral lesions 2 cm or less in size. Bilateral groin dissection is indicated for larger lesions, for central lesions, or in the presence of gross disease in the ipsilateral groin. If the groin contains 1 or more clinically positive lymph nodes, the groin dissection is performed before administration of radiotherapy.

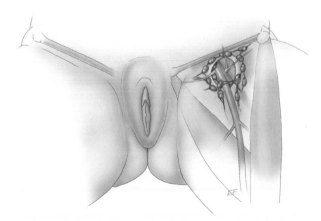

FIGURE 27-8. The inguinofemoral lymph nodes are located below the fascia of Scarpa and drain into the deep femoral nodes through the fossa ovalis.

| Box 27-7 | Master Surgeon's Corner |

- Deep femoral lymph nodes are located medial to the femoral vein. In dissecting these nodes, there is no need to remove the fascia lateral to the femoral vein where there is risk of injuring the femoral nerve.
- The great saphenous vein enters the common femoral vein near where the deep external pudendal artery crosses the common femoral vein from its origin on the medial side of the femoral artery. This artery should be clipped or ligated prior to the dissection around the saphenous vein.
- Dissection in the superficial compartment should be deep to the level of the superficial inferior epigastric artery cephalad to the inguinal ligament. This ensures adequate blood supply to the skin and minimizes the risk of flap necrosis.
- There are no deep femoral nodes distal to the fossa ovalis (or the insertion of the saphenous vein into the femoral vein). Dissection distal to this site is not necessary.

Preoperative Preparation

All patients should have a thorough examination with careful inspection of the inguinal regions. Although vulvar cancer is a surgically staged disease, preoperative evaluation with a computed tomography scan may also be helpful in detecting occult disease. Positron emission tomography and magnetic resonance imaging have also been evaluated, but they usually do not obviate the need for surgical dissection.[9]

Operative Procedure

Initial Steps

General or regional anesthesia is required, and the patient is placed in modified dorsal lithotomy position. Adequate exposure to the lower abdomen is obtained by not flexing the hips until the groin dissection is complete. Allen stirrups are usually used. If only a groin dissection is to be performed, the patient can be positioned supine, with the legs in a frog-leg position with the hips abducted and externally rotated and the knees flexed 90 degrees. Prophylactic antibiotics are given prior to the skin incision, and a catheter is placed in the bladder after the patient is prepped and draped.

Incision

Incisions separate from the vulvectomy are most commonly used (Figure 27-9), but for large laterally placed vulvar tumors, the incisions can be combined in a "butterfly" configuration. The superficial inguinal lymphadenectomy removes lymph nodes that lie superficial to the cribriform fascia of the medial thigh and the inguinal ligament. The anterior superior iliac spine and the pubic tubercle are identified, and the groin incision is made 2 cm above and parallel to the inguinal ligament. The incision is carried through

the full thickness of skin and the subcutaneous tissues to the aponeurosis of the external oblique muscle.

Superficial Nodal Dissection

Allis forceps are applied to the dermal surface of the upper skin incision to provide traction, and the fat pad is removed from 3 to 4 cm above the inguinal ligament and 3 to 4 cm medial to the anterior superior ischial spine. Care must be taken not to dissect too close to the skin because this will devascularize the skin and may lead to flap necrosis. The medial border of the dissection is the pubic tubercle and the adductor longus muscle. Once the fat pad containing superficial inguinal nodes is cleared off the external oblique aponeurosis and mobilized off the lower margin of inguinal ligament, the dissection proceeds inferiorly toward the deep fascia of the thigh to create the caudal skin flap (Figure 27-10). The dissection is performed in a lateral to medial direction, and the superficial circumflex iliac and superficial inferior epigastric vessels are identified and cauterized or ligated as they penetrate the cribriform fascia. Anteromedially, the long saphenous vein is identified and may be preserved by carefully dissecting the surrounding lymphatic tissue for its branches (Figure 27-11). If it is divided, it should be ligated with a transfixing stitch of permanent suture.

Deep Nodal Dissection

If deep femoral lymphadenectomy is performed, the dissection is taken deeper into the femoral triangle

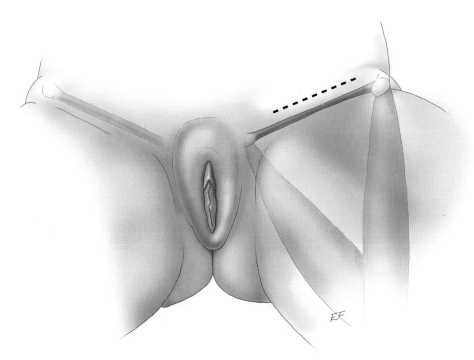

FIGURE 27-9. Incision for inguinofemoral lymph node dissection, 2 cm above and parallel to the inguinal ligament.

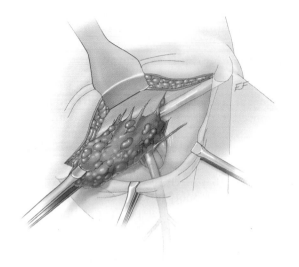

FIGURE 27-10. Completion of the upper and medial portions of the inguinofemoral lymph node dissection.

beneath the cribriform fascia by incising the fascia over the femoral artery near the inguinal ligament and continuing inferiorly just below the saphenous vein. Dissecting medially involves dissection or ligation of the deep external pudendal artery and greater saphenous vein. This exposes the femoral triangle, bounded medially by the adductor longus muscle and laterally by the sartorius muscle. Superiorly, the inguinal ligament forms the base of the triangle. The floor of the triangle is made of the pectineus and iliopsoas muscles. The deep nodes are located medial to the femoral

vein and continue cephalad beneath the inguinal ligament into the pelvis as the external iliac nodal chain. Cloquet node is the most superior deep inguinal node and is variably present. The deep nodes can be removed in continuity with superficial groin nodes if desired. The sartorius muscle may be transposed to cover the defect in the deep fascia and to protect the femoral vessels. The sartorius muscle is transected from its tendinous attachment to the anterior spine, rotated medially, and sutured to the inguinal ligament just above the femoral vessels. If the deep dissection is medial to the femoral artery, however, transposition is not usually necessary. It is also possible to remove the deep nodes by placing traction on the lymphovascular fatty tissue above the cribriform fascia, further minimizing the risk to the femoral vessels.[10] The skin is closed with staples or interrupted vertical mattress sutures. A closed suction drain is brought out laterally above the groin and secured.

Box 27-8	Caution Points

- When dissecting lateral to medial in the superficial compartment, the superficial inferior epigastric, circumflex iliac and external pudendal vessels may be encountered twice, near the skin and at their origin from the femoral vessels. They should be cauterized or ligated at each location.
- Small branches of the saphenous vein are encountered during the medial part of the deep dissection and should be ligated.
- Lymphatic drainage often increases several days after surgery when the patient begins to ambulate more. Low output in the hospital can be misleading.

Postoperative Care

Patients usually remain in bed for 24 to 48 hours, and deep vein thrombosis prophylaxis should be maintained at least during the hospital stay. Position and ambulation will often be dictated by the extent of the vulvar dissection if performed. The suction drainage is continued until incision is healed and the dissected space is obliterated. The drain output is carefully monitored. Because lymphatic drainage often increases several days after surgery, most patients should go home with the drains in place. The incision over the skin flap is inspected for signs of necrosis or infection. A lymphocyst increases the risk of skin necrosis. The staples and drains can usually be removed in 10 to 14 days.

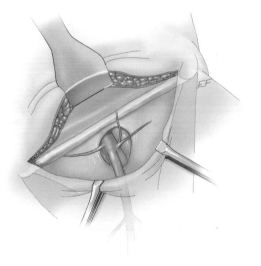

FIGURE 27-11. Preservation of the saphenous vein during inguinofemoral lymph node dissection.

CHAPTER 27

Box 27-9	Complications and Morbidity

- Intraoperative bleeding secondary to venous or arterial tear
- Wound separation/breakdown, skin flap necrosis
- Wound cellulitis
- Lymphedema
- Lymphangitis
- Hematoma, seroma, lymphocyst formation
- Decreased sensation over the medial thigh
- Venous thromboembolism

SENTINEL LYMPH NODE DISSECTION

Procedure Overview

The sentinel lymph node (SLN) is defined as the first node that receives drainage from a primary tumor. Assessment of the SLN has recently been introduced into the treatment of early-stage squamous cell vulvar cancer in an attempt to limit morbidity while providing an accurate assessment of regional nodes. Levenback et al[11,12] began developing the SLN mapping technique for vulvar cancer in 1993 using isosulfan blue dye based on the technique described for cutaneous melanoma. However, the combination of a radioactive tracer and blue dye is the most accurate technique for SLN detection and frozen-section analysis. In addition, ultrastaging of the nodal sample minimizes the need for reoperations and decreases the risk of false negatives. In early-stage vulvar cancer, the groin recurrence rate is low with a negative SLN, and survival is excellent. However, the procedure requires a multidisciplinary approach, and the authors recommended that the procedure should be performed at least 5 to 10 times a year to maintain competence.

All patients with SLN metastases require additional treatment to the groin, independent of the size of metastasis in the SLN, and currently, this includes inguinofemoral lymphadenectomy.[13]

Box 27-10	Master Surgeon's Corner

- The isosulfan blue dye should be given intradermally at the junction of the tumor and normal tissue at least 10 minutes before the groin incision is made.
- Any lymph node that exhibits blue dye or radioactivity is biopsied.
- The SLN biopsy is performed before the excision of the primary vulvar lesion.

Preoperative Preparation

Preoperative examination and imaging are recommended to rule out gross nodal involvement. A computed tomography scan can detect local and distant disease.

If the radioisotopes are used, a preoperative radiolymphoscintigram is performed to detect the localization of the SLN(s). This image is used to guide the site and size of the incision and to localize the SLN. The procedure requires peritumoral injection with technetium 99m radioisotope bound to nanoparticles. Using a 27-guage needle, 0.1 to 0.5 mCi of the radiolabeled colloid is injected intradermally at the leading edge of the vulvar lesion 2 to 4 hours preoperatively. Radiocolloid tracer is transported to the SLN and is identified with a gamma counter applied to the patient. The time interval for maximum tracer accumulation in SLN is 1.5 hours after injection, and it remains there for at least 2 to 6 hours after injection.

Operative Procedure

Injection of Blue Dye

Both radioisotope and blue dye are used to help in accurate localization of the SLN. Lithotomy position is required to delineate the primary vulvar lesion. General or regional anesthesia is required to obtain adequate access to the vulva and groin region. The injection of blue dye is given intradermally in the operating room at least 10 minutes before the groin incision is made. Approximately, 4 mL of isosulfan blue dye is injected circumferentially at the junction of the tumor and normal tissue (Figure 27-12). The dye reaches the lymph node through microlymphatics in

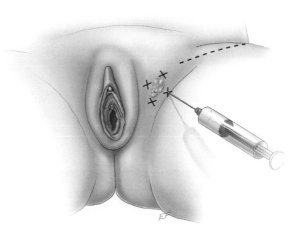

FIGURE 27-12. Sentinel lymph node biopsy; circumferential injection of isosulfan blue dye around tumor site.

about 5 minutes, and the median stain time of dye in the SLN is 21 minutes.

Isolation of SLN

The intraoperative handheld gamma probe is used to accurately localize the SLN in the operating room, using 10-fold higher measured radiation than the basal count at the primary injection site as a cutoff. After the SLN is detected and marked, a small incision is made in the groin, parallel to inguinal ligament, directly over the point of maximum radiation count. The fatty lymphatic tissue is carefully dissected through the area until blue-stained lymphatic channels and lymph node(s) are visualized. Visualization of isosulfan blue dye and increased radioisotope counts detected with gamma counter facilitate the identification of the SLN. Any lymph node that exhibits blue dye or radioactivity is biopsied. After removal of the first node, the gamma counter is used to assess the remainder of the groin node basin. This indicates whether the correct node has been removed or if there is another SLN. Nodes are usually re-examined with the probe ex vivo to confirm radioactivity. SLNs are sent for pathologic evaluation as separate specimens. The resultant groin incision is closed transversely with interrupted 2-0 or 3-0 delayed-absorbable sutures. After node dissection, the appropriate vulvar operation is performed.

Box 27-11 | **Caution Points**

- SLN procedure is not recommended for tumors larger than 4 cm or multifocal lesions.
- Suspicious inguinal adenopathy is a contraindication to SLN dissection.
- Inability to evaluate the groins, particularly in a patient with a larger primary tumor or a midline tumor, is a contraindication to SLN.

Postoperative Care

Care relates primarily to the concurrent vulvar surgery. Drains are usually not necessary, and patients can ambulate the day of surgery.

Box 27-12 | **Complications and Morbidity**

- Wound complication (infection or lymphocyst)
- Lymphedema
- Sensory deficit
- Allergy to isosulfan blue dye

UPPER VAGINECTOMY

Procedure Overview

An upper vaginectomy is most often performed for high-grade vaginal dysplasia (vaginal intraepithelial neoplasia [VAIN] stage 2 or 3) and carcinoma in situ or early invasive stage I vaginal cancer (see Chapter 10). This is usually after hysterectomy but may be performed for lesions in the posterior upper third of the vagina with the uterus intact. Two-year cure rates approach 90%. Occult invasion has been seen in up to 12% of upper vaginectomies performed for VAIN.[14] Alternative treatments such as vaginal 5-fluorouracil and laser vaporization have been used with lower success rates and have the disadvantage of not providing a tissue specimen for pathologic evaluation. Upper vaginectomy has also been performed using a loop electrosurgical excision procedure. High success rates with minimal morbidity have been reported in small series.[15]

Box 27-13 | **Master Surgeon's Corner**

- Prior radiation therapy and postmenopausal status may make Lugol iodine ineffective in delineating lesions because the entire vagina will not be glycogenized.
- When excising the vaginal cuff, especially after radiation therapy, the dissection should proceed posterior to anterior. Entry into the peritoneum is not a major problem and may facilitate identification of the bladder.
- Full-thickness excision of vaginal mucosa is required to rule out invasion. Entry into the subvaginal spaces facilitates this.
- Giving 5 mL of indigo carmine after induction of anesthesia will color the urine blue and make an inadvertent injury to the bladder or ureters more apparent. This is more useful after hysterectomy.

Preoperative Preparation

All patients should undergo colposcopic evaluation of the entire vagina and cervix (if present) and careful inspection of the external genitalia. No special bowel preparation or antibiotics are necessary. Vaginal retractors and long instruments (forceps, needle holders, Allis clamps, and long knife handle) are required. Electrocautery and suction are also helpful. Patients should be informed of the risk of bladder or rectal injury and dyspareunia.

Operative Procedure

Initial Steps

Lithotomy position is required, and "candy cane" stirrups provide the best access for the surgeon and

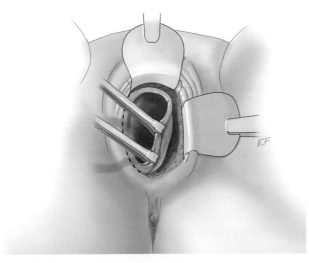

FIGURE 27-13. Upper vaginectomy after prior hysterectomy.

assistants, although Allen stirrups may also be used. Bladder catheterization is only required if the patient has a distended bladder or large cystocele. Lugol iodine applied to vagina is helpful to delineate the lesions, and 3% acetic acid may help identify hyperkeratotic lesions. General or regional anesthesia is usually required to obtain adequate access to the entire vagina.

Incision and Dissection

The lesion should be infiltrated with a dilute lidocaine and epinephrine solution (eg, 1% lidocaine with 1:100,000 epinephrine) and then circumscribed using a #11 blade. Stay sutures may be placed to help elevate the margins. The incision should be through the full thickness of the vaginal wall and should enter into the subvaginal spaces in proximity to the lesion (vesicovaginal, rectovaginal, pararectal, or paravesical). The edges of the lesion are grasped with Allis clamps, and the procedure can be completed with sharp-curved scissors or the scalpel (Figure 27-13). If there was a prior hysterectomy for cervical dysplasia, the vaginal cuff often must be excised. The resultant vaginal defect is closed transversely with interrupted 2-0 or 3-0 delayed-absorbable sutures.

● Injury to the bladder or entry into the peritoneum is most likely to occur when excising the vaginal cuff after a hysterectomy. Both injuries can be repaired vaginally, but cystoscopy should be available to ensure a ureteral injury does not occur during bladder repair.

Postoperative Care

Bladder catheterization is not required unless an injury has occurred. Most patients can be discharged on the day of surgery. Light vaginal bleeding may occur for 2 to 4 weeks, and patients should be instructed not to place anything in the vagina for at least 4 weeks, when they should be seen for a postoperative visit. Strenuous exercise should be avoided until then as well. For extensive resections or entry into the peritoneum, intercourse should be avoided for 6 to 8 weeks.

RADICAL VAGINECTOMY

Procedure Overview

A radical vaginectomy is most often performed for an early invasive stage I vaginal cancer in the upper vagina in combination with an abdominal radical hysterectomy (see Chapter 25). This approach was commonly used for diethylstilbestrol-associated clear cell carcinomas of the cervix and upper vagina.[16] Radical vaginectomy may also be performed for treatment of primary vaginal cancer (especially distal lesions) or recurrent cervical cancer in the vagina after prior hysterectomy.[17] However, when cervical cancer recurs after definitive radiotherapy (external beam and brachytherapy), a pelvic exenteration is usually required. In rare instances, radical vaginectomy, with or without hysterectomy, can be used for vaginal melanoma. Although radiation therapy is considered the standard treatment for stage II vaginal cancer, one series has reported encouraging results using neoadjuvant chemotherapy followed by radical vaginal resection.[18] Similar to radical hysterectomy, a nerve-sparing approach can be performed.[19]

| Box 27-16 | Master Surgeon's Corner |

- Most vaginal cancers occur in the upper posterior vagina, making them potentially treatable with an extended radical hysterectomy with subtotal vaginectomy.
- Entry into the pararectal and paravesical spaces both abdominally and vaginally facilitates the dissection and minimizes blood loss. A combined approach helps to delineate the distal vaginal margins.
- Dissection in the rectovaginal septum and vesicovaginal space is critical to avoid injury to the rectum and bladder. This can be facilitated by hydrodissection with saline or a dilute solution of lidocaine with epinephrine (see Upper Vaginectomy section).
- Distal vaginal lesions should include dissection of inguinal lymph nodes. SLN techniques have not been adequately studied but may be applicable.

Preoperative Preparation

All patients should undergo colposcopic evaluation of the entire vagina and cervix (if present) and careful inspection of the external genitalia. Although experience is limited, based on evidence for cervical cancer, computed tomography/positron emission tomography scan may be the best approach to exclude lymphatic or distant metastasis. Magnetic resonance imaging may be helpful in characterizing the lesion's local extent and relation to bladder and rectum. Cystoscopy and proctoscopy are also useful to rule out local extension to these organs. A mechanical bowel preparation is helpful. Based on experience with hysterectomy, prophylactic antibiotics should be used, as well as deep vein thrombosis prophylaxis. Bladder catheterization is required. If there is a vaginal phase, special vaginal retractors and long instruments (forceps, needle holders, Allis clamps, and knife handle) are required. If an upper vaginectomy is combined with an abdominal radical hysterectomy, the equipment is identical as for radical hysterectomy (see Chapter 25). Patients should be informed of the risk of bladder or rectal injury and dysfunction. Depending on what reconstructive techniques are chosen, a shortened or strictured vagina and dyspareunia are common.

Operative Procedure

Initial Steps

If an abdominal radical hysterectomy with an extended vaginectomy is performed, the supine position may be adequate. The lithotomy position using Allen stirrups is required if a vaginal approach is performed exclusively or if a vaginal approach is used in combination with an abdominal hysterectomy. General and/or regional anesthesia is usually required to obtain adequate access to the abdomen and entire vagina.

Abdominal Approach

If a combined abdominal-vaginal approach is used to perform a radical hysterectomy with extended radical vaginectomy, the procedure begins as a standard type III radical hysterectomy (see Chapter 25). This can be performed using a vertical or transverse skin incision and may also use laparoscopic or robotic techniques. A pelvic lymphadenectomy should be performed first and suspicious lymph nodes sent for frozen-section analysis. An inguinal-femoral lymph node dissection is indicated for distal vaginal lesions. The parametrial dissection should continue all the way to the pelvic floor, and the rectovaginal septum needs to be dissected all the way to the perineum (Figure 27-14).

Perineal Approach

From below, a circumferential vaginal incision should be made through the full thickness of the vaginal wall and should enter into the subvaginal spaces at least 2 cm distal to the lesion. The edges of the posterior vagina should be grasped with Allis or Chrobak forceps and elevated so that the rectovaginal septum can be dissected cephalad until the posterior cul-de-sac is reached. As the dissection proceeds in a cephalad direction, the avascular pararectal spaces can be entered laterally to further mobilize the vagina (Figure 27-15). Care should be taken not to injure the levator muscles during this dissection because troublesome bleeding will ensue. The uterosacral ligaments may be encountered near the apex of the vagina, and these can be cauterized or clamped and cut at the border of the rectum. Allis forceps should then be placed on the anterior vagina, and dissection should proceed in the vesicovaginal space until the anterior cul-de-sac is reached. If the patient has had a hysterectomy, there is no separate anterior and posterior cul-de-sac. During the anterior dissection, the paravesicle spaces should be entered and the ureters should be identified by palpation. The connective tissue attaching the bladder and ureter to the vagina or cervix (the bladder pillars) needs to be cut to free the ureter from the specimen. If the connective

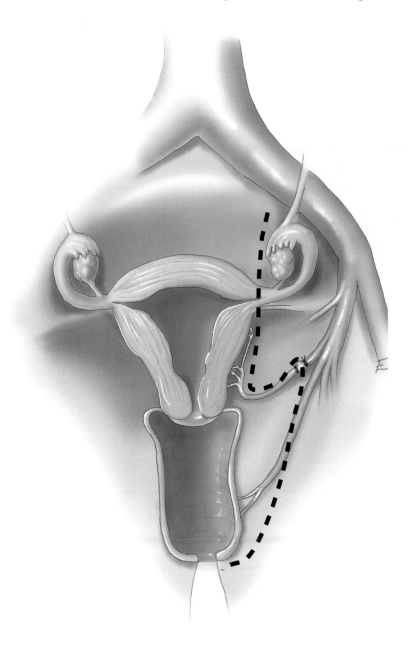

FIGURE 27-14. Radical vaginectomy using a combined abdominal and perineal approach.

tissue lateral to the vagina (paracolpos and parame-trium) has not been dissected from above, this should be clamped as lateral as possible and cut. Entry into the cul-de-sac is then performed to either excise the entire vaginal specimen or complete the extended radi-cal hysterectomy.

Reconstruction will depend on the amount of vagina removed and the wishes of the patients. Rectus abdom-inis and gracilis myocutaneous flaps can be used as for a pelvic exenteration (see Chapter 32C). In some cases, for small mid to lower vaginal lesions, partial vaginec-tomy may be performed and repaired with local trans-position flaps.

Box 27-17 | **Caution Points**

- Entry into the pararectal spaces from below should be above where the levator muscles attach to the perineal muscles. Dissection too low or too lateral will result in troublesome bleeding from the levator muscles.
- Injury to the bladder or ureter is more likely to occur when excising the vaginal cuff after a hysterectomy. Cystoscopy and ureteral catheterization before surgery may facilitate the dissection and help avoid injury.

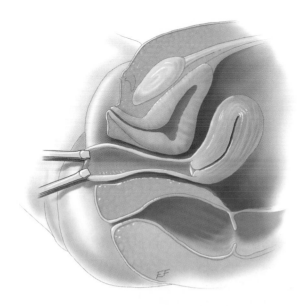

FIGURE 27-15. Radical vaginectomy, sagittal view.

Postoperative Care

Bladder catheterization is required for 1 to 2 weeks, and a postvoid residual urine should be measured after the catheter is removed. Patients should continue deep vein thrombosis prophylaxis for at least until discharge. Light vaginal bleeding may occur for 2 to 4 weeks, and patients should be instructed not to place anything in the vagina for at least 4 weeks, when they should be seen for a postoperative visit. Strenuous exercise should be avoided for up to 3 months.

Box 27-18	Complications and Morbidity

- Bladder injury resulting in fistula
- Bladder dysfunction (initially retention, but overactivity can develop later)
- Rectal injury resulting in infection or fistula
- Vaginal shortening and stenosis resulting in dyspareunia

Vaginal Reconstruction

When vaginectomy is performed at the time of exenterative surgery, gracilis or rectus abdominis myocutaneous flaps are commonly used for reconstruction. However, when vaginectomy is performed for dysplasia or cancer without removal of the bladder and/or rectum, there is usually less room for those bulky flaps. In that case, transposition flaps are more useful. Vaginal reconstruction using transposition flaps is described in Chapter 32C.

REFERENCES

1. Morley GW. Surgery for vulvar cancer. In: Nichols DH, ed. *Gynecologic and Obstetric Surgery*. St. Louis, MO: Mosby-Year Book, Inc.; 1993:286-296.
2. Rettenmaier MA, Berman ML, Disaia PJ. Skinning vulvectomy for the treatment of multifocal vulvar intraepithelial neoplasia. *Obstet Gynecol*. 1987;69:247-250.
3. Way S. Carcinoma of the vulva. *Am J Obstet Gynecol*. 1960;79: 79692-79697.
4. Stroup A, Harlan LT. Demographic, clinical, and treatment trends among women diagnosed with vulvar cancer in the U.S. *Gynecol Oncol*. 2008;108(3):577-583.
5. Groenen SMA, Timmers PJ, Burger CW. Recurrence rate in vulvar carcinoma in relation to pathological margin distance. *Int J Gynecol Cancer*. 2011;20:869-873.
6. Landrum LM, Lanneau GS, Skaggs VJ, et al. Gynecologic Oncology Group risk groups for vulvar carcinoma: improvement in survival in the modern era. *Gynecol Oncol*. 2007;106: 521-525.
7. Disaia PJ, Creasman WT, Rich WM. An alternative approach to early cancer of the vulva. *Am J Obstet Gynecol*. 1979;133: 825-830.
8. Gonzalez Bosquet J, Magrina JF, Gaffey TA, et al. Long-term survival and disease recurrence in patients with primary squamous cell carcinoma of the vulva. *Gynecol Oncol*. 2005;97: 828-833.
9. Stehman FB, Ali S, Disaia PJ. Node count and groin recurrence in early vulvar cancer: a Gynecologic Oncology Group study. *Gynecol Oncol*. 2009;113:52-56.
10. Selman TJ, Luesley DM, Acheson N, Khan KS, Mann CH. A systematic review of the accuracy of diagnostic tests for inguinal lymph node status in vulvar cancer. *Gynecol Oncol*. 2005;99: 206-214.
11. Levenback C, Burke TW, Morris M, et al. Potential applications of intraoperative lymphatic mapping in vulvar cancer. *Gynecol Oncol*. 1995;59:216-220.
12. Levenback C, Burke TW, Gershenson D, et al. Intraoperative lymphatic mapping for vulvar cancer. *Obstet Gynecol*. 1994;84: 163-167.
13. Oonk MH, van Hemel BM, De Hullu JA, et al. Size of sentinel-node metastasis and chances of non-sentinel-node involvement and survival in early vulvar cancer: results from GROINSS-V, a multicentre observational study. *Lancet Oncol*. 2010;11(7): 646-652.
14. Indermaur MD, Martino MA, Fiorica JV, Roberts WS, Hoffman MS. Upper vaginectomy for the treatment of vaginal intraepithelial neoplasia. *Am J Obstet Gynecol*. 2005;193: 577-581.
15. Fanning J, Manahan KJ, McLean SA. Loop electrosurgical excision procedure for partial upper vaginectomy. *Am J Obstet Gynecol*. 1999;181:1382-1385.
16. Herbst AL. Behavior of estrogen-associated female genital tract cancer and its relation to neoplasia following intrauterine exposure to diethylstilbestrol (DES). *Gynecol Oncol*. 2000;76: 147-156.
17. Pierluigi BP, Manci N, Bellati F, et al. Vaginectomy: a minimally invasive treatment for cervical cancer vaginal recurrence. *Int J Gynecol Oncol*. 2009;19:1625-1631.
18. Pierluigi BP, Filippo B, Francesco P, et al. Neoadjuvant chemotherapy followed by radical surgery in patients affected by vaginal carcinoma. *Gynecol Oncol*. 2008;111:307-311.
19. Raspagliesi F, Ditto A, Nartinelli F, et al. Nerve sparing radical vaginectomy. *Int J Gynecol Oncol*. 2009;19:794-797.

28 Lymphadenectomy

Lisa A. dos Santos and Nadeem R. Abu-Rustum

INTRODUCTION

Surgical staging including lymph node dissection is the cornerstone of treatment of early-stage endometrial and ovarian malignancies. In 1988, surgical staging replaced clinical staging for endometrial cancer, due to inherent underreporting of metastatic disease distribution in the clinical staging system. Comprehensive staging guides treatment planning for subsequent chemotherapy and/or radiation therapy. In the setting of advanced or recurrent disease, lymph node dissection may be undertaken for the purpose of removing bulky tumor. Although cervical cancer is staged clinically, lymph node dissection plays a role in the management of early-stage tumors.

The lymphatic drainage of the uterus, tubes, and ovaries follows the blood supply of these organs and includes the pelvic lymph node basins as well as the aortic lymph nodes (Figure 28-1). Depending on the site of malignancy and the clinical indications, lymph node dissection may be undertaken in some or all of these basins, either unilaterally or bilaterally.

PELVIC LYMPH NODE DISSECTION

Procedure Overview

Box 28-1	Master Surgeon's Corner

● Adequate exposure and identification of anatomic structures are crucial to avoid injury to adjacent structures of the pelvic sidewall.

● Proper development of the paravesical and pararectal spaces is an essential step prior to beginning the process of removing lymph nodes.

● Appropriate use of hemostatic clips and vessel-sealing devices (ie, limiting the use of monopolar cautery and blunt dissection) may reduce the risk of lymphorrhea.

Indications and Historical Perspective

There is a generalized lack of standardization in the technique of pelvic lymphadenectomy in gynecologic cancer that is apparent in both the literature and surgical practice. With the exception of sentinel lymph node mapping, the total number of lymph nodes removed is most often used as a surrogate for the radicality and completeness of the procedure. Cibula and Abu-Rustum[1] recently attempted to clarify and standardize the terminology and anatomic basis for the procedure, proposing a new anatomically based classification system for pelvic lymphadenectomy. In this system, a complete systematic lymphadenectomy or "type III dissection" includes the removal of all fatty lymphatic tissue from the predicted areas of high incidence of lymph nodes with metastatic involvement. This comprehensive procedure is described later in this chapter and includes dissection of the 5 main anatomic regions of the pelvic lymphatic drainage: external iliac, obturator, internal iliac, common iliac, and presacral lymph nodes. In certain circumstances, more limited dissection may

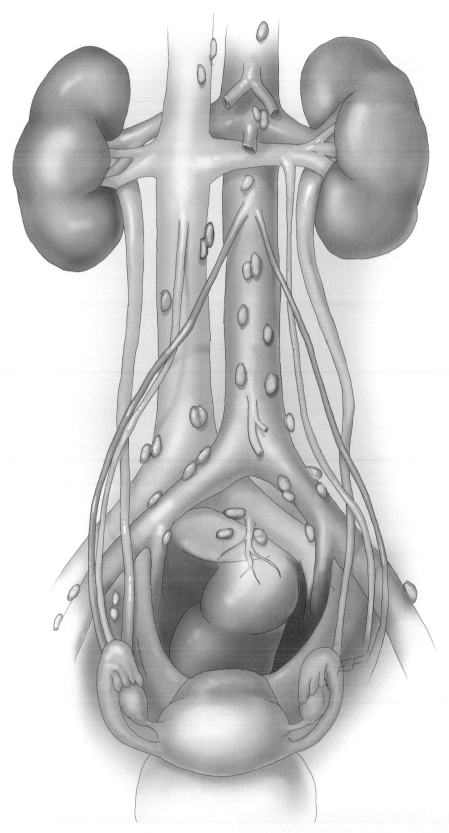

FIGURE 28-1. Pelvic and aortic lymph node basins. (Redrawn, with permission, from Chi DS, Bristow RE, Gallup DG. Surgical principles in gynecologic oncology. In: Barakat RR, Markman M, Randall ME, eds. *Principles and Practice of Gynecologic Oncology*. Baltimore, MD: Lippincott Williams & Wilkins; 2009:270.)

be indicated, such as sentinel lymph node biopsy, excision of only bulky nodes, or lymph node sampling.

Several operative approaches may be used for the pelvic lymph node dissection. It is often performed via laparotomy at the time of open hysterectomy or laparoscopically at the time of total laparoscopic hysterectomy or laparoscopic-assisted vaginal hysterectomy. In some cases, it is performed as part of a secondary staging procedure, which often may be accomplished laparoscopically. In addition, the technique of pelvic sentinel lymph node mapping may be used in selected cases. The equipment required varies by the operative approach, as described later.

Preoperative Preparation

Patient Evaluation and Work-Up

Prior to surgery, the patient should undergo a complete history and physical, complete blood count, basic metabolic panel, coagulation profile, pregnancy test, electrocardiogram, and chest radiograph (when indicated by the patient's age).

Consent Considerations

In addition to the standard risks of general anesthesia and abdominal surgery, a discussion of procedure-specific risks is warranted, including chronic lymphedema, lymphocele potentially requiring further medical or surgical treatment, and injury to adjacent nerves, vascular structures, and the ureter.

Patient Preparation

A preoperative bowel preparation may be helpful to decompress the bowel and facilitate exposure. Epidural anesthesia may be offered for open procedures, which may optimize postoperative pain control while reducing the adverse effects of intravenous opioid analgesia. As with any open procedure, a single dose of prophylactic antibiotics should be administered intravenously within 60 to 120 minutes of the initial skin incision.

Operative Procedure

Box 28-2	Caution Points

- Careful placement of lateral retractors without exertion of excessive pressure on the psoas muscle will avoid potential injury to the femoral nerve.

- Careful identification of the genitofemoral and obturator nerves is essential to avoid injury, and the use of electrocautery should be minimized in close proximity to these fine nerve structures.
- Retraction on the external iliac vein during the obturator dissection must be applied gently to avoid intimal injury and minimize the risk of subsequent deep vein thrombosis.
- Careful dissection is particularly important in the obturator space to avoid bleeding from the corona mortis.

Open Pelvic Lymph Node Dissection

The procedure may be performed in the supine position, although it is usually combined with hysterectomy requiring the dorsal lithotomy position. A Foley catheter is placed. While a pelvic lymph node dissection may sometimes be adequately performed through an extended transverse incision (eg, Maylard or Cherney), maximal exposure is obtained with a vertical midline approach, particularly in the obese patient or if dissection of the deep common iliac lymph nodes is required. Standard laparotomy equipment is required for an open dissection, including a self-retaining retractor (eg, Bookwalter). In addition to standard instrumentation, Penfield dissectors may be useful in cases with adherent lymphadenopathy (Figure 28-2).

Opening the Pelvic Peritoneum
The round ligament is clamped and divided, and the umbilical ligament is isolated. Working parallel to the round ligament, the peritoneum is incised with Metzenbaum scissors or electrocautery in a linear fashion between the round ligament and the umbilical ligament to the reflection of the anterior abdominal wall.

Development of the Paravesical Space
The umbilical ligament is retracted medially to facilitate blunt dissection of the paravesical space, exposing the external iliac nodes, obturator space, and ventral aspect of the hypogastric vessels.

Identification of the Ureter
The ureter should be clearly identified as it crosses the bifurcation of the common iliac artery into the internal and external iliac artery, and courses along the medial leaflet of the broad ligament. A vessel loop may be placed around the ureter for gentle retraction and continued identification throughout the procedure.

Development of the Pararectal Space
The peritoneal incision is extended cephalad along the psoas muscle, lateral and parallel to the infundibulopelvic ligament. Next, the infundibulopelvic ligament

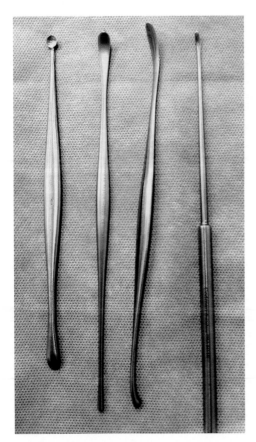

FIGURE 28-2. Penfield dissectors.

(if not already divided) and ureter are retracted medially, and the hypogastric artery is identified. The pararectal space is then developed bluntly, retracting the rectum medially and providing access to the hypogastric nodes and obturator space.

External Iliac Lymph Node Dissection

The dissection begins with the external iliac lymph nodes. A Singley (ringed) forceps may be used to gently grasp the lymphatic tissue without fracturing the nodes. Sharp or blunt dissection with Metzenbaum scissors is used to isolate small blood vessels and lymphatic channels, which are secured with hemostatic clips and divided. The lateral border of the dissection is the genitofemoral nerve. Moving from lateral to medial, the nodal tissue is dissected first from the psoas muscle and then the external iliac vessels, taking care to protect the genitofemoral nerve and the external iliac artery and vein. The cephalad limit of the external iliac dissection is the bifurcation of the common iliac artery, and the caudal limit is the deep circumflex iliac vein, a branch of the external iliac vein that is usually seen coursing anteriorly over the external iliac artery. Lymph nodes caudal to the deep circumflex iliac vein predominantly drain the lymphatics of the

lower extremity, and their removal may increase the risk of lymphedema.

Obturator and Hypogastric Lymph Node Dissection

The obturator and hypogastric lymph nodes may be accessed from a medial or a lateral approach, and many surgeons use a combined approach. Beginning with a medial approach, the external iliac vein is gently pulled laterally with a vein retractor, and the nodal package posterior to the vein is grasped with the Singley forceps. Gentle dissection is used to identify the obturator nerve, and the nodal package between the vein and nerve is dissected free. Next, additional nodes may be removed from below the nerve. Care should be taken to avoid injury to the obturator vessels and anastomotic obturator or pubic veins, which may sometimes be encountered in the distal portion of the obturator space. This area has been referred to as the "corona mortis," or ring of death, due to the potentially treacherous plexus formed by variable anastomotic veins that are often found linking the obturator and external iliac venous systems. A 4-part "ring" may be formed by the external iliac vein, hypogastric vein, obturator vein, and anastomotic obturator or pubic vein (Figure 28-3).

The hypogastric nodes may then be dissected from the proximal portion of the umbilical ligament, moving cephalad over the hypogastric artery and the origin of the uterine artery. Finally, the external iliac vessels are bluntly mobilized medially from the psoas muscle, allowing access to the obturator space from a lateral approach, to remove any remaining nodal tissue from behind and beneath the vessels, particularly near the common iliac artery bifurcation.

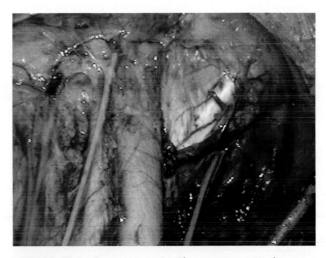

FIGURE 28-3. Corona mortis. The anastomotic obturator or pubic vein is seen crossing the distal obturator space and entering the left external iliac vein.

Common Iliac Lymph Node Dissection

In a type III pelvic lymph node dissection as described by Cibula and Abu-Rustum,[1] the common iliac dissection includes removal of the superficial and deep common iliac lymph nodes. The common iliac lymph nodes receive lymphatic vessels from 2 major lymphatic trunks draining the uterus and cervix. A superficial trunk enters the pelvis via the femoral canal, courses along the ventral aspect of the external iliac vessels, receives branches from the parametrium, and continues along the ventral aspect of the common iliac artery (Figure 28-4). On the right side of the pelvis, these lymphatics continue toward the precaval and interaortocaval regions; on the left side of the pelvis, they continue to the left para-aortic region.

A deep trunk also enters the pelvis via the femoral canal but follows a more medial course, surrounding the obturator nerve and receiving parametrial lymphatics before entering the common iliac area (Figure 28-5). This deep trunk then divides into 2 branches. A lateral branch courses between the common iliac vein and the psoas muscle, forming the deep common iliac nodes before entering the paracaval region. A medial branch tunnels beneath the common iliac vessels to the medial aspect of the vessels and enters the presacral area, forming the presacral nodes, before coursing toward the interaortocaval and preaortic regions.

The common iliac dissection begins with careful removal of the superficial common iliac lymph nodes

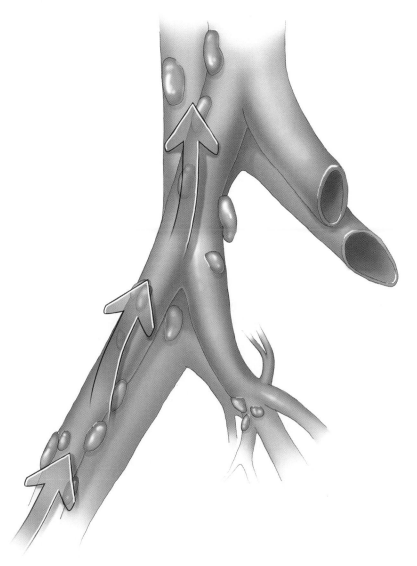

FIGURE 28-4. Pelvic lymphatic drainage: the superficial lymphatic trunk. (Redrawn, with permission, from Cibula D, Abu-Rustum NR. Pelvic lymphadenectomy in cervical cancer: surgical anatomy and proposal for a new classification system. *Gynecol Oncol.* 2010;116:33-37.)

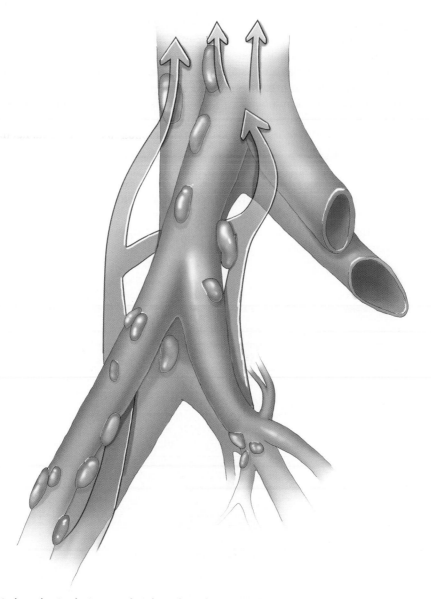

FIGURE 28-5. Pelvic lymphatic drainage: the deep lymphatic trunk. (Redrawn, with permission, from Cibula D, Abu-Rustum NR. Pelvic lymphadenectomy in cervical cancer: surgical anatomy and proposal for a new classification system. *Gynecol Oncol.* 2010;116:33-37.)

from the ventral and lateral surfaces of the common iliac artery and vein. Next, the deep common iliac lymph nodes (formed by the lateral branch of the deep lymphatic trunk) are identified between the common iliac vein and the psoas muscle. These are carefully removed. The cephalad limit of the dissection is the aortic bifurcation, and the lateral border is the psoas muscle. The floor of the dissection will expose the lumbosacral trunk and the obturator nerve.

Presacral Lymph Node Dissection

The presacral lymph nodes are found on the anterior surface of the sacrum between the common iliac veins and receive lymphatics from the medial branch of the

deep lymphatic trunk. These lymph nodes are carefully removed, with particular care taken to avoid injury to the left common iliac vein.

Laparoscopic Transperitoneal Pelvic Lymph Node Dissection

The patient is placed in the dorsal lithotomy position with the legs placed in Allen stirrups. A Foley catheter is inserted, and an orogastric tube is placed by the anesthesiologist to provide gastric decompression. After initial trocar placement, the patient is placed in steep Trendelenburg position. Suggested equipment for the laparoscopic approach includes a 10-mm blunt port, two 5-mm trocars, a 5/10-mm trocar, 5- and 10-mm laparoscopic clip appliers, 5-mm graspers, and a 10-mm lymph node spoon. For dissection, we use a monopolar cautery device; a vessel-sealing device is also used. The procedure may be performed using a variety of available monopolar cautery devices for dissection and a vessel-sealing device.

Trocar Placement

Using an open laparoscopy technique, a blunt 10-mm trocar is placed in the umbilicus, and the abdomen is insufflated (Figure 28-6). Under direct visualization, two 5-mm trocars are placed in the right and left lower quadrants, at a point approximately 1 cm superior to and 1 cm medial to the anterior superior iliac spine. Care should be taken to avoid injury to the inferior epigastric vessels. A 5/10-mm trocar is placed in the suprapubic area, carefully avoiding injury to the bladder. Individual trocar size and placement may vary depending on planned concurrent procedures, choice of instrumentation, the patient's habitus, and prior surgical history.

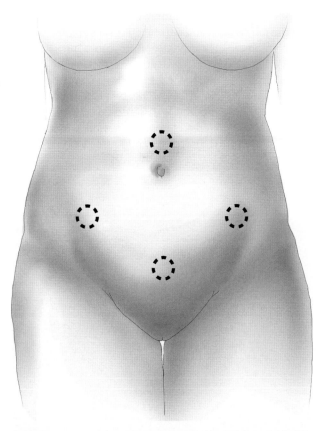

FIGURE 28-6. Trocar placement for laparoscopic pelvic and aortic lymph node dissection. (Redrawn, with permission, from Abu-Rustum NR, Sonoda Y. Transperitoneal laparoscopic staging with aortic and pelvic lymph node dissection for gynecologic malignancies. *Gynecol Oncol.* 2007;104[suppl]:S5-S8.)

Development of the Paravesical Space

Using the surgeon's chosen instrument, the round ligament is divided, and the umbilical ligament is isolated. Working parallel to the umbilical ligament, the peritoneum is incised in a linear fashion between the round ligament and the umbilical ligament to the reflection of the anterior abdominal wall. Gentle medial traction is then applied to the umbilical ligament, and the paravesical space is developed with a blunt instrument.

Development of the Pararectal Space

The ureter should be clearly identified as it crosses the bifurcation of the common iliac artery and courses along the medial leaflet of the broad ligament. The peritoneal incision is extended cephalad along the psoas muscle, parallel to the infundibulopelvic ligament. Next, the infundibulopelvic ligament (if not already divided) and ureter are retracted medially, the hypogastric artery is identified, and the pararectal space is developed bluntly, retracting the rectum medially and providing access to the hypogastric nodes and obturator space.

External Iliac Lymph Node Dissection

The dissection begins with the distal common iliac lymph nodes, lateral to the common iliac artery, and moving caudal to the external iliac lymph nodes. Laparoscopic graspers are used to protect the ureter medially and provide gentle traction on the nodal package. The monopolar cautery device may be used as both a blunt dissector and a cautery device to isolate small blood vessels and lymphatic channels, which are secured with hemostatic clips and divided. Larger vessels may be transected with a vessel-sealing device. Moving from lateral to medial, the nodal tissue is dissected first from the psoas muscle and then the external iliac vessels, taking care to protect the genitofemoral nerve and the external iliac artery and vein. The caudal limit of the dissection is the deep circumflex iliac vein, a branch of the external iliac vein that is usually seen coursing anteriorly over the artery. The nodes may be removed atraumatically from the abdomen using a 10-mm laparoscopic spoon.

Obturator and Hypogastric Lymph Node Dissection

The obturator nodal package, located posterior to the external iliac vein, is grasped gently and retracted medially. Gentle blunt dissection is used to identify the obturator nerve, and the nodal package between the vein and nerve is dissected free, using clips and cautery as necessary to divide small vessels and lymphatics. Additional nodes may be removed from below the nerve, taking extreme care to avoid injury to the obturator vessels and potential anastomotic pelvic veins, which may sometimes be encountered in the distal portion of

CHAPTER 28

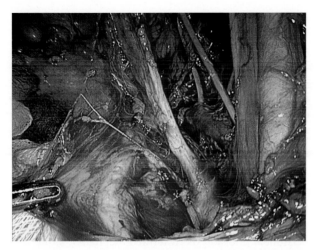

FIGURE 28-7. Completed laparoscopic pelvic lymph node dissection. The completed dissection of the right pelvis exposes the ureter, medial aspect of the external iliac vessels, ventral aspect of the hypogastric vessels, and superior part of the obturator space, exposing the obturator vessels and nerve.

the obturator space. The hypogastric nodes may then be dissected from the proximal portion of the umbilical ligament, near the origin of the uterine artery. Finally, the iliac vessels are gently dissected medially off of the psoas muscle, allowing lateral access to the obturator space to remove any residual nodal tissue. The specimen is removed using the laparoscopic spoon.

The completed dissection of the pelvis exposes the ureter, medial aspect of the external iliac vessels, ventral aspect of the hypogastric vessels, and superior part of the obturator space, exposing the obturator vessels and nerve (Figure 28-7).

Sentinel Lymph Node Mapping and Dissection

The technique of sentinel lymph node mapping in early-stage cervical and uterine malignancy may be used in selected cases.[2] A cervical blue dye injection is administered in the operating room prior to beginning the case. This may be performed at the time of examination under anesthesia, or it may be performed after skin preparation and draping. Although methylene blue 1% solution may be used, we generally use isosulfan blue 1% (Lymphazurin), a sterile aqueous solution packaged in 5-mL vials that requires no refrigeration or special preparation. Mild adverse reactions to isosulfan blue may occur in a small number (< 1%) of patients, consisting of localized swelling or pruritus of the neck, abdomen, hands, or feet. Severe anaphylactic reactions are rare but have been reported with similar compounds. Use is contraindicated in patients with a known hypersensitivity to

phenylethane compounds. A transient idiosyncratic decrease in the pulse oximeter reading is common immediately after the injection and represents detection of the blue dye in the circulation rather than actual hypoxemia. Blue-tinged urine is frequently noted for up to 24 hours after surgery.

The cervical injection may be performed with a spinal needle, and a tenaculum placed on the anterior lip of the cervix may be used for traction. A total of 4 mL of blue dye is injected into the cervical stroma, with 2 mL injected at each of the 3 o'clock and 9 o'clock positions. It is important to inject the dye into the cervical stroma, with approximately 1 mL injected deeply and 1 mL injected superficially. This approach avoids excessive staining of the bladder flap and targets the parametrial lymphatic drainage. If gross cervical tumor is present, the dye should be injected into the cervical stroma adjacent to the lesion.

The procedure then continues as planned, either via laparoscopy or laparotomy. The lymph node mapping is usually visible transperitoneally upon entering the pelvis, and the sentinel lymph node dissection is then performed in an expeditious manner to avoid excessive dissipation of the dye. The pelvic sidewalls are opened in the usual manner, the ureter is identified, and the paravesical and pararectal spaces are developed. Blue lymphatic channels are often seen coursing along the uterine vessels and crossing the hypogastric artery before draining into the external iliac and hypogastric lymph nodes (Figure 28-8). The first blue node noted along the drainage pathway is removed and designated as the sentinel node. Additional blue nodes may sometimes be identified and designated as secondary sentinel lymph nodes.

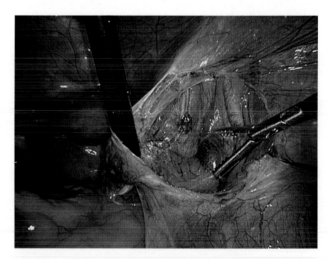

FIGURE 28-8. Pelvic sentinel lymph node mapping. A sentinel right external iliac lymph node is identified in the usual location medial to the external iliac vessels and ventral to the hypogastric vessels.

AORTIC LYMPH NODE DISSECTION

Procedure Overview

Box 28-3	Master Surgeon's Corner

- The goal of the operation is to remove all lymphatic tissue from around and between the abdominal aorta and IVC, which can only be accomplished by first exposing and isolating these vessels and securing control of the surrounding vasculature.
- Familiarity with potential variations in vascular anatomy of the retroperitoneum facilitates safe dissection.
- Using the ventral surface of the aorta as the midline, a "split-and-roll" technique is used to define and dissect the lateral aortic nodes in a medial to lateral fashion.

Indications and Historical Perspective

Dissection of the aortic lymph nodes is often indicated in the surgical staging of endometrial, cervical, and ovarian malignancies, as well as in cases of clinically apparent adenopathy and recurrent disease. In the staging of endometrial and cervical cancer, the dissection is generally carried to the level of the inferior mesenteric artery (IMA). In ovarian cancer, the cephalad limit of dissection is generally the renal vessels. The extent of dissection in a particular case is individualized. The technique of complete open retroperitoneal lymph node dissection is described later in this section. In some cases, such as staging of endometrial and cervical cancer, a more limited dissection may be performed.

Three surgical approaches may be used. Open dissection is used in cases where there are other indications for laparotomy (eg, concurrent procedures, extensive adhesions, patient habitus) or when a complete retroperitoneal lymph node dissection is indicated. In appropriately selected patients, transperitoneal laparoscopic aortic dissection may be used. A third approach is laparoscopic extraperitoneal dissection, which combines the benefits of laparoscopy with those of extraperitoneal dissection (feasibility despite intraperitoneal adhesions and decreased risk of bowel injury and future adhesion formation). This approach is most commonly used in the surgical staging and treatment planning of patients with locally advanced cervical cancer but may be used in other select patients as well.

Preoperative Preparation

Considerations for preoperative preparation are similar to those listed for a pelvic lymph node dissection. In cases where a complete retroperitoneal lymph node dissection to the level of the renal vessels is planned, bowel preparation is essential to provide adequate bowel decompression in order to achieve optimal exposure. In cases where a laparoscopic extraperitoneal lymph node dissection is planned, preoperative imaging should be performed to evaluate the retroperitoneal vascular anatomy, because correct identification of anatomic landmarks with limited exposure is particularly crucial to the success and safety of the procedure.

Operative Procedure

Box 28-4	Caution Points

- Limit monopolar cautery and blunt dissection in lymphatic basins to decrease lymphorrhea, chylous ascites, and lymphocyst formation.
- In a complete retroperitoneal dissection, meticulous identification and control of the lumbar vessels is essential to avoid potential hemorrhage.
- Meticulous use of hemostatic clips is particularly important around the left renal vein to secure the prominent lymphatics in that region.
- In a laparoscopic extraperitoneal lymph node dissection, it is crucial to avoid premature perforation of the peritoneum at the beginning of the procedure and to fenestrate the peritoneum at the conclusion of the procedure.

Open Aortic Lymph Node Dissection

Anatomy of the Retroperitoneum

A thorough anatomic understanding of the lymphatic drainage surrounding the aorta and inferior vena cava (IVC) will guide the extent of necessary dissection and facilitate lymph node removal while avoiding injury to adjacent structures (Figure 28-9). The aortic lymph nodes may be generally divided into 3 subgroups. The preaortic nodes drain the gastrointestinal tract to the level of the midrectum. The lateral aortic nodes (right and left) drain the iliac systems and therefore the pelvic viscera. The retroaortic nodes do not drain a particular area. Hence, the lateral aortic lymph nodes are most relevant to the staging and treatment of gynecologic malignancies. There are typically 15 to 20 lateral aortic nodes per side. These occupy the space bordered by the aorta medially, the medial aspect of the psoas

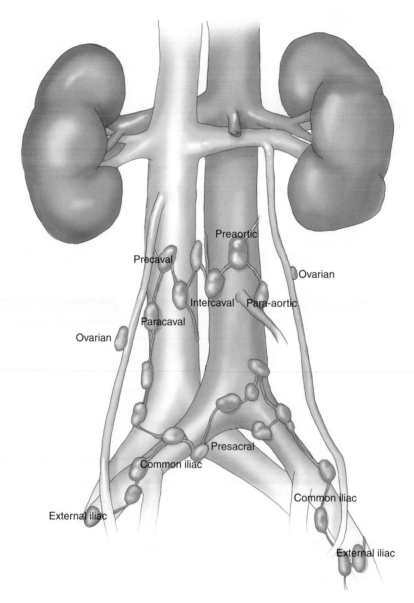

FIGURE 28-9. Lymphatic anatomy of the retroperitoneum. (Redrawn, with permission, from Zivanovic O, Abu-Rustum NR, Sheinfeld J. Retroperitoneal lymph node dissection. In: Levine DA, Barakat RR, Abu-Rustum NR, eds. *Atlas of Procedures in Gynecologic Oncology.* London, UK: Informa Healthcare; 2008:118, Figure 6.1.)

muscle laterally, the lumbar spine posteriorly, the diaphragmatic crura cephalad, and the aortic bifurcation caudad.

In the staging of endometrial and cervical cancer, the lateral aortic nodes are usually dissected to the level of the IMA. This artery arises from the anterior aspect of the aorta approximately 3 to 4 cm above the aortic bifurcation and provides perfusion to the descending colon and rectum. Caudal to the IMA, several pairs of lumbar arteries arise from the posterolateral surface of the aorta. The middle sacral artery arises from the posterior surface of the aorta just above the bifurcation.

The lymphatic drainage of the ovaries courses along the ovarian vessels toward their origin from the aorta approximately 5 to 6 cm above the bifurcation and 2 to 3 cm below the renal vessels. Therefore, the surgical staging of ovarian cancer requires dissection of the lateral aortic nodes from the aortic bifurcation cephalad to the level of the renal vessels. The ovarian arteries cross the ureters as they course toward the pelvis. Anomalies of the uterine arteries are not uncommon, and they may arise from aberrant locations of the aorta or directly from the renal arteries. The renal arteries arise from the aorta at the level of L2. The right renal artery normally crosses dorsal to the IVC.

The venous drainage of the para-aortic area is also variable and must be carefully identified to avoid unnecessary hemorrhage. The right ovarian vein most commonly inserts directly into the IVC approximately 1 cm below the right renal vein, but may insert into the right renal vein. The left ovarian vein follows a course close to the ureter and inserts into the left renal vein. Several pairs of lumbar veins insert into the IVC and may drain into additional ascending lumber veins that drain into the left renal vein. The left renal vein normally crosses beneath the superior mesenteric artery and ventral to the aorta to insert into the IVC. The renal veins drain into the IVC at the level of L2.

Procedure

A complete retroperitoneal lymph node dissection requires a midline abdominal incision extending from the pubic symphysis to the xiphoid process. The falciform ligament is ligated, divided, and excised to facilitate exposure and wound closure. Abdominal wall retraction may be accomplished with a self-retaining retractor such as the Bookwalter. For optimal exposure, we use 2 Balfour-type retractors, 1 placed in the pelvis and 1 placed in the abdomen, combined with a Goligher-type retractor positioned over the patient's head and used to gently retract the exteriorized bowel. The goal of the operation is to remove all lymphatic tissue from around and between the abdominal aorta and IVC, which can only be accomplished by first exposing and isolating these vessels and securing control of the surrounding vasculature.

Exposing the Retroperitoneum. The dissection begins on the right side, with incision of the peritoneum overlying the right common iliac artery. This may be an extension of the pelvic lymph node dissection, or it may be performed first. A right angle clamp or forcep is used to elevate the peritoneum, and the peritoneum is incised with Metzenbaum scissors or electrocautery. The ureter should be clearly identified as it courses lateral to the vena cava and crosses the bifurcation of the common iliac artery into the internal and external iliac artery; it should be retracted laterally. The peritoneal incision is carried cephalad to the duodenum, which is mobilized superiorly to expose the left renal vein. The left ureter is mobilized bluntly and retracted laterally. Sharp and blunt dissection is then used to dissect the avascular plane lateral to the root of the mesentery, until the third portion of the duodenum is reached at the ligament of Treitz.

The small bowel and right colon are then mobilized. This is accomplished by incising the white line of Toldt along the right paracolic gutter and using sharp and blunt dissection to lift the right colon and small bowel off of the right renal fascia. Next, the fibroadipose tissue anterior to the left renal vein and between the undersurface of the duodenum and pancreas is clipped and divided. Completing this process allows adequate exposure to the retroperitoneum, as the small and large bowel may then be elevated and exteriorized, covered with moist laparotomy sponges, and placed on the chest. Two wide Deaver-type retractors can be attached to the Goligher-type retractor and used to gently hold the bowel in place on the chest wall, taking care not to place excessive traction.

The bilateral ureters are then identified and gently retracted laterally with vessel loops. Blunt dissection is used to develop a plane between the left colon mesentery and the left aortic lymphatic tissue. The right ovarian vessels are identified, and the right ovarian vein is ligated and divided at its insertion into the vena cava. The right ovarian artery is ligated and divided at its origin from the right anterior surface of the aorta.

Right Aortic Lymph Node Dissection. Using sharp and blunt dissection with Metzenbaum scissors, the lymphatic tissue overlying the right common iliac artery is elevated and dissected. Small blood vessels and lymphatic channels are carefully identified, secured with hemostatic clips, and divided. The incision is carried cephalad along the ventral surface of the aorta to the level of the origin of the IMA. Using a "split-and-roll" technique, the right para-aortic lymphatic tissue bundle is then mobilized from medial to lateral. The majority of the nodes are found in the aortocaval region and overlying the IVC. The lateral limit of the dissection is the fat plane on the lateral border of the IVC.

Special care is taken to identify and ligate the so-called "fellow's vein," a small perforating vein from the lymph nodes usually found inserting into the anterior surface of the vena cava just above the caval bifurcation. Failure to perform this step may result in inadvertent tearing of the vessel and significant bleeding. Similarly, control of the lumbar veins is essential to the safe removal of the lymphatic tissue residing lateral to and behind the IVC. The IVC may be gently rolled laterally and medially to identify these veins inserting into the posterolateral surface of the vessel. These are carefully isolated, doubly ligated with suture, and transected.

Left Aortic Lymph Node Dissection. The incision is continued along the ventral surface of the aorta. Using a "split-and-roll" technique, the lymphatic tissue is carefully elevated and mobilized from the ventral and lateral surface of the aorta. The lumbar arteries are identified, doubly ligated with suture, and divided. This step is essential to allow safe removal of all lymphatic tissue residing lateral to and behind the aorta. The posterior limit of the dissection is the anterior spinous ligament. Working from caudad to cephalad, the lymphatic tissue surrounding the aorta and vena cava is removed until the level of the renal veins is reached.

In the left lateral aortic area, the left ovarian artery is identified at its origin from the aorta, doubly ligated, and divided. With the lymph node specimen on gentle lateral traction, the lymphatic tissue immediately lateral to the aorta is then divided. Remaining lumbar vessels arising from the left posterolateral surface of the aorta are identified and carefully divided, working from the left common iliac artery to the level of the left renal vein. The left ovarian vein is identified, doubly ligated, and divided near its insertion into the left renal vein. Lymphatic tissue is carefully dissected from the undersurface of the left renal vein and renal artery. Meticulous use of hemostatic clips to secure the prominent lymphatics in this area is essential to reduce the risk of lymphorrhea and chylous ascites. The left aortic nodal specimen is then removed.

Interaortocaval Lymph Node Dissection. Attention is turned to the interaortocaval lymph nodes, residing between the great vessels. Working from caudad to cephalad, these are carefully resected from the level of the aortic bifurcation to the level of the left renal vein. Hemostatic clips are used to secure and divide the lymphatics as they course underneath the renal vein.

Right Common Iliac Lymph Node Dissection. Finally, attention is returned to the right side, and any remaining lymphatic tissue lateral to the right common iliac artery and IVC is carefully dissected and removed. The completed retroperitoneal lymph node dissection results in full exposure of the aorta, IVC, and left renal vessels (Figure 28-10).

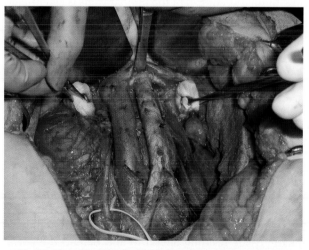

FIGURE 28-10. Completed open retroperitoneal lymph node dissection.

Laparoscopic Transperitoneal Aortic Lymph Node Dissection

The setup for the laparoscopic transperitoneal aortic lymph node dissection is similar to the laparoscopic pelvic lymph node dissection described earlier. The patient is placed in the dorsal lithotomy position with the legs secured in Allen stirrups. A Foley catheter is inserted, and an orogastric tube is placed by the anesthesiologist to provide gastric decompression. After initial trocar placement, the patient is placed in steep Trendelenburg position. Suggested equipment for the laparoscopic approach includes a 10-mm blunt port, two 5-mm trocars, a 5/10-mm trocar, 5- and 10-mm laparoscopic clip appliers, 5-mm graspers, and a 10-mm lymph node spoon. The procedure may be performed using a variety of available monopolar cautery devices for dissection and a vessel-sealing device. In a procedure that includes both pelvic and aortic dissection, the aortic lymph node dissection is performed first, before turning attention to the pelvis.

Trocar Placement

Using an open laparoscopy technique, the blunt 10-mm trocar is placed in the umbilicus, and the abdomen is insufflated. Under direct visualization, the 5-mm trocars are placed in the right and left lower quadrants, at a point approximately 1 cm superior to and 1 cm medial to the anterior superior iliac spine. Care should be taken to avoid injury to the inferior epigastric vessels. A 5/10-mm trocar is placed in the suprapubic area, carefully avoiding injury to the bladder. Individual trocar size and placement may vary depending on planned concurrent procedures, choice of instrumentation, the patient's habitus, and prior surgical history.

Surgeon Positioning

The right-handed surgeon stands on the patient's right side, holding in the right hand a dissecting monopolar cautery device placed through the 10-mm umbilical trocar and in the left hand a grasper placed through the right lower quadrant 5-mm trocar. The assistant stands on the patient's left side. The assistant's left hand holds the camera placed in the 5/10-mm suprapubic trocar, and the assistant's right hand holds a grasper placed through the left lower quadrant 5-mm trocar.

Right Aortic Lymph Node Dissection

The laparoscopic aortic lymph node dissection begins with the right lateral aortic nodes, which overlie the IVC. Using the 2 graspers, the peritoneum overlying the right common iliac artery is elevated and incised with monopolar cautery. This incision is carried cephalad to the level of the duodenum and then carried caudad to the level of the sacrum.

Attention is turned first to the right lateral peritoneal leaflet created by this incision. Using a combination of blunt dissection and monopolar cautery, the surgeon develops the plane between the peritoneal leaflet and the lymph nodes overlying the IVC. The psoas muscle, ureter, IVC, and duodenum are identified.

The removal of lymphatic tissue begins at the lateral border of the right common iliac artery. The assistant may use the closed laparoscopic grasper to protect the ureter laterally. The surgeon uses a grasper to provide gentle traction on the nodal package. The monopolar cautery device may be used as both a blunt dissector and a cautery device to isolate small blood vessels and lymphatic channels, which are secured with hemostatic clips and divided. Larger vessels may be transected with a vessel-sealing device. The dissection is carried cephalad to the desired level, usually to the border of the duodenum near the insertion of the right ovarian vein into the IVC. The duodenum may be gently protected by the assistant, who grasps the peritoneal edge immediately caudal to the duodenum and retracts it superiorly. Hemostatic clips are particularly important at the superior border of the dissection. Particular care is taken to identify and ligate the so-called "fellow's vein," a small perforating vein from the lymph nodes usually found inserting into the anterior surface of the vena cava just above the caval bifurcation (Figure 28-11). The lymph node specimen is removed from the abdomen using the laparoscopic spoon.

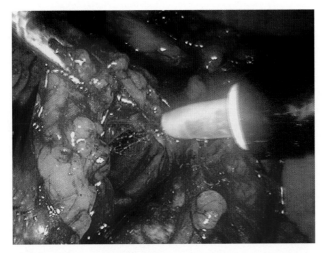

FIGURE 28-11. Identification of the fellow's vein. (Reproduced, with permission, from Sonoda Y, Barakat RR. Laparoscopic staging procedures. In: Levine DA, Barakat RR, Abu-Rustum NR, eds. *Atlas of Procedures in Gynecologic Oncology.* London, UK: Informa Healthcare; 2008:159, Figure 11.13a.)

Left Aortic Lymph Node Dissection

The superior extent of the peritoneal incision is extended in a transverse fashion along the duodenum toward the insertion of the left renal vein. This allows development of the left lateral peritoneal leaflet, exposing the left lateral aortic area. The IMA is identified at its origin from the ventral surface of the aorta approximately 2 cm above the aortic bifurcation. The left common iliac artery is identified. Using a grasper in the surgeon's left hand, the IMA is elevated. Using the surgeon's right hand instrument, blunt dissection is used to identify the left ureter and left psoas muscle in the window created by the elevated IMA. These 2 structures define the lateral limit of the dissection. Using a grasper, the assistant elevates the nodal package while the surgeon removes the nodes using a combination of blunt dissection, monopolar cautery, and hemostatic clips.

Interaortocaval Lymph Node Dissection

Attention is then turned to the interaortocaval nodes, which are resected in a similar manner. If the extent of dissection requires left para-aortic dissection cephalad to the IMA, the incision below the duodenum is extended further laterally along the left renal vessels. The dissection is carried cephalad to the IMA, working immediately lateral to the aorta, removing lymphatic tissue up to the level of the left renal vein. Hemostatic clips are particularly important to secure the prominent lymphatics at the superior border of the dissection, caudal to the renal vein. The specimen is removed.

Presacral Lymph Node Dissection

The presacral lymph nodes may be removed following completion of the left aortic dissection. The peritoneal incision is extended over the left common iliac vein, which is located immediately caudal to the aortic bifurcation. The lymphatic tissue in this area is carefully dissected, paying close attention to avoid injury to the vein.

The completed dissection exposes the aorta, vena cava, IMA, and common iliac vessels (Figure 28-12).

Laparoscopic Extraperitoneal Aortic Lymph Node Dissection

The setup for the laparoscopic extraperitoneal aortic lymph node dissection is similar to the laparoscopic pelvic lymph node dissection described earlier. The patient is placed in the dorsal lithotomy position with the legs placed in Allen stirrups. A Foley catheter is inserted, and an orogastric tube is placed by the anesthesiologist to provide gastric decompression. After initial trocar placement, the patient is placed in steep Trendelenburg

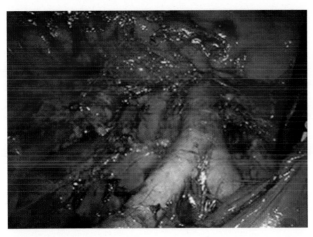

FIGURE 28-12. Completed laparoscopic aortic lymph node dissection.

position. Suggested equipment for the laparoscopic approach includes a 10-mm blunt port, two 5-mm trocars, a 5/10-mm trocar, 5- and 10-mm laparoscopic clip appliers, 5-mm graspers, and a 10-mm lymph node spoon. The procedure may be performed using a variety of available monopolar cautery devices for dissection and a vessel-sealing device.

Diagnostic Laparoscopy

Prior to beginning the extraperitoneal procedure, a transperitoneal diagnostic laparoscopy is performed. One trocar is placed in the umbilicus, and one is placed in the right lower quadrant to allow insertion of a bowel grasper. The abdomen and pelvis are evaluated for evidence of peritoneal disease or bulky adenopathy. If necessary, a third trocar may be placed in the suprapubic area to assist with lysis of adhesions or retraction of the bowel.

Trocar Placement

A 15-mm incision is made in the left lower quadrant, 3 to 4 cm medial to the left anterior superior iliac spine. Two accessory trocars are eventually placed, one 10-mm trocar in the left midaxillary line and one 5-mm trocar in the anterior axillary line approximately 5 cm below the costal margin (Figure 28-13).

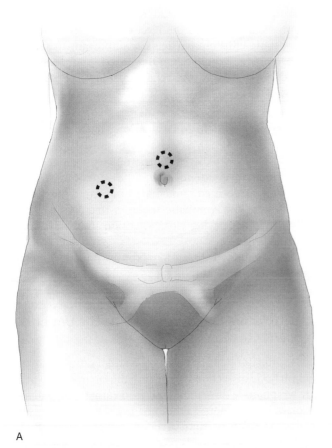
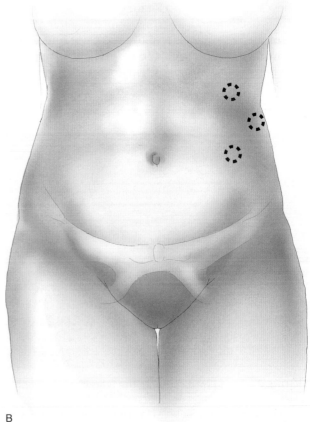

A   B

FIGURE 28-13. Laparoscopic extraperitoneal lymph node dissection: port placement guide. A. Trocar placement for diagnostic laparoscopy. **B.** Trocar placement for extraperitoneal aortic lymph node dissection.

Manual Dissection

The extraperitoneal space is developed using blunt dissection with a finger inserted through the 15-mm incision medial to the left anterior superior iliac spine. After traversing the abdominal fascia and muscle layer, the plane between the muscles and peritoneum is carefully developed bluntly without perforating the peritoneum. This step may be performed under direct laparoscopic visualization, using the camera inserted in the umbilical trocar. After identifying the psoas muscle and left common iliac artery, the peritoneum is further mobilized off of the anterior abdominal wall muscles, working in a cephalad direction.

Placement of Additional Trocars

After ensuring sufficient separation of the peritoneum from the muscle layer, the accessory trocars are carefully placed under direct manual guidance with the surgeon's finger. Inadvertent puncture of the peritoneum at this point must be avoided, because it will make successful extraperitoneal insufflation impossible. Finally, the surgeon's finger is removed and a balloon port is placed through the incision into the extraperitoneal space, under laparoscopic guidance. The extraperitoneal space is then insufflated with carbon dioxide gas in the usual fashion (Figure 28-14).

Identification of the Psoas Muscle

The psoas muscle is identified, and additional mobilization of the peritoneum off the psoas muscle may be accomplished under direct visualization using laparo-

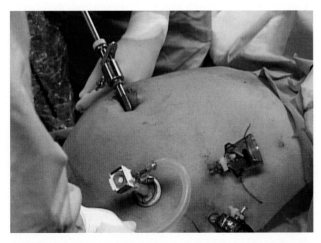

FIGURE 28-14. Laparoscopic extraperitoneal lymph node dissection: final port placement. (Reproduced, with permission, from Sonoda Y, Querleu D, Leblanc E. Extraperitoneal lymph node dissection. In: Levine DA, Barakat RR, Abu-Rustum NR, eds. *Atlas of Procedures in Gynecologic Oncology*. London, UK: Informa Healthcare; 2008:251, Figure 16.4.)

scopic instruments. Using sharp and blunt dissection, the psoas muscle itself is then mobilized ventrally and laterally, releasing it from the underlying tissue, including the renal fascia. The mobilization creates space for the nodal dissection and creates a recessed area for dependent drainage of blood and irrigation fluid away from the dissection bed.

Identification of the Vasculature

The left common iliac artery is identified using blunt dissection. The left ureter and left ovarian vessels are left attached to the peritoneum, and they are therefore elevated off of the common iliac artery as the peritoneum is mobilized from the artery using blunt dissection. The artery is traced cephalad until the aortic bifurcation is identified. Working carefully in a cephalad direction, the IMA is identified, as well as the sympathetic trunk, which is most easily identified in this area coursing on the lateral surface of the aorta. Continuing cephalad, the dissection is carried to the level of the left renal vein.

Left Aortic Dissection

The left common iliac nodes and left lateral aortic nodes are carefully dissected using laparoscopic graspers, a monopolar or bipolar cautery instrument, and a vessel-sealing device. Hemostatic clips are applied as needed, particularly in the area of prominent lymphatics immediately caudal to the left renal vein. The lymphatic tissue is removed from the lateral aspect of the aorta, remaining ventral to the sympathetic trunk. Care is taken to avoid injury to the lumbar veins and the azygos vein. The left ovarian artery must also be carefully identified at its origin from the aorta 2 to 3 cm below the renal vessels.

Right Aortic Dissection

The right aortic dissection begins with identification of the right ureter, which is protected laterally using a closed grasper. The right ovarian artery is identified and divided (if desired) at its origin from the aorta 2 to 3 cm caudal to the right renal vessels. The right common iliac and right aortic nodes are carefully dissected free, avoiding injury to the vena cava and right ureter. Small perforators from the vena cava to the nodal package (eg, the so-called "fellow's vein") must be carefully identified and divided. Avulsion of these vessels may cause hemorrhage. The interaortocaval and presacral nodes may then be dissected, with care taken to avoid injury to the left common iliac vein and middle sacral vein.

Completion of Dissection

The limits of the laparoscopic extraperitoneal dissection are the left renal vein cephalad and the common

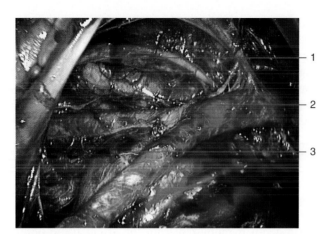

FIGURE 28-15. Completed laparoscopic extraperito-neal aortic lymph node dissection. 1 = Right common iliac artery; 2 = Aorta; 3= Left common illiac artery. (Repro-duced, with permission, from Sonoda Y, Querleu D, Leblanc E. Extraperitoneal lymph node dissection. In: Levine DA, Barakat RR, Abu-Rustum NR, eds. *Atlas of Procedures in Gynecologic Oncology.* London, UK: Informa Healthcare; 2008:255, Figure 16.15b.)

iliac arteries caudad (Figure 28-15). If radiation therapy is planned, the lower limit of the dissection is marked with clips to assist the radiation oncologist with treat-ment planning. At the conclusion of the procedure, it is essential to fenestrate the peritoneum along the left paracolic gutter, allowing postoperative lymphatic fluid to drain into the peritoneal cavity, thus reducing post-operative symptomatic lymphocele formation.

INGUINOFEMORAL LYMPH NODE DISSECTION

Procedure Overview

Box 28-5   Master Surgeon's Corner

- From lateral to medial, the contents of the femoral triangle include the femoral nerve, femoral artery, femoral vein, empty space, and lymph nodes (N-A-V-E-L).
- Palpation of the femoral triangle is essential to the proper identification of the femoral artery and adjacent landmarks.
- In sentinel lymph node dissection, any residual radioactivity in the dissection bed after sentinel node removal must be pursued with further dissection, because more than 1 sentinel node may be present.

Indications and Historical Perspective

Inguinofemoral lymph node dissection is most com-monly indicated in the staging and treatment of vulvar malignancy. Occasionally, it may be performed for sur-gical resection of clinically apparent nodal involvement by other gynecologic malignancies. The use of sentinel lymph node mapping in primary vulvar malignancy has been evaluated in 2 prospective trials and may be appropriate in selected cases.[3]

Preoperative Preparation

Considerations for preoperative preparation are simi-lar to those listed earlier for pelvic and aortic lymph node dissections, except that bowel preparation is not necessary. The consent discussion with the patient should include special emphasis on the elevated risk of lower extremity lymphedema after inguinofemoral dissection. Pre- or postoperative instruction regarding lymphedema prevention and management is recom-mended.

The procedure is usually performed in conjunction with vulvar resection requiring the dorsal lithotomy position. The legs are secured in Allen stirrups, and the bilateral groins are prepped and draped using ster-ile technique. The legs are positioned with the knees bent and the thigh only slightly flexed at the hip, providing adequate exposure of the entire groin area. The inguinofemoral lymph node dissection is gener-ally performed first, with skin closure performed prior to potential contamination of the field by the vulvar portion of the procedure. Required instrumentation includes skin retractors and an electrocautery device. If sentinel lymph node mapping is planned, preopera-tive injection with radioisotope is performed, and blue dye is injected in the operating room as described later in this section.

Operative Procedure

Box 28-6   Caution Points

- Care is taken to keep the subcutaneous fat attached to the skin, because making the flaps too thin may lead to skin necrosis.
- Meticulous isolation and clipping of lymphatic channels will reduce postoperative lymphocele formation.
- Control of the saphenous vein and its tributaries is essential to reduce troublesome bleeding during the medial portion of the dissection.

Inguinofemoral Lymph Node Dissection

Creation of Flaps

The procedure begins with palpation of the groins to identify any clinically apparent adenopathy. If sentinel lymph node injection has been performed, the gamma probe is used to localize the sentinel lymph nodes. These assessments may guide the location of the skin incision, which is generally 8 to 10 cm long and parallel to the inguinal ligament. The skin edges are elevated with skin hooks, and a plane is created between the subcutaneous adipose tissue and the underlying lymphatic tissue. This may be accomplished with sharp dissection using a scalpel or electrocautery. Care is taken to keep the subcutaneous fat attached to the skin, because making the flaps too thin may lead to skin necrosis.

Identification of Landmarks

The limits of the dissection are identified. The medial boundary of dissection is the lateral border of the adductor longus muscle. This muscle is palpated, and the incision is carried down to the level of its fascia. The lateral boundary of dissection is the medial border of the sartorius muscle, which is easily identified. The cephalad boundary is the mons pubis and pubic tubercle medially, and the aponeurosis of the external oblique muscle laterally.

Superficial Lymph Node Dissection

The dissection begins at the cephalad boundary, near the inguinal ligament. The fat pad containing the superficial lymph nodes is elevated from the aponeurosis of the external oblique muscle. Working from cephalad to caudad, the fat pad is mobilized inferiorly to the edge of the inguinal ligament. The dissection is accomplished using sharp and blunt dissection, with electrocautery and hemostatic clips applied as needed. Medially, the external inguinal ring and superficial external pudendal vessels are identified. Laterally, the superficial circumflex iliac vessels are identified. From lateral to medial, the contents of the femoral triangle include the femoral nerve, femoral artery, femoral vein, and lymph nodes.

Deep Lymph Node Dissection: Femoral Artery

The femoral nerve is identified laterally, emerging caudad to the inguinal ligament. Working toward the femoral triangle, the superficial dissection is carried deeper by incision of the cribriform fascia overlying the common femoral artery. The artery may be identified by palpation. This incision is carried along the ventral aspect of the artery. The superficial external pudendal artery may be encountered at its origin from the femoral artery at the most medial and cephalad area of the dissection. This vessel should be ligated and divided. Other branches of the femoral artery may be encountered, including the superficial epigastric artery and the superficial circumflex iliac artery.

Deep Lymph Node Dissection: Femoral Vein

The nodal package is elevated and the dissection is continued from lateral to medial, freeing the lymphatic tissue from the ventral surface of the femoral vein. The greater saphenous vein drains into the common femoral vein near the cephalad limit of the dissection, at the point where the superficial external pudendal artery crosses the common femoral vein. The greater saphenous vein is skeletonized approximately 1 to 2 cm from its insertion. It is doubly ligated with permanent suture and divided at its insertion into the common femoral vain. Care is taken not to compromise the lumen of the common femoral vein as this suture is placed. Small tributaries of the saphenous vein are carefully identified and ligated as they are encountered during the medial portion of the deep lymph node dissection. Any remaining attachments of the specimen to the dissection bed are carefully divided, and the specimen is removed. The completed dissection exposes the structures of the femoral triangle (Figure 28-16).

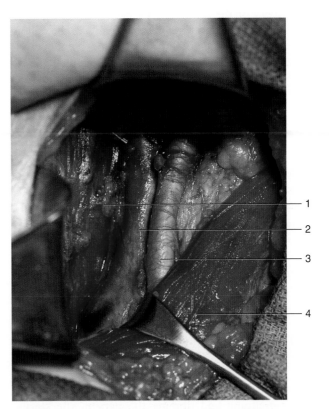

FIGURE 28-16. Femoral triangle. 1 = adductor longus muscle; 2 = left femoral vein; 3= left femoral artery; 4 = Sartorius muscle. (Reproduced, with permission, from Gemignani ML. Surgery for carcinoma of the vulva. In: Levine DA, Barakat RR, Abu-Rustum NR, eds. *Atlas of Procedures in Gynecologic Oncology*. London, UK: Informa Healthcare; 2008:52, Figure 3.24.)

Completion of the Dissection

The dissection bed is irrigated and inspected for hemostasis. Hemostatic clips are placed on small vessels and lymphatics as needed. If desired, the sartorius muscle may be transposed over the vessels at this point in the procedure. The muscle is transected with electrocautery at its tendinous attachment to the anterior superior iliac spine, and it is transposed medially over the vessels. The proximal portion of the muscle is then sutured to the inguinal ligament and pectineal fascia using interrupted delayed-absorbable sutures. The subcutaneous tissue is reapproximated with interrupted delayed-absorbable sutures, and the skin incision is closed with staples.

Inguinofemoral Sentinel Lymph Node Mapping

Sentinel lymph node mapping in vulvar malignancy uses a combined approach with both radioisotope and blue dye used to localize the sentinel lymph nodes.

Radioisotope Injection

The radioisotope injection may be given the morning of surgery or the day prior. Filtered technetium 99m sulfur colloid is used, with 0.1 to 0.5 mCi of the colloid injected at the edge of the vulvar lesion. A preoperative lymphoscintigram is performed approximately 2 to 6 hours after the injection. This study may identify both the laterality and number of sentinel lymph nodes, thus assisting in preoperative planning. In the operating room, after positioning the patient, the gamma probe is used to localize the sentinel node in the groin, and radioactivity counts are measured at this site as well as at the primary injection site. The groin site of maximal radioactivity is marked.

Blue Dye Injection

The injection of blue dye is performed in the operating room after the induction of anesthesia. Approximately 4 mL of isosulfan blue dye (described earlier) is injected circumferentially around the lesion in an intradermal fashion, at the junction of tumor and the normal surrounding skin. Deeper cutaneous injection may be added in the case of a large lesion. Injection directly into the lesion is not effective.

Intraoperative Localization

After prepping and draping the patient, the sterile-draped gamma probe is used to confirm the location of the sentinel node at the previously marked groin site.

Skin Incision

A small incision is made directly over the area of maximal radioactivity, parallel to the inguinal ligament. If a

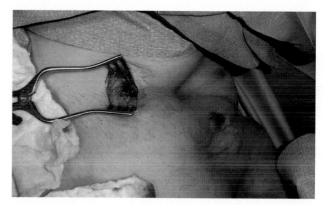

FIGURE 28-17. Inguinofemoral sentinel lymph node mapping.

full inguinofemoral lymphadenectomy is planned, this incision may be extended later.

Dissection of the Sentinel Node

The fatty tissue surrounding the lymph nodes is carefully dissected, identifying the blue lymphatic channels leading to the sentinel lymph node. The gamma probe is used to guide the dissection until the blue-stained sentinel node is found (Figure 28-17). The node is carefully dissected free from the surrounding tissue and removed. Any node that exhibits radioactivity, regardless of color, is also removed. The gamma probe is used to obtain ex vivo counts of all nodes removed, and the color and radioactivity status of each resected node are recorded.

Postexcision Radioactivity Counts

The lymphatic basin is checked for radioactivity after the sentinel node is removed, and any area of residual radioactivity is pursued with dissection. Residual lymphatic basin counts should be reduced 4- to 10-fold over the initial counts in the groin.

Completion of the Dissection

The skin incision may be closed with absorbable sutures. Alternatively, if an inguinofemoral lymphadenectomy is planned, the incision is extended at this point, and the dissection is performed as described earlier.

POSTOPERATIVE CARE

Standard postoperative care is required after lymphadenectomy. Although the historical literature reports the use of intraperitoneal drains after lymph node dissection, recent data do not support their routine placement in the absence of other factors, such as unusual concern for delayed bleeding, infection, or lymphorrhea, or concurrent procedures requiring drain placement. In contrast, drains are routinely placed in the groin after inguinofemoral lymph node dissection and left in place until lymphatic fluid output becomes minimal. This practice reduces the occurrence of inguinal lymphocele, which can lead to pain, infection, and wound breakdown.

| Box 28-7 | Complications and Morbidity |

- Hemorrhage: Excessive bleeding is a potential issue during any lymph node dissection and is best avoided by meticulous dissection, identification of vascular structures, and use of hemostatic clips where indicated.
- Nerve injury: Several nerves lie in close proximity to the vascular supply and lymphatic drainage of the gynecologic organs. Knowledge of the anatomic location of these structures is essential, and they must be carefully identified and protected. Symptoms of nerve injury may vary in duration and severity. In general, injury of the genitofemoral nerve causes numbness and paresthesia of the medial thigh without motor deficit. Injury of the obturator nerve causes weakness in abduction of the thigh.
- Lymphocele: Postoperative lymphocele formation is very common and is frequently an asymptomatic finding on postoperative imaging of the abdomen and pelvis. In some instances, however, the fluid collections may cause persistent pain or fever, necessitating drainage. This can usually be accomplished by interventional radiology.
- Chylous ascites: Persistent large-volume lymphorrhea may cause clinically significant ascites. This occurs most commonly following extensive aortic lymph node dissection and, in some cases, may require drainage by paracentesis. The risk of chylous ascites is reduced by meticulous identification and clipping of lymphatic vessels.
- Venous thromboembolism: Patients undergoing lymph node dissection for malignancy are at elevated baseline risk for deep vein thrombosis. This risk is further increased by excessive manipulation of the venous vasculature during the dissection, which may cause trauma to the vessel wall. Therefore, care should be taken to retract veins gently and for short periods of time to reduce the risk of injury.
- Lymphedema: The incidence of lymphedema following lymph node dissection varies by procedure. Several factors contribute to an elevated risk, including obesity, pre-existing venous stasis or lymphedema, prior limb surgery, and radiation treatment.

REFERENCES

1. Cibula D, Abu-Rustum NR. Pelvic lymphadenectomy in cervical cancer: surgical anatomy and proposal for a new classification system. *Gynecol Oncol.* 2010;116:33-37.
2. Abu-Rustum NR, Khoury-Collado F, Gemignani ML. Techniques of sentinel lymph node identification for early-stage cervical and uterine cancer. *Gynecol Oncol.* 2008;111(suppl):S44-S50.
3. Levenback C. Update on sentinel lymph node biopsy in gynecologic cancers. *Gynecol Oncol.* 2008;111(suppl):S42-S43.

Staging Procedures

29

Summer B. Dewdney and Matthew A. Powell

PROCEDURE OVERVIEW

- Complete surgical staging including lymph node dissection, omentectomy, appendectomy, and staging biopsies should be performed for all patients with apparent early-stage epithelial ovarian carcinomas because nearly a third of patients will have metastatic disease that was not appreciated visually or by palpation.
- The extent of surgical staging for endometrial carcinoma remains controversial as to when pelvic and/or para-aortic lymph nodes should be removed. Surgeons managing patients with endometrial carcinoma should be prepared for the possibility of performing these procedures in all cases.
- Accurate and complete surgical staging is a crucial part of managing patients with gynecologic malignancies and allows for appropriate informed discussions regarding further interventions and accurate risk stratification of patients on clinical trials.

Indications

Currently, ovarian and endometrial carcinomas are recommended to be surgically staged cancers by the International Federation of Obstetrics and Gynecology (FIGO). This requires removal of the primary site and any area of spread or potential spread when possible. Surgical staging is a crucial portion of the treatment for these gynecologic malignancies. Accuracy and completeness of staging ensures objective data, which helps guide appropriate administration of adjuvant therapies and development of clinical trials.

Historical Perspective

For patients with ovarian cancer, Young et al[1] established the importance of surgical staging. These investigators performed systematic restaging on 100 patients and showed a 31% rate of upstaging after patients were fully surgically staged, which included multiple peritoneal biopsies and removal of pelvic and para-aortic lymph nodes. In addition, 77% of these 31 patients actually had stage III disease. Prior to this study, the staging of ovarian cancer was either not performed or relied on bipedal lymphangiography, intravenous pyelography, barium enemas, and peritoneoscopy (laparoscopy). Today, in early-stage ovarian cancer, comprehensive staging as defined by the National Cancer Institute–sponsored Gynecologic Oncology Group (GOG) includes a systematic evaluation and biopsies to determine a need for adjuvant therapy. In advanced-stage ovarian cancer, an attempt at optimal cytoreduction is the standard of care and is addressed in detail elsewhere in this text.

Prior to 1988, endometrial cancer was clinically staged through uterine sounding and imaging to determine possible spread. It was treated with a combination of preoperative radiation followed by surgery.

CHAPTER 29

The GOG helped transition from clinical staging to surgical staging through a prospective cohort that underwent a staging surgery; the GOG found surgical staging to be more beneficial to patients.[2] In 1988, FIGO changed the staging to a surgical-pathologic system which has not been changed until recently.[3] In 2009, FIGO updated the staging of endometrial cancer. Most recently, a GOG prospective randomized controlled trial (LAP2) showed that a laparoscopic approach to endometrial cancer shows no difference in detecting advanced-stage disease compared with an open approach.[4]

Vulvar and vaginal cancer staging is discussed elsewhere in this text.

Expected Clinical Outcomes

The primary purpose of a staging procedure is to provide an accurate account of the extent of disease to determine the need for further therapy. In addition, a universal staging system allows comparison of the outcomes of patients between institutions and countries. Interpretable results from clinical trials evaluating adjuvant therapies rely on accuracy and completeness of the surgical staging of the enrolled patients. Thus, some patients can often be excluded from participation from clinical trials due to improperly performed cancer surgery.

PREOPERATIVE PREPARATION

Patient Evaluation and Work-Up

All patients who are undergoing a surgical evaluation need a preoperative work-up for their comorbidities as determined by the surgery team and anesthesia.

According to the National Comprehensive Cancer Network (NCCN), if a patient is suspected of having ovarian cancer, it is necessary to obtain a family history and, depending on results, consider family history evaluation with genetics. A complete physical examination including an abdominal/pelvic examination is performed, and evaluation of any gastrointestinal symptoms is pursued if clinically indicated. Imaging with an ultrasound and/or abdominal/pelvic computed tomography with chest imaging is usually indicated. Laboratory tests that are typically obtained include a CA-125 or other tumor markers as clinically indicated, complete blood count (CBC), and chemistry profile with liver function tests.[5]

For endometrial cancer, initial evaluation includes a pathology review of the endometrial sample. Patients who are less than 50 years old may need genetic counseling if they have a significant family history and/or selected pathologic risk features. This can occur after surgery as well. The NCCN also recommends a CBC, chest x-ray, and current cervical cytology.[6]

Consent Considerations

Consent is permission, granted by the patient to the surgeon, to make a diagnostic or therapeutic intervention on the patient's behalf.[7] To be valid, the patient must be informed. For all staging procedures, it is important that the patient is aware of risks, benefits, and alternatives to the procedure being done. The risk of most staging procedures is low, for example taking random peritoneal biopsies and washings, but higher risk may be associated with performing lymph node dissection (discussed in Chapter 28) for early-stage endometrial cancer. The risk of lymphedema and other adverse effects of lymph node removal should be discussed with the patient.

Patient Preparation

In the past, bowel preparation has been used to decrease intraluminal fecal mass, presumably to decrease the bacteria load in the bowel. It has been used widely in general surgery and in gynecology oncology. Despite the widespread use of bowel preparation, there are limited data on its effectiveness. Multiple randomized controlled trials have shown no benefit of a mechanical bowel preparation. A Cochrane review analyzing 13 randomized controlled trials with 4777 participants found no difference in patient outcomes between patients who had a mechanical bowel preparation and patients who did not.[8] We do not routinely use bowel preparations in our patients; there is no proven benefit with level I evidence, and bowel preparations are expensive, uncomfortable, and unpleasant for patients. There is still debate about the uses of bowel preparation in patients with planned left colon resections. Special considerations should also be made for patients with partial obstructions or chronic constipation.

Antimicrobial prophylaxis to reduce surgical site infection has been clearly established. For our endometrial cancer cases that are unlikely to involve any bowel, we use cefazolin for prophylaxis as per the American College of Obstetrics and Gynecology (ACOG) recommendations for hysterectomies. For patients undergoing ovarian cancer staging, we often use cefoxitin, which is recommend for bowel surgeries and which may be more appropriate given ovarian cancer involvement of the bowel and need for bowel resections for cytoreduction.

According to American College of Chest Physicians guidelines, for gynecologic patients undergoing major surgical procedures for either benign disease or malignancy, venous thromboembolism (VTE) prophylaxis with chemical or mechanical prophylaxis is necessary.[9]

The duration of VTE prophylaxis for patients undergoing major gynecologic procedures is at least until hospital discharge, and one should consider extending prophylaxis for higher risk patients. Almost all patients undergoing surgical staging for a gynecologic malignancy are considered higher risk patients, especially if over age 60 years. The ENOXACAN II trial showed that 40 mg of enoxaparin preoperatively and continued for 4 weeks postoperatively significantly decreased VTEs.[10] At our institution, we give postoperative, prolonged, prophylactic low molecular weight heparin to these patients after discharge for home administration.

Required Instrumentation

Instrumentation for staging procedures includes standard instruments. In addition, we have found electrosurgical vessel-sealing devices to be very useful for omentectomies and other surgical staging procedures. These electrosurgical devices have been shown to be safe and effective both in laparotomy and laparoscopic procedures.[11-15]

OPERATIVE PROCEDURE

Box 29-2	Caution Points

- Appropriate patient positioning to allow for both planned and any possible additional procedures is crucial.
- Access to the primary tumor and staging procedures can be performed via a laparoscopic approach or an open approach.

Positioning

The patient is placed in either supine or dorsal lithotomy position depending on surgeon preference and the need for access to the perineum, bladder, and/or rectum. If lithotomy position is used, it is very important to take extra caution in positioning to ensure no pressure points or hyperextension of joints. The risk of nerve injury is higher in this position. In robotic or laparoscopic cases when there is a need for steep Trendelenburg positioning, care must be taken if shoulder braces are used because there is a risk of brachial plexus injury. We recommend not using shoulder braces, but instead a gel pad and chest straps, all with appropriate padding.

Abdominal Entry

A midline vertical skin incision is made using the electrosurgical device or a scalpel. The subcutaneous fat and fascia are then incised with either instrument to match the overlying skin incision. The fascia then is gently dissected off the rectus muscle to identify the linea alba. Once identified, the underlying peritoneum is grasped and entered. It may be necessary to extend this incision depending on the malignant potential of the mass or if the surgery is for endometrial cancer and there is disease outside of the uterus. The incision will need to be extended to the umbilicus and, most of the time, around the umbilicus to gain adequate exposure for exploration and for a para-aortic lymph node dissection if indicated. The inferior facial and peritoneal incision needs to be to the pubic bone with avoidance of injury to the bladder. A retractor is then used for adequate exposure; we often use a Bookwalter or Balfour with a C-arm (or third arm).

Exploration

Exploration of the abdominopelvic cavity follows a stepwise progression based on the potential peritoneal and retroperitoneal patterns of dissemination of ovarian and endometrial cancers (Figure 29-1). All peritoneal surfaces including the paracolic gutters, the surface of both diaphragms, and the serosa and mesentery of the gastrointestinal tract should be visualized and palpated for evidence of metastatic disease. This includes "running" the entire length of the small bowel from the ileocecal junction to the ligament of Treitz and large intestine. Both diaphragms should be palpated in addition to the liver, gallbladder, spleen, and kidneys. The pelvic and para-aortic lymph node bed should be palpated for grossly enlarged nodes. Ideally, the palpation of lymph nodes should occur after the opening of the retroperitoneal spaces to directly identify the nodal tissue. The omentum should be carefully inspected.

Cytologic Washings

The volume of any free peritoneal fluid (ascites) should be noted and sent for cytology. If there is no free fluid present, then washings will be obtained from the pelvis, paracolic gutters, and infradiaphragmatic area for ovarian cancer staging using approximately 50 to 100 mL of normal saline. In endometrial cancers, peritoneal washings for cytologic examination are obtained by irrigating the pelvis with warm saline (Figure 29-2). Washings for endometrial cancer are no longer part of the surgical staging criteria per the new FIGO 2009 guidelines, but they are still recommended to be obtained and results reported.

Peritoneal Biopsies

If there is no evidence of disease beyond the ovary, peritoneal biopsies must be performed for ovarian cancer. In addition, peritoneal biopsies should be done

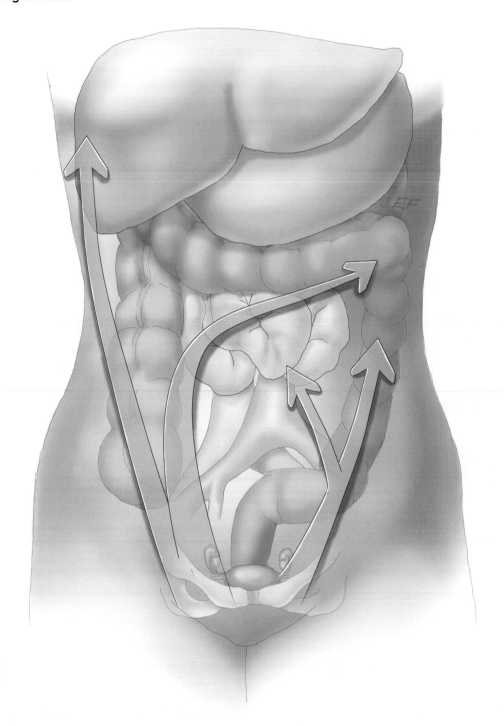

FIGURE 29-1. Abdominal exploration proceeds in a stepwise fashion and follows the peritoneal and retroperitoneal pattern of dissemination.

for high-grade endometrial cancer. These can be done by grasping the peritoneal surface with an Allis clamp and using Metzenbaum scissors or electrocautery to remove a sampling of the peritoneal surface (Figure 29-3). The following areas should be biopsied:

1. Posterior cul-de-sac
2. Anterior cul-de-sac (vesical peritoneum)
3. Right and left pelvic sidewalls
4. Right and left paracolic gutters
5. Right diaphragm peritoneum

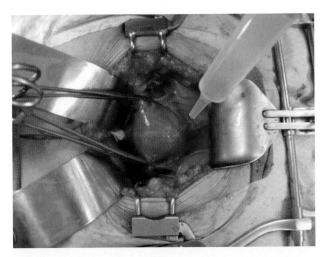

FIGURE 29-2. Pelvic washings to obtain cytologic specimen.

Biopsy or scraping of the right diaphragm is done in the setting of early-stage ovarian cancer and high-grade endometrial cancer staging. This can be done with a spatula to send for cytology or direct biopsy of the serosal covering of the diaphragm.

Omentectomy

An avascular plane between the transverse colon and the infracolic omentum is identified and entered (Figure 29-4). The omentum is detached from the transverse colon, usually only requiring electrocautery. It is then detached from the gastrocolic omentum usually with serial pedicles, clamping with Kelly clamps, and then cutting and tying these pedicles. In addition, a bipolar electrosurgical sealing device can be used and is safe and efficient in performing this procedure. An infracolic omentum is sufficient for early-stage ovarian cancer and high-grade endometrial cancer.

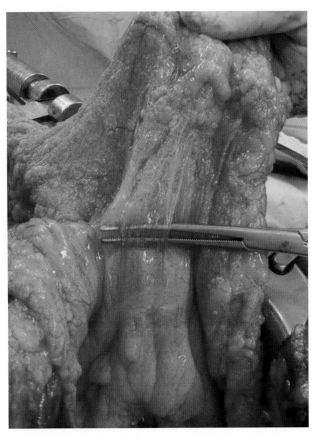

FIGURE 29-4. Infracolic omentectomy: clamp demonstrating avascular plane.

Extended Omentectomy (Gastrocolic Omentectomy)

If there is any suspicious area within the gastric omentum (area between stomach and transverse colon), then the entire gastrocolic omentum should be removed (Figure 29-5).

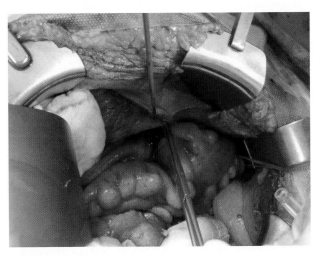

FIGURE 29-3. Pelvic peritoneal biopsy.

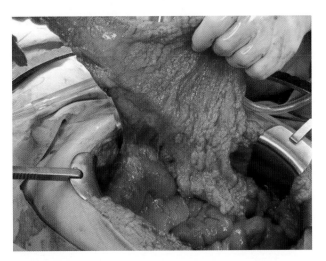

FIGURE 29-5. Complete gastrocolic omentectomy.

Bilateral Pelvic and Para-Aortic Lymphadenectomy

Lymphadenectomy is discussed in detail in Chapter 28.

Appendectomy

At times during an ovarian cancer staging surgery or an endometrial cancer staging surgery, the appendix may be removed. It can be removed for a variety of reasons including possible tumor involvement or inflammation. In addition, when a primary ovarian tumor is found to be a mucinous subtype on frozen section pathology, it is important to remove the appendix to exclude a primary appendiceal neoplasm. Often, the mucinous histology seen in the ovary will be a metastasis from an appendiceal origin (or a gastrointestinal origin).

A Babcock is used to grasp the appendix atraumatically to lift it up on tension. Next, the mesoappendix is identified, which holds the blood supply to the appendix, the appendiceal artery. The mesentery including the artery is then isolated, doubly clamped, and suture ligated.

The appendix is then free of its attachments and can be freely lifted up to identify the base. The base is then clamped with a straight hemostat, crushed, and then moved up a few millimeters toward the specimen. A free tie (delayed-absorbable or permanent) can then be used to ligate the crushed portion. Once this is done, a knife is used to transect below the clamp, which ensures no spillage of bowel contents into the operative field (Figure 29-6). The appendiceal stump can be buried with a Z-stitch or a purse-string suture. Some surgeons will cauterize the stump, and some do not bury it; no method has been shown to be more beneficial than the others.

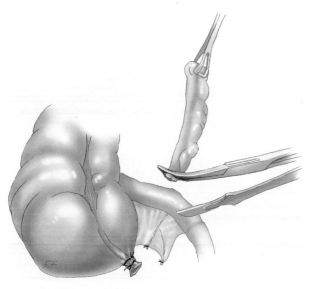

FIGURE 29-6. Appendectomy.

Closure and Final Steps

At the conclusion of the surgery, the fascia is closed using #1 loop polydioxanone (PDS) in a mass closure fashion including all of the abdominal wall layers. Prior to closure, all pedicle sites should be reinspected to ensure hemostasis.

POSTOPERATIVE CARE

Box 29-3	Complications and Morbidity

- Patients with gynecologic malignancies are in the highest risk category of having a pulmonary embolism or deep vein thrombosis.
- Bowel obstruction from adhesions may occur in the first 7 to 21 days postoperatively.
- Unrecognized serosal bowel injury can present as peritonitis in the first 72 hours postoperatively.

Diet and activity after a surgical staging depend on the extent of surgery performed and will need to be adjusted to the individual patient. In the majority of patients, it is important to have them ambulating the day of surgery or the first day after surgery. Traditionally, many surgeons will delay oral fluids and/or food immediately postoperative. However, the evidence does not fully support this style of management. A Cochrane review of 14 randomized controlled trials including 1224 patients undergoing gastrointestinal surgery indicates that earlier feeding may reduce the risk of postsurgical complications, and the authors found no obvious advantage of keeping patients NPO (nothing by mouth).[16] In addition, another Cochrane review showed that early feeding after major abdominal gynecologic surgery is safe but associated with an increased risk of nausea and reduction in the length of hospital stay.[17]

Discharge planning is an important part of a patient's hospital stay. It is necessary to evaluate for possible needs at home after discharge. Discharge planning and optimizing home health care will become increasingly important to contain costs of hospital stays and surgeries for gynecologic cancer patients.

REFERENCES

1. Young RC, Decker DG, Wharton JT, et al. Staging laparotomy in early ovarian cancer. *JAMA*. 1983;250:3072-3076.
2. Creasman WT, Morrow CP, Bundy BN, et al. Surgical pathologic spread patterns in endometrial cancer: a Gynecologic Oncology Group study. *Cancer*. 1987;60:2035-2041.

3. Mutch DG. The new FIGO staging system for cancer of the vulva, cervix, endometrium and sarcomas. *Gynecol Oncol.* 2009; 115:325-328.

4. Walker JL, Piedmonte MR, Spirtos NM, et al. Laparoscopy compared with laparotomy for comprehensive surgical staging of uterine cancer: Gynecologic Oncology Group study LAP2. *J Clin Oncol.* 2009;27:5331-5336.

5. National Comprehensive Cancer Network guidelines version 2.2011. Epithelial ovarian cancer/fallopian tube cancer/primary peritoneal cancer. Accessed June 29, 2011.

6. National Comprehensive Cancer Network guidelines version 2.2011. Uterine neoplasms. Accessed June 29, 2011.

7. Carson RA. Ethics in surgery. In: Townsend CM, Beauchamp RD, Evers BM, Mattox KL, eds. *Sabiston Textbook of Surgery.* 18th ed. Philadelphia, PA: Saunders; 2008.

8. Guenaga KF, Matos D, Wille-Jorgensen P. Mechanical bowel preparation for elective colorectal surgery (review). *Cochrane Database Syst Rev.* 2009;1:CD001544.

9. Geerts WH, Bergqvist D, Pineo GF, et al. Prevention of venous thromboembolism: American College of Chest Physicians evidence-based clinical practice guidelines (8th edition). *Chest.* 2008;133:S381-S453.

10. Bergqvist D, Agnelli G, Cohen AT, et al. Duration of prophylaxis against venous thromboembolism with enoxaparin after surgery for cancer. *N Engl J Med.* 2002;346:975-980.

11. Hefni MA, Bhaumik J, El-Toukhy T, et al. Safety and efficacy of using the LigaSure vessel sealing system for securing the pedicles in vaginal hysterectomy: randomised controlled trial. *BJOG.* 2005;112(3):329-333.

12. Cronje HS, de Coning EC. Electrosurgical bipolar vessel sealing during vaginal hysterectomy. *Int J Gynaecol Obstet.* 2005; 91:243-245.

13. Hagen B, Eriksson N, Sundset M. Randomised controlled trial of LigaSure versus conventional suture ligature for abdominal hysterectomy. *BJOG.* 2005;112:968-970.

14. Slomovitz BM, Ramirez PT, Frumovitz M, et al. Electrothermal bipolar coagulation for pelvic exenterations. *Gynecol Oncol.* 2006;102(3):534-536.

15. Kriplani A, Garg P, Sharma M, et al. A review of total laparoscopic hysterectomy using LigaSure uterine artery-sealing device: AIIMS experience. Lower extremity neuropathies associated with lithotomy positions. *Anesthesiology.* 2000;93(4): 938-942.

16. Andersen HK, Lewis SJ, Thomas S. Early enteral nutrition within 24h of colorectal surgery versus later commencement of feeding for postoperative complications. *Cochrane Database Syst Rev.* 2006;4:CD004080.

17. Charoenkwan K, Phillipson G, Vutyavanich T. Early versus delayed oral fluids and food for reducing complications after major abdominal gynaecologic surgery. *Cochrane Database Syst Rev.* 2007;4:CD004508.

Cytoreductive Procedures

Edward J. Tanner III, Fady Khoury-Collado, and Dennis S. Chi

PROCEDURE OVERVIEW

Ovarian cancer is one of the few solid tumors in which surgical cytoreduction is indicated for advanced metastatic disease. The most common indication for cytoreductive surgery is suspected or confirmed advanced-stage ovarian cancer. In selected cases, cytoreductive surgery is indicated for other advanced or recurrent gynecologic cancers. The goal of the cytoreductive surgery, defined in terms of the diameter of the largest residual implant, has evolved over the last 3 decades. Although leaving no residual tumor larger than 1 cm is currently defined as "optimal," maximal survival benefit is associated with removal of all gross tumor. Therefore, the goal should be to attempt removal of all visible disease (complete cytoreduction). The available surgical techniques have similarly evolved during the same period to achieve this goal

and now include upper abdominal procedures, tumor ablation techniques, and radical pelvic surgery.

Whether performed for primary or recurrent tumors or following neoadjuvant therapy, the same surgical principles and techniques of cytoreductive surgery discussed in this chapter are applicable.

PREOPERATIVE PREPARATION

Cytoreduction procedures are often lengthy and complex and carry the potential for significant intra- and postoperative morbidities. The patient needs to be evaluated thoroughly to assess whether she is able to tolerate such procedures, to optimize any underlying medical condition, and to plan postoperative care.

As in any patient assessment, the initial step is to take a detailed history, not only of the complaint that led to the suspicion or diagnosis of advanced ovarian cancer, but also of any associated symptoms that can indicate the existence or severity of associated comorbidities. Specifically, any respiratory symptoms should be investigated, because multiple etiologies can coexist. These can be related to the diagnosis of ovarian cancer (eg, pleural effusion, ascites) or simply denote the presence of a medical comorbidity (eg, chronic lung disease, cardiac disease) that either needs to be optimized prior to surgery or may contraindicate an extensive surgery. The presence of nausea and vomiting, abdominal distention, and difficulty with bowel movements may indicate bowel obstruction. A history of recent significant weight loss can point to potential malnutrition. If severe malnutrition is confirmed on laboratory evaluation, preoperative parenteral nutrition should be considered.

A detailed physical examination should specifically look for findings that denote the extent of disease or the underlying condition of the patient, or even suggest a different or coexistent primary malignancy (eg, breast examination, rectal examination). The abdomen is examined closely for ascites, which can cause significant abdominal distention, compromising the respiratory status of the patient and for which a simple paracentesis can provide immediate and significant relief. In the pelvis, a bimanual examination assesses the extent of pelvic disease and gives a reasonable idea about the likelihood of the requirement for a rectosigmoid colon resection.

Routine preoperative testing includes a complete blood count, coagulation studies, metabolic panel including albumin, renal and liver function tests, and an electrocardiogram. Tumor markers, although not mandatory, are commonly obtained as baseline values. Occasionally, they can suggest a different primary malignancy.

Imaging typically includes a computed tomography (CT) scan of the chest, abdomen, and pelvis. A chest radiograph is an acceptable alternative to chest CT. A CT scan of the chest, however, can determine the presence of enlarged mediastinal lymph nodes and pleural tumor deposits, in addition to moderate to large pleural effusions. If the CT demonstrates thoracic disease, an intrathoracic cytoreduction is attempted first.[1] The CT of the abdomen and pelvis helps determine the extent of disease in the abdomen and will assist in the counseling and planning for the procedure.

The patient is informed about the main goal of the surgery and the potential procedures required to achieve complete or optimal cytoreduction. A realistic description of the length and complexity of the procedure, associated complications, need for intensive care monitoring, and expected recovery time is discussed, including the possibility of requiring a temporary or permanent stoma. Transfusion of blood and blood products is frequently needed, and any objections to their use on behalf of the patient should be clearly defined, because this can impact the safety of the planned procedure. At the same time, the possibility of aborting the debulking procedure based on intraoperative findings is discussed.

Patients are instructed to shower the night before or the morning of surgery. Mechanical bowel preparation is not mandatory but is given according to the surgeon's preference. Prophylactic antibiotics are routinely given, typically cefotetan 2 g, within 1 hour prior to skin incision, with repeated doses given as needed (eg, prolonged surgeries, increased blood loss). Prophylactic antibiotics are discontinued within 24 hours of the operation. Required surgical instrumentation includes a fixed self-retaining retractor (eg, Bookwalter) and electrosurgical unit; automated gastrointestinal stapling devices, an argon beam coagulator, and a vessel-sealing cutting device are highly recommended.

OPERATIVE PROCEDURE

Box 30-2	Caution Points

- Avoid injury to the hepatic veins when mobilizing the liver.
- Avoid injury to the transverse mesocolon and the middle colic artery during entry into the lesser sac during omentectomy.
- Avoid excessive traction on the omentum at the splenic flexure, which can create splenic capsular tears.
- Identify the ureters clearly (eg, tag with vessel loops) at all times during the pelvic part of the procedure.

Pneumatic compression devices must be in place and functioning prior to the induction of anesthesia. The dorsal lithotomy position, using Allen stirrups (Allen Medical Systems, Cleveland, OH), is preferred over the supine position because it allows for bimanual examination to determine the extent of tumor involvement in the posterior cul-de-sac and provides access and exposure to the pelvis when performing a rectosigmoid resection and reanastomosis (Figure 30-1). After positioning the patient, the stirrups are rotated into the position they will remain in during surgery to ensure that no undue pressure is exerted on the legs during prolonged periods.

Following positioning, a vertical midline incision is marked from above the xiphoid process to the pubic symphysis. The locations of possible chest tubes and intraperitoneal catheter reservoirs are marked, if anticipated. Antiseptic preparation of the skin follows and is applied from the nipple line to mid thighs. After draping the patient, a sterile catheter is placed in the bladder.

Cytoreductive Procedures

Abdominal Entry

Entry into the abdominal cavity is best achieved through a midline vertical incision from the pubic symphysis to the xiphoid process. Abdominal entry may be hindered by adherence of omental disease to the anterior abdominal wall, although this can be excised without difficulty or bowel injury. If ascites is anticipated, the peritoneum is tented up and entered through a small opening. Fenestrated suction catheters can then be inserted and fluid evacuated in a controlled fashion.

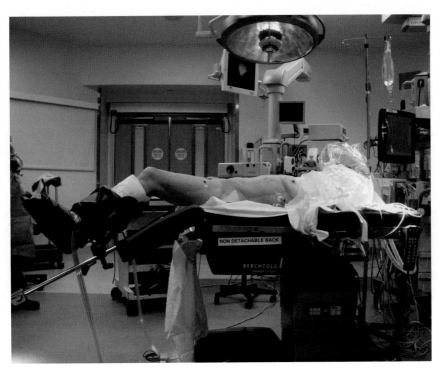

FIGURE 30-1. Patient positioning.

A fixed-arm, self-retaining retractor (eg, Bookwalter or Omni) is then placed, and a survey of the abdominal cavity is performed to determine the feasibility of resection. Lateral retractor blades should be placed carefully to avoid femoral nerve injury caused by psoas muscle compression.

Omentectomy

In ovarian cancer, the omentum is a frequent site of tumor metastases, which can vary from microscopic implants to total replacement of the omentum by an "omental cake." Therefore, omentectomy is part of staging and debulking procedures. An infracolic omentectomy is usually sufficient for staging purposes, whereas a supracolic omentectomy is performed when the gastrocolic omentum is involved with tumor. The omentectomy starts by reflecting the omentum cephalad and to the dorsal reflection onto the transverse colon (Figure 30-2). If the omentum is attached to the abdominal wall by tumor implants, it usually can be easily released bluntly or with electrocautery dissection.

The omental dissection starts in the avascular part of the posterior leaf, a few millimeters from the transverse colon serosa, at a level where omental tissue is not replaced by tumor. Using electrocautery, the posterior leaf of the omentum is incised, and with the use of traction and counter traction, the omentum is kept under tension as the incision is extended toward the splenic and hepatic flexures. Where the tumor is

adherent to the bowel serosa, sharp dissection with Metzenbaum scissors is used. The lesser sac is entered and inspected for the presence of disease through the space between the anterior and posterior leafs of the omentum. The anterior leaf of the omentum can be taken at any time during the dissection, progressively detaching the omentum from the underlying transverse colon. If tumor implants on the omentum extend

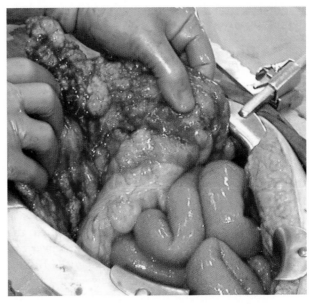

FIGURE 30-2. Omental cake reflected cephalad.

laterally to the hepatic and/or splenic flexures, these will need to be mobilized to be able to remove the disease in its entirety. As the omental dissection proceeds toward the splenic flexure, caution should be exercised when placing tension on the omentum, because excessive traction can lead to a splenic capsular tear and troublesome bleeding.

As the dissection proceeds, it is important not to lose the orientation and the direction of the dissection, which can easily happen due to the redundant layers of the omentum. In this context, frequent examination of the transverse mesocolon is critical to avoid an inadvertent injury to the middle colic vessels. When omental vessels are encountered, they can be secured with clamps and ties or using a vessel-sealing device. The right and left gastroepiploic vessels and the intervening gastroepiploic vessels are divided. In rare cases, the tumor densely infiltrates the transverse colon to a point where no plane of dissection can be created without entering the serosa of the bowel. In this case, removing the omental tumor requires a contiguous en bloc resection of involved segment of the colon. The decision whether to proceed with the resection depends on the overall spread of the disease, the extent of the colon segment to be resected, and the likelihood of achieving the cytoreductive goal.

If the supracolic omentum is involved with tumor, a gastrocolic omentectomy is performed. The gastrocolic omentum is divided from its attachment to the greater gastric curvature, and the vessels arising from the gastric arcade are systematically secured. Caution should be exercised at this level to avoid injury to the stomach. It is commonly recommended to decompress the stomach for 24 hours after surgery to avoid bleeding from the vessels secured along the greater curvature of the stomach. We have not routinely followed this practice and have not experienced any incidents of postoperative bleeding.

Right Upper Quadrant Cytoreduction

In patients with advanced ovarian cancer undergoing primary or secondary cytoreductive surgery, the right upper quadrant is a frequent site of disease. The right diaphragm frequently harbors metastatic disease, which can range from superficial peritoneal implants to full-thickness infiltrating tumors. Due to their proximity, the peritoneum covering Morrison's pouch and Gerota's fascia is also a frequent site of disease. Tumor implants can also involve the liver surface, the gallbladder, the porta hepatis, and less often, the liver parenchyma. Superficial disease on the liver can be ablated with the argon beam coagulator (ABC) or other ablative devices or superficially excised along with Glisson's capsule. More extensive liver disease should not be considered an impediment to primary cytoreduction but will frequently require the assistance of an hepatobiliary surgeon (eg, partial liver resections, cholecystectomy, dissection of the porta hepatis). The details of these latter procedures will not be discussed in this chapter. We will instead focus on the procedures most commonly used in cytoreduction of disease in the right upper quadrant, which can be safely incorporated, with appropriate training, into the skill set of the gynecologic oncologist with interest in cytoreductive surgery. We will describe mainly the mobilization of the right lobe of the liver and removal of right diaphragm disease, because the right side is the most commonly affected. When the left diaphragm is involved, a similar approach can be used.

Liver Mobilization

The liver is attached to the anterior abdominal wall by the falciform ligament. The free edge of the falciform ligament contains the round ligament—a remnant of the left umbilical vein. The bare area of the liver, located on its posterior surface in direct contact with the diaphragm, is limited by the coronary ligaments anteriorly and posteriorly and the triangular ligaments laterally.

Liver mobilization is an indispensable initial step in cytoreduction of the right upper quadrant. When omitted, the extent of diaphragm disease is often underestimated. In addition, regardless of the modality for cytoreduction used (eg, tumor ablation, peritonectomy, diaphragm resection), exposure is less than ideal if the liver is not mobilized. The patient, typically in the lithotomy position for the debulking procedure, is rotated to a "right upper quadrant up" position, which is a combination of a reverse Trendelenburg position with inclination of the operating table to the patient's left side. Self-retaining retractors (eg, Bookwalter, Omni, Goligher) are used to elevate the ribs and expose the diaphragm. The primary surgeon stands either between the legs of the patient or to the patient's left side.

For mobilization of the liver, the free edge of the falciform ligament containing the round ligament is divided first (Figure 30-3). A suture ligature placed on the lower edge can be used to aid in downward traction on the liver. The liver is separated from its attachment to the anterior abdominal wall as the falciform is divided, close to its liver attachment, in a cephalad direction until its peritoneal layers divide laterally to form the right and left anterior coronary ligaments (Figure 30-4). The dissection continues along the right coronary ligament (Figure 30-5). This dissection can be performed sharply or with electrocautery, the critical point being the identification and avoidance of injury to the right hepatic vein and inferior vena cava. Depending on the adequacy of exposure and

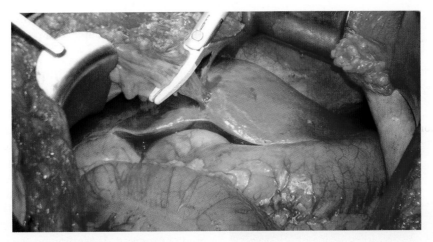

FIGURE 30-3. Division of round ligament of liver.

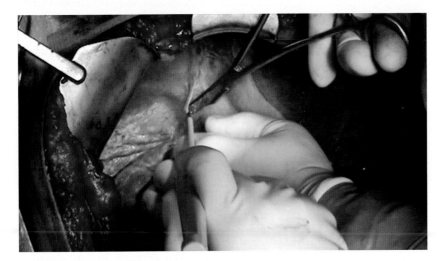

FIGURE 30-4. Division of falciform and coronary ligaments.

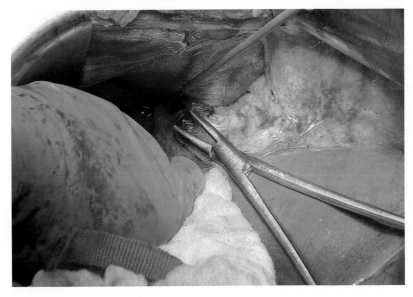

FIGURE 30-5. Division of right coronary ligament.

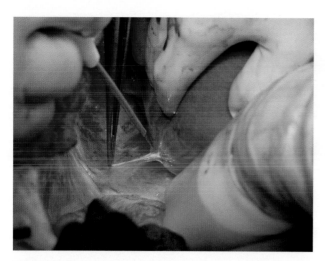

FIGURE 30-6. Division of right triangular ligament.

the amount of disease present, the dissection of the coronary ligament may continue for a variable amount of length, until it becomes more appropriate to start the dissection laterally by dividing the right triangular ligament and proceed medially (Figure 30-6). The dissection proceeds on either side until the bare area of the liver is exposed. The mobilization of the right lobe of the liver is completed by freeing the right posterior coronary ligament. The different steps of the mobilization do not necessarily follow the same order in every case; the sequence of steps is dictated by the amount of disease and the ease of exposure. Once the bare area is exposed, the liver is gently retracted medially and inferiorly, exposing the entire right diaphragm, Morrison's pouch, and Gerota's fascia (Figure 30-7).

At this time, optimal exposure of the right diaphragm is achieved and the extent of disease is inspected and

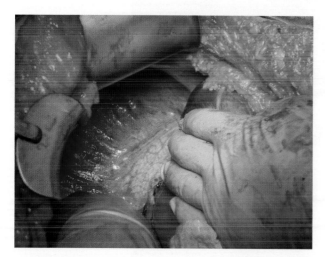

FIGURE 30-7. Exposure of bare area of the liver after liver mobilization.

palpated to assess for the depth of invasion of tumor implants into the diaphragm muscle.

Diaphragm Peritonectomy

Several reports have demonstrated the feasibility and improved outcome associated with cytoreduction of disease of the diaphragm.[2,3] After inspection of the diaphragm peritoneum, the area to be excised is outlined. The peritoneal incision usually starts at the level of the costal margin and proceeds posteriorly until all the area involved with tumor is released from the underlying diaphragm muscle (Figure 30-8). During this part, the peritonectomy will alternate between lateral and medial progress, depending on the situation.

Several techniques to separate the peritoneum from the underlying muscle have been described, and the surgeon can use whichever technique he or she feels is the most appropriate in each situation. The simplest form is to grasp and put under tension the incised peritoneal edge with several clamps (eg, ring forceps or Allis clamps) and to separate the underlying muscle bluntly by exerting pressure posteriorly and cephalad using a sponge stick. This technique works well when the tumor implants do not infiltrate deeply. In areas where the peritoneal layer is adherent to the muscle (central tendon of the diaphragm, deeper implants), blunt dissection may not be appropriate, and other forms of dissection need to be used. Electrocautery or the ABC can be used to aid in the dissection (Figure 30-9).

The detachment of the involved diaphragm peritoneum will proceed in this way, alternating techniques and direction until all the involved peritoneum is removed (Figure 30-10). Small-vessel bleeding from branches of the phrenic artery and vein often occurs during this dissection and can be controlled with electrocautery, the ABC, or a vessel-sealing device. Once the peritonectomy is completed, the integrity of the diaphragm is verified with a "bubble test"—the right upper quadrant is filled with saline, and the patient is given a maximal inspiration. Bubbles indicate a connection with the pleural cavity. The site of bubbling is identified, and interrupted sutures are placed. The technique for repair of larger defects is described in the following section.

Diaphragm Resection

Tumor implants firmly adherent to the diaphragm muscle are indicative of muscle invasion or full-thickness involvement and require partial diaphragm resection to clear the tumor. In patients who undergo video-assisted thoracic surgery, full-thickness diaphragm involvement and the presence of pleural implants can be directly visualized and the extent of diaphragm resection planned accordingly. Occasionally, preoperative

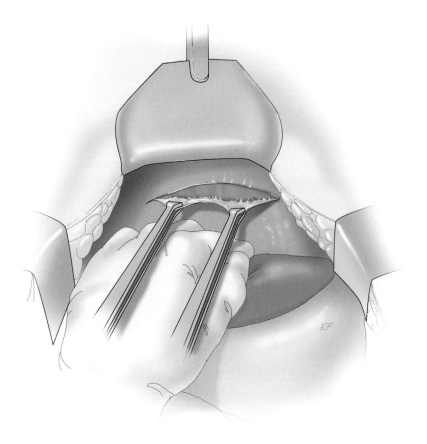

FIGURE 30-8. Diaphragm peritonectomy incision.

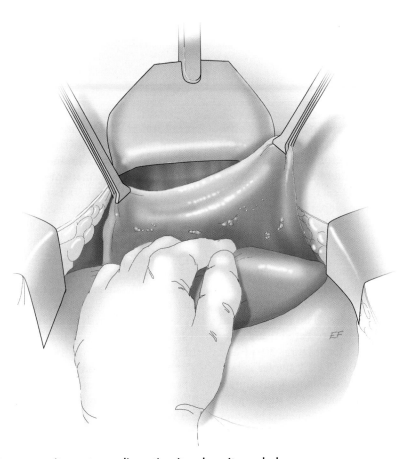

FIGURE 30-9. Diaphragm peritonectomy dissection in subperitoneal plane.

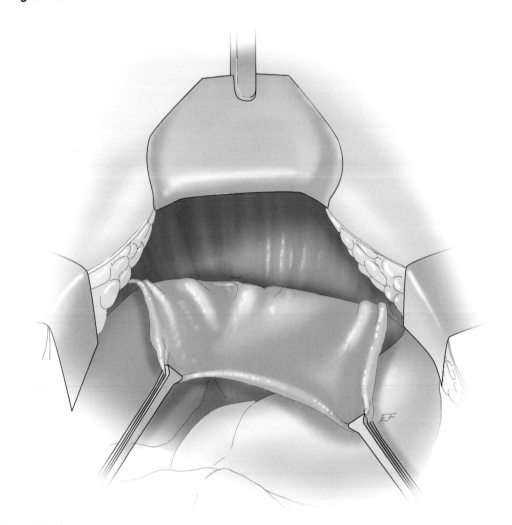

FIGURE 30-10. Diaphragm peritonectomy exposure of muscle.

imaging can point to full-thickness diaphragm involvement. The right phrenic nerve innervates the right diaphragm, entering on the superomedial surface and branching immediately in a radial fashion. Therefore, resections that extend medially carry a higher risk of nerve injury and postoperative diaphragm paralysis.

From the abdominal side, which is by far the most common approach to diaphragm resection, palpation of the involved area can help in identifying the area to be resected. The anesthesiologist is notified about imminent entry into the pleural space with the resultant pneumothorax. When the pleural cavity is entered, the lung is visualized and avoided. The area involved with tumor is outlined and can be resected using electrocautery or an Endo GIA stapler (Figures 30-11 and 30-12). An advantage of the Endo GIA stapler is better delineated edges, which are easier to approximate and suture, with a lesser likelihood of the suture pulling through the muscle because the staple line provides a resistant line of support. The Endo GIA or TA stapling devices (both from Covidien, Mansfield, MA) can occasionally be used in a single step to excise a

small lesion while tenting down the diaphragm. Even diaphragm defects as large as 10 cm can be primarily closed without undue tension using interrupted figure-of-eight permanent sutures (1-0 polypropylene) (Figures 30-13 and 30-14). A single or looped running suture has also been used successfully.[4,5] When the defect is too extensive for a tension-free primary closure, a polytetrafluoroethylene patch can be sutured in place with a running suture, starting at the medial edge.

To prevent postoperative pneumothorax and pleural effusion, air and fluid need to be evacuated from the pleural cavity as the diaphragm defect is closed. A commonly used technique includes passing of a 14- to 16-French red Robinson catheter through the diaphragm defect into the pleural cavity as the closure of the defect is coming to an end (final 1-2 cm). A purse-string or figure-of-eight suture is placed loosely through the diaphragm muscle to surround this remaining connection with the pleural space. As the patient is given several maximal inspirations followed by a Valsalva maneuver, the Robinson catheter, while placed under gentle suction or under a water seal, is

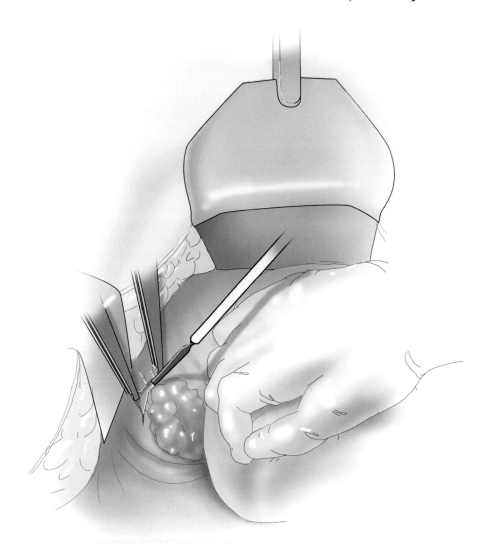

FIGURE 30-11. Full-thickness diaphragm resection using the electrosurgical unit.

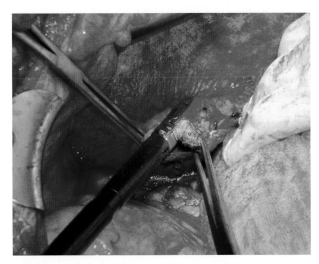

FIGURE 30-12. Full-thickness diaphragm resection using the Endo GIA stapler.

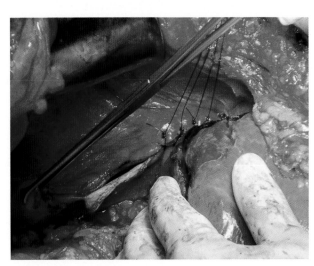

FIGURE 30-13. Diaphragm closure with interrupted stitches.

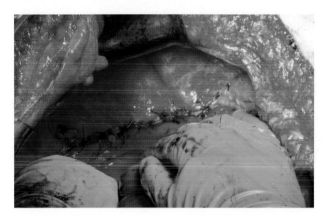

FIGURE 30-14. Completed diaphragm closure.

removed as the suture is tightened. Persistent pneumothorax is evaluated using the previously described "bubble test." Alternatively, a chest tube can be placed in the pleural cavity, with minimal morbidity, under direct visualization of the pleural space through the diaphragm opening, and it will effectively drain air and fluid from the pleural space for the first few postoperative days (Figure 30-15).

Left Upper Quadrant

The left upper quadrant is a frequent site of metastatic disease in advanced ovarian cancer, with disease involving the spleen, stomach, distal pancreas, and transverse colon. Recent retrospective evidence suggests that even in the setting of extensive upper abdominal disease, optimal cytoreduction improves survival, and this can be achieved with acceptable morbidity.[6]

Adequate exposure to the left upper quadrant requires a vertical midline incision. Exposure can be further enhanced by initially addressing extensive omental disease to facilitate visualization of important

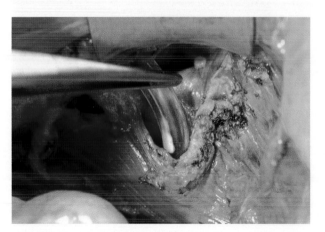

FIGURE 30-15. Chest tube placed under direct visualization.

vascular structures and viscera in the left upper quadrant. The posterior leaf of the omentum is initially divided, allowing access to the lesser sac. Once the lesser sac is entered, the omental cake and stomach can be reflected anteriorly so that a thorough exploration of the distal pancreas, splenic hilum, porta hepatis, and celiac trunk can be performed. This allows for a more accurate estimation of disease resectability.

Partial Transverse Colectomy

If no plane between the involved omentum and transverse colon can be achieved, en bloc transverse colectomy and omentectomy may be required. To perform an en bloc resection of the transverse colon and omentum, the lesser sac is first entered superiorly by dividing the gastrocolic ligament. The gastrocolic ligament is transected with a vessel-sealing device along the entire length of the greater curvature of the stomach. The surgeon must ensure that this dissection does not extend into the underlying transverse colon mesentery because this may compromise blood supply to the anastomosis site. The transverse colon is fully mobilized by dividing the hepatocolic and splenocolic ligaments, with care to avoid avulsing the blood supply to the spleen. The location of the bowel resection is then determined (Figure 30-16). The integrity of the marginal artery of Drummond should be confirmed by transillumination prior to completing the resection. This will ensure that the reapproximated ends of proximal and distal transverse colon will have an adequate blood supply. Otherwise, the distal end of the anastomosis should occur distal to the splenic flexure in the descending colon. After dividing the colon with a GIA (gastro-intestinal anastomosis) stapling device, the transverse colon mesentery is transected with a vessel-sealing device, and the specimen is removed en bloc (Figure 30-17).

Once the specimen has been excised, the colon can be further mobilized by incising the peritoneum overlying the paracolic gutters (white line of Toldt) and reflecting both limbs of the proposed anastomosis medially. Once the proposed anastomosis is mobilized adequately to ensure the absence of tension, a side-to-side (Figure 30-18) or end-to-end bowel anastomosis can be performed, as stated elsewhere in the chapter; however, the remainder of the upper abdomen dissection should be performed prior to completion of the anastomosis. If an anastomosis cannot be achieved due to tension, a diverting ascending colostomy can be performed, although in our experience, this is rarely necessary.

Splenectomy

Splenectomy is required to achieve optimal cytoreduction in approximately 10% of patients with advanced

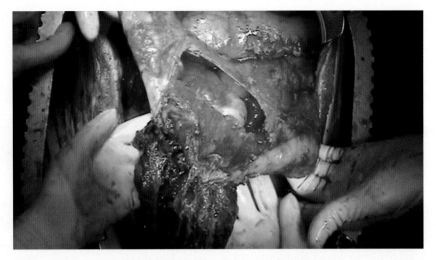

FIGURE 30-16. Partial transverse colectomy: delineation of extent of resection.

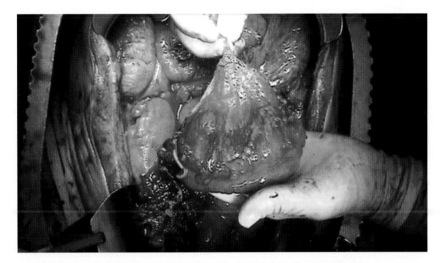

FIGURE 30-17. Partial transverse colectomy specimen with "wedge" of mesentery.

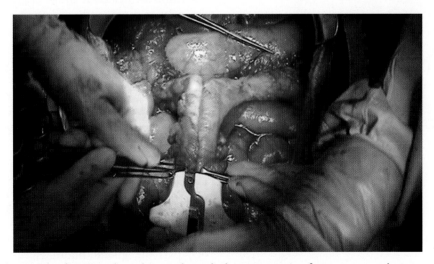

FIGURE 30-18. Side-to-side, functional, end-to-end stapled anastomosis of transverse colon.

ovarian cancer.[7] Splenic involvement can occur due to direct tumor extension or hematogenous metastasis, although the former is more likely. An anterior or posterior approach can be performed; the choice of approach depends on the distribution of disease in the left upper quadrant, and a combination of techniques may be required in some cases.

The anterior approach to splenectomy is most useful if the anterior attachments of the spleen are free from tumor, as often occurs when the splenic hilum is involved by tumor without direct extension of disease from the omentum. After entering the lesser sac, the stomach is retraced medially so that the gastrosplenic ligament and associated vessels can be sequentially divided with a vessel-sealing device. The gastrosplenic ligament is divided carefully to avoid including the posterior gastric wall in the specimen. If the spleen is free from adhesions laterally, a posterior approach may be initiated prior to dividing the splenic vessels. If the lateral attachments are involved by tumor, the splenic vessels are controlled first. To do so, the spleen can be gently lifted anteriorly so that the demarcation between the tail of the pancreas and splenic hilum is identified. This step prevents inadvertent resection of the pancreatic tail in the splenectomy specimen. The splenic artery is isolated and double ligated with nonresorbable silk sutures. The splenic vein is then ligated separately to allow for drainage of the venous reservoir in the organ following arterial ligation and to prevent formation of arteriovenous fistula (Figure 30-19). Anterior and medial mobilization of the spleen allows

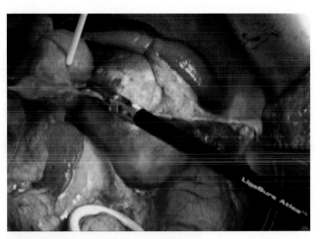

FIGURE 30-20. Splenectomy: hilar tumor requiring posterior approach.

for division of the posterior and lateral lienorenal ligament. If the left hemidiaphragm is involved by tumor, the spleen can be resected en bloc with the diaphragm specimen.

If there is extensive omental infiltration of the splenic hilum, a posterior approach to splenectomy may be preferable (Figure 30-20). The patient is placed "left side up" to allow the surgeon operating from the patient's right side easier access to the left upper quadrant. The spleen is then retracted medially, and the lienorenal ligament is divided. The splenic vessels should be visible medially, although division of the splenophrenic ligaments may be required to allow for additional medial and anterior retraction of spleen and improved visualization. After identifying the tail of the pancreas, the splenic vessels are sequentially isolated and ligated, as stated previously (Figure 30-21). After dividing these vessels, the lesser sac can be accessed and the spleen rotated medially out of the incision. This should allow for posterior visualization of the gastrosplenic ligament and short gastric vessels, which can now be more easily skeletonized and divided.

Once the spleen has been removed, the splenic vascular pedicles are inspected and reinforced as necessary. If the tail of the pancreas is injured inadvertently, this area can be reinforced with a continuous layer of delayed resorbable 3-0 sutures. Following a splenectomy, a closed-suction drain is placed in the splenic bed prior to closure of the abdomen to assess for postoperative pancreatic leaks.

Distal Pancreatectomy

The distal pancreas may occasionally be involved in patients with advanced ovarian cancer. This most often occurs when omental disease extends posteriorly past the splenic hilum. Access to the tail of the pancreas requires full exposure of the lesser sac. The

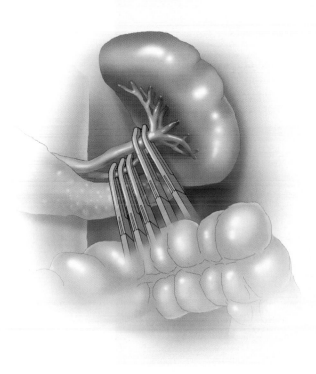

FIGURE 30-19. Splenectomy: anterior approach.

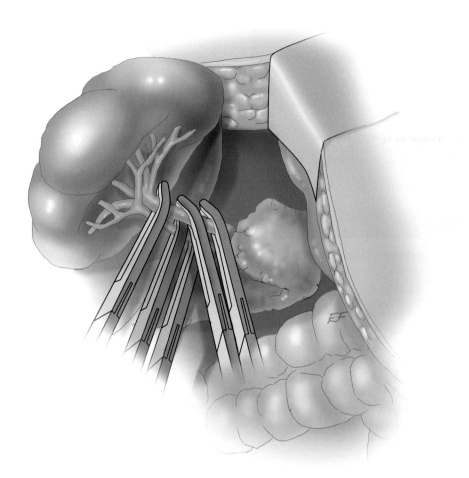

FIGURE 30-21. Splenectomy: posterior approach.

gastrosplenic ligament and short gastric vessels are sequentially incised along the greater curvature of the stomach so that the posterior borders of the lesser sac, including the pancreas and splenic hilum, are visualized. The peritoneum overlying the inferior border of the pancreas is incised from just proximal to the involved portion toward the splenic hilum, with care to avoid the underlying inferior mesenteric vein. The splenic artery is then identified on the superior border of the pancreas, ligated, and transected, as previously described. The previously identified splenic vein can then be ligated and transected separately. A vascular load (2.5-mm) Endo GIA stapler is then used to transect the pancreas (Figure 30-22). We frequently place a 2-0 delayed-resorbable running suture layer along the entire length of the transected pancreas. A closed-suction drain should be placed in the left upper quadrant to monitor for pancreatic leak.

Partial Gastrectomy

When omental metastasis involves the supracolic omentum, the tissue plane between the greater curvature of the stomach and omentum usually remains intact. Occasionally, there is direct extension into the gastric body. If optimal cytoreduction is achievable, a partial gastrectomy should be considered. To do so, involved

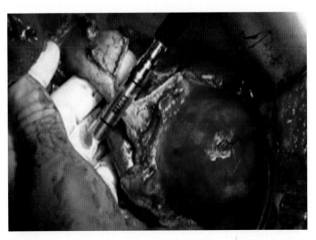

FIGURE 30-22. Distal pancreatectomy using an Endo GIA stapler.

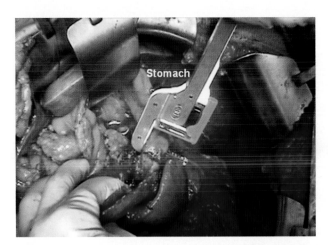

FIGURE 30-23. Partial gastrectomy using a TA stapler.

portions of the gastrocolic and gastrosplenic ligaments are ligated with a vessel-sealing device to allow for better access to the posterior gastric body within the lesser sac. Once the posterior border of the gastric body is freely mobilized, a large TA or GIA stapling device can be passed above the involved portion of the greater curvature, and the involved portion is removed (Figure 30-23). The suture line is then reinforced with a second layer of 3-0 silk interrupting imbricating sutures, and the stomach is decompressed by nasogastric tube placement for at least 24 hours postoperatively.

Pelvis

The pelvis is often obliterated by multiple and/or confluent tumor nodules in patients with advanced epithelial ovarian cancer, such that removal of the pelvic viscera and surrounding peritoneum is often necessary to achieve a minimal residual disease state. Over the last 40 years, these en bloc resections have been referred to in a number of ways (ie, radical oophorectomy, modified posterior exenteration, low anterior resection), but essentially, all refer to en bloc excision of the uterus, cervix, bilateral fallopian tubes and ovaries, rectosigmoid colon, and pelvic peritoneum. Several recent analyses have shown that these procedures can be performed safely while increasing the rate of optimal cytoreduction.[8] Patients who undergo modified posterior exenteration for advanced ovarian cancer have a low rate of complications related to the procedure. Overall, the rate of colorectal anastomotic leak/fistula is 2.1%, and the mortality rate is only 0.8%.[9]

The first step in the modified posterior exenteration is a circumscribing peritoneal incision around the pelvic viscera and extending cranially along the psoas muscles (Figure 30-24). If a rectosigmoid resection is required, the left lateral incision may be extended along the line of Toldt as far as the splenic flexure to allow for adequate mobilization of the descending colon in anticipation of a tension-free rectal anastomosis. All pelvic disease should be incorporated into the specimen, if possible; thus, a lateral peritoneal incision is preferred. If the round ligaments are obscured by peritoneal implants, they can be identified retroperitoneally after the lateral peritoneal incision has been made (Figure 30-25). The pararectal space is then developed, and the ureter and ovarian vessels are identified. After dissecting the ureters off of the medial leaf of the broad ligament, vessel loops are passed under the ureters to allow for future identification and lateral traction, as necessary. The ureters are then skeletonized from the pelvic brim to the tunnel of Wertheim. The infundibulopelvic ligaments can then be transected and ligated with suture or a vessel-sealing device (eg, LigaSure vessel sealer; Covidien).

The round ligaments are then divided as close to their attachment along the pelvic sidewall as possible, and the anterior pelvic peritoneum is incised along the pubic symphysis to the midline. The paravesical space is then developed down to the cardinal ligaments. The anterior pelvic peritoneum is grasped with Allis clamps along the midline and retracted cranially to allow for electrocautery dissection between this layer and the bladder dome (Figure 30-26). This dissection is then carried inferiorly to the pubocervical fascia (Figures 30-27 and 30-28). Occasionally, bladder wall invasion is encountered and may require full-thickness bladder resection. In this event, careful consideration must be taken to avoid unrecognized resection of the bladder trigone, because this requires a more complex bladder reconstruction, with possible ureteral reimplantation.

The uterine pedicles are skeletonized, ligated, and divided at the level of the ureters (Figure 30-29). The ureters are then unroofed from the bladder pillars, allowing lateral reflection away from the specimen. The bladder is then dissected off of the vagina approximately 2 to 3 cm distal to the cervical junction, and an anterior colpotomy is performed 1 to 2 cm distal to the cervical junction using electrocautery. This location can be better identified by performing a bimanual examination or inserting a sponge-stick or end-to-end anastomosis sizer into the anterior vagina. The colpotomy is then extended laterally, using Heaney clamps to secure and suture ligate the vaginal angles (Figure 30-30). Alternatively, a vessel-sealing device (eg, LigaSure) can be used to easily divide the vagina, with excellent hemostasis. The posterior wall of the vagina is then incised with electrocautery and the rectovaginal septum entered (Figure 30-31). At this point, the extent of surgical resection is dependent on the amount of tumor involvement in the posterior cul-de-sac (type I vs. type II modification).

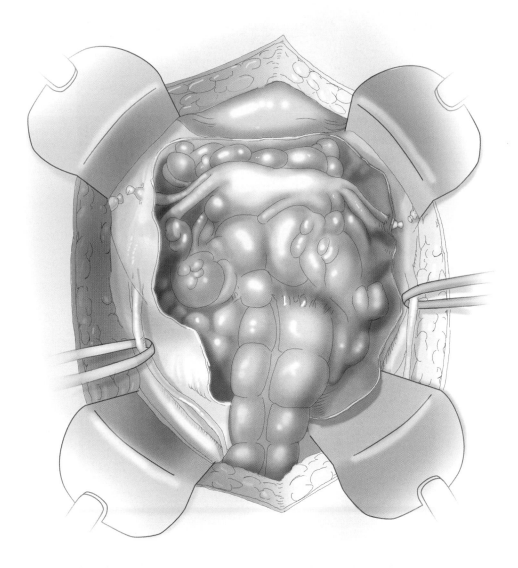

FIGURE 30-24. Modified posterior exenteration: circumscribing pelvic peritoneal incision.

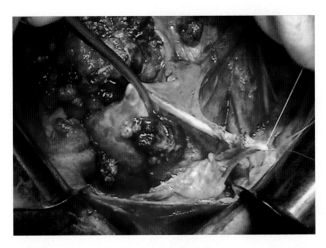

FIGURE 30-25. Modified posterior exenteration: ligation of round ligament.

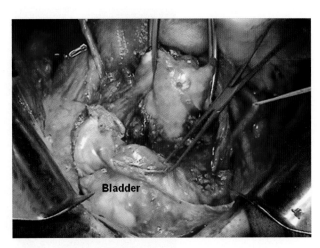

FIGURE 30-26. Modified posterior exenteration: anterior pelvic peritoneum grasped with Allis clamp.

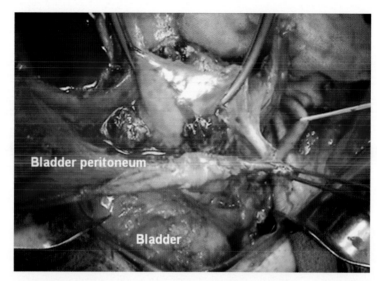

FIGURE 30-27. Modified posterior exenteration: anterior peritoneum raised.

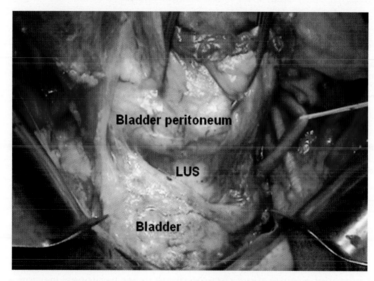

FIGURE 30-28. Modified posterior exenteration: pubocervical fascia exposed. LUS, lower uterine segment.

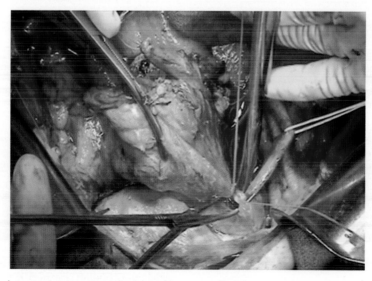

FIGURE 30-29. Modified posterior exenteration: uterine artery ligation.

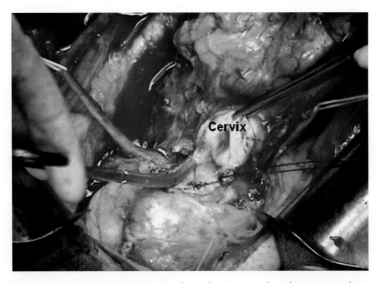

FIGURE 30-30. Modified posterior exenteration: vaginal angles secured with Heaney clamps.

In the type I modification, the rectum can be spared if uninvolved by tumor. The posterior cul-de-sac peritoneum is incised at the level of the previously ligated infundibulopelvic ligaments and extended along the lateral pelvic gutters. This incision is carried caudally and toward the midline so that the peritoneum of the posterior cul-de-sac and paraovarian fossa can be included in the specimen. Tumor and underlying peritoneum may require sharp dissection to be separated from the underlying rectal serosa (Figure 30-32). If a small rectal defect (<2 cm) is inadvertently created or required to resect limited tumor implants, the colotomy can be repaired with a single layer of inverting interrupted 3-0 polypropylene sutures. Excision of the posterior cul-de-sac is extended toward the rectovaginal septum incision created anteriorly, allowing for the specimen to be removed en bloc.

In the type II modification, the rectosigmoid colon is removed with the uterus and ovaries due to complete obliteration of the posterior pelvis or extensive serosal implants along the rectosigmoid (Figure 30-33). The rectosigmoid colon can be divided with a GIA stapling device at any location from the pelvic brim to the splenic flexure, as required, to achieve optimal cytoreduction; however, 2 to 3 cm of uninvolved colon should be available proximal to the planned transection site. Following colon transection, the peritoneum of the mesentery is incised laterally to join the pelvic peritoneal incision of the pelvic dissection, with care to avoid the underlying ureters. The sigmoid mesentery is then incised and transected with suture ligation or a vessel-sealing device perpendicular to the long axis of the sigmoid for several centimeters prior to passing caudally and parallel to the long axis of the sigmoid at

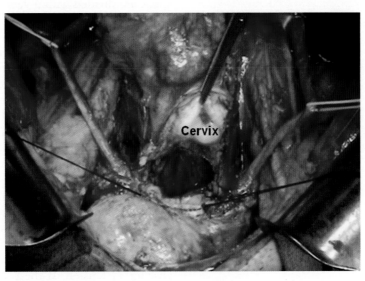

FIGURE 30-31. Modified posterior exenteration: posterior vaginal entry.

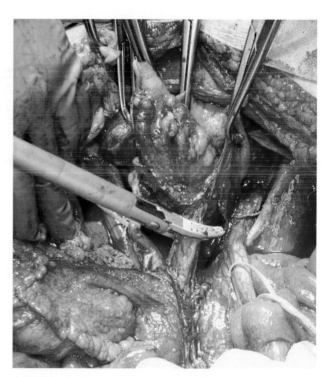

FIGURE 30-34. Transection of rectosigmoid colon mesentery.

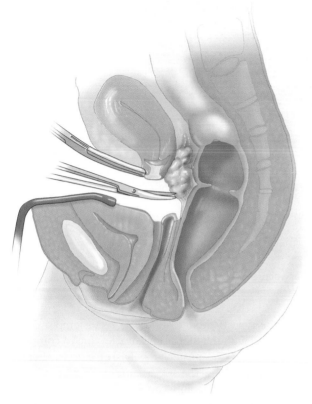

FIGURE 30-32. Modified posterior exenteration: type I modification.

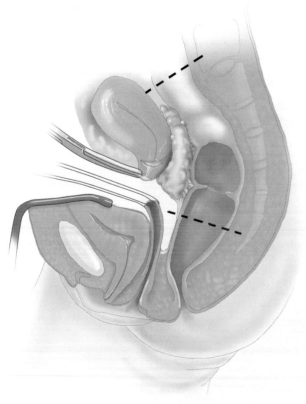

FIGURE 30-33. Modified posterior exenteration: type II modification.

the pelvic brim to ensure removal of involved mesenteric lymph nodes (Figure 30-34). The superior rectal artery and vein are identified and ligated during this dissection. Care must be taken to avoid transection of the left colic artery during any part of the procedure so that adequate blood supply to the descending colon is maintained.

The pararectal space is then entered at the pelvic brim, and the rectum is dissected off of the underlying presacral fascia with a combination of blunt dissection and a vessel-sealing device. The rectal pillars that represent the posterior and lateral borders of the presacral space are divided with a vessel-sealing device. At this point, the posterior cul-de-sac and the rectum should be completely freed posteriorly to the level of rectovaginal septum incision created anteriorly. The specimen can be lifted ventrally and the remaining mesorectal fat cleared off of the site of rectal resection (Figure 30-35). The rectal resection is most easily performed with a TA stapler 2 to 3 cm distal to the most distal extent of rectal tumor involvement (Figure 30-36). Prior to firing the TA stapler, the surgeon must ensure that the ureters are not incorporated into the resection. Following rectal transection, the specimen should be completely detached and can be passed off the field.

Rectal reanastomosis is most easily performed using an end-to-end stapling technique, to be described in detail later in this chapter. Successful rectal reanastomosis requires an adequate blood supply in the absence of tension. If these conditions do not exist,

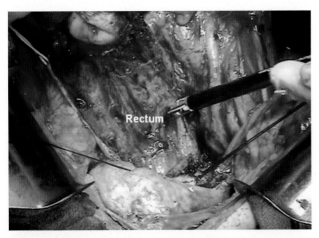

FIGURE 30-35. Division of mesorectum using vessel-sealing device.

anastomotic leak may occur. Management of this complication will be discussed later in this chapter. To avoid anastomotic leaks, mobilization of the sigmoid colon is often required. Several techniques may be used to aid in this process, including the following:

1. Transect the attachments between transverse colon and the infracolic omentum or splenic flexure.
2. Mobilize the descending colon and associated mesentery medially.
3. Open the lesser sac and divide the gastrocolic ligament to allow for mobilization of the splenic flexure.
4. Open the descending colon mesentery and ligate individual vessels of the descending colon including the left colic artery. This procedure is not feasible if collateral circulation from the marginal artery of Drummond has previously been ligated or is functionally absent, as is the case in approximately 5% of the population.

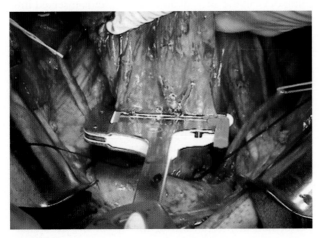

FIGURE 30-36. Transection of proximal rectum using TA stapler.

5. Ligate the inferior mesenteric vein inferior to the pancreas, allowing for greater descent of the mesentery.

If an adequate blood supply cannot be ensured or any degree of tension is suspected in the anastomosis, diverting loop ileostomy or colostomy should be considered. Although diversion will not prevent the formation of an anastomotic leak, it will usually prevent peritonitis caused by dissemination of stool throughout the abdominal cavity. This risk must be weighed against the inconvenience of a temporary ostomy for the patient and potential for exclusion for clinical trials in patients who desire early reversal of their anastomosis.

Intestinal Surgery

Cytoreductive surgery for ovarian cancer requires resection of all large-volume disease. Because ovarian cancer may involve any peritoneal surface, small bowel and colon implants are frequently encountered. Although full-thickness bowel wall invasion is uncommon, it can be difficult to remove tumor implants on the bowel wall without injuring underlying tissues. Thus, bowel resection is often required to achieve optimal cytoreduction. In our experience, approximately 35% of patients with stage III or IV disease will require large bowel resection, and 5% will require small bowel resection during primary cytoreductive surgery.[7] Although there are no prospective data, most retrospective analyses suggest that bowel resections can be performed safely and may improve survival in patients with advanced-stage disease if resection results in optimal cytoreduction.[9] If optimal cytoreduction cannot be safely achieved, bowel resection should only be performed at time of exploratory laparotomy if impending bowel obstruction is encountered. In this section, we will review the intestinal procedures frequently encountered during ovarian cancer surgery.

There are several techniques for bowel resection and anastomosis. The incorporation of surgical stapling devices has greatly decreased the time required to perform these procedures without a negative impact on patient safety. In general, any intestinal anastomosis should: (1) be tension free, with an adequate blood supply; (2) have an adequate lumen to allow for passage of intestinal contents; and (3) be hemostatic and secure. Surgical techniques used for bowel resection depend on the location of disease (ie, ileum, right colon, or rectosigmoid) and the lumen of the bowel to be reanastomosed (ie, distal ileum, colon, or rectum). The most commonly performed procedures involve the resection of the distal ileum, cecum, and ascending colon or of the sigmoid and rectum. Due to the unreliable blood supply to the distal 10 cm of ileum, resection of this segment requires incorporation of the cecum to facilitate adequate blood supply of the anastomotic site. Regardless of the type of bowel resected or anastomosis required, this can generally be achieved with either hand-sewn or stapled techniques.

Bowel Resection

Bowel transection is most easily achieved with a GIA stapling device. The advantage of this device is the simultaneous transection and closure of the bowel lumen. In the case of small bowel resections, the bowel wall is transected at a slight angle, allowing a greater length of the mesenteric edge of the bowel segment to be retained to ensure adequate transmural blood supply to the antimesenteric border of the anastomosis. A wedge of the associated mesentery is then divided, with care to avoid the distal branches of the superior mesenteric artery supplying the distal small bowel segments. This is facilitated with the use of a vessel-sealing device. Resection of underlying bulky (diameter ≥ 1 cm) mesenteric adenopathy must be considered if optimal cytoreduction is to be achieved.

Bowel Anastomosis Techniques

Hand-Sewn Anastomosis

Given the simplicity and speed of using bowel stapling devices, hand-sewn anastomoses are usually reserved for small bowel resections in which the length of adjacent uninvolved bowel is not adequate for the use of a stapling device or if there is significant bowel wall edema. A 2-layer closure, using 3-0 silk or polypropylene for both layers, is generally preferred for the hand-sewn technique. To accommodate the discrepancy in bowel lumen between the distal ileum and ascending colon, a Cheatle incision may be made in the antimesenteric surface of the small bowel to increase its diameter prior to reanastomosis. The transected bowel ends are first reapproximated with bowel clamps, and a row of interrupted imbricating Lambert sutures is placed in the posterior wall of the seromuscular layer. The bowel clamps are removed, and the staple line is excised. A continuous full-thickness stitch is then passed close to the posterior mucosal edges. Once the corner of the posterior edge has been reached, the needle is passed to the outside of the anterior bowel wall, and the remaining anterior inner layer is closed by passing the needle full thickness outside-in and then inside-out (Connell stitch). The anterior seromuscular layer is then closed with interrupted sutures similar to the outer posterior layer and the mesenteric defect repaired with care to avoid ligation of the underlying mesenteric vessels. Although a single-layer closure can be used for both small bowel and colonic anastomoses, this technique is generally reserved only for colonic reanastomosis at the time of obstruction and has not been shown to be beneficial over stapling techniques.

Stapled Anastomosis

Stapled anastomoses can be performed quickly and safely under most circumstances. The 3 primary techniques are the end-to-end, end-to-side, and side-to-side anastomoses. The decision to use hand-sewn versus stapled techniques is often based on cost, time, and surgeon preference.

A stapled end-to-end anastomosis (EEA) is generally performed to reapproximate 2 ends of colon, as is often encountered following rectal resection at the time of posterior exenteration, or, less commonly, to reapproximate the right and left colon following en bloc resection of the transverse colon and omentum. After both limbs of bowel have been transected with a stapling device, the anvil of an EEA stapler is inserted into one end of the colon. During rectal resection, this is usually the proximal loop of sigmoid. The anvil is secured with a polypropylene purse-string suture placed by hand or with the assistance of a purse-string applicator. The EEA stapler is then inserted into the distal bowel segment through colotomy (made several centimeters away from the proposed anastomosis) or by passing the stapler into the rectum in the case of a rectal resection (Figure 30-37). The EEA trocar is then passed through the prior staple line and the anvil attached. The EEA stapler is then fired and removed, creating a new bowel lumen. If a colotomy was performed to accommodate the EEA stapler, this may be closed with a TA stapling device, with care to avoid narrowing the bowel lumen by creating a staple line perpendicular to the bowel lumen. Following the completion of the anastomosis, an adequate seal can be confirmed by filling the pelvis with water and distending the rectum with air. A proctoscope can be used to directly visualize the intraluminal staple line, if desired.

An end-to-side stapled anastomosis is usually performed to reapproximate 2 loops of bowel of different diameter, as is the case after an ileocecal resection. After both limbs of bowel have been transected with a stapling device, the anvil of an EEA stapler is inserted into the proximal loop of ileum, and a purse-string suture is placed, as previously described. The lumen of the distal loop of colon is then opened to accommodate the EEA stapler. The EEA trocar is then advanced through the antimesenteric wall of the colon and the anvil attached. The EEA stapler is then fired and removed, creating the new bowel lumen. The open end of colon is then closed with a TA stapling device, and the mesenteric defect is reapproximated. As an alternative to the end-to-end technique for rectal reanastomosis following modified posterior exenteration, a rectal "J-pouch" can be created by anastomosing the distal rectum to a detubularized loop of sigmoid colon, with the sigmoid anastomosis performed at the bottom of the "J" of the detubularized loop. To allow for adequate evacuation of stool, the length of pouch should be limited to 5 cm or less.

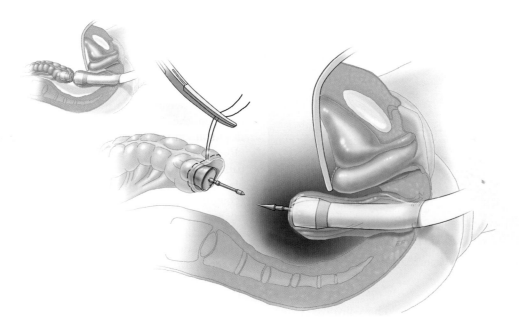

FIGURE 30-37. Stapled circular end-to-end anastomosis (CEEA) of colon to rectum.

Under most circumstances, a side-to-side (functional end-to-end) stapled technique is preferred for reanastomosis of 2 small bowel segments or to reapproximate the distal ileum to ascending colon if an end-to-side technique is not performed. Following bowel resection, the antimesenteric edges of the transected bowel are placed side by side, and the antimesenteric corners are incised. Stay sutures may be placed along the antimesenteric surface of the planned anastomosis to prevent misalignment of the bowel segments and prevent tension along the staple line. The 2 arms of the GIA stapling device are inserted into the holes created in the staple line, and the GIA stapler is fired to create a new intestinal lumen (Figure 30-38). Prior to firing the stapler, the surgeon must ensure that the mesenteric edges of the bowel are not incorporated into the staple line to avoid devascularization. The stapler is removed and the remaining defect closed with a TA stapler. Prior to closure of the luminal defect, the staple lines of the new intestinal lumen are offset to prevent intraluminal adhesions or devascularization that may occur at an area incorporating multiple staple lines. Regardless of the technique used, patency of the bowel lumen must be confirmed by pinching the anastomosis between the thumb and index finger following completion of the anastomosis.

Tumor Ablation

Intraoperative tumor ablation techniques are commonly used in ovarian cancer surgery and play an important role in achieving the cytoreductive goal while reducing the need for major organ resections. Ovarian cancer commonly presents with innumerable tumor implants in the abdominal cavity, and achieving complete cytoreduction requires their meticulous removal. In this setting, the most commonly used ablative tools are the ABC and the Cavitron Ultrasonic Surgical Aspirator (CUSA).

Argon Beam Coagulator

Electrosurgical ablation of tumor implants using the ABC is especially useful to eradicate tumors from

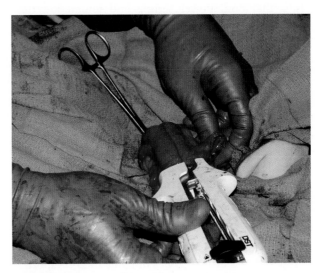

FIGURE 30-38. Small bowel anastomosis.

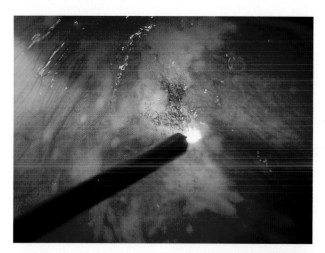

FIGURE 30-39. Argon beam coagulator for tumor ablation.

areas where the alternative would have involved extensive resections, in which the morbidity and long-term consequences can be significant (eg, diffuse small bowel mesenteric implants, diaphragm) (Figure 30-39). In addition to tumor ablation, the ABC has a hemostatic effect, and its utility has been demonstrated in surgeries associated with extensive blood loss.[10]

The ABC uses a beam of inert argon to conduct unipolar current in a noncontact, directed fashion. The energy transmitted (40-150 W) is in the same range as standard monopolar electrocautery. The electrical current is initiated only when the tip is within 10 mm of the target tissue. The current spreads out on the tissue surface with a more homogeneous distribution of energy than standard electrocautery. In addition to tissue destruction, the argon displaces the blood and debris from the immediate operative field and coagulates vessels up to 2 to 3 mm in diameter; therefore, good visibility is maintained while it is used.[11]

A consistent finding in experimental animal models is that both power setting and interaction time increase the amount of tissue damage. Application to the bowel serosa should be avoided; in a canine model, a 40-W application for 1 second reached the muscularis propria in 50% of cases. At 3 seconds, damage extended into the submucosa, and at 5 seconds, full-thickness injury had occurred in all cases. In addition, delayed (5-7 days after the injury) bowel perforation at 50% of the application sites occurred with 3-second applications.[12] Therefore, if the ABC is applied inadvertently for a period longer than 1 second, the area of bowel injured should be oversewn or resected, and the patient should be closely monitored in the postoperative period for signs and symptoms suggesting bowel perforation.

The depth of destruction produced by the ABC is composed of 3 distinct zones of tissue injury: vaporization (immediate tissue/current interface), carbonized

eschar, and coagulative necrosis (deepest layer).[11] It increases from 1.7 mm to 5.5 mm as the power setting of the ABC (60, 80, and 100 W) and the interaction time between the ABC and the tissue (1, 3, and 5 seconds) increase. An important finding is that at all power settings and interaction intervals, the ratio between the depth of coagulative necrosis and the depth of carbonized eschar is relatively constant and close to 1. This means that for any thickness of visible tumor destroyed (the carbonized eschar part), there is an equivalent amount of deeper tissue also destroyed (coagulative necrosis part), even if it appears grossly normal.

Typically, 60- to 80-W settings are used for small nodules and implants on the bowel mesentery. Higher power settings (100-110 W) can safely be used for larger tumor plaques and for disease located on the diaphragm, liver, and abdominal peritoneum.[11]

Cavitron Ultrasonic Surgical Aspirator

The ultrasonic surgical aspirator consists of a handpiece with a high-frequency (23,000 Hz) ultrasonic vibrator, which destroys tissue by cavitation, and an irrigation and aspiration system, which cleans the operative field and cools the tip of the instrument.[13] The tip is hollow, and broken pieces of tumor are aspirated with saline through the handpiece. Cavitation induces selective tissue fragmentation: Tissue with a high water content (eg, fat, muscle, carcinoma) is destroyed easily, whereas tissue with a high content of collagen and elastic fibers (eg, blood vessels, nerves, ureters, serosa) is more difficult to damage. The amplitude of vibration controls the excursion of the instrument tip and the depth of tissue disruption. The amplitude setting most commonly used for tumor resection is 0.7 to 0.8 (210-240 µm). The tissue removed can be used to establish a histologic diagnosis.[14,15]

The CUSA has been used to remove tumor nodules from the diaphragm, liver surface, major vessels, ureters, and bowel and bladder serosa.[13,16] It does not seem to be associated with a higher incidence of operative complications. However, the dissection and removal of tumor can be tedious and time consuming. Increased operative time may be offset if extensive dissection and reconstruction required by standard techniques are avoided by using the CUSA.[15]

An increased risk of coagulopathy with extended use of the CUSA has been suggested, but this was not confirmed by other studies, and this is probably related to the surgery itself rather than the use of the CUSA.[13,17] Ultrasonic cell destruction, combined with continuous irrigation, causes a cloud of fine droplets above the surgical field,[18] which has been shown to carry tumor cells. Although this may not be a concern in advanced cases with widely disseminated disease, the CUSA should be used with caution when resecting isolated tumors (eg, isolated recurrence).[18,19]

Final Steps and Closure

After the completion of optimal cytoreductive surgery, an intraperitoneal catheter may be inserted prior to incision closure (see Chapter 33). Prior to closure, the abdominal cavity is irrigated copiously with warm saline, and a meticulous survey of all operative surfaces to ensure hemostasis is performed. Antiadhesion barriers (eg, hyaluronic acid–carboxymethylcellulose barrier; Seprafilm, Genzyme, Cambridge, MA) may be placed in the pelvis and along the anterior abdomen at this point. These products should not be placed near bowel anastomoses due to an increased risk of anastomotic leak. Suction drains, though not mandatory, can be placed according to the surgeon's preference and extent and type of surgery.

Careful attention during abdominal wall closure is necessary to reduce the already high risk of ventral hernia and wound infection in patients undergoing laparotomy for cytoreductive surgery. Closure of the abdominal fascia is performed using a continuous delayed-absorbable monofilament suture (Polydioxanone [PDS]), with a suture-to-wound length of at least 4:1. Randomized data support the placement of fascial sutures close to the fascial edge (5-8 mm), with care to avoid inclusion of extra fat and muscle that may devascularize and increase the risk of ventral hernia and infection.[20] Subcutaneous fat is then irrigated and reapproximated with polyglactin sutures if greater than 2 cm in depth.

POSTOPERATIVE CARE

| Box 30-3 | Complications and Morbidity |

- Monitor patients for development of pleural effusion if diaphragm peritonectomy/resection is performed; obtain chest radiograph in postanesthesia care unit and daily, as needed.
- Acute shortness of breath in the postoperative setting is not uncommon, and a quick diagnosis is essential because treatment is different according to the etiology and can be lifesaving. Among the common etiologies, the differential diagnoses include pulmonary embolism, large pleural effusion, and hospital-acquired pneumonia.
- Anastomotic leaks should be ruled out in cases of unexplained persistent febrile morbidity or leukocytosis.

Patients who have undergone extensive cytoreductive surgery require close monitoring, especially during the first 24 hours postoperatively. Many patients will have received large quantities of crystalloid, colloid, and blood products intraoperatively. In the setting of malnutrition, ascites, and pre-existing medical comorbidities, the management of postoperative fluid shifts often requires the close attention of the intensive care unit (ICU) or a step-down unit. Elderly patients, patients with medical comorbidities, and patients having undergone intestinal surgery are more likely to require ICU care.[21]

To ensure rapid return of bowel function, early refeeding should be encouraged in patients who have not undergone bowel resection or those who have undergone a diverting loop ileostomy. In patients who have undergone colon resection, we generally begin feeding clear liquids on the second postoperative day and advance to a low-residue diet as tolerated. In cases with concern for a tenuous anastomosis, conservative refeeding with solid food initiated at the onset of flatus can be considered, although data regarding its benefit are lacking.

Postoperative ileus is also a common complication in patients who have undergone extensive abdominal surgery and can occur as late as several days after the patient has resumed bowel function. Delayed onset of nausea and vomiting is suspicious of ileus/small bowel obstruction as well as abdominal abscess even in the absence of fever or leukocytosis. Usually, postoperative ileus can be managed with bowel rest and nasogastric decompression if nausea and vomiting are persistent with bowel rest.

Early ambulation is an important part of the recovery process following cytoreductive surgery, potentially reducing the rates of postoperative ileus and thromboembolic events. Regional anesthesia results in improved pain control and facilitates early ambulation. Physical therapy may be necessary to assist patients in the early postoperative period and assess the need for additional rehabilitation after discharge. This is especially important in elderly patients.

Most patients will have a bladder catheter placed for several days after surgery to monitor urine output. Urine output should be monitored closely as an indicator of intravascular fluid status. In the author's experience, failure to begin spontaneous diuresis within 7 days of surgery is suggestive of a postoperative infection or anastomotic leak as most patients will begin to have reduction in the "stress response" that results in salt retention by the kidneys. In patients with resection of bladder peritoneum implants, we recommend leaving the Foley catheter in place for 5 to 7 days after surgery, and even longer if bladder resection is required. In these patients, a trial of void is generally recommended after catheter removal. Although urinary retention occurs in less than 10% of patients with epidural anesthesia to control laparotomy pain, we generally do not remove the Foley catheter until the epidural is removed, which usually occurs when the patient has tolerated a regular diet for 24 hours.

In patients who have intraperitoneal drains placed along the splenic bed following splenectomy with or without distal pancreatectomy, drain output should be measured daily, and if it increases or persists, it should be checked for amylase to evaluate for an unrecognized pancreatic leak. Amylase levels 3-fold higher than found in the serum may be suggestive of an unrecognized pancreatic leak. Management should include drain placement (if not already present) and close monitoring for signs of sepsis. If drain output and leukocytosis improve, the patient can resume a regular diet. Somatostatin can decrease fistula output but has not been shown to shorten the time to closure of the fistula.

Most patients should receive prophylactic anticoagulation with low molecular weight heparin starting on the first day after surgery if there are no concerns about active bleeding. This should continue throughout the hospitalization and should be considered for the first month after surgery in an outpatient setting to reduce the risk of postoperative thromboembolic events.

Patients who are scheduled to undergo cytoreductive surgery for suspected advanced ovarian cancer should be counseled by the operating surgeon about a number of short- and long-term complications that may affect their ability to care for themselves after surgery. This should include the potential for discharge with unanticipated stomas, urinary catheters, peritoneal drains, and wound infections. Discharge planning should begin several days prior to discharge, with a thorough assessment of all potential homecare needs. Patients occasionally require placement in rehabilitation facilities. Elderly patients and those who have enduring immobilization during a prolonged intensive care unit stay are most at risk for needing rehabilitation placement.

REFERENCES

1. Diaz JP, Abu-Rustum NR, Sonoda Y, et al. Video-assisted thoracic surgery (VATS) evaluation of pleural effusions in patients with newly diagnosed advanced ovarian carcinoma can influence the primary management choice for these patients. *Gynecol Oncol.* 2010;116(3):483-488.

2. Montz FJ, Schlaerth JB, Berek JS. Resection of diaphragmatic peritoneum and muscle: role in cytoreductive surgery for ovarian cancer. *Gynecol Oncol.* 1989;35(3):338-340.

3. Aletti GD, Dowdy SC, Podratz KC, Cliby WA. Surgical treatment of diaphragm disease correlates with improved survival in optimally debulked advanced stage ovarian cancer. *Gynecol Oncol.* 2006;100(2):283-287.

4. Silver DF. Full-thickness diaphragmatic resection with simple and secure closure to accomplish complete cytoreductive surgery for patients with ovarian cancer. *Gynecol Oncol.* 2004;95(2): 384-387.

5. Finley DJ, Abu-Rustum NR, Chi DS, Flores R. Reconstructive techniques after diaphragm resection. *Thorac Surg Clin.* 2009;19(4):531-535.

6. Zivanovic O, Sima CS, Iasonos A, et al. The effect of primary cytoreduction on outcomes of patients with FIGO stage IIIC ovarian cancer stratified by the initial tumor burden in the upper abdomen cephalad to the greater omentum. *Gynecol Oncol.* 2010;116(3):351-357.

7. Chi DS, Eisenhauer EL, Zivanovic O, et al. Improved progression-free and overall survival in advanced ovarian cancer as a result of a change in surgical paradigm. *Gynecol Oncol.* 2009;114(1):26-31.

8. Houvenaeghel G, Gutowski M, Buttarelli M, et al. Modified posterior pelvic exenteration for ovarian cancer. *Int J Gynecol Cancer.* 2009;19(5):968-973.

9. Hoffman MS, Zervose E. Colon resection for ovarian cancer: intraoperative decisions. *Gynecol Oncol.* 2008;111(suppl 2): S56-S65.

10. Bristow RE, Montz FJ. Complete surgical cytoreduction of advanced ovarian carcinoma using the argon beam coagulator. *Gynecol Oncol.* 2001;83(1):39-48.

11. Bristow RE, Smith Sehdev AE, Kaufman HS, Montz FJ. Ablation of metastatic ovarian carcinoma with the argon beam coagulator: pathologic analysis of tumor destruction. *Gynecol Oncol.* 2001;83(1):49-55.

12. Go PM, Bruhn EW, Garry SL, Hunter JG. Patterns of small intestinal injury with the argon beam coagulator. *Surg Gynecol Obstet.* 1990;171(4):341-342.

13. van Dam PA, Tjalma W, Weyler J, et al. Ultraradical debulking of epithelial ovarian cancer with the ultrasonic surgical aspirator: a prospective randomized trial. *Am J Obstet Gynecol.* 1996;174(3):943-950.

14. Thompson MA, Adelson MD, Jozefczyk MA, et al. Structural and functional integrity of ovarian tumor tissue obtained by ultrasonic aspiration. *Cancer.* 1991;67(5):1326-1331.

15. Rose PG. The cavitational ultrasonic surgical aspirator for cytoreduction in advanced ovarian cancer. *Am J Obstet Gynecol.* 1992;166(3):843-846.

16. Eisenkop SM, Nalick RH, Wang HJ, Teng NN. Peritoneal implant elimination during cytoreductive surgery for ovarian cancer: impact on survival. *Gynecol Oncol.* 1993;51(2):224-229.

17. Donovan JT, Veronikis DK, Powell JL, et al. Cytoreductive surgery for ovarian cancer with the Cavitron Ultrasonic Surgical Aspirator and the development of disseminated intravascular coagulation. *Obstet Gynecol.* 1994;83(6):1011-1014.

18. van Dam PA, Coppens M, van Oosterom AT, et al. Is there an increased risk for tumor dissemination using ultrasonic surgical aspiration in patients with vulvar carcinoma? *Eur J Obstet Gynecol Reprod Biol.* 1994;55(2):145-147.

19. Nahhas WA. A potential hazard of the use of the surgical ultrasonic aspirator in tumor reductive surgery. *Gynecol Oncol.* 1991;40(1):81-83.

20. Millbourn D, Cengiz Y, Israelsson LA. Effect of stitch length on wound complications after closure of midline incisions: a randomized controlled trial. *Arch Surg.* 2009;144(11):1056-1059.

21. Brooks SE, Ahn J, Mullins CD, Baquet CR. Resources and use of the intensive care unit in patients who undergo surgery for ovarian carcinoma. *Cancer.* 2002;95(7):1457-1462.

Minimally Invasive Surgery

Pedro T. Ramirez, Michael Frumovitz, and Pedro F. Escobar

INTRODUCTION

Minimally invasive surgery is currently considered a safe and viable option in the management of most gynecologic malignancies. Compared to standard laparotomy, laparoscopic or robotic surgery is associated with lower blood loss and transfusion rates, lower intraoperative complication rates, decreased analgesic requirements in the immediate postoperative period, shorter length of hospitalization, lower postoperative complication rates, quicker return of bowel function, and improved short-term quality of life.

This chapter provides an overview of the standard laparoscopic procedures and robotic surgery. Details on the preoperative evaluation and postoperative care of patients undergoing the procedures described and specific steps for the more commonly performed procedures are provided. Because the anatomical dissections are the same as for open procedures (see Chapters 25 and 26), the illustrations and figures are limited to those aspects specific to the minimally invasive surgical approach.

LAPAROSCOPIC SURGERY

Cervical Cancer

Laparoscopic Radical Hysterectomy

Procedure Overview
Since the initial publications by Nezhat et al[1] and Canis et al,[2] several retrospective studies have documented the safety and feasibility of total laparoscopic radical

hysterectomy (TLRH), with a major complication rate of just 5%.[3] In a study by Frumovitz et al,[4] the authors compared 35 women who had undergone TLRH to 54 women who had open radical hysterectomy (ORH) and found significantly less blood loss, shorter length of hospital stay, and increased operative time for the TLRH group. Transfusion rates were low in both groups (15% for ORH vs. 11% for TLRH). Intraoperative and postoperative noninfectious complications were the same for both groups, but the ORH group had a significantly higher postoperative infectious complication rate than the TLRH group (53% vs. 18%, respectively). These complications included postoperative febrile morbidity, wound cellulitis, urinary tract infections, pneumonia, and intra-abdominal abscesses.

In evaluating oncologic outcomes, it appears that there is equivalency between TLRH and ORH. In their large series of 295 women who underwent TLRH, Chen et al[3] reported overall disease-free survival rates of 95% for women with stage IA disease and 96% for women with stage IB disease.

Box 31-1	Master Surgeon's Corner

- Proper patient positioning with steep Trendelenburg will facilitate pelvic exposure and dissection.
- Develop the avascular paravesical and pararectal spaces early in the course of operation to facilitate exposure to the parametria for ureteral dissection.

Preoperative Management

Patients with early-stage cervical cancer scheduled for a radical hysterectomy should routinely undergo a chest x-ray and blood type and cross. The use of other imaging modalities such as computed tomography (CT) or magnetic resonance imaging (MRI) scans is not recommended, unless there is evidence to suspect metastatic disease.

All patients should undergo bowel preparation 1 day prior to surgery and receive antibiotic prophylaxis on the day of surgery. The choice of bowel preparation used by the authors is HalfLytely (polyethylene glycol), and the antibiotic regimen most frequently recommended is cefoxitin 2 g intravenously. Although there is no standard regimen for thromboembolic prophylaxis, patients should either undergo administration of subcutaneous heparin (5000 U) preoperatively or have compression devices used during the procedure and subsequently until ambulation.

Surgical Technique

Initial Steps. After induction of general anesthesia, the patient is placed in the low lithotomy position using Allen stirrups. Typically, the patient's arms are tucked at her sides. Care must be taken to protect the patient's hands and fingers when the foot of the table is raised or lowered (Figure 31-1). Monitors are placed at the foot of the table.

After the patient is prepared and draped, a Foley catheter is placed under sterile conditions. A sterile speculum is then placed into the vagina, and a single-toothed tenaculum is used to grasp the anterior lip of the cervix. A uterine manipulator is placed. The preferred uterine manipulator used by the authors is the V-Care manipulator (Conmed Endosurgery, Utica, NY).

Incision Placement. A 12-mm Xcel Bladeless Trocar (Ethicon Endo-Surgery, Cincinnati, OH) that incorporates a 0-degree laparoscope is placed at the level of the umbilicus and introduced into the abdominal cavity under direct visualization. In patients with a prior midline incision, the initial entry into the abdominal cavity is made approximately 2 cm below the left costal margin at the level of the midclavicular line to avoid injury to bowel adherent to the anterior abdominal wall. Once the trocar has been safely introduced into the abdominal cavity, the cavity is insufflated. The intra-abdominal pressure is maintained at 16 mm Hg. Two additional 5- or 12-mm Xcel Bladeless Trocars are placed in the right and left lower quadrants, and an additional 5-mm Xcel Bladeless Trocar is inserted in the midline above the pubic symphysis (Figure 31-2).

Retroperitoneal Exploration. The pelvis and abdomen are thoroughly explored to rule out intraperitoneal disease. The bowel is then mobilized into the upper abdomen, and the round ligaments are transected bilaterally. An incision is made in the peritoneum over the psoas muscle immediately lateral to the infundibulopelvic ligament. The infundibulopelvic ligament is retracted medially to permit identification of the ureter. The iliac vessels are also exposed at this time. The lymph-bearing tissue is then probed to rule out any obvious metastatic disease to the pelvic lymph nodes. Any suspicious nodes are removed and sent for frozen-section examination. Barring obvious lymph node metastasis, the pelvic lymph node dissection is completed after the radical hysterectomy.

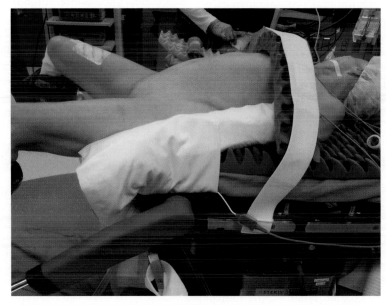

FIGURE 31-1. Patient positioning for laparoscopic surgery.

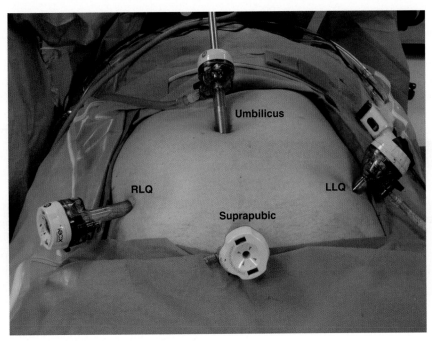

FIGURE 31-2. Trocar placement for standard laparoscopic procedures. LLQ, left lower quadrant; RLQ, right lower quadrant.

Parametrial and Bladder Dissection. The paravesical space is dissected by following the external iliac vessels distally and placing medial traction on the superior vesical artery. The pararectal space is identified by dissecting between the internal iliac vessels and the lateral aspect of the ureter. Once these spaces have been created, one can easily identify the uterine vessels. After identification, the uterine vessels are transected at the point of origin from the internal iliac vessels. The uterine artery and vein are transected together. The bladder peritoneum is incised across the anterior aspect of the uterus and dissected down off the cervix. The bladder should be mobilized to below the level of the cup of the uterine manipulator to assure there is an adequate surgical margin of at least 1 to 2 cm. This can be performed by pushing the uterine manipulator cephalad with the uterus straight along its axis. We take particular care at this point in the procedure to completely separate the bladder fibers from the anterior vagina because this facilitates closure of the vaginal cuff at the end of the procedure.

The ureters are separated from their medial attachments to the peritoneum. The parametrial tissue is mobilized medially over the ureters. The ureters are unroofed to the point of their insertion into the bladder bilaterally. The lateral aspect of the vesicouterine ligament is then divided, and the bladder is further mobilized inferiorly to ensure adequate vaginal margins. The uterus is anteflexed using the uterine manipulator, and blunt graspers are used to apply counter traction across the posterior cul-de-sac. The peritoneum above the sigmoid colon and rectum is then incised, exposing

the rectovaginal space. The attachments between the rectum and the vagina are cut in the midline, exposing the uterosacral ligaments. The uterosacral ligaments are then divided.

Circumferential Vaginotomy and Closure. Once the previously described procedures are complete, the cervix is now free of all its vascular and suspensory attachments, and the specimen can be removed. A circumferential incision is made into the vagina along the ring of the uterine manipulator. The specimen is completely separated from the upper vagina and removed. The vaginal cuff is sutured laparoscopically.

Box 31-2   Caution Points

- Ensure that the patient's legs are properly positioned and the hands protected to avoid inadvertent injury.
- Maintain direct visualization of the ureter when using thermal energy for parametrial dissection and division of vascular pedicles.

Postoperative Management
Patients undergoing laparoscopic radical hysterectomy are routinely placed on a demand intravenous analgesic pump and an oral analgesic regimen. All patients are ordered a regular diet on the evening of surgery. A Foley catheter is left in place postoperatively for a total of 5 to 7 days. A trial of void is attempted at that time, and if the postvoid residual is less than 150 mL, the catheter

is removed. If the patient fails the voiding trial, then the catheter is left in place for another week. We do not routinely recommend thromboembolic prophylaxis postoperatively in patients undergoing minimally invasive surgery. A study by Nick et al[5] in patients undergoing laparoscopic surgery showed that the rate of a deep venous thromboembolism or pulmonary embolism was 0.7%.

| Box 31-3 | Complications and Morbidity |

- Ureteral or bladder injury (1%-3%)
- Delayed recovery of bladder function
- Port site hematoma or hernia

Laparoscopic Staging for Locally Advanced Cervical Cancer

Procedure Overview

Surgical staging of patients with locally advanced cervical cancer remains controversial. An open transperitoneal approach is associated with high morbidity and mortality secondary to bowel complications, particularly when surgery is followed by radiotherapy. An extraperitoneal approach by laparotomy has been shown to decrease the complication rate from 30% to 2% compared with the transperitoneal approach.[6]

As many as 22% of patients with stage IB2 to IV cervical cancer and negative para-aortic lymph nodes on preoperative CT or combined positron emission tomography (PET)/CT imaging will be found to harbor metastatic disease in the para-aortic nodes when submitted to laparoscopic extraperitoneal staging.[7] These findings strongly argue for the consideration of surgical staging in patients with locally advanced cervical cancer for diagnostic purposes. In addition, LeBlanc et al[8] found a therapeutic effect from surgical staging of locally advanced cervical cancer. In their study of 184 patients with stage IB2 to IVA cervical cancer, they found that women with microscopic metastatic disease to the para-aortic lymph nodes had the same survival as women who had pathologically negative lymph nodes.

| Box 31-4 | Master Surgeon's Corner |

- Detection of microscopic metastatic para-aortic nodal disease will facilitate disease-directed radiation therapy field selection for patients with locally advanced cervical cancer.
- Both transperitoneal and extraperitoneal laparoscopic staging techniques are preferable to open laparotomy for preradiation treatment staging of cervical cancer.
- Carefully mark out planned incision sites according to anatomic landmarks.

Preoperative Management

Patients scheduled to undergo surgical staging of locally advanced cervical cancer routinely undergo a PET/CT imaging evaluation. Alternatively, a CT scan of the chest, abdomen, and pelvis is recommended. Patients should have no evidence of metastatic disease prior to undergoing surgery. Routine bowel preparation, antibiotic prophylaxis, and thromboembolic prophylaxis are recommended.

Surgical Technique

Initial Steps. The patient is placed in a supine position under general anesthesia with the right arm adducted and secured and the left arm placed at a right angle to the patient. A 5-mm endoscope is placed at the inferior margin of the umbilicus. The abdominal and pelvic cavities are inspected for intraperitoneal metastatic disease.

Development of Extraperitoneal Space. If the intraperitoneal inspection is clear, a 15-mm incision is made 3 to 4 cm medial and superior to the left anterior iliac spine. The skin, fascia, transverse muscles, and deep fascia are incised, with care taken not to open the peritoneum. The surgeon's left forefinger is introduced in the incision to free the peritoneal sac from the deep surface of the muscles of the abdominal wall under laparoscopic monitoring. A 10-mm balloon-tip trocar is then placed in the extraperitoneal space of the flank. The retroperitoneum is insufflated to a pressure not exceeding 15 mm Hg. At the same time, the peritoneal cavity is deflated. The laparoscope is then introduced through the balloon-tip trocar. A second 10-mm trocar is then introduced into the extraperitoneal space. The penetration point is located in the midaxillary line under the subcostal margin approximately 5 cm cephalad to and 3 to 4 cm lateral to the initial point. A 5-mm trocar is then placed 3 to 4 cm cephalad to this second 10-mm trocar (Figure 31-3).

Removal of Common Iliac and Para-Aortic Nodes. The dissection is performed bilaterally from the level of the common iliac vessels to the level of the left renal vein (Figure 31-4). When there is evidence of grossly positive lymph nodes, these are sent to pathology for frozen-section evaluation. If metastatic disease is confirmed, the laparoscopic procedure is aborted. At the completion of the procedure, all patients have an incision performed in the peritoneum overlying the left paracolic gutter to minimize the likelihood of development of postoperative lymphocysts. If a patient is found to have a grossly positive node, then the incision on the peritoneum is not performed. This is to reduce the potential of spread of disease to the peritoneal cavity. No drains are placed at the completion of surgery.

CHAPTER 31

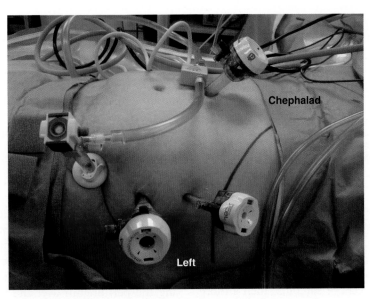

FIGURE 31-3. Trocar placement for extraperitoneal para-aortic lymphadenectomy.

| Box 31-5 | Caution Points |

- Careful blunt dissection is required to avoid entering the peritoneal cavity when developing the extraperitoneal space.
- Ensure that the ureters are under direct visualization when using thermal energy to dissect nodal tissue.

Postoperative Management

This procedure is routinely performed as an outpatient procedure. No drains are placed at the completion of surgery. Most patients are placed on an oral analgesic regimen and are discharged from the hospital once they have voided and tolerated a regular diet. Generally,

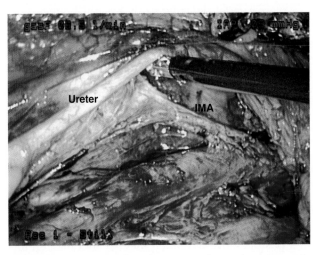

FIGURE 31-4. Completed extraperitoneal para-aortic lymphadenectomy. IMA, inferior mesenteric artery.

patients are able to start treatment with chemotherapy and radiation within 14 days from their surgery.

| Box 31-6 | Complications and Morbidity |

- Vascular injury
- Ureteral injury
- Retroperitoneal lymphocyst formation

Uterine Cancer

Simple Hysterectomy and Staging

Procedure Overview

The introduction of minimally invasive surgery as a treatment option for women with endometrial cancer began in the early 1990s with multiple reports of laparoscopic-assisted vaginal hysterectomy and lymph node staging. In 1996, the Gynecologic Oncology Group opened LAP2, a randomized controlled trial assigning patients to laparoscopy or laparotomy in a 2:1 ratio. Upon completion, 2516 patients were evaluable.[9]

As expected, operative time was longer in the laparoscopy group versus the laparotomy group (204 minutes vs. 104 minutes, respectively), but hospital length of stay was shorter (3 days vs. 4 days, respectively). Only 52% of patients who underwent laparoscopy stayed for more than 2 days compared to 94% of patients who had a laparotomy. There was no difference in intraoperative complications between the 2 groups, although 26% of patients in the laparoscopy group required conversion to laparotomy. Grade 2 or greater postoperative complications were significantly higher in the laparotomy group compared to the laparoscopy group (21% vs. 14%, respectively).

Box 31-7	Master Surgeon's Corner

- Laparoscopic hysterectomy and staging for endometrial cancer are feasible in the majority of patients, including the obese and morbidly obese.
- Procedural success is dependent on achieving steep Trendelenburg position with adequate exposure to the abdominal retroperitoneum.

Preoperative Management

Patients with a diagnosis of endometrial cancer routinely undergo a chest x-ray evaluation prior to surgery. If the patient has a preoperative diagnosis of a high-risk type of endometrial cancer such as papillary serous carcinoma, clear cell, or sarcoma, then a more extensive evaluation such as a CT or MRI scan of the abdomen and pelvis is recommended.

Surgical Technique

Laparoscopic Hysterectomy. The patient setup and port placement for a simple hysterectomy are the same as those described earlier for a radical hysterectomy. Once all ports have been placed and the patient is in steep Trendelenburg position, the procedure is started by coagulating and transecting the round ligaments. While the assistant places lateral traction on the right round ligament, the surgeon holds the medial aspect of the round ligament, and the peritoneum over the external iliac vessels is opened to expose the retroperitoneal space. The ureter is identified. The infundibulopelvic ligament is then transected. While placing upward traction on the uterus, the uterine vessels are skeletonized.

The same procedure is performed on the left side. Care must be taken to dissect the reflection of the colon off the left infundibulopelvic ligament to assure an adequate distance between bowel and the instrument coagulating the left infundibulopelvic ligament. Similarly, the left uterine vessels are skeletonized. Attention is then placed on mobilizing the bladder peritoneum inferiorly. This is performed while placing upward traction on the uterus.

The uterine vessels are coagulated and transected bilaterally. The pedicles of the descending branches of the uterine vessels are then coagulated and cut. Once the reflection of the ring of the uterine manipulator is visualized, a colpotomy is performed circumferentially around the demarcation of the ring, and the specimen is removed vaginally. The vaginal cuff is then sutured closed by laparoscopy.

Lymph Node Dissection. In patients requiring a lymph node dissection, the pelvic lymphadenectomy is performed by removing all lymph node–bearing tissue along the pelvic vessels. The most cephalad point of the dissection is the common iliac vessels, and the distal margin is the circumflex iliac vessels. Inferiorly, the margins of dissection extend to the obturator nerve, and the medial margins are the internal iliac vessels.

To perform a para-aortic lymphadenectomy, it is recommended that all monitors are moved to a location near the patient's right and left shoulder. The surgeon stands on the patient's left side, and the assistant stands on the patient's right side. The surgeon holds a grasper in his or her left hand through the suprapubic port and a coagulating-cutting device in the right hand through the left lower quadrant port. The assistant holds a grasper in his or her right hand through the right lower quadrant port and the camera in the left hand at the umbilicus. The procedure is started by transecting the peritoneum over the bifurcation of the aorta medial to the right ureter. While the assistant places upward and lateral traction on the peritoneum, the surgeon develops a space above the inferior vena cava and the right ureter to identify the lateral boundary of dissection, the psoas muscle. The lymphatic tissue over the vena cava is removed to the level of the insertion of the right gonadal vein. The left para-aortic nodes are retrieved by placing lateral traction on the peritoneum, identifying the left ureter, and subsequently removing all the lymphatic tissue below the inferior mesenteric artery. Dissection of the lymph nodes above the inferior mesenteric artery is more challenging and requires excellent exposure to minimize injury to the renal vessels. The peritoneum is further mobilized laterally; the lymphatic tissue is then removed to the level of the left renal vessels.

Box 31-8	Caution Point

- If a uterine manipulator is used, it should be placed under direct laparoscopic visualization to avoid inadvertent uterine perforation and spillage of malignant cells into the peritoneal cavity.

Postoperative Management

Patients undergoing laparoscopic simple hysterectomy and staging are routinely placed on a demand intravenous analgesic pump and an oral analgesic regimen. All patients are ordered a regular diet on the evening of surgery. A Foley catheter is left in place until the morning after surgery. The use of thromboembolic prophylaxis postoperatively is not routinely recommended. Patients are usually discharged home on the first postoperative day when they are ambulating, tolerating a regular diet, and voiding spontaneously.

Box 31-9	Complications and Morbidity

- Ureteral or bladder injury (1%-3%)
- Conversion to laparotomy (7%-26%)

ROBOTIC SURGERY

The da Vinci Surgical System (Intuitive Surgical, Sunnyvale, CA) was approved by the Food and Drug Administration for gynecologic indications in 2005. Introduction of this robotic surgical system has addressed many of the obstacles of conventional laparoscopy including lack of depth perception, limited range of motion, unstable camera, and a steep learning curve. The da Vinci system provides 3-dimensional visualization, improved dexterity with 7 degrees of freedom mimicking the surgeon's actual wrist movements, restoration of proper hand-eye coordination, and an ergonomic position.

Cervical Cancer

Robotic Radical Hysterectomy

Procedure Overview

Since the initial report of robotic radical hysterectomy in 2006 by Sert and Abeler,[10] a number of other investigators have reported on the safety and feasibility of this approach in the management of patients with early-stage cervical cancer. Magrina et al[11] compared 3 groups of patients who underwent radical hysterectomy: robotic, laparoscopy, and laparotomy. The authors concluded that surgical outcomes in the robotic and laparoscopy groups were similar and that these procedures

were preferable to laparotomy. Blood loss and length of hospital stay were similar for the 2 minimally invasive groups and were reduced significantly when compared with laparotomy. There were no significant differences in complications between the 3 groups.

Recently, Cantrell et al[12] evaluated survival outcomes for women who underwent robotic type III radical hysterectomy for cervical cancer. The authors assessed progression-free survival (PFS) and overall survival (OS) as their primary end points. Comparison was made to a group of historical open radical hysterectomies. The authors found that at 3 years, there was no statistically significant difference in PFS or OS between the 2 groups.

Preoperative Management

The preoperative evaluation and postoperative management of patients undergoing robotic radical hysterectomy are the same as those described earlier for laparoscopic radical hysterectomy.

Surgical Technique

Initial Steps. The patient is placed in the semilithotomy position using the Allen stirrups (Allen Medical, Acton, MA) with the arms loosely tucked to each side. Foam padding is used to protect both arms and legs. The patient is placed on her back directly on an antiskid foam material (Figure 31-5). Two monitors are located at each side of the operating table at the level of the patient's knees. The robotic tower and the tower containing the electrosurgical generators are positioned lateral to the patient's right foot. The da Vinci column may be positioned between the patient's feet or to the side of the patient (side-docking) to allow ample access to the vagina.

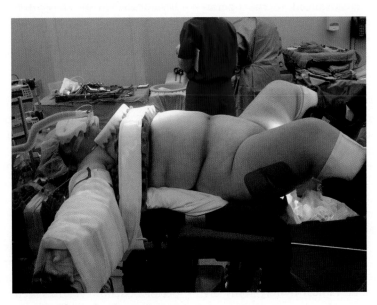

FIGURE 31-5. Patient positioning for robotic surgery.

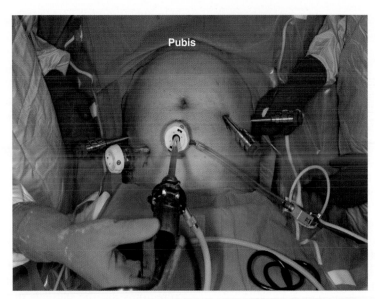

FIGURE 31-6. Routine trocar placement for robotic surgery.

Trocar Placement. A 12-mm Xcel trocar is placed approximately 2 cm below the left costal margin. This trocar will be used by the assistant during the case. The patient is then placed in steep Trendelenburg position, and the abdomen is inspected for any evidence of metastatic disease. If none is found, then a 12-mm transumbilical trocar is introduced under direct visualization. Three 8-mm trocars, specific for the da Vinci robotic system, are placed. The first is placed 8 to 10 cm lateral to the assistant trocar on the left side. The second is placed 8 to 10 cm lateral and to the right of the umbilical trocar, and the third is placed 8 to 10 cm lateral to the right abdominal robotic trocar (Figure 31-6). Similar to the laparoscopy approach, we use a V-Care uterine manipulator.

The robotic column is advanced to the operating table and placed between the patient's feet. The robotic arms are attached to each robotic trocar, and the robotic instruments are introduced. An EndoWrist Precise bipolar grasper (Intuitive Surgical) is used in the left robotic arm. An EndoWrist monopolar scissors (Intuitive Surgical) is used in the right robotic arm. An EndoWrist Cardiere grasper (Intuitive Surgical) is placed in the fourth robotic arm. For vaginal cuff closure, the monopolar scissors is replaced by an EndoWrist needle holder (Intuitive Surgical).

Radical Hysterectomy. The steps of the radical hysterectomy by the robotics approach are the same as those for the laparoscopic radical hysterectomy described earlier.

Postoperative Management

Patients undergoing robotic radical hysterectomy are routinely placed on a demand intravenous analgesic pump and an oral analgesic regimen. All patients are ordered a regular diet on the evening of surgery. A Foley catheter is left in place postoperatively for a total of 5 to 7 days. A trial of void is attempted at that time, and if the postvoid residual is less than 150 mL, the catheter is removed. If the patient fails the voiding trial, then the catheter is left in place for another week. Routine use of thromboembolic prophylaxis is not recommended.

Robotic Radical Trachelectomy

Procedure Overview

Radical trachelectomy is performed in selected patients diagnosed with early-stage cervical cancer who wish to preserve their fertility. Since the procedure was first described by Dargent et al[13] in 1994, numerous reports have documented the safety and feasibility of the vaginal approach.[14,15] Alternatively, the procedure may also be performed successfully via the abdominal approach.[16,17]

Persson et al[18] were the first to report on the robotic approach in performing fertility-sparing surgery in patients with gynecologic malignancies. Since that time, others have added their experience to the published literature.[19] To date, there is a paucity of data regarding whether the robotics approach is equivalent to the open or vaginal approach with regard to oncologic and obstetrical outcomes.

Preoperative Management

Patients considered for robotic radical trachelectomy are counseled regarding the option of radical hysterectomy. A formal infertility evaluation is not routinely performed; however, this is encouraged in patients who have been unsuccessful in prior pregnancy attempts.

In the preoperative counseling, it is also important to stress the fact that approximately 30% of patients scheduled to have a radical trachelectomy will not be able to conceive due to factors such as lymph node positivity, close (< 5 mm) surgical margins, or the need for adjuvant radiation therapy postoperatively.

All patients undergo a routine chest x-ray to rule out the possibility of spread of disease to the chest. An MRI of the pelvis is recommended to evaluate the extent of the tumor in the cervix and assure that the tumor does not extend to the upper endocervical margin because this could increase the likelihood of having to convert to a radical hysterectomy. In addition, this imaging study allows for evaluation of the pelvic lymph nodes to determine whether there is any suspicion of lymph node metastases. A preoperative pregnancy test should be performed on the day of surgery.

Surgical Technique

Initial Steps. The patient is placed in the dorsal lithotomy position. A V-Care manipulator is placed in the uterus for manipulation. Once the manipulator is placed, attention is focused on the abdominal part of the procedure. Trocar placement is as described earlier for the robotic radical hysterectomy.

Retroperitoneal Dissection and Division of Uterine Vessels. First, an incision is made over the round ligament, and the peritoneum lateral to the infundibulopelvic ligament is opened bilaterally. The paravesical and pararectal spaces are then developed. The ureters are then separated from the peritoneum down to where they enter the lateral parametrial tissue. The level of resection of the parametria is as follows: The ureters are dissected from the parametria and mobilized completely to the bladder after division of the anterior and posterior vesicouterine ligaments. The peritoneum over the bladder is then incised, and the bladder is mobilized inferiorly over the anterior vaginal wall. The uterine vessels are transected bilaterally at their origin and dissected over the ureters bilaterally. The anterior vesicouterine ligaments are then divided.

Excision of Cervix and Closure. The peritoneum over the rectovaginal space is then incised, and the uterosacral ligaments are divided bilaterally. While upward traction is placed on the vaginal cuff, a circumferential incision is made approximately 2 cm below the vaginal stump. The V-Care manipulator is then removed. The specimen is then held by the parametria bilaterally using graspers. A monopolar scissors is used to amputate the cervix, leaving approximately 1 cm of residual cervical stump. The specimen—including cervix, bilateral parametria, and upper vaginal margin—is then removed through the vagina. The specimen is then sent for frozen-section evaluation. The endocervical

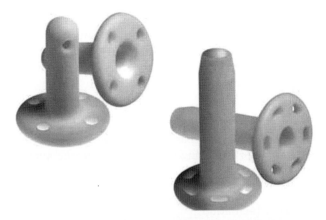

FIGURE 31-7. Smit sleeve used for radical trachelectomy.

margin should be tumor free at least 10 mm from the level of the tumor. A Smit sleeve cannula (Nucletron, Columbia, MD) (Figure 31-7) is then introduced vaginally and placed into the uterus by using the robotic graspers. The Smit sleeve is secured to the uterus with 3-0 chromic sutures. We use the Smit sleeve cannula to decrease the potential for scarring of the residual cervix. It is usually left in the uterus for approximately 2 to 4 weeks. A cerclage is placed using 0 Ethibond suture, and the uterus is sutured to the upper vagina using 0 Vicryl sutures placed using the EndoWrist Mega Needle driver. The cerclage is placed abdominally using the robotic system. The pelvic lymphadenectomy is performed bilaterally using the same anatomical landmarks as for a radical hysterectomy.

Postoperative Management

Patients undergoing robotic radical trachelectomy have a similar plan of management as patients undergoing a radical hysterectomy. An intravenous analgesic pump and an oral analgesic regimen are ordered. A regular diet is ordered on the evening of surgery. A Foley catheter is left in place postoperatively for a total of 5 to 7 days. A trial of voiding is attempted at that time, and if the postvoid residual is less than 150 mL, the catheter is removed. If the patient fails the voiding trial, then the catheter is left in place for another week. Routine use of thromboembolic prophylaxis is not recommended. The Smit sleeve is removed approximately 4 weeks postoperatively.

Robotic Extraperitoneal Para-Aortic Staging

Procedure Overview

The robotics approach has also been reported in the setting of surgical staging of patients with locally advanced cervical cancer prior to chemotherapy and radiation. The first series published on the robotics approach in this setting was by Vergote et al.[20] In that

CHAPTER 31

series, the authors reported on 5 patients who underwent the procedure. The median body mass index of the group was 24.4 kg/m² (range, 19.3-28.8 kg/m²). The median number of lymph nodes retrieved was 9 (range, 7-12 nodes).

Preoperative Management

The preoperative preparation for robotic extraperitoneal para-aortic staging is the same as for the laparoscopic approach.

Surgical Technique

Incision Placement and Development of Extraperitoneal Space. Under direct visualization through an umbilical port, a small incision is made 3 cm medial to the anterior superior iliac spine. The extraperitoneal space is developed by finger dissection of the peritoneum over the psoas muscle and left flank. A 10- to 12-mm Spacemaker Plus Dissector System (US Surgical, Norwalk, CT) is inserted 3 cm medial to the anterior superior iliac spine. The obturator with a balloon is inserted in a craniolateral direction through the trocar, and the balloon is inflated to its maximum. An 8-mm robotic trocar is inserted through the 10- to 12-mm Spacemaker Plus Dissector System. The 12-mm optical trocar is introduced through the patient's left flank along the posterior axillary line, 10 cm cranial, and lateral, from the caudal robotic trocar. A second 8-mm robotic trocar is placed 10 cm cranial, and medial, to the laparoscope, immediately below the left costal margin and in line with the caudal robotic trocar. The assistant trocar is inserted immediately adjacent to the anterior superior iliac spine, equidistant between the laparoscope and the caudal robotic trocar. A 30-degree laparoscope (InSite Vision System; Intuitive Surgical) is used.

Lymph Node Dissection. A retroperitoneal lymphadenectomy is performed including the left external iliac, presacral, and bilateral common iliac pelvic nodes and the aortic nodes from the aortic bifurcation to the renal vessels. For the removal of the presacral and common iliac nodes, the laparoscope is rotated 45 degrees counterclockwise, which provides additional instrument reach by avoiding collision of the robotic arms with the scope.

Postoperative Management

This procedure is routinely performed as an outpatient procedure. No drains are placed at the completion of surgery. Most patients are placed on an oral analgesic regimen and are discharged from the hospital once they have voided and tolerated a regular diet. Generally, patients are able to start treatment with chemotherapy and radiation within 14 days from their surgery.

Uterine Cancer

Simple Hysterectomy and Staging

Procedure Overview

Robotic surgery has also been shown to provide similar benefits as laparoscopic surgery when performing standard simple hysterectomy, bilateral salpingo-oophorectomy, and staging. In the largest series to date, Lowe et al[21] evaluated perioperative outcomes and learning curve characteristics from a multi-institutional experience with robotic surgical staging for endometrial cancer. Four hundred five patients were identified, with a mean age of 62.2 years and a mean body mass index of 32.4 kg/m². The mean operative time was 170.5 minutes, and the mean estimated blood loss was 87.5 mL. The mean lymph node count was 15.5, and the mean hospital stay for all patients was 1.8 days. An intraoperative complication occurred in 3.5% of the patients, and conversion to laparotomy occurred in 7%. The rate of postoperative complications was 14.6%.

Preoperative Management, Surgical Technique, and Postoperative Management

Preoperative preparation for patients scheduled to undergo a robotic simple hysterectomy and staging is the same as for laparoscopic hysterectomy. The patient setup, port placement, and instrumentation for the robotic simple hysterectomy are the same as for the robotic radical hysterectomy. The steps for this procedure and postoperative management are the same as those described for a laparoscopic simple hysterectomy.

SUMMARY

Minimally invasive surgery currently encompasses multiple modalities that allow the surgeon and the patient versatility in the surgical approach for the management of gynecologic malignancies. Laparoscopic surgery remains the foundation of the minimally invasive approach and should be a priority in the training of fellows and residents. Robotic surgery provides a more technologically advanced platform, enhancing surgeon dexterity, visualization, and comfort while at the same time offering equivalent or improved results compared with laparoscopy.

REFERENCES

1. Nezhat CR, Burrell MO, Nezhat FR, et al. Laparoscopic radical hysterectomy with para-aortic and pelvic node dissection. *Am J Obstet Gynecol.* 1992;166:864-865.
2. Canis M, Mage G, Wattiez A, et al. Does endoscopic surgery have a role in radical surgery of cancer of the cervix uteri? *J Gynecol Obstet Biol Reprod (Paris).* 1990;19:921.

3. Chen Y, Xu H, Li Y, et al. The outcome of laparoscopic radical hysterectomy and lymphadenectomy for cervical cancer: a prospective analysis of 295 patients. *Ann Surg Oncol.* 2008;15:2847-2855.

4. Frumovitz M, dos Reis R, Sun CC, et al. Comparison of total laparoscopic and abdominal radical hysterectomy for patients with early-stage cervical cancer. *Obstet Gynecol.* 2007;110:96-102.

5. Nick AM, Schmeler KM, Frumovitz M, et al. Risk of thromboembolic disease in patients undergoing laparoscopic gynecologic surgery. *Obstet Gynecol.* 2010;116:956-961.

6. Berman ML, Lagasse LD, Watring WG, et al. The operative evaluation of patients with cervical carcinoma by an extraperitoneal approach. *Obstet Gynecol.* 1977;50:658-664.

7. Ramirez PT, Jhingran A, Macapinlac H, et al. Laparoscopic extraperitoneal para-aortic lymphadenectomy in locally advanced cervical cancer: a prospective correlation of surgical findings with PET/CT findings. *Cancer.* 2011;117:1928-1934.

8. Leblanc E, Narducci F, Frumovitz M, et al. Therapeutic value of pretherapeutic extraperitoneal laparoscopic staging of locally advanced cervical carcinoma. *Gynecol Oncol.* 2007;105:304-311.

9. Walker JL, Piedmonte MR, Spirtos NM, et al. Laparoscopy compared with laparotomy for comprehensive surgical staging of uterine cancer: Gynecologic Oncology Group Study LAP2. *J Clin Oncol.* 2009;27:5331-5336.

10. Sert BM, Abeler VM. Robotic-assisted laparoscopic radical hysterectomy (Piver type III) with pelvic node dissection: case report. *Eur J Gynaecol Oncol.* 2006;27:531-533.

11. Magrina JF, Kho RM, Weaver AL, et al. Robotic radical hysterectomy: comparison with laparoscopy and laparotomy. *Gynecol Oncol.* 2008;109:86-91.

12. Cantrell LA, Mendivil A, Gehrig PA, et al. Survival outcomes for women undergoing type III robotic radical hysterectomy for cervical cancer: a 3-year experience. *Gynecol Oncol.* 2010;117:260-265.

13. Dargent D, Brun JL, Roy M, et al. Pregnancies following radical trachelectomy for invasive cervical cancer. *Gynecol Oncol.* 1994;52:105. Abstract.

14. Plante M. Radical vaginal trachelectomy: an update. *Gynecol Oncol.* 2008;111:S105-S110.

15. Hertel H, Kohler C, Grund D, et al. Radical vaginal trachelectomy (RVT) combined with laparoscopic pelvic lymphadenectomy: prospective multicenter study of 100 patients with early cervical cancer. *Gynecol Oncol.* 2006;103:506-511.

16. Ungar L, Palfalvi L, Hogg R, et al. Abdominal radical trachelectomy: a fertility-preserving option for women with early cervical cancer. *Br J Obstet Gynaecol.* 2005;112:366-369.

17. Nishio H, Fujii T, Kameyama K, et al. Abdominal radical trachelectomy as a fertility-sparing procedure in women with early-stage cervical cancer in a series of 61 women. *Gynecol Oncol.* 2009;115:51-55.

18. Persson J, Kannisto P, Bossmar T. Robot-assisted abdominal laparoscopic radical trachelectomy. *Gynecol Oncol.* 2008;111:564-567.

19. Ramirez PT, Schmeler KM, Malpica A, et al. Safety and feasibility of robotic radical trachelectomy in patients with early-stage cervical cancer. *Gynecol Oncol.* 2010;116:12-15.

20. Vergote I, Pouseele B, Van Gorp T, et al. Robotic retroperitoneal lower para-aortic lymphadenectomy in cervical carcinoma: first report on the technique used in 5 patients. *Acta Obstet Gynecol.* 2008;87:783-787.

21. Lowe MP, Johnson PR, Kamelle SA, et al. A multiinstitutional experience with robotic-assisted hysterectomy with staging for endometrial cancer. *Obstet Gynecol.* 2009;114:236-243.

Pelvic Exenteration

A. Total Pelvic Exenteration

Barbara A. Goff and Howard G. Muntz

PROCEDURE OVERVIEW

Total pelvic exenteration is a surgical procedure that involves the en bloc removal of female reproductive organs, rectosigmoid colon, and lower urinary tract. It may include a perineal phase to remove the urethra, vagina, and anus. Modifications can be made depending on tumor location and size.

The first series of pelvic exenterations was published in 1948 by Alexander Brunschwig for the palliative treatment of advanced pelvic malignancies.[1] Although the operative mortality in this group of 22 patients was 23%, there were also several long-term survivors, indicating potential benefit beyond palliation. The original operation included implanting both ureters into the colon to produce a wet colostomy; however, this resulted in significant problems with hyperchloremic acidosis, pyelonephritis, and renal failure. In 1956, Bricker[2] published a technique of using a closed loop of ileum as a bladder substitution. Over the past 50 years, there have been many advances in perioperative care such as blood products, antibiotics, intensive care support, and surgical techniques such as retractors, cautery, and staplers that now allow for a variety of vaginal reconstructions and urinary conduits that can reduce the impact this procedure has on quality of life.[3-10] As a result, pelvic exenteration is now considered a safe and feasible procedure that can cure selected patients for whom there are no other treatment options. In modern series, operative mortality ranges from 0% to 5%, and 5-year survival rates range from 39% to 53% depending on the specific indications for the exenteration.[3-7] Patient selection, patient preparation, surgical technique, and postoperative care can have a major impact on the outcome for patients undergoing this operation.

Indications

The main indication for pelvic exenteration is the central persistence or recurrence of cervical, vaginal, or vulvar cancer after primary radiation or chemoradiation. Central recurrence is defined as the absence of both pelvic sidewall involvement and distant disease. Some have advocated the use of exenteration for primary treatment of stage IVA cervical cancer; however, with modern chemoradiation, this has become uncommon. Long-term survival after exenterative surgery in women with pelvic failure after surgery and radiation for endometrial cancer or sarcomas has also been reported.[11,12] Extensive radiation injury to bladder, vagina, and/or rectum, especially if patients have evidence of significant necrosis with fistula formation, is another potential indication for exenteration.[7]

Exenterative surgery to resect centrally recurrent pelvic cancer is only rational in the absence of metastatic disease. Para-aortic nodal involvement is generally considered an absolute contraindication for exenteration. If pelvic lymph nodes are found to be the only site of metastatic disease, then patients can still be considered surgical candidates, although long-term cure rates will only be about 15%.[13] Palliative exenteration (documented extrapelvic disease with no expectation for cure) should be performed only if there is a high likelihood for significant improvement in quality of life, because 70% of patients will experience major complications.[6,8] In general, pelvic side-wall involvement is a contraindication to performing an exenteration, but with laterally extended endopelvic resections[14] or intraoperative radiation therapy,[15,16] selected patients can also be considered candidates for exenteration. Common selection criteria include the following: (1) a central pelvic malignancy potentially curable by exenteration; (2) absence of local or distant metastases; (3) medical and psychological fitness to withstand exenterative surgery; and (4) ability for postoperative self-care. The likelihood of discovering metastatic disease or an unresectable pelvic tumor at exploratory surgery and abandoning exenterative surgery is 30% to 50%, depending on preoperative selection criteria (eg, tumor size).

Classification of Exenteration

Pelvic exenteration includes 3 basic variations (Figure 32A-1). Total pelvic exenteration consists of en bloc removal of the gynecologic organs, bladder, and rectosigmoid colon. Anterior exenteration is a combination of radical hysterectomy-vaginectomy and cystectomy, and posterior exenteration is a combination of radical hysterectomy-vaginectomy and rectosigmoid colectomy. Pelvic exenteration can also be classified according to the extent of tissue resection and associated anatomical alteration (Figure 32A-2). A type I, or supralevator, exenteration is indicated for lesions confined to the upper pelvis without involvement of the lower one-half of the vagina. A type II, or infralevator, exenteration is the most commonly performed variation and includes visceral resection below the levator ani muscles with limited resection of the levator muscles and urogenital diaphragm. Rarely, a type III exenteration (infralevator with vulvectomy) is required for tumor extension to the vulva or perineum and includes resection of the urogenital diaphragm.

Expected Clinical Outcomes

Table 32A-1 shows clinical outcomes of the most contemporary series of pelvic exenterations.[3-7] Long-term disease-free survival ranges from 30% to 60% depending on nodal and margin status, time from initial radiation to recurrence, size of the lesion, and primary disease site.[3-10] Factors that have not been shown to impact survival are age and subsequent treatment following

exenteration. Operative mortality is quite low (0%-5%) and is usually a result of sepsis with multiorgan failure, pulmonary embolism, or cardiac events.

Surgical morbidity with pelvic exenteration can be substantial. The median estimated blood loss ranges from 1290 to 2500 mL, and 70% to 85% of patient will require blood transfusions. Median operative time is approximately 8 hours but varies widely depending on the reconstructive procedures that are done following the exenteration. The average length of stay following exenteration is 15 to 28 days. Major morbidity is seen in 30% to 50% of patients. The most common complications seen with exenterations include infection, abscess, anastomotic leaks, wound dehiscence, thromboembolic events, ileus, bowel obstruction, secondary bleeding, and cardiovascular events.[3-10]

Box 32A-1	Master Surgeon's Corner

- If a perineal phase is needed, have 2 surgical teams.
- Ligation of the anterior division of the internal iliac artery, once resectability has been determined, can reduce blood loss.
- In patients who are heavily irradiated, the use of flaps can significantly reduce the risk of infection and fistula formation.

PREOPERATIVE PREPARATION

Patient Evaluation and Work-up

A thorough preoperative assessment is mandatory. Assuming only physiologically fit and psychologically sound patients are being evaluated, the key factors for consideration include histologic confirmation of recurrent disease, resectability of the recurrent tumor, and absence of metastatic disease.

Because radiation necrosis can mimic the appearance of recurrent cancer (and vice versa), an examination under anesthesia should be performed with multiple biopsies, including deep Tru-cut biopsies. Directed biopsies obtained with interventional radiology guidance may be required.

Resectability of a centrally recurrent pelvic tumor is not always predictable. The triad of ipsilateral leg edema, sciatic pain, and ureteral obstruction is almost always associated with sidewall extension and unresectability. Evaluation of disease resectability can be aided by pelvic magnetic resonance imaging and positron emission tomography/computed tomography. However, in the setting of fibrosis, infection, and fistula

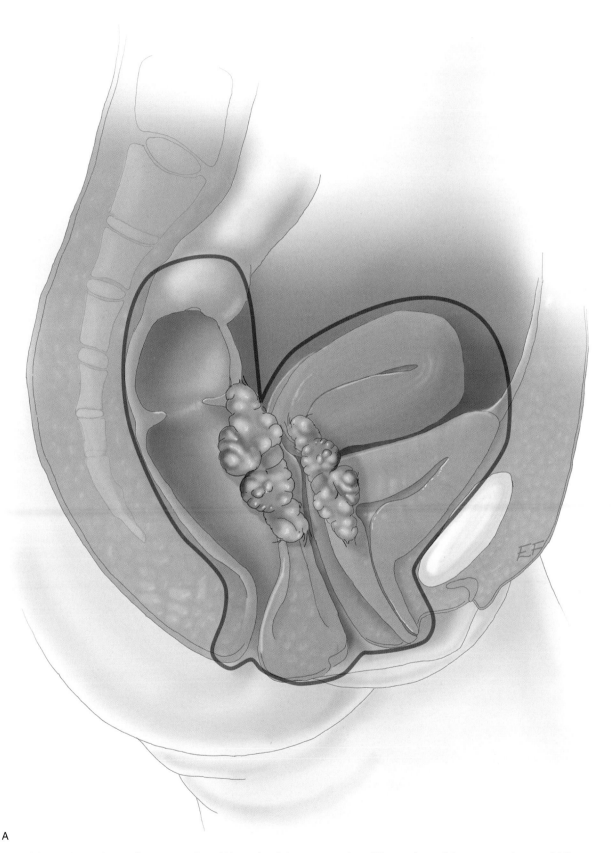

A

FIGURE 32A-1. Variations of exenteration: (A) total pelvic exenteration; **(B)** anterior pelvic exenteration; and **(C)** posterior pelvic exenteration.

B

FIGURE 32A-1. (Continued)

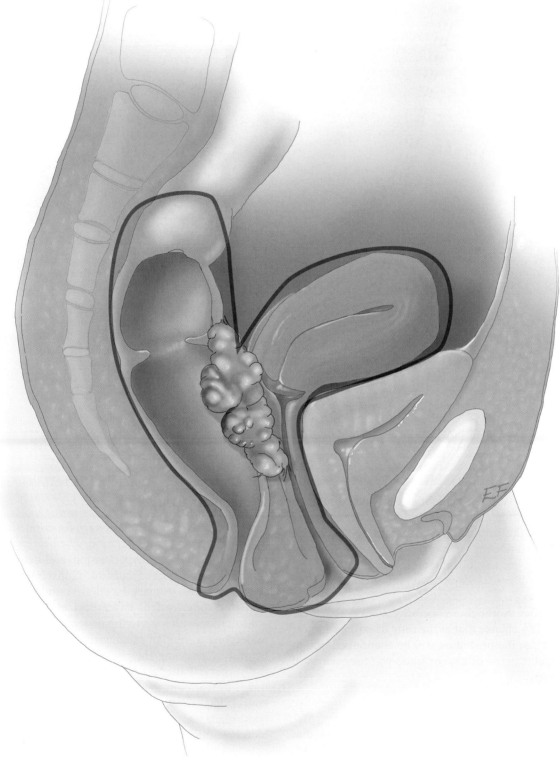

C

FIGURE 32A-1. *(Continued)*

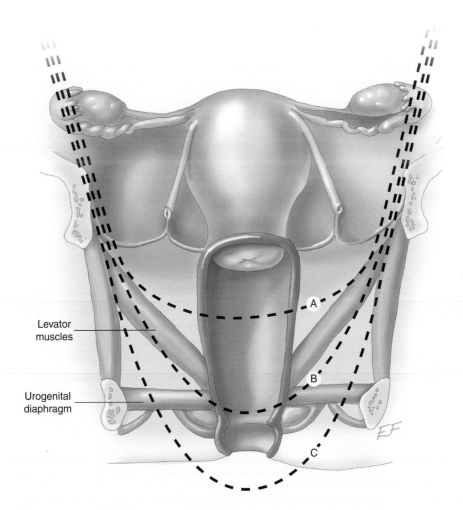

FIGURE 32A-2. Classification of pelvic exenteration: (A) supralevator exenteration; **(B)** infralevator exenteration; and **(C)** infralevator exenteration with vulvectomy.

formation, all of these modalities can have significant false-positive rates.[17-20] Examination under anesthesia is often the best way for a surgeon to determine sidewall involvement. If there is any question about resectability because of sidewall involvement, patients should be offered surgical exploration and possible exenteration.

Even after thorough preoperative assessment, there is still a 30% chance that at the time of exploration for exenteration, the procedure will be abandoned due to unresectable pelvic disease or small-volume peritoneal metastases.[20]

Consent Considerations

Patients should understand there is a 30% chance that the operation will not be completed,[20] and even if completed, cure rates vary widely (30%-60%).[3-10] Patients need to be counseled about the loss or severe alteration of bladder, rectal, and sexual function, as well as potential emotional distress.[21,22]

Patient Preparation

Nutritional status and pulmonary function should be optimized prior to exenteration. Medical comorbidities, such as diabetes, hypertension, and heart disease, should be under good control. Consultation with a stoma therapist to mark location(s) and review function is recommended. Psychological evaluation and consultation with a surviving patient having previously undergone a similar exenterative procedure may be helpful in assessing the patient's emotional readiness for surgery. Patients should undergo a mechanical bowel preparation the day before surgery and receive appropriate antibiotic and thromboembolic prophylaxis. Placement of a central line and having adequate blood product availability are also advised.

Required Instrumentation

Instrumentation for exenteration varies according to surgeon preference but should include a self-retaining

Levator muscles

Urogenital diaphragm

Table 32A-1 Clinical Outcomes of Pelvic Exenteration

Series	Berek et al[3] 2005 (N = 75)	Goldberg et al[4] 2006 (N = 103)	Maggioni et al[5] 2009 (N = 106)	McLean et al[7] 2010 (N = 44)	Fotopoulou et al[6] 2010 (N = 47[a])
Median procedure duration, hours	7.8	NR	8.1	9.5	5.4
Mean EBL, mL	2500	NR	1240	2497	NR
Postoperative mortality	3/75	1/103	0	1/44	4/47
Transfusions	4.9 U	NR	62%	86%	5 U
Length of hospitalization, days	23.4	NR	21.6	15	29
Survival	39%	47%	53%	52%	53%[b]
Complications					
Infection	86%	71%	NR	68%	NR
Fistula	27%	28%	NR	2%	NR
Intestinal obstruction	33%	9%	NR	18%	NR
Early complications	NR	NR	44.8%	NR	70%
Late complications	NR	NR	48.5%	NR	NR

EBL, estimated blood loss; NR, not reported; U, median number of units.
[a]Twenty-two cases done for palliation.
[b]Median follow-up was 7 months.

retractor such as a Bookwalter, bowel staplers, ureteral stents, vaginal stents, and stoma appliances. Electrothermal bipolar coagulation instruments, such as the vessel-sealing and cutting device LigaSure, can decrease the need for suturing, decrease surgical time, and reduce intraoperative blood loss.[7]

OPERATIVE PROCEDURE

Anesthesia and Positioning

General anesthesia is mandatory; an epidural catheter can be placed for postoperative pain management. Patients are placed in a low dorsal lithotomy position in Allen or Yellow Fin stirrups, and the surgical preparation should extend from the nipple line to the knees to ensure adequate access for use of abdominal or lower extremity–based myocutaneous flaps for pelvic reconstruction.

Surgical Exploration and Evaluation of Para-aortic Lymph Nodes

A generous midline incision is made, taking into account the potential need for abdominal flap creation and stoma placement, and normal anatomy restored. A thorough exploration is performed to evaluate for intraperitoneal malignancy or other distant metastasis, and suspicious lesions are sent for frozen-section analysis. A self-retaining retractor is placed, para-aortic lymph node basins are explored (see Chapter 28) and dissected, and specimens are sent for frozen-section analysis while attention is directed toward developing the pelvic phase of the operation. Involvement of para-aortic lymph nodes would be a contraindication to proceeding.

Opening the Pelvic Sidewall and Evaluation of Pelvic Lymph Nodes

The pelvic sidewalls are opened by incising the round ligaments and mobilizing the broad ligament medially and developing the pararectal and paravesical spaces. The external iliac and obturator lymph nodes are dissected (see Chapter 28), and any suspicious nodes are sent for frozen-section analysis. With the lymph nodes removed and the paravesical and pararectal spaces developed, the pelvic sidewalls can now be directly assessed for involvement. To verify the absence of sidewall extension, a finger is inserted in the paravesical space, and a finger is inserted into the pararectal space, and the intervening tissue of the cardinal ligament is palpated down to the pelvic floor to evaluate the proximity of tumor to the pelvic wall.

Bladder Mobilization and Development of Retropubic Space

The peritoneal incision is extended along the posterior border of the symphysis pubis, and the retropubic space of Retzius is developed using a combination of blunt and sharp dissection down to the pelvic floor. The anterior pelvic dissection proceeds laterally, resulting in unification of the retropubic space and the bilateral paravesical spaces.

Rectum Mobilization and Development of Presacral Space

Following the anterior pelvic dissection, the ureters are fully mobilized down the cardinal ligament and held with Vessi-loops for traction. The peritoneal incision is extended medially into the posterior pelvis toward the sigmoid mesentery. The pararectal spaces are extended posteriorly and medially underneath the sigmoid mesentery to develop the presacral (retrorectal) space, working in the avascular plane anterior to the sacrum. The absence of sacral involvement should

be verified by confirming the ability to lift the rectosigmoid colon out of the sacral hollow. This is the last decision point to abandon the exenteration before dividing the bowel and ureters.

Division of Rectosigmoid Colon and Ureters; Unification of Pelvic Spaces

The rectosigmoid colon is divided using a linear stapling device (eg, gastrointestinal anastomotic), and the sigmoid mesentery is taken down between clamps or using a vessel-sealing and cutting device (eg, LigaSure); the inferior mesenteric vascular pedicle is clamped, divided, and secured with suture ligatures (see Chapter 30). The presacral space is then developed down to the pelvic floor. The ureters are ligated and divided at least 2 cm from the central pelvic tumor mass. The proximal ureters and sigmoid colon can be packed out of the operative field until the reconstructive phase. At this point, the pelvic spaces are unified with the exception of the cardinal ligaments and anterior division of the internal iliac vessels (Figure 32A-3).

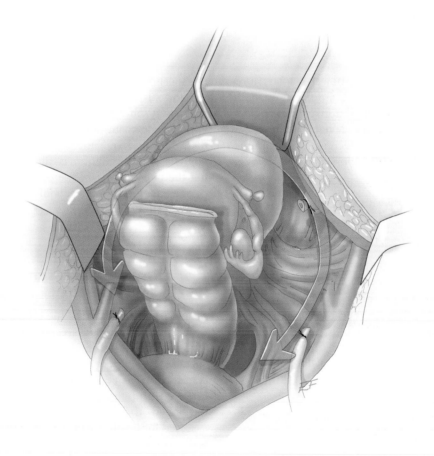

FIGURE 32A-3. Initial phase of total pelvic exenteration. The retropubic space is extended laterally to reach continuity with the paravesical spaces, and the presacral space is extended laterally to reach continuity with the pararectal spaces.

Division of Cardinal Ligaments

The central pelvic tumor specimen is placed on contralateral traction with the surgeon's fingers or straightened Heaney retractors used to expose the pelvic sidewall. The internal iliac vessels are often indistinguishable as separate structures in a previously radiated field but lie within the tissue of the cardinal ligament. Working from the pelvic brim toward the pelvic floor, the cardinal ligament tissue is serially clamped at the pelvic sidewall, divided, and secured with suture ligatures (Figure 32A-4). If the internal iliac artery and vein are identifiable, they can either be preserved and the uterine vascular pedicle divided at its origin, or resected en bloc. If sacrificed, the internal iliac vessels should be individually secured with vascular clamps and divided a short distance from the pelvic wall to

allow for an adequate pedicle in the event of unexpected hemorrhage. Division of the internal iliac arteries may limit neovagina reconstructive options (see Chapter 32C). Posteriorly, the mesorectum and rectal pillars are divided between clamps or taken down to the pelvic floor using a vessel-sealing and cutting device (eg, LigaSure). The exposure and dissection are duplicated on the contralateral side.

Supralevator Exenteration: Final Extirpative Steps

The final extirpative phase of a supralevator exenteration begins by placing posterior traction on the central specimen exposing the anterior pelvis. The Foley catheter can be palpable within the urethra. The surrounding

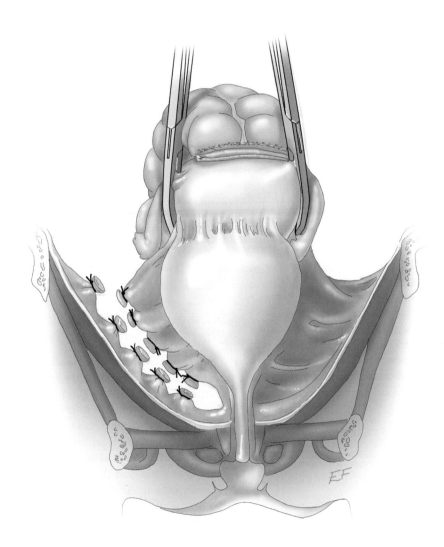

FIGURE 32A-4. Total pelvic exenteration. The cardinal ligaments (with or without the internal iliac vessels) are resected at the level of the pelvic wall down to the levator muscles of the pelvic floor for a supralevator exenteration; the levator muscles are included in the resection for infralevator exenteration.

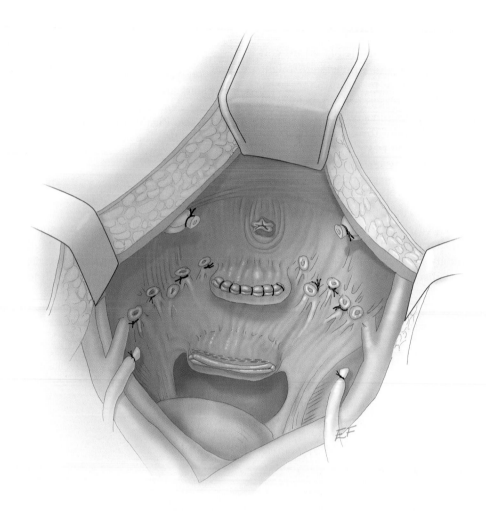

FIGURE 32A-5. Total supralevator pelvic exenteration: extirpation of the specimen with resulting pelvic defect.

paravesical tissue is taken down to the pelvic floor, and the urethra is divided using the electrosurgical blade. The vagina can be cross-clamped and divided or circumscribed using the electrosurgical blade at the level of the pelvic floor. The distal rectum is divided using a linear stapling (eg, transverse anastomosis) device (see Chapter 30), and the specimen is removed (Figure 32A-5). A laparotomy pack is placed in the pelvis to tamponade any small bleeding sites while the specimen is inspected to ensure grossly negative resection margins.

Infralevator Exenteration: Resection of Levator Muscles

For an infralevator exenteration, a second surgical team begins the perineal phase when the abdominal dissection reaches the level of the levator muscles. The central pelvic tumor specimen is placed on countertraction, and the electrosurgical blade is used to incise

the levator muscle plate circumferentially at least 2 cm lateral to the area of tumor extension (Figure 32A-6).

Infralevator Exenteration: Perineal Phase and Specimen Removal

The second surgical team outlines the planned perineal resection to encompass a variable extent of vulvectomy tailored to the extent of tumor involvement (Figure 32A-7). The subcutaneous dissection is developed in the paravesical and pararectal spaces cephalad, using a combination of clamps with suture ligatures and the electrosurgical blade. The abdominal surgeon can place a hand in the pelvis to help guide the perineal dissection. After the perineal phase has reached the fascial plane of the pelvic floor, 4 potential spaces are developed: the suprapubic and presacral spaces and the right and left paravaginal spaces (Figure 32A-8). These potential spaces are separated by 5 pedicles: 2 pubourethral, 2 rectal pillar, and the posterior anococcygeal. These pedicles are clamped, divided, and

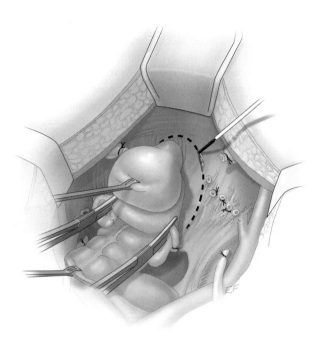

FIGURE 32A-6. Total infralevator pelvic exenteration: resection of levator muscle plate.

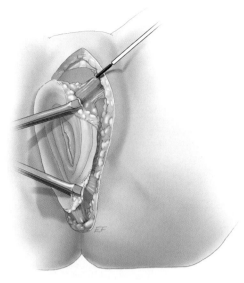

FIGURE 32A-8. Total infralevator exenteration. The suprapubic, paravaginal, and presacral spaces are developed to define the pubourethral, rectal pillar, and anococcygeal pedicles.

secured with suture ligatures. Circumferential dissection results in complete detachment of the specimen, which can be removed abdominally or vaginally (Figure 32A-9).

Closure and Final Steps

The simplest and most expedient way to close the perineum is for the second surgical team to perform a layered closure of the deep pelvic and perineal tissues (Figure 32A-10). Reconstruction of the urinary tract should be performed next according to the patient's desires and available surgical options (see Chapter 32B). Due to the large amount of dead space left after an

exenteration, a neovagina, a rectus flap, or an omental flap is needed to fill the pelvis and bring in tissue with a good blood supply. Our recommendation, even in women who do not want a neovagina, is that a rectus flap be placed into the pelvis and an omental J-flap placed on top of it (see Chapter 32C).

Once the vaginal, pelvic, and urinary reconstructions are performed, attention is directed to the intestinal tract. Re-establishing intestinal continuity should be undertaken with caution, because the risk of anastomotic dehiscence or leak is as high as 50% after radiation. After tolerance-dose pelvic radiation, our preference is to perform end colostomy at the time of total or posterior pelvic exenteration. The colostomy

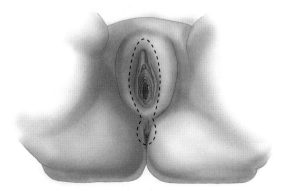
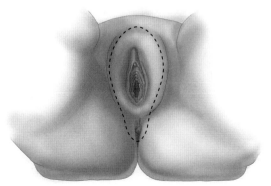

FIGURE 32A-7. Total infralevator exenteration. The extent of the perineal resection is tailored to the degree of lower vaginal or vulvar involvement with tumor.

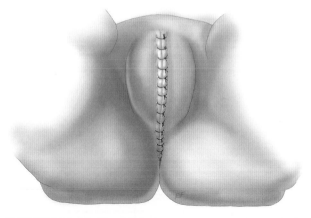

FIGURE 32A-9. Total infralevator exenteration: pelvic defect.

is usually the final procedure prior to closing. A 2- to 3-cm circular piece of skin is removed from the site of the stoma (see Chapter 30). The subcutaneous tissue is dissected to the fascia, and a cruciate incision is made in the anterior abdominal wall fascia so that the rectosigmoid can easily be brought through the anterior abdominal wall. Retraction of the colon back into the abdomen is prevented by carefully placing sutures between the fascia and proximal bowel. Additional sutures can also be placed on the peritoneal side. The stoma should be matured to the skin in a rosebud fashion (skin to

FIGURE 32A-10. Total infralevator exenteration: simple closure of the pelvic floor.

proximal bowel to distal bowel edge) once the abdomen is closed to prevent any fecal contamination.

Prior to closing the abdomen, the operative site should be copiously irrigated and hemostasis confirmed. The abdomen and pelvis should be adequately drained to promote wound healing. There will be extensive third spacing and small urinary leaks from the conduit, so adequate drainage is essential. The wound should be closed in a mass closure with delayed absorbable or permanent suture.

Box 32A-2 Caution Points

- During the perineal phase, have the abdominal surgical team guide the dissection to ensure the lateral margins are adequate.
- Do not disrupt presacral veins when dissecting the rectum off the sacral promontory and sacral hollow.
- Dissect ureters as low in the pelvis as possible so there is adequate length for anastomosis.

Anterior Exenteration

If only the bladder, urethra, uterus, cervix, and vagina need to be removed and the rectum can be spared, then the posterior part of the dissection is modified. For an anterior exenteration, the peritoneum between the rectum and vagina is incised and the rectovaginal septum developed. The entire vaginal tube can be mobilized in a combined abdominal and perineal approach if the entire vagina needs to be taken, or a portion of the posterior vagina can be left in place if margins are adequate.

Posterior Exenteration

With a posterior exenteration, the anterior part of the exenteration is modified. The ureters are dissected to their entry into the bladder, similar to a radical hysterectomy. The dissection between the vagina and bladder is taken down to the perineal dissection or until there are adequate margins around the cancer. The entire vaginal tube can be taken if needed, or a portion of the anterior vagina can be left if the margins are adequate. Posterior exenterations for central recurrence following radiation are not often performed because of the high likelihood of bladder dysfunction and urinary fistulization when the rectum, vagina, and cervix are removed. In addition, because of the damage to the hypogastric plexus that enervates the bladder, many patients will require some type of catheter drainage to facilitate bladder emptying.

POSTOPERATIVE CARE

It is common for many patients to require an intensive care unit stay for 24 to 48 hours after surgery to manage large blood loss, transfusion, and fluid shifts. Postoperative pain is best managed with patient-controlled epidural analgesia. Total parenteral nutrition can be started to help facilitate adequate nutrition and wound healing. Early feeding can be initiated, although prolonged ileus may prevent this. Venous thromboembolism prophylaxis should be continued during the entire hospitalization; some authors recommend a total of 4 weeks of medical prophylaxis. Ambulation is usually begun by day 2 to 3.

Drains should remain in place for approximately 7 to 10 days and may be discontinued when the output is less than 100 mL in a 24-hour period. If there is concern about ureteral leakage, the fluid in the drain can be sent for creatinine. A creatinine from drain fluid that is significantly higher than the serum value is indicative of a leak. If there is a leak, with adequate drainage and ureteral stenting, the leak will usually heal.

Complications following an exenteration will occur in approximately 50% of patients. Wound infections, pelvic abscess requiring drainage, anastomotic leaks, bowel obstruction, fistula, venous thrombosis, and other medical complications are the most common.

Box 32A-3 Complications and Morbidity

- Major bleeding is the most common intraoperative complication. Adequate blood should be available. Be prepared to give platelets and fresh frozen plasma if bleeding is significant.
- Thromboembolic complications are common in the perioperative period. Both mechanical and medical prophylaxis should be used.
- Infectious complications are very common. Patients need redosing of intraoperative antibiotics secondary to large blood loss and extended time of the surgery.
- In patients who are malnourished, preoperative oral or total parenteral nutrition (TPN) should be given until the prealbumin level is in the normal range. Postoperative TPN is usually given to all patients to promote healing and prevent anastomotic leaks.
- Abscesses and anastomotic leaks are common complications. Placement of drains at the time of surgery can reduce these complications. Postoperative abscesses or leaks can also be managed conservatively by interventional radiology.

REFERENCES

1. Brunschwig A. A complete excision of pelvic viscera for advanced carcinoma: a one-stage abdominoperineal operation with end colostomy and bilateral ureteral implantation into the colon above the colostomy. *Cancer.* 1948;1:177-183.
2. Bricker EM. Bladder substitution after pelvic evisceration. *Surg Clin North Am.* 1950;30:1511-1512.
3. Berek JS, Howe C, Lagasse LD, Hacker NF. Pelvic exenteration for recurrent gynecologic malignancy: survival and morbidity analysis of the 45-year experience at UCLA. *Gynecol Oncol.* 2005;99:153-159.
4. Goldberg GL, Sukumvanich P, Einstein MH, Smith HO, Anderson PS, Fields AL. Total pelvic exenteration: The Albert Einstein College of Medicine/Montefiore Medical Center Experience (1987 to 2003). *Gynecol Oncol.* 2006;101:261-268.
5. Maggioni A, Roviglione G, Landoni F, et al. Pelvic exenteration: ten-year experience at the European Institute of Oncology in Milan. *Gynecol Oncol.* 2009;114:64-68.
6. Fotopoulou C, Neumann U, Kraetschell R, et al. Long-term clinical outcome of pelvic exenteration in patients with advanced gynecologic malignancies. *J Surg Oncol.* 2010;101:507-512.
7. McLean K, Zhang W, Dunsmoor-Su RF, et al. Pelvic exenteration in the age of modern chemoradiation. *Gynecol Oncol.* 2011;121:131-134.
8. Spahn M, Weiss C, Bader P, et al. The role of exenterative surgery and urinary diversion in persistent or locally recurrent gynecologic malignancy: complications and survival. *Urol Int.* 2010;85:16-22.
9. Guimarães GC, Baiocchi G, Ferreira AC, et al. Palliative pelvic exenteration for patients with gynecological malignancies. *Arch Gynecol Obstet.* 2011;283:1107-1112.
10. Marnitz S, Dowdy S, Lanowska M, et al. Exenterations 60 years after first description: results of a survey among US and German gynecologic oncology centers. *Int J Gynecol Cancer.* 2009;19:974-977.
11. Barakat RR, Goldman NA, Patel DA, et al. Pelvic exenteration for recurrent endometrial cancer. *Gynecol Oncol.* 1999;75:99-102.
12. Morris M, Alvarez RD, Kinney WK, Wilson TO. Treatment of recurrent adenocarcinoma of the endometrium with pelvic exenteration. *Gynecol Oncol.* 1996;60:288-291.
13. Fleisch MC, Panthe P, Beckman MW, et al. Predictors of long-term survival after interdisciplinary salvage surgery for advanced or recurrent gynecologic cancers. *J Surg Oncol.* 2007;95:476-484.
14. Höckel M. Laterally extended endopelvic resection (LEER)—Principles and practice. *Gynecol Oncol.* 2008;111:S13-S17.
15. Stelzer KH, Koh WJ, Greer BE, et al. The use of intraoperative radiation therapy in radical salvage for recurrent cervical cancer: outcome and toxicity. *Am J Obstet Gynecol.* 1995;172(6):1881-1886.
16. Martinez-Monge R, Jurado M, Aristu JJ, et al. Intraoperative electron beam radiotherapy during radical surgery for locally advanced and recurrent cervical cancer. *Gynecol Oncol.* 2001;82(3):538-543.
17. Popovich MJ, Hricak H, Sugimura K, Stern JL. The role of MR imaging in determining surgical eligibility for pelvic exenteration. *Am J Roentgenol.* 1993;160:525-531.
18. Husain A, Akhurst T, Larson S, et al. A prospective study of the accuracy of 18-fluorodeoxyglucose positron emission tomography (18FDG PET) in identifying sites of metastasis prior to pelvic exenteration. *Gynecol Oncol.* 2007;106:177-180.
19. Lai CH, Huang KG, See LC, et al. Restaging of recurrent cervical carcinoma with dual-phase [18F]fluoro-2-deoxy-D-glucose positron emission tomography. *Cancer.* 2004;100:544-552.

CHAPTER 32

20. Miller B, Morris M, Rutledge F, et al. Aborted exenterative procedures in recurrent cervical cancer. *Gynecol Oncol*. 1993;50: 94-99.
21. Hawighorst-Knapstein S, Schonefussrs G, Hoffmann SO, Knapsteinn PG. Pelvic exenteration: effects of surgery on quality of life and body image. A prospective longitudinal study. *Gynecol Oncol*. 1997;66:495-500.
22. Ratliff CR, Gershenson DM, Morris M, et al. Sexual adjustment of patients undergoing gracilis myocutaneous flap vaginal reconstruction in conjunction with pelvic exenteration. *Cancer*. 1996;78:2229-2235.

B. Urinary Diversions

Thomas C. Krivak and Paniti Sukumvanich

PROCEDURE OVERVIEW

The utilization of urinary diversion and creation of urinary conduits have been developed and modified with the principal of maintaining a quality of life in the patients undergoing radical surgery for treatment of recurrent gynecologic cancer or complications from previous therapy.[1-5] Initially, Brunschwig used a "wet colostomy" (ie, an ureterosigmoidostomy) as a means to provide urinary diversion. This procedure unfortunately led to high rates of pyelonephritis and renal failure, which limited the utility of such a procedure. In subsequent years, Bricker described using the terminal ileum for diverting the urinary stream, whereas Rowland described using the large bowel as the reservoir for the urinary diversion. These 2 later techniques decreased the complication rate and had acceptable postoperative complications, thus making such procedures more widely used in patients undergoing pelvic exenteration.

Urinary diversions may be necessary in cases where there is obstruction of the ureters due to pelvic tumor growth or complications of radiation therapy (eg, radiation fibrosis or genitourinary fistula), or as part of a curative exenterative procedure. Depending on the clinical situation, the methods for urinary diversion may range from incontinent diversions, such as percutaneous nephrostomy tubes or ileal conduit, to continent urinary diversion, such as a large bowel continent urinary diversion.

The gynecologic oncology surgeon should carefully evaluate the clinical scenario in order to choose the most appropriate treatment, given the variety of methods available for urinary diversion. In cases where an exenteration is not being performed, one should also consider whether a nonpermanent diversion such as a percutaneous nephrostomy would suffice in place of permanent diversion. Another clinical scenario issue to consider is whether or not the procedure is for curative intent or palliation of symptoms. In cases where the procedure is needed as part of a pelvic exenteration procedure, the main point to consider is whether it should be a continent or incontinent urinary diversion.

An example of a patient who would be an ideal candidate for continent colon urinary diversion would be a patient with an anterior cancer recurrence undergoing an anterior exenteration.[6-12] A continent diversion in this case would provide the patient with a better cosmetic result because only a small ostomy for catheterization of the continent reservoir will be present on her abdomen. Conversely, in a patient with a central recurrence and distant disease who has a large vesicovaginal fistula requiring urinary diversion, one should consider a percutaneous nephrostomy placement or noncontinent small bowel conduit, because this may have a better impact on her quality of life. This chapter will focus on the various methods for urinary diversion and the management of complications that can ensue from such procedures.

Box 32B-1	Master Surgeon's Corner

- Avoid using any tissue that shows signs of significant radiation changes.
- Obtain a mucosal-to-mucosal ureteroileal anastomosis to decrease risk of anastomotic leaks.
- Obtain adequate spatulation with the ureteroileal anastomosis to decrease risk of strictures.
- Be sure to have an adequate protrusion of the stoma above the abdominal wall skin level.
- Ensure that the small bowel conduit is secured with the direction of bowel peristalsis toward the stoma.

PREOPERATIVE PREPARATION AND INDICATIONS

The 4 main issues to consider in the preoperative planning phase of the procedure are as follows:

1. Determining the degree of renal function
2. Determining the type of urinary diversion

3. Obtaining informed consent
4. Determining the location of the stoma

Determining the Degree of Renal Function

Prior to performing a procedure that can have significant long-term consequences, it is important to determine that the patient's kidneys are indeed functional. Laboratory tests such as serum electrolytes, blood urea nitrogen (BUN), and creatinine levels should be obtained to assess baseline renal function. If there has been any evidence of long-term obstruction, then one should consider a renal ultrasound and nuclear renal scan. Radiographic studies, such as a radionucleotide or renal Lasix scan, are important to obtain because a normal BUN or creatinine level does not always imply that both kidneys are functional. This should be done to ensure that a urinary diversion is not performed on a nonfunctioning kidney. Generally, a nonfunctioning kidney is confirmed by a less than 5% total glomerular filtration rate of one kidney. When a nonfunctioning kidney is encountered, a nephrectomy should be taken considered as part of the surgical procedure to avoid chronic pyelonephritis.

Determining the Type of Urinary Diversion

Urinary diversions can be divided into 2 types: permanent and temporary (ie, percutaneous nephrostomy). In a patient who is a poor surgical candidate and in whom the goal of any surgical intervention is palliation, one should consider the placement of percutaneous nephrostomy tubes. Such a procedure can provide relief of symptoms due to obstruction and fistulas with a minimum of morbidity. This technique may also allow the patient to regain her renal function as well as undergo antegrade passage of stents at a later time. This may be a temporary or permanent type of diversion based on patient prognosis. Another indication for percutaneous nephrostomy tube placement is a patient with ureteral strictures, because such treatment may allow for passage of a ureteral stent as well as balloon catheters for dilatation. In a patient undergoing definitive treatment with a pelvic exenteration, a permanent urinary diversion such as an incontinent ileal conduit or continent conduit would be indicated. In general, a patient who is undergoing a total exenteration is a good candidate for an ileal conduit.[12-14] Continent conduits can be considered for patients undergoing an anterior exenteration because the cosmetic result with a small stoma may be more appealing to the patient.

Obtaining Informed Consent

It is important to thoroughly explain the risks and benefits of any permanent urinary diversion procedure. Such counseling is often done in conjunction with the discussion on the expected outcomes, utility, and risks of the pelvic exenteration procedure. Patients have to be aware of the lifestyle changes that will be required, such as long-term care of the colostomy and urostomy or the care required for continent large bowel urinary diversion (self-catheterization). Complication rates reported in the literature for ileal conduits include a ureteral-ileal anastomosis postoperative leak rate of 5% to 10%, postoperative pyelonephritis risk of 5% to 20%, chronic pyelonephritis risk of 5% to 10%, parastomal hernia risk of less than 5%, stomal stenosis in continent conduits risk of 5% to 15%, nephrolithiasis risk of 5% to 10%, and a risk of chronic renal sufficiency.[5,7,8,11,15]

Determination of the Location of the Stoma

Determining the placement of the stoma will often depend on what other procedures are being done at the same time. It is recommended that the patient should have a preoperative consultation with an enterostomal therapist to help with markings for the stoma. It should be kept in mind that locations that are at the level of the umbilicus are not ideal, as the waistbands of women's pants are often placed at that level. Any stoma should be placed at a least 8 to 10 cm away from the midline incision, either above or below the umbilicus, not in a skin crease and clear of any bony prominences. Patients should be evaluated while standing and supine to ensure the location is ideal in both positions.

OPERATIVE PROCEDURE

Noncontinent Urinary Diversion: Ileal Conduit

Ureteral Mobilization

Care should be taken with dissection of the ureters from the retroperitoneal space. Often, this dissection can be quite difficult due to radiation fibrosis. One should gently handle the ureters because they can easily be devascularized. In general, it is recommended to excise any portion of the ureter that shows signs of extensive radiation fibrosis and to use a portion of the ureter that is out of the radiated field. One should also try to conserve as much of the periureteral tissue as possible without completely stripping the ureter because this will also help to prevent devascularization of the ureter. Isolation of the ureters may begin with a pericolic gutter peritoneal incision in order to dissect from lateral to medial. This will allow for identification of the important vascular structures that are close to the ureter such as the infundibulopelvic ligament. The cecum and the ascending colon will also need to be mobilized as part of the right ureteral dissection. The left ureteral dissection can be done along with the rectosigmoid colon mobilization. The ileal conduit stoma is typically placed in the right lower quadrant. As such, the left ureter will need to be mobilized for a distance of approximately 15 cm to allow it to be brought underneath the inferior mesenteric artery and sigmoid colon mesentery to reach the conduit. Because the right ureter has a shorter path to travel to the conduit, it usually must be mobilized for a distance of 10 cm or so to ensure a tension-free anastomosis. One might need more or less dissection; the amount dissected should allow for a tension-free anastomosis to the conduit. Once the dissection has been performed, the ureters should be ligated with 2-0 silk ties. This will lead to dilatation of the ureters and will allow for easier placement of the ureteral stents, facilitating the ureteroileal anastomosis. The amount of time the ureters are ligated should be monitored, because the ureters cannot be ligated for longer than 3 to 4 hours due to the development of electrolyte abnormalities. The anesthesiologist should be notified of the ureteral ligation in order to allow for fluid optimization during this portion of the procedure.

Isolation of Small Bowel Segment

Once the ureters have been dissected and ligated, the next step is selecting the ileal segment to be used for the conduit. The ileal segment for the conduit should be at least 15 cm away from the ileocecal valve and should be a nonmottled, well-vascularized, healthy-appearing segment of bowel. Approximately 12 to 18 cm of bowel is typically required for an ileal conduit. The actual length required may depend on numerous factors such as whether a Turnbull loop will be needed or the segment is long enough to allow for a tension-free anastomosis with the ureters. The segment of ileum should not be too long, because redundancy can lead to postoperative electrolyte abnormalities from absorption of electrolytes from a long segment of ileum. Once the segment of ileum has been identified, one should ensure that there is adequate blood supply by elevating the distal ileum and transilluminating the mesentery. If good blood supply is identified, then a segment of ileum 15 cm away from the ileocecal valve is marked and tagged with a Penrose drain, and a proximal segment is measured between 12 and 20 cm in length for the proximal and distal ends of the ileal conduit. In an obese patient, an additional 5- to

10-cm segment should be considered to allow for the Turnbull loop. The Turnbull loop stoma allows for a longer segment of small bowel to traverse the abdominal wall without compromising vascular supply. Once the bowel has been marked and tagged with a Penrose drain, the proximal and distal portions may be isolated and divided using a GIA-60 stapler. A series of 3-0 silk horizontal mattress sutures are used to oversew the staple line at the proximal end of the conduit, where the ureters will be connected, in order to decrease contact of the staple line with urine and reduce the risk of nephrolithiasis.

Stoma Creation

Once the ileal loop has been isolated, the skin aperture is created, and the stoma is formed (Figure 32B-1). The layers that will need to be excised are the skin, the subcutaneous tissue, the anterior rectus sheath, the rectus muscle, the posterior rectus sheath, and the peritoneum. Ideally, the skin site will have been marked preoperatively to avoid any bony prominences, prior abdominal scars, and abdominal creases. Pulling up a piece of skin with a Kocher clamp and cutting across should result in a 2- to 2.5-cm small circumferential incision. Remove all the fatty tissue down to the anterior rectus sheath. Be sure to place tension on the anterior and posterior rectus sheath by pulling medially on the fascia through the midline incision, and then make a cruciate incision through the rectus sheath, rectus muscle, and underlying peritoneum using an electrosurgical unit (Bovie) device. The skin incision may need to be larger if a loop stoma (Turnbull loop) is going to be created. Care should be taken not to damage any of the surrounding structures, such as the inferior epigastric vessels, during this process. The aperture should accommodate 2 fingers to pass through easily. The distal end of the ileal conduit is then grasped by a Babcock clamp that has been passed through the aperture, and the conduit is then brought up to the skin. At this point, the surgeon must ensure that the bowel mesentery is not strangulated or twisted and that the direction of intestinal peristalsis is pointed toward the efferent limb of the conduit. Once the conduit has been safely pulled through the skin, Allis clamps are placed on the corners below the prior staple line. The staple line is excised, and copious irrigation should be performed to ensure that small bowel contents are removed completely. The ileal segment should be re-evaluated to ensure that there is adequate length for the ureteral-ileal anastomosis.

Creation of the stoma is done by placing 4 equally spaced 3-0 Vicryl sutures first 1 cm from the skin edge, then approximately 4 cm from the stoma opening, and finally through the opening of the stoma to facilitate eversion ("rosebud") of the stoma. It is extremely

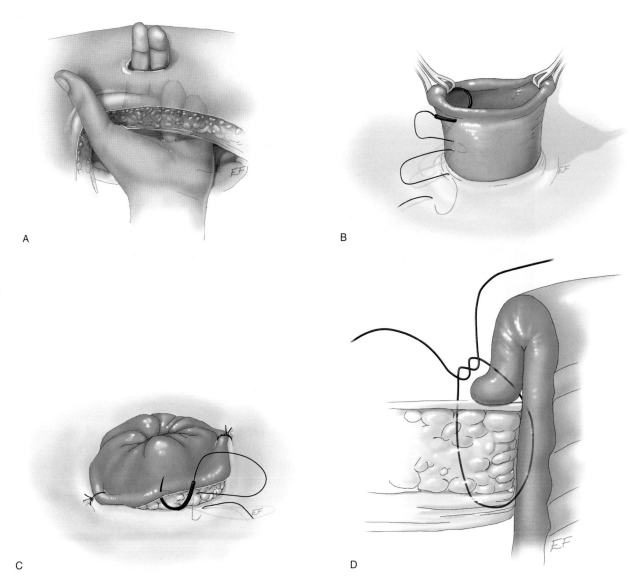

FIGURE 32B-1. Creation of the urinary conduit stoma. (A) Creation of the stoma aperature. **(B), (C), (D)** 'Rosebud' stoma creation.

important to ensure that there is adequate eversion of the stoma, because low-profile stomas can make it very difficult for appliances to be placed around the stoma, thus allowing for caustic urinary leak on the skin. Care should also be taken not to ligate critical vascular supply within the mesentery so as not to devascularize the distal end of the conduit. The stoma should be pink and healthy and not blue with compromised blood supply. The ileal conduit is then fixed to the posterior rectus sheath using several 3-0 Vicryl sutures to decrease the risk of parastomal hernia.

Ureteroileal Anastomoses

The distal ureters should be incised and spatulated to allow for placement of the ureteral stent. Care should be taken not to make the opening too large because

this can lead to reflux (the opening should be no larger than 1 cm). Once this has been completed, the screw-on tip of a metal Yankauer suction is removed, and it is then placed down through the stoma into the conduit to the location where the left ureter will be anastomosed to the conduit (Figure 32B-2). It is usually easiest to perform the left ureteral anastomosis first. A 1-cm incision is created with a #15 blade on ileum over the tip of the Yankauer to allow the suction tip to protrude. A guide wire is placed through the Yankauer and fed through the ureter. A single-J, 6- or 7-French ureteral stent is passed over the guide wire through the ureter into the kidney. Palpation of the ureter should be done while the stent is being passed to make sure the stent is placed up into the kidney. The ureter is then sutured into the conduit using a series of 5 to 8 interrupted 4-0 polydioxanone sutures on a vascular

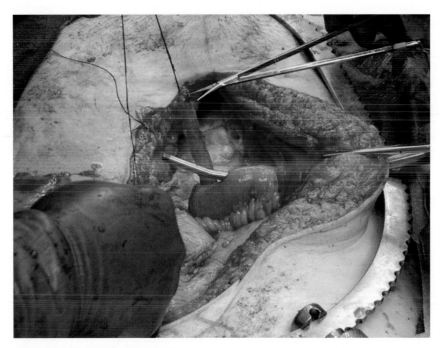

FIGURE 32B-2. Yankauer suction tip used to facilitate placing ureteral stent guide wire.

needle placed circumferentially. Care should be taken to go from the mucosa of the ureter to the mucosa of the ileum to achieve a mucosa-to-mucosa anastomosis. The ureter should be sutured in such a way that the knot is on the outside of anastomosis. The surgeon should be careful not to place too many sutures with this anastomosis, as this can compromise the blood flow and

prevent adequate healing of the anastomotic site. The left ureter should not be kinked, and the anastomosis should be tension-free (Figure 32B-3). Once the left ureteral-ileal anastomosis is complete, a 1-0 chromic suture should be placed through-and-through the ileal conduit, piercing through the stent to prevent any stent migration during the immediate postoperative

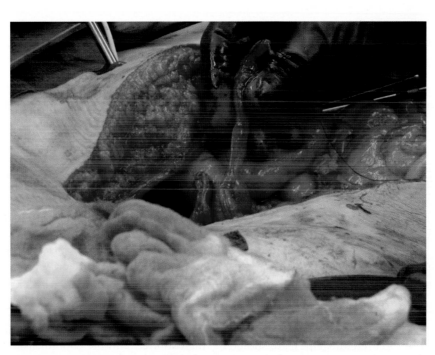

FIGURE 32B-3. Tension-free ureteroileal anastomosis.

period. The procedure is repeated for the right ureter. Both anastomoses should be water-tight and tension-free without ureteral angulation, strictures, or twisting. A water-tight seal of the ureteral-ileal anastomosis can be confirmed by insufflating the conduit with a diluted indigo carmine blue solution. The stents should be flushed, and urine production from the stents should be confirmed. The distal ends of the ureteral stents emerging from the efferent end of the conduit should be trimmed to an appropriate length to fit within the urinary appliance and may be sutured to the peristomal skin as an additional measure to prevent migration during the postoperative period.

Re-establish Intestinal Continuity

After completion of the conduit, intestinal continuity is re-established via a side-to-side functional end-to-end enteroenterostomy using the divided ends of ileum. The anastomosis is performed anterior to the ileal conduit. The anastomosis is done in the usual manner using GIA-60 and TA-60 stapling devices. The mesenteric defect is closed with a series of interrupted 3-0 Vicryl sutures to prevent an internal bowel hernia. When closing the mesenteric defect, avoid constricting the mesenteric blood supply to the ileal conduit. Finally, the proximal end of the conduit should be secured to the sacral promontory with several 2-0 or 3-0 delayed-absorbable sutures to prevent migration and creation of tension on the ureteral anastomoses (Figure 32B-4). A closed-suction drain (eg, Jackson-Pratt) is placed in the dependent pelvis. Postoperatively, an abdominal film should be obtained to confirm proper ureteral stent location.

Noncontinent Ileal Conduit: Alternatives and Modifications

Alternatives to the ileal conduit include a transverse colon conduit and a double-barrel wet stoma.[16-21] An advantage of the transverse colon noncontinent conduit is that it provides a large-caliber segment of bowel that has not been irradiated and may be used when the small bowel has been heavily irradiated. The double-barrel wet colostomy (ureters implanted directly into an end colostomy segment) has the advantage of a single stoma but is less than ideal due to the risk of ascending kidney infections. This procedure may be a viable option for patients who may have difficulty with care of 2 stomal sites.

There are several modifications of the previously described ileal conduit construction. In the technique of Leadbetter, the proximal end of the conduit is sutured to the sacral promontory, and both ureters are brought to the midline for the anastomosis of the

intestinal segment. This allows for a more vertically oriented ileal conduit than the transverse oriented conduit of the Bricker method.[5,17] The Turnbull loop stoma can provide adequate blood supply and less compromise of the mesentery for patients who are obese or have had prior complications of ileal conduits such as stomal strictures.[18-20]

A modification of the ileal conduit to help reduce ureteral-ileal anastomotic complications has been described by Barbieri et al[21] in which a small linear incision is made in the ileal segment and the ureteroileal anastomoses created under direct visualization. The reported stricture rate was less than 2%, and the complications from making a linear incision along the small bowel conduit were minimal.

POSTOPERATIVE CARE

Box 32B-2	Complications and Morbidity

- Early Complications
  - Anastomotic leak (5%-10%)
  - Stoma retraction, necrosis
  - Low urine output
  - Infection (5%-20%)
- Late Complications
  - Ureteroileal anastomotic stenosis (10%-15%)
  - Stoma stenosis or hernia (5%-15%)
  - Chronic pyelonephritis (5%-10%)
  - Renal insufficiency

The immediate postoperative period should be focused on detecting early complications related to the urinary conduit, such as ureteroileal anastomotic leak and complications with the stoma. Urine leak will be heralded by an increase in pelvic drainage output and a markedly elevated creatinine level in the drain effluent. Conservative management with percutaneous nephrostomy drainage is the preferred management and frequently allows spontaneous closure in the absence of severely irradiated tissues. Extensive necrosis of the stoma that extends below the skin line requires surgical revision. The differential diagnosis for low urine output includes insufficient volume replacement, ureteroileal anastomotic leak, a defect in the proximal conduit stump, ureteral obstruction (kinking, stent occlusion), and improper stent position. Persistently low urine output after volume repletion should be evaluated with a computed tomography (CT) urogram. The closed-suction pelvic drain should be left in place until the output is less than 50 to 100 mL per 24-hour period. The ureteral stents can be removed

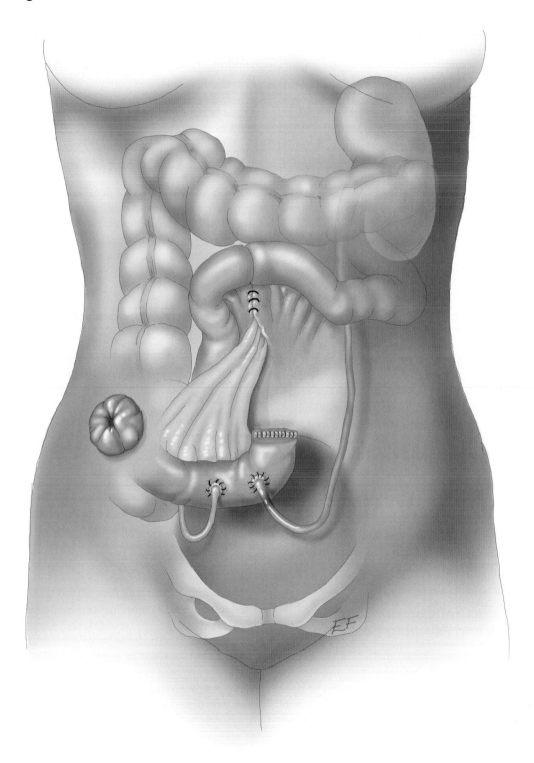

FIGURE 32B-4. Completed ileal conduit.

6 to 12 weeks postoperatively after confirmation of anastomotic integrity by intravenous pyelogram or CT urogram. Long-term surveillance should include periodic renal ultrasound (or CT imaging) to evaluate for hydronephrosis and stone formation as well as regular renal function testing. Delayed ureteroileal anastomosis stenosis can often be managed by percutaneous balloon dilatation. Stomal stenosis or parastomal hernia will require conduit revision and/or relocation.

RIGHT COLON CONTINENT URINARY DIVERSION

Procedure Overview

Box 32B-3   Master Surgeon's Corner

- Appropriate patient selection and preoperative counseling should be done to ensure that the patient will be able to self-catheterize and flush the conduit in the immediate postoperative time frame.
- Transilluminate the colonic mesentery to ensure adequate blood supply to the isolated bowel segment.
- Test the "tightness" of the ileocecal valve placation before fixation of the conduit to the abdominal wall.
- The ileal segment of the conduit should be as short as possible to avoid kinking and difficulty with catheterization.

There are a number of variations on the continent urinary conduit (pouch) using both large and small bowel segments. The most commonly used procedure in gynecologic oncology, and the focus of this section, uses a detubularized segment of right (ascending) colon and distal ileum, with the ileocecal valve serving as the continence mechanism. In most cases, a continent urinary diversion is chosen when the exenterative patient does not require concurrent diversion of the fecal stream (eg, end colostomy). Although formation of an end colostomy is not an absolute contraindication to continent urinary diversion, the cosmetic advantages are largely mitigated. Continent urinary diversions require more intensive maintenance and attention than their noncontinent counterparts. The ideal candidate would be a patient who requires an anterior exenteration or a total pelvic exenteration with a rectosigmoid resection than can have low anterior anastomosis accomplished safely. This will allow

for the patient to have no appliances on the anterior abdominal wall.

Preoperative Preparation

Preoperative evaluation and counseling are similar to what has been described for incontinent small bowel urinary diversion. However, preoperative assessment for a continent urinary diversion must include detailed counseling and education regarding the care and maintenance of the urinary pouch as well as an appraisal of the patient's ability and motivation for self-care. Any history of prior radiation therapy should be reviewed, with careful attention to the potential damage to the terminal ileum and/or ascending colon. Reconstruction of the urinary tract must consider the totality of the exenterative procedure, including the available length and viability of intestinal tract as well as modifications of the abdominal wall that may be required for vaginal reconstruction.

Operative Procedure

Preparation of the Right Colon

The most common bowel segment used for continent urinary diversion in gynecologic oncology surgery is the right colon with terminal ileum, with minor variations on this theme having been described as the "Miami pouch" or the "Indiana pouch."[22-26] The general principles of a typical right colon continent urinary diversion are described in this section.

After completion of the extirpative phase of the operation, the ureters are adequately mobilized as described previously for the ileal conduit. The small bowel is mobilized by incising the base of the small bowel mesentery up to the ligament of Treitz. The cecum, ascending colon, and transverse colon are mobilized by dividing along the white line of Toldt, taking down the hepatic flexure, and dividing the gastrocolic ligament. The mesenteric blood supply to the terminal ileum and proximal colon should be carefully preserved. In general, a 26- to 30-cm segment of colon is required to create the right colon pouch. The mesentery of the right colon and transverse colon is transilluminated to identify the right colic and middle colic vascular pedicles. The proximal transverse colon is divided using a GIA stapler just proximal to the middle colic vascular pedicle, and the mesentery is "back-cut" down to its base, proximal and parallel to the middle colic vascular pedicle, to achieve maximum mobility. The distal ileum is divided using a GIA stapler approximately 12 to 15 cm from the ileocecal valve.

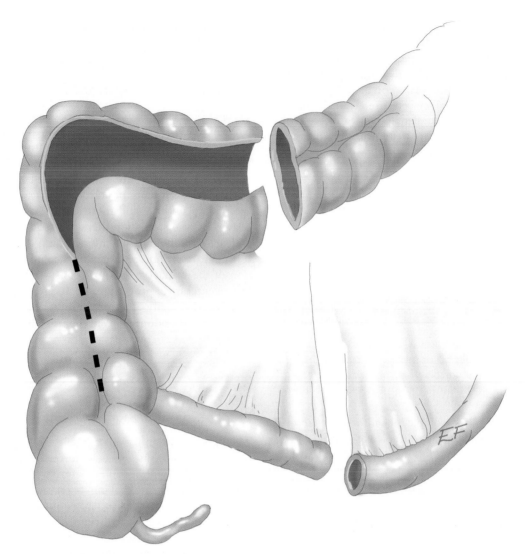

FIGURE 32B-5. Detubularization of the right colon segment for construction of urinary pouch.

The isolated segment of right colon is then detubularized by incising along the tenia omentalis (anteriormost tenia) from the proximal transverse colon down to the cecum using the electrosurgical unit, and the bowel lumen is copiously irrigated (Figure 32B-5). If not done previously, appendectomy should be performed. The segment of right colon is then folded over on itself to form a detubularized intestinal "pouch." The posterior "wall" of the pouch is approximated using a 2-layer closure of running 3-0 Vicryl suture. It is often easiest to place the outer (imbricating) layer prior to the inner (full-thickness, mucosa-to-mucosa) layer. The anterior "wall" of the pouch is then approximated in a similar fashion, leaving a large enough opening in the cecum to facilitate constructing the ureterocolic anastomoses. For the anterior closure, the inner (mucosa-to-mucosa) layer should be placed first, followed by the outer (imbricating) layer.

Creation of the Continence Mechanism

The distal ileal segment should be trimmed to a length 3 to 4 cm longer than the thickness of the abdominal wall to allow for "rosebudding" of the stoma with the ileocecal valve juxtaposed to the abdominal wall peritoneum. The ileal segment is then tapered to facilitate straight-line catheterization by placing a 14- or 16-French Robinson catheter into the lumen, grasping the mesenteric border with several Babcock clamps (incorporating the Robinson catheter), and firing 1 or 2 applications of the GIA stapling device along the antimesenteric border of ileum to excise the redundant lumen (Figure 32B-6). With the red Robinson catheter still in place, the ileocecal valve is then plicated using 3 or 4 imbricating stitches of 2-0 or 3-0 silk sutures placed along the antimesenteric border (Figure 32B-7). At this juncture, the Robinson catheter should be

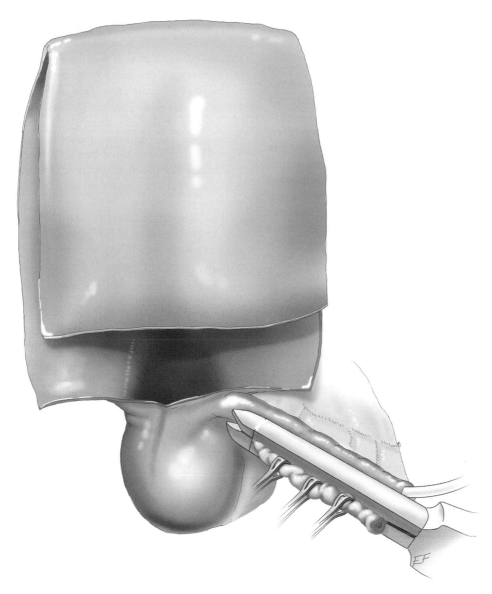

FIGURE 32B-6. Tapering of the ileal segment.

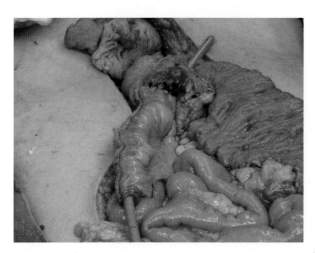

FIGURE 32B-7. Plication of the ileocecal valve continence mechanism.

withdrawn and reinserted several times to ensure that the plicated ileocecal valve is tight enough to ensure continence yet still able to be easily intubated by the pliable Robinson catheter.

Creation of Stoma Site

Maximum mobility of the right colon pouch should be confirmed, and an appropriate stoma site in the right lower quadrant should be selected that will allow a tension-free approximation of the distal ileal segment to the skin. The ileal segment is passed through the stoma aperture to test the "fit," and then returned to the abdominal cavity. The stoma will be created in the same fashion as described earlier for an ileal conduit.

Ureterocolic Anastomosis and Closure of the Pouch

The base of the right colon pouch should lie tension-free in the right lower quadrant. The left ureter is mobilized above the pelvic brim and brought beneath the inferior mesenteric artery to reach the posterior wall of the pouch, generally the cecum or proximal ascending colon. The right ureter will be anatomically closer to the base of the pouch and requires less mobilization. It is easier to perform the right ureterocolic anastomosis first. An appropriate site is selected on the posterior wall of the pouch that will allow a tension-free anastomosis for the right ureter, and a small defect is created in the colonic wall at this site over a Mixter or tonsil clamp using the electrosurgical unit. The clamp is then used to grasp the suture on the ligated end of the right ureter, and the ureter is brought into the base of the pouch. The distal ureter is trimmed obliquely and spatulated, as previously described, and a 6- or 7-French double-J ureteral stent is passed up to the level of the renal pelvis. A direct mucosa-to-mucosa anastomosis is created using 6 to 8 interrupted stitches of 4-0 delayed-absorbable monofilament suture, and the stent is transfixed to the colonic mucosa using a through-and-through stitch of 1-0 chromic suture. A 3-0 delayed-absorbable monofilament suture is passed through the distal end of the double-J ureteral stent and passed down the ileal segment and out the efferent end to be used for later extraction of the stent.

The same procedure is repeated for the left ureter (Figure 32B-8). It is advisable to use different color sutures passed through the distal ends of the right and left ureteral stents to facilitate accurate identification at the time of stent extraction. Alternatively, an antireflux mechanism can be constructed by tunneling the ureters under the muscularis of the colon for a distance of 2 cm and then placating over this with 4-0 Vicryl suture. Care must be taken when constructing this antireflux mechanism to ensure the ureters have adequate spatulation and opening so that there are no ureteral strictures.

The Robinson catheter should be replaced by a 14- or 16-French 3-way Foley catheter. The anterior closure of the pouch base is completed, and the efferent ileal segment (with Foley catheter and ureteral extraction sutures protruding) is brought through the abdominal wall to the stoma site (Figure 32B-9). The anterior wall of the pouch should be secured to the peritoneum of the anterior abdominal wall to ensure that the ileocecal valve continence mechanism is juxtaposed to the anterior abdominal wall and that redundancy of the ileal segment will not be created by the pouch "settling" into the pelvis. The "rosebud" stoma is created in the same fashion as for an ileal conduit. The pouch is filled with 400 to 500 mL of a dilute methylene blue solution, through the irrigating port of the 3-way Foley catheter, and inspected for any areas of leakage. The ureteral stent extraction sutures are secured to the skin 1 to 2 cm away from the

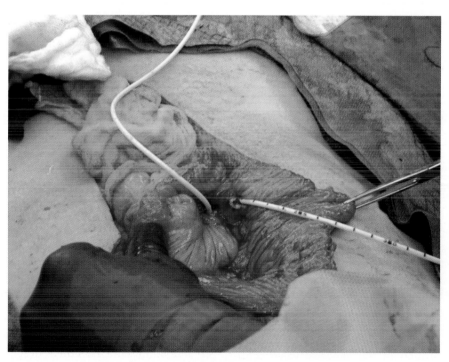

FIGURE 32B-8. Ureteral anastomosis to the colonic urinary pouch.

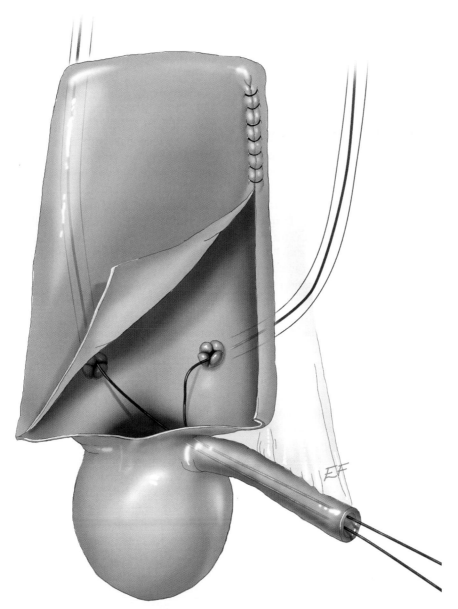

FIGURE 32B-9. Final stages of completing colonic urinary pouch.

stoma using a Mayo needle, and the Foley catheter is attached to drainage. Prior to closure of the abdomen, a closed-suction drain (eg, Jackson-Pratt) is placed in the dependent pelvis.

Re-establish Intestinal Continuity

Intestinal continuity is re-established by creating a side-to-side functional end-to-end enterocolostomy between the distal ileum and midtransverse colon using the GIA and TA stapling devices. The intervening mesenteric defect is closed with a series of interrupted sutures, with care taken not to constrict the blood supply to the right colon urinary pouch.

Postoperative Care

Box 32B-4	Complications and Morbidity

- Early Complications
  - Anastomotic leak
  - Catheter obstruction from thick mucus
  - Difficulty catheterizing pouch
  - Infection
- Late Complications
  - Anastomotic stricture, hydronephrosis
  - Chronic renal insufficiency
  - Nephrolithiasis

The management of a continent pouch postoperatively is more complex than managing a noncontinent ileal conduit. An abdominal film should be obtained in the postoperative period to confirm stent position, and stoma condition should be assessed daily. The 3-way Foley catheter should be irrigated with 60 to 120 mL of saline solution every 3 to 4 hours until mucus production decreases (usually 10-14 days). The Foley catheter is drained to gravity in between irrigations. The differential diagnosis of low urine output includes the same entities as for ileal conduit, as well as a blocked Foley catheter due to thick colonic mucus production. An abdominal ultrasound can detect an overdistended pouch. Increased frequency of irrigation should remedy this problem. The Foley catheter can be removed on postoperative day 10, and the patient is instructed in self-catheterization using an 18- to 22-French catheter. Self-catheterization should be performed every 4 hours initially, with frequent use of irrigation until mucus production subsides. The frequency of catheterization can gradually be decreased. Ideally, maximum pouch capacity will be at least 500 mL, and the patient should have to self-catheterize no more than 4 or 5 times per day, although this is highly individualized.

Three to 6 weeks postoperatively, an intravenous pyelogram or CT urogram should be obtained to confirm pouch integrity. Removal of the ureteral stents is accomplished by cutting the ureteral stent extraction sutures attached to the peristomal skin and pulling out one stent at a time. The same precautions and surveillance for long-term complications and electrolyte abnormalities observed for the ileal conduit apply to care of the continent colonic conduit.

A pouchogram should be ordered 4 to 5 weeks postoperatively and in 3 to 6 months to evaluate the size of the pouch. If there are any abnormalities noted or if the patient is having any difficulty with significant residual after catheterization, additional postoperative care should include evaluation with an intravenous pyelogram, pouchogram, serum electrolytes, and renal ultrasound and nuclear medicine scans to ensure that the pouch and renal function and upper urinary tracts stay within normal limits. It should also be noted that it is very difficult to assess urine culture status and that treatment of pyelonephritis would need to be based on clinical symptoms such as back pain, leukocytosis, and febrile episodes.

The complications are similar to those with an ileal conduit and can be divided into early complications and late complications. Complications include urinary leakage, low urine output, and small bowel obstruction similarly seen with other urinary diversion procedures. Ureteral anastomotic leaks may occur, as well as leaks from the pouch. Such complications should initially have nonsurgical interventions such as placement of drains via interventional radiology and percutaneous nephrostomy drainage to safely manage these complications because the ileal conduit will resolve and heal on its own.[22-26] It should be noted that if there is urine extravasation on a pouchogram done within the early postoperative period, conservative management should be the initial treatment. Such treatment includes drainage with a Jackson-Pratt drain placed within the pelvis, percutaneous nephrostomy drainage, and continuation with ureteral stents. One should also make sure that a ureteral anastomotic leak is not present. Urinomas need to be not only diverted, but also drained to ensure adequate healing. With urinomas or pelvic abscesses, this acute inflammatory process will cause significant edema and inflammation and may lead to ureteral strictures. It is extremely important that the patient is able to self-catheterize and get good emptying of the pouch. The Malecot drain should stay in place until this has been demonstrated. Hyperchloremic metabolic acidosis is a complication that can be seen with continent urinary diversions, especially a large continent urinary diversion due to absorption of solute. If this occurs, depending on the severity of the issue, the patient may need to self-catheterize more often or be managed with sodium bicarbonate supplementation. If the problem continues, the patient may need a conversion to a noncontinent urinary diversion with placement of a catheter along with a stomal bag.

In a recent review by Ramirez et al[7] from the MD Anderson Cancer Center, complications of continent urinary diversion using the ileal colonic segment were studied. The most common complications postoperatively included febrile episodes, pneumonia bacteremia, postoperative ileus, wound complications such as infections and wound disruption, prolonged intubations, anastomotic leak, pelvic abscess, and deep venous thrombosis. Complications related to the continent conduit reservoir included stomal strictures, acute renal failure, ureteral colonic anastomosis strictures, and anastomotic leaks. Late complications occurring after more than 60 days included chronic pyelonephritis, urinary stomal strictures, nephrolithiasis, the pouch basically being incontinent, ureteral strictures, acute renal failure, and fistula development. It should be noted that of the patients in this study, 18 were without evidence of disease at follow-up, 13 had died of disease, 7 had died from other causes, and 2 were alive with disease. In the patients who had long-term follow-up, 36 of 40 reported normal continent function after management of their complications.

It should be highlighted that these complications should be managed conservatively and reoperation is reserved for patients who fail conservative measures. Conservative management procedures include ureteral dilatation and percutaneous nephrostomy tube drainage for management of ureteral stenosis and urinary leaks. The need for reimplantation of ureters may be very challenging, and if the stricture is due to ischemia, reoperation with a radiated ureter again may lead to further stricture development. If there is an incompetent ileocecal valve, this incompetence results from high pressure spikes, and it may be necessary to consider reoperation for ureteral reimplantation and creation of a new pouch or conversion to a noncontinent diversion. An additional long-term complication may be the development of nephrolithiasis and pouch stones. The longer patients have these pouches, the more these complications may be seen, and management will depend on renal function and symptoms.

REFERENCES

1. Estape R, Mendez LE, Angioli R, Penalver M. Urinary diversion in gynecologic oncology. *Surg Clin N Am.* 2001;81(4): 781-797.

2. Lambrou NC, Pearson JM, Averette HE. Pelvic exenteration of gynecologic malignancy: indications, and technical and reconstructive considerations. *Surg Oncol Clin N Am.* 2005;14(2): 289-300.

3. Goldberg GL, Sukumvanich P, Einstein MH, Smith HO, Anderson PS, Fields AL. Total pelvic exenteration: The Albert Einstein College of Medicine/Montefiore Medical Center Experience (1987 to 2003). *Gynecol Oncol.* 2006;101(2): 261-268.

4. Berek JS, Howe C, Lagasse LD, Hacker NF. Pelvic exenteration for recurrent gynecologic malignancy: survival and morbidity analysis of the 45-year experience at UCLA. *Gynecol Oncol.* 2005;99(1):153-159.

5. Morrow CP, Curtin JP. Surgery on the urinary tract. In: Morrow CP, Curtin JP, eds. *Gynecologic Cancer Surgery.* New York, NY: Churchill Livingstone; 1996:279.

6. Goldberg JM, Piver MS, Hempling RE, et al. Improvements in pelvic exenteration: factors responsible for reducing morbidity and mortality. *Ann Surg Oncol.* 1998;5(5):399-406.

7. Ramirez PT, Modesitt SC, Morris M, et al. Functional outcomes and complications of continent urinary diversions in patients with gynecologic malignancies. *Gynecol Oncol.* 2002;85(2): 285-291.

8. Mirhashemi R, Im S, Yazdani T. Urinary diversion following radical pelvic surgery. *Curr Opin Obstet Gynecol.* 2004;16(5): 419-422.

9. Houvenaeghel G, Moutardier V, Karsenty G, et al. Major complications of urinary diversion after pelvic exenteration for gynecologic malignancies: a 23-year mono-institutional experience in 124 patients. *Gynecol Oncol.* 2004;92(2):680-683.

10. Evans B, Montie JE, Gilbert SM. Incontinent or continent urinary diversion: how to make the right choice. *Curr Opin Urol.* 2010;20:421-425.

11. Silver DF, Ashwell TR. Choices in creating continent urostomies following pelvic exenteration for gynecologic malignancies. *Gynecol Oncol.* 2001;82(3):510-515.

12. Wheeless CR. Recent advances in surgical reconstruction of the gynecologic cancer patient. *Curr Opin Obstet Gynecol.* 1992;4(1):91-101.

13. Stanhope CR, Symmonds RE, Lee RA, et al. Urinary diversion with us of ileal and sigmoid conduits. *Am J Obstet Gynecol.* 1986;155(2):288-292.

14. Karsenty G, Moutardier V, Lelong B, et al. Long-term follow-up of continent urinary diversion after pelvic exenteration for gynecologic malignancies. *Gynecol Oncol.* 2005;97(2): 524-528.

15. Katkoori D, Samvedi S, Adiyat KT, Soloway MS, Manoharan M. Is the incidence of uretero-intestinal anastomotic stricture increased in patients undergoing radical cystectomy with previous pelvic radiation? *BJU Int.* 2010;105(6):795-798.

16. Golda T, Biondo S, Kreisler E, et al. Follow-up double-barreled wet colostomy after pelvic exenteration at a single institution. *Dis Colon Rectum.* 2010;53(5):822-829.

17. Kouba E, Sands M, Lentz A, Wallen E, Pruthi RS. A comparison of the Bricker versus Wallace ureteroileal anastomosis in patients undergoing urinary diversion for bladder cancer. *J Urol.* 2007;178(3):945-949.

18. Chechile G, Klein EA, Bauer L, Novick AC, Montie JE. Functional equivalence of end and loop ileal conduit stomas. *J Urol.* 1992;147(3):582-586.

19. Winter WE, Krivak TC, Maxwell GL, et al. Modified technique for urinary diversion with incontinent conduits. *Gynecol Oncol.* 2002;86(3):351-353.

20. Elkas JC, Berek JS, Leuchter R, Lagasse LD, Karlan BY. Lower urinary tract reconstruction with ileum in the treatment of gynecologic malignancies. *Gynecol Oncol.* 2005;97(2): 685-692.

21. Barbieri CE, Schwartz MJ, Boorjian SA, Lee MM, Scherr DS. Ureteroileal anastomosis with intraluminal visualization: technique and outcomes. *Urology.* 2010;76(6):1496-1500.

22. Ngioli R, Zullo MA, Plotti F, et al. Urologic function and urodynamic evaluation of urinary diversion (Rome pouch) over time in gynecologic cancers patients. *Gynecol Oncol.* 2007;107(2):200-204.

23. Penalver MA, Angioli R, Mirhashemi R, Malik R. Management of early and late complications of ileocolonic continent urinary reservoir (Miami Pouch). *Gynecol Oncol.* 1998;69(3):185-191.

24. Penalver MA, Bejany DE, Averette HE, et al. Continent urinary diversion in gynecologic oncology. *Gynecol Oncol.* 1989;34(3):274-288.

25. Wilson TG, Moreno JG, Weinberg A, Ahlering TE. Late complications of the modified Indiana pouch. *J Urol.* 1994; 151(2):331-334.

26. Rowland RG, Kropp BP. Evolution of the Indiana continent urinary reservoir. *J Urol.* 1994;152(6):2247-2251.

C. Vaginal and Vulvar Reconstruction

Leigh G. Seamon and Jay W. Carlson

VAGINAL RECONSTRUCTION

Indications for Vaginal Reconstruction

Following the extirpative phase of radical pelvic surgery for gynecologic, urologic, or colorectal malignancies, neovaginal creation is an important aspect of pelvic floor reconstruction. In addition to optimizing potential sexual function, pelvic reconstruction serves to close anatomical dead space and introduce new vascular supply to an often previously irradiated and devascularized area. The reconstruction results in improved wound healing, decreased fistula formation, reduced postoperative seroma and abscess formation, and improved quality of life.[1-8] Although surgical times may be longer in patients undergoing primary vaginal reconstruction, pelvic abscesses and small bowel fistulas are reduced compared to patients without neovaginal reconstruction (0%-7% vs. 20%-27% and 3% vs. 20%, respectively).[2,3] Other authors report a reduction in intestinal fistula rates from 16% to 5% with reconstruction and no increase in operative time with the use of 2 surgical teams.[1,9-11]

Some patients may not desire a neovagina for intercourse; however, the reduced perioperative morbidity associated with myocutaneous flap neovascularization should be considered when counseling patients for reconstruction. A knowledge of various reconstructive techniques is an essential component in the gynecologic surgeon's operative armamentarium.[12] The main goals and principles of vaginal reconstruction are outlined in Table 32C-1.

Classification of Vaginal Defects Following Exenteration

A formal classification system for vaginal defects following extirpative surgery was proposed by Cordeiro et al[13] to facilitate an algorithm for vaginal reconstruction (Figure 32C-1). In this system, partial vaginal removal is considered a type I defect, whereas circumferential vaginal resection is a type II defect. Type I (partial) vaginal defects are further separated into type IA defects, described as anterior or lateral vaginal wall defects, and type IB defects, described as removal of only the posterior vaginal wall. Circumferential defects (type II) are subdivided into type IIA, removal of the upper two-thirds of the vagina, and type IIB, total vaginectomy.[13]

The surgeon must be prepared to perform the optimal procedure for the specific situation accounting for individual preoperative and postoperative variables.[12] Rather than using a specific algorithm, we have used this anatomical classification system, acknowledging its limitations, to propose various methods for surgical reconstruction according to anatomical defect.

Classification of Surgical Procedures for Vulvovaginal Reconstruction

Reconstruction can be generally classified according to procedure type: grafts or flaps. Grafts are further subdivided into split-thickness, full-thickness, and anastomosed grafts. Flaps are usually named by the location of the donor site and are described as random skin flaps, axial pattern skin flaps, fasciocutaneous flaps,

Table 32C-1 Goals and Principles of Vaginal Reconstruction at the Time of Pelvic Exenteration

1. Appropriately counseled patient and family using a multidisciplinary approach
2. Reconstruction should:
   a. Provide immediate restoration of anatomic function
   b. Improve operative outcomes by:
      i Facilitating primary healing
      ii Closing anatomic dead space
      iii Decreasing fistula formation
      iv Reducing postoperative seromas and abscess formation
   c. Have acceptable morbidity and operative time
   d. Have donor site selected that has similar characteristics to vaginal tissue, is expendable, and is transferable with acceptable morbidity
3. Method of reconstruction
   a. Appropriately planned preoperatively to meet the above goals accounting for patient variables such as history of previous radiation, comorbidities, and patient body mass index
   b. Alternative plan in the event of unanticipated findings or surgical misadventure

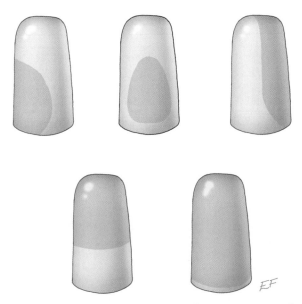

FIGURE 32C-1. Anatomical classification system for vaginal defects following extirpative surgery. (Redrawn, with permission, from Pusic AL, Mehrara BJ. Vaginal reconstruction: an algorithm approach to defect classification and flap reconstruction. *J Surg Oncol.* 2006;94(6):515-521.)

myocutaneous flaps, or intestinal flaps (Table 32C-2). Additionally, the procedures can be classified according to donor site (distant vs. local), blood supply (none, random, or a specific artery), and type of sensory innervation (sensate vs. nonsensate).

General Preoperative Preparation for Vaginal Reconstruction

During the preoperative phase, the goals and objectives of vaginal reconstruction are reviewed with the patient. For the patient and the supporting family, a multidisciplinary approach with psychiatry, enterostomal therapy nurses, and a patient who has previously undergone a similar procedure may be beneficial.[12,14] Consultation with anesthesia and reservation of a critical care bed are also essential steps in preoperative planning. Additionally, it is important to consult with radiation oncology regarding previous radiation doses and fields and discuss any planned intraoperative or postoperative radiation because this may have important implications for reconstruction and flap selection.[14,15] The gynecologic surgeon must have a

Table 32C-2 Classification of Reconstructive Vulvovaginal Procedures

	Donor Site	Blood Supply	Sensory Innervation	Ref
Grafts				
Split-thickness skin graft	Distant	NA	Recipient site	14,15
Full-thickness skin graft	Distant	NA	Recipient site	16
Buccal mucosa graft	Distant	NA	Recipient site	17
Random skin flaps				
Limberg flaps[a]	Local	Random	S3,4 dermatomes	18
Pubolabial V-Y amplified advancement flap[b]	Local	Random	L1,2;S3,4 dermatomes	19
Medial thigh V-Y advancement flap, with or without gracilis muscle	Local	Random	L2; S3,4 dermatomes	20,21
Gluteal V-Y advancement flap, with or without gluteus maximus muscle	Local	Random	S2-4 dermatomes	22,23
Axial pattern skin flaps				
Anterior labial flap[c]	Local	Descending branch of superficial external pudendal artery	NA	24
Posterior labial flap[c]	Local	Posterior labial artery (terminal branch of internal pudendal artery)	NA	25
Mons pubis flap[d]	Local	Superficial external pudendal artery	NA	26
Groin flap	Local	Superficial circumflex Iliac artery	NA	27,28

(Continued)

Table 32C-2 Classification of Reconstructive Vulvovaginal Procedures (Continued)

	Donor Site	Blood Supply	Sensory Innervation	Ref
Fasciocutaneous flaps				
Pudendal thigh flaps[e]	Local	Perineal terminal branches of internal pudendal artery	Superficial perineal branches of pudendal nerve; perineal branches of posterior cutaneus nerve of thigh	29,30
Anterolateral thigh flap	Distant	Lateral circumflex femoral artery	Lateral femoral cutaneous nerve	31
Medial thigh flap	Distant	Branch of superficial femoral artery	Anterior cutaneous branches of femoral nerve	32
Muculocutaneous flaps				
Rectus femoris flap	Distant	Lateral circumflex femoral artery	Anterior cutaneous branches of femoral nerve	33
Tensor fasciae latae flap	Distant	Lateral circumflex femoral artery	Lateral femoral cutaneous nerve	34
Vastus lateralis flap	Distant	Lateral circumflex femoral artery	Lateral femoral cutaneous nerve	35
Gluteal thigh flap[f]	Distant	Terminal branches of inferior gluteal artery	Posterior cutaneous nerve of thigh	36
Gracilis flap	Distant	Medial circumflex femoral artery	Anterior cutaneous branches of femoral nerve; cutaneous branch of obturator nerve	37
Short gracilis flap	Distant	Terminal branches of obturator artery	Cutaneous branch of obturator nerve	38
Rectus abdominis flap[g]	Distant	Deep Inferior epigastric artery	NA	39
Deep Inferior epigastric perforator flap	Distant	Deep Inferior epigastric artery	NA	40,41
Bowel flaps				
Ileum flap	Distant	Ileal artery	NA	42
(ileo)caecum flap	Distant	Ileocolic artery	NA	43
Sigmoid-colon flap	Distant	Sigmoid-colon artery	NA	44

NA = not applicable.[a]Rhomboid flaps. [b]V-Y amplified sliding flap from pubis. [c]Bulbocavernosus flap, Martius flap. [d]Superficial external pudendal artery flap. [e]Lotus petal flap, gluteal fold (sulcus) flap, Singapore flap. [f]Gluteus maximus flap. [g]Vertical rectus abdominis flap (VRAM) or transverse rectus abdominis flap (TRAM).
Reprinted, with permission, from Hockel M, Dornhofer N. Vulvovaginal reconstruction for neoplastic disease. *Lancet Oncol.* 2008;9(6):559-568.

well-thought-out approach to both the extirpative and reconstruction phases with contingency plans based on the operative events or surgical findings.

General preoperative preparation for vaginal reconstructive procedures is similar for vulvar surgeries. If the patient has undergone a previous abdominal procedure or has severe peripheral vascular disease and a rectus myocutaneous flap is planned, a review of the operative report or a preoperative arteriogram may be required to ensure the patency of the inferior epigastric artery. When reconstruction is performed immediately following an exenteration, we recommend preoperative stomal site marking. Given the radicality of exenterative procedures and the reconstruction, it is the authors' preference to instruct the patient to undergo a chlorhexidine shower/wash and prepare the bowel. Patients are instructed to drink clear liquids the day prior to surgery and use a cathartic solution over 2 to 4 hours. Perioperative prophylactic antibiotic must include a spectrum of coverage for bowel organisms. In the preoperative holding area, the patient is given heparin 5000 units subcutaneously 2 hours prior to surgery. If vaginal reconstruction accompanies an exenterative procedure, the patient is typed and crossed for 4 units of packed red blood cells.

Positioning and Planning

The patient is placed in dorsal low lithotomy position with support of the lower leg (Allen stirrups; Hill-Rom Holdings, Inc., Batesville, IN) with the coccyx slightly overhanging the end of the operating room table. Positioning may be best accomplished with the patient in slight Trendelenburg to simulate perineal access for the extirpative and reconstructive phases because any slight intraoperative cephalad shift may impede exposure. The potential donor site(s) is (are) marked with a permanent pen. Regardless of the planned procedure, the entire abdomen is prepped from the midnipple line to the pubic symphysis, covering the midaxillary line, and inguinal regions. Prepping this area, as well as the lateral thigh and both legs from below the knee to the perineum, will allow for the preparation of multiple donor sites if required. Additionally, the perineum, including the anus, buttocks, and posterior anal/coccygeal area, is thoroughly prepped, and a Foley catheter is placed.

To expedite total operative length, a second surgical team is beneficial to concomitantly perform the vulvovaginal extirpative and reconstruction phases. If a rectus myocutaneous flap is planned, harvesting the flap and rotating it into the pelvis is typically the first reconstructive step initiated immediately after the resection is completed. This allows a second surgical team to tubularize the flap and suture the neovagina in place. This procedural order also prevents potential disruption of the urinary/fecal diversion as well as stomal site misplacement caused by flap harvesting and abdominal wall mobilization required to close the donor-site defect.

Reconstruction for Type I (Partial) Vaginal Defects

Skin Grafts With an Omental Flap

Free skin grafts are classified into 3 categories: split-thickness skin grafts (STSGs), full-thickness skin grafts (FTSGs), and anastomosed grafts. This chapter will focus only on STSGs and FTSGs. These 2 grafts

depend on the spontaneous development of vascular supply and intimate contact between the graft and the recipient site. The host site should be free of infection and remain immobile until neovascularization occurs. This requires strict bed rest for 2 to 3 days postoperatively with the blood supply remaining tenuous until approximately 7 days postoperatively.

Split-Thickness Skin Grafts

Procedure Overview

Box 32C-1	Master Surgeon's Corner

- STSG with an omental flap is most useful for coverage of partial vaginal (type I) defects.
- Meticulous hemostasis must be achieved.
- The STSG must be well applied to the vaginal stent to ensure complete "take."

After the pelvic extirpative phase, an STSG with an omental flap as its base can be used for partial vaginal removal (type IA or IB) or for circumferential defects (type IIA or IIB), particularly when the pelvis does not allow room for a myocutaneous flap, such as in an obese patient, or when a coloproctostomy (low rectal anastomosis) is performed (Figure 32C-2). This technique for neovaginal reconstruction following pelvic exenteration was first reported by Berek and colleagues, who modified the McIndoe-Banister vaginoplasty by using omentum to create the anterior and lateral vaginal walls.[16,17] Wheeless modified Berek's procedure by using the omentum as a cylindrical neovaginal wall lined by an STSG.[18,19] Since these initial reports, other authors affirmed the feasibility of this procedure or further modified the technique by eliminating the STSG and substituting a polyglycolic acid mesh or an acellular dermal allograft for type IA (anterior wall) vaginal defects.[20-23] Additionally, use of fibrin tissue adhesive (Tisseel VH fibrin sealant; Baxter, Deerfield, IL) with or without vacuum-assisted closure (V.A.C. Therapy System; KCI, San Antonio, TX) may improve STSG viability and is further described in the section on STSG for vulvar reconstruction.[16,24-26] Although STSG combined with omental cylinder is feasible for type II defects following exenteration, we believe it is not well suited for large defects in previously irradiated fields, where we prefer a myocutaneous flap such as the rectus myocutaneous flap described later.

Preoperative Preparation

Skin grafting requires careful selection of the donor site. The patient should be encouraged to wear shorts or other similar clothing to assist with defining

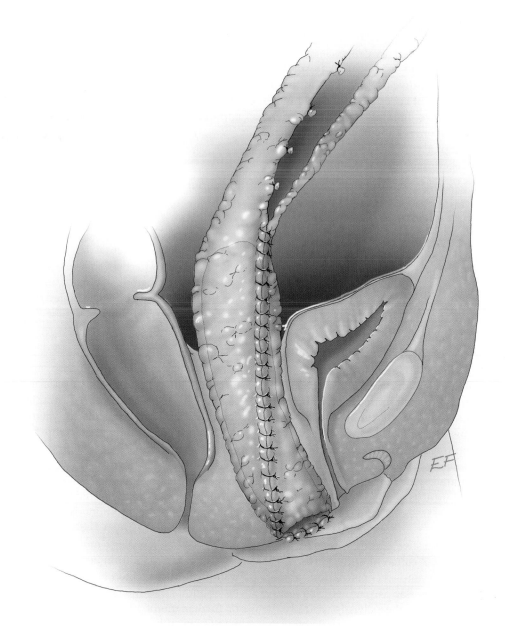

FIGURE 32C-2. Split-thickness skin graft with omental flap for neovaginal reconstruction.

donor-site concealment boundaries.[27] For a more cosmetic result, several authors advocate using the inner thigh or the buttocks versus the lateral or anterior thigh as the donor site; however, the skin on the inner thigh is generally thinner (0.016 in) than skin on the buttocks or lateral/anterior thigh (0.018 in), and the dermatome should be adjusted accordingly.[27]

Operative Procedure

Preparing the Omental Flap for STSGs. First, the lesser sac is entered, as is done for an omentectomy. The omentum is freed from the transverse colon and colonic mesentery and harvested from the stomach's greater curvature by securing the right gastroepiploic vessels and its gastric branches. The left gastroepiploic vessels are spared and supply blood to the omental flap. It is important to adequately mobilize the omentum in order to obtain the desired pedicle. The omental J-flap is placed out of the way until the reconstructive phase when it is placed lateral to the descending colon along the left colic gutter. It is recommended to delay suturing the proximal omentum to the gutter until the omental cylinder and graft with vaginal stent are placed in the pelvis. This maximizes manipulation and utilization of the omental flap.

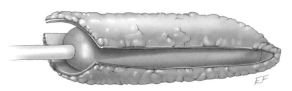

FIGURE 32C-3. Split-thickness skin graft with the dermis facing outward over a vaginal mold. (Adapted from Kusiak JF, Rosenblum NG. Neovaginal reconstruction after exenteration using an omental flap and split-thickness skin graft. *Plast Reconstr Surg.* 1996;97(4):775-781.)

Harvesting the STSG and Placing the Graft Over a Vaginal Stent. Prior to sterile prepping, the donor site is marked to allow a 10 × 20 cm STSG. A region at least this size is needed to accommodate the 20% passive contraction that is expected with STSG. A 10 × 20 cm STSG is harvested from the donor site using an air-powered dermatome set to 13 to 19/1000 of an inch (0.013-0.019) and the graft meshed in a ratio of 1.5:1. If the graft is taken from the buttocks, this is done prior to the laparotomy, and the graft is stored. A thin layer of thrombin spray (or diluted 100-fold Tisseel) is placed on the donor site and covered with a clear occlusive dressing such as Tegaderm (3M, St. Paul, MN) or petrolatum-impregnated gauze followed by a pressure dressing. The STSG is placed over a vaginal stent (Adjustable Vaginal Stent; Mentor Corporation, Santa Barbara, CA) with the dermis facing outward. The STSG is sutured together using undyed interrupted 3-0 polyglycolic acid suture (Figure 32C-3).

Wrapping the STSG and Mold in the Distal Omental Flap and Placement in the Pelvis. The graft and mold are placed into the distal portion of the omental flap, which is made into a cylinder. The lateral rolled margins and apex/cephalad portion are sutured without compromising the vascular supply using interrupted and mattress 3-0 polyglycolic acid sutures, respectively. The apical sutures prevent the vaginal mold and graft from migrating deep into the pelvis. The STSG-covered stent and omental cylinder are placed in the pelvis, taking care not to distort the orientation of the omental cylinder. The distal omentum is sutured to the vaginal introitus.

The proximal omental flap is sutured along the left lateral gutter and to the iliopectineal line to create a "pelvic lid" preventing bowel prolapse into the pelvis. If there is not enough omentum to create the lid, the omental lid can be augmented with polyglycolic acid mesh. Transverse monofilament sutures (2-0 nylon) placed through the labia serve to secure the stent and prevent expulsion. It is recommended that the patient be taken back the operating room in 7 to 10 days for stent removal under sedation.

Postoperative Care

Box 32C-2	Complications and Morbidity

- Graft "take" is re-evaluated on postoperative day 7 to 10 to assess viability.
- Necrotic tissue should be resected at this time.
- Total graft failure requires repeat skin grafting or use of a myocutaneous flap.
- Vaginal stenting should continue until sexual activity or for a period of 1 year.

The patient should remain at complete bed rest for 2 to 3 days postoperatively. On day 7 to 10 following the procedure, the patient returns to the operating suite for vaginal stent removal, donor-site dressing change, and fitting of a soft Silastic vaginal mold. The mold is placed inside a condom, and the condom is changed daily. For patient comfort and to prevent expulsion, the length of the mold should not protrude from the introitus. The patient is instructed to insert the stent for 20 to 30 minutes 3 times a day and while asleep at night. The patient returns to the office 2 to 4 weeks after stent removal for inspection of the neovagina. Sexually active patients may discontinue the vaginal mold after 3 to 6 months and resume intercourse. Otherwise, it is recommended that the stenting continue for 1 year.

Full-Thickness Skin Grafts

Procedure Overview

FTSGs include the epidermal and dermal skin layer versus only the epidermal layer with STSG. The main advantage of FTSGs over STSGs is reduction in secondary contracture, which translates into decreased risk of neovaginal stenosis and less time required for vaginal stenting. Additionally, the donor site of FTSGs heals in a more cosmetic fashion due to primary closure, whereas the STSG requires secondary healing. However, the disadvantages of FTSG over STSG include hair growth, increased primary contraction rates (up to 50% vs. 20% with STSG), a potentially higher infection risk, and longer healing time (14 days vs. 7-10 days with STSG).[27]

Preoperative Preparation

The patient is prepared as described earlier for STSG. Prior to prepping the skin, an 8 × 16 to 17 cm hairless, elliptical donor site is marked in the groin region adhering to Langer's lines (Figure 32C-4). Some authors recommend bilateral groin grafts measuring 7 × 15 cm each, whereas others recommend a graft that is 3 times longer than wide, allowing nice donor-site approximation.[28]

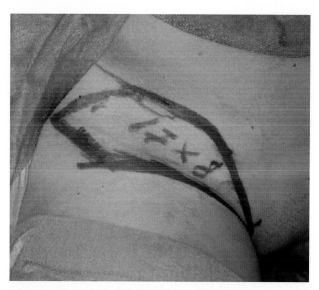

FIGURE 32C-4. Donor site for a full-thickness skin graft for vaginal reconstruction. (Reproduced, with permission, from Hallberg H, Holmstrom H. Vaginal construction with skin grafts and vacuum-assisted closure. *Scand J Plast Reconstr Surg Hand Surg.* 2003;37(2):97-101.)

Consideration may be given to preoperative donor-site depilation to avoid hair growth.

Operative Procedure and Postoperative Care

The previously marked donor site is incised, the graft is harvested and moistened with saline, and the subcutaneous adherent fat is removed with curved scissors. The FTSG is meshed if required, and the donor site is closed primarily. The graft is then sutured around a vaginal mold and placed into the pelvic cavity, and the free edges are sutured to the introitus. A suprapubic catheter will avoid potential urethral necrosis from the vaginal mold placing pressure on the Foley catheter. Postoperative care is similar to STSG; however, because the FTSG is less prone to secondary contracture, vaginal stenting is only needed for 3 to 6 months.

Mesh or Allograft Omental Flaps

Procedure Overview

Alternatives to using autologous grafts for vaginal reconstruction include use of polyglycolic acid mesh and acellular dermal allografts in combination with an omental flap. This technique is best suited for partial vaginal wall defects (type I defects). The advantages to this approach include that there is readily available material, decreasing the operative time and avoiding donor-site issues including potential infection, postoperative pain, and scar formation. The basic principles of the procedure are similar to STSG, as described earlier.

Preoperative Preparation

Patients should be informed that a skin substitute will help recreate the vaginal wall and that the possibility of an infection or reaction to this material exists. Materials used for neovagina reconstruction after exenteration includes a woven mesh (Vicryl; Ethicon Inc., Cornelia, GA) and a regenerative tissue matrix (AlloDerm; LifeCell Corp., The Woodlands, TX).[21-23] Although Vicryl mesh is made from polyglycolic acid and is absorbable, AlloDerm is procured from human cadaver skin and processed to allow a foundation for neoangiogenesis and epithelialization without an inflammatory response.[29] These acellular dermal allografts are generally 2.06 to 3.30 mm thick and meshed 1:1 (LifeCell).

Operative Procedure and Postoperative Care

The omental flap is prepared, and an acellular dermal allograft is selected (6 × 16 cm or 4 × 12 cm), rehydrated in sterile saline for 5 minutes, and trimmed to fit the defect. If used for a type II defect, the 6 × 16 cm piece is chosen and folded over a vaginal stent to create a cylinder. Alternatively, 2 pieces of 4 × 12 cm grafts are trimmed and sutured together. The allograft is placed over the vaginal mold, sutured to the omental bed (or cylinder for type II defects), and placed in the pelvis. The allograft is then sutured into the remaining vaginal wall or the introitus, if a total exenteration is performed.

Alternatively, for type I defects, a polyglycolic acid mesh with omental flap can be considered. The mesh is trimmed to size, fit over a vaginal stent, and sutured into the remaining vagina with a running 3-0 polyglycolic acid suture. The postoperative care is similar to STSGs.

Reconstruction for Type II (Circumferential) Vaginal Defects

Circumferential vaginal defects following exenterative procedures usually require reconstructive flaps. Flap selection will depend on the size of the defect, the functional effect on both the recipient and donor sites, and operator experience. Although no single flap is suitable in all situations for neovaginal reconstruction, we prefer the vertical rectus abdominis flap when feasible due to its bulk, reliability, and minimal donor-site morbidity and incorporation into the midline incision.[9,30-32]

Skin Flap Classification

Skin flaps include the epidermis, dermis, and subcutaneous tissue, whereas fasciocutaneous flaps incorporate the underlying fascia in addition to the epidermis, dermis, and subcutaneous tissue. A myocutaneous flap also incorporates the underlying muscle. Myocutaneous flaps that are supplied by a single artery (tensor fascia lata), a dominant pedicle plus 1 or more minor vessels (gracilis), or 2 dominant vessels (rectus abdominis) are considered type I, type II, or type III flaps, respectively.

A simplified classification divides flaps into groups according to blood supply: cutaneous/random pattern, arterial/axial pattern, island, and free flaps.[33] Cutaneous flaps or random pattern skin flaps rely on subdermal vascularization, whereas a single subcutaneous vessel supplies arterial or axial pattern flaps. Flaps whose pedicle consists of only the vessels are termed island flaps. Free flaps are harvested from distant sites and require microvascular anastomoses compared to local flaps, which are derived from skin adjacent to the recipient site. Local flaps are further characterized by the manner in which the donor site arrives at the recipient site: transposition, rotation, or advancement. A transposition flap further describes that it has been tunneled under or passed over a normal tissue bridge. Flaps that are rotated in an arc to reach the recipient site are rotational flaps, whereas flaps that arrive at the recipient site by mobilization in a relatively straight line are called advancement flaps.

Posterior Labial Artery/Pudendal Thigh Fasciocutaneous/Singapore Flaps

Procedure Overview

Box 32C-3	Master Surgeon's Corner

- The pudendal thigh flap is a sensate, axial pattern, fasciocutaneous flap that is useful for covering vaginal defects or neovagina creation with bilateral flaps.
- Flap size can be tailored to patient anatomy.
- The underlying adductor fascia is raised with the flap, and labial "tunnel" pressure is avoided to ensure viability.

In 1989, Wee and Joseph[34] from Singapore first described the neurovascular pudendal thigh fasciocutaneous flap for vaginal reconstruction. The pudendal thigh flap is a sensate, axial pattern, fasciocutaneous flap that is vascularized by the posterior labial artery, a terminal branch of the superficial perineal artery, which is derived from the internal pudendal artery. Anastomosis with the deep external pudendal artery, a branch of the femoral artery, provides additional blood supply. Because the main supply to the flap is the posterior labial artery, the Singapore flap may not be viable if hypogastric artery ligation is performed during the extirpative phase.

Posteriorly, the flap is innervated by both the pudendal nerve via its posterior labial branches and the perineal rami of the posterior cutaneous nerve of the thigh. Anteriorly, the genitofemoral and ilioinguinal nerves supply sensation; however, these nerves are often denervated on harvesting of the flap. Thus, there is only sensation in the lower neovagina.

The advantages of the Singapore flap include technical simplicity, hidden scars for enhanced cosmesis with minimal donor-site morbidity, less bulk than myocutaneous flaps, a natural vaginal angle, sensation similar to the inner thigh and perineum, and no requirement for postoperative vaginal stenting or use of dilators. A disadvantage with the flap is the limited experience with concurrent exenteration or for radiation necrosis. Bilateral flaps are required for neovaginal creation, and additional chronic problems with the Singapore flap include vulvar pain, vaginal discharge, hair growth, and flap prolapse. Thus, we do not favor this operation for reconstruction of type II vaginal defects following exenteration. Nonetheless, the Singapore flap is a useful tool in the surgical armamentarium as a single flap for complex rectovaginal fistula repair and vulvar and perineal reconstruction.

Preoperative Preparation

The patient is prepped for the operating room as previously described.

Operative Procedure

Marking the Pudendal Thigh Donor Site. The hair overlying the groin, perineum, and labia is shaved with clippers. The ischial tuberosity is located because this is where the flap's vascular supply emerges. A bilateral horn-shaped 4 to 6 × 9 to 16.5 cm flap is marked with a permanent pen just lateral to the hair-bearing labia majora and to the medial corner of the femoral triangle (Figure 32C-5). The posterior skin margin is at the level of the fourchette, and the flap is centered on the groin crease. The flap width and length depend on defect size and the patient's anatomy. Bilateral larger flaps are needed for neovaginal recreation following total pelvic exenteration, but a unilateral smaller flap may suffice for creating 1 vaginal wall following an anterior or posterior exenteration.

Harvesting the Pudendal Thigh Flap. An incision is carried down on each side through the subcutaneous tissue to the deep fascia, except at the flap's base. The underlying deep fascia and epimysium of the adductor muscle are incised and raised with the distal flap, but not at the base. The fascia is intermittently sutured to the skin flap to prevent inadvertent vessel shearing during manipulation.

To allow 70- to 90-degree transposition to meet the opposing flap, the posterior flap margin/base on each

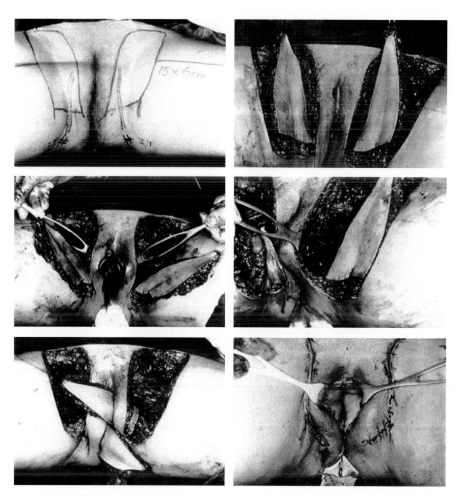

FIGURE 32C-5. Pudendal thigh myocutaneous flap. For neovaginal creation, a 5 to 6 × 14.5 to 16.5 cm flap is marked bilaterally centered on the groin crease. The flaps are harvested, tunneled under the labia, and sutured into place. (Reproduced, with permission, from Wee JT, Joseph VT. A new technique of vaginal reconstruction using neurovascular pudendal-thigh flaps: a preliminary report. *Plast Reconstr Surg.* 1989;83(4):701-709.)

side is incised only through the dermis and subcutaneous tissue to a 1- to 1.5-cm depth and undermined 4 cm parallel to the skin. This creates a subcutaneous pedicle for rotation that contains the neurovascular supply. A suture is placed at the tip of the flap to assist with maneuvering the flap under the labia.

Tunneling the Pudendal Thigh Flap Versus Dividing the Labia. Once each flap is raised, the labia are mobilized off the pubic rami and perineal membrane. The labia should be elevated sufficiently to allow passage of the flap, creating a bridge. Each flap is transposed 70 to 80 degrees and passed under the labia to meet the contralateral flap. Some authors recommend removing the epidermis of the buried part of the flap.[35] Alternatively, the labia are divided and the flaps rotated into place. This modification eliminates tunnel pressure on the vascular supply, potentially increasing flap viability, and is recommended if using this flap after exenteration.

Suturing the Pudendal Thigh Flap and Deep Fixation. In the midline, the flap is sutured to the contralateral flap creating a vaginal tube. The posterior flap junction is sutured first, followed by the anterior junction. The tube is invaginated and the apex fixed securely to the sacrum or retropubic/obturator fascia with a nonabsorbable suture, and the neovaginal opening is sutured to the introitus/labia minoral mucocutaneous junction. Drains are placed in the donor sites and the pelvis. Each donor site is closed primarily.

Postoperative Care

Box 32C-4   Complications and Morbidity

- Vulvar pain, vaginal discharge, hair growth, and flap prolapse are potential complications.
- Flap prolapse can be prevented by securing the neovaginal tube to the sacrum or obturator fascia.
- Flap viability should be assessed daily.

The perineal area and lower vaginal tube are inspected for viability on daily rounds. Although no stents or dilators are required in the perioperative period for most fasciocutaneous or myocutaneous flaps, we prefer to leave a mold in place to prevent possible agglutination of the neovagina. The mold is removed on postoperative day 2 or 3.

Bulbocavernosus Myocutaneous Flap, or Martius Flap

Procedure Overview

In 1928, Martius first described a bulbocavernosus flap for large urethrovaginal and vesicovaginal fistulas in which the skin was left in situ.[36] The bulbocavernosus flap can include the overlying dermis and epidermis and be used for partial neovaginal construction following supralevator exenteration. The flap is a sensate, axial pattern flap that can be mobilized as an island or transposition flap. This flap also works well as a secondary flap to augment another flap. The neurovascular supply of the bulbocavernosus flap is derived from the pudendal artery and nerve. Like the Singapore flap, the Martius flap may be nonviable if the internal iliac artery is sacrificed during the extirpative phase. The advantages include surgical simplicity, minimal and acceptable donor-site morbidity, minimal blood loss, and less disfigurement than other flaps. It is a sensate island flap and seems to have a minimal impact on vaginal intercourse; however, some patients will experience pain, loss of sensation, or paresthesias over the donor site. Due to the location of the flap, hair is retained and could be the source of chronic vaginal discharge.[37] Another disadvantage is that the Martius flap is shorter than other myocutaneous flaps and requires compliance with postoperative dilation.[38]

Preoperative Preparation and Operative Procedure

Marking the Martius Donor Site. The patient is prepared for vaginal reconstructive surgery as previously described. The flap is marked for maximum width and length, yet still allowing for primary closure. The flap is designed overlying the bilateral labia majoral fat pad with the superior margin at the clitoral level or just slightly superiorly, while the inferior margin is marked at the perineal body. The medial and lateral margins are bounded by the sulcus between the labia minora and majora and the lateral edge of the labia majora, respectively. The patient's anatomy determines the flap's length (8-10 cm) and width (4-7 cm).

Harvesting the Martius Flap. The flap is harvested by sharply incising the medial margin, freeing the labia minora and introitus from the underlying labial fat pad. The subcutaneous tissue is dissected to the pubic

ramus. Next, the tissue under the bulbocavernosus muscle is carefully undermined laterally mobilizing the bulbocavernosus pad. Note that the vascular supply, the perineal branch of the pudendal artery, is at risk at this point in the dissection as it enters the inferior margin of the pedicle. The skin along the lateral and superior margin is incised and the subcutaneous tissue is dissected. Finally, the flap is harvested by incising the posterior margin. The flap is mobilized on the inferior pedicle and ready for transposition. The same procedure is carried out on the opposite side.

Tunneling the Martius Flap. A bridge is made in the paravaginal tissue by elevating the remaining 3 to 4 cm of vagina away from the pubic ramus. The flap is passed through this window into the pelvis (Figure 32C-6). A stay suture at the tip of the flap may help transpose the flap into position and avoid shearing the cutaneous portion.

Suturing the Martius Flap. The flap is made into a vaginal tube using interrupted sutures. First, the posterior aspect of the neovagina is sutured onto the vaginal cuff. Next, the flaps are sewn together to complete the posterior wall of the neovagina. The anterior portion of the neovaginal flap is sutured to the anterior vaginal cuff as well as to the contralateral flap. The apex of the neovagina is closed with interrupted sutures, and an omental flap is placed in the pelvis (Figure 32C-7). For stabilization of the neovagina, the flap is secured laterally to the levator muscle pedicles. A vaginal mold is placed in the neovagina and removed on postoperative day 3 or 4, after which time a 3-cm Silastic rod is fitted. Drains are placed in the donor sites, and these sites are closed primarily.

Postoperative Care

Postoperative care is similar to that for the pudendal thigh fasciocutaneous flap; however, the Martius flap is shorter than the pudendal thigh flap and requires meticulous use of a dilator as described for STSG.

Bilateral Gracilis Myocutaneous Flap

Procedure Overview

Box 32C-5	Master Surgeon's Corner

- Obesity and concurrent rectal anastomosis are relative contraindications to the gracilis flap because of its bulk.
- The gracilis flap may be used to cover combination vulvovaginal defects with a single flap.
- To ensure flap viability, the skin island should be shorter than the muscle length, and excessive rotation of the flap should be avoided.

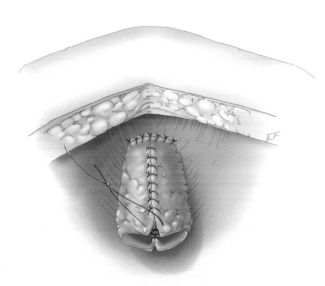

FIGURE 32C-6. Bulbocavernosus myocutaneous (Martius) flap for vaginal reconstruction. The bilateral flaps are marked, harvested, tunneled into position. (Adapted from Green AE, Escobar PF, Neubaurer N, Michener CM, Vongruenigen VE. The Martius flap neovagina revisited. *Int J Gynecol Cancer.* 2005;15(5):964-966.)

FIGURE 32C-7. Bulbocavernosus myocutaneous (Martius) flap for vaginal reconstruction. The bilateral flaps are tabularized and sutured to the remaining vagina or introitus. (Adapted from Green AE, Escobar PF, Neubaurer N, Michener CM, Vongruenigen VE. The Martius flap neovagina revisited. *Int J Gynecol Cancer.* 2005;15(5):964-966.)

McCraw originally developed the gracilis flap for vaginal reconstruction in 1976 with several modifications described by Berek and Copeland.[10,18,39] Neovaginal creation after total exenteration (type II vaginal defect) requires bilateral gracilis flaps, whereas unilateral flaps may suffice following partial exenteration (type I vaginal defect). The long gracilis flap is considered a type II flap with 1 dominant pedicle, the medial circumflex femoral artery (a branch of the deep femoral artery), and 1 or 2 other minor vessels that are generally sacrificed when harvesting the full flap. In contrast, a short gracilis flap is supplied by the terminal branches of the obturator artery and may be used for vaginal reconstruction as long as the hypogastric and obturator arteries remain intact. The short gracilis is an excellent flap for vulvar reconstruction. Both the short and long gracilis flaps maintain good to fair pressure and touch sensibility as well as some muscle contractility via the intact obturator nerve.[39]

The advantages of gracilis myocutaneous neovaginal formation compared to no definitive reconstruction at the time of exenteration include an overall decrease in complication rate, prevention of bowel herniation, decreased fistulization rates, improved primary healing, reduced fluid loss from the denuded pelvic cavity, decrease in hospital stay, and an adequate portal for cancer surveillance. Due to the bulk of bilateral flaps, the gracilis is not suitable if a low rectal anastomosis is planned. Additionally, obesity is considered a relative contraindication to the procedure given the increased risk of flap necrosis.[10]

Unfortunately, bilateral flaps are required for neovaginal recreation, and they lead to unsightly scars and are associated with high rates of prolapse (18%), painful intercourse (18%), excessive vaginal secretions (28%) or dryness (33%), and complaints of neovaginal size.[40] Although there are notable disadvantages to the gracilis over the rectus flap (see later section on vertical rectus abdominis myocutaneous flaps), the gracilis flap is preferred when the rectus cannot easily rotate into the defect such as those involving the lower vagina, introitus, or vulva, particularly with an intact vaginal apex.[30]

Preoperative Preparation and Operative Procedure

Marking the Gracilis Donor Site. The patient is placed in lithotomy, positioning the knee in less than 45 degrees of flexion and the hips at 45 degrees of abduction with 15 degrees of flexion. A line is drawn from the pubic tubercle at the adductor longus tendon insertion to the medial tibial condyle where the semitendinosus tendon inserts. The elliptical flap is outlined posterior to this line and is generally 12 cm (range, 8-14 cm) in length and 6 cm (range, 4-7 cm) in width.[10] The cutaneous portion above this line is supplied by perforating branches of the sartorius muscle and is at risk for marginal skin necrosis if harvested with the gracilis.[39] The gracilis can support a cutaneous island 2 cm above and 4 cm below the muscle. Although the size can be adjusted intraoperatively to fit the defect, the skin overlying the distal third of the gracilis (near the medial tibial condyle) is at highest risk for sloughing because the distal vascular pedicles are often sacrificed during flap mobilization. The entire gracilis muscle will remain viable, but harvesting the entire skin paddle should be avoided. After the flap is marked, the entire thigh must be prepped from below the knee to the perineum including the buttocks. The flap is harvested as an island flap.

To avoid harvesting the wrong flap, Morrow and Curtin[27] prefer to design the skin island after anatomically locating the course of the gracilis. First, the semitendinosus tendon is easily palpable at the posterior medial tibial condyle and marked. Next, a 2- to 3-cm incision is made superior to the marked site and represents the area overlying the gracilis tendon insertion. Dissection is carried through the subcutaneous tissue and fascia lata until the gracilis tendon is isolated. An instrument is passed beneath the tendon, and the tendon is placed on tension clearly outlining the gracilis muscle's path (Figure 32C-8). The skin paddle is then centered over the muscle.

Harvesting the Gracilis Flap. The dissection is begun by incising the skin along the anterior boundary down to the level of the fascia lata. The adductor longus tendon is identified immediately anterior to the incision. The adductor longus tendon fascia is incised, elevated with the gracilis flap, and retracted medially. This will expose the adductor brevis muscle and possibly the neurovascular pedicle. The vascular pedicle is invested in the facial layer emerging from the adductor longus and brevis muscles approximately 5 to 10 cm from the insertion of the gracilis on the pubic ramus.

Centering the skin paddle over the muscle is critical to avoiding skin necrosis. Dissection is continued to the distal apex taking care to harvest the gracilis muscle enveloped in its fascia. Exposure of the muscle without its facial envelope suggests the wrong plane.[27] To prevent shearing, sutures are sequentially placed as the fascia is incised to secure the fascia to the skin (Figure 32C-9). Distally, the gracilis muscle is transected with electrocautery and elevated off the underlying fascia.

Posteriorly, the dissection continues, exposing the bare abductor magnus and brevis, and is carried out to meet the apex of the skin island near the pubic ramus.

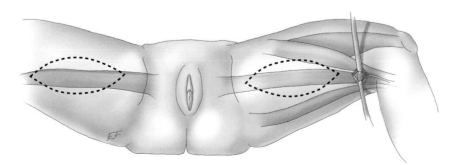

FIGURE 32C-8. Identification of the gracilis tendon insertion at the medial tibial condyle.

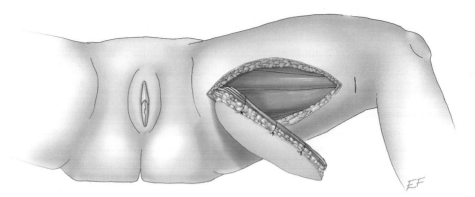

FIGURE 32C-9. The gracilis muscle is harvested, and the proximal portion remains attached to the pubic ramus. AB, adductor brevis muscle; AL, adductor longus muscle; AM, adductor magnus muscle.

During this dissection, the neurovascular pedicle is reidentified with a sterile Doppler. If shorter gracilis flaps are planed and mobilization is an issue, the vascular pedicle may be sacrificed with little or no flap necrosis due to primary vascularization from the obturator artery.[10]

Tunneling the Gracilis Flap for Vaginal Reconstruction.
After the island flap is completely elevated, a capacious subcutaneous tunnel is developed forming a labial skin bridge between the flap incision and the pelvic cavity. The adequacy of this space cannot be overemphasized

because the most common cause of flap failure is compression in the tunnel.[41] The flap is rotated 180 degrees posterior on its pedicle, which is clockwise around the left pedicle and counterclockwise around the right pedicle, and placed gently through the tunnel into the pelvis. Alternatively, it can be rotated anteriorly 90 degrees to fill perineal defects.

Suturing the Gracilis Flap. Each flap margin and apex is sewn to its contralateral flap creating a vaginal tube with the flap's skin forming the neovaginal walls (Figure 32C-10). The complex is gently lifted into the

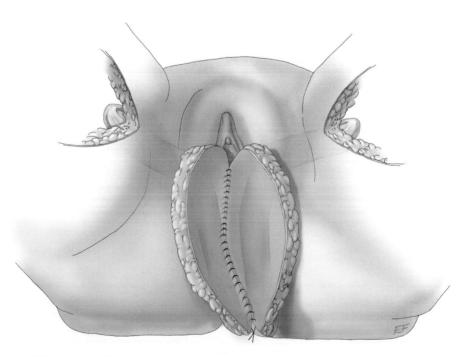

FIGURE 32C-10. The bilateral gracilis flaps are rotated into place, and the posterior wall of the neovagina is approximated with sutures.

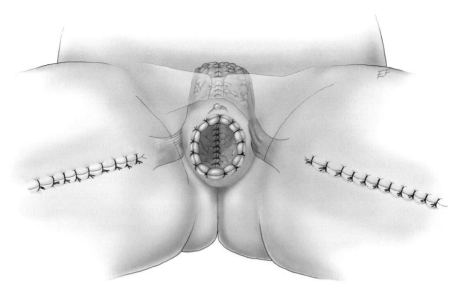

FIGURE 32C-11. The tubularized gracilis flaps are situated within the pelvis and secured in place. Donor sites are closed primarily.

pelvis, and the skin edges are sutured to the introitus. We prefer to suture the neovagina to the levator and retropubic fascia when feasible to help reduce neovaginal prolapse. A vaginal mold is sutured to the labial folds and removed on postoperative day 2 or 3. An omental flap is harvested to form a pelvic lid and prevent bowel herniation into the pelvis. A pelvic drain is recommended to reduce fluid accumulation around the flap.

The donor sites are carefully closed primarily with several vertical mattress sutures and multiple interrupted sutures or staples, avoiding compression of the gracilis vascular pedicle (Figure 32C-11). The legs are wrapped with bandages, again avoiding pressure in the proximal portion near the vascular pedicle.

Postoperative Care

> **Box 32C-6** **Complications and Morbidity**
>
> - The gracilis flap may be subject to flap prolapse and result in vaginal secretion and painful intercourse.
> - Flap viability should be assessed daily.
> - The most common cause of flap necrosis is compromised vascular supply due to angulation during rotation.

The patient is not restricted in ambulation. The vaginal mold is removed on postoperative day number 2 or 3 without the further use of molds or dilators.

Vertical Rectus Abdominis Myocutaneous (VRAM) Flap and Extended VRAM Flap

Procedure Overview

> **Box 32C-7** **Master Surgeon's Corner**
>
> - VRAM flap size and orientation can be tailored to the patient's anatomy and reconstructive needs.
> - Viability of the ipsilateral inferior epigastric artery must be confirmed.
> - The VRAM flap should be harvested early in the reconstructive phase to facilitate planning of additional reconstructive procedures (urinary and bowel diversions).
> - A fascial substitute may be required to ensure a tension-free closure of the donor site.

Due to its reliability, single donor site with incorporation into the primary incision with minimal donor site morbidity, 360-degree arc of rotation, no requirement for postoperative dilation, and technical ease, the rectus abdominis myocutaneous flap is the preferred flap for neovaginal recreation. Tobin and Day first described the use of distally based rectus flaps for vulvar and vaginal reconstruction with several modifications described by others.[9,31,42] It is a paralyzed, non-sensate flap due to motor and sensory denervation that occurs during harvesting. As a type III flap, the blood supply is reliable with 2 dominant arteries and other smaller musculocutaneous perforators. The dominant blood supply for the proximal and distal rectus flap is derived from the superior and inferior epigastric vessels, respectively. The inferior epigastric artery is a branch of the external iliac artery, whereas the superior epigastric artery is derived from the internal thoracic artery, a branch of the subclavian artery.

The rectus abdominis flap can be raised in a vertical, transverse, or diagonal fashion for complete vaginal reconstruction (type IIA or IIB defects), partial vaginal reconstruction (type IA or IB defects), or other inguinal or perineal defects. It is distally based and requires patent inferior epigastric vessels. Although raising a transverse rectus abdominis myocutaneous flap is suitable, this flap requires harvesting the skin island perpendicular to the previously made vertical midline skin incision. The diagonally extended vertical rectus abdominis myocutaneous (VRAM) flap (also known as the oblique rectus abdominis musculocutaneous [ORAM] flap) has the advantage of a longer skin island due to anastomoses between the epigastric perforators and the superficial intercostal arteries, which also communicate with the superficial epigastric artery and the cutaneous branches of the lateral deep and superficial circumflex iliac arteries. Based on our experience, the anticipated maximum width and length of the diagonally extended VRAM (ORAM) are 10 to 15 cm and 10 cm, respectively. We prefer the ORAM flap for neovaginal reconstruction due to its width, versatility, and ease of flap inset compared to the conventional VRAM.

We recommend harvesting the rectus flap as the first step of the reconstructive phase. After the flap is raised and rotated into the pelvis, the first surgical team can continue with other abdominal procedures, such as the ileal conduit formation and colostomy while the second surgical team completes the perineal reconstruction. Elevating the rectus flap first allows for optimal stomal placement and reduces potential disruption of the conduit and colostomy. These flaps may be harvested from either side.

The main advantages of the rectus flap over the gracilis flap for neovaginal reconstruction include a lower rate of flap necrosis (5%-9% vs. 10%-38%), single donor site incorporated into the primary incision compared to 2 donor sites with unpleasant scar formation, and perhaps a decreased rate of vaginal prolapse (1.5% vs. up to 18%). Although current sexual function studies regarding postexenterative vaginal reconstruction are limited, 50% to 85% of patients report intercourse after rectus neovaginal reconstruction.[31]

The rectus myocutaneous flap may not be well suited for morbidly obese patients or those with extremely thick abdominal walls. Other disadvantages include mild stenosis (up to 18% of patients) correctable with dilation, potential for difficult abdominal closure with up to 23% of patients requiring mesh closure, and a 3% fascial dehiscence rate.[31] Absolute contraindications include occlusion of the ipsilateral inferior epigastric vessel and ipsilateral previous Maylard incision or stoma placement.[31]

Preoperative Preparation

We recommend a preoperative arteriogram in patients with severe peripheral vascular disease or previous abdominal surgery to ensure inferior epigastric patency and an intraoperative sterile Doppler to confirm patency prior to raising the flap.

Operative Procedure

Harvesting the VRAM Flap. The donor site for the rectus flap is outlined prior to prepping the patient, as shown in Figure 32C-12. The skin island is incised with the scalpel and the dissection carried down to the fascia. The lateral edge of the anterior rectus fascia is incised, and the lateral edge of the rectus muscle is identified and isolated. Care must be taken to harvest the entire rectus muscle. Next, the superior boundary of the flap and rectus is identified, and the rectus muscle is elevated from the posterior rectus sheath, clamped, transected, and suture ligated. The posterior rectus sheath is preserved.

The previously made anterior rectus sheath incision is continued in such a fashion to mirror a smaller version of the skin flap. Stay sutures are placed at 3- to 4-cm intervals between the anterior rectus fascial cut edge and the skin paddle to stabilize the flap and avoid shearing during manipulation. The dissection is continued to the arcuate line. Below the arcuate line, the muscle is raised with the peritoneum, and the entire rectus sheath is preserved. The inferior epigastric vessels enter the flap posteriorly and laterally at approximately 4 to 6 cm above the pubic symphysis. If additional length is required, the vascular pedicle can be skeletonized and the rectus muscle developed completely to its tendinous insertion.

Tunneling the VRAM Flap. With the flap sufficiently mobilized, the skin island is rotated directly into the hemostatic pelvis and placed under the pubic symphysis (Figure 32C-13). The skin island should easily reach the perineum without tension on the vascular pedicle or muscle or shearing the flap. If tension is noted, the rectus muscle should be further mobilized. At this point, the other surgical team can begin the urinary conduit, colostomy, or other planned reconstructive procedures.

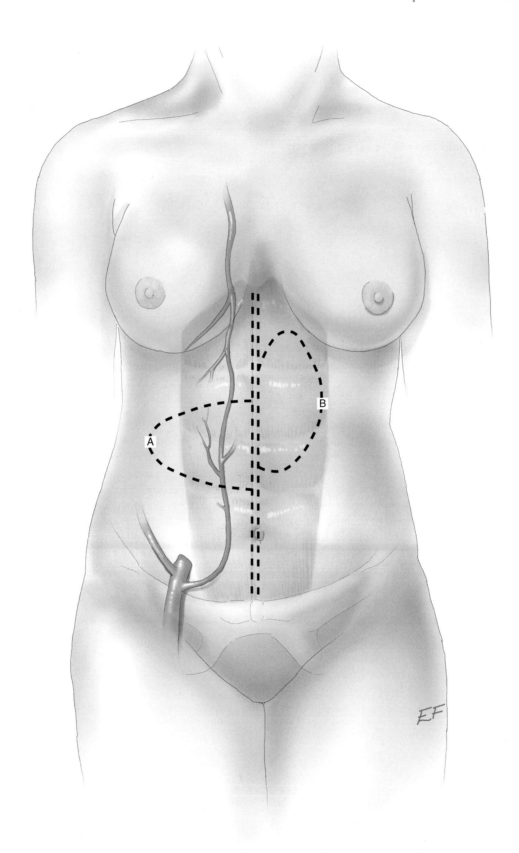

FIGURE 32C-12. The rectus abdominis myocutaneous flap is outlined on a transverse (Flap A) or vertical (Flap B) axis.

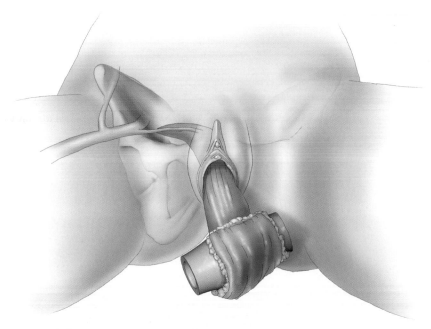

FIGURE 32C-13. The rectus abdominis myocutaneous flap is harvested, tubularized, and rotated into position in the pelvis.

Suturing the VRAM Flap. The skin island is tubularized into a vaginal cone with the skin paddle facing the inside, forming the neovagina. The skin edges are sutured together with interrupted absorbable suture (Figure 32C-14). The neovagina subcutaneous tissue is secured to the levator ani and retropubic fascia. The neovaginal opening is sutured to the introital skin edge. A vaginal mold is sutured to the labial folds and removed on postoperative day 2 or 3. An omental flap is harvested to form a pelvic lid and to prevent bowel herniation into the pelvis.

Attention is turned to closing the donor site. This occasionally requires bilateral mobilization of the subcutaneous tissue to the midaxillary line, vertical mattress sutures, or rarely a mesh. The donor site should be mobilized completely prior to finalizing stoma and drain sites to avoid misplacement. If a urinary conduit is performed, 2 drains are placed in the pelvis. One drain is placed above the neovagina flap, and another drain is placed near the conduit ureteral anastomosis. Additional drains may be placed in the subcutaneous tissue to drain the donor site.

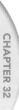

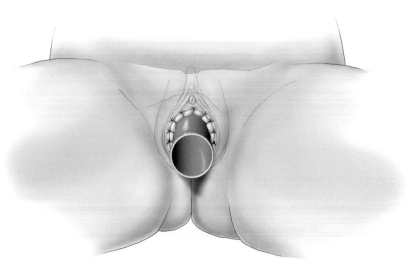

FIGURE 32C-14. A vaginal mold is placed in the neovagina.

Postoperative Care

Box 32C-8	Complications and Morbidity

- The donor site should be monitored vigilantly to ensure its integrity.
- Bowel or urinary diversion stomas placed in the reconstructed abdominal wall should be monitored for prolapsed or peristomal herniation.
- The most common cause of flap necrosis is compromised vascular supply due to angulation during rotation.

The patient is not restricted in ambulation. The vaginal mold is removed on postoperative day 2 or 3 without the further use of molds or dilators.

VULVAR RECONSTRUCTION

Indications for Vulvar Reconstruction

The primary goal of the vulvar reconstructive effort is to maximize the healing at the surgical site. The cosmetic appearance, while extremely important, is a secondary goal of this reconstructive effort. Flaps can be used to obliterate dead space, bring new vascularity to an area that has frequently received radiation, and allow for primary closure while improving body self-image and allowing for sexual function. The success of the primary reconstructive procedure is inversely related to the complexity of deformity and the flap design.[43] Age greater than 60 years, weight greater than 80 kg, tobacco abuse, and vascular disease also confound reconstructive efforts.[44]

Perioperative Considerations for Vulvar Reconstruction

Thromboembolic prevention should be used for all patients. Standard antibiotic prophylaxis can be prescribed for the abdominal or pelvic portion of the case, with consideration given for a redosing of the antibiotic at the time of the skin incisions for the reconstructive portion of the procedure.

In addition to the general anesthetic, the preoperative placement of an epidural may be helpful in providing excellent pain management for: (1) the primary surgical site, (2) the potential donor sites required during the reconstructive phase, and (3) the 48 to 72 hours of bed rest potentially required postoperatively.

The dorsal low lithotomy position using stirrups to support the heel and lower leg is the preferred position for most flaps. In general, the lower extremity should be partially abducted to provide adequate access to the perineal region.

The lower extremities should be prepped to below the knee to allow the option of using a combination of potential flaps for the reconstructive phase. Consider sewing the anus closed with a purse-string suture to minimize contamination during these procedures. If the bladder and urethra are retained, prolonged transurethral (>24 hours) or suprapubic bladder drainage may be required for these patients given the extent of surgery performed and the localized periurethral swelling that may ensue.

STSG for Vulvar and Perineal Reconstruction

The principles of STSGs for vaginal reconstruction are identical for vulvar reconstruction.

Preoperative Care and Operative Procedure

Preoperative care and marking the donor site for STSGs are the same as previously described for vaginal reconstruction.

Harvesting the STSG and Placing on the Vulva

The STSG is usually harvested from the inner thighs or buttocks using an air-powered dermatome. The dermatome is set to a thickness of 13 to 19/1000 of an inch, and the graft is meshed (normally 1.5:1) and trimmed to fit the defect. Fibrin sealants such as Tisseel have been used to increase the graft success rate.

The graft is secured with 3-0 or 4-0 absorbable sutures. The recipient site is then covered with a pressure dressing over petrolatum-impregnated gauze, or a vacuum-assisted closure device (VAC) may be used (Figure 32C-15). If a wound VAC is used over an STSG,

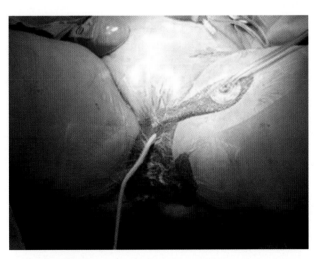

FIGURE 32C-15. Vacuum-assisted closure device (VAC) over the vulvar wound.

the recommended pressure is 100 mm Hg on an intermittent setting. The VAC is generally removed on postoperative day 3 or 4. A liquid diet is recommended until it is removed. The patient will be able to pass flatus with the VAC in place, but sometimes, it requires earlier removal for a bowel movement. The utilization of a hydrocolloid dressing (DuoDERM; ConvaTec, Skillman, NJ) around the anus and nongrafted areas may be helpful in facilitating a leak-free system.[24]

Postoperative Care

The patient remains at complete bed rest for 3 days postoperatively or while the VAC is in place. A Foley catheter is recommended. Activity should be restricted to walking for the first 2 weeks.

Rhomboid Transposition Flap

Procedure Overview

The rhomboid transposition flap is an extremely useful and versatile flap for vulvar reconstruction. The first description of this type of transposition flap is credited to Limberg, who in 1946 described closure of a parallelogram with 60- and 120-degree angles with a transposition flap named for him. This flap derives its vascular supply from the underlying subcutaneous tissue and does not require a myofascial incision. The underlying subcutaneous portion of the flap should be at least 1.0 to 1.5 cm thick. Because the flap derives its blood supply from the subcutaneous tissue, the flap base may be oriented posteriorly or anteriorly depending on the shape of the vulvar defect and the perceived best closure. In general, this flap is for a smaller defect, with the ideal flap being 4 to 6 cm across the base.[45]

Preoperative Preparation

The patient is prepped for the operating room as previously described. There are no unique requirements for this flap.

Operative Procedure

Marking the Donor Site for the Rhomboid Flap

The skin site next to the vulvar defect is marked and measured. The practical flap is limited to about 4 × 4 cm, with larger flaps being technically possible but associated with some breakdown and subsequent granulation. The origin of the incision should be slightly more posterior than the midpoint of the vulvar defect (Figure 32C-16). The flap should be 0.5 cm larger than the measured surgical defect because this allows for some normal contraction and closure with less tension.

A similar-sized flap may be required on the opposite side depending on the vulvar defect.

Mobilizing the Rhomboid Flap

The original irregular defect is converted to a rhomboid with 60- and 120-degree angles. The parallelogram has a long diagonal and a short diagonal (Figure 32C-17). A line is drawn extending from the short diagonal with a length equal to the short diagonal. A line is then drawn from the end of the first line with a length equal to and parallel to one of the adjacent sides of the defect. Flap elevation should be in the subcutaneous plane to preserve the dermal-subdermal plexus of vessels. At least 1.0 to 1.5 cm of subcutaneous tissue must be attached to the flap. The flap is then transposed and the mucosal edge approximated to the edge of the flap with a 3-0 absorbable suture. The donor site edges are undermined and closed in layers with 3-0 absorbable suture for the deep dermal layer and 4-0 absorbable monofilament suture for the subcuticular closure.

Securing the Rhomboid Flap in Place

The flap is secured with interrupted 3-0 absorbable sutures (Figure 32C-18). A single nonabsorbable 2-0 monofilament suture is used to secure the flap at the perineal body if there is any perceived tension. Given the extent of the undermining required, larger flaps may benefit from the placement of a subcutaneous drain for the first 3 postoperative days to help reduce the incidence of hematomas, seromas, and infection. Alternatively, a VAC may be placed over the vulvar area and removed on postoperative day 3.

Postoperative Care

For a posterior flap in the perianal area, a liquid diet is recommended for the first 3 days. If a VAC was used, a liquid diet is also recommended until the device is removed. The patient will be able to pass flatus with the VAC in place, but it usually requires removal for a bowel movement.

V-Y Advancement Flap

Procedure Overview

Simple sliding V-Y or axial advancement flaps are very reliable primary flaps for smaller vulvar defects. Occasionally, these flaps may be used as secondary flaps to augment a primary flap. In general, the V-Y flaps can be used to primarily close more extensive vulvar defects than a rhomboid flap. V-Y advancement flap advantages include sensation, reliable blood supply, and concealed scars on the gluteal fold.

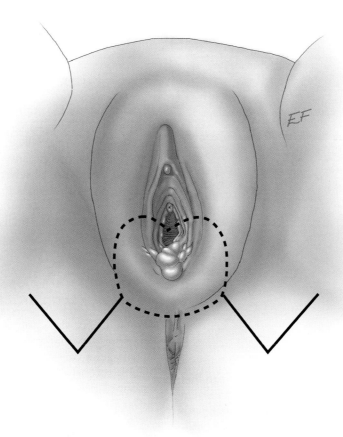

FIGURE 32C-16. Bilateral rhomboid flaps are designed to cover a posterior vulvar defect. (Redrawn, with permission, from Burke TW, Morris M, Levenback C, Gershenson DM, Wharton JT. Closure of complex vulvar defects using local rhomboid flaps. *Obstet Gynecol.* 1994;84(6):1043-1047.)

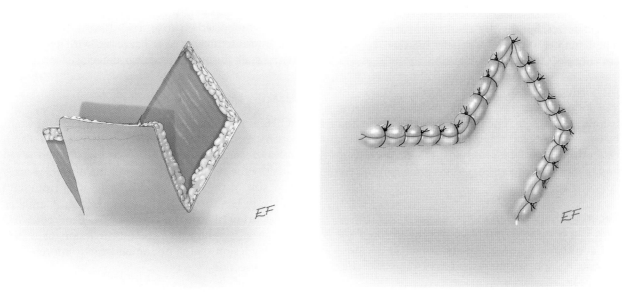

FIGURE 32C-17. The defect is converted to a parallelogram with angles of 60 and 120 degrees, and the flap is designed accordingly. (Adapted from Morrow CP, Curtin JP. Reconstructive surgery. In: Morrow CP, Curtin JP, eds. *Gynecologic Cancer Surgery.* Philadelphia, PA: Churchill Livingstone; 1996:323-380.)

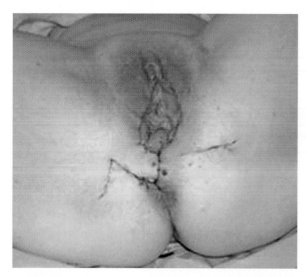

FIGURE 32C-18. The rhomboid flap rotated and secured over the vulvar defect.

Preoperative Preparation

The general preoperative preparation is similar to that for the flaps described earlier. The unique requirement for this flap is to be sure the patient is positioned with the coccyx on the end of the table, giving partial exposure to the gluteus.

Operative Procedure

Marking the Donor Site for the V-Y Advancement Flap

The flap is marked with the apex of the "V" on the gluteal fold. The base of the triangular flap is centered on the vulvar wound (Figure 32C-19). The size is dependent on the defect, but may be 12 to 15 cm across the base. The length of this flap is usually between 10 and 15 cm (Figure 32C-20).

Mobilizing the V-Y Flap

The incision is carried through the skin to the underlying muscle fascia. The flap mobilization is facilitated by incising and elevating the underlying muscular fascia both proximally and distally. The flap is advanced and the leading edge trimmed to fit the contour of the vulvovaginal defect.

Securing the V-Y Flap in Place

This flap is sutured into place with interrupted 2-0 or 3-0 absorbable sutures. The donor defect is closed in a linear fashion, forming the base of the "Y" (Figure 32C-21).

Postoperative Care

The postoperative care is similar to described earlier for other vulvar reconstructive procedures. If the flap

is in close proximity to the anus, consider a liquid diet and bed rest for the first 3 postoperative days.

Pudendal Thigh Flap (Singapore Flap)

In addition to its utility for vaginal reconstruction, the pudendal thigh flap, or Singapore flap, is another potential option for vulvar, vaginal, or perineal reconstruction. The preoperative care and steps of marking and harvesting are reviewed earlier. To allow rotation to close the vulvar defect, the posterior medial base may require a minimal amount of triangular cutaneous excision. This avoids a pucker at the rotation base. The postoperative care is the same.

Myocutaneous Flaps for Vulvar and Perineal Reconstruction

Myocutaneous flaps are more complicated than cutaneous or fasciocutaneous flaps, but they have the advantage of covering large vulvoperineal defects with reliable reconstruction. In addition to the specific flaps described below, the rectus flap is another option for vulvar reconstruction. The rectus flap, harvested from the rectus abdominis muscle as described earlier for vaginal reconstruction, may be transposed under a mons skin bridge and used on the anterior or lateral vulva, or even in the inguinal area (Figure 32C-22).

Martius Flap

The Martius transposition island skin flap may also be used to repair vulvar defects. The stalk is harvested to allow sufficient length to reach the defect. The paddle may be mobilized on an anterior base if the defect is in the anterior vulvar area or harvested with a posteriorly based stalk for posterior vulvar defects.

Gracilis Myocutaneous Flap

Whereas the long gracilis is frequently used for vaginal reconstruction, the short gracilis is an excellent flap for vulvar reconstruction. The short gracilis flap is supplied by the terminal branches of the obturator artery. The size of the short gracilis flap varies from 12 to 14 cm in length and 5 to 7 cm in width. A unilateral flap is primarily used in vulvar or perineal reconstruction in a patient with a recurrent lesion or a bulky primary lesion that is not amendable to more conservative resection.

Tensor Fascia Lata Flap

Procedure Overview

The tensor fascia lata flap was commonly used for vulvar reconstruction in the era of the en bloc radical

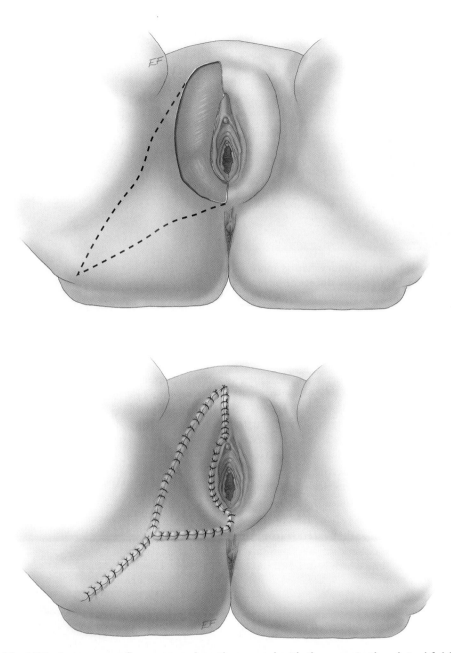

FIGURE 32C-19. The V-Y advancement flap centered on the wound with the apex in the gluteal fold. (Adapted, with permission, from Lee PK, Choi MS, Ahn ST, Oh DY, Rhie JW, Han KT. Gluteal fold V-Y advancement flap for vulvar and vaginal reconstruction: a new flap. *Plast Reconstr Surg.* 2006;118(2):401-406.)

vulvectomy with bilateral inguinal lymphadenectomy, or the butterfly incision. This radical resection was associated with an extremely high postoperative morbidity and wound separation. Now that most vulvectomies are performed through separate incisions, the utilization of this flap has declined. Nevertheless, it remains an option for inguinal, anterior, and lateral vulvar reconstruction. The tensor fascia lata muscle originates at the anterior superior iliac spine and extends distally down the lateral thigh into the fascia lata. This myocutaneous flap derives its vascular supply from the lateral femoral circumflex artery, which usually arises from the profunda femoral artery and enters the muscle approximately 6 to 8 cm caudal of the spine. The flap, with its unique blood supply, may support a pedicle up to 40 cm in length and 15 cm in width.[46] The tensor fascia lata is innervated by the superior gluteal nerve that enters the muscle posteriorly and deep to the vascular pedicle. The cutaneous portion is innervated by the lateral cutaneous branch of the 12th thoracic nerve as well as the lateral cutaneous nerve of the thigh.

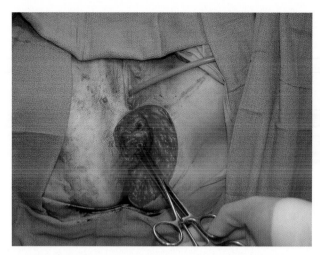

FIGURE 32C-20. The V-Y advancement flap is marked for closure of a large posterior vulvar defect after resection of vulvar melanoma. (Photo contributed by Drs. Mark Morgan, Sara Kim, and Sameer Patel.)

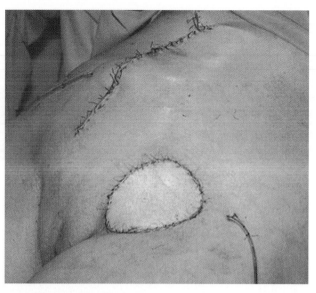

FIGURE 32C-22. The rectus abdominis myocutaneous flap mobilized and secured over the left groin area.

Operative Procedure

Marking the Tensor Fascia Lata Donor Site. The marking and measuring for this flap start at the site of vascular insertion, approximately 8 cm caudal to the superior iliac spine (Figure 32C-23). The measuring then extends medially to the most inferior aspect of the perineal defect to determine the length of the flap required. Next, the anterior border of the flap is defined by drawing a line from the anterior superior iliac spine to the lateral tibial condyle. The posterior border is determined from a line that extends from the greater trochanter to the knee, ending approximately 5 cm cephalad to the knee. The width is determined by

the inguinal and vulvar defect size but is usually from 5 to 8 cm. The length is also based on the size of the defect plus an extra centimeter to allow for contraction during mobilization.

Mobilizing the Tensor Fascia Lata Flap. The outlined flap is incised to the fascia. The base of this flap should be wider than the cutaneous portion. Care should be taken to maintain the vascular pedicle as it enters the flap between the rectus femoris and vastus lateralis.

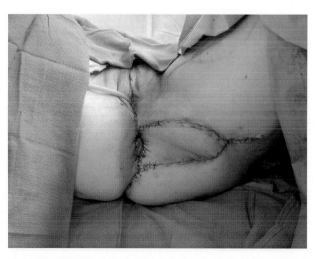

FIGURE 32C-21. The V-Y advancement flap is sutured into place. (Photo contributed by Drs. Mark Morgan, Sara Kim, and Sameer Patel.)

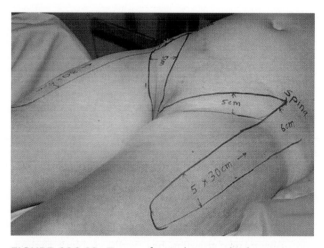

FIGURE 32C-23. Tensor fascia lata marked out preoperatively. (Reprinted, with permission, from Knapstein PG, Frieberg V. Reconstructive operations of the vulva and vagina. In: Knapstein PG, Frieberg V, Sevin BU, eds. *Reconstructive Surgery in Gynecology.* New York, NY: Thieme Medical Publishers; 1997:11-70.)

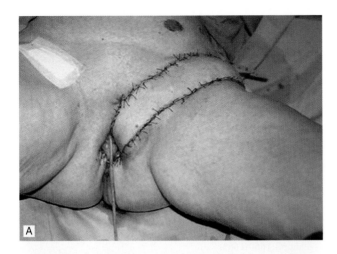

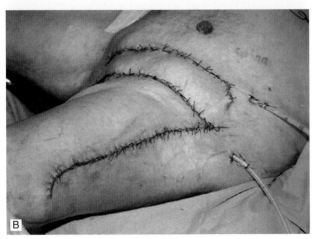

FIGURE 32C-24. (A and B) Tensor fascia lata mobilized and secured in defect. (Reprinted, with permission, from Knapstein PG, Frieberg V. Reconstructive operations of the vulva and vagina. In: Knapstein PG, Frieberg V, Sevin BU, eds. *Reconstructive Surgery in Gynecology.* New York, NY: Thieme Medical Publishers; 1997:11-70.)

The skin should be secured to the fascia with interrupted 2-0 or 3-0 absorbable sutures to prevent shearing during mobilization.

Securing the Tensor Fascia Lata Flap. Once harvested, this flap is transposed medially along the groin and vulvar areas to fill the surgical defect. The flap is secured with interrupted 2-0 absorbable sutures (Figure 32C-24, A and B). Undermining the subcutaneous defect margins along the entire length is required to facilitate donor site closure. The donor site is closed with staples. A subcutaneous drain is placed in the donor site.

Postoperative Care
Ice packs to the donor site may be helpful in reducing edema and surgical site pain for the first 48 hours.

However, ice to the flap itself may compromise perfusion and increase morbidity. It is the authors' preference to keep the vulvar wound as dry as possible.

REFERENCES

1. Miller B, Morris M, Gershenson DM, Levenback CL, Burke TW. Intestinal fistulae formation following pelvic exenteration: a review of the University of Texas M. D. Anderson Cancer Center experience, 1957-1990. *Gynecol Oncol.* 1995;56(2): 207-210.
2. Jurado M, Bazan A, Alcazar JL, Garcia-Tutor E. Primary vaginal reconstruction at the time of pelvic exenteration for gynecologic cancer: morbidity revisited. *Ann Surg Oncol.* 2009;16(1): 121-127.
3. Jurado M, Bazan A, Elejabeitia J, Paloma V, Martinez-Monge R, Alcazar JL. Primary vaginal and pelvic floor reconstruction at the time of pelvic exenteration: a study of morbidity. *Gynecol Oncol.* 2000;77(2):293-297.
4. Mirhashemi R, Averette HE, Lambrou N, et al. Vaginal reconstruction at the time of pelvic exenteration: a surgical and psychosexual analysis of techniques. *Gynecol Oncol.* 2002;87(1):39-45.
5. Soper JT, Berchuck A, Creasman WT, Clarke-Pearson DL. Pelvic exenteration: factors associated with major surgical morbidity. *Gynecol Oncol.* 1989;35(1):93-98.
6. Scott JR, Liu D, Mathes DW. Patient-reported outcomes and sexual function in vaginal reconstruction: a 17-year review, survey, and review of the literature. *Ann Plast Surg.* 2010;64(3): 311-314.
7. Abbott DE, Halverson AL, Wayne JD, Kim JY, Talamonti MS, Dumanian GA. The oblique rectus abdominal myocutaneous flap for complex pelvic wound reconstruction. *Dis Colon Rectum.* 2008;51(8):1237-1241.
8. Hawighorst-Knapstein S, Schonefussrs G, Hoffmann SO, Knapstein PG. Pelvic exenteration: effects of surgery on quality of life and body image—A prospective longitudinal study. *Gynecol Oncol.* 1997;66(3):495-500.
9. Sood AK, Cooper BC, Sorosky JI, Ramirez PT, Levenback C. Novel modification of the vertical rectus abdominis myocutaneous flap for neovagina creation. *Obstet Gynecol.* 2005; 105(3):514-518.
10. Copeland LJ, Hancock KC, Gershenson DM, Stringer CA, Atkinson EN, Edwards CL. Gracilis myocutaneous vaginal reconstruction concurrent with total pelvic exenteration. *Am J Obstet Gynecol.* 1989;160(5 Pt 1):1095-1101.
11. Rutledge FN, Smith JP, Wharton JT, O'Quinn AG. Pelvic exenteration: analysis of 296 patients. *Am J Obstet Gynecol.* 1977;129(8):881-892.
12. Fowler JM. Incorporating pelvic/vaginal reconstruction into radical pelvic surgery. *Gynecol Oncol.* 2009;115(1):154-163.
13. Cordeiro PG, Pusic AL, Disa JJ. A classification system and reconstructive algorithm for acquired vaginal defects. *Plast Reconstr Surg.* 2002;110(4):1058-1065.
14. Pusic AL, Mehrara BJ. Vaginal reconstruction: an algorithm approach to defect classification and flap reconstruction. *J Surg Oncol.* 2006;94(6):515-521.
15. del Carmen MG, Eisner B, Willet CG, Fuller AF. Intraoperative radiation therapy in the management of gynecologic and genitourinary malignancies. *Surg Oncol Clin N Am.* 2003;12(4):1031-1042.
16. Dainty LA, Bosco JJ, McBroom JW, Winter WE 3rd, Rose GS, Elkas JC. Novel techniques to improve split-thickness skin graft viability during vulvo-vaginal reconstruction. *Gynecol Oncol.* 2005;97(3):949-952.
17. McIndoe AH, Banister JB. An operation for the cure of congenital absence of the vagina. *J Obstet Gynaecol.* 1938;45:490-494.

18. Berek JS, Hacker NF, Lagasse LD. Vaginal reconstruction performed simultaneously with pelvic exenteration. *Obstet Gynecol.* 1984;63(3):318-323.

19. Wheeless CR Jr. Neovagina constructed from an omental J flap and a split-thickness skin graft. *Gynecol Oncol.* 1989;35(2):224-226.

20. Kusiak JF, Rosenblum NG. Neovaginal reconstruction after exenteration using an omental flap and split-thickness skin graft. *Plast Reconstr Surg.* 1996;97(4):775-781.

21. Esrig D, Freeman JA, Stein JP, Elmajian DA, Lytton B, Skinner DG. New technique of vaginal reconstruction following anterior exenteration. *Urology.* 1997;49(5):768-771.

22. Elaffandi AH, Khalil HH, Aboul Kassem HA, El Sherbiny M, El Gemeie EH. Vaginal reconstruction with a greater omentum-pedicled graft combined with a vicryl mesh after anterior pelvic exenteration. Surgical approach with long-term follow-up. *Int J Gynecol Cancer.* 2007;17(2):536-542.

23. Stany MP, Sunde J, Bidus MA, Rose GS, Elkas JC. The use of acellular dermal allograft for vulvovaginal reconstruction. *Int J Gynecol Cancer.* 2010;20(6):1079-1081.

24. Hallberg H, Holmstrom H. Vaginal construction with skin grafts and vacuum-assisted closure. *Scand J Plast Reconstr Surg Hand Surg.* 2003;37(2):97-101.

25. Bhathena HM. Vacuum-controlled condom stent for vaginal reconstruction. *J Gynecol Surg.* 1996;12:117-121.

26. Adamson CD, Naik BJ, Lynch DJ. The vacuum expandable condom mold: a simple vaginal stent for McIndoe-style vaginoplasty. *Plast Reconstr Surg.* 2004;113(2):664-666.

27. Morrow CP, Curtin JP. Reconstructive surgery. In: Morrow CP, Curtin JP, eds. *Gynecologic Cancer Surgery.* Philadelphia, PA: Churchill Livingstone; 1996:323-380.

28. Akn S. Experience with neovaginal construction using the full-thickness skin graft in vaginal agenesis. *Ann Plast Surg.* 2004;52(4):391-396.

29. Lattari V, Jones LM, Varcelotti JR, Latenser BA, Sherman HF, Barrette RR. The use of a permanent dermal allograft in full-thickness burns of the hand and foot: a report of three cases. *J Burn Care Rehabil.* 1997;18(2):147-155.

30. Soper JT, Secord AA, Havrilesky LJ, Berchuck A, Clarke-Pearson DL. Comparison of gracilis and rectus abdominis myocutaneous flap neovaginal reconstruction performed during radical pelvic surgery: flap-specific morbidity. *Int J Gynecol Cancer.* 2007;17(1):298-303.

31. Smith HO, Genesen MC, Runowicz CD, Goldberg GL. The rectus abdominis myocutaneous flap: modifications, complications, and sexual function. *Cancer.* 1998;83(3):510-520.

32. Casey WJ 3rd, Tran NV, Petty PM, Stulak JM, Woods JE. A comparison of 99 consecutive vaginal reconstructions: an outcome study. *Ann Plast Surg.* 2004;52(1):27-30.

33. Daniel RK. Letter: toward an anatomical and hemodynamic classification of skin flaps. *Plast Reconstr Surg.* 1975;56(3):330-332.

34. Wee JT, Joseph VT. A new technique of vaginal reconstruction using neurovascular pudendal-thigh flaps: a preliminary report. *Plast Reconstr Surg.* 1989;83(4):701-709.

35. Monstrey S, Blondeel P, Van Landuyt K, Verpaele A, Tonnard P, Matton G. The versatility of the pudendal thigh fasciocutaneous flap used as an island flap. *Plast Reconstr Surg.* 2001;107(3):719-725.

36. Martius J, McCall M, Bolton KA. Operations for urinary incontinence. In: MM., KAB., eds. *Operative Gynecology.* Boston, MA: Little Brown; 1956.

37. Hatch KD. Neovaginal reconstruction. *Cancer.* 1993;71(4 suppl):1660-1663.

38. Green AE, Escobar PF, Neubaurer N, Michener CM, Vongruenigen VE. The Martius flap neovagina revisited. *Int J Gynecol Cancer.* 2005;15(5):964-966.

39. McCraw JB, Massey FM, Shanklin KD, Horton CE. Vaginal reconstruction with gracilis myocutaneous flaps. *Plast Reconstr Surg.* 1976;58(2):176-183.

40. Ratliff CR, Gershenson DM, Morris M, et al. Sexual adjustment of patients undergoing gracilis myocutaneous flap vaginal reconstruction in conjunction with pelvic exenteration. *Cancer.* 1996;78(10):2229-2235.

41. Mathes SJ, Nahai F. *Clinical Applications for Muscle and Musculocutaneous Flaps.* St. Louis, MO: CIV Mosby; 1982.

42. Tobin GR, Day TG. Vaginal and pelvic reconstruction with distally based rectus abdominis myocutaneous flaps. *Plast Reconstr Surg.* 1988;81(1):62-73.

43. Reid R. Local and distant skin flaps in the reconstruction of vulvar deformities. *Am J Obstet Gynecol.* 1997;177(6):1372-1383.

44. Soper JT, Rodriguez G, Berchuck A, Clarke-Pearson DL. Long and short gracilis myocutaneous flaps for vulvovaginal reconstruction after radical pelvic surgery: comparison of flap-specific complications. *Gynecol Oncol.* 1995;56(2):271-275.

45. Burke TW, Morris M, Levenback C, Gershenson DM, Wharton JT. Closure of complex vulvar defects using local rhomboid flaps. *Obstet Gynecol.* 1994;84(6):1043-1047.

46. Chafe W, Fowler WC, Walton LA, Currie JL. Radical vulvectomy with use of tensor fascia lata myocutaneous flap. *Am J Obstet Gynecol.* 1983;145(2):207-213.

Ancillary Procedures

Joan L. Walker

INTRAPERITONEAL CATHETER AND PORT PLACEMENT

Procedure Overview

The placement of an intraperitoneal (IP) catheter and access port should ideally occur at the time of resection and staging for advanced-stage ovarian cancer confined to the peritoneal cavity. This requires the preoperative expectation that cancer will be found and subsequent consent for planned chemotherapy on a clinical trial or using chemotherapy delivered to the peritoneal cavity. The ease of removal of the device makes it a better choice to place an IP port at initial surgery rather than to have to schedule a second surgery to implant the device.

Alternatively, the device can be placed at an interval procedure using interventional radiologic techniques, laparoscopy, or a 2- to 4-cm laparotomy incision in the right or left lower quadrant. It is preferred to avoid the previous midline incision, when trying to introduce the catheter into the peritoneal cavity.

Preoperative Preparation

The location of the planned device port should not interfere with the patient's undergarments or her sleeping position. The size of the port relative to the size of the patient may cause discomfort and require altering the choice of devices. The nursing staff must be able to palpate the port, and it must be secured to a platform, such as the fascia overlying the ribs, to prevent complications during insertion of the Huber needle.

The operating room staff must have the device available, as well as 2-0 prolene sutures, Huber needles, and heparin 100 units/mL for flushing. The patient must be sterile and draped from the nipples to the middle thighs and laterally to the posterior axillary line.

The preferred device is a subcutaneously implanted port attached to a silicone catheter. Do not use products with Dacron cuffs. A Bardport silicone peritoneal catheter 14.3 French is the preferred device, and it has been Food and Drug Administration approved for use in IP therapy. The 9.6-French, single-lumen intravenous (IV) access device, also made of silicone, can be substituted if the peritoneal catheter is not available. The firmness of the catheter prevents kinking, and the silicone prevents adherence to peritoneal structures so the catheter can be withdrawn without difficulty.[1,2]

Operative Procedure

Laparotomy

The port pocket is created by making a 5- to 6-cm incision 3 finger-breadths above the lower costal margin, at the midclavicular or anterior axillary line, and 4 prolene sutures are placed in the fascia overlying the ribs and through the port to stabilize the device to this platform (Figure 33-1). A long tonsil clamp is tunneled subcutaneously (just above the rectus fascia) to approximately the level of the umbilicus and then through the fascia, muscle, and peritoneum to grasp the nonfenestrated end of the catheter, which pulled it into the port pocket (Figure 33-2). The 2 ends of the catheter are trimmed so that approximately 15 cm of catheter is located within the peritoneal cavity and the tip is not

673

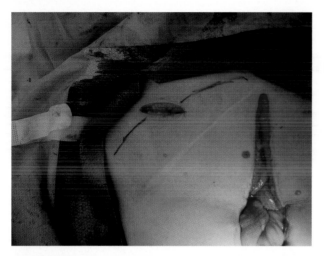

FIGURE 33-1. Intraperitoneal port placement: incision above left costal margin.

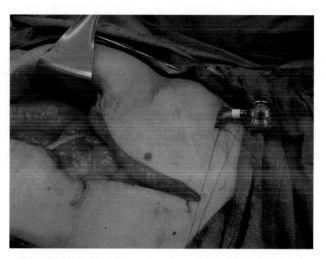

FIGURE 33-3. Intraperitoneal port placement: fixation of port reservoir.

long enough to reach the bladder or vagina. The catheter should not be left between the transverse colon and the abdominal wall, because it is likely to be entrapped in adhesions between those 2 structures due to the omentectomy. The catheter is attached to the port and fixed in place with 2-0 prolene sutured to fascia overlying ribs (Figure 33-3). The port pocket is closed in 2 layers with 3-0 absorbable suture and flushed with 100 units/mL of heparin to document that the system functions prior to leaving the operating room.

Mini-Laparotomy

An IP port can be placed as an interval procedure remote from the primary debulking operation via mini-laparotomy. The port pocket is created as described earlier. Entry into the peritoneal cavity should be

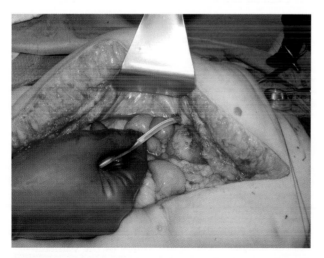

FIGURE 33-2. Intraperitoneal port placement: tunneling of catheter.

away from previous midline wound and avoid areas of bowel resections or extensive dissection. Free peritoneal space is generally available overlying the cecum and is often the ideal site for incision to obtain entry into the peritoneal cavity. After identifying the peritoneal cavity, under direct visualization, the catheter is drawn through the full thickness of the peritoneum, muscle, and fascia into the subcutaneous tissue. The catheter is then pulled through the subcutaneous tissue layer above the fascia into the port pocket, trimmed to length, sutured, and positioned as described earlier. Every layer of the peritoneum, fascia, and skin should be closed individually at the mini-laparotomy site to avoid leakage. The device should not be used for at least 24 hours.

Laparoscopy

Either right or left upper quadrant entry techniques can be used for laparoscopic IP port placement. The stomach should be aspirated with an oral gastric tube or nasogastric tube prior to initiating the procedure. Open laparoscopic techniques or mini-laparotomy may prove to be more advantageous when adhesions are expected. Blind Veress needle technique in the left upper quadrant should only be undertaken if knowledge of the anatomy in that location indicates it is free of adhesions or if ascites is present and ultrasound guidance can be used. A 5-mm trocar is placed 2 to 3 finger-breadths below the costal margin in the midclavicular line. The laparoscope is inserted and used to guide placement of a second 5-mm port. The IP catheter is inserted through the lower trocar under direct visualization and the trocar removed over the catheter (Figure 33-4). The port pocket is then created overlying the fascia of the lower ribs as described earlier,

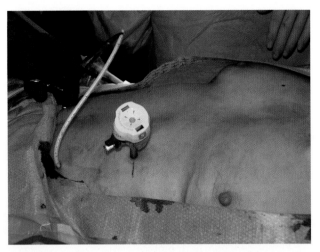

FIGURE 33-4. Laparoscopic intraperitoneal port placement.

and the catheter is pulled from the lower insertion site with a long tonsil up into the port pocket. The catheter is trimmed to proper length, attached to the port, and sutured to the fascia overlying the ribs with 2-0 prolene sutures. The port and catheter are flushed with 10 mL of heparin 100 units/mL using a Huber needle, and the port pocket is closed in 2 layers.

Postoperative Care

Complications are categorized into port access problems, inflow obstruction, abdominal pain, infections, and leaking into wound, bowel lumen, or bladder or out of the vagina. The expected complication rate is 10%.

Difficulty accessing the port or inflow obstruction is evaluated by fluoroscopy with infusion of a small amount of dilute solution of IV contrast dye. Surgical correction of the device can be considered, but usually the device is removed and IV chemotherapy is given. Successful correction is dependent on the cause being a mechanical problem, rather than a patient-specific problem, such as adhesions.

A fever in an IP chemotherapy patient can be evaluated by irrigating and aspirating saline from the port to send to microbiology, for cell count and culture, to look for evidence of peritoneal or catheter infection. Cellulitis surrounding an IP port is rarely treated with antibiotics alone; the port and catheter are generally removed. Leaking around the port or subcutaneous tissues is often an indication of inflow obstruction or intra-abdominal adhesions surrounding the catheter with retrograde flow of fluid back into the port pocket. Fluoroscopy will usually be diagnostic.

The device leaking into the vagina, bladder, or bowel is generally corrected by percutaneous removal of the catheter. Fistulas do not always occur as a result,

and a laparotomy is not generally needed, unless the patient appears to have peritonitis, free air, or a urinoma. Complaints of diarrhea or incontinence of urine with IP chemotherapy administration should be investigated with contrast dye to determine a potential communication between bowel, bladder, peritoneum, and infusion with the catheter.

INTRAPERITONEAL PORT REMOVAL

Procedure Overview

An IP port can be removed either in the operating room under sedation and local anesthesia or as an office procedure using only local anesthetic. It is best to remove these devices as soon as their useful life is over, so a complication will not interfere with the patient's quality of life.

Preoperative Preparation

The patient should not be neutropenic or thrombocytopenic, and medications that inhibit platelet function should be withheld. A list of equipment needed for office removal is provided in Table 33-1.

Operative Procedure

Sterile skin preparation is first, followed by placement of a disposable sterile drape with a perforation at the site of the port. The skin surrounding the port pocket is infiltrated with 1% lidocaine. A skin incision is made overlying the port through old scar. The adipose tissue is dissected down to the palpable port where the catheter is attached. A dense fibrinous sheath is found

Table 33-1 Equipment Needed for Intraperitoneal Port Removal

List of equipment needed:
   Sterile field prep and drape
   Mayo stand and sterile cover
   Scalpel
   Mayo scissors
   Hemostats
   Needle driver
   Forceps
   Retractors
   Lidocaine
   3-0 Vicryl SH needle
   4-0 Vicryl PS-2 needle
   Electrocautery is optional

over the port and the catheter, and this sheath has to be incised without cutting the catheter itself. A hemostat is used to undermine the catheter and pull it up and out of the abdomen, and this is used for traction. The port is elevated, and the 4 prolene sutures are cut, while cutting through the fibrinous sheath surrounding the port, and the port and catheter are removed. The port pocket is closed in 2 layers.

Postoperative Care

A prescription for narcotics is often given, but nonsteroidal pain medications are generally adequate. Covering the incision for 24 hours is all that is required.

MANAGEMENT OF INTRAOPERATIVE HEMORRHAGE

Procedure Overview

The effective management of unexpected intraoperative hemorrhage includes the creation of an adequate incision, ensuring good retraction, and optimizing exposure and lighting. The identification of important landmarks and the use of reliable surgical dissection planes will help to minimize blood loss. Depending on the origin of blood loss, a variety of hemorrhage control techniques are at the surgeon's disposal.

Preoperative Preparation

Most patients undergoing surgery for gynecologic cancer should be considered a potential risk for major hemorrhage. Anticipation of such situations and proper preparation are key to effective management. An emergency vascular surgical tray of standard topical hemostatic agents (Table 33-2) should be readily available, as well as vessel loops and long hemoclip appliers; for obese patients, an extra long lighted retractor set (St. Mark Deep Pelvic Lighted Retractor), extra long suction, and a laparoscopic clip applier are helpful. Rapid notification plans for anesthesia, nursing, blood bank and surgical assistance from trauma, and vascular or general surgery should be in place. Coagulopathy, hypothermia, and dilutional problems, due to the use of excessive crystalloid for blood pressure support when blood is not available, should be avoided.

Operative Procedure

Standard trauma surgery practice is to put a dry lap in all quadrants and work from the most likely site of hemorrhage outward, applying manual pressure on the bleeding site until proper exposure and isolation can be obtained.

Rapid decision making is often the key to successful outcomes. Considerations include adequacy of the

Table 33-2 Hemostatic Agents for Topical Application

Thrombin:
  Bovine
    JMI; King Pharmaceuticals, Inc., Bristol, TN
  Human pooled
    Evithrom; Johnson & Johnson, Summerville, NJ
  Recombinant
    Recothrom; ZymoGenetics, Inc., Seattle, WA

Fibrin Sealants: Vascular Surgery
  Fibrinogen, aprotinin, human thrombin, bovine thrombolysis inhibitor
    Tisseel VH; Baxter Healthcare Corp., Westlake Village, CA
  Fibrinogen, human thrombin
    Evicel; Johnson & Johnson
  Thrombin and fibrinogen spray
    CoSeal; Baxter Healthcare

Liquid Topical Agents
  Gelatin matrix (thrombin can be added [not included]; saline is included)
    Surgiflo; Johnson & Johnson
  Gelatin granules and thrombin
    Floseal; Baxter Healthcare

Mechanical
  Gelatin
    Gelfoam; Pharmacia & Upjohn, Kalamazoo, MI
    Surgifoam; Johnson & Johnson
  Gelatin sponge plus pooled human thrombin
    Gelfoam Plus; Baxter Healthcare
  Collagen
    Avitene flour and sheets; Davol-Bard, Warwick, RI
  Cellulose
    Surgicel (original; fibrillar; nu-knit); Ethicon-360, Johnson & Johnson
  Polysaccharide spheres
    Arista; Medafor, Minneapolis, MN

Special Intravascular Replacement
  Factor VIIa, recombinant; Nova Seven, Novo Nordisk, Bagsværd, Denmark
    Approved for postpartum hemorrhage after replacement with packed red blood cells and fresh frozen plasma and cryoprecipitate
  Cryoprecipitate, factor VIII, von Willebrand factor (vWF), fibrinogen, factor XIII, fibronectin, etc
    Indications: low fibrinogen (≤100 mg/dL)
      Tissue plasminogen activator reversal
      Massive transfusion (>10 units packed red blood cells)
      Uremic bleeding
      Tissue sealant (fibrin glue)
      von Willebrand disease

incision, measures necessary to obtain proximal and distal control of a vascular injury, need for temporary compression of the aorta, and need for additional personnel (eg, vascular surgeon). Significant vascular injuries encountered during laparoscopy should be tamponaded while preparations are made for laparotomy. Ideally, laparotomy equipment is available in the room for every laparoscopic surgery.

Control of Abdominal Hemorrhage

Bleeding from left para-aortic dissection may require a modified Mattox maneuver (Figure 33-5) in which mobilization of the left colon and splenic flexure toward the midline and separation of the colon mesentery from Gerota fascia exposes of the aorta, left kidney, ureter, and renal vessels. Anatomic identification of all structures is most efficient by following the left ureter and left ovarian vein cephalad to their insertions into the kidney and the renal vein on the left and vena cava on the right.

Vena cava lacerations should be adequately exposed before repair is attempted, and the Cattell-Braasch maneuver (Figure 33-6), which mobilizes the right colon with the cecum, ascending colon, and hepatic flexure at the white line of Toldt and reflects the colon

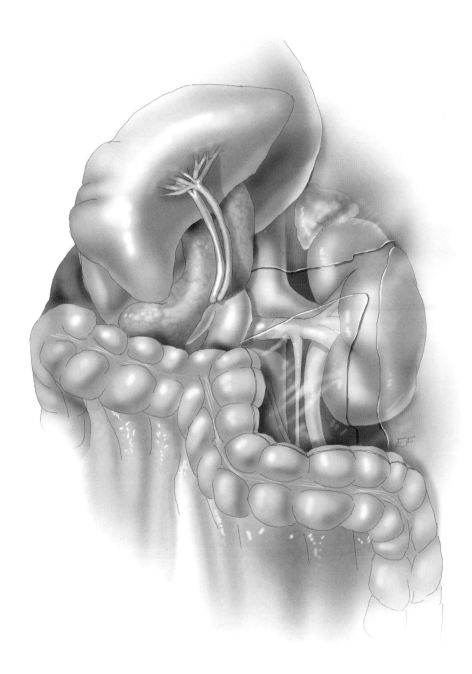

FIGURE 33-5. Modified Mattox maneuver. Mobilization of the left colon and spleen allows visualization of the left renal vessels and aorta.

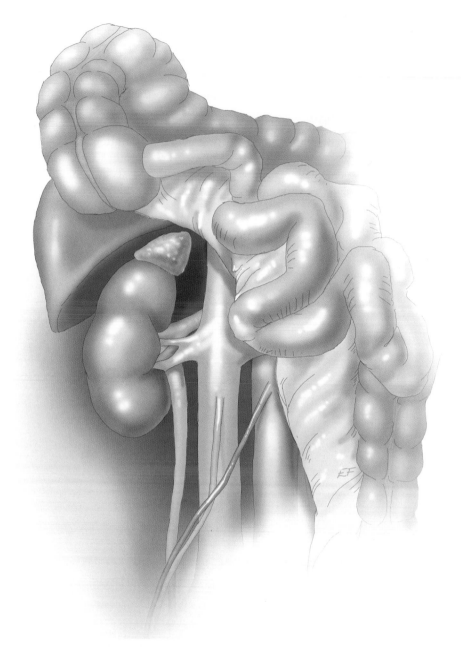

FIGURE 33-6. Cattell-Braasch maneuver: dissection of the cecum, ascending colon, and hepatic flexure at the white line of Toldt and reflecting the colon and the base of the mesentery medially and superiorly to achieve exposure of vena cava, aorta, right ureter, right kidney, and renal vessels.

and the base of the mesentery medially and superiorly, may be necessary. This maneuver allows excellent exposure of the vena cava, aorta, right ureter, right kidney, and renal vessels. If the laceration is more cephalad, the Kocher maneuver should be performed, which mobilizes the duodenum and posterior aspect of the head of the pancreas. Compression proximal and distal to the injury allows for a controlled closure of the laceration. Small injuries to the vena cava may be controlled with the application of 1 or 2 vascular hemoclips. Alternatively, an Allis or Satinsky clamp can be used to approximate the laceration, while a 4-0

or 5-0 prolene continuous running suture is used to reapproximate the vascular edges.

Lacerations of the splenic capsule during omentectomy can be controlled with thrombin-soaked gel foam, fibrin glue, or Floseal and Surgicel. Splenectomy is an alternative when these maneuvers fail.

Control of Pelvic Hemorrhage

General Measures

Pelvic hemorrhage is one of the most difficult areas of bleeding to control, particularly if bleeding is multifocal and exposure is limited. Packing with tamponade is usually the best initial strategy for unanticipated major pelvic blood loss. Anesthesia should be notified and the institutional massive hemorrhage protocol initiated. Once adequate resources have been mobilized, the packs are removed, and a systematic approach is undertaken to explore IP structures and the retroperitoneal spaces to locate and control the source of bleeding. The ureters should always be clearly identified and mobilized away from the field of dissection. Development of the pararectal and paravesical spaces facilitates exposure of the major retroperitoneal vasculature. Bleeding sites should be controlled individually; hemoclips or sutures should never be placed blindly into the pelvic sidewall.

Bleeding from the external iliac vein is usually easily controlled by grasping with a Satinsky or bulldog clamp or Allis clamp. Proximal and distal control can also be achieved by occlusion with sponge sticks (Figure 33-7). Alternatively, the vessel can be systematically approached by surrounding the vein distally and proximally with a Potts loop (wrapping a vessel loop twice around the vein and applying gentle elevation). The vein may have a laceration on top by avulsion of the circumflex iliac or on the underside by the accessory obturator vein. Suturing the defect is less likely to decrease the lumen diameter compared with using a hemoclip; however, the clip applied parallel to

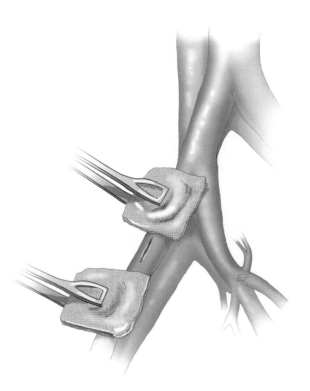

FIGURE 33-7. Occlusion of external iliac vein to localize and repair vascular injury.

the vein is faster when feasible. Small defects can be grasped with smooth forceps, elevated, and controlled with a single hemoclip or 2 hemoclips placed in the shape of a "V." Alternatively, a series of figure-of-eight stitches with 4-0 or 5-0 prolene suture on a vascular needle should be adequate. If the defect is long, a running 5-0 prolene suture is used. Deep venous thrombosis is common after intimal injury and repair and should be prevented with anticoagulation as soon as feasible; early diagnosis postoperatively with Doppler imaging is recommended.[3]

The obturator space under the external iliac vein may be a site of bleeding during the dissection of lymph nodes from this region. This space may be approached from between the psoas muscle and the external iliac vessels to visualize the obturator nerve and vessels while the source of bleeding is secured. Alternatively, the medial approach using the paravesical space can be used to identify the obturator nerve and the hypogastric artery and vein. Bleeding from veins retracting into obturator foramen should stop with pressure or Gelfoam soaked in thrombin or the use of Floseal. An accessory obturator vein is present in 24% of patients and is located on the inferior surface of the external iliac vein. Control of bleeding from this vessel requires that the external iliac vein be rotated laterally for adequate exposure.

Hypogastric vein bleeding and lateral pelvic hemorrhage constitute another very difficult surgical dilemma. The preferred approach is to achieve adequate visualization of the bleeding vessel and control it with hemoclips or sutures. Use of hemostatic agents and pressure is secondary.

Bleeding from the presacral space and associated venous plexus can be life threatening. Hemostatic agents such as thrombin, Nu Knit and Fibrillar Surgicel, and Floseal with manual pressure are usually effective in controlling bleeding unless a large laceration has occurred. Suturing in the presacral space is notoriously unsuccessful. A bleeding friable vein can be coated with Floseal; then Fibrillar Surgicel is applied on top of Floseal and pressure is held for 10 to 15 minutes. In the event of failure of hemostatic agents and pressure, sterile thumb tacks placed into the sacrum on top of the Gelfoam or Surgicel may be considered. The indication for sterile thumb tacks is for control of localized severe hemorrhage from the presacral area. This technique should only be used when other techniques are ineffective. The bleeding can only be effectively controlled by this technique if it can be localized by manual compression with a surgeon's fingers or sponge stick. Contraindications include bleeding greater than 2 cm from the midline and bleeding that appears to originate from the sacral neural foramina or ureter, rectum, or vagina. The above techniques are unlikely to control presacral bleeding in the face of systemic coagulation disorder. In such circumstances, packing the pelvis and using the guiding principles of "damage control surgery" with temporary closure, resuscitation in the intensive care unit, and reoperation are more likely to be life saving. Interventional radiology is also helpful in many of these situations. Return to the operating room is planned in 24 to 48 hours to remove the packing after resuscitation and stabilization.

Hypogastric Artery Ligation (Ligation of the Anterior Division of the Internal Iliac Artery)

Hypogastric artery ligation can be used to control hemorrhage from any gynecologic surgery complicated by bleeding from the central pelvis or parametria due to small vessel injury. The procedure is effective for arterial bleeding from the vaginal apex and in the broad ligament. It is not effective for venous oozing anywhere in the pelvis. Bilateral hypogastric artery ligation was first performed by Howard A. Kelly at the Johns Hopkins Hospital in 1894 as an emergency measure to control pelvic bleeding in a patient undergoing hysterectomy for cervical cancer.[4] The effectiveness of hypogastric artery ligation is predicated on the resulting decrease in arterial pulse pressure distal to the site of ligation and is dependent on successful prevention of collateral circulation beyond the ligature via branches of the posterior division of the hypogastric artery (iliolumbar, lateral sacral, and superior gluteal arteries).[5] The posterior division arises within 5 cm of the common iliac artery bifurcation in 95% of cases.[6]

As such, the point of ligation should be at least 5 cm distal to the common iliac artery bifurcation.

The technique is safest after development of the pararectal and paravesical spaces to visualize the entire pelvic vasculature and ureter. The common iliac, external iliac, and hypogastric vasculature should be visually confirmed and a point on the hypogastric artery at least 5 cm distal to the common iliac artery bifurcation selected for placement of the ligature. The hypogastric vein lies lateral and deep to the hypogastric artery and should be carefully avoided. The hypogastric artery is carefully dissected by passing a right angle clamp beneath it, working from lateral to medial without injuring the underlying vein. This is accomplished by pushing the artery medially and ventrally as the tips are advanced from lateral to medial around the artery toward the midline. The tips must not be pushed laterally into the vein. The hypogastric artery is ligated with a 1-0 or 2-0 silk suture (Figure 33-8). There is no need to place a transfixion stitch or to divide the artery once ligated.

At the conclusion of the procedure, one must be cautious to evaluate the remainder of the abdomen for unsuspected injuries or bleeding and removal of all instruments and packing. If the patient cannot be adequately resuscitated, rapid abdominal closure after packing for tamponade of bleeding may be the best decision. Damage control surgery is, on occasion, the best choice with the expectation that reoperation in 24 to 48 hours is the safest plan.

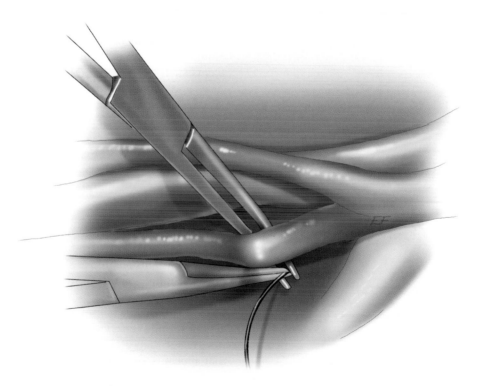

FIGURE 33-8. Hypogastric artery ligation.

WOUND MANAGEMENT AND VACUUM-ASSISTED CLOSURES

Primary Abdominal Closure (Clean and Clean/Contaminated)

The patient factors and surgical factors affecting the risk of wound infection, seroma, hernias, fascial dehiscence, and evisceration should be considered for every gynecologic oncology procedure. Obesity, advanced age, diabetes, cancer, and poor nutrition are common comorbidities that compromise wound healing.

The mass closure of fascia can be performed as an interrupted technique (Smead-Jones) or a modified continuous running suture. Monofilament delayed-absorbable suture in a continuous or interrupted mass closure (#1 polydioxanone or Maxon) has become the technique preferred by most surgeons, but it may be appropriate to use permanent monofilament suture (#2 nylon) in very high-risk individuals or when a hernia is already present.[7-9]

Alternative Abdominal Wall Closures

Intra-abdominal sepsis and contaminated wounds are indications for alternative strategies for abdominal wall closures. Primary routine fascial closure is appropriate for the stable patient defined as follows: normothermic; without coagulopathy or bleeding; not acidotic; and the source of the infection has been isolated and permanently treated. In these circumstances, the wound should be irrigated, a closed suction drainage system is placed, the abdominal wall is approximated using a mass closure, and a wound vacuum device is applied to the adipose layer for secondary closure. The risk of fascial necrosis and unseen infections can be eliminated by leaving the adipose and skin open and frequently evaluated.

Uncontrollable hemorrhage requiring packing and the presence of gross abdominal sepsis are indications for damage control surgery or open abdomen management.[10] Phase I in damage control surgery is control of the hemorrhage and/or the contamination. The unfinished surgery may require packing to be left in place to control bleeding, or delay of the hysterectomy that did not get performed or the tumor that was not removed. In the case of intra-abdominal sepsis, the bowel injury or perforation may have been temporarily stapled across without completing the anastomosis or bringing up a stoma. Hemorrhage, once under control, or packed, requires a rapid running mass closure suture of the abdominal wall and covering the wound. This approach prevents retraction of the fascia and thus provides a better opportunity for complete abdominal wall closure in 24 hours when the patient is completely resuscitated. Intra-abdominal sepsis may result

in intra-abdominal compartment syndrome, and the open abdomen approach has become recognized as an alternative to abdominal wall closure under certain circumstances, including lactic acidosis, coagulopathy, and hypothermia. Isolation of the source of infection, warm irrigation, drainage, and an open abdomen dressing for 24 hours constitute the operative plan. Retraction of the fascia is a major complication of this approach, and therefore, rapid (<48 hours) return to the operating room for fascial closure is required.

Phase II in damage control surgery is a rapid transfer to the intensive care unit for resuscitation and allowing time for patient warming, correction of acidosis, correction of coagulopathy, ventilation, blood pressure, and fluid management. Monitoring of intra-abdominal pressure and careful attention to the early diagnosis of abdominal compartment syndrome will help determine the timing of future abdominal explorations and wash out procedures.

Phase III in damage control surgery is a return trip to the operating room in 24 to 48 hours for completion of previously postponed surgical steps, including removal of packing, control of bleeding, reanastomosis of bowel, maturation of stomas, intra-abdominal wash out, placement of drains, and exploration for viable versus necrotic tissue and unrecognized injuries. A major goal of the second operation should be closure of the abdominal fascia, and when not feasible, traction on the fascia must be instituted to allow for future closure when there is a reduction of intra-abdominal swelling and edema. A wound vacuum is generally applied to the adipose layer. Postoperatively, the patient needs to be observed for development of intra-abdominal compartment syndrome.

Open Abdomen Wound Management Systems

The basic concept of open abdomen wound management systems is to provide closed-suction drainage to the intra-abdominal compartment, protect the intra-abdominal contents with a thin plastic sheet, cover the wound with sterile towels or sponges, and then apply an adhesive dressing over the entire abdomen. A commercially available kit, the ABThera (Kinetic Concepts, Inc., San Antonio, TX), provides the prepackaged materials to manage this situation (Figure 33-9). The missing component is the traction on the fascia. The fascia must be primarily closed, closed within 24 hours, or have continuous traction on it to prevent the permanent retraction, which makes future abdominal closure impossible. Closure of the fascia is generally attempted daily or the wound may never reapproximate.[11] The ABRA abdominal wall closure device (Canica Design, Inc., Almonte, Ontario, Canada) was developed to assist with fascial closure when edematous bowel and

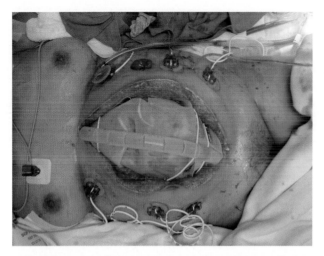

FIGURE 33-9. ABThera open wound management system and ABRA fascial closure system (incision open).

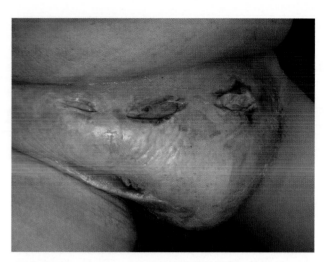

FIGURE 33-11. Necrotizing fasciitis of the vulva.

increased intra-abdominal pressure require fascial closure to be delayed over a number of days (Figures 33-9 and 33-10).

Vacuum-Assisted Closure Device (Negative-Pressure Wound Therapy)

Negative-pressure wound technology protects the surrounding skin while assisting with control of moisture and promoting granulation tissue development and wound closure in the adipose tissue below the skin level. Indications in gynecologic oncology for negative-pressure wound therapy (vacuum-assisted closure [VAC]) include planned secondary closure of open wounds in contaminated or septic cases and secondary closure of wounds opened after seroma or wound infections. In the setting of necrotizing fasciitis of the abdominal wall or vulva (Figure 33-11), the wound

VAC device can be a valuable tool after all necrotic tissue has been debrided. Wound assessments every 24 hours must occur for a few days after the initial debridement, and then less frequent changes can occur. Contraindications include settings where there is devitalized tissue, tumor in the wound, potential fistula underlying wound, vascular graft, vessels, nerves, or exposed organs. Infection should be controlled prior to application of the device.

The surrounding skin must be clean and dry, and Mastisol liquid adhesive is applied to the skin prior to sealing the wound. The negative-pressure wound therapy systems (wound VAC devices) include a sponge that is cut to fit to the depth, width, and length of the wound and an adhesive barrier that covers the sponge and provides and air-tight seal to the skin (Figure 33-12). The vacuum tubing is attached to the foam, which is attached to the provided collection device and vacuum

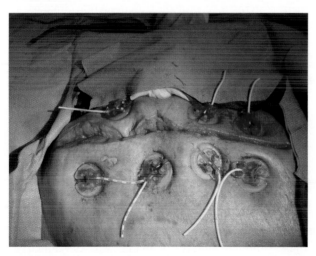

FIGURE 33-10. ABRA fascial closure system (incision closed).

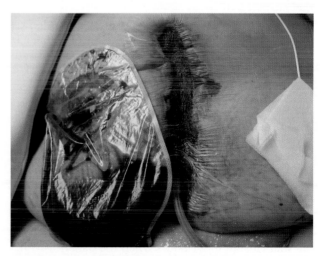

FIGURE 33-12. Wound vacuum system.

control for the fluids produced by the wound. Sponge consists of an open-pore polyurethane ether foam sponge, which is then covered with a semiocclusive adhesive cover and attached to the fluid collection system and the suction pump. The dressings are changed at least every 3 days and whenever the vacuum seal is lost.

REFERENCES

1. Walker JL, Armstrong DK, Huang HQ, et al. Intraperitoneal catheter outcomes in a phase III trial of intravenous versus intraperitoneal chemotherapy in optimal stage III ovarian and primary peritoneal cancer: a Gynecologic Oncology Group study. *Gynecol Oncol.* 2006;100:27-32.
2. Markman M, Walker JL. Intraperitoneal chemotherapy of ovarian cancer: a review, with a focus on practical aspects of treatment. *J Clin Oncol.* 2006;24(6):988-994.
3. Quan RW, Gillespie DL, Stuart RP, et al. The effect of vein repair on the risk of venous thromboembolic events: a review of more than 100 traumatic military venous injuries. *J Vasc Surg.* 2008;47(3):571-577.
4. Kelly HA. Ligation of both internal iliac arteries for hemorrhage in hysterectomy for carcinoma uteri. *Bull Johns Hopkins Hosp.* 1894;5:53-54.
5. Burchell RC. Physiology of internal iliac artery ligation. *J Obstet Gynaecol Br Commonw.* 1968;75: 642-651.
6. Bleich AT, Rahn DD, Wieslander CK, Wai CY, Roshanravan SM, Corton MM. Posterior division of the internal iliac artery: Anatomic variations and clinical implications. *Am J Obstet Gynecol.* 2007;197:658:e1-e5.
7. O'Dwyer PJ, Courtney CA. Factors involved in abdominal wall closure and subsequent incisional hernia. *Surgeon.* 2003;1(1):17-22.
8. Hodgson NCF, Malthaner RA, Østbye T. The search for an ideal method of abdominal fascial closure. A meta-analysis. *Ann Surg.* 2000;231(3):436-442.
9. Colombo M, Maggioni A, Parma G, et al. A randomized comparison of continuous versus interrupted mass closure of midline incisions in patients with gynecologic cancer. *Obstet Gynecol.* 1997;89(5, Pt 1):684-689.
10. Sugrue M, D'Amours SK, Joshipura M. Damage control surgery and the abdomen. *Injury.* 2004;35(7):642-648.
11. Pliakos I, Papavramidis TS, Mihalopoulos N, et al. Vacuum-assisted closure in severe abdominal sepsis with or without retention sutured sequential fascial closure: a clinical trial. *Surgery.* 2010;148(5):947-953.

Page references followed by *f* indicate figures; page references followed by *t* indicate tables.